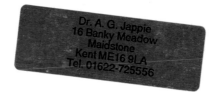

INTENSIVE CARE MANUAL

To my family – Lala, Kazia and Stefan – and to Millar Forbes, a friend from whom I learned vision.

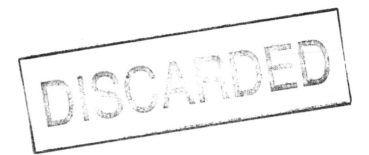

INTENSIVE CARE MANUAL

FOURTH EDITION

Edited by

T E Oh

MB BS, MD, FRCP, FRCPE, FRACP, FRCA, FANZCA, FFICANZCA, FHKAM

Professor and Chairman
Department of Anaesthesia and Intensive Care
Chinese University of Hong Kong
Prince of Wales Hospital
Shatin, Hong Kong

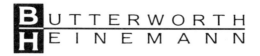

BUTTERWORTH
HEINEMANN

Butterworth-Heinemann
Linacre House, Jordan Hill, Oxford OX2 8DP
A division of Reed Educational and Professional Publishing Ltd

ℛ A member of the Reed Elsevier plc group

OXFORD   BOSTON   JOHANNESBURG
MELBOURNE   NEW DELHI   SINGAPORE

First published 1979
Reprinted 1981
Second edition 1985
Reprinted 1986
Reprinted 1988
Third edition 1990
Reprinted 1991
Fourth edition 1997

British Library Cataloguing in Publication Data
A catalogue record for this book is available from
the British Library

Library of Congress Cataloguing in Publication Data
A catalogue record for this book is available from
the Library of Congress

ISBN 0 7506 2358 6

Composition by Genesis Typesetting, Rochester, Kent
Printed and bound in Great Britain by The Bath Press, Bath

Contents

Contributors

Cindy S. T. Aun MB BS, MD, FRCA, FANZCA, FHKAM.
Professor, Department of Anaesthesia and Intensive Care, Chinese University, Prince of Wales Hospital, Shatin, Hong Kong.

Rinaldo Bellomo MB BS, MD, FRACP.
Specialist in Intensive Care, Department of Anaesthesia and Intensive Care, Austin Hospital, Heidelberg, Melbourne, Victoria, Australia.

Andrew Bersten MB BS, MD, FANZCA, FFICANZCA.
Deputy Director, Department of Critical Care Medicine, Flinders Medical Centre, Bedford Park, Adelaide, South Australia, Australia.

Julian F. Bion MB BS, MD, MRCP(UK), FRCA.
Senior Lecturer in Intensive Care Medicine, Department of Anaesthesia and Intensive Care, University of Birmingham, Queen Elizabeth Hospital, Edgbaston, Birmingham, UK.

Judith M. Branch MB BS, FANZCA.
Staff Specialist, Department of Anaesthesia, St Vincent's Hospital, Darlinghurst, Sydney, New South Wales, Australia.

Thomas A. Buckley MB ChB, FANZCA, FFICANZCA, FHKAM.
Consultant, Honorary Clinical Lecturer, Department of Anaesthesia and Intensive Care, Chinese University, Prince of Wales Hospital, Shatin, Hong Kong.

Po Tong Chui MB BS, FANZCA, FHKAM.
Consultant, Honorary Clinical Lecturer, Department of Anaesthesia and Intensive Care, Chinese University, Prince of Wales Hospital, Shatin, Hong Kong.

Geoffrey M. Clarke MB BS, DA RCPS, FRCA, FANZCA, FFICANZCA.
Head, Intensive Care Unit, Royal Perth Hospital, Perth, Western Australia, Australia; Dean, Faculty of Intensive Care, Australian and New Zealand College of Anaesthetists.

D. Jamie Cooper BM BS, FRACP, FANZCA, FFICANZCA.
Head, Trauma ICU, Assistant Director, Intensive Care Unit, Alfred Hospital, Prahran, Melbourne, Victoria, Australia.

Lester A. H. Critchley BMedSci (Hons), MB ChB, FFARCSI, FHKAM.
Associate Professor, Department of Anaesthesia and Intensive Care, Chinese University, Prince of Wales Hospital, Shatin, Hong Kong.

James L. Derrick MB BS, FANZCA.
Honorary Clinical Lecturer, Department of Anaesthesia and Intensive Care, Chinese University, Prince of Wales Hospital, Shatin, Hong Kong.

Geoffrey J. Dobb BSc (Hons), MB BS, MRCP(UK), FRCA, FANZCA, FFICANZCA.
Senior Specialist, Intensive Care Unit, Royal Perth Hospital, Perth, Western Australia, Australia.

Karl D. Donovan MB BCh, FRCP(I), FRACP.
Senior Specialist, Intensive Care Unit, Royal Perth Hospital, Perth, Western Australia, Australia.

Alan W. Duncan MB BS, FRCA, FANZCA, FFICANZCA.
Director, Intensive Care Unit, Princess Margaret Hospital for Children, Subiaco, Perth, Western Australia, Australia.

Malcolm M. Fisher MB ChB, MD, FRCA, FANZCA, FFICANZCA.
Head, Intensive Therapy Unit, Royal North Shore Hospital, St Leonards, Sydney, New South Wales, Australia.

A. Millar Forbes MB ChB, FRCPE, FRCA, FANZCA, FFICANZCA.
Senior Specialist, Department of Intensive Care, Sir Charles Gairdner Hospital, Nedlands, Perth, Western Australia, Australia.

Ross C. Freebairn BHB, MB ChB, DipObs, FANZCA, FFICANZCA.
Lecturer, Department of Anaesthesia and Intensive Care, Chinese University, Prince of Wales Hospital, Shatin, Hong Kong.

Martyn A. H. French MB ChB, MD, MRCP(UK), FRCPath, FRACP.
Clinical Immunologist, Department of Clinical Immunology, Royal Perth Hospital, Perth, Western Australia, Australia.

Fred J. E. Gilligan MB BS, Dip D Hyperb Med, FANZCA, FFICANZCA.
Director, Retrieval and Resuscitation, Department of Anaesthesia and Intensive Care, Royal Adelaide Hospital, Adelaide, South Australia, Australia.

Tony Gin BSc, MB ChB, MD, FRCA, FANZCA, FHKAM.
Professor, Department of Anaesthesia and Intensive Care, Chinese University, Prince of Wales Hospital, Shatin, Hong Kong.

Charles D. Gomersall BSc, MB BS, MRCP(UK), FRCA.
Assistant Professor, Department of Anaesthesia and Intensive Care, Chinese University, Prince of Wales Hospital, Shatin, Hong Kong.

Daniel Hanley MD.
Co-Director, Neurological Neurosurgical ICU, Department of Anesthesia, Johns Hopkins University Hospital, Baltimore, Maryland, USA.

Don G. A. Harrison MB BS, FANZCA, MHPEd.
Head, Cardiothoracic ICU, Department of Anaesthesia, St Vincent's Hospital, Darlinghurst, Sydney, New South Wales, Australia.

Felicity H. Hawker MB BS, FRCA, FANZCA, FFICANZCA.
Director, Intensive Care Unit, Cabrini Hospital, Malvern, Melbourne, Victoria, Australia.

Robert Henning BSc(Med), MB BS, DCH, FRCA, FANZCA, FFICANZCA.
Senior Specialist, Intensive Care Unit, Royal Children's Hospital, Parkville, Melbourne, Victoria, Australia.

David R. Hillman MB BS, FANZCA.
Senior Staff Specialist, Department of Pulmonary Physiology, Sir Charles Gairdner Hospital, Nedlands, Perth, Western Australia, Australia.

Bernard Hockings MB BS, MD, FRACP.
Director, Coronary Care Unit, Royal Perth Hospital, Perth, Western Australia, Australia.

James P. Isbister BMedSc, MB BS, FRACP, FRCPA.
Head, Department of Haematology, Royal North Shore Hospital, St Leonards, Sydney, New South Wales, Australia.

Alice Jones Cert(Phty), MPhil, MSc(Ed), FACP.
Assistant Professor, Department of Rehabilitation Sciences, Hong Kong Polytechnic University, Kowloon, Hong Kong.

Gavin M. Joynt MB ChB, FCA(SA), FCA(CritCare).
Associate Professor, Department of Anaesthesia and Intensive Care, Chinese University, Prince of Wales Hospital, Shatin, Hong Kong.

James A. Judson MB ChB, FANZCA, FFICANZCA.
Clinical Director, Department of Critical Care Medicine, Auckland Hospital, Auckland, New Zealand.

Keith Klugman BSc(Hons), MB BCh, DTM&H, MMed, FFPath(SA), PhD.
Professor and Head, Department of Microbiology, South African Institute of Medical Research, University of The Witwatersrand, Johannesburg, Republic of South Africa.

Geoffrey J. Knight MB BS, FRACP.
Staff Specialist, Intensive Care Unit, Princess Margaret Hospital for Children, Subiaco, Perth, Western Australia, Australia.

Ashok B. Kumar MB BS, FRACR, FRCR.
Consultant, Department of Radiology, Sir Charles Gairdner Hospital, Nedlands, Perth, Western Australia, Australia.

Richard P. Lee MB BS, FANZCA, FFICANZCA.
Senior Specialist, Department of Intensive Therapy, St Vincent's Hospital, Darlinghurst, Sydney, New South Wales, Australia.

Jeffrey Lipman MB ChB, FCA(SA), FCA(CritCare).
Director, Intensive Care Unit, Baragwanath Hospital; Associate Professor, Department of Anaesthesia, University of The Witwatersrand, Johannesburg, Republic of South Africa.

Brian L. Lloyd MB BS, PhD, FRACP, FACC.
Cardiologist, Department of Cardiovascular Medicine, Sir Charles Gairdner Hospital, Nedlands, Perth, Western Australia, Australia.

Frederic T. A. Lovegrove MBA, MB BS, FRACP.
Physician in Nuclear Medicine, Department of Nuclear Medicine, St John of God Hospital, Subiaco, Perth, Western Australia, Australia.

John S. M. Low MA, BM BCh, FRCA, FHKAM.
Professor, Department of Anaesthesia and Intensive Care, Chinese University, Prince of Wales Hospital, Shatin, Hong Kong.

Colin J. McArthur BHB, MB BS, FANZCA, FFICANZCA.
Staff Specialist, Department of Critical Care Medicine, Auckland Hospital, Auckland, New Zealand.

Sharon McKinley RN, PhD.
Professor of Critical Care Nursing, University of Technology, Sydney, Royal North Shore Hospital, St Leonards, Sydney, New South Wales, Australia.

Neil T. Matthews MB BS, FANZCA, FFICANZCA.
Director, Intensive Care Unit, Adelaide Children's Hospital, North Adelaide, South Australia, Australia.

John A. Myburgh MB BCh, DA(SA), FANZCA, FFICANZCA.
Deputy Director, Intensive Care Unit, Department of Anaesthesia and Intensive Care, Royal Adelaide Hospital, Adelaide, South Australia, Australia.

Warwik D. Ngan Kee BHB, MB ChB, FANZCA.
Associate Professor, Department of Anaesthesia and Intensive Care, Chinese University, Prince of Wales Hospital, Shatin, Hong Kong.

Teik E. Oh MB BS, MD, FRCP, FRCPE, FRACP, FRCA, FANZCA, FFICANZCA, FHKAM.
Professor of Anaesthesia and Intensive Care, Chinese University; Chief of Service, Department of Anaesthesia and Intensive Care, Prince of Wales Hospital, Shatin, Hong Kong.

Garry D. Phillips BSc(Med), MB BS, FACEM, FANZCA, FFICANZCA.
Professor of Anaesthesia and Intensive Care, Flinders University; Chairman, Department of Anaesthesia, Flinders Medical Centre, Bedford Park, Adelaide, South Australia, Australia.

William B. Runciman BMedSc, MB BS, PhD, FRCA, FANZCA, FFICANZCA.
Professor of Anaesthesia and Intensive Care, Adelaide University; Chairman, Department of Anaesthesia and Intensive Care, Royal Adelaide Hospital, Adelaide, South Australia, Australia.

John Sanderson MB BS, MD, FRCP, FACC, FHKAM.
Professor, Department of Medicine, Chinese University, Prince of Wales Hospital, Shatin, Hong Kong.

John D. Santamaria MB BS, MD, FRACP.
Director, Intensive Care Unit, St Vincent's Hospital, Fitzroy, Melbourne, Victoria, Australia.

Caros D. Scheinskestel MB BS, FRACP, DipDHM.
Deputy Director, Intensive Care Unit and Hyperbaric Service, Alfred Hospital, Prahran, Melbourne, Victoria, Australia.

Frank A. Shann MB BS, MD, FRACP.
Professor of Critical Care Medicine, University of Melbourne. Director, Intensive Care Unit, Royal Children's Hospital, Parkville, Melbourne, Victoria, Australia.

Timothy G. Short MB ChB, MD, FANZCA, FHKAM.
Associate Professor, Department of Anaesthesia and Intensive Care, Chinese University, Prince of Wales Hospital, Shatin, Hong Kong.

George A. Skowronski MB BS (Hons), MRCP(UK), FRACP.
Senior Specialist, Intensive Care Unit, St George Hospital, Kogarah, Sydney, New South Wales, Australia.

Joseph Sung MB BS, PhD, MRCP(UK), FHKAM.
Associate Professor, Department of Medicine, Chinese University, Prince of Wales Hospital, Shatin, Hong Kong.

Paul K. Swan MB BS, FANZCA, FFICANZCA.
Consultant, Department of Anaesthesia, King Fahad National Guard Hospital, Riyadh, Saudi Arabia.

Jukka Takala MD, PhD.
Director, Critical Care Research Program, Department of Intensive Care, Kuopio University Hospital, Kuopio, Finland.

Ian K. S. Tan MB BS, MRCP(UK), FANZCA, FFICANZCA.
Lecturer, Department of Anaesthesia and Intensive Care, Chinese University, Prince of Wales Hospital, Shatin, Hong Kong.

Walter R. Thompson MB BS, DObst, FANZCA, FFICANZCA.
Head, Department of Intensive Care, Sir Charles Gairdner Hospital, Nedlands, Perth, Western Australia, Australia.

James Tibballs BMedSc (Hons), MEd, MB BS, FANZCA, FFICANZCA.
Deputy Director, Intensive Care Unit, Royal Children's Hospital, Parkville, Melbourne, Victoria, Australia.

David V. Tuxen MB BS, MD, FRACP, DHM.
Director, Department of Intensive Care and Hyperbaric Medicine, Alfred Healthcare Group, Prahran, Melbourne, Victoria, Australia.

John Ulatowski MD, PhD.
Co-Director, Neurological Neurosurgial ICU, Department of Anesthesia, Johns Hopkins University Hospital, Baltimore, Maryland, USA.

Alnis E. Vedig MB BS, FANZCA, FRACP, FFICANZCA.
Head, Department of Critical Care Medicine, Flinders Medical Centre, Bedford Park, Adelaide, South Australia, Australia.

John W. N. Weeks MB BS, FANZCA, FFICANZCA.
Senior Specialist, Intensive Care Unit, Royal Perth Hospital, Perth, Western Australia, Australia.

Lindsay I. G. Worthley MB BS, FRACP, FANZCA, FFICANZCA.
Senior Consultant, Department of Critical Care Medicine, Flinders Medical Centre, Bedford Park, Adelaide, South Australia, Australia.

Gordon H. M. Yau MB BS, FRCA, FAMS, FHKCA.
Specialist Anaesthetist; previously Senior Lecturer, Department of Anaesthesia, National University of Singapore, National University Hospital, Singapore.

Karl K. Young MB BS, FANZCA, FFICANZCA, FHKAM.
Honorary Clinical Lecturer, Department of Anaesthesia and Intensive Care, Chinese University, Prince of Wales Hospital, Shatin, Hong Kong.

Robert J. Young MB BS, FANZCA, FFICANZCA.
Associate Professor, Department of Anaesthesia and Intensive Care, Chinese University, Prince of Wales Hospital, Shatin, Hong Kong.

Acknowledgements

I wish to express my sincere thanks to the many individuals, authors, journal editors, and publishers who have made it possible for me to complete this 4th edition. Their contributions are gratefully acknowledged in the relevant pages. I also thank my wife Lala, my teenagers Kazia and Stefan, Butterworth-Heinemann, Nancy my secretary and all my Department staff, and my colleagues for their unfailing support. I am also grateful to the Chinese University of Hong Kong for a grant from the Vice-Chancellor's Discretionary Fund for Excellence.

T.E. Oh

Preface

This 4th edition follows the successful format of the previous three – rapid access to lucid information on the practical management of diseases and problems in an Intensive Care Unit as well as on subjects relevant to critical care medicine. Each chapter has again been planned to be self-contained, with cross-referencing between chapters. The manual is produced as a comprehensive handbook. It is not intended to be a reference tome, although topics are covered fairly extensively and sufficiently for most clinical situations.

New material in this edition present recent advances and additional chapters. The new chapters contribute to critical care aspects of nursing, infections, oxygenation, and organ transplantation, and to paediatric intensive care. Some chapters have been assigned to different sections, and there are new sections on environmental injuries, pharamcological considerations, and transplantation.

The specialty of critical care medicine is now mature, with societies, qualifications, specialist recognition, and career infrastructures founded and implemented in many countries. Critical care personnel, other health professionals, and students have found past editions of the book useful. I am confident that they will find this edition likewise.

Teik Oh
Hong Kong, March 1996

Part I

Organization aspects

1	# Design and organization of intensive care units

TE Oh

An intensive care unit (ICU) is a specially staffed and equipped hospital ward dedicated to the management of patients with life-threatening illnesses, injuries or complications. It has been suggested that the ICU developed from the postoperative recovery room or the poliomyelitis epidemic in the early 1950s, when the use of long-term artificial ventilation resulted in reduced mortality. However, modern intensive care or critical care medicine is not limited to postoperative care or mechanical ventilation. It is a specialty which evolved from the experience of respiratory and cardiac care, physiological organ support and coronary care units (CCUs, which were established in the early 1960s).[1] Benefits of centralizing special equipment, staff and facilities to treat critically ill patients and to avert complications (or reduce their severity) became recognized. The 1970s saw a heightened interest in intensive care, with research into the patho-physiological processes, treatment regimens and outcomes of the critically ill, and the founding of specialty journals, training programmes and qualifications dedicated to intensive care.[2–4] Intensive care today is a separate specialty,[5] and while some period of training in an ICU is valuable to all specialties, it can no longer be regarded as part of anaesthesia, chest medicine, general surgery or any acute discipline.

Economics of intensive care[6]

Utilization of ICUs increased markedly in developed countries in the 1970s and early 1980s (e.g. annual increases of 8% in USA and 4.8% in Canada).[7] This inevitably necessitates economic considerations. There are *fixed costs* in any ICU which are irrelevant to the workload and patient outcome. Salaries make up the bulk of fixed costs (up to 80%). *Variable costs* depend on patient admissions and the services rendered (e.g. investigations, monitoring and procedures). In both fixed and variable costs, there are components which are related to patient care (*direct costs*) and those which are not, e.g. hotel or administration expenditures (*indirect costs*).

Provision of intensive care services relates to *supply* and *demand*. Supply of resources to ICUs comes from government funds, private fees and insurance payments. Rising costs have resulted in restrictions on supply through reduced hospital budgets (implicit rationing) and payments for services (explicit rationing). Some countries have adopted a prospective payment system based on diagnosis-related groups (DRGs) introduced in the USA in 1983. However, DRG reimbursements for certain ICU patients fall short of actual costs. Demand for ICU services is related to demography, economy and technology, but can also be doctor generated (see the section on operational policies, below). An ICU bed costs three times more per day than an acute ward bed,[7] and the ICU uses 8% of the total hospital budget (14–20% in USA).[7,8] Total ICU costs per patient of US$22 000 in the USA (1978)[9], and A$1375 in Australia (1986)[10] have been reported.

Role of the ICU

The definition and delineation of roles of hospitals in a region or area are necessary to rationalize services and optimize the use of resources. Each ICU should similarly have its role in the region defined, which should support the defined duties of its hospital. In general, district and general hospitals require ICUs which involve only monitoring and close observation. An ICU which uses complex management and requires investigative back-up should be located in a large tertiary referral hospital of the region. Three levels of ICUs can thus be classified.[11]

Level I – district hospital

A level I ICU has a role in small district hospitals. It may also be called a high-dependency unit, rather than an ICU. Such a unit allows for close nursing observation and electrocardiogram (ECG) monitoring. Immediate resuscitation is possible, but only short-term (e.g. less than 24 h) ventilation should be undertaken.

Level II – general hospital

A level II ICU is located in larger general hospitals. It is capable of undertaking more prolonged ventilation, and has a resident doctor and access to physiotherapy, pathology and radiological facilities at all times. More complex forms of life support (e.g. dialytic therapies), invasive monitoring (e.g. intra-cranial pressure monitoring) and investigations (e.g. computed tomography scans) would not normally be provided. It should support the role of its hospital (e.g. area trauma centre).

Level III – tertiary hospital

A level III ICU is located in a major tertiary referral hospital. It should provide all aspects of intensive care required by its referral role. The unit is staffed by specialist intensivists with trainees, critical care nurses, allied health professionals and clerical and scientific staff. The support of complex investigations and imaging, and by specialists of all disciplines required by the referral role of the hospital, is available at all times.

Type, size and site of an ICU[6,11–14]

Health-planning policies may rationalize services by hospitals within a geographical region, so as not to duplicate expensive services unnecessarily. Hence, within each classification, an ICU may not be able to provide intensive care for all subspecialties, or may need to be more oriented towards a particular area of expertise (e.g. neurosurgery, cardiac surgery, burns or trauma). Also, an institution may organize its intensive care beds into multiple units, under separate management by single-discipline specialists, i.e. medical ICU, surgical ICU, burns ICU, etc. While this may be appropriate in certain hospitals, Australasian experience has favoured the development of general multidisciplinary ICUs. Thus, with the exception of dialysis units, CCUs and neonatal ICUs, critically ill patients are admitted to the hospital's multidisciplinary ICU and managed by specialist intensivists (or paediatric intensivists in paediatric hospitals). There are good economic and operational arguments for a multidisciplinary ICU as against separate medical or surgical ICUs.[6] Duplication of some equipment and services is avoided. Critically ill patients develop the same pathophysiological pro-cesses no matter whether they are classified as medical or surgical, and they require the same approaches to support vital organs. The problems of critically ill patients are not confined to their primary disease.

Single-discipline doctors lack the experience and expertise to deal with the complexities of multiorgan failure.

The number of ICU beds in a hospital usually ranges from 1 to 4 per 100 total hospital beds.[6,7,15] This depends on the role and type of ICU. Multidisciplinary ICUs require more beds than single-specialty ICUs, especially if high-dependency beds are not available elsewhere in the hospital. ICUs with fewer than four beds are considered not to be cost-effective, whereas those with over 20 non-high-dependency beds may be difficult to manage.

The ICU should be sited in close proximity to relevant acute areas, i.e. operating rooms, emergency department, CCU, labour ward and acute wards, and to investigational departments (e.g. radiology and organ imaging and pathology laboratories). Critically ill patients are at risk when they are moved (see Chapter 3). There should be sufficient numbers of lifts, and these, with doors and corridors, should be spacious enough to allow easy passage of beds and equipment – vital points often ignored by planning experts.

Design of an ICU[12,14]

There should be a single entry and exit point, attended by the unit receptionist. Through traffic of goods or people to other hospital areas must never be allowed. An ICU should have areas and rooms for public reception, patient management and support services (Table 1.1).

Patient areas

Each patient bed area requires a minimum floor space of 18.5 m² (200 ft²), with single rooms being larger, to accommodate patient, staff and equipment without overcrowding. The ratio of single-room beds to open-ward beds depends on the role and type of the ICU. Single rooms are essential for isolation cases and – less importantly – privacy for conscious long-stay patients. Positive/negative-pressure air conditioning for single isolation rooms is expensive and of unproven value.

Bedside service outlets should conform to local standards and requirements (including electrical safety and emergency supply). Three oxygen, two air, four suction and 16 power outlets with a bedside light are optimal for a level III ICU. How the services are supplied (e.g. from floor column, wall-mounted or bed-pendent) depends on individual preferences, as each design has its pros and cons. There should be room to place or attach additional portable monitoring equipment, and as much as possible equipment should be kept off the floor. Space for charts, syringes, sampling tubes, pillows, suction catheters and patient personal belongings is best arranged in bed dividers. Lead-lining these dividers

Table 1.1 Physical design of a major intensive care unit

Reception area
Reception foyer
Waiting room for visitors (with telephones and beverage facilities)
Distressed ('crying')/interview room
Overnight relatives' room

Patient areas
Open multi-bed ward(s)
Single-bed isolation rooms
Central nurse station (including drugs storage)
Specialized rooms/beds if necessary, for:
    Procedures/minor surgery (e.g. tracheostomy)
    Haemodialysis
    Burns
    Use of bypass or intra-aortic balloon pump machines

Storage and utility areas
Monitoring and electrical equipment
Respiratory therapy equipment
Disposables and central sterilizing supplies
Linen
Stationery
Fluids, vascular catheters and infusion sets
Non-sterile hardware (e.g. drip stands and bed rails)
Clean utility
Dirty utility
Equipment sterilization

Technical areas
Laboratory
Workshop for repairs, maintenance and development

Staff areas
Lounge/rest room (with facilities for meals)
Changing rooms
Toilets and showers
Offices
Doctors' on-call rooms
Seminar/conference room

Other support areas
Cleaners' room
Plant room/alcove

will help minimize X-ray radiation risks to staff and patients.

All central staff and patient areas must have large clear windows. Lack of natural light and windowless ICUs give rise to patient disorientation and increased stress to all. Since critical care nursing is at the bedside, staffing a central nurse station is less important than in a CCU. Nevertheless, the station should be sited so as to allow all patients to be seen. This station usually houses a central monitor, drugs cupboard, drugs/specimens refrigerator, telephones, laboratories-linked computer and patient records. Sufficient numbers of non-splash hand-wash basins should be built close to all beds and one for each single room. At least one multi-display X-ray viewer is needed in each multi-bed ward. Proper facilities for haemodialysis, such as filtered water, should be incorporated.

Storage and supporting services areas

Most ICUs lack storage space. Storage areas should total a floor space of about 25–30% of all the patient and central station areas. Frequently used items (e.g. intravenous (IV) fluids and giving sets, sheets, dressing trays, etc.) should be located closer to patients than infrequently used or non-patient items (e.g. more sophisticated monitoring devices).

Floor areas for supporting services (Table 1.1) should make up about 20–25% of the patient and central station areas. Clean and dirty utility rooms must be separate, each with its own access. Disposal of soiled linen and waste must be catered for, including contaminated items from infectious patients. Facilities for estimating blood gases, electrolytes, haemoglobin, haematocrit and osmolality, with a microscope being available, are usually sufficient for the unit laboratory. Larger ICUs may require a satellite pharmacy within the unit. A good communication network of phones or intercoms is vital to locate and inform staff quickly. A special paging code, such as 1111, will enable instant summoning of ICU staff in emergencies. Adequate arrangements for offices, doctor on-call rooms, staff lounge (with food and drinks facilities), wash rooms and teaching complete the unit.

Equipment

The quantity and level of equipment will depend on the role and type of ICU. Level I and II ICUs will obviously require less than a level III unit (Table 1.2). For example, a two-channel bedside monitor should suffice for a small district hospital ICU, whereas a major teaching hospital ICU should be equipped with monitors able to display at least four physiological signals. Monitoring devices and ventilators are discussed in Chapters 27, 28 and 95–97. Equipment should be chosen by experienced intensivists, as often expensive but inappropriate or unsuitable equipment is bought by inept or less knowledgeable people.

Staffing[2,14,16]

The level of staffing also depends on the type of hospital. A large hospital ICU requires a large team of people (Table 1.3).

Medical staff

Career intensivists are the best senior medical staff to be appointed to the ICU.[2,4] The ICU director is one of such specialists. Less preferable are ICUs staffed by specialists from other disciplines (such as anaesthesia or medicine) who often have clinical commitments elsewhere.

Junior medical staff in the ICU may be intensive care trainees, but should ideally also include trainees

Table 1.2 Equipment in a major intensive care unit

Monitoring
Bedside and central monitors
12-lead ECG (paper) recorder
Intravascular and intracranial pressure-monitoring devices
Cardiac output computer
Pulse oximeters
Pulmonary function monitoring devices
Expired carbon dioxide analysers
Cerebral function/EEG monitor
Patient/bed weighers
Temperature monitors
Enzymatic blood glucose meters

Radiology
X-ray viewers
Portable X-ray machine
Image intensifier

Respiratory therapy
Ventilators – bedside and portable
Humidifiers
Oxygen therapy devices and airway circuits
Intubation trolley (airway control equipment)
Airway devices
Manual self-inflating resuscitators
Fibreoptic bronchoscope
Anaesthetic machine

Cardiovascular therapy
Cardiopulmonary resuscitation trolleys
Defibrillators
Temporary transvenous pacemaker
Intra-aortic balloon pump
Infusion pumps and syringes

Dialytic therapy
Haemodialysis machine
Peritoneal dialysis equipment
Continuous haemofiltration sets

Laboratory
Blood-gas analyser
Selective ion (electrolyte) electrode analysers
Osmometer
Haematocrit centrifuge
Thromboelastograph
Microscope

Hardware
Dressing trolleys
Drip stands
Bed restraints
Heating/cooling blankets
Pressure distribution mattresses
Sterilizing equipment (e.g. autoclave and glutaraldehyde bath)

ECG = Electrocardiogram; EEG = electroencephalogram.

Table 1.3 Staff of a major intensive care unit

Medical
Director
Staff specialist intensivists
Junior doctors

Nurses
Nurse managers
Nurse specialists
Nurse educators
Critical care nurse trainees

Allied health
Physiotherapists
Pharmacist
Dietician
Social worker
Respiratory therapists

Technicians

Secretarial
Secretary
Ward clerk

Radiographers

Support staff
Orderlies
Cleaners

Nursing staff

The level of nursing staffing will also depend on the type of ICU. Major ICUs should have a majority of their nurses experienced in critical care nursing. Courses or training programmes in critical care are valuable if creditable. The actual total numbers of nurses for an ICU must take into account night shifts and annual, sick, or study leave. At all times, all critically ill patients must have one-to-one nursing. Occasionally, very unstable patients requiring complex therapy (e.g. dialytic therapy) require two nurses most of the time. Practical staff numbers can be derived from work statistics and types of patients.[14] (see Chapter 5).

Allied health

Major ICUs should have 24-h access to physiotherapists and radiological services. Access to other therapists, dieticians and social workers should also be available. A dedicated ward clinical pharmacist is invaluable. Respiratory therapists are allied health personnel trained in, and responsible for, the equipment and clinical aspects of respiratory therapy – a concept well-established in North America, but not the UK, Europe and Australasia. Technicians, either as members of the ICU staff, or seconded from biophysics departments, are necessary to service, repair and develop equipment.

of other acute disciplines (e.g. anaesthesia, medicine and surgery). For a level II or III ICU, it is imperative that junior doctors are adequately supervised, with specialists being readily available.

Other staff

Provision should be made for adequate secretarial support. Transport and lifting orderly teams will reduce physical stress and possible injuries to nurses and doctors. If no mechanical system is available to transport specimens to the laboratories (e.g. air-pressurized chutes), sufficient and reliable manual labour must be provided to do this day and night. Contact is made with the local chaplains, priests or officials of all religions, when there is need for their services. Their role in counselling and consoling distressed relatives is invaluable (see below).

Operational policies[6,13,14]

Clear-cut administrative policies are vital to the functioning of an ICU. An *open* ICU has unlimited access by multiple doctors who are free to admit and manage their patients. A *closed* ICU has admission, discharge and referral policies under the control of intensivists. Improved cost benefits are likely with a closed ICU and patient outcome may be better, especially if the intensivists have full clinical responsibilities.[17–19]

Some ICUs, particularly in countries without qualifications or training programmes in intensive care, adopt a management-in-consultation policy. A team (usually anaesthetists) looks after the day-to-day and emergency aspects, but co-manages the patients with the referring specialists. Whilst laudably democratic, lines of responsibility at times are unclear, and acquisition of knowledge or experience may not be optimal. Regardless of whoever is in charge, lines of management must be delineated for all staff members, and their job descriptions defined. The director must have final overall authority of all staff and their actions, although in other respects each group may be responsible to their respective hospital heads, e.g. director of nursing.

Policies for the care of patients should be formulated. They should be unambiguous, periodically reviewed, and all staff should be familiar with them. Certain policies are universally applicable, e.g. antibiotic policies and compulsory hand-washing before and after examining patients. Others depend more on local situations and personal beliefs, e.g. donning gowns and over-shoes before entering the ICU – a ritual not proven to reduce cross-infection.

Quality assurance, continuing education and research

The measurement and improvement of quality of care are very much applicable to intensive care. Quality assurance programmes in the ICU can be considered under three headings:

1 *Structure* – documentation must be available to show that the ICU functions according to its operational guidelines and conforms to policies of training and specialist bodies (e.g. staffing establishment and levels of supervision). Data on clinical workload and case mix should be collected.
2 *Clinical process* – audits of clinical performance are conducted as peer review meetings, clinical–pathological conferences and critical incident reporting. A critical incident is as an event which has or would have led to patient morbidity or mortality.[20] Analysis of reports will alter practice to improve care.
3 *Outcome* – quality of care in terms of outcome is difficult to measure. Mortality rates are not useful. The acute physiology and chronic health evaluation II (APACHE II) illness severity scoring system (see Chapter 2) can be used across countries.[21,22] Its multivariate analysis model has been used to compare performance in terms of actual versus predicted death rates.[21,22] Data on quality of life of survivors are difficult to collect and assess.

ICUs should also have ongoing academic programmes. Apart from clinical reviews (see above), meetings to review journals and new developments should be held regularly. Teaching programmes must be instituted for trainees, nurses and other health care workers who must be encouraged to develop their quality assurance programmes. Research has to be pursued.

Ethics in intensive care[23,24]

Ethics in patient care, research and conduct towards colleagues must be scrupulously upheld. ICUs with their high-technological and life support systems are vulnerable to legal, moral and ethical controversies of euthanasia or overenthusiastic treatment, and extreme opposite convictions which are represented by 'right-to-life' and voluntary euthanasia groups. Difficulties are caused by public misconceptions of medical practices and different interpretations of terminology, which are not helped by irresponsible public media. Some institutions have ethics committees which arbitrate on disagreements concerning withdrawal of treatment, but they should not replace clinician decision-makers. Ethical issues in the ICU can be different from those in other health care areas, e.g. palliative care wards.

Euthanasia[25–28]

The acceptance of death by the diagnosis of brain death from brainstem function tests is now well-established (see Chapter 45). Terminating life support on a patient with proven brain death should no longer have any legal or ethical implications. Euthanasia can be defined as *a direct act to terminate* life *with primary intent* and can be viewed as three types:

1 voluntary euthanasia, or intentional killing of those who have expressed a competent, freely made wish to be killed;
2 professionally assisted suicides;
3 non-voluntary euthanasia, or homicide by agreement of all parties except the subject, who may or may not survive intensive therapy, when death is not imminent (e.g. newborns with congenital defects and ventilated patients with chronic, debilitating diseases).

There is much debate on euthanasia.[25–28] Advocates of euthanasia argue that it is morally justified in certain cases, as the ultimate outcome is 'good' and 'best' for the patient. In the ICU scenario, assisted suicide is not a consideration. Non-voluntary euthanasia is, technically, murder. Requests for voluntary euthanasia in the ICU are rare. None the less, such acts are illegal and cannot be ethically justified.

Withdrawal or withholding of treatment[29–33]

The withdrawal or withholding of treatment which sustains or prolongs life has been unfortunately called 'passive euthanasia'[34] a term which is misleading.[35] Allowing a patient to die by withdrawing failed treatment, or forgoing treatment judged to be of no benefit, when death is usually inevitable albeit not always invariable – is not euthanasia, as the intentions are different. None the less, difficulties lie with the assessment of survival probability (see Chapter 2), decision-making and the concepts of autonomy and paternalism.

Autonomy versus paternalism[36]

The principle of *autonomy* dictates that the individual controls his or her own life and destiny; doctors must therefore respect and follow the patient's wishes. This presupposes that the patient can rationally determine his or her best treatment option. *Paternalism* allows the doctor to make decisions for, and in the best interests of, the patient. It presupposes that the doctor 'always knows best'. Arguments against autonomy are that the doctor has a better knowledge of the disease process, societal interests (i.e. efficient use of health resources) should override individual rights, and the patient, in acute illness, may not be rational to exercise control. None the less, most institutions now recognize the rights of competent patients to refuse treatment. The practice of autonomy in the ICU is even more difficult with incompetent patients.

Incompetent patients

If ICU patients are incapacitated to make decisions, surrogates, usually relatives, become involved in decision-making. However, decisions may be influenced by grief, guilt, greed or other feelings or motives. US legislation since November 1991, requires hospitals to inform all patients on admission of their rights to make an advanced treatment declaration or to appoint a decision-making surrogate.[32] As these *living wills* are made in advance without knowing the nature of one's future incapacitation (or indeed that it will occur), they lack precision. For example, a 'no life support' *living will* would prevent effective management of diabetic or anaphylactic shock, both treatable conditions with potentially excellent outcomes. Consequently, difficulties in interpretation of *living wills* arise.[37] The legal status of the *living will* and surrogate-signed documents are present in some American states, but are largely untested outside the USA.

Patients in a *postanoxic persistent vegetative state* (PVS), although incompetent, are not close to death. As they are not brain-dead, they are able to breathe spontaneously, and indeed are able to live for years with good care. Recently, high court decisions in the USA, UK, Canada and New Zealand permitted doctors (upon the family's request) to withdraw nutrition and hydration in PVS patients.[32–34] Thus the right to forgo unwanted treatment in incompetent patients, even without the presence of a terminal illness, has been established. None the less, patients in PVS should be discharged to the wards once spontaneous ventilation is established, and not managed in the ICU.

Practical considerations

There are few institutional guidelines but no societal and legal accords on the practice of ethical principles in the ICU. The following may be helpful practical considerations.

1 Caring for the patient and family should take precedence over all-out preservation of life *per se*.
2 The wishes of a competent patient (or, if incompetent, as clearly expressed in a *living will*) to refuse treatment must be respected. Alternative treatment modes should be explored. If the patient's rationality is in question, steps are deferred or his or her wishes may be overridden *initially*.
3 If a patient is incompetent, surrogates in priority are spouses, adult offspring, parents and the nearest living relative. Parents are always surrogates for incapacitated paediatric patients.
4 It is proper to withdraw or forgo treatment which has failed or has complications that outweigh benefits when the prognosis is grave, and when the quality of life is not expected to be acceptable to

the patient. Withdrawal of treatment is not abandonment of treatment.

5. A consensus on the withdrawal of treatment should be reached amongst medical and nursing staff, after consideration of ethical factors. This medical decision must be explained with the relatives but *without putting the burden of decision-making* on them. Discussions must be recorded. The decision should be reviewed and re-evaluated.

6 There are no moral differences between categories of treatment, such as to withdraw antibiotics but to continue hydration. Nevertheless, treatment should preferably not be withdrawn so that a single step results rapidly in death (e.g. disconnection from ventilators). Reduction or discontinuation of inotropic drugs and supplemental oxygen are common first steps. It is imperative that the patient must be free from pain and discomfort. Opioids and sedatives must be given liberally, even though they may hasten death through respiratory depression.

7 Effective communication between the ICU team and the patient's family must be established (see below). Families, especially in some cultures, frequently request continuation of inappropriate, futile treatment. Further discussions to achieve consensus should be held, but limited care may be continued initially.

Handling relatives[38]

ICU care must include sensitive handling of patients' relatives. Family members undergo at various times feelings of fear, anxiety, disbelief, incomprehension, denial, anger, guilt, and 'why me?' The ICU environment of equipment, alarms, patients and constant activity can be hostile and frightening. Antagonism and frustration can build up through concern for their critically ill loved ones, failure by staff to provide explanations, and an inhospitable physical environment (e.g. hours of waiting in corridors). Attention must be paid to the following considerations in handling relatives.

Effective communication

One senior doctor (specialist or senior registrar/resident) should be identified as the ICU representative to liaise with a particular family. He or she should identify, by consensus, a spokesperson for the family to whom information is normally conveyed. An ICU nurse, preferably the one caring for the patient, is a valuable member in discussions with the family. Relatives feel less daunted in the presence of a nurse, who helps in explanations and consoling distressed members. Children should not be excluded in discussions.

In each interview, the intensivist must ascertain what the family already knows or has been told. Any misinformation or misconceptions must be rectified. When providing explanations, simple, clear, consistent terms must be used. Stressed relatives shut out bad news and can misunderstand or misinterpret what was said. Honesty is best; if death is probable or imminent, say so. Failure to inform about grave prognosis and changes in condition give an impression of uncaring and incompetent staff. The intensivist should show empathy and avoid cliches, false sympathy and patronage. One should listen, encourage questions and expect a spectrum of emotions from any family member. Worried, grieving relatives can be abusive as well as tearful. They should be enabled to cry and accept reality. Assurances that measures to relieve pain and suffering are being given to their loved one must be made. Culture permitting, touch (e.g. holding hands of distressed members) should be appropriately applied. Request for organ donation must be made by an experienced specialist, and at an appropriate time, usually after conformation of brain death. The time, date and discussion of each interview should be recorded.

Physical environment

Interviews should be conducted in a private, suitably furnished, dedicated room. Tissues, tea/coffee and a telephone must be available, and relatives should have access to toilets and a cafeteria. An availability of hospital short-term accommodation for those who live far away is helpful. Visiting hours must be liberal, if not round the clock. Entry of children into the ICU would be at the discretion of the family and staff. If relatives have to wait for a prolonged period while the patient is undergoing treatment, a staff member should explain the delay.

Other supportive measures

Contact with a social worker, counsellor, priest or religious minister should be arranged if appropriate. Sedatives may need to be prescribed for some family members. Follow-up counselling may be required. Emotional support for staff may be necessary and is also important. If death occurs, the family should be allowed privacy to mourn, and to view, touch and hold the deceased. Whether children should view the patient after death is best decided by the family.

References

1 Editorial (1988) Twenty five years of coronary care. *Lancet* **ii**:830–831.

2 Policy Document (IC2) (1994) *The Duties of an Intensive Care Specialist in Hospital with Approved Training Posts*. Melbourne: Australasian and New Zealand College of Anaesthetists.

3 National Institutes of Health (1983) Consensus Development Conference on Critical Care Medicine. *Crit Care Med* **11**:466–469.

4 Policy Document (IC3) (1994) *Guidelines for Hospitals*

Seeking Approval of Training Posts in Intensive Care. Melbourne: Australasian and New Zealand College of Anaesthetists.

5 Dudley HAF (1987) Intensive care: a specialty or a branch of anaesthetics? *Br Med J* **294**:459–460.

6 Oh TE (1994) The development, utilization, and cost implications of intensive care medicine – strategies for the future. In: Tinker J, Browne D and Sibbald W (eds) *Critical Care – Standards, Audit and Ethics.* London: Edward Arnold, pp.11–20.

7 Jacobs P and Noseworthy TW (1991) National estimates of intensive care utilization and costs: Canada and the United States. *Crit Care Med* **18**:1282–1286.

8 Singer DE, Carr PL, Mulley AG and Thibault GE (1983) Rationing intensive care – physician responses to a resource shortage. *N Engl J Med* **309**:1155–1160.

9 Cullen DJ, Keene R, Waternoux C, Kunsman JM, Caldera DL and Peterson H (1984) Results, changes, and benefits of intensive care for critically ill patients: update 1983. *Crit Care Med* **12**:102–106.

10 Slatyer MA, James OF, Moore PG and Leeder SR (1986) Costs, severity of illness and outcome in intensive care. *Anaesth Intens Care* **14**:381–389.

11 Policy Document (ICI) (1994) *Minimum Standards for Intensive Care Units.* Melbourne: Australasian and New Zealand College of Anaesthetists.

12 Task Force on Guidelines, Society of Critical Care Medicine (1988) Recommendations for critical care unit design. *Crit Care Med* **16**:796–806.

13 Task Force on Guidelines, Society of Critical Care Medicine (1988) Recommendations for intensive care unit admission and discharge criteria. *Crit Care Med* **16**:807–808.

14 *Standards for Intensive Care Units* (1983) London: Intensive Care Society (UK).

15 Miranda DR and Langrehr D (eds) (1986) *The ICU: A Cost–Benefit Analysis.* International Congress Series 709. Amsterdam: Excerpta Medica.

16 Task Force on Guidelines, Society of Critical Care Medicine (1988) Recommendations for services and personnel for delivery of care in a critical care setting. *Crit Care Med* **16**:809–811.

17 Knaus WA, Draper EA, Wagner DP and Zimmerman JE (1986) An evaluation of outcome from intensive care in major medical centers. *Ann Intern Med* **104**:410–418.

18 Brown JJ and Sullivan G (1989) Effect on ICU mortality of a full-time critical care specialist. *Chest* **96**:127–129.

19 Groeger JS, Strosberg MA, Halpern NA *et al.* (1992) Descriptive analysis of critical care units in the United States. *Crit Care Med* **20**:846–863.

20 Short TG, O'Reagan A, Lew J and Oh TE (1993) Critical incident reporting in an anaesthetic department quality assurance programme. *Anaesthesia* **48**:3–7.

21 Zimmerman JE, Knaus WA, Judson JA *et al.* (1988) Patient selection for intensive care: a comparison of New Zealand and United States hospitals. *Crit Care Med* **16**:318–326.

22 Oh TE, Hutchinson RC, Short S, Buckley TA, Lin ES and Leung D (1993) Verification and use of the acute physiology and chronic health evaluation scoring system in a Hong Kong intensive care unit. *Crit Care Med* **21**:698–705.

23 Paris JJ and Reardon FE (1991) Moral, ethical, and legal issues in the intensive care unit. *J Intens Care Med* **6**:175–195.

24 Lundberg D (1993) Ethical considerations in the intensive care unit. *Curr Opin Anaesthesiol* **6**:306–308.

25 van der Maas PJ, van Delden JJM, Pijnenborg L and Looman CWN (1991) Euthanasia and other medical decisions concerning the end of life. *Lancet* **338**:669–674.

26 Pollard BJ (1991) Medical aspects of euthanasia. *Med J Aust* **154**:613–616.

27 van der Wal and Dillmann RJM (1994) Euthanasia in the Netherlands. *Br Med J* **308**:1346–1349.

28 Ethics Committee, Royal Australasian College of Physicians (1993) *Ethics: Voluntary Euthanasia. Issues Involved in the Case For and Against.* Sydney: Royal Australasian College of Physicians.

29 Task Force on Ethics of the Society of Critical Care Medicine (1990) Consensus report on the ethics of forgoing life-sustaining treatments in the critically ill. *Crit Care Med* **18**:1435–1439.

30 Fisher MM and Raper RF (1990) Withdrawing and withholding treatment in intensive care. *Med J Aust* **153**:217–229.

31 American Thoracic Society (1991) Withholding and withdrawing life-sustaining therapy. *Ann Intern Med* **115**: 478–485.

32 Jennett B (1992) Letting vegetative patients die. *Br J Med* **305**:1305–1306.

33 Pollard BJ (1991) Withdrawing life-sustaining treatment from severely brain-damaged persons. *Med J Aust* **154**:559–561.

34 Safar P and Winter P (1990) Helping to die. *Crit Care Med* **18**: 788–789.

35 House of Lords Select Committee in Medical Ethics (1994) *Report.* London, HMSO.

36 Pollard BJ (1993) Autonomy and paternalism in medicine. *Med J Aust* **159**:797–801.

37 Heintz LL (1988) Legislative hazard: keeping patients living against their wills. *J Med Ethics* **14**: 82–86.

38 McLauchlan CAJ (1990) ABC of trauma. Handling distressed relatives and breaking bad news. *Br Med J* **301**: 1145–1149.

2 | Severity and outcome of critical illness

JF Bion

A remarkable reduction in mortality was achieved in the polio epidemic in Copenhagen over 40 years ago, by ventilating victims with respiratory failure and centralizing such care.[1] This achievement contributed to the development of intensive care medicine, now well-established in many countries. However, intensive care is an expensive facility.[2,3] In the USA, it consumes around 1.5% of the gross national product and 15% of the hospital budget[3] (see Chapter 1). Intensive care given to non-survivors costs twice as much survivors.[4] A major determinant of this wasted expenditure is prognostic uncertainty.[5] Heterogeneous case mix, small sample sizes and difficulty in measuring severity of illness have hindered research on outcome prediction.

A major advance was the introduction in 1981 of a new measure of severity of illness, which took into account the problems of case-mix variation – the acute physiology and chronic health evaluation (APACHE) scoring system.[6-8] This defines severity of illness in terms of physiological derangement, and mortality risk is closely related to the extent of interference with homeostatic mechanisms. It became possible to describe objectively how sick a patient was across a range of diagnostic groups, and give a numerical estimate of the risk of death. Since then, considerable work has been undertaken to improve the accuracy of this and other measures of severity of illness.

Factors influencing outcome

Critical illness implies failure of one or more vital organ systems. The four main determinants of outcome from critical illness are described below.

Physiological reserve

This includes the presence or absence of chronic disease, functional limitation of specific organ systems, immunoparesis, cancer and age. Age has an inconsistent relationship with mortality, because *chronological age* is an easily measured surrogate for *biological age*, which varies according to individual and population health status. Age should never be used as the sole criterion for making therapeutic decisions. Physiological reserve is difficult to measure, because it is often occult, only becoming manifest in response to physiological stress and tissue injury.

Reserve is important because it may determine susceptibility to critical illness. Accurate measures of reserve would identify patients at risk, and enable preventive action to be taken. Limited reserve (whether measured as chronic disease or impaired quality of life before the acute illness) is the main factor affecting quality and duration of survival following hospital discharge from intensive care.[9]

Severity of acute illness

This is the most important determinant of outcome, and can be described in physiological, anatomical or functional terms, or a combination of these. The extent to which acute illness affects physiological or functional variables depends on the balance between the gravity of the applied stress and the patient's physiological reserve. Physiological disturbance is one of the most useful measures of severity of acute illness because health and homeostasis are so closely linked.

Diagnosis

Diagnosis contains implicit information about susceptibility to specific therapy and hence prognosis. Survival rates at similar severity bands vary markedly between patients with different diagnoses (e.g. sepsis, heart failure and diabetic ketoacidotic coma).[10] However, a specific diagnosis must not distract attention from whole patient considerations, since making an accurate diagnosis is difficult in a patient with multiple co-morbidities. For example, patients with haematological malignancies or following bone marrow transplantation who require urgent mechanical ventilation for acute respiratory failure have low survival rates (less than 5%), but the same patients requiring elective mechanical ventilation following a surgical procedure have a much better prognosis.

Diagnosis is not an exact science. One alternative is to use weighting for organ-system failures either alone[11] or in conjunction with physiological methods.[12] Another is to examine change in physiology with treatment, and systems which do this[12,13] perform as well as diagnostic weighting. In the APACHE III system,[7] change in score with time provides additional prognostic power.[14] However, while diagnosis may be less important for measurement of severity of illness, it is needed to explain variations in outcome related to pathophysiological irreversibility or end-stage single organ-system failure (e.g. chronic lung disease).

Therapy

Therapeutic specificity is important (see above). Another determinant of outcome is the timing of treatment. Delay in treatment increases the risks of multiple organ failure[15] and death.[16] However, if treatment is given before ICU admission, physiologically based measurement systems will underestimate the severity of the illness, because data will be collected after treatment has started to improve physiological values. This effect is called lead-time bias.[17]

Accuracy of severity measurement

All systems of measurement need to be compared with some external and independent standard. This is usually mortality, because it is easy to verify and sufficiently frequent to be useful (8–40%).[18] Scoring systems are generally constructed by identifying (either by clinical consensus or statistical analysis) variables which are best related to mortality. Weights are then attributed to those variables to generate a score or a probability using logistic regression. The system must then be applied to an independent patient population for validation. Two main techniques to assess accuracy and compare different systems are receiver–operator characteristic (ROC) curves[18] and goodness-of-fit tests.[19] ROC curves are constructed by plotting the true-positive (sensitivity) and true-negative (specificity) rates for different values (cut-off points) of the severity score. In laboratory terms, the cut-off point is the value at which the test becomes positive. However, in severity measurement there is no such clear break point between values for survivors and non-survivors, only gradations of risk. The area under the curve is a measure of the overall predictive power of the system. The sensitivity and specificity of the system at different cut-off points are calculated using a standard two-by-two table of predicted versus actual outcomes. Sensitivity (predicting death) is calculated as the number of correctly predicted non-survivors divided by the total number of deaths, and specificity (predicting survival) as the number of correctly

predicted survivors divided by the total number of survivors. The area under the ROC curve allows comparison of overall accuracy of different scoring systems.

Outcome

Most studies refer to hospital and not ICU mortality, but recording both may help identify potential deficiencies in ward care or in admission and discharge policies.[20] Death is only one possible outcome, however, and morbidity, functional disability and quality of survival (and indeed, quality of dying) should be considered as well. Documenting long-term survival is important. Evidence suggests that patients may need to be followed for up to 4 years.[21] The sickness impact profile (SIP) and Uniscale have been used as measures of function and life quality respectively, in a questionnaire study of 140 of 254 survivors from intensive care.[4] The worst outcomes were associated significantly with the highest therapeutic intervention scoring system (TISS) scores (see below) and total costs of hospital stay, and to a lesser extent with APACHE II score. Chronic health status before admission also predicted life quality and survival following discharge. Hence, prior limited physiological reserve places constraints on the extent of recovery, while the severity of acute physiological disturbance only determines the quality of survival when it is extreme and prolonged. The main determinant of hospital mortality is severity of the acute illness. Prior chronic ill health is the main determinant of death after hospital discharge. Prior quality of life determines quality of survival afterwards. The implication is that predictions about potential quality of survival should be based on careful history-taking and not on the assistance of scoring systems.

Methods of severity measurement

Many of these in ICU are intended for specific diagnostic groups. The best known can broadly be classified as physiological, clinical or therapeutic, in terms of data used for their construction. Data collection may be laborious, and subject to significant error. Automated data collection is now available for many physiological variables, but does not avoid the problem of data selection and validation.

APACHE II and III

This is a standard to compare other systems. APACHE II[7] has been validated in many countries. The 34 variables in the original version[6] were selected by clinical consensus, and then refined for APACHE II by statistical techniques to 12 physiological variables, with additional weighting for pre-existing chronic disease related to urgency of admission and age.[10] APACHE III[8] has been developed in a multicentre study of 17 440 patients in the USA. It employs 17 physiological variables and a revised version of the Glasgow coma scale (GCS; see below) based on eye-opening and excluding verbal responses. Only those chronic diseases or co-morbidities which affect the patient's immune status appear to influence outcome, and the effect is only seen in emergency admissions. Chronic disease and age contribute 15% to total mortality risk, the rest being acute physiology. The worst physiological values during the first 24 h of intensive care are used, except for neurological assessment (to avoid misclassifying sedated patients as suffering from neurological disease). The sum of the weighted values provides a score which can be used to stratify patients by severity group. However, calculation of risk of individual patients requires a predictive equation using weights for diagnosis and treatment location before admission. This predictive equation is proprietary to APACHE Medical Systems and is not in the public domain. APACHE III demonstrates modest improvement in predictive power (ROC curve area 0.9) over APACHE II, which was already good (ROC 0.85).

APACHE-related systems

The simplified acute physiology score (SAPS),[22,23] the Riyadh intensive care programme (RIP)[12] and the sickness severity score (SSS)[13] systems are based on the APACHE method. None of these use diagnostic weights. RIP and SSS are dynamic scoring systems using change in score over time as a substitute for diagnostic weighting.

SAPS

SAPS has recently been updated as SAPS II[23] in an international study of 19 124 patients, in conjunction with a revision of the mortality probability model (MPM; described below). The first version of SAPS[22] incorporated 14 variables and excluded chronic health data, diagnoses and measures of oxygenation. It did not provide probabilities of survival. SAPS II employs 12 physiological variables with additional weights for age, type of admission and three underlying diseases – acquired immunodeficiency syndrome (AIDS), metastatic malignancies or haematological malignancy. Urine output has better predictive power than creatinine which has therefore been excluded, and the simpler Pao_2/FiO_2 ratio is used for ventilated patients (as it is for the SSS), rather than the $A-aDo_2$ of the APACHE score or weights for mechanical ventilation from the earlier SAPS. Probability of survival is obtained from a graph which plots score against probability using logistic regression. SAPS II performs well as a predictor of outcome for groups of patients (ROC curve area 0.86).

RIP

RIP[12] uses trend analysis of APACHE II scores in association with weighting for organ-system failures, and examines both the absolute score and the rate of change to generate predictions of outcome. A recent single-centre study[24] reported that, of 560 non-survivors at 90 days, 137 were predicted to die; 6 of these patients actually survived.

MPM

MPM was originally called the mortality prediction model,[25] and has undergone multicentre revision to MPM II[26] in the same study as SAPS II. The first version[25] employed 11 binary variables (requiring 'yes/no' responses) selected not by clinical consensus, but by multiple logistic regression analysis. MPM II generates direct estimates of risk of death on admission and at 24 h using 15 binary variables, which include emergency admission, mechanical ventilation, cardiopulmonary resuscitation, renal failure, cirrhosis, cancer, coma, heart rate and systolic blood pressure. Like SAPS, SSS and RIP, it does not require detailed diagnostic information. MPM II has similar prognostic power to SAPS II, with ROC curve areas around 0.83. It is the only method validated for use at the time of ICU admission. Since it is treatment-independent, it may be more useful for triage decisions than physiologically based methods.

Organ-system failures (OSFs)

OSFs are superficially attractive because of their apparent simplicity, ease of application and relevance to clinical practice. The number and duration of OSFs (using physiological definitions independent of therapy except for mechanical ventilation) are closely related to outcome.[11] However, difficulty lies with providing definitions which recognize varying degrees of failure without excessive complexity or oversimplification, and which avoid undue dependence on therapeutic interventions.

GCS[27]

GCS is a well-accepted method of assessing neurological responses and conscious level 6 h or more after head injury. Paediatric versions are available.[28] Its original function was to provide a common descriptive language, which it does well. Weights were subsequently attached to the various components of the scale (from 3 = no motor, verbal or ocular responses, to 15 = normal). This, however, implies an equivalence between the various responses, which is not strictly valid. The GCS was designed for assessing coma following trauma, and not for functional metabolic deficits or therapeutic sedation. It is used in conjunction with the Glasgow outcome scale,[29] which defines five levels of quality of outcome, from death or persistent vegetative state to good recovery. In predicting outcome from hypoxic–ischaemic coma, recursive partitioning has been employed, and simple classification trees have been produced[30] using pupillary light reflexes and motor responses.

TISS[31]

TISS is based on the premiss that therapeutic intensity defines severity of illness. While this is partly true, the relationship is non-linear,[32] and subject to variations in clinical practice. A score of 1–4 points is awarded to each of 70 nursing and medical procedures. A version is available for high-dependency care.[33] The system is more useful for assessing expenditure than severity. Considerable variation in the way TISS is applied is likely, and inter-ICU comparisons should be preceded by detailed staff training in its use. A simple alternative is weighted hospital days,[34] by which the cost of bed-days is calculated as a multiple of ordinary ward bed-days; the first ICU day for a medical patient is worth 3 ordinary ward bed-days, and 2 thereafter.

Injury severity score (ISS), trauma score (TS) and TRISS

The abbreviated injury scale (AIS) is an ordinal ranking system which attaches values to injuries of increasing severity affecting each of six anatomical areas. Summing the squared values for each area gives a linear relationship between score and outcome: this is the ISS.[35] It can be calculated retrospectively at death or discharge, and is therefore best used for audit purposes. The TS[36] is a simple physiological system designed for field use, which sums coded values for three intervals of the GCS, and five intervals of systolic blood pressure and respiratory rate. Combining the ISS and the TS gives an anatomical and physiological index of severity of injury – the TRISS method.[37]

Applications of severity measurement

Applications of severity measurement include stratification for research, controlling for case mix, auditing quality and cost-efficacy of care, and facilitating clinical decision-making by providing estimates of mortality risk. Many of these are interrelated.

Research

Prior stratification by risk of death is essential for clinical intensive care research, and may help to identify subsets of patients who may benefit or be harmed by new treatments. For example, by using ISS, it was possible to show that excess mortality in trauma patients could not be attributed to increased severity of injury,[38] thus directing attention to the

potent adrenocortical suppressant effect of etomidate infusions (see Chapter 78).

Audit of performance

Severity measurement has been used to analyse aspects of structure, process and outcome of intensive care medicine.[39] Of particular importance is the assessment of efficacy, which means obtaining the greatest number of survivors within each risk band. Severity scoring permits calculation of expected mortality rates, which can then be compared with actual mortality rates to generate a mortality ratio, either within specific severity bands, or averaged for comparing different ICUs or different countries.[40] A ratio in excess of 1.0 suggests a performance below average, and lower than 1.0 above average. However, use of mortality ratios has problems. In an early APACHE II study of 13 hospitals, ICUs with the highest observed:expected mortality ratios (i.e. worst performance) had the poorest standards of organization and communication,[41] but this relationship cannot be demonstrated in the APACHE III study by the same workers.[42] Mortality ratios based on physiological systems may not be accurate descriptors of performance for several reasons. Poor care may be masked because the resulting increase in abnormal physiological variables produces a higher calculated risk and actual mortality rates; mortality rato is thus unchanged.[43] Lead-time bias may result in falsely low predicted mortality rates.[17] Dishonest or inaccurate data acquisition may result in higher scores and artificially good mortality ratios. Mortality ratios are also likely to be normally distributed, and subject to regression to the mean. A range of ratios may therefore be expected in any comparison between ICUs or countries, and random variation may occur between study periods. Cross-validation using different scoring systems may be useful, but there is considerable variation in outcome prediction at the individual patient level.[44] Mortality ratios, while useful, should be interpreted with caution.

Clinical decisions from outcome prediction

Measures of severity of illness are calibrated against the frequency (hence probability or risk) of a specific outcome in groups of patients. They do not, and cannot, provide predictions for individual patients. Probabilities are continuous variables; predictions are dichotomous. A 50% probability of death may identify a sick patient population, but does not tell us whether an individual patient is one of the 50 in every 100 within that risk band who will live, or one of the 50 who will die. Indeed, a 50% probability means that the system is maximally uncertain about the outcome at the level of the individual patient. Even the 100% mortality band does not tell us the outcome for the next patient. It simply tells us that given current therapy, survival of patients this sick is unprecedented.

This does not mean that severity measurements cannot be used for audit or to assist in clinical decision-making. In general terms, scoring systems perform better than clinical judgement in predicting outcome. Scoring systems are now based on much larger numbers of patients than any intensivist is likely to see in clinical practice. Aggregated information can therefore be used to tell us to what extent our particular patient resembles the group. Nevertheless, scoring systems should be used in the same way as diagnostic laboratory tests – to inform but not substitute for clinical judgement. Scoring systems need not necessarily be used to favour withdrawal of treatment. They may also provide better than expected prognoses, and thereby encourage continuing treatment. Outcome prediction has been shown to alter management in patients with head injury; a 39% reduction in specified aspects on intensive care was seen in patients predicted to have the worst outcome, and overall outcome or length of stay was not affected.[45] No scoring system has yet been developed for triage purposes to determine access to intensive care, with the possible exception of birth weight in neonatal intensive care.[46]

References

1 Lassen HCA (1953) A preliminary report on the 1952 epidemic of poliomyelitis in Copenhagen with special reference to the treatment of acute respiratory insufficiency. *Lancet* i:37–41.

2 Bion J (1994) Cost containment: Europe. The United Kingdom. *New Horizons* 2:341–344.

3 Chalfin DB and Fein AM (1994) Cost-containment in the United States. Critical care medicine in managed competition and a managed care environment. *New Horizons* 2:275–282.

4 Sage WM, Rosenthal MH and Silverman JF (1986) Is intensive care worth it? An assessment of input and outcome for the critically ill. *Crit Care Med* 14:777–782.

5 Detsky AS, Stricker SC, Mulley AG and Thibault GE (1981) Prognosis, survival, and the expenditure of hospital resources for patients in an intensive-care unit. *N Engl J Med* 305:667–672.

6 Knaus WA, Zimmerman JE, Wagner DP, Draper EA and Lawrence DE (1981) APACHE – acute physiology and chronic health evaluation: a physiologically based classification system. *Crit Care Med* 9:591–603.

7 Knaus WA, Draper EA, Wagner DP and Zimmerman JE (1985) APACHE II: a severity of disease classification system. *Crit Care Med* 10:818–829.

8 Knaus WA, Wagner DP, Draper EA *et al.* (1991) The APACHE III prognostic system. Risk prediction of hospital mortality for critically ill hospitalized adults. *Chest* 100:1619–1636.

9 Yinnon A, Zimran A and Hershko C (1989) Quality of life and survival following intensive medical care. *Quart J Med* 264:347–357.

10 Wagner DP, Knaus WA and Draper EA (1986) Physiologic abnormalities and outcome from acute disease. Evidence for a predictable relationship. *Arch Intern Med* 146:1389–1396.

11 Knaus WA, Draper EA, Wagner DP and Zimmerman JE (1985) Prognosis in acute organ-system failure. *Ann Surg* 202:685–693.

12 Chang RWS, Jacobs S and Lee B (1988) Predicting outcome among intensive care unit patients using computerised trend analysis of daily APACHE II scores corrected for organ system failure. *Intens Care Med* 14:558–566.

13 Bion JF, Aitchison TC, Edlin SA and Ledingham IMcA (1988) Sickness scoring and response to treatment as predictors of outcome from critical illness. *Intens Care Med* 14: 167–172.

14 Wagner DP, Knaus WA, Harrell FE, Zimmerman JE and Watts C (1994) Daily prognostic estimates for critically ill adults in intensive care units: results from a prospective, multicentre, inception cohort analysis. *Crit Care Med* 22:1359–1372.

15 Henao FJ, Daes JE and Dennis RJ (1991) Risk factors for multiorgan failure – a case control study. *J Trauma* 31:74–80.

16 Purdie JM, Ridley SA and Wallace PM (1990) Effective use of regional intensive care units. *Br J Med* 300:79–81.

17 Dragsted L, Jorgensen J, Jensen N-H *et al.* (1989) Interhospital comparisons of patient outcome from intensive care: importance of lead-time bias. *Crit Care Med* 17:418–422.

18 Altman DG and Bland JM (1994) Diagnostic tests 3: receiver operating characteristic plots. *Br Med J* 309:188.

19 Rowan KM, Kerr JH, Major E, McPherson K, Short A and Vessey MP (1993) Intensive Care Society's APACHE II study in Britain and Ireland – II: Outcome comparisons of intensive care units after adjustment for case mix by the American APACHE II method. *Br Med J* 307:977–981.

20 Bion J (1993) Outcomes in intensive care. *Br Med J* 307:953–954.

21 Ridley S and Plenderleith L (1994) Survival after intensive care. Comparison with a matched normal population as an indicator of effectiveness. *Anaesthesia* 49:933–955.

22 Le Gall JR, Loirat P, Alperovitch A *et al.* (1984) A simplified acute physiology score for ICU patients. *Crit Care Med* 12:975–977.

23 Le Gall J-R, Lemeshow S and Saulnier F (1993) A new simplified acute physiology score (SAPS II) based on a European/North American multicentre study. *J Am Med Assoc* 270:2957–2963.

24 Atkinson S, Bihari D, Smithies M *et al.* (1994) Identification of futility in intensive care. *Lancet* 344:1203–1206.

25 Lemeshow S, Teres D, Avrunin JS and Gage RW (1988) Refining intensive care unit outcome prediction by using changing probabilities of mortality. *Crit Care Med* 16:470–477.

26 Lemeshow S, Teres D, Klar J, Avrunin JP, Gehlbach SH and Rapoport J (1993) Mortality probability models (MPM II) based on an international cohort of intensive care unit patients. *J Am Med Assoc* **270**:2478–2486.

27 Teasdale G and Jennett B (1974) Assessment of coma and impaired consciousness. A practical scale. *Lancet* **ii**:81–84.

28 Reilly PL, Simpson DA and Thomas L (1988) Assessing the conscious level in infants and young children: a paediatric version of the Glasgow Coma Scale. *Child Nerv Syst* **4**:30–33.

29 Murray GD (1986) Use of an international data bank to compare outcome following severe head injury in different centres. *Statist Med* **5**:103–112.

30 Levy DE, Caronna J, Singer BH, Lapinski RH, Frydman H and Plum F (1985) Predicting outcome from hypoxic–ischemic coma. *J Am Med Assoc* **253**:1420–1426.

31 Cullen DJ, Civetta JM, Briggs BA and Ferrara LC (1974) Therapeutic intervention scoring system: a method for quantitative comparison of patient care. *Crit Care Med* **2**:57–60.

32 Zimmerman JE, Shortell SM, Rousseau DM *et al.* (1993) Improving intensive care: observations based on organisational case studies in nine intensive care units: a prospective, multicentre study. *Crit Care Med* **21**:1443–1451.

33 Cullen DJ, Nemeskal AR and Zaslavsky AM (1994) Intermediate TISS: a new therapeutic intervention scoring system for non-ICU patients. *Crit Care Med* **22**:1406–1411.

34 Rapoport J, Teres D, Lemeshow S and Gehlbach S (1994) A method for assessing the clinical performance and cost-effectiveness of intensive care units: a multicentre inception cohort study. *Crit Care Med* **22**:1385–1391.

35 Baker SP, O'Neil B, Haddon W and Long W (1974) The injury severity score: a method for describing patients with multiple injuries and evaluating emergency care. *J Trauma* **14**:187–196.

36 Champion HR, Sacco WJ, Carnazzo AJ, Copes W and Fouty WJ (1981) Trauma score. *Crit Care Med* **9**:672–676.

37 Boyd CR, Tolson MA and Copes WS (1987) Evaluating trauma care: the TRISS method. *J Trauma* **27**: 370–378.

38 Watt I and Ledingham IMcA (1984) Mortality amongst multiple trauma patients admitted to an intensive therapy unit. *Anaesthesia* **39**:973–981.

39 Bion JF (1994) Audit and quality assurance in critical care. In: Dobb GJ, Bion J, Burchardi H and Dellinger RP (eds) *Current Topics in Intensive Care.* London: WB Saunders, pp. 218–242.

40 Oh TE, Hutchinson RC, Short S, Buckley TA, Lin ES and Leung D (1993) Verification and use of the acute physiology and chronic health evaluation scoring system in a Hong Kong intensive care unit. *Crit Care Med* **21**:698–705.

41 Knaus WA, Draper EA, Wagner DP and Zimmerman JE (1986) An evaluation of outcome from intensive care in major medical centers. *Ann Intern Med* **104**:410–418.

42 Zimmerman JE, Shortell SM, Rousseau DM *et al.* (1993) Improving intensive care: observations based on organisational case studies in nine intensive care units: A prospective, multicentre study. *Crit Care Med* **21**:1443–1451.

43 Boyd O and Grounds RM (1993) Physiological scoring systems and audit. *Lancet* **341**:1573.

44 Lemeshow S (1994) Individual outcome prediction: the case for and against. *Reanim Urgences* **3**:223–227.

45 Murray LS, Teasdale GM, Murray GD *et al.* (1993) Does prediction of outcome alter patient management? *Lancet* **341**: 1487–1491.

46 Powell TG and Pharoah POD (1987) Regional neonatal intensive care: bias and benefit. *Br Med J* **295**:690–692.

3 | Transport of the critically ill

JE Gilligan

Critically ill patients have absent or small physiological reserves. Moving such patients presents major problems,[1,2] and adverse physiological changes arising during transport can be life-threatening. Thus transport of critically ill patients requires careful planning and strict attention to detail. Although guidelines are available,[3] it remains a commonly neglected area of intensive care.[4,5] The principles of achieving safe transport are encompassed in the five Ps:

1 *planning* (including communications);
2 *personnel* (i.e. correct number and skill mix of staff involved in transport);
3 *properties* (i.e. equipment used in transportation);
4 *procedures* (i.e. measures to stabilize the patient before transport, and continuation of resuscitative care in transit;
5 *passage* (i.e. choice of route and transport mode).

Categories of transport operations

Transport of critically ill patients involves intra-hospital (*intramural*) movements and outside-hospital (*extramural*) movements. The latter operations may be *primary* (pre-hospital) transport of the patient from the site of accident to the first hospital; *secondary* (interhospital) transport between hospitals; or long-distance or international transport.[6,7] Other patient transport categories include neonatal and paediatric transport, and moving ICU patients in a fire threat (see below).

Intra-hospital (intramural) transport[8]

In the setting of intensive care, intra-hospital transport is required for patients coming to the ICU from the emergency department, operating rooms and general wards, and ICU patients being moved for diagnostic or therapeutic interventions, or being discharged to areas of less intensive care. Intra-hospital transport is usually relatively elective, but a need for urgency (e.g. moving to the operating rooms for emergency surgery) must also be anticipated. The transport itself must be justified. Whatever the benefits of proposed interventions, they must outweigh the risks of moving the critically ill patient and those posed by the procedures themselves. To warrant moving the patient, diagnostic interventions should result in changes in patient management, or confirm that current therapy is correct and thus rule out a new and potentially dangerous course of treatment.

Planning

Planning should first formulate a protocol, which must be made widely known and available. The protocol should strive for care during intra-hospital transport to equate with that in the ICU or recovery ward. A precise time for the movement should be decided and a best route planned. Faulty arrangements subject patients to prolonged, unnecessary trips and waiting in corridors.

Personnel

Key personnel for each transport event should be identified, depending on the patient to be moved. Transport teams should consist of *combinations* of a nurse, an orderly, a respiratory therapist and a doctor. Each team must be familiar with the equipment, and be sufficiently experienced with securing airways, ventilation of the lungs, resuscitation and other anticipated emergency procedures. Inexperienced or unskilled staff may not recognize or deal with problems.[2] A dedicated transport team could be considered, if transport of critically ill patients or of special cases (such as neonates) is a frequent event. Tasks are apportioned accordingly.

Properties

Dedicated transport equipment must be able to function in the intervention area (e.g. a magnetic resonance imaging room), and facilities for remote patient monitoring should be available. Gas and electrical supplies at the destination must be present and compatible. No equipment should be placed on the patient or carried by staff; specially designed receptacles (e.g. bed frames)[9] or transport trolleys are useful.

The level of equipment required depends on the stability of the patient. Basic monitoring of electrocardiogram (ECG) heart rate and blood pressure is necessary for all patients (except perhaps for well-recovered patients being discharged to the wards). Respiratory monitoring, a pulse oximeter, a defibrillator and a suctioning device should be available for ventilator-dependent or unstable patients. A portable ventilator delivers a more consistent ventilation than a manual resuscitator bag, which, none the less, must also be available. A mounted ICU ventilator, with gas and battery power for 1–2 h offers the best option. Positive end-expiratory pressure (PEEP) values are used to maintain PEEP or continuous positive airways pressure (CPAP). Automated non-invasive blood pressure monitors and infusion pumps are highly recommended. Emergency drugs, analgesics, sedatives, muscle relaxants and equipment to secure the airway must be available, and are best carried in a dedicated crash box. Spare battery packs for electrical devices must be available. All equipment must be readily accessible and regularly checked.

Procedures

The transport team must be freed from other duties. Receiving staff at the destination must be notified, and the arrival time clearly understood. All equipment must be checked (Table 3.1). Final preparations of the patient are made (e.g. giving bolus doses of muscle relaxants or sedatives, replacing an empty fluid or blood bag, and ensuring that prescribed inotropes are being infused). The status of the patient is checked before transport begins (Table 3.2). Transport preparations must not overshadow or neglect the patient's fundamental care and treatment.

Passage

The patient bed and linked devices must be able to enter lifts (elevators) and pass through all doorways *en route*. If the bed cannot be wheeled to the destination, the patient is moved on a trolley, but this is often inadequate for carriage of equipment. Care must be taken to avoid injury to patient and staff when shifting the patient from bed to trolley.[10] Lifts should be secured beforehand. Relatives, visitors and media personnel should be shepherded, so as not to obstruct the bed or trolley. Abrupt movements and vibrations should be minimized. Adequate communication facilities during transit and at the destination must be available. The status of the patient

must be checked at intervals. Any change in the patient's condition, unexpected event or critical incident must be recorded.

Extra-hospital (extramural) operations

Pre-hospital (primary) transport

Intensivists may need to assist emergency services staff in the pre-hospital transport of critically ill patients

Table 3.1 Intra-hospital transport – pre-departure equipment and document checklist

The ECG monitor functions properly; set alarm limits
The non-invasive BP monitor (if available) functions properly; set alarm limits
The pulse oximeter (if available) functions properly; set alarm limits
The capnograph (if available) functions properly; set alarm settings
The manual resuscitation bag functions properly
The ventilator (if available) functions properly; set respiratory variables
The ventilator disconnect alarm (if available) functions properly
The suction device functions properly
Oxygen ($\pm$ air) cylinders are full
A spare oxygen cylinder is available
Airway and intubation equipment are all available and working
Emergency drugs, analgesics, sedatives and muscle relaxants are all available
Additional drugs are made available if indicated
Spare intravenous fluids or blood are available if needed
Spare batteries are available for all battery-powered equipment
Chest clamps (if an underwater chest drain is present) are available
Patient notes, X-rays, necessary forms (especially the informed consent form) are available

ECG = Electrocardiogram; BP = blood pressure.

Table 3.2 Patient status checklist

Airway is secured and patent
Ventilation is adequate; respiratory variables are appropriate
All equipment alarms are switched on
PEEP/CPAP (if set) and Fio_2 levels are correct
All drains (urinary, wound, underwater seal) are functioning and secured
Underwater seal drain is not clamped
Venous access is adequate and patent
Intravenous drips and infusion pumps are functioning properly
Patient is safely secured on trolley
Vital signs are charted

PEEP = Positive end-expiratory pressure; CPAP = continuous positive airways pressure; Fio_2 = inspired oxygen concentration.

as a result of vehicular accidents, mass disasters and rescue operations (e.g. cliff falls). A disaster is an adverse event which overwhelms regional medical resources. The rate of arrival of injured patients to a hospital overwhelms facilities more than the total number of patients *per se*. Thus controlled movement of patients to a selected range of hospitals is desirable. Acute hospitals should be prepared to mobilize a medical team as part of their response to a disaster. Counter-disaster medicine is relatively basic. Hence equipment taken and procedures done are designed to 'do the greatest good for the greatest number'. Details of on-site care are beyond the scope of this chapter, but medical teams need to triage and treat patients before moving them.

Inter-hospital (secondary) transport

This involves transport from a rural or district hospital to a major centre[11,12] or a specialized unit (e.g. neonatal or obstetric).[13,14] Special mobile intensive care teams and services may be required (e.g. accompanying neonatologist or obstetrician).

International/long-distance transport

Operations over considerable distances (e.g. > 3000 km) produce additional requirements.[7] Jet aircraft, especially commercial airliners, are commonly used. The team, patient and equipment may need 15 passenger seats.[7] Military transport aircraft (e.g. Hercules C 130) is spacious, noisy, pressurized and slower than commercial aircraft. Commercial airliners commonly have 28 V DC power, but not all carriers permit its use. Non-dedicated aeromedical aircraft may lack connections to utilize 28 V DC power. Patients must be stable enough to travel. In cases of acute myocardial infarction, medical transport at 2 weeks is considered valid.[15]

Immigration requirements, accommodation, availability of supplies *en route* and legal status of the staff and medications carried should be resolved beforehand. The transport team is away for a protracted time, and should be sufficient for 12 h shifts. Time zones may be crossed, and charting of data should be done on home hospital time. In general, medical teams need to provide their own equipment and electrical power. Electrical and gas adaptors are needed to overcome incompatible connections. Waste disposal (e.g. syringes, needles, dressings and body wastes) needs to be considered.

Conduct of extra-hospital transport

Planning

Coordination and good communication between the evacuation/retrieval and ambulance teams and staff at both ends of the trip are vital. Poor communication limits detailed information dissemination, and specialist staff may not be able to assess a critical situation adequately. A phone and facsimile link[11,12] will provide advice to local personnel on resuscitation and managing the critically ill patient pending arrival of the evacuation/retrieval team.

Personnel

Transport staff require diagnostic and resuscitative skills. Advanced Trauma Life Support (ATLS)[16] or in Australasia, Emergency Management of Severe Trauma (EMST)[17] certification is recommended. Familiarity of safety procedures, effects on patient and crew and other factors (e.g. communications) relating to the transport mode used is necessary.

Motion sickness, eustachian tube obstruction or other disorders may affect patient and staff. Personnel particularly vulnerable to motion sickness should avoid transport missions. The most effective medication against motion sickness is hyoscine hydrobromide (scopolamine),[18,19] taken 4 h prior to travel; transdermal patches may take 8 h to act.[20] Side-effects are sedation, dry mouth and dystonia.

Properties (Table 3.3)

General considerations[21,22]

Bedside equipment must be secured during all phases of transport. The medical pack (Table 3.3) should not exceed 40 kg. A single stretcher for both air-borne and road transport is preferred. A reflecting space blanket offers better weather protection than conventional bedding; alternatively a transparent plastic sheet over bedding is used. Appropriate equipment to protect staff from infected material is necessary (e.g. disposable gloves and gowns, eye protection, a sharps bin, and non-needle injection systems).

Transport monitors and devices are generally battery-powered. Newer batteries have improved endurance; over 6 h or twice the anticipated travel time is desirable. Commonly used nickel–cadmium (NiCd) rechargeable cells need to be discharged completely before recharging, to prolong endurance.[23] Sealed lead-acid batteries have similar endurance, but should be kept fully charged,[24] as periodic exhaustion will shorten their life. Wet-cell lead acid batteries are unsafe.

Battery power in compact monitors may range up to 10 A/h at 12 V, and monitors use as little as 0.2 A. Supplementary power should be available as spare batteries, a larger storage battery, or from the vehicle's DC system. Motor vehicles are equipped for 12 V DC and airplanes for 28 V DC (with 12 V also available in some). Access to both power sources can be achieved with a standard three-pin Cannon connection which utilizes either voltage without adjustment (socket MS 310 2E 20–19S).[22] Devices should also be able to utilize domestic power sources (240 V 50 Hz AC in Australia),

Table 3.3 Mobile intensive care equipment for extramural transport

Circulatory drugs
Inotropes
α- and β-blockers
Atropine (anticholinergic)
Neostigmine (cholinergic)
Antiarrhythmics
Antihypertensives/vasodilators

Intravenous fluids
Hartmann's normal saline, 5% dextrose, etc.
Polygeline (Haemaccel) or similar.

Blood products as required for specific missions
Blood (usually O negative)
Normal serum albumin
Blood products (factors II, VII, IX, X)
Anti-haemophilic factor, cryoprecipitate
Platelets

Renal agents
Diuretics (loop and osmotic)

Allied drugs
Potassium
Magnesium
Sodium bicarbonate 8.4%
Calcium chloride
Glucose, hypertonic

Antibiotics
Penicillin, others as needed

Coagulation drugs
Heparin
Vitamin K_1
Thrombolytic agents

Uterine agents
Oxytocics
Tocolytics

Steroids

Respiratory
Bronchodilators

Nervous system drugs
Opioids
Opioid and other antagonists
Anticonvulsants
Sedatives
Neuromuscular blockers
Antiemetics
Local anaesthetic agents
General anaesthetic agents (usually intravenous)

Nutrients
Parenteral nutrition required on some long-distance medevacs

Respiratory equipment
Airways (Guedel)

Ventilation bag (self-inflating) and masks
Ventilator (compact) and spare exhale valve
Simple spirometer
Intubation equipment
   Endotracheal tubes and adaptors
   Introducer
   Magill forceps, artery forceps
   Laryngoscopes, blades, globes, batteries
   Bronchoscopes, rigid, battery handle-type
   Suction device, Yankaeur handle, catheters
   Cricothyrotomy equipment, tracheostomy tubes
Laryngeal masks
Pleural drainage
   Catheters, trocars, cannulae, scalpel
   Howard Kelly forceps
   Heimlich valves
   Wound drainage bags
Suture material with attached needle
Nebulizer

Circulatory equipment
Monitor/defibrillator
Multiple parameter monitor
Pulse oximeter
Electronic blood pressure measurement (invasive/non-invasive)
Sphygmomanometer cuff and clock
Venous cannulae (peripheral and central)
Intravenous fluids and pressurization sleeve
Arterial cannulae
Non-distensible tubing; bubble isolator or transducer (if equipped for arterial monitoring)
Infusion pump
Giving sets (including those for intravenous pumps)
Syringes, needles, non-needle injection system

Gastrointestinal equipment
Nasogastric tube
Drainage bag

Renal equipment
Urinary catheters and collecting bags

General equipment
Lightweight stretcher (e.g. Scoop)
and requisite mattress (e.g. vacuum type)
Spare batteries for electronic devices, or
facility to utilize aircraft power supply
Nasal decongestant (ear clearance in aircraft)
Torch
Writing equipment, including skin crayon
Labels – medication and name
Clothing shears
Adhesive tape
Antiseptic (e.g. povidone-iodine)
Reflecting (space) blanket

especially for recharging their batteries. Some air ambulances can provide 240 V AC power, generated via inverters.[25]

Potential interference of aircraft navigational radiofrequency by electronic medical devices and equipment carried by medical teams should be determined. Radios and mobile phones have caused such problems,[26-28] and digital devices are more troublesome than analogue systems.

Haemodynamic equipment

Combined ECG monitor/defibrillator devices are usual. Pulse oximetry enables Sao_2 and pulse rate to be read non-invasively. It can be used with sphygmomanometer cuff inflation to monitor blood pressure (BP), but may give faulty readings in vasoconstricted states.[29] Screen displays may be hard to read in transit, and alarm signals may not be audible. Communication head sets[30] may be adapted to relay monitor sound signals. Similarly, BP measurement by auscultation is difficult in transit. Systolic pressure measurement with an aneroid sphygmomanometer and pulse palpation remains the commonest technique. Non-invasive BP recorders are heavy and tend to over-read when mean BP is low.[31] An arterial line gives the most reliable recording in transit. Mean BP can be simply displayed using a heparin-filled line connected via a membrane isolator to an aneroid sphygmomanometer. Compact multifunction monitors are available, providing non-invasive and invasive recordings of ECG, Sao_2, end-tidal carbon dioxide, physiological pressures and temperature.

Intracardiac catheters and transvenous pacing wires require electrical isolation. Many battery-powered monitors and devices have built-in 'front end' isolation, which should protect the patient against microshock. External cutaneous pacing is feasible in short-term transport. If counterpulsation (intra-aortic balloon pump) is used, the transport vehicle needs to be large and the machine secured against dislodgement.

Respiratory equipment

Accompanying staff must have ready access to the patient's head during transit to enable endotracheal intubation in emergencies. When mechanical ventilation is necessary, ventilators are superior to manual ventilation. Electrically powered ventilators require heavy batteries and are not popular. A compact gas-driven, fluid logic portable ventilator is commonly used (e.g. Oxylog, ULCO; see Chapter 27). Air-entrainment (Fio_2 0.5) will minimize oxygen use. For children, an extra pressure-limiting valve may be needed. Transport ventilators have limitations, and a larger, AC-electrically driven ICU ventilator may be needed for patients with severe lung disease (with an inverter to generate AC from vehicular DC).

PEEP valves should operate in any spatial orientation, and an intermittent mandatory ventilation (IMV) valve may be needed in some patients. If CPAP is required, a low-flow balloon 'clapper-board' system is preferred. However, such patients may be better transported fully ventilated. Humidification is best achieved by heat and moisture exchangers. Suction devices are battery-powered, foot-operated or Venturi-driven.[32] Patients on extracorporeal membrane oxygenation present major problems; few transported cases have been documented.

The source of medical oxygen in aircraft must be separate from that for emergency cabin decompression. Carrying double the expected consumption for each patient allows for unexpected contingencies. Aeromedical transport commonly uses cylinder oxygen supplies,[33] as other options have limited use. Most portable gas regulators do not have self-seal outlets. Disconnection from a ventilator hose when gas is flowing may cause disruption of the regulator, which will fail when the hose is reconnected. Ball flow meters must be aligned vertically (but not gauge flow meters). At altitude, with reduced cabin pressure, the volume delivered slightly exceeds flow meter reading.

Other equipment

A rectal or oesophageal thermistor probe and electronic display to measure temperature are required. Tympanic membrane measurement is an alternative.[34,35] Mercury thermometers can be unsafe, as spilt mercury from breakage is hazardous.

Drainage systems or facilities for urinary, wound and nasogastric catheters are necessary. Apart from fluid balance charting and patient comfort, catheter drainage will minimize the expansion of entrapped gas at altitude (e.g. gastric distension; see below).

Plaster shears should be carried against possible tissue and vascular compression, when limbs are splinted. Such limbs may swell during long-distance transport (especially if dependent) and should be elevated.

Dialytic therapies are usually suspended during patient transport. However, in long-distance transport, continuous haemofiltration/haemodiafiltration techniques may be necessary (see Chapter 39) and such equipment must be available. Peritoneal dialysis may need to be continued. If so, mechanical ventilation may be necessary if breathing becomes compromised by abdominal distension.

Useful biochemical monitoring equipment includes reflectance blood glucose meters and dry chemistry systems[36] (e.g. Boehringer Mannheim Refletron and Kodak DT 60) for estimating haemoglobin, Na^+, K^+, Cl^-, urea, creatinine, glucose, bilirubin, cholesterol and liver enzymes.

Procedures

Patient assessment at the pick-up site is followed by the A,B,Cs of resuscitation (airway, breathing and circulatory control), plus correction of major thermal and biochemical disorders. A low threshold to endotracheal intubation should be adopted, as this is difficult in a transport vehicle if the patient later deteriorates. Vital, urgent data (e.g. arterial blood gases or X-rays) should be obtained before departure, and cross-matched blood checked. Potentially violent or restless patients may constitute a hazard to themselves and others, and are sedated or judiciously restrained.[37]

A chest intercostal drain is best attached to a Heimlich flutter valve draining into a vented plastic bag. Underwater seal drainage systems are awkward to transport, but are sometimes used in long-distance transport. Clamping the drainage tube when lifting the patient risks producing a tension pneumothorax, when a bronchopleural fistula is present.

Intravenous (IV) lines are inserted (preferably away from joints) and secured well. Central venous lines may be necessary. Luer-lock junctions reduce disconnection risks. Pressor infusion sleeves are indicated for emergency volume replacement. Alternatively, plastic air-free infusion bags can be wedged under the patient's buttock. IV bolus drugs are prepared and labelled well beforehand. If parenteral nutrition is ceased, rebound hypoglycaemia should be prevented by infusing 10% glucose and the blood glucose monitored. Infusion pumps give better control of drug and fluid administration during transit.

Passage

Designs of road and air transport facilities should comply with general requirements (Table 3.4).[38] Road

Table 3.4 Ideal requirements for a transport modality

Adequate safety of operation

No abrupt movements in any axis

Sufficient room for at least one critically ill patient, and supporting team, with an attendant at the head end

Adequate supply of energy and medical gases for life support systems

Adequate lighting and internal climate control, including cabin pressurization

Tolerable noise and vibration levels

Adequate restraint devices for stretchers, occupants and equipment

Easy embarkation and disembarkation of patient

A stretcher suitable for all phases of transport, obviating the need for changing stretchers between vehicles

Minimal secondary transport (e.g. road transport in air evacuation)

Adequate speed

Effective communication systems

transport is used for metropolitan areas, but less frequently for rural-to-city transfers. Aircraft are essential in most emergency medical systems, with indications for both helicopters and fixed-wing aircraft. Helicopters allow rapid deployment and mobility and can be landed near an accident site. Their operational altitude is less than in fixed-wing aircraft and cabins are not pressurized. Flight speed is around 120 nautical mph, with an operating radius of 200 km. They are used for major accidents[39] in rural or outer city areas (usually within a flight radius of 30–100 km), but are also used for inter-hospital transport in some major cities. Fixed-wing aircraft commonly operate for ranges 150–1500 km, and require adequate landing facilities. Planes commonly used are twin-engined, giving an acceptable payload. Speeds of turboprop and jet aircraft are 240 and 500 nautical mph respectively.

Positioning the patient transversely produces the least inertial change in body fluids, but few aircraft have the necessary width to allow this. There is little clinical difference in lengthwise positioning head or feet first,[40] but the former enables more effective restraint during deceleration.

There are potential problems encountered in transit. The patient stretcher may be incompatible between vehicles or poorly anchored. Loading the stretcher on to the vehicle may be difficult. Adverse weather and environment will affect staff, patient and equipment. Ambient temperature reduces approximately 2°C per 1000 ft of altitude – at 10 000 ft external temperature is 0°C.[41] Turbulence, bright sunlight and darkness in flight may cause discomfort. Low-frequency vibration (<20 Hz) is potentially damaging to various organs.[42–44] Vibration and noise will accentuate fatigue. Noise and daylight may render monitors and alarms temporarily inaudible and unreadable. Equipment may become dislodged from their anchorage (e.g. webbing belts).

One major problem is the effect of decreasing atmospheric pressure with increasing altitude (Fig. 3.1). Aircraft cabin pressurization is relative – commonly maintained at 630 mmHg (84 kPa), equivalent to an altitude of 1550 m (5000 ft; Fig. 3.1), when the actual altitude may be up to 12 500 m (40 000 ft). Pressurized cabin pressure at sea level pressure (760 mmHg, 101 kPa) requires a flight restricted to an altitude of 4900–8200 m (16 000–27 000 ft). Air ambulances, chartered executive jets and military aircraft may fly at this lower, less efficient (and bumpier) altitude, but this is impractical for jet airliners. Altitude causes:

1 *Reduced partial pressure of oxygen:* oxygen supplementation needs to be increased.
2 *Increased gas volumes in enclosed spaces:* volumes of endotracheal tube cuffs, inflated pneumatic antishock garment (PASG) suits and pneumatic splints will increase. Air enclosed in drip chambers will cause gravity-regulated IV rates to vary. Monitoring and correcting for these changes are

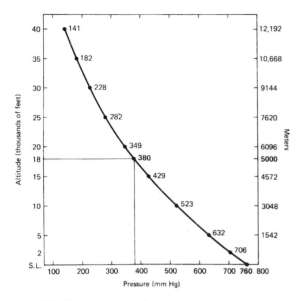

Fig. 3.1 Altitude and atmospheric pressure.

Medical air is necessary to regulate the F_{IO_2} precisely, minimizing risks of retrolental fibroplasia.

Transport of the diving-injury patient[46]

Patients with decompression sickness or arterial gas embolism are intolerant of even low (100–200 m) altitude, because bubble expansion exacerbates clinical effects. For air-borne retrieval, most diving-accident patients are given 100% oxygen by facemask, and evacuated by rapid flight at sea-level cabin pressure to a major hyperbaric unit. Alternatively, transportable hyperbaric chambers are taken to the site,[47] but this cumbersome mode presents problems of loading and lack of space.

Movement of ICU patients in a fire threat

The greatest cause of death in fires is smoke inhalation and carbon monoxide and cyanide poisoning (see Chapter 72). Consequently, should a fire arise in or close to the ICU, staff should first move spontaneously breathing patients. Ventilated patients have their compressed gas supply, and are transferred last, by which time smoke infiltration may have subsided. Lifts should not be used.

necessary. Expansion of air in body cavities is reduced by denitrogenation (breathing 100% oxygen before and during flight), and is applied to patients with gut distension, blocked sinuses and intracranial air. Entrapped air in penetrating eye injuries, with raised intraocular pressure from vomiting, coughing, straining or hypoxia, may discharge globe contents at altitude. This can be minimized by eye binding, antiemetics, sitting the patient upright, providing 100% oxygen therapy,[45] and flying at the lowest effective altitude.

Patients with potentially life-threatening effects from altitude (e.g. with gas embolism, decompression sickness, and severe hypoxaemia despite breathing 100% oxygen) will need to be transported at sea-level cabin pressure.

Special transport operations

Transport of the neonate[13]

Incubators are bulky (often weighing 80 kg), and consume around 200 W power (using AC or DC) for thermal homeostasis and around 20 W for monitoring. Use of the transport vehicle's medical gases and electrical energy reduces the number of gas cylinders carried and conserves battery power.

References

1 Gentleman D and Jennett B (1981) Hazards of inter hospital transfer of comatose head injured patients. *Lancet* **2**:853–855.
2 Braman S, Dunn S, Amico CA and Millman RP (1987) Complications of intrahospital transport in critically ill patients. *Ann Intern Med* **107**:469–473.
3 Australian and New Zealand College of Anaesthetists and Australian College of Emergency Medicine (1992) *Minimum Standards for Transport of the Critically Ill (P23).* Melbourne: ANZCA.
4 Gilman J (1987) Carrier and vendor selection. In: Hackel A (ed.) *Critical Care Transport.* International Anesthesiology Clinics. Boston: Little, Brown, pp. 117–137.
5 Bion JF, Wilson IH and Taylor PA (1988) Transporting critically ill patients by ambulance: audit by sickness scoring. *Br Med J* **296**:170–174.
6 Gunby P (1989) Winged medical care ranges worldwide. *J Am Med Assoc* **244**:420–427.
7 Merlone S and Hackel A (1987) Care of patients during long distance transport. In: Hackel A (ed.) *Critical Care Transport.* International Anesthesiology Clinics. Boston: Little, Brown, pp. 105–116.
8 Oh TE (1995) *Intrahospital Transport of the Critically Ill Patient.* International Task Force on Anaesthesia Safety. Seattle: Communicore.
9 Wishaw K, Munford B and Roby H (1990) The Careflight stretcher bridge: a compact mobile intensive

care unit. *Anaesth Intens Care* **18**:234–245.

10 Standards Association of Australia (1987) *Guide to the Lifting and Moving of Patients. Part 1 – Safe Manual Lifting and Moving of Patients 1982. Part 2 – Selection and Use of Mechanical Aids for Patient Lifting and Moving.* AS 2596.1-1982 and AS 2569.2-1987. Sydney: SAA.

11 Gilligan JE, McCleave DJ, Nicholson B *et al.* (1977) Retrieval of the critically ill in South Australia: a coordinated approach. *Med J Aust* **2**:849–855.

12 Waydhas C, Schneck G and Duswald KH (1995) Deterioration of respiratory function after intrahospital transport of critically ill surgical patients. *Intensive Care Med* **21**:784–789.

13 James AG (1995) Neonatal resuscitation, stabilisation and emergency neonatal transportation. *Intens Care World* **11**:53–57.

14 Bolan JC (1990) Indications for maternal transport. In: McDonald MG and Miller M (eds) *Emergency Transport of the Perinatal Patient.* Boston: Little, Brown.

15 Roby H (1993) Air transport of patients post acute myocardial infarction. Proceedings of the International Society of Aeromedical Services, Sydney. ISAS, Arncliffe, NSW. *ISAS News* **5**:15–16.

16 American College of Surgeons (1988) *Advanced Trauma Life Support Course.* Chicago: ACS.

17 Royal Australasian College of Surgeons (1989) *Emergency Management of Severe Trauma. Course Manual.* Melbourne: RACS.

18 Wood CD (1979) Antimotion sickness and antiemetic drugs. *Curr Therapeutics* **20**:155–168.

19 Brand JJ (1966) Drugs used in motion sickness. *Pharmacol Rev* **18**:895–924.

20 Levy GD and Rapaport MH (1985) Transderm scopolamine efficacy related to time of application prior to the onset of motion. *Aviat Space Environ Med* **56**:591–593.

21 Standards Association of Australia (1986) *Guide to the Safe Use of Electricity in Patient Care.* AS 2500-1986. Sydney: SAA.

22 International Society of Aeromedical Services (Australian chapter) (1993) *Aeromedical Standards.* Arncliffe: ISAS (Australasia).

23 Health Devices Alerts (1985) *Defibrillator/monitors, Battery Powered (11-129).* 1985.8.2. Plymouth Meeting Pennsylvania: ECRI.

24 Health Devices Alerts (1987) *Gates Rechargeable Lead Acid Batteries.* 1987.16.6. Plymouth Meeting Pennsylvania: ECRI, 1987.

25 Standards Association of Australia (1985) *Electrical Installations – Patient Treatment Areas of Hospitals and Medical and Dental Practices.* AS 3003-1985. Sydney: SAA.

26 Levy B (1995) *Analogue or Digital? Mobile Communications.* Sydney: Austcom Publishing.

27 Editorial: Mobile telephone interference with devices (1994) *Australian Therapeutic Device Bulletin* 1.2–4.

28 Editorial (1993) Cellular telephones and radio transmitters – interference with clinical equipment. *Health Devices* **22.8.9**:416–418.

29 Clayton D, Webb RK, Ralston AC, Duthie D and Runciman WB (1991) A comparison of 20 pulse oximeters under conditions of poor perfusion. *Anaesthesia* **46**:3–10.

30 Weien R (1992) Helmets and helmet mounted systems. In: *Proceedings of the Conference on Helicopter Survival.* Buckinghamshire, UK: Intavox training conferences.

31 Rutten AJ, Ilsley AH, Skowronski GA and Runciman WB (1986) A comparative study of mean arterial blood pressure using automatic oscillometers, arterial cannulation and auscultation. *Anaesth Intens Care* **14**:58–65.

32 Australian Standard (1992) Medical suction equipment. Part 1 (AS 2120.1): electrically powered suction equipment – safety requirements. Part 2 (AS 2120.2): manually powered suction equipment. Part 3 (AS 2120.3): suction equipment powered from a vacuum or pressure source. Sydney: Standards Australia.

33 McNeil EL (1983) Sources of oxygen. In: McNeil EL (ed.) *Airborne Care of the Ill and Injured.* New York: Springer-Verlag, pp. 107–111.

34 Ferrara-Lov R (1991) A comparison of tympanic and pulmonary artery measures of core temperature. *J Post Anesth Nursing* **6**:10–11.

35 Green MM and Danzi DF (1989) Infra-red tympanic thermography in the emergency department. *J Emerg Med* **7**:437–440.

36 Steinhausen RL and Price CP (1985) Principles and practice of dry chemistry systems. In: Price CP and Alberti KGMM (eds) *Recent Advances in Clinical Biochemistry*, no 3. Edinburgh: Churchill Livingstone, pp. 273–295.

37 Jones DR (1980) Aeromedical evacuation of psychiatric patients; historical review and present management. *Aviation Space Environment Med* **61**:709–714.

38 Sub-Committee Report: Road ambulance design (1990) *Stretcher Security.* Proceedings of the Convention of Australian Ambulance Authorities. Canberra: AAA.

39 Baxt WG and Moody P. The impact of a physician as part of the aeromedical prehospital team in patients with blunt trauma. *J Am Med Assoc* **257**:3246–3250.

40 McNeil EL (1983) Orientation and posture. In: McNeil EL (ed.) *Airborne Care of the Ill and Injured.* New York: Springer-Verlag, pp. 65–68.

41 Thom T (1992) *Meteorology and Navigation. The Pilot's Manual Series.* Williamstown, Vic: Aviation Theory Centre P/L.

42 Von Gierke H and Goldman DE (1976) Effects of shock and vibration on man. In: Harris CM and Crede CE (eds) *Shock and Vibration Handbook*, 2nd edn. New York: McGraw Hill, pp. 1–56.

43 Floyd WN, Broderson AB and Goodno JF (1973) Effect of whole body vibration and peripheral nerve conduction time in the rhesus monkey. *Aerospace Med* **67**:281–284.

44 Clark JG, Williams JD, Hood WB *et al.* (1967) Initial cardiovascular response to low frequency whole body vibration in humans and animals. *Aerospace Med*

38:464–468.

45 Hyldegaard O and Madsen J (1994) Effect of air, heliox and oxygen breathing on air bubbles in aqueous tissues in the rat. *Undersea Hyperbaric Medicine* **21**:413–424.

46 Edmonds C, Lowry C and Pennefather J (eds) (1992) *Diving and Subaquatic Medicine*, 3rd edn. Oxford: Butterworth-Heinemann.

47 Gilligan JE, Gorman DF and Millar I (1988) Use of an airborne recompression chamber and transfer under pressure to a major hyperbaric facility. In: Shields TG (ed) *Proceedings of the XIV Meeting of the European Undersea Biomedical Society*. Aberdeen: European Undersea Biomedical Society.

4 Physiotherapy in intensive care

A Jones

The use of chest physiotherapy was first documented in 1901,[1] and has been widely applied to treat pulmonary disorders since 1954.[2] Despite extensive research, some optimal modalities remain debatable, due to non-standardized research designs. Although reports in the ICU setting are limited, chest physiotherapy has a significant role in the overall care of the intensive care patient.[3-6]

Rationale for physiotherapy

The immobilized critically ill patient suffers muscle deconditioning and an increased risk of deep vein thrombosis. Artificial airways and inadequate humidification increase mucus production, decrease ciliary activity[7] and increase the risk of nosocomial infection through contamination of the lower airways. Mechanical ventilation leads to decreased functional residual capacity (FRC), atelectasis, decreased lung compliance, ventilation/perfusion ($\dot{V}/\dot{Q}$) mismatch,[8] and increased dead space:tidal volume ratio. Thus, the goals of physiotherapy treatment in the ICU are to maximize musculoskeletal performance and to maintain or improve cardiopulmonary function (by promoting mucociliary clearance, sputum expectoration and alveolar expansion).[4,9]

Staffing levels and service hours

An ICU should provide a 24-h physiotherapy cover.[10-14] This is usually provided by day and evening shifts and an on-call night service. Costs of a 24-h service will be balanced by savings from shorter patient-days in ICU, resulting from fewer complications and faster recovery. The number of physiotherapists required in an ICU depends on the nature of the ICU and the patient workload. Some duties will overlap with those of respiratory therapists in institutions with this job classification. Frequency of physiotherapy treatments should be tailored to individual needs, but patients are usually treated twice daily, with each treatment lasting 15–45 min.[3] Assuming an average treatment time of 30 min, a full-time physiotherapist is required for every six ICU beds in level II and III ICUs (see Chapter 1).

Treatment modalities

Planning and assessment

A physiotherapy programme involves a cycle of problem identification, planning, treatment and evaluation of effectiveness (Fig. 4.1). Identification of precise problems in a patient and accurate analysis and interpretation of assessment findings are thus important.

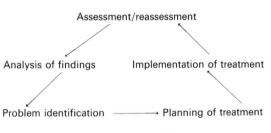

Fig. 4.1 Physiotherapy programme cycle

Positioning and postural drainage

Correct positioning is an integral part of physiotherapy management to remove secretions and improve $\dot{V}/\dot{Q}$ matching. The supine position significantly decreases FRC.[15] The patient should be positioned sitting upright or lying on one side, and not supine or sitting slumped.[16]

Gravity-assisted postural drainage facilitates drainage of secretions from a specific lung area, and is recommended mainly for patients with excessive

Table 4.1 Conditions requiring special consideration during postural drainage

Severe hypertension
Acute myocardial infarction, angina, cardiac arrhythmias
Congestive cardiac failure, pulmonary oedema
Raised intracranial pressure
Cerebral or aortic aneurysms
Dyspnoea
Oesophageal operations, hiatus hernia, regurgitation
Eye surgery
Peritoneal dialysis, haemodialysis, haemofiltration
Ascites, abdominal distension

secretions. Each drainage position should be maintained for 10 min.[17] Certain conditions require caution or a modified technique (Table 4.1)[12] – e.g. head-down positioning may increase cerebral blood volume and intracranial pressure (ICP) in head-injured patients.[18]

Positioning is a simple but often neglected technique for maximizing lung ventilation. In spontaneously breathing normal subjects, ventilation is preferentially distributed to the base (dependent part) of the lung. Mechanical ventilation, however, reverses preferential ventilation to the (non-dependent) apex. Since perfusion is preferentially distributed to the base, spontaneous breathing achieves better $\dot{V}/\dot{Q}$ matching. Hence, to improve ventilation to an affected part of the lung during spontaneous breathing, it seems reasonable to position the part downwards. However, studies have reported improved oxygenation in spontaneous breathing *and* mechanically ventilated patients with unilateral lung disease, when positioned with the good lung down.[19–22] This position also facilitates secretion drainage and lung re-expansion of the affected lung.

In neonates, the more compliant chest wall exerts a compression force on the dependent lung; ventilation is better in the non-dependent area.[23] Oxygenation in neonates with unilateral lung disease may be improved with the affected lung placed downwards.

Positioning for optimal V/Q matching may be more unpredictable in patients with bilateral lung disease. The side–decubitus position may provide better oxygenation. Changing from supine to prone can often improve oxygenation, due possibly to removal of retained secretions.[24,25]

Improved alveolar expansion in different parts of the lungs is accomplished by frequent alternate changes of side–decubitus positions. Extra care is required when changing the position of an intubated patient. The patient should be disconnected momentarily from the ventilator during turning, and manually 'bagged' whilst the ventilator circuit is prepared.

Percussion and vibration

Percussion is the clapping of the chest with cupped hands at a frequency of about 5 Hz.[4] The mechanical waves of energy produced are believed to be transmitted through the chest wall to loosen airway mucus.[26] Percussion vibrates alveoli, alveolar ducts and bronchioles, and may also promote gas flow through collateral and small airways. Vibration is fine shaking of the chest during expiration, and is usually combined with chest wall compression. These techniques are often used in conjunction with postural drainage to facilitate removal of secretions.

Percussion by itself will not increase mucociliary clearance[27] or sputum expectoration.[28] It may cause a decrease in FEV_1[29] and induce hypoxaemia,[30] but these adverse effects can be prevented if breathing control and thoracic expansion exercises are incorporated into the treatment programme.[31] Percussion should not be performed over bare skin nor cause pain; facial expressions should be observed during treatment. Consequences of pain are muscle splinting and increased work of breathing and oxygen consumption, which are particularly important during ventilator weaning.

Breathing control, forced expiration technique and autogenic drainage

Breathing exercises aim to assist basal lung re-expansion in spontaneously breathing patients. Deep breathing increases the alveolar–pleural pressure difference, thereby increasing collateral flow between an atelectatic segment and open airways.[4] Thoracic expansion exercises[7] with inspiratory hold (i.e. breath-holding for 3 s) are used to increase tidal volume and augment alveolar expansion. This breathing pattern accommodates the different time constants of 'fast' and 'slow' alveoli[15] to promote more uniform gas distribution, and has been shown to decrease the incidence of postoperative atelectasis.[32] Incentive spirometry was designed to encourage sustained voluntary inspiration with an open glottis. The patient can practise the breathing exercise regularly without a physiotherapist being present. However, incentive spirometry is no better than conventional physiotherapy programmes in reducing hospital stay or pulmonary complications.[33] In patients with hyperinflated lungs, incentive spirometry and inspiratory hold may be contraindicated.

The forced expiration technique (FET) uses 1–2 forced expiratory huffs combined with breathing control.[7] Utilizing the equal pressure point principle, a forced expiration from mid to low lung volume may help shift secretions from distal to more proximal airways.[34,35] Huffing is performed with an open glottis, and generates a lower intrathoracic pressure compared to coughing. This technique may be preferred in patients with pain or bronchomalacia.

Autogenic drainage is a technique which varies tidal volume through controlled breathing to enhance mucus mobilization.[36,37] It has been used mainly in Europe, and further investigation is required to agree on a standard procedure which will achieve a favourable effect.

Manual inflation (bagging)

Manual inflation or bagging delivers manually controlled tidal volumes to the intubated patient with a manual resuscitator. Indications for bagging are:

1 to increase alveolar oxygenation with an increased inspired oxygen (Fio_2). This is normally employed before and after tracheal suctioning;
2 to correct atelectasis. The patient's lungs are inflated with a large tidal volume, and inflation is maintained for a few seconds before the bag is slowly released. This presumes to improve alveolar gas distribution via collateral flow;
3 to mobilize secretions. The patient's lungs are inflated with a large tidal volume, and the bag is released quickly to create a high alveolar–mouth pressure gradient and a fast expiratory flow. This technique simulates a cough (or more correctly a huff) which shifts secretions to more proximal airways for suctioning;
4 to hyperventilate to lower $Paco_2$ in certain cases (e.g. to lower ICP).

Bagging has been shown to increase total static compliance in ventilated patients by 16%.[38] Oxygen saturation is also significantly improved. Chest wall compression with bagging produces a significantly higher maximal expiratory flow[39] than bagging alone. Ideally, bagging should be performed by two physiotherapists – one performing manual ventilation, and the other synchronized chest wall vibration and compression (compression should start at the beginning of bag release). Suctioning may be undertaken by a nurse or the non-ventilating physiotherapist. Precautions required for suctioning must be considered before implementing this technique.[14]

Manual resuscitators commonly used for bagging include the Hope, Ambu self-inflating bag, Mapleson-C circuit, and Laerdal[3] (see Chapter 27). Clinical performance of bagging circuits may differ from those of bench tests.[40,41] The main determinant to choose a bagging circuit is the familiarity of the therapist with the circuit.[41] The Laerdal bag is easy and safe to use, produces a reliable expiratory flow, and can be recommended for physiotherapists less experienced with the bagging procedure.

Intermittent positive-pressure breathing (IPPB)

IPPB in spontaneously breathing patients may be achieved with a Mark 7 or 8 Bird respirator. Claimed benefits are efficient delivery of bronchodilators, increased secretion mobilization, re-expansion of alveoli and decreased work of breathing. However, good scientific basis for its use is lacking, and use of IPPB has markedly decreased since the 1970s.

Non-invasive intermittent positive-pressure ventilation (NIPPV)

NIPPV delivers intermittent positive-pressure ventilation without tracheal intubation, using face or nasal masks.[42,43] (see Chapter 26). The role of the physiotherapist in NIPPV is to ensure patient comfort and optimize alveolar ventilation. Provided training is adequate, NIPPV can be satisfactorily managed by physiotherapists, respiratory therapists and ICU nurses.[44,45] Physiotherapists should be aware of the potential uses of NIPPV (e.g. in the initial postintubation period).

Continuous positive airway pressure (CPAP) and positive expiratory pressure (PEP)

CPAP maintains a positive pressure during both the inspiratory and expiratory phases of spontaneous breathing (see Chapter 26). It can be delivered to an intubated patient or to a non-intubated patient via a face or nasal mask. The main benefits of CPAP are increased FRC, reduced work of breathing and prevention of dynamic airway collapse during expiration.[46] Nasal CPAP has a significant role in the management of obstructive sleep disorder.[47] The effect of CPAP in improving lung function in postoperative patients has been established.[48,49] Periodic application of CPAP after extubation or in postoperative patients with decreased ventilation is now a regular adjunct to conventional physiotherapy treatment. There are no absolute contraindications, but mask pressure is a major concern. CPAP should be applied with caution in patients with head injury, and is contraindicated in those with skull fractures.[50]

A PEP mask system consists of a facemask and a one-way valve to which a variable expiratory resistance is attached. Airway transmural pressure in the central and peripheral airways is increased. The PEP mask is recommended for recruitment or re-expansion of obstructed alveoli and mobilization of peripheral secretions.[51] Use of a PEP mask for 30 breaths every hour is an effective prophylactic treatment against atelectasis in the postoperative patient.[52] The frequency and duration of treatment should be tailored to individual needs.

Flutter valve

The Flutter VRP1 is another PEP device recently introduced to physiotherapy. This simple device consists of a mouthpiece and a valve compartment. The latter has a stainless steel ball sitting on a circular canal which is housed with a perforated cover. Expiration into the mouthpiece causes movement of the ball, which generates a vibrating effect on endobronchial positive pressure. This vibrating effect is believed to assist in mucus elimination. Flutter VRP1 significantly increased the amount of sputum expectorated in patients with cystic fibrosis.[53] However, no advantages were seen with this valve in post-thoracotomy patients,[54] and it failed to improve peak flow or FEV_1 in patients with moderately severe asthma.[55] Its use as an adjunct to physiotherapy requires further evaluation.

Exercises

Exercises are important to maintain blood circulation, sensory input, joint range and muscle length and strength. These effects can be achieved by passive, assisted active or active exercises. Exercises will increase pulmonary ventilation, and limb movement has been used to increase pulmonary volume. Passive mobilization of the limbs of an unconscious or semi-conscious patient should attempt to stretch muscles to full length and maintain maximal joint range. Patients should be encouraged to sit up or out of bed as soon as they are able to. Assisted active or active exercises should be practised, provided they do not unnecessarily increase work of breathing. Extra precautions are taken when exercising patients on inotropic support or with pulmonary oedema, as they may not have sufficient cardiovascular reserve to comply.[14]

Mobilization is the most effective way to improve and maintain cardiopulmonary function. Patients on mechanical ventilation can be sat out of bed or mobilized using portable ventilators or manual bagging. A rollator walking frame allows shoulder girdle support, improves pulmonary reserve, and is ideal for exercise tolerance training. Monitoring of oxygen saturation with a pulse oximeter (Spo_2) provides useful assessment of progress. A conservative approach should be taken when exercising a patient with pulmonary hypertension, right ventricular hypertrophy and cor pulmonale, because hypoxia induced by exercise may cause acute decompensation. Hypoxaemia induced by exercise may also trigger ventricular arrhythmias.[9] During exercise, the patient's Spo_2 should not fall by more than 5% or below 80%.[56]

Special considerations

A physiotherapy programme should be tailored to the individual patient. Patients are not identical, and the condition of a patient may change between visits. Each patient may require special considerations at different stages of his or her illness.

Weaning

Weaning occurs when a patient receiving mechanical ventilation is judged to be able to resume spontaneous breathing. Common modes of mechanical ventilation used for weaning include intermittent mandatory ventilation, pressure support ventilation, T-piece weaning and CPAP (see Chapter 26). As a member of the ICU team, the physiotherapist should assist in fulfilling the team strategy for weaning.

During weaning, the patient's intrinsic drive to breathe should be maintained.[57] The physiotherapist can reinforce breathing by using a bagging circuit to 'train' the patient to breathe spontaneously. However, supported breaths must be given according to the patient's need. Weaning will be adversely affected by haemodynamic instability, sepsis, agitation and disordered mentation. The physiotherapist should thus ensure that physiotherapy techniques during weaning do not affect haemodynamic stability. Hyperinflation of the lungs with an inspiratory pause by bagging may cause an increase in right ventricular volume and a decrease in right ventricular ejection fraction.[58] Although exercise is important, unreasonable increases in a patient's oxygen consumption must be avoided during weaning. Careful monitoring of the patient's haemodynamic status, arterial oxygenation and subjective feelings is essential during treatment. Finally, patient anxiety is also important. The physiotherapist must incorporate both verbal (i.e. clear explanation) and non-verbal communication skills (e.g. touch and eye contact) to allay anxiety.

Acute respiratory distress syndrome (ARDS)

This is a condition with altered alveolar membrane permeability and unstable surfactant, resulting in atelectasis, alveolar flooding, impaired oxygen uptake and hypoxaemia and, possibly, lung fibrosis and death (see Chapter 29). Sputum retention is rarely a problem in these patients. Physiotherapy is usually directed towards positioning for maximal gas exchange and limb exercises (avoiding any increase in oxygen consumption). As lung compliance is decreased in ARDS, bagging at higher airway pressures is required. This is only undertaken if there is a demonstrable benefit (e.g. improved arterial oxygenation and breath sounds after bagging), because of the risk of barotrauma. If positive end-expiration pressure is used, precautions are taken to ensure that it is not discontinued during treatment (e.g. by disconnecting the circuit).

Acute head injury

Management of a patient with acute head injury includes maintaining cerebral perfusion pressure above 80 mmHg (10.6 kPa) or ICP below 20 mmHg (2.7 kPa). The head-down position increases cerebral blood volume, and theoretically should be avoided in head-injury patients. Whether this position actually increases ICP remains controversial.[59,60] An increased ICP may result from obstructed cerebral venous return, and the physiotherapist should ensure that the patient's neck position is neutral during treatment. Suctioning, coughing and bagging with an inspiratory pause may also increase ICP, and should be performed with caution.[14,61] Hyperventilation lowers Pa_{CO_2} and ICP, but Pa_{CO_2} should be maintained above 25 mmHg (3.33 kPa) to avoid cerebral ischaemia.[61]

ICU environment

The ICU can be frightening for patients, non-ICU staff and visitors. If a patient is to be admitted to the ICU after elective surgery, a preoperative visit to the ICU is psychologically helpful. For patients who require to remain intubated postoperatively, communication protocols between the patient and the physiotherapist should be discussed. The rationale for physiotherapy care and the expectations of the patient should be clearly explained preoperatively.

At the ICU bedside, vital signs and ventilation parameters should be checked before treatment, continuously monitored during treatment, and reassessed at the end of treatment. Before leaving a patient, the physiotherapist must ensure that all alarms are reactivated, all vital signs are stable and that a conscious patient feels comfortable and secure.

References

1 Ewart W (1901) The treatment of bronchiectasis and of chronic bronchial affections by posture and respiratory exercises. *Lancet* 2:70–72.

2 Thoren L (1954) Post-operative pulmonary complications: observations on their prevention by means of physiotherapy. *Acta Chirur Scand* 107:193–205.

3 Jones AYM, Hutchinson RC and Oh TE (1992) Chest physiotherapy practice in intensive care units in Australia, the UK and Hong Kong. *Physiotherapy Theory Pract* 8:39–47.

4 Mackenzie CF (1989) Physiological changes following chest physiotherapy. In: Mackenzie CF (ed.) *Chest Physiotherapy in the Intensive Care Unit*, 2nd edn. Baltimore, MD: Williams & Wilkins, pp. 215–250.

5 Mackenzie CF and Shin B (1985) Cardiorespiratory function before and after chest physiotherapy in mechanically ventilated patients with post-traumatic respiratory failure. *Crit Care Med* 13:483–486.

6 Mackenzie CF and Shin B, Hadi F and Imle PC (1980) Changes in total lung/thorax compliance following chest physiotherapy. *Anesth Analg* 59: 207–210.

7 Pryor J (1992) Mucociliary clearance. In: Ellis E and Alison J (eds) *Key Issues in Cardiorespiratory Physiotherapy*. Oxford, UK: Butterworth-Heinemann, pp. 105–130.

8 West JB (1992) *Pulmonary Physiology – The Essentials*, 4th edn. Baltimore, MD: Williams & Wilkins, pp. 180–193.

9 Alison J and Ellis E (1992) Pulmonary limitations to exercise performance. In: Ellis E and Alison J (eds) *Key Issues in Cardiorespiratory Physiotherapy*. Oxford, UK: Butterworth-Heinemann, pp. 131–157.

10 Intensive Care Society (1983) *Standards for Intensive Care Units*. Department of Health and Social Security (DHSS) document. London: BioMedica.

11 Society of Critical Care Medicine – Task Force on Guidelines. Recommendations for intensive care unit admission and discharge criteria. *Crit Care Med* 16:807–811.

12 Jacob W (1990) Physiotherapy in the ICU. In: Oh TE (ed.) *Intensive Care Manual*, 3rd edn. Sydney: Butterworths, pp. 22–27.

13 Ntoumenopoulos G and Greenwood K (1991) Variation in the provision of cardiothoracic physiotherapy in Australian hospitals. *Aust J Physiotherapy* 37:29–36.

14 Hough A (1991) *Physiotherapy in Respiratory Care – A Problem Solving Approach*. London: Chapman & Hall, pp. 143–165.

15 Nunn JF (1987) *Applied Respiratory Physiology*, 3rd edn. London: Butterworths, pp. 23–45.

16 Jenkins SC, Soutar SA and Moxham J (1988) The effects of posture on lung volumes in normal subjects and in patients pre- and post-coronary artery surgery. *Physiotherapy* 74:492–496.

17 Webber BA (1988) *The Brompton Hospital Guide to Chest Physiotherapy*, 5th edn. London: Blackwell Scientific Publications.

18 Marini JJ, Tyler MI, Hudson LD, Davis BS and Huseby JS (1984) Influence of head-dependent positions on lung volume and oxygen saturation in chronic air-flow obstruction. *Am Rev Respir Dis* 129:101–105.

19 Dhainaut JF, Bons J, Bricard C and Monsallier JF Improved oxygenation in patients with extensive unilateral pneumonia using the lateral decubitus position. *Thorax* 35:792–379.

20 Ibanez J, Raurich M, Abizanda R *et al.* (1981) The effect of lateral positions on gas exchange in patients with unilateral lung disease during mechanical ventilation. *Intensive Care Med* 7:321–324.

21 Remolina C, Khan AU, Santiago TV and Edelman NH (1981) Positional hypoxemia in unilateral lung disease. *N Engl J Med* 304:523–525.

22 Rivara D, Articio H, Arcos J and Hiriart C (1984) Positional hypoxemia during artificial ventilation. *Crit Care Med* 12:436–438.

23 Davies H, Kitchman R, Gordon I and Helms P (1985) Regional ventilation in infancy – reversal of adult pattern. *N Engl J Med* 313:1626–1628.

24 Pichl MA and Brown MS (1976) Use of extreme position changes in acute respiratory care. *Crit Care Med* 4:13–15.

25 Gattinoni L, Pelosi P, Vitale G, Pesanti A, D'Andrea L and Mascheroni D (1991) Body position changes redistribute lung computed-tomography density in patients with acute respiratory failure. *Anesthesiology* 74:15–23.

26 Pavia D (1990) The role of chest physiotherapy in mucus hypersecretion. *Lung* 168(suppl): 614–621.

27 van der Schans CP, Piers DA and Postma DS. Effect of manual percussion on tracheobronchial clearance in

patients with chronic airflow obstruction and excessive tracheobronchial secretion. *Thorax* 41:448–452.

28 Webber BA, Parker RA and Hofmeyr JL (1985) Evaluation of self percussion during postural drainage using the forced expiration technique. *Physiotherapy Practice* 1:42–45.

29 Campbell AH, O'Connell JM and Wilson F (1975) The effect of chest physiotherapy upon the FEV$_1$ in chronic bronchitis. *Med J Aust* 1:33–35.

30 McDonnell T, McNicholas WT and Fitzgerald MX (1986) Hypoxaemia during chest physiotherapy in patients with cystic fibrosis. *Irish J Med Sci* 155:345–348.

31 Pryor JA, Webber BA and Hodson ME (1990) Effect of chest physiotherapy on oxygen saturation in patients with cystic fibrosis. *Thorax* 45:77.

32 Ward RJ, Danziger F, Bonica JJ, Allen GD and Bowes J (1966) An evaluation of post-operative respiratory maneuvers. *Surg Gynecol Obstet* 123:51–54.

33 Hall JC, Tarala R, Harris J, Tapper J and Christiansen K (1991) Incentive spirometry versus routine chest physiotherapy for prevention of pulmonary complications after abdominal surgery. *Lancet* 337:953–956.

34 West JB (1990) *Respiratory Physiology – The Essentials*, 4th edn. Baltimore, MD: Williams & Wilkins, p. 109.

35 Nunn JF (1987) *Applied Respiratory Physiology*, 3rd edn. London: Butterworths, pp. 46–71.

36 Kraemer R, Zumbuhl C, Rudeberg A, Lentze MJ and Chevaillier J (1986) Autogene Drainage bei Patienten mit zytischer Fibrose. *Pädistrische Praxis* 33: 223–232.

37 David A (1991) Autogenic drainage – the German approach. In: Pryor JA (ed.) *Respiratory Care*. London: Churchill Livingston, pp. 65–78.

38 Jones AYM, Hutchinson RC and Oh TE (1992) Effects of bagging and percussion on total static compliance of the respiratory system. *Physiotherapy* 78:661–666.

39 MacLean D, Drummond G, Macpherson C, McLaren G and Prescott R (1989) Maximum expiratory airflow during chest physiotherapy on ventilated patients before and after the application of an abdominal binder. *Intensive Care Med* 15:396–399.

40 Jones AYM, Jones RDM and Bacon-Shone J (1991) A comparison of expiratory flow rates in two breathing circuits used by chest physiotherapists. *Physiotherapy* 77:593–597.

41 Jones A, Hutchinson R, Lin E and Oh T. Peak expiratory flow rate produced with the Laerdal and Mapleson C circuits. *Aust Physio J* 38:211–215.

42 Restrick LJ, Scott AD, Ward EM, Feneck RO, Cornwell WE and Wedzicha JA (1993) Nasal intermittent positive-pressure ventilation in weaning intubated patients with chronic respiratory disease from assisted intermittent, positive-pressure ventilation. *Respiratory Med* 87:199–204.

43 Fernandez R, Blanch LI, Valles J, Baigorri F and Artigas A (1993) Pressure support ventilation via face mask in acute respiratory failure in hypercapnic COPD patients. *Intensive Care Med* 19: 456–461.

44 Bott J, Carroll MP, Conway JH *et al.* (1993) Randomised

controlled trial of nasal ventilation in acute ventilatory failure due to chronic obstructive airways disease. *Lancet* 341:1555–1557.

45 Pennock B, Crawshaw L and Kaplan P (1994) Noninvasive nasal mask ventilation for acute respiratory failure – institution of a new therapeutic technology for routine use. *Chest* 105:441–444.

46 Petrof BJ, Legare M, Goldberg P, Milic-Emili J and Gottfried SB (1990) Continuous positive airway pressure reduces work of breathing and dyspnea during weaning from mechanical ventilation in severe chronic obstructive airway disease. *Am Rev Respir Dis* 141:281–289.

47 Shivaram U, Cash ME and Beal A (1993) Nasal continuous positive airway pressure in decompensated hypercapnic respiratory failure as a complication of sleep apnea. *Chest* 104:770–774.

48 Heitz M, Holzach P and Dittmann M (1985) Comparison of continuous positive airways pressure and blowing bottles on functional residual capacity after abdominal surgery. *Respiration* 48:277–284.

49 Linder KH, Lotz P and Ahenfeld FW (1987) Continuous positive airways pressure on functional residual capacity vital capacity and its subdivisions. *Chest* 92:66–70.

50 Young AER and Nevin M (1994) Tension pneumocephalus following mask CPAP. *Intensive Care Med* 20:83.

51 Falk M and Andersen JB (1991) Positive expiratory pressure (PEP) mask. In: Pryor JA (ed.) *Respiratory Care. International Perspectives in Physical Therapy*. Singapore: Churchill Livingstone, pp. 51–63.

52 Ricksten SE, Bengtsson A, Soderberg C, Thorden M and Kvist H (1986) Effects of periodic positive airway pressure by mask on postoperative pulmonary function. *Chest* 89:774–781.

53 Konstan MW, Stern RC and Doershuk CF (1994) Efficacy of the Flutter device for airway mucus clearance in patients with cystic fibrosis. *J Pediatrics* 124:689–693.

54 Chatham K, Marshall C, Campbell I and Prescott R (1993) The Flutter VRP1 device for post-thoracotomy patients. *Physiotherapy* 79:95–98.

55 Swift G, Rainer T, Saran R, Campbell I and Prescott R (1994) Use of Flutter VRP1 in the management of patients with steroid-dependent asthma. *Respiration* 61: 126–129.

56 Cropp GJ, Pullano TP, Cerny FJ and Nathanson IT (1982) Exercise tolerance and cardiorespiratory adjustments at peak work capacity in cystic fibrosis. *Am Rev Respir Dis* 126:211–216.

57 Conway JH, Hitchcock RA, Goderey RC and Carroll MP (1993) Nasal intermittent positive pressure ventilation in acute exacerbations of chronic obstructive pulmonary disease – a preliminary study. *Respiratory Med* 87:387–394.

58 Jardin F, Brun-Ney D, Hardy A, Aegerter P, Beauchet A and Bourdarias JP (1991) Combined thermodilution and two-dimensional echocardiographic evaluation of right ventricular function during respiratory support with PEEP. *Chest* 99:162–168.

59 Mitchell PH, Mauss NK, Ouna J *et al.* Relationship of

nurse/patient activity and ICP variation. In: Shulman K, Marmarou A and Miller JP (eds) *ICP IV*. New York: Springer-Verlag, pp: 565–568.

60 Artru F, Linossier JP, Baisson D and Eyssette M (1983) Prevention et traitement par posture ventrale declive des pneumopathies chez les traumatises craniens en assistance ventilatoire, influence sur la pression intra-cranienne. *Agressologie* **24**:245–247.

61 Ada L, Canning C and Paratz J (1990) Care of the unconscious head-injured patient. In: Ada L and Canning C (eds) *Key Issues in Neurological Physiotherapy*. Oxford, UK: Butterworth-Heinemann, pp. 249–287.

5 | Critical care nursing

S McKinley

Nursing in intensive care is concerned with provision of life support, monitoring critical illness in patients and their responses to interventions, and prevention of complications, particularly nosocomial infections. It is also concerned with patient comfort, understanding and cooperation, and family information, understanding and support. As such, the requirements of nursing in the ICU are for organized, knowledgeable staff in adequate numbers, well-organized care delivery and, overlaying all, good teamwork. The concerns above are also those of medical and allied health clinicians in varying degrees, and a well-coordinated multidisciplinary effort is needed to address them.

Nursing staff establishment and rostering

Staff establishment

The size of the nursing staff establishment (i.e. the number of nurses on the roster) of an ICU depends primarily on the number of beds in the unit. As an absolute minimum, the establishment and rostering must provide for at least two registered nurses (RNs) in the ICU at all times, including staff meal times. This is essential to provide emergency cardiopulmonary resuscitation, a requirement for even a level I ICU (see Chapter 1). Clearly, the nurse staffing of level II and level III ICUs will need to exceed this absolute minimum, even for small four-bed units. The standard in Australia has generally been to have one nurse (usually an RN, see below) per patient per shift, for adult patients with endotracheal tubes, with or without mechanical ventilation. This standard has been argued and accepted on the basis of patient safety, with patients being at risk of respiratory and cardiac arrest if accidentally extubated or disconnected from the ventilator. Often such patients have complex problems and therapies which keep their nurse fully occupied for the shift. Staff establishments for level II and III ICUs have, therefore, usually been calculated on the basis of one nurse per occupied bed per shift. Larger units (e.g. more than six beds) add one RN per shift in an 'in charge' or team leader role, on top of this.

Although relatively crude, somewhat arbitrary decisions about how many beds will be staffed at ratios of one nurse to one patient (1:1) and one nurse to two patients (1:2) have to date been the main bases for calculating ICU nursing staff establishments. The establishment is expressed as a total number of full-time equivalent (FTE) or equivalent full-time (EFT) positions, which may be filled by all full-time or a mixture of full and part-time staff. Table 5.1 illustrates a way of calculating the required number of nursing staff for a 10-bed ICU with average 90% patient occupancy and a 1:1 ratio per occupied bed. The basic calculation (A) assumes EFT staff are working 8 h/day, 5 days a week, and indicates that the ICU needs 5.3 EFT positions per occupied bed. If employees work 38 h per week, rather than 40, column B shows that 5.6 EFT positions are needed per occupied bed. Column C shows the EFT in A adjusted for a night shift of 10 h rather than 8 h. If four high-dependency beds were to be added to the unit, two at 1:1 and two at 1:2 staffing ratio, an additional three nurses would be needed per shift, affecting the required EFT as shown in column D. The specific entitlements of employees (e.g. full-time hours per week and leave entitlements) should be confirmed with human resources staff in nursing administration and/or the personnel department. Once the basic formula is established, adjustments to it can be readily made. For example, the addition of a second team-leader position in scenario D above affects the required EFT as shown in column E of the table.

The use of 12-h shifts is still uncommon in Australian ICUs, but is seen in North America[1] and in some other areas of Australian nursing, e.g. mental health. Potential advantages of 12-h shifts include reduction of personal disturbances related to working a mixture of shifts within a few days and minimization of night duty.

Table 5.1 Nurse staff establishment:
Example of establishment calculations for 10-bed ICU, 90% occupancy, 1:1 nurse–patient ratio

	EFT/week	*B*	*C*	*D*	*E*
A 3 shifts/day @ 8 h; 1 EFT = 5/shifts per week (40 h)					
1 Calculate total number of shifts needed per week:					
10 beds @ 90% occupancy (9 patients) need 9 staff					
plus 1 team leader = 10 shifts					
10 shifts @ 3/day = 30 shifts/day					
30 shifts/day × 7 = 210 shifts/week					
Add nurse manager @ 5 shifts = 215 shifts/week					
2 Divide number of shifts needed per week by 5(215/5)	43.00	(+2.15)	(+3.58)		
	43.00	45.15	46.58	55.60	58.40
3 Adjust 2 for annual leave entitlements*, e.g.	(+3.31)	(+3.47)	(+3.58)	(+4.28)	(+4.49)
4 week/EFT per year = 4/52 = 7.69%	46.31	48.62	50.16	59.88	62.43
4 Adjust 2 for other leave entitlements* (e.g. sick,	(+1.72)	(+1.81)	(+1.86)	(+2.22)	(+2.34)
compassionate, long service, study), e.g. 4%/EFT/year†	48.03	50.43	52.02	62.10	65.22
5 Calculate EFT per occupied bed	5.33	5.60	5.78	4.78	5.02

A = Basic calculations; B = 38-hour week; C = 10-hour night shift; D = additional four beds, two at 1:1, two at 1:2 nurse:patient ratios; E = D plus team leaders.
EFT = Equivalent full-time.
*Seek advice from nursing administration/personnel department re rates for leave entitlements.
†Calculate as proportion of EFT in 2, then add to EFT in 3.
Notes
B Adjustment for 38-h week = +2 h/EFT = +5%/EFT per week prior to leave entitlements.
C Adjustment for 10-h night shift = +2 h per day = +8.33%/EFT per week, prior to leave entitlements.
D Addition of four beds, two at 1:1, two at 1:2 staffing ratios* anticipated occupancy 100% = +3 staff/shift = 9 shifts/day, prior to calculating shifts/week and leave entitlements.
E Scenario D plus extra team leader on afternoon and night shifts (2 shifts/day).

Patient dependency and case-mix classifications

There are contentious issues in basing nurse staffing on unproved patient safety requirements and arbitrary staffing ratios. In particular, there is uncertainty about staff requirements for patients who are not intubated or ventilated and those with manifest need for more than one nurse per shift. Actual establishment levels are therefore often set by negotiation as much as formula. A more sound approach would be to group patients into classes according to reliable estimates of the amount of nursing time required, using a patient–nurse dependency or nursing acuity system.[1,2] A retrospective analysis of the number of patients in each class over, for example, a 12-month period, will yield the total nursing time required. This can be used in conjunction with the average occupancy rate for the period to project more accurately the required nursing establishment for a unit. Such patient dependency systems must include all nursing time, i.e. that spent on direct patient care, patient-related indirect care, and other activities not directly related to specific patients, such as unit administration.

Some work on patient dependency systems for ICU has been reported,[3] but they are not in routine use in Australasia. However, the imminent use of case-mix information for administrative purposes in intensive care[4] may provide an alternative scientific approach. Case-mix classification systems group together patients who have similar clinical characteristics and require similar amounts of hospital resources,[5] the best known being diagnosis-related groups (DRGs). Information from case-mix classifications has many administrative uses, e.g. analysis of the quality of a service, costing of services, and full or partial funding of a service. The average amount of nursing time required according to case-mix class can be measured,[6] including that for the patients' stay in ICU.[7] As long as these measures are reliable, retrospective data can then be used in conjunction with a unit's case-mix profile to project its required nursing establishment.

Derivation of ICU nursing establishment levels by any of the above methods must still take into account patient safety requirements. The minimum number of staff required in an emergency must be available at all times, and other safety conditions (e.g. one RN per paralysed ventilated patient or one RN per ventilated patient in a single room) must be provided for.

Skill mix

Australian ICUs usually have a predominantly RN staff, many of whom have formal intensive care or critical care nursing qualifications. The use of enrolled nurses is limited, because they are proscribed by the nurse registering authorities from carrying out many routine intensive care nursing functions, e.g. intravenous administration of drugs. Allocation of enrolled nurses to direct patient care would require additional supervisory RNs, and therefore an overall increase in the nursing establishment numbers.

Auxiliary staff such as ward assistants, orderlies and ward clerks are required to assist with activities which do not require qualified staff, and with heavy physical work. The numbers of such personnel depend on the size and workload of the unit. They should be sufficient to relieve nursing staff of the need to do routine clerical, housekeeping and courier work. Auxiliary staff are additional to the nursing staff establishment levels outlined above. They may or may not be directly responsible to the nurse manager of the ICU, although arguably such a line of reporting would be optimal for cohesion and teamwork. There have been reports from North America of the use of auxiliary staff as 'nurse extenders' in direct patient care,[8] partly in response to a shortage of RNs in ICUs. While this strategy might be the best solution in a crisis, its permanent institution is likely to perpetuate RN shortages. Use of such unqualified personnel in direct patient care would entail a still greater amount of supervision by RNs, and greater still establishment numbers. The efficiency of using non-RN staff in the direct care of ICU patients is dubious, because of its fragmentation of nursing care and increased overall staffing requirements. A staff of competent RNs is likely to be the leanest and provide the best continuity of care. These issues are worthy of administrative research.

Amongst the staff on the roster there needs to be sufficient RNs with intensive/critical care nursing certificates or diplomas (see the section on education, below). Efforts to define standards for this[9] are ultimately arbitrary rather than empirical, and may be unrealistic for many units. There usually will be a mixture of RNs with critical care training plus a range of experience, and RNs without certificates or diplomas, some of whom are undertaking specialist training if available. The nurse manager of the unit should have a critical care certificate or diploma, as should the RN in charge of each shift. As the complexity and size of the ICU increase, so too should the number of staff with critical care training. In the absence of any empirical basis for specific recommendations about desirable numbers of critical care-trained staff, suggestions based on experience are shown for a range of units in Table 5.2. The inclusion of first-year graduate RNs on the ICU roster is controversial, and should only be done when the unit has an effective orientation programme and adequate numbers of critical care-trained staff to advise and assist them.

While many ICUs achieve the above desirable staffing levels and skill mix much of the time, most

Table 5.2 Recommended proportions of critical care-trained registered nurses (RNs)

Unit	Number of critical care-trained RNs per shift	Number of EFT positions (approximate)
Level I: 4 beds	1 each shift	5.7
Level II: 6 beds	3 each day shift 2 evening/night shifts	12.8
Level III: 10 beds	4 each shift, plus 1 EFT nurse manager	23.8

EFT = Equivalent full-time.

units from time to time cannot manage do so. When this occurs, there is a need for careful judgement and negotiation between the nursing and medical managers of the unit as to how the situation is best managed. The major consideration must be the well-being of the patients, but the demands on the available staff – nursing and medical – should not be lightly dismissed. The goal should be to keep as many beds as possible available for the care of critically ill patients without putting them at increased risk and without producing working conditions which cause staff attrition.

Rostering

Good rostering is essential to ensure that the available staff establishment and skill mix are of maximum benefit to patient care. The main goal is to distribute the available staff numbers and skills according to patient requirements. In units with a large elective surgical case load, scheduling of operating lists will be a major factor in determining this. If a patient dependency system is in use, analysis of past trends in nursing workload may suggest which shifts or days of the week need more or less staff. ICUs, however, generally have unpredictable fluctuations in workload. The goal then is to distribute the available staff across the 21 shifts of the week, perhaps weighting in favour of the morning shift in busy level II and III units. The assignment of staff to shifts should be done according to broad categories of training and experience. For example these might be:

1 critical care-trained, up to 12 months' experience;
2 critical care-trained, more than 12 months' experience;
3 critical care course student;
4 RN without critical care certificate/diploma.

Categories could also be determined by designated positions, e.g. clinical nurse specialist and associate charge nurse. The proportion of staff in each category in the establishment should be reflected as much as possible on each shift.

The secondary aim of rostering is to be as equitable as possible in the assignment of staff, especially to evening, weekend and night shifts. Staff should have roster requests granted as much as possible, so long as they do not jeopardize patient safety or discriminate against other staff. Self-rostering is popular, with staff negotiating amongst themselves to provide the coverage specified by the nurse manager (or delegate). Surveillance is required to ensure that personal preferences of staff do not compromise balanced and equitable rostering. Because of the many factors involved, repeated manipulation of shift assignments and recalculation of numbers are needed to arrive at the best possible roster, particularly when the staff establishment is large. This is very time consuming and computerized rostering packages can be used to speed up the process. The nurse manager however retains accountability for the adequacy of staffing on each shift as determined by the roster.

Organization of nursing care

The organization of nursing care includes the assignment of staff to patients and the use of documentation tools in delivering care.

Approaches to care delivery

The predominant approach to assigning nurses to patients in Australian ICUs has been to assign staff on a shift-by-shift basis. This has the advantage of best matching the skills of staff on a shift to the needs of patients in the unit at that time. Staff assignment could be assisted by a reliable patient dependency system, especially when more than one nurse is needed for some patients. However, in staff assignment, discretion is usually required in matching a nurse's skill to a patient's need, rather than in the number of staff to be assigned to a patient, and a patient dependency system is not helpful in this.

Team nursing and primary nursing, which have had surges of popularity at different times, have not been widely adopted in Australian ICUs. Primary nursing would involve a patient being cared for by the same nurse (when on duty) for the duration of the patient's stay in ICU. It would be logistically difficult, if not impossible, to adopt primary nursing for all patients in a unit. It could perhaps be done for selected patients in whom continuity of care is particularly important. Team nursing involves the same team of staff working together on the same shifts, e.g. for a week at a time. Again, this would be logistically difficult. Both the team and primary nursing approaches would compromise the ability to match staff to patients' needs on a shift-by-shift basis.

Documentation tools

Documentation tools used to assist in the organization and delivery of nursing care have included nursing care plans and nursing assessment tools. Their use is endorsed and promoted in the nursing literature and in nursing education programmes. In practice, the use of nursing care plans is variable. This appears to relate to the expertise of the staff in a particular unit. Where staff are largely proficient or expert in their field of practice, nursing care plans are reduntant,[10] whereas staff new to an area benefit from the guidance in organizing their work. Care plans can also be valuable when continuity of care is crucial, e.g. dressing of burns or difficult wounds and management of psychological problems, as well as for tracking routine line/tube changes.

The use of tools to assess patients systematically and routinely is also variable. However, their use has much more practical value than that of nursing care plans. Documentation of nursing assessment of patients, especially on admission to ICU, is essential to:

1 systematically identify patient problems which require nursing care;
2 provide a record for the use of other staff;
3 provide legal evidence of nursing assessment.

The system by which nursing assessment is organized is discretionary. For example, it could be done according to body systems with additional categories for social and psychological problems, or according to an integrated nursing conceptualization of physiological, social and psychological domains.[11] The former lends itself to a combined medical and nursing problem list, which both disciplines use in combined patient progress notes. The latter assists in distinguishing the contribution of nursing to patient care in ICU and is recommended if policy prohibits combined progress notes.

Systems known as case management or managed care have been widely adopted in North American.[12,13] Managed care involves the use of documentary tools known as critical paths or clinical management plans. Clinical management plans document key interventions which should take place, and outcomes which should be achieved, during a patient's course in hospital, as well as the time at which they should occur.[14] The successful implementation of managed care with clinical management plans has been reported in an open-heart surgery unit in Australia; the clinical management plan replaced the nursing care plan and was integrated with the nursing assessment form and patient problem list.[14] Tools such as clinical management plans or critical paths appear not to have been adopted in general intensive care but are worthy of evaluation for selected patients.

The advent of computerized clinical information systems (see Chapter 95) offers great potential for the automation of routine nursing recording. In addition to the automatic storing of trends in parameters being electronically monitored, thus eliminating the need for duplicate manual recording, these systems can automate and improve accuracy in charting of fluid balance, drug administration and a range of other functions.

Education

Formal education for intensive/critical care nursing can be described under specialist training programmes, orientation and continuing education. Formal education implies a teaching and learning process. A goal of formal education however should be to engender career-long learning in the nurse. Educational opportunities and qualifications are inherently linked to career progression.

Specialist nurse training programmes

Hospital-based post-basic courses in intensive care and related critical care areas have been the mainstay in preparation for specialty nursing in Australian practice, with most states offering intensive care and/or coronary care or cardiothoracic courses in the 1980s.[15] The courses were often approved by the state nurse-registering authorities and their graduates were and still are sought after. Post basic courses were directed towards developing clinical proficiency in the units in which they were based, and were highly successful in this. They contributed to good management of critical care patients, whether or not the nursing contribution to this was evident. The courses also assisted greatly in the recruitment of staff, with RNs often attracted to a hospital or unit by the courses it offered.

With the completion of the transfer of pre-registration nursing education programmes from hospitals to universities, there is now a trend for post-registration education for specialty practice to be at postgraduate level in universities. Increasing numbers of critical care graduate diplomas and graduate certificates are being offered.[16] The impetus for change to tertiary education for nursing specialization is from several sources. It is seen by some as a natural progression from tertiary undergraduate preparation and an opportunity to develop broader professional abilities, as well as clinical proficiency. Strained hospital finances jeopardized the continued funding of post-basic courses, which were relatively expensive, while universities have incentives to expand their graduate programmes and student numbers. Another impetus is the provision of access to higher education for hospital-trained RNs who would not otherwise be given entry to graduate programmes. It is possible in most universities for nurses with very good academic achievement in graduate diploma programmes to gain entry to a masters degree by coursework programme, even if they do not have an undergraduate degree.

Some specialty graduate programmes are offered only at the graduate diploma level and integrate specialty practice subjects with generic graduate study, e.g. research. Others offer a graduate certificate course which concentrates on clinical practice. Some graduate certificates articulate with a further programme of generic graduate subjects, thereby allowing students who have the aptitude and desire to go on to a graduate diploma. Many of the graduate programmes are joint initiatives between a university nursing faculty or school and one or several hospitals. Input from the two parties varies, as do the funding arrangements. In addition to graduate nursing courses sponsored partly or fully by hospitals some universities offer government-funded places for students. Students usually pay at least a small part of the cost of their courses.

Whether critical care graduate courses are at the certificate or diploma level, the learning which occurs during clinical practice in the units continues to be central to producing proficient clinical practitioners. Planned, graduated experience with patients with increasingly complex problems, with access to qualified and experienced staff for guidance and assistance when necessary, leads to the knowledge gained from doing. The role of the critical care qualified nursing staff in using teaching opportunities which arise in patient care continues to be essential to student learning, above and beyond any formal nurse educator staff who might be available to the students.

The intended outcomes of graduate diploma programmes are:

1 specialist RNs who are clinically proficient across critical care units both within a hospital and in different hospitals;
2 clinical nurses who can evaluate the clinical applicability of research findings and develop practice based on research;
3 graduates able to provide clinical leadership and participate in collegial practice with doctors and other professionals;
4 identification of the nursing contribution to good patient management in critical care units.

Graduate certificates are likely to contribute to the first of the above outcomes and thereby increase on the established contribution to good patient care made by hospital post-basic courses. It is too early yet to determine if university graduate preparation for specialist nursing practice in critical care will achieve its intended outcomes or maintain the side benefit of attracting staff to particular units. However, it is likely that graduate programmes will be retained and evolve to ensure their viability.

Orientation programme

All RNs joining the staff of an ICU should be offered a programme which is designed to orient them to that particular unit. This applies equally to first-year graduate nurses, to qualified and highly experienced critical care nurses, and to those in between.

While a range of approaches to orientation of new staff may be seen, the recommended approach is the use of preceptors[17] in combination with competency-based orientation.[18] In this approach, new staff are linked with a preceptor, preferably an RN with critical care qualifications and more experienced than the new staff member. The preceptor works with new RNs to establish their present level of knowledge and clinical competence in the care of patients in that unit. In competency-based orientation, essential competent practice specific to the unit's patient population, organization and policies, is specified as behavioural objectives. The new staff member may demonstrate competence in achieving most objectives or may be a relative novice, e.g. a recent graduate or from another nursing specialty, and be able to achieve few objectives on starting. A personalized learning programme to assist them towards achieving competence in the outstanding objectives is planned with input from the nursing manager, who is accountable for the care given by the RN, and perhaps with help from a nurse educator if available. The timing of assessments to review progress should be included in the plan, the time frame varying according to entry level.

Some units are able to have new staff work with another staff member in a 'doubling' capacity for several shifts, rather than immediately taking sole responsibility for patients. Ironically, the autonomy for nursing managers to choose to use their staffing budgets in this way is increasing at a time when budget constraints militate against it. If it is possible, new staff members should work with their preceptor on those shifts. *Ad hoc* doubling with different staff members, without systematic assessment and competency-based objectives, is inferior to the approach recommended here.

Integral in this approach is the need for new staff members to take responsibility for their own learning, with assistance from the preceptor in planning and achieving it. Learning resources available within the unit may include in-service lectures, self-directed learning packages, computer-assisted learning packages, unit protocols, policy manuals and videos. A major learning resource in the unit is planned experience in caring for particular types of patients, with access to guidance from experienced staff when it is needed, and later review with the preceptor. Various internal and external continuing education opportunities can also be built into the individual's competency-based orientation programme.

Continuing education

Continuing education refers to the continual updating and extension of the knowledge needed to carry out one's practice. It is primarily the responsibility of the individual practitioner. ICUs and hospitals provide opportunities to access learning, e.g. units often have multidisciplinary rounds, clinical meetings and in-service lectures, while hospitals often run staff development and other nursing education programmes at little or no cost to their own staff, and most have some sort of fund to give financial support to attend external educational meetings and courses. The critical care professional organizations offer continuing education ranging from local nursing updates to high-quality multidisciplinary meetings at the state and national levels. Participation in the activities of the professional organizations also provides access to information about international continuing education opportunities.

Research

The increase in research activity in intensive care nursing in Australia is evidenced by the programmes and abstracts of the annual scientific meeting on intensive care. For example, there were seven nursing research papers in 1984[19] compared to 30 in 1994, generally of very good quality.[20] The major objectives now must be to increase the very low rate of journal publication of this research, and to increase the reading and evaluation of published research, so that practice is scientifically based. Both of these objectives are likely to be assisted by the increased tertiary education of critical care nurses which is occurring. The course-work graduate diplomas and masters degrees referred to above will contribute to the latter, while nursing research training at the honours, masters and doctoral level will contribute to both.

Review of the published research on clinical practice topics should be integrated into the quality improvement processes of critical care nurses. Examples of practices found in such reviews by clinical nurses to have questionable scientific bases include the installation of saline prior to endotracheal suctioning, the frequency of tracheostomy tube changes, and the use of polyurethane dressings and antiseptic ointment on central venous catheter insertion sites. On the other hand, lack of familiarity with the abundant nursing research on the needs of families of critically ill patients is indicated by proposals for further descriptive investigation of the topic, rather than development and investigation of nursing interventions to meet families' needs.

The conduct of quality research and attainment of scholarship skills in research degrees will assist in critical care nursing research being published. However, nursing managers can also provide some time to clinical nurses to work on their research. This is less necessary for data collection, as this can often be done around clinical work once a project is underway, but is often crucial to the success of the writing stages of the project. Applications for ethics approval and funding may be managed in the researchers' own time, but preparation of journal manuscripts appears to be virtually unachievable without work-time free from clinical demands. Nursing and hospital managers can also assist nursing research by facilitating access in the clinical areas to computerized research indexes which are necessary to the preparation of research proposals and of publications for research journals.

The ethics of including patients and others in research which is not published, and therefore made available for practice, is dubious. Even if nurses are not involved in conducting research, they should be acquainted with the requirements for ethical research. The relevant Australian guidelines are the *Statement on Human Experimentation and Supplementary Notes*; supplementary note no. 2 refers specifically to patients unable to give informed consent,[21] a situation common in intensive care. Ethical issues particular to qualitative research methods, increasingly popular in nursing, are canvassed in a (draft) information paper on the subject.[22]

References

1 Schulmerich S (1991) Twenty-four hour staffing. In: Birdsall C (ed.) *Management Issues in Critical Care*. St Louis: Mosby-Year Book, pp. 155–168.

2 Birdsall C (1991) Patient classification. In: Birdsall C (ed.) *Management Issues in Critical Care*. St Louis: Mosby-Year Book, pp. 131–154.

3 Ferguson L (1992) Using the therapeutic intervention scoring system to quantify nursing care. Paper presented at the 17th Australian and New Zealand Scientific Meeting on Intensive Care, Auckland, New Zealand.

4 Daffurn K (1994) Intensive care and DRGS – where are we up to? *Aust Crit Care* **7**:13.

5 Hindle D (1994) Funding intensive care in the DRG age: an overview. *Aust Crit Care* **7**:8–11.

6 Ferguson L and Picone D (1994) *Casemix and Nursing Management*. National Casemix Education Series, no.8. Canberra: Department of Human Services and Health

7 Commonwealth Department of Human Services and Health (1994) *Critical Care Costing Study Hospital Reference Manual*. Adelaide: KPMG Peat Marwick.

8 Manthey M (1990) Definitions and basic elements of a patient care delivery system with an emphasis on primary nursing. In: Mayer G, Madden M and Lawrenz E (eds) *Patient Care Delivery Models*. Rockville MD: Aspen, pp. 201–211.

9 *Minimum Standards for Intensive Care Units* (1994) Faculty of Intensive Care, Australian and Zealand College of Anaesthetists. Melbourne: FICANZCAF.

10 Benner P (1984) *From Novice to Expert: Excellence and Power in Clinical Nursing Practice*. San Francisco: Addison-Wesley.

11 Guzzetta C (1989) Developing a nursing data base prototype from the unitary person framework. In: Guzzetta C, Bunton S, Prinkey L, Sherer A and Seifert P (eds) *Clinical Assessment Tools for Use With Nursing Diagnoses*. St Louis: CV Mosby, pp. 6–22.

12 Zander K (1988) Nursing case management: resolving the DRG paradox. *Nursing Clin North Am* **23**:503–520.

13 Olivas G, Del Togno-Armanasco V, Erickson J and Harter S (1989) Case management: a bottom-line care delivery model. Part 2. Adaptation of the model. *J Nursing Admin* **19**:12–17.

14 Kingsland S, Smith P and McKinley S (1994) Introduction of managed care plans in a cardiac surgery unit. *Contemporary Nurse* **3**:189–194.

15 Commonwealth Department of Health (1985) *Post Basic Nursing Courses in Australia*, 7th edn. Canberra: Australian Government Publishing Services.

16 Lord M (ed.) (1993) *Directory of Higher Education Courses 1994*. Sydney: New Hobson Press.

17 Fiore-Lopez N (1991) Career development. In: Birdsall C (ed.) *Management Issues in Critical Care*. St Louis: Mosby, pp. 3–20.

18 Mackin J, Watts D and Birdsall C (1991) Competency based orientation. In: Birdsall C (ed.) *Management Issues in Critical Care*. St Louis: Mosby, pp. 169–187.

19 Programme (1984) The Ninth Australian and New Zealand Scientific Meeting on Intensive Care. Perth:

20 *Conference Handbook* (1994) 19th Australian and New Zealand Scientific Meeting on Intensive Care, Sydney.

21 National Health Medical Research Council (1992) *Statement on Human Experimentation and Supplementary Notes*. Canberra: Australian Government Publishing Service.

22 National Health Medical Research Council (1994) *Ethical Aspects of Qualitative Methods in Health Research: An Information Paper for Institutional Ethics Committees*. Canberra: Australian Government Publishing Service.

Part II

Acute coronary care

6 Acute myocardial infarction

BEF Hockings and KD Donovan

Coronary artery disease (CAD) accounts for over 30% of all deaths in western industrialized society.[1] Acute myocardial infarction (MI) is a common medical emergency, and suspected MI is one of the most frequent causes of hospital and ICU admission; diagnosis is confirmed in approximately one-third.[2]

Aetiology

The majority of patients with acute MI have atheromatous deposits in the walls of their coronary arteries. Major risk factors for the development of coronary artery atheroma are increased plasma low-density lipoprotein (LDL) and low high-density lipoprotein (HDL) cholesterol concentrations, smoking, hypertension and a family history with a first-degree relative having angina or MI aged < 55 years. Despite the strong association of these risk factors with CAD, the majority of patients who present with MI do not possess any of them.[3] Other recognized risk factors for the development of CAD are given in Table 6.1.

Many risk factors can be modified. There is good evidence that lowering plasma cholesterol, stopping smoking and adopting a more active lifestyle can all help prevent the development of CAD.[4–6] Although there is clear benefit from treating hypertension in terms of stroke reduction, the impact on CAD is less clear.[7]

Occasionally, acute MI without underlying coronary artery atherosclerosis can be caused by a dissecting aortic aneurysm, polyarteritis nodosa, coronary emboli, coronary artery spasm, ergotamine administration or cocaine abuse.

Pathophysiology

Acute MI occurs when coronary blood flow falls below a certain critical level required to maintain myocardial cell viability. Most often, this is a total cessation of flow associated with an occlusive thrombus. Atheromatous plaques within the walls of the coronary artery may fissure, and bleeding into the wall of the plaque can cause a sudden increase in plaque size, obstructing the lumen of the artery.[8,9] Intraluminal thrombosis may occur and propagate from the plaque, sometimes resulting in total occlusion of the vessel. Platelets and coronary artery spasm are involved in the causation of acute MI, but their precise role remains unclear.

The interrupted supply of oxygenated blood to myocardial cells results in loss of function, cellular disruption, thinning and softening of the affected myocardium, and later fibrosis and ventricular remodelling. If the infarcted area is of sufficient size, left ventricular (LV) systolic function is impaired, stroke volume falls and ventricular filling pressures rise, not infrequently leading to hypotension and pulmonary congestion. The hypotension may impair coronary perfusion pressures and exacerbate the myocardial ischaemia. LV diastolic function is also affected by MI; initially infarcted muscle is softened, leading to an increase in ventricular compliance, but as fibrosis takes place, compliance is subsequently decreased. With time, there is often expansion of the infarcted segment and compensatory hypertrophy of unaffected myocardial cells occurs (i.e. ventricular remodelling) which can affect overall ventricular function and prognosis.[10]

Clinical presentation

History

Typically, the pain of acute MI is severe, constant and retrosternal, spreading across the chest and lasting for more than 20 min. There may be radiation to the throat and jaw, down the ulnar aspect of both arms and to the interscapular area. The pain is often accompanied by sweating, nausea, pallor, dyspnoea and anxiety. Even if the pain is not excruciating, patients often report a feeling of impending doom.

Table 6.1 Risk factors for coronary artery disease

Major factors	Other influences
Abnormal lipids	Increasing age
Elevated total cholesterol concentration	Male sex
Elevated plasma LDL concentration	Increased plasma fibrinogen
Low plasma HDL concentration	Increased plasma viscosity
Smoking	Raised white cell count
Hypertension	Increased plasma triglyceride concentration
Family history (<55 years)	Lack of physical activity
Diabetes	Hyperhomocysteinaemia

LDL = Low-density lipoprotein; HDL = high-density lipoprotein.

Prodromal symptoms of a similar but milder nature occur in 20–60% of patients in the days preceding the infarct.[11,12] The pain may sometimes be atypical, occasionally beginning in the epigastrium (which presents a possible misdiagnosis as an abdominal condition). Aortic dissection and pericarditis are two important differential diagnoses. The pain of MI probably represents ongoing ischaemia, and the term 'myocardium infarcting' has been suggested to emphasize the need to relieve the ischaemia (for which the pain is a marker) and thus prevent ongoing muscle damage.

Atypical or silent presentations are common; 20–60% of non-fatal infarctions are unrecognized at onset.[13,14] Silent infarction is more common in patients with diabetes or hypertension[13] and is often followed by silent ischaemia.

Physical examination

Apart from obvious signs of distress, examination of patients with acute MI is often unremarkable. Heart rate and blood pressure are often normal, but pulse rate may vary from a marked bradycardia to a tachycardia. With more severe infarction and extensive myocardial injury, signs of heart failure and even shock may be apparent. Auscultation of the heart may be normal, but a fourth heart sound is common, whereas a third heart sound usually indicates a large infarction with extensive muscle damage. A systolic murmur may be present and may be transient or persistent. These murmurs usually result from mitral regurgitation, either due to papillary muscle dysfunction or LV dilatation. An infarct-related ventricular septal defect can give rise to a similar systolic murmur, and is an important complication of acute MI which needs to be recognized early and treated surgically. Pericardial friction rubs occur frequently with infarction but are usually transient. With infarction of the right ventricle, there may be marked elevation of the jugular venous pressure, although cardiogenic shock caused by extensive LV dysfunction can also increase central venous pressure. The latter setting will usually have associated hypotension and marked pulmonary venous congestion.

Investigations

Routine diagnostic technique

Electrocardiogram (ECG)

Despite potential problems with interpretation, a 12-lead ECG is the most useful investigation because it can be performed simply and quickly. Elevation of the ST segments occurs within minutes of the onset of infarction and is usually evanescent; pathological Q waves (>40 ms in duration or >25% of the height of the ensuing R wave) may take hours or even days to develop. These ECG changes of infarction usually persist indefinitely, but may regress in a minority of patients, and the ECG can even return to normal.[15–17] Depression of the ST segment and T-wave inversion are non-specific changes. Serial ECG changes are often more helpful, as changes with time are more likely to indicate acute infarction. A single normal ECG tracing cannot exclude infarction, although if two tracings 30 min apart are normal, there is <10% chance of MI. Even if infarction has occurred, the prognosis for these patients is excellent.

Acute MI is often classified on the basis of the ECG into Q-wave and non-Q-wave infarctions. Diagnosis of non-Q-wave infarction relies on a combination of the history, increased serum cardiac enzymes and ECG changes. These infarctions are usually associated with smaller amounts of myocardial damage, but substantial amounts of heart muscle may still be at risk. Therefore patients with non-Q-wave infarction are often considered for coronary angiography prior to hospital discharge.

The ECG can localize the area of heart muscle damage (Table 6.2; Figs 6.1–6.4), although indication

Table 6.2 Electrocardiogram changes in infarct location

Location	Changes	Figure
Anterior	Changes in I, aVL, V2–V4	Fig. 6.1
Inferior	Changes in II, III, aVF	Fig. 6.2
True posterior	Tall R waves in V1	Fig. 6.3
Right ventricular	Changes in V4R	Fig. 6.4

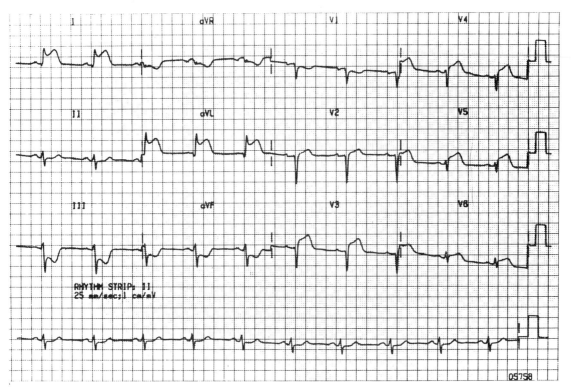

Fig. 6.1 Acute anterior myocardial infarction with ST elevation in I, aVL, V3–V6. There is ST depression in the inferior leads (II, III and aVF).

of the infarction site is not uniformly accurate. Often, the infarction involves more than one discrete region of myocardium; e.g. anteroseptal involves changes in I, aVL, V1–V3; anterolateral I, aVL, V5 and V6; extensive anterior V1–V6; inferolateral II, III, aVF, V5, V6; high lateral aVL plus high precordial leads (the same horizontal distribution as standard precordial levels but placed one or two interspaces higher). The coronary arteries are shown in Figure 6.5. Anterior MI usually results from occlusion of the left anterior descending artery; inferior, true posterior and right ventricular (RV) infarction result from occlusion of the right coronary or circumflex arteries.

Certain ECG features such as left bundle branch block,[18] Wolff–Parkinson–White syndrome or presence of a previous infarction may make it difficult to diagnose acute MI and ECG criteria, but the clinical presentation and serial cardiac enzyme estimations will usually clarify the situation.

It is important to recognize RV infarction and ST segment elevation in the right precordial leads; V4R, especially, is relatively sensitive and specific for RV infarction.[18–22] A routine V4R lead should be obtained (by placing the usual V4 lead in an equivalent position on the right anterior chest wall) in all patients with suspected acute MI. The RV muscle mass is small in comparison to the left, but RV infarction has a clinical significance disproportionate to the amount of myocardium damaged, with a relatively poor prognosis.[18,19] Such patients may need to be considered for acute angioplasty.

Serum enzymes

Irreversibly damaged myocardial cells release a number of enzymes into the circulation which can be measured by biochemical assays. Interpretation of the results should account for varying time delays for the enzymes to appear in serum (Fig. 6.6) and for other enzyme sources (Table 6.3).

Diagnostic accuracy can be improved by assaying isoenzymes. Creatine kinase (CK) has three isoenzymes – MM found in skeletal muscle, MB in heart and BB in brain. The presence of CK-MB in the plasma usually indicates myocardial necrosis, although it is found in small quantities in the small intestine, tongue, diaphragm, uterus and prostate. Trauma or surgery to these organs can also result in CK-MB release into plasma. Myocardial necrosis is usually the source of CK-MB when the isoenzyme exceeds 5% of an abnormally raised total CK, or when the CK-MB mass >9 units and the index [(CK-MB µg/l/total CK units/l) × 100] is greater than 2.5. Lactic dehydrogenase

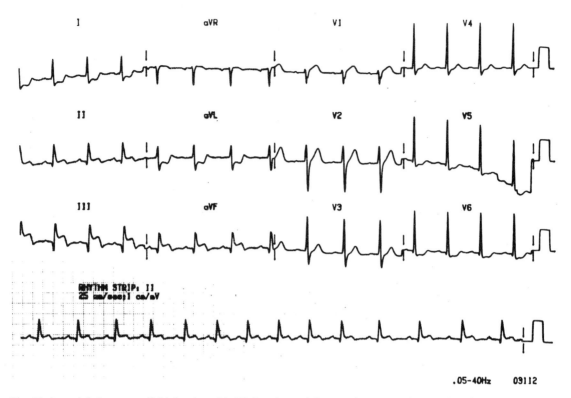

Fig. 6.2 Acute inferior myocardial infarction with ST elevation and Q waves in II, III and aVF. There is ST depression in I, aVL, V5 and V6.

(LDH) has five isoenzymes and the heart contains principally LD_1. A rise in this subfraction or an increase in the $Ld_1:Ld_2$ ratio greater than 1.0 indicates myocardial necrosis.[23]

The peak concentration of enzymes detected in plasma points to the size of the MI, but coronary reperfusion (either spontaneous or induced by thrombolytic therapy or angioplasty) results in a high early peak.[24,25] Measurement of isoenzymes should be reserved for problem cases, and not requested routinely because of the expense involved.

Other investigations

Echocardiography

Echocardiography can detect regional wall motion abnormalities and thinning of the myocardium (which are consequences of MI) but cannot differentiate acute from pre-existing changes. Mural thrombus formation overlying a region of wall motion abnormality is common in acute anterior MI, and can be identified by echocardiography.[26]

Radionuclide studies

Radionuclide angiography, perfusion scintigraphy, infarct-avid scintigraphy and positron emission tomo-graphy can all be used to help diagnose acute MI and assess infarct size and LV function.[27–31] Routine use of these techniques is not necessary, but a technetium pyrophosphate uptake 'hot spot' scan of the myocardium can be helpful in detecting myocardial necrosis if the diagnosis is uncertain. These scans are best performed 24–72 h post-infarction.

Coronary angiography and left ventriculography

In the appropriate clinical setting, coronary angiography will usually identify a culprit artery subtending a region of wall motion abnormality. These investigations are reserved for patients in whom percutaneous transluminal coronary angioplasty (PTCA) is proposed to re-establish flow to the infarcted myocardium.

Management of acute MI

Pre-hospital care

Death in the first few hours following MI is usually due to ventricular fibrillation (VF), and the patient is extremely vulnerable during this time. Many ambulances are equipped with a defibrillator and respond

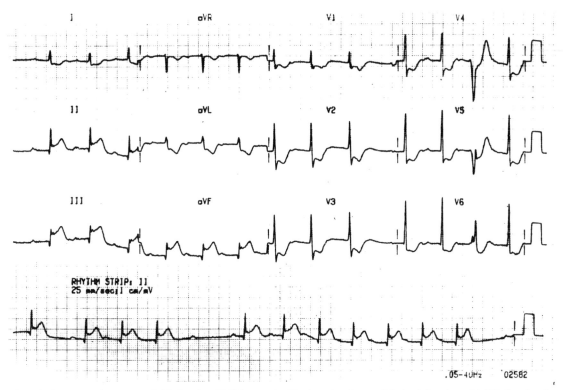

Fig. 6.3 True posterior myocardial infarction. Tall R wave in V1. Associated acute inferior infarction with ST elevation in II, III and aVF (and ST depression in leads I, aVL and across the chest leads). The patient is in sinus rhythm with first-degree atrioventricular block and episodes of Wenckebach block.

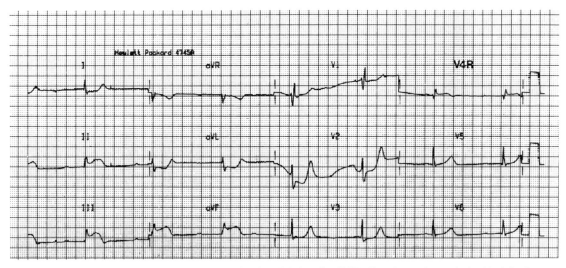

Fig. 6.4 Inferior infarction with right ventricular infarction (ST elevation V4R). Complete atrioventricular block is also present.

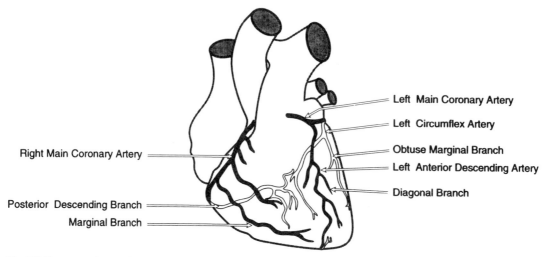

Fig. 6.5 Coronary artery anatomy

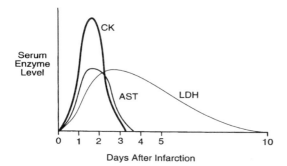

Fig. 6.6 Serum enzyme changes after acute myocardial infarction. CK = Creatine kinase; AST = asparate transaminase; LDH = lactic dehydrogenase.

Table 6.3 Non-cardiac sources of serum enzymes

Creatine kinase
Intramuscular injections, defibrillation, exercise, muscle disease, trauma, convulsions, hypothyroidism, cerebral infarction, alcoholism, diabetes mellitus, pulmonary embolism.

Aspartate transaminase
Most hepatic or muscle diseases, intramuscular injections, pulmonary embolism, shock

Lactic dehydrogenase
Haemolysis, leukaemia, liver disease, renal disease, various neoplasms, pulmonary embolism, myocarditis, skeletal disease, shock

quickly. However, if early access to a defibrillator is not possible, it may be appropriate to transfer the patient to the nearest hospital by private car. Pre-hospital thrombolytic therapy has been used, but does not provide any advantage over prompt

administration on hospital arrival (<15 min), if transport time to the hospital is short. Protocols have been devised to 'fast track' patients for thrombolytic therapy on arrival at hospital (Fig 6.7). Thrombolytic therapy should be given in the emergency department and not in the coronary care unit (CCU) or ICU, as the latter significantly delays treatment.

Immediate hospital care (Table 6.4)

1 *Cardiac monitoring* (usually established in the ambulance) is continued or started.
2 *Oxygen*: via a facemask is continued or given.
3 *ECG (12-lead)* is taken as soon as possible while a brief history is obtained and physical examination performed.
4 *Aspirin* 160 mg[32] should be given routinely to all patients with suspected MI on arrival at hospital (see below).
5 *Thrombolytic therapy*: a priority of management is to decide quickly whether the patient is to receive aspirin and/or thrombolytic therapy (see below).
6 *Acute angioplasty,* if available, should be considered, particularly for patients:
  (a) with contraindications to thrombolytic therapy,
  (b) presenting within 4 h of a large anterior MI:
  (c) in whom MI may be due to a vein graft occlusion:
  (d) with cardiogenic shock.[33] This last group has a poor prognosis even when treated with thrombolytic therapy.
7 *Pain relief* should be provided. Ongoing pain is a symptom of infarcting myocardium and intravenous (IV) nitroglycerine and IV β-blockade may be helpful, but often IV opioids are required.
8 *β-Adrenergic blockers* should be commenced as soon as possible (usually after thrombolytic therapy

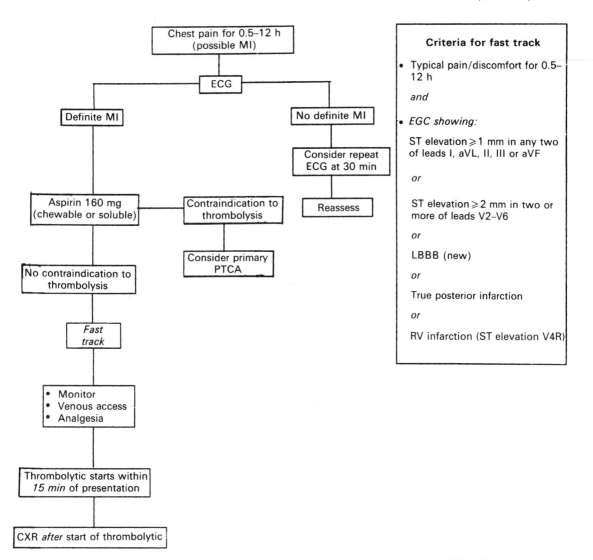

Fig. 6.7 Plan of management for suspected acute myocardial infarction (MI) in the early phase. ECG = Electrocardiogram; PTCA = percutaneous transluminal coronary angioplasty; CXR = chest X-ray, LBBB = left bundle branch block; RV = right ventricular.

has been given; Table 6.5). Survival is probably improved with early IV β-blockade.[34,35] There may be other benefits such as a decreased incidence of VF, decreased cardiac rupture, relief of chest pain and decreased infarct size. β-Blockers are contraindicated in patients with severe heart failure, hypotension, bradycardia, second- or third-degree atrioventricular block, or asthma. Even if IV β-blockade is not used acutely, oral β-blockers should be administered for most patients as soon as possible after admission to CCU/ICU, as long-term survival is improved.[35] Atenolol

50–100 mg daily, metoprolol 50–100 mg b.d. or timolol 10 mg b.d.[36] are commonly used.

Thrombolytic therapy[37]

Thrombolytic therapy should be considered as a matter of urgency for all patients presenting within 12 h after the onset of acute MI. Major trials[32,38] have shown improved LV function and survival when patients with acute MI are treated with thrombolytic agents. Benefits appear to be critically linked to the time of treatment after the onset of

Table 6.4 Immediate care of the patient with suspected acute myocardial infarction (MI)

Immediate (diagnosis, assessment and early treatment must be concurrent)
Cardiac monitor/12-lead ECG
Defibrillator (immediately available)
Brief history/examination (usually < 5 min)
Venous access
Continue oxygen via mask
Pain relief

Then (when history and ECG indicate probable MI), unless contraindicated
Aspirin (chewable or soluble 160 mg)
Thrombolysis
β-Adrenergic blockers (usually after thrombolysis)

ECG = Electrocardiogram.

Table 6.5 Intravenous β-blockade in acute myocardial infarction (MI)

Include
All patients with suspected MI (prolonged chest pain and ECG changes)

Exclude
Asthma or severe chronic obstructive lung disease
Already receiving β-blockers, verapamil or diltiazem
Heart rate < 50 beats/min
Systolic blood pressure < 100 mmHg (13.3 kPa)
Severe heart failure (breathless at rest, crepitations above lower scapula)
Atrioventricular block – second- or third-degree

β-Blocker administration (the earlier the better)
Atenolol 5 mg IV over 5 min. Stop if heart rate < 40 beats/min or any other contraindication develops (e.g. hypotension)

After 10 min, if heart rate ≥ 60 beats/min, give further 5 mg atenolol IV over 5 min. Stop if heart rate < 40 beats/min or any other contraindication develops

10 min after the second IV dose of atenolol, if heart rate ≥ 40 beats/min, give atenolol 50 mg orally, followed by a further 50 mg 12 h later. Atenolol should be continued orally if tolerated at 50–100 mg/day

ECG = Electrocardiogram; IV = intravenous.

Table 6.6 Thrombolysis in acute myocardial infarction (MI)

No contraindications (see Table 6.7)
Ischaemic chest pain (> 30 min, < 6–12 h)
ECG
  ST elevation ≥ 1 mm in two or more of leads I, aVL, III or aVF or ≥ 2 mm in two or more of leads V2–V6.
  Left bundle branch block (new)
  True posterior MI
    Tall R in V1 (with ST depression)
    Exclude other causes of tall R wave (e.g. right bundle branch block, right ventricular hypertrophy, Wolff–Parkinson–White syndrome)
    Right ventricular infarction (ST elevation V4R)

ECG = Electrocardiogram.

Table 6.7 Contraindications to thrombolytic therapy

Major contraindicatotions
Trauma or surgery within 10 days
Active internal bleeding
Recent (within 2 months) stroke, intracranial or intraspinal surgery
Recent head trauma or known intracranial neoplasm
Blood pressure > 200/120 mmHg after relief of pain
Possible aortic dissection
Possible pericarditis
Pregnancy

Relative contraindications
Recent central venous puncture
Recent arterial puncture (non-compressible vessel)
Peptic ulcer
History of haemorrhagic stroke
Known bleeding diathesis or current use of anticoagulants
Prolonged or traumatic cardiopulmonary resuscitation
Significant liver dysfunction
Prior exposure to streptokinase or APSAC (alteplase or urokinase can be given)
Severe diabetic retinopathy

*APSAC = Anisoylated plasminogen–streptokinase activator complex.

Table 6.8 Complications of thrombolytic therapy

Complication	Incidence
Allergic reactions	1–7%
Hypotension	4–10%
Bleeding	
Minor*	15–30%
Major†	0.5%

*Mainly at vascular puncture sites.
†Haemorrhagic stroke or bleeding requiring transfusion.

symptoms. Most studies show significant mortality benefits if this interval is under 6 h (and if under 1 h, mortality is reduced by about 50%). The late assessment of thrombolytic efficacy (LATE) study indicated that there may be benefits even with an interval of up to 12 h.[39] Benefit is potentially greater for patients with larger infarcts; small infarctions have no significant benefit.[38] Indications, contra-indications and complications of thrombolytic therapy are listed in Tables 6.6–6.8 respectively.

Thrombolytic agents

Streptokinase

Streptokinase is the most widely used agent. It binds to plasminogen indirectly to activate the proenzyme plasminogen, with resultant lysis of clot by plasmin (Fig. 6.8). Antibodies formed to streptokinase can limit its effectiveness or cause severe allergic reactions, if second or subsequent treatments are given (3 or more days after the initial dose). There is general agreement that streptokinase should not be administered again within 2 years.[41] Some even recommend that repeat treatment should never be given. It is the agent of choice for patients presenting with acute MI within 12 h, who have not had treatment previously. The dosage regimen is given in Table 6.9.

Anisoylated plasminogen–streptokinase activator complex (APSAC)

This modified active plasminogen–streptokinase complex was developed for single IV bolus administration. Apart from this, it has no clear advantage over streptokinase, and is considerably more expensive.

Alteplase (previously tissue plasminogen activator, t-PA).

This is an endogenous enzyme found in vascular endothelium, but is synthesized using DNA techniques.

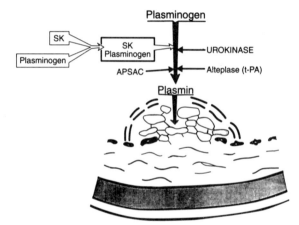

Fig. 6.8 Activation of proenzyme plasminogen by thrombolytic agents with lysis of the platelet fibrin clot by plasmin. SK = Streptokinase; APSAC = anisoylated plasminogen–streptokinase activator complex; t-PA = tissue plasminogen activator.

Like urokinase, alteplase activates plasminogen (Fig. 6.8). The alteplase molecule has a binding site for fibrinogen, allowing preferential attachment to a clot and subsequent lysis, without causing global activation of plasminogen. Despite this theoretical advantage, some systemic plasminogen activation occurs with the clinical doses used, and bleeding complications are not lessened when compared to streptokinase. The recent GUSTO trial,[40] however, showed a small mortality reduction (6% alteplase:7% streptokinase). Alteplase is 10 times more expensive than streptokinase and appears to have a slightly higher bleeding tendency (including an increased stroke rate). Transient antibody formation has occurred in under 0.5% of patients, and repeat dosing is possible, unlike streptokinase or APSAC. Alteplase is the agent of choice for patients who have previously received streptokinase, or who are aged 55–75 years, or present with an anterior infarction within 4 h of the onset of symptoms.[40] Dosage details are given in Table 6.9.

Urokinase

Urokinase is a serine protease that converts plasminogen to active plasmin. It has similar effectiveness to streptokinase, but because of its prohibitive cost it is not routinely used. With the smaller doses required for intracoronary thrombolysis, urokinase is a cost-effective strategy when a thrombolytic agent is indicated during coronary angiography or angioplasty.

Adjunctive agents used with thrombolysis[40–43] (Table 6.10)

Aspirin

Aspirin helps prevent reocclusion after successful clot lysis, and has a clear benefit when combined with streptokinase.[32] In the ISIS-2 trial,[32] mortality was reduced 25% with streptokinase alone, 23% with

Table 6.9 Dosage of streptokinase and alteplase (tissue plasminogen activator or t-PA)

Dosage of streptokinase
1.5 million units in 250 ml of 0.9% NaCl given over 60 min

Dosage of alteplase (t-PA)	Pump rate	Volume infused (1 mg/ml)
15 mg bolus over 2 min *then*	450 ml/h for 2 min	15 ml
45 mg over 30 min *then*	90 ml/h for 30 min	45 ml
40 mg over 1 h *then* flush line with:	40 ml/h for 1 h	40 ml
50 ml 0.9% NaCl	40 ml/h	50 ml

Note: 'Time is muscle' – the earlier the thrombolytic agent is given, the greater chance of preserving myocardium. A physician should be present during administration of the bolus.

Table 6.10 Anticoagulation post myocardial infarction (MI)

	Anterior MI		Inferior MI
	Large	*Small*	
Streptokinase	High-dose SC heparin plus warfarin	Low-dose SC heparin	Low-dose SC heparin
Alteplase (t-PA)	IV heparin for 24 h then high-dose SC heparin plus warfarin	IV heparin for 24 h then low-dose SC heparin	IV heparin for 24 h then low-dose SC heparin
No thrombolytic therapy	High-dose SC heparin plus warfarin	Low-dose SC heparin	Low-dose SC heparin

SC = Subcutaneous; IV = intravenous; t-PA = tissue plasminogen activator.
High-dose = Maintain activated partial thromboplastin time at approximately twice normal (60–85 s); low-dose = heparin 7500 units b.d. or 5000 units t.d.s. subcutaneously.

aspirin alone and 42% with combined streptokinase and aspirin therapy. There is no definitive data on use with alteplase, but aspirin use is now recommended with all thrombolytic agents, although optimal dose and starting times have not been defined. Currently, aspirin 160 mg is given orally, as soon as possible after the onset of symptoms.[32]

Heparin

Heparin blocks the action of thrombin and helps prevent reocclusion. Heparin administration following alteplase therapy has been shown to be beneficial; early vessel patency rates were reduced by up to 50% when heparin was not given.[40,41] It is recommended that heparin be started concurrently with alteplase and continued for at least 24 h. There are no studies showing unequivocal benefit for heparin following streptokinase therapy. None the less, it is currently recommended that heparin be commenced 6–12 h after the streptokinase infusion.[42,43]

Hirudin

Hirudin and other potent highly specific thrombin inhibitors are currently being investigated.[44]

Haemostatic monitoring

Blood should be taken prior to thrombolytic therapy, for haemoglobin, haematocrit, platelet count, thrombin time, activated partial thromboplastin time (APTT) and prothrombin time (PT) estimations. During infusion of thrombolytic agents, coagulation tests and measures of fibrinolytic activity do not reliably predict efficacy of therapy or risk of bleeding, and are not usually performed. When heparin is used with alteplase and streptokinase (see above), APTT is kept at 60–85 s.

Treatment of bleeding complications

With thrombolytic therapy, there is an increased risk of bleeding in females, older patients and those with low body weight or hypertension. Most bleeding episodes are relatively minor and can be controlled by simple measures without transfusion therapy. Often, the bleeding is from vascular puncture sites amenable to locally applied pressure. About 4% of patients will need surgical control of bleeding from vessel puncture sites.[41] If the bleeding site is not obvious, stool and gastric aspirate need to be examined for blood, and the possibility of retroperitoneal haemorrhage considered (particularly if a femoral artery puncture had been performed). If bleeding is haemodynamically significant, thrombolytic and anticoagulation agents should be discontinued, although most bleeding occurs after the completion of thrombolytic agent infusion. Reversal of heparin with protamine should be considered if the bleeding is massive or intracranial. One mg of protamine is usually given for every 80–100 units of heparin administered within the preceding 4 h, but the APTT should be monitored closely. Protamine administration is not without risk (see Chapter 89).

A small number of cases require transfusion. Fibrinogen depletion is most marked 3–5 h after thrombolytic therapy, and cryoprecipitate is likely to be of benefit. Usually 10 units are given initially and may need to be repeated. Fresh frozen plasma followed by platelet transfusion is also recommended. Blood loss is corrected with fresh whole blood if available, or with packed red cells. In life-threatening haemorrhage, cryoprecipitate, fresh frozen plasma and empirical platelet administration are warranted. Under these circumstances, aminocaproic acid and aprotinin have been used, but they carry a risk of precipitating coronary rethrombosis. Whilst they prevent further fibrinolysis, they do not correct the hypocoagulable state that is the immediate cause of bleeding.

Antiarrhythmic drugs

Antiarrhythmic drugs such as lignocaine are no longer administered routinely following MI because of possible complications. Even though IV lignocaine does reduce the incidence of VF, mortality is unaffected because of an increased incidence of asystole.[35,45,46] If VF occurs only within the first 48 h of infarction, long-term antiarrhythmic therapy is not usually indicated. See below for the indications to use lignocaine.

Complications of MI

Arrhythmias

Some form of rhythm disturbance occurs in nearly all patients following acute MI (Table 6.11), and is particularly likely to occur within the first few hours of chest pain. Management of arrhythmias depends on the haemodynamic status of the patient. Precipitating or aggravating factors, such as hypoxia or acid–base disturbances, should be corrected. Every effort should be made to maintain the serum potassium in the high normal range.

1 *Ventricular ectopic beats (VEBs)* occur in nearly all patients with acute MI and generally do not require treatment. β-Blockers may abolish VEBs and prevent VF.
2 *VF and ventricular tachycardia (VT)* VF or VT in haemodynamically unstable patients requires immediate DC cardioversion. Prophylactic lignocaine to prevent the occurrence of VT/VF is no longer recommended.[35,47] Lignocaine is now used to treat sustained monomorphic VT (provided the patient is haemodynamically stable). Lignocaine is also used short-term (e.g. 24 h) to prevent recurrence of VT/VF should they occur. Sotalol IV is an alternative to lignocaine. Bretylium IV may be useful in refractory VF or VT.

3 *Accelerated idioventricular rhythm (AIVR)* Sometimes inappropriately called slow VT, this is common in patients with inferior MI, where it is usually associated with sinus bradycardia. It is usually benign and treatment is rarely necessary. Occasionally atropine, which increases the sinus node discharge rate, may be necessary.
4 *Atrial fibrillation (AF)* may not require treatment if the patient is not symptomatic or haemodynamically compromised. IV β-blocker or amiodarone (up to 7 mg/kg over 30 min) can be used to slow the ventricular rate. Digoxin may be the treatment of choice when heart failure is present. There is, however, no evidence that digoxin is beneficial in restoring sinus rhythm, although it is effective in slowing the ventricular rate.
5 *Atrial flutter* associated with acute MI is difficult to treat. Drug therapy is usually ineffective, although a short acting β-blocker (e.g. esmolol) can be used cautiously to control the ventricular response in patients without significant heart failure or haemodynamic compromise. Most patients will revert spontaneously to sinus rhythm over time. Should this not occur, rapid atrial pacing or synchronized DC cardioversion may be necessary.
6 *AV nodal and AV re-entry tachycardia (AVNRT and AVRT)* are uncommon. Adenosine is the treatment of choice. Verapamil should be avoided, especially in patients with heart failure.
7 *Bradyarrhythmias* Temporary pacing is indicated for all symptomatic bradycardias. Atropine, or occasionally isoprenaline, can be used for immediate treatment, whilst pacing is being instituted or if temporary pacing is unavailable. The increased availability of external temporary cardiac pacing has largely obviated the need to consider prophylactic temporary pacing for patients with various types of intraventricular block. Complete heart block secondary to inferior MI usually recovers within a few days, and has a good prognosis, but temporary pacing is required if the ventricular rate is slow and associated with haemodynamic compromise. Permanent pacing is rarely necessary. Complete heart block secondary to anterior infarction is usually related to extensive muscle damage affecting all three fascicles of the intracardiac conducting system, and has a poor prognosis. Although there is little evidence that pacing improves the long-term prognosis, temporary pacing is usually instituted, and if the patient survives the acute episode, permanent pacing is considered.

Table 6.11 Frequency of arrhythmias in patients with acute myocardial infarction (MI)

Arrhythmia	Frequency (%)
Ventricular premature beats	Almost universal
Ventricular tachycardia*	9–25
Ventricular fibrillation*	8–19
Accelerated idioventricular rhythm	9
Atrial fibrillation/flutter	9–14
AV nodal/AV re-entry tachycardia	3–4
AV block (first- or second-degree)	13
Complete AV block (third-degree)	7

AV = Atrioventricular.
* Life-threatening ventricular arrhythmias are 10–20 times more common in the first few hours after acute MI. The incidence of primary ventricular fibrillation seems to have decreased over recent years.[47]

Cardiac failure

Cardiac failure is treated with diuretics and nitrates (primarily to reduce preload), and inotropic support may be necessary (see Chapter 13). Hypotension secondary to RV infarction (these patients have a markedly elevated jugular venous pressure with little or no pulmonary congestion) should be managed by volume loading, usually with the aid of a Swan–Ganz catheter to maintain an optimal LV filling pressure at around 16–18 mmHg (2.1–2.4 kPa). Diuretics will often cause haemodynamic deterioration. Angiotension-converting enzyme (ACE) inhibitors are recommended for all patients with significant LV dysfunction, and are usually started early following infarction.[48–52] Captopril 3 mg t.d.s. can be used initially if the blood pressure is $\geqslant 100$ mm Hg (13.3 kPa) systolic; the dose is gradually increased. By the time of discharge, a longer-acting ACE inhibitor can be used.

Cardiogenic shock[33]

Mortality from cardiogenic shock remains very high at around 80% despite medical advances.[53] Conventional treatment with vasopressors, inotropic agents and intra-aortic balloon pump are temporizing measures, which are futile without definitive therapy (see Chapter 15). Direct coronary angioplasty has been shown to result in significantly improved survival for selected patients,[54–56] and – with coronary artery bypass grafting – may be the best available treatment.[53] Patients under 65 years, with a first infarction, and with intervention within 24 h, are likely to offer the best results. Definitive proof that these expensive strategies improve survival is being researched.[57]

Reinfarction

This occurs in up to 10% of patients following MI within the first few weeks. It is often due to reocclusion of a reperfused artery in the original area of infarction, but can occasionally be due to occlusion of a different coronary artery.

Cardiac rupture

Rupture of the interventricular septum is usually associated with a large infarction, and is often heralded by a new systolic murmur. Initially, the murmur may be soft and the patient may not be haemodynamically compromised. Definitive diagnosis can be made non-invasively using Doppler echocardiography or by Swan–Ganz catheterization (step-up in pulmonary artery compared to right atrial oxygen saturation) or occasionally angiography. Almost always, there is progressive deterioration in the patient's condition, and survival without cardiac surgery is rare. Surgical repair is considered as soon as the diagnosis is made.

Rupture of part of the papillary muscle resulting in severe mitral regurgitation may occur with relatively small infarctions. This diagnosis should be considered whenever a patient has heart failure disproportionate to the size of the infarction, even if a significant murmur cannot be heard.

Rupture of the free wall of the left ventricle results in acute cardiovascular collapse and electro-mechanical dissociation. Occasionally, a free wall rupture will be contained by the pericardium and a false aneurysm will be formed, which may be amenable to surgical repair.

Thromboembolism

Thrombus formation overlying the infarcted myocardium is common (it occurs in up to 30% of patients following anterior MI). Systemic embolization occurs in 5.5%, usually within the first 10 days, but is uncommon following inferior MI. Patients with large anterior infarctions should be heparinized and given warfarin at the same time. Warfarin can be withdrawn at discharge if no LV thrombus is seen on echocardiography. However, there is evidence for an improved prognosis when warfarin is continued.[58,59]

Cardiac dilatation and left ventricular aneurysm formation

Patients with large infarcts develop thinning of the affected myocardium, with stretching and dilatation of the ventricle, and sometimes frank aneurysm formation. ACE inhibitors appear to limit dilatation, help preserve LV function,[60,61] and improve prognosis.[48–52]

Postinfarction angina

This condition is an indication for early coronary angiography with a view to myocardial revascularization.

Dressler's syndrome (post myocardial injury syndrome)

This is now an uncommon syndrome, thought to be an immunopathic response to myocardial necrosis. It is characterized by pleuropericardial pain, fevers, friction rubs and a high blood sedimentation rate. The condition is managed with high-dose aspirin or non-steroidal anti-inflammatory agents, but is often persistent for several weeks; recurrences within a 12-month period are common.

Ongoing care of patients recovering from acute MI (Fig. 6.9)

Bed rest is recommended for the first 48 h after infarction, although toilet privileges can be allowed. Low-dose heparin (5000 units t.d.s. or 7500 units b.d. subcutaneously) is administered to prevent deep venous thrombosis, until the patient is mobile. There is often associated psychological stress, and patients need repeated reassurance and explanation of their condition. Use of minor tranquillizers is sometimes helpful. Aspirin and β-blocking drugs are continued.

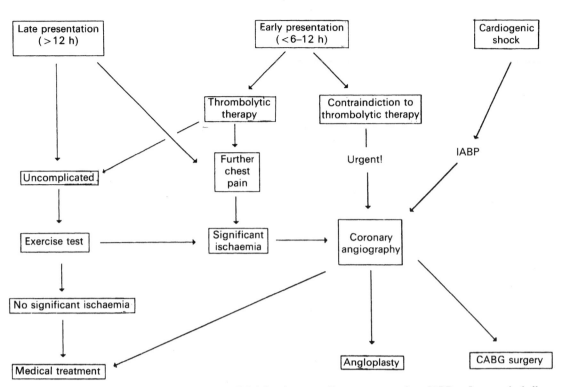

Fig. 6.9 Hospital management of acute myocardial infarction according to presentation. IABP = Intra-aortic balloon pump.

ACE inhibitors are recommended for patients with large infarcts and should be started early (see below).

1 *Aspirin* should be taken unless there are strong contraindications. Evidence for long-term benefits of aspirin comes from meta-analysis of trial data. Most trials have used high doses (300–600 mg/day). There is limited information on lower doses (100–160 mg/day) despite being commonly used.

2 *Warfarin* is currently given to patients with a large anterior MI (see above).

3 *β-Blockers*, when used following MI, have been shown to decrease mortality, reinfarction rate, incidence of VF and cardiac rupture. Decrease in sudden death after MI has only been documented with non-selective β-blockers,[36] despite the widespread use of selective β-blockers (e.g. metoprolol and atenolol).

4 *ACE inhibitors*[62] attenuate ventricular remodelling after MI, and possibly decrease the number of ischaemic events and reinfarctions. Reduced mortality following acute MI has been reported, especially in high-risk patients (e.g. with large anterior infarcts and significant LV dysfunction).[48–52,62] About 50–60 lives are saved per 1000 patients treated. Benefit is more modest in patients without significant impairment of LV function – about 5 lives are saved per 1000 patients treated.

Oral ACE inhibitors should be started during the acute phase of MI, perhaps within the first 24 h, provided there are no contraindications (e.g. hypotension). Therapy should continue in all patients with LV impairment, particularly those with extensive anterior MI.

5 *Amiodarone* in low doses (200 mg daily) may reduce mortality,[35] but results of definitive controlled trials are still awaited. At present amiodarone cannot be recommended as routine therapy.

6 *Magnesium* The LIMIT II trial[63] suggested a beneficial effect with IV magnesium administered early (<4 h) following acute MI, but the confidence limits were wide (1–43%) and the results only just reached statistical significance. The much larger ISIS-4 trial[49] did not demonstrate any effect, and hence routine administration of magnesium is not currently recommended.

7 *Nitrates* The recent GISSI-3[48] and ISIS-4[49] trials failed to demonstrate any beneficial effect on mortality when transdermal or oral nitrates were prescribed following acute MI. At present, it seems appropriate to use IV nitrates when there is continuing chest pain, especially when systemic hypertension and/or pulmonary oedema is present. However, long-term treatment is not indicated unless there is postinfarction angina.

8 *Calcium antagonists* There are possibly minor

benefits in terms of secondary protection, when diltiazem[64] or verapamil[65] are used for patients with non-Q-wave infarction and no evidence of cardiac failure. However, adverse effects have been described when dihydropyridine agents, particularly nifedipine, were administered to patients following infarction.[66-68]

9 *Lipid-lowering drugs* The recent 4S trial[69] showed that lowering cholesterol concentrations following MI resulted in a decrease in mortality and subsequent MI rate. All patients with an abnormal lipid profile following MI should be considered for lipid-lowering therapy, either by dietary measures or with pharmacological therapy if the former is unsuccessful.

Post MI investigations

Stress testing

Many centres perform submaximal stress testing (to a heart rate of about 120 beats/min), prior to hospital discharge, for patients with an uncomplicated course. Other centres delay stress testing until 3–6 weeks postinfarction, when a maximal symptom-limited stress test is performed. Some institutions perform both predischarge submaximal stress testing and maximal testing at a later stage. If stress testing shows evidence of inducible myocardial ischaemia, coronary angiography should be considered.

Echocardiography

Echocardiography is a useful investigation following MI to assess LV function[70] and to look for intraventricular thrombus.[26] The investigation is also helpful to look for RV infarction or complications of MI, such as acute mitral regurgitation,[71] ventricular septal defect,[53] pericardial effusion, or even subacute rupture of the ventricle.

Coronary angiography

Patients who have evidence of ongoing myocardial ischaemia, with recurrence of chest pain with or without associated ECG changes, are usually considered for coronary angiography prior to hospital discharge. Elective angiography is considered for patients with evidence of inducible myocardial ischaemia (from stress testing).

Outcome of MI

The in-hospital mortality from acute MI has been steadily decreasing over the past two decades from 15–30% in the 1970s, to approximately 10% in 1980, and now to around 8% in the 1990s.[40,72-77] Despite improved mortality, 60% of all deaths occur within the first hour (often from VF), and usually before reaching a medical facility. Modern management of acute MI has undoubtedly contributed to decreased mortality, but further significant reduction in mortality must come from management strategies within the first hour of the onset of symptoms.

References

1 Sutherland JE, Persky VW and Brody JA (1990) Proportionate mortality trends: 1950 through 1986. *J Am Med Assoc* **264**:3178–3184.

2 National Center for Health Statistics (1987) Utilization of short stay hospitals, United States 1987. *Vital Health Stat* **31**:197.

3 Heller RF, Chinn S, Tundstall Pedoe HD and Rose G (1984) How well can we predict coronary heart disease? Findings in the United Kingdom heart disease prevention project. *Br Med J* **88**:1409–1411.

4 Rossouw JE, Lewis B and Rifkind BM (1990) The value of lowering cholesterol after myocardial infarction. *N Engl J Med* **323**:1112–1119.

5 Kannel WB (1978) Hypertension, blood lipids and cigarette smoking as co-risk factors for coronary heart disease. *Ann NY Acad Sci* **304**:128–139.

6 Slattery ML, Jacobs DR Jr and Nichaman MZ (1989) Leisure time physical activity and coronary heart disease death. The US railroad study. *Circulation* **79**:304–311.

7 Yusuf S, Wittes J and Friedman L (1988) Overview of results of randomized clinical trials in heart disease II. Unstable angina, heart failure, primary prevention with aspirin, and risk factor modification. *J Am Med Assoc* **260**:2259–2263.

8 Davies MJ and Thomas AC (1985) Plaque fissuring – the cause of acute myocardial infarction, sudden ischaemic death, and crescendo angina. *Br Heart J* **53**:363–373.

9 Falk E (1989) Morphologic features of unstable athero-thrombotic plaques underlying acute coronary syndrome. *Am J Cardiol* **63**:114E–120E.

10 Pfeffer MA and Braunwald E (1990) Ventricular remodelling after myocardial infarction. *Circulation* **81**:1161–1172.

11 Alonzo AM, Simon AB and Feinleib M (1975) Prodromata of myocardial infarction and sudden death. *Circulation* **52**: 1056–1062.

12 Muller DWM, Topol EJ, Califf RM *et al.* (1990) Relationship between antecedent angina pectoris and short-term prognosis after thrombolytic therapy for acute myocardial infarction. *Am Heart J* **119**:224–231.

13 Margolis JR, Kannel WF, Feinleib M *et al.* Clinical features of unrecognised myocardial infarction: silent and symptomatic. Eighteen year follow-up: the Framingham study. *Am J Cardiol* **32**:1–7.

14 Yano K and MacLean CJ (1989) The incidence and prognosis of unrecognised myocardial infarction in the Honolulu, Hawaii, heart program. *Arch Intern Med* **149**:1528–1532.

15 Jaarsma W, Visser CA, Van Eenige J and Roos JP (1987) Left ventricular wall motion with and without Q wave

disappearance after acute myocardial infarction. *Am J Cardiol* **59**:516–518.

16 Coll S, Betriu A, De Flores T *et al.* (1988) Significance of Q-wave regression after transmural acute myocardial infarction. *Am J Cardiol* **61**:739–742.

17 Haiat R, Worthington FX, Castellanos A and Lemberg L (1971) Unusual normalisation of the electrocardiogram on the 6th day of myocardial infarction. *J Electrocardiol* **4**:363–368.

18 Berger PB, de Zwaan C, Brugada P, Coenegracht JM and Wellens HJJ (1990) Inferior myocardial infarction. High risk subgroups. *Circulation* **81**:401–411.

19 Zehender M, Kasper W, Kauder E *et al.* (1994) Eligibility for and benefit of thrombolytic therapy in inferior myocardial infarction: focus on the prognostic importance of right ventricular infarction. *J Am Coll Cardiol* **24**:362–369.

20 Lopez-Sendon J, Coma-Canella I, Alcasena S *et al.* (1985) Electrocardiographic findings in acute right ventricular infarction. Sensitivity and specificity of electrocardiographic alterations in right precordial leads V4R, V3R, V1, V2, and V3. *J Am Coll Cardiol* **6**:1273–1279.

21 Sgarbosa EB, Pinski SL, Barbagelata A *et al.* (1996) Electrocardiographic diagnosis of evolving acute myocardial infarction in the presence of left bundle branch block. *New Engl J Med* **334**:481–487.

22 Robalino BD, Whitlow PL, Underwood DA and Salcedo EE (1989) Electrocardiographic manifestations of right ventricular infarction. *Am Heart J* **118**:138–144

23 Lee TH and Goldman L (1986) Serum enzyme assays in the diagnosis of acute myocardial infarction. *Ann Intern Med* **105**:221–223.

24 Ong L, Reiser P, Coromilas J *et al.* (1983) Left ventricular function and rapid release of creatine kinase MB in acute myocardial infarction: evidence for spontaneous reperfusion. *N Engl J Med* **309**:1–6.

25 Blanke H, von Hardenberg D, Cohen M *et al.* (1984) Patterns of creatine kinase release during acute myocardial infarction after nonsurgical reperfusion. Comparison with conventional treatment and correlation with infarct size. *J Am Coll Cardiol* **3**:675–680.

26 Spirito P, Bellotti P, Chiarella F *et al.* (1985) Prognostic significance and natural history of left ventricular thrombi in patients with acute anterior myocardial infarction: a two-dimensional echocardiographic study. *Circulation* **72**:774–780.

27 Co-operating investigators from the MILIS study group (1985) Electrocardiographic, enzymatic and scintigraphic criteria of acute myocardial infarction as determined from study of 726 patients (MILIS study). *Am J Cardiol* **55**:1463–1468.

28 Gibson RS, Taylor GJ, Watson DD *et al.* (1981) Predicting the extent and location of coronary artery disease during the early post-infarction period by quantitative thallium-201 scintigraphy. *Am J Cardiol* **47**:1010–1019.

29 Khaw BA, Gold JK, Yasuda T *et al.* (1986) Scintigraphic quantification of myocardial necrosis in patients after intravenous injection of myosin-specific antibody. *Circulation* **74**:501–508.

30 Hashimoto K, Jambara H, Fudo T *et al.* (1988) Non-Q wave versus Q wave myocardial infarction: regional myocardial metabolism and blood flow assessed by positron emission tomography. *J Am Coll Cardiol* **12**:88–93.

31 Johnson LL, Seldin DW, Becker LC *et al.* (1989) Antimyosin imaging in acute transmural myocardial infarction: results of a multicenter clinical trial. *J Am Coll Cardiol* **13**:27–35.

32 ISIS 2 collaborative group (1988) Randomized trial of intravenous streptokinase, oral aspirin, both or neither among 17 187 cases of suspected acute myocardial infarction: ISIS 2. *Lancet* **2**:349–360.

33 Califf RM and Bengtson JR (1994) Cardiogenic shock. *N Engl J Med* **330**:1724–1730.

34 ISIS-1 (First International Study of Infarct Survival) collaborative group (1986) Randomized trial of intravenous atenolol among 16 027 cases of suspected acute myocardial infarction. ISIS-1. *Lancet* **2**:57–62.

35 Teo KK, Yusuf S and Furberg CD (1993) Effects of prophylactic antiarrhythmic drug therapy in acute myocardial infarction: an overview of results from randomised trials. *J Am Med Assoc* **270**:1589–1595.

36 The Norwegian multicentre study group (1981) Timolol induced reduction in mortality and reinfarction in patients surviving acute myocardial infarction. *N Engl J Med* **304**:801–807.

37 Anderson HV and Willerson JT (1993) Thrombolysis in acute myocardial infarction. *N Engl J Med* **329**:703–709.

38 Gruppo Italiano per lo Studio della Streptochinasi Nell'infarcto Miocardico (GISSI) (1986) Effectiveness of intravenous thrombolytic treatment in acute myocardial infarction. *Lancet* **1**:397–401.

39 LATE study group (1993) Late assessment of thrombolytic efficacy (LATE) study with alteplase 6–24 hours after onset of acute myocardial infarction. *Lancet* **342**:759–766.

40 The GUSTO angiographic investigators (1993) The effects of tissue plasminogen activator, streptokinase, or both on coronary-artery patency, ventricular function, and survival after acute myocardial infarction. *N Engl J Med* **329**:1615–1633.

41 Task Force on the Management of Acute Myocardial Infarction of the European Society of Cardiology (1996) Acute myocardial infarction: prehospital and inhospital management. *Eur Heart J* **17**:43–63.

42 Hsia J, Hamilton WP, Kleiman N *et al.* (1990) The heparin–aspirin reperfusion trial (HART): a randomized trial of heparin versus aspirin adjunctive to tissue plasminogen activator-induced thrombolysis in acute myocardial infarction. *N Engl J Med* **323**:1433–1437.

43 Beich SD, Nichols T, Schumacher R *et al.* (1989) The role of heparin following coronary thrombolysis with tissue plasminogen activator (t-PA). *Circulation* **80** (supp II):113.

44 Lee VL for the TIM16 investigators. Initial experience with hirudin and streptokinase in acute myocardial infarction: results of the thrombolysis in acute myo-

cardial infarction (TIMI) 6 trial. *Am J Cardiol* **75**:7–13.

45 Wyse DG, Kellen J and Rademaker AW (1988) Prophylactic versus selective lidocaine for early ventricular arrhythmias of myocardial infarction. *J Am Coll Cardiol* **12**:507–513.

46 Hine LK, Laird N, Hewitt P and Chalmers TC (1989) Meta-analytic evidence against prophylactic use of lidocaine in acute myocardial infarction. *Arch Intern Med* **149**:2694–2698.

47 Antman EM and Berlin JA (1992) Declining incidence of ventricular fibrillation in myocardial infarction: implications for the prophylactic use of lignocaine. *Circulation* **86**:764–773.

48 GISSI-3 (1994) Effects of lisinopril and transdermal glyceryl trinitrate singly and together on 6-week mortality and ventricular function after acute myocardial infarction. *Lancet* **343**:1115–1122.

49 ISIS-4 (Fourth International Study of Infarct Survival) collaborative group (1995) A randomised trial assessing early oral captopril, oral mononitrate, and intravenous magnesium sulphate in 58 050 patients with suspected acute myocardial infarction. *Lancet* **345**:669–685.

50 The Acute Infarction Ramipril Efficacy (AIRE) study investigators (1993) Effect of ramipril on mortality and morbidity of survivors of acute myocardial infarction with clinical evidence of heart failure. *Lancet* **342**:821–828.

51 Pfeffer MA, Braunwald E, Moye LA *et al.* Effect of captopril on mortality and morbidity in patients with left ventricular dysfunction after myocardial infarction: results of the survival and ventricular enlargement trial. *N Engl J Med* **327**:669–677.

52 Ambrosini E, Borghi C, Magnani B for the Survival of Myocardial Infarction Long-term Evaluation (SMILE) study investigators (1995) The effect of the angiotensin-converting enzyme inhibitor Zofenopril on mortality and morbidity after anterior myocardial infarction. *N Engl J Med* **332**:80–85.

53 O'Neill WW (1992) Angioplasty therapy of cardiogenic shock: are randomized trials necessary? *J Am Coll Cardiol* **19**:915–917.

54 Moosvi AR, Khaja F, Villanueva L *et al.* (1992) Early revascularization improves survival in cardiogenic shock complicating acute myocardial infarction. *J Am Coll Cardiol* **19**: 907–914.

55 Hibbard MD, Holmes DR, Bailey KR *et al.* (1992) Percutaneous transluminal coronary angioplasty in patients with cardiogenic shock: reports on therapy. *J Am Coll Cardiol* **19**:639–646.

56 Lee L, Erbel R, Brown TM *et al.* Multicentre registry of angioplasty therapy of cardiogenic shock: initial and long-term survival. *J Am Coll Cardiol* **17**:599–603.

57 Hochman JS, Boland J, Sleeper LA *et al.* (1995) Current spectrum of cardiogenic shock and effect of early revascularisation on mortality. Results of an international registry. *Circulation* **91**:873–881.

58 Turpie AGG (1990) Anticoagulant therapy after acute myocardial infarction. *Am J Cardiol* **65**:20C–23C.

59 Smith P, Arnesen H and Holme I (1990) The effect of

60 Pfeffer MA, Lamas GA, Vaughan DE *et al.* (1988) Effect of captopril on progressive ventricular dilatation after anterior myocardial infarction. *N Engl J Med* **319**:80–86.

61 Sharp N, Smith H, Murphy *et al.* (1991) Early prevention of left ventricular dysfunction after myocardial infarction with angiotensin-converting-enzyme inhibition. *Lancet* **337**:872–876.

62 Pfeffer MA (1995) ACE inhibition in acute myocardial infarction. *N Engl J Med* **332**:116–120.

63 Woods KL, Fletcher S, Roffe C *et al.* (1992) Intravenous magnesium sulphate in suspected acute myocardial infarction: (LIMIT-2). *Lancet* **339**:1553–1558.

64 Gibson RS, Boden WE, Theroux P *et al.* Diltiazem and reinfarction in patients with non-Q wave infarction. *N Engl J Med* **315**:423–429.

65 The Danish study group on verapamil in myocardial infarction (1990) Effect of verapamil on mortality and major events after acute myocardial infarction (the Danish verapamil infarction trial II – DAVIT II). *Am J Cardiol* **66**: 779–785.

66 Muller JE, Morrison J, Stone PH *et al.* (1984) Nifedipine therapy for patients with threatened and acute myocardial infarction: a randomized, double-blind, placebo controlled comparison. *Circulation* **69**: 740–747.

67 Erbel R, Pop T, Meinertz T *et al.* (1988) Combination of calcium channel blocker and thrombolytic therapy in acute myocardial infarction. *Am Heart J* **115**:529–538.

68 Report of the Holland interuniversity nifedipine/metoprolol trial (HINT) research group (1986) Early treatment of unstable angina in the coronary care unit: a randomized, double-blind, placebo-controlled comparison of recurrent ischaemia and thrombolytic therapy in patients treated with nifedipine or metoprolol or both. *Br Heart J* **56**:400–413.

69 The Scandinavian Simvastatin survival study group (1994) Randomized trial of cholesterol lowering in 4444 patients with coronary heart disease: the Scandinavian Simvastatin survival study (4S). *Lancet* **344**:383–388.

70 Weiss JL, Bulkley BH, Hutchins GM and Mason SJ (1981) Two-dimensional echocardiographic recognition of myocardial injury in man: comparison with postmortem studies. *Circulation* **63**:401–408.

71 Donaldson RM and Ballester M (1982) Echocardiographic visualization of the anatomic causes of mitral regurgitation resulting from myocardial infarction. *Postgrad Med J* **58**:257–263.

72 Cairns JA, Singer J, Gent M *et al.* (1989) One year mortality outcomes of all coronary and intensive care unit patients with acute myocardial infarction, unstable angina or other chest pain in Hamilton, Ontario, a city of 375 000 people. *Can J Cardiol* **5**:239–246.

73 Pell S and Fayerweather WE (1985) Trends in the incidence of myocardial infarction and in associated mortality and morbidity in a large employed population, 1957–83. *N Engl J Med* **312**:1005–1011.

74 Gomez-Martin O, Folsom AR, Kottke KE *et al.* (1987)

Improvement in long-term survival among patients hospitalized with acute myocardial infarction, 1970–1980. *N Engl J Med* **316**:1353–1359.

75 Beaglehole R (1986) Medical management and the decline in mortality from coronary heart disease. *Br Med J* **292**:33–35.

76 Kuller LH, Traven ND, Rutan GH *et al.* (1989) Marked decline of coronary heart disease mortality in 35–44 year-old white men in Allegheny County, Pennsylvania. *Circulation* **80**:261–266.

77 Naylor CD and Chen E (1994) Population-wide mortality trends among patients hospitalised for acute myocardial infarction: the Ontario experience 1981–1991. *J Am Coll Cardiol* **24**:1431–1438.

7 Cardiopulmonary resuscitation

TE Oh

Cardiac arrest is the cessation of cardiac mechanical activity with no clinical cardiac output. If immediate cardiopulmonary resuscitation (CPR) is not started, death or serious cerebral damage will result. Hospital staff generally lack competent CPR skills.[1] How CPR training should best be implemented is unclear.[1] None the less, ICU staff should promote CPR training and be the driving force behind a hospital's resuscitation team.

Causes

Cardiac arrest may result from intrinsic pump failure, or from an arrhythmia. The causes of cardiac arrest are varied (Table 7.1). In adults, the commonest cause is primary ischaemic disease. Precipitating factors in critically ill patients are hypoxia, circulatory failure and acid–base and electrolyte imbalance.

Clinical presentation

Cardiac arrest may or may not be witnessed. The victim is unresponsive with an absent pulse. Cyanosis, absent breathing and convulsions may be present.

Table 7.1 Common causes of cardiac arrest

Primary: sudden cessation of cardiac function
Myocardial ischaemia: ventricular fibrillation
Heart disease ⎫
Electric shock ⎬ ventricular fibrillation
Drugs, e.g. potassium ⎭ and asystole
Secondary: non-intrinsic cardiac causes
Asphyxia, hypoxia, hypercarbia
Exsanguination
Central nervous system failure
Metabolic/electrolyte disorders
Temperature extremes
Toxins
Acute anaphylaxis

Spontaneous breathing and pupil size are irrelevant to the diagnosis.[2] Cardiac arrest is usually associated with any of four rhythms: ventricular fibrillation (VF), pulseless ventricular tachycardia (VT), asystole or electromechanical dissociation (EMD). VF is the commonest primary arrhythmia and may be preceded by pulseless VT (of which treatment is identical). Asystole is the primary arrhythmia in up to 25% of in-hospital arrests. EMD refers to absent mechanical activity despite a coordinated ECG waveform and is diagnosed infrequently.

Management[3–6]

As preventive measures, continuous ECG monitoring will detect life-threatening arrhythmias, and adverse factors are corrected. CPR consists of *basic life support* (i.e. maintaining an airway and supporting breathing and the circulation without special equipment other than an airway device)[3,4] and *advanced cardiac life support* (i.e. definitive treatment with drugs and DC shock).[5–7]

Basic life support

The airway, breathing and circulation must be assessed before initiating active intervention; this can be achieved by the ABC of resuscitation.

Airway

A patent airway is secured. Vomitus or debris from oropharynx is removed. A Guedel's airway may be inserted.

Breathing

Mouth-to-mouth breathing is started. To minimize gastric distension and the risk of pulmonary aspiration, a slow inspiratory time (1.5–2.0 s) and a low inflation pressure (<20 cm H_2O (2 kPa); the oesophageal opening pressure in anaesthetized adults) are used.[3] Cricoid pressure (Sellick's manoeuvre) is extremely useful. About 10–12 breaths/min should be delivered.

Cardiac compression or external cardiac massage (ECM)

A precordial thump may terminate a witnessed or monitored cardiac arrest, but is not recommended in basic life support for unwitnessed arrests.[4] ECM is started, depressing the lower half of the sternum 4–5 cm in an adult. Blood flow during ECM is postulated to be due to either compression of the heart between the sternum and the spine to eject blood (cardiac pump mechanism) or raised intrathoracic pressure forcing forward flow which is maintained by venous valves; the heart acts as a passive conduit (thoracic pump mechanism).[8] Both mechanisms are probably involved.

ECM produces only 10–33% of pre-arrest cardiac output. Blood is directed mostly to the brain and upper trunk. Flow to the brain is reduced 50–90% of normal, to the myocardium 20–50% of normal, and to the abdomen and lower extremities less than 5% of normal.[8] Coronary perfusion occurs primarily during the relaxation (diastole) phase of ECM, and coronary perfusion pressures above 15 mmHg (2 kPa) are associated with successful resuscitation.[9] Thus ECM must aim to achieve adequate diastolic and mean blood pressures. Short quick jabs are ineffective. A compression phase equal in time to the relaxation phase is recommended.[10] ECM is continued at a rate (not absolute number of compressions) of 80/min, but 60–100/min is acceptable. Single rescuers should pause to ventilate once after every 15 ECM cycles, and after every five cycles if there are two rescuers.

Advanced cardiac life support

Protocols

The American Heart Association (AHA), European Resuscitation Council (ERC), and Australian Resuscitation Council (ARC) recommend guidelines and protocols to manage VF (and pulseless VT), asystole, and EMD (Figs 7.1 and 7.2).[5–7] All protocols are similar in stressing early defibrillation and advanced care. A precordial thump is recommended for VF and asystolic arrests, especially if witnessed. This conversion of mechanical to electrical energy may revert 40% of VT and 2% of VF cases.[11] The three ERC protocols have loops or cycles of activity consisting of giving 1 mg adrenaline, 10 sequences of 5:1 ECM/ventilation, and advanced airway care and venous access (Fig. 7.1).[6] Rapid defibrillation for VF and pulseless VT is emphasized; three DC shocks should be given in quick succession within 30–45 s while administration of antiarrhythmic drugs is delayed.[6] ARC protocols are more conventional.[7]

Their simplified single flowchart presents sequential management steps (Fig 7.2). Present AHA guidelines are detailed and comprehensive,[5] but are too complex for practical use. EMD is included under a broader term of pulseless electrical activity. Regimens for higher doses of adrenaline are included, and early transcutaneous pacing for asystole is recommended. Regardless of which protocol is used, rhythm and pulse should be checked after each DC shock, without delaying defibrillator recharging or delivering the next shock. Normal ECG complexes do not always indicate effective cardiac output.

Advanced airway care

The trachea is intubated after the first DC shocks. Once intubation is achieved, ventilation can proceed without pause in ECM or regard for the ECM cycle. Oxygen is given when available. Some manual resuscitator bags cannot deliver adequate concentrations of oxygen.[12,13] High oxygen concentrations generally cannot be achieved without a reservoir bag in series (see Chapter 27). Resuscitators with a soft feel on inflation can help the operator to assess the patient's lung compliance. Less satisfactory alternatives to tracheal intubation include use of the laryngeal mask, oesophageal obturator airway, combitube and pharyngeal tracheal airway. These devices and percutaneous surgical cricothyrotomies and tracheostomies are discussed in Chapter 23. Other means of achieving ventilation by personnel unskilled in intubation are:

1 *Resuscitator bag-mask ventilation:* Use by two operators, one to hold the mask and the other to inflate the bag, is recommended to achieve a leak-proof seal on the face.[5]
2 *Alternatives to mouth-to-mouth breathing:* Direct contact between rescuer and patient is eliminated, although there are no documented cases of cross-infection with human immunodeficiency virus (HIV) or hepatitis B virus from CPR. The devices include facemasks for mouth-to-mask breathing (e.g. Laerdal pocket mask) and face shields. Mouth-mask ventilation has been reported to be superior to resuscitator bag-mask ventilation, due to the rescuer's use of two hands to seal the mask and the larger gas volume from the lungs.[14,15] Supplemental oxygen can be given through the mask. Face shields are barrier sheets covering the victim's nose and mouth, with a filter or valve to divert exhaled gas away from the rescuer. Their efficacy and usefulness remain to be established.

Cardiac compression

Techniques which raise intrathoracic pressure, e.g. simultaneous ventilation/compression, abdominal binding with compression, and use of the pneumatic

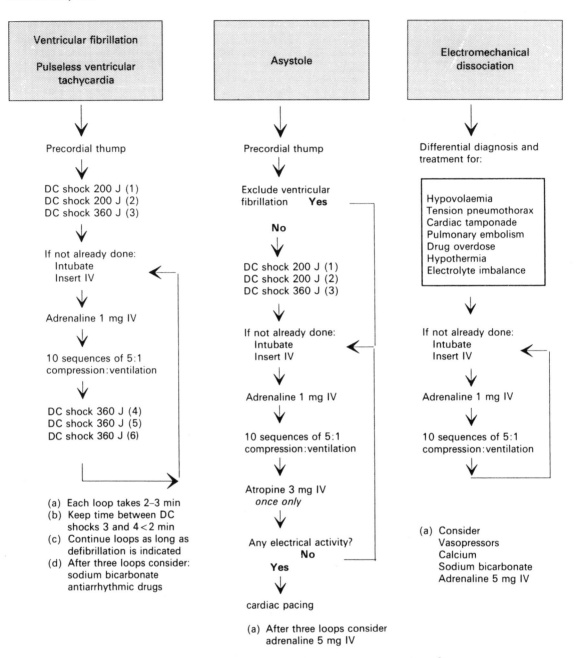

Fig. 7.1 European Resuscitation Council advanced cardiac life support protocols or algorithms.[6]

antishock garment, are not recommended.[8] Interposed abdominal counterpulsation CPR (IAC-CPR, i.e. abdominal compression during the relaxation phase of ECM)[16] and active compression–decompression CPR[17] require further outcome studies.

Open heart massage is rarely necessary, but may be indicated in trauma arrests, e.g. associated with penetrating chest wounds, severe chest crush injuries, haemothorax and cardiac tamponade.

Drugs

Drugs should be given whenever possible through a central vein. However, peripheral venous cannulation is rapid and does not interfere with CPR. Drugs given into a peripheral vein should be propelled by a bolus of 20 ml saline to promote entry into the circulation. Endobronchial administration is less preferable as absorption is unpredictable.[18,19] If this route is used,

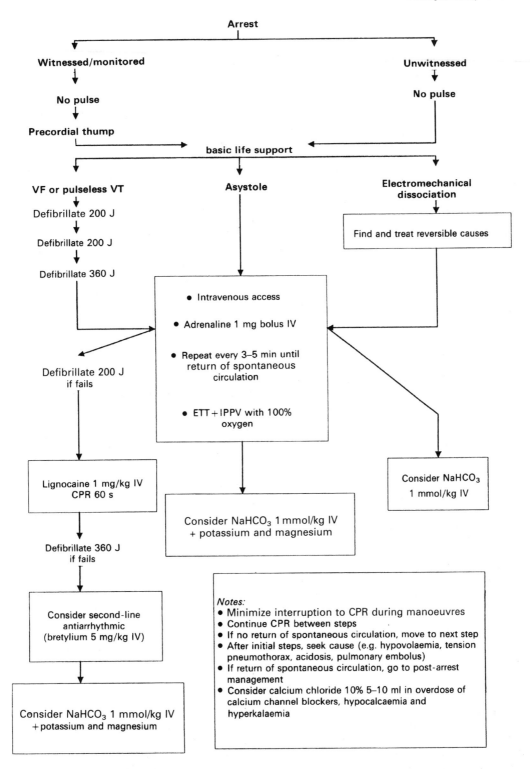

Fig. 7.2 Advanced life support flowchart – Australian Resuscitation Council.[7] VF = Ventricular fibrillation; VT = ventricular tachycardia; IV = intravenous; ETT = endotracheal tube; IPPV = intermittent positive-pressure ventilation; CPR = cardio-pulmonary resuscitation.

a dose 2.0–2.5 times that for the IV route, diluted to 10 ml with saline,[5,6,20] is instilled via a catheter down the trachea, followed by forceful lung hyperinflations. Intracardiac drug administration is still recommended by some[21] but advantages, if any, are countered by potential myocardial injury and interruption of CPR. Drugs used in CPR are:

1 *Adrenaline:* 1 mg (1 ml of 1:1000 or 10 ml 1:10 000) is given. Efficacy lies entirely in its α-adrenergic properties, as peripheral vasoconstriction increases diastolic pressure and coronary perfusion. Its β-adrenergic properties are potentially deleterious.[22] Adrenaline does not enhance defibrillation or improve success.[23] The value of high doses (5–18 mg) is conflicting[8] but a 5-mg dose should be considered if response is lacking, especially if asystole persists.[6] Other strong α-adrenergic catecholamines (methoxamine, phenylephrine or dopamine) appear equally effective in CPR.[8]

2 *Sodium bicarbonate* should not be given routinely. Bicarbonate causes sodium overloading and hyperosmolality (with cellular oedema), paradoxical cerebral acidosis, myocardial depression, depressed cardiac contractility and metabolic alkalosis with tissue deprivation of oxygen.[24,25] It should be given slowly (up to 50 mmol) only in prolonged arrests or if hyperkalaemia is present. Knowledge of arterial blood-gas values is desirable, although they do not accurately reflect tissue acid–base status. Bicarbonate may be judiciously repeated. The standard 8.4% solution should be issued only in 100 ml (100 mmol) containers. Other buffering agents, e.g. THAM, Carbicarb and Tribonate, have no advantages.

3 *Antiarrhythmic agents*[26–28] (see Chapter 9): Routine use of lignocaine to treat VF is inappropriate. It raises the threshold and energy requirements for defibrillation and is associated with post-defibrillation asystole.[29] *Lignocaine* 1.0–1.5 mg/kg should be given if VF persists, followed by an infusion of 2–4 mg/min. *Procainamide* (250–500 mg IV over 5–10 min) can be used if lignocaine is contraindicated. *Bretylium tosylate* is given if lignocaine fails, as a slow bolus of 5 mg/kg. *Amiodarone* 5 mg/kg IV over 5–10 min may be used but its role in CPR is not as established. No drug has been proven to be more superior than the others in refractory VF.

4 *Atropine:* 0.3–1.0 mg IV is cautiously given for symptomatic bradyarrhythmias. A single large 3-mg dose to block vagal tone fully is recommended for asystolic arrest.

5 *Isoprenaline:* 50–100 μg IV, followed by a titrated rate infusion of 2 mg in 500 ml 5% dextrose, is only given as a temporary measure if symptomatic bradycardia is not controlled by atropine.

6 *Calcium* should not be routinely given because of possible harm in cerebral ischaemia (see Chapter 44). It is reserved for EMD victims

associated with hypocalcaemia, hyperkalaemia or calcium antagonist medication. Usual dose is IV 10 ml of 10% calcium chloride.

7 *Magnesium and potassium:* No evidence exists to support their use in CPR.

End-tidal CO$_2$ and echocardiography

End-tidal CO$_2$ can be used to monitor effectiveness of CPR. CO$_2$ excretion during CPR is flow-rather than ventilation-dependent. During low flows, alveolar dead space is large and end-tidal CO$_2$ is very low. As cardiac output increases, more alveoli are perfused and end-tidal CO$_2$ rises. Successful CPR is seen with an end-tidal CO$_2$ over 20 mmHg (2.66 kPa) and values below 10 mmHg (1.33 kPa) predict death.[30] Transoesophageal echocardiography during CPR can provide continuous cardiac imaging without interrupting resuscitation, but its role in this area requires evaluation (see Chapter 21).

Ethics of resuscitation

If CPR has not resulted in satisfactory cardiac output or rhythm after an appropriate period (e.g. up to 60 min), resuscitation should be discontinued. This decision should be made by the team leader. CPR is futile in many patients, e.g. those with advanced terminal cancer or severe heart or lung disease. Guidelines not to resuscitate have been proposed.[31–33] CPR should be withheld if previously refused by a competent patient; if resuscitation is considered not in the best interests of an incompetent patient; and if CPR is judged to be futile. However, in practice such considerations can be complex.[32]

Outcome

Complications of CPR include fractured ribs, flail chest and pneumothorax. Cerebral oedema, cerebrovascular accidents and renal failure are some sequelae in survivors. No specific post-arrest treatment can be recommended, apart from maintaining stable cardiac output, oxygenation, normocarbia and electrolyte balance (see Chapter 44).

Cardiac arrest victims may survive the resuscitation, but the survival to hospital discharge rate is 18% with a 1-year survival rate of 12.5%.[34] The success rate has not changed over 30 years.[35] Prediction of survivors is unreliable.[36] Mortality is higher with chronic debilitating illness, unwitnessed arrest, arrest outside hospital or in poorly staffed areas, elderly victims, asystole or EMD, and the onset and quality of CPR.[37] To understand CPR outcome better, standardized collection of data is imperative, and the Utstein-style template[38] is strongly recommended. CPR in children is discussed in Chapter 101.

References

1 Dent THS and Gillard JH (1993) Cardiopulmonary resuscitation: effectiveness, training and survival. *J R Coll Physicians Lond* **27**:354–355.

2 Campbell IT and Swan G (1993) Guidelines and training in cardiopulmonary resuscitation. *Lancet* **341**:470–471.

3 American Heart Association (1992) Standards for cardiopulmonary resuscitation and emergency cardiac care. Adult basic life support. *J Am Med Assoc* **268**:2184–2198.

4 Basic Life Support Working Party of the European Resuscitation Council (1992). Guidelines for basic life support. *Resuscitation* **24**:103–110.

5 American Heart Association (1992) Standards for cardiopulmonary resuscitation and emergency cardiac care. Adult advanced cardiac life support. *J Am Med Assoc* **268**:2199–2241.

6 Advanced Life Support Working Party of the European Resuscitation Council (1992) Guidelines for advanced life support. *Resuscitation* **24**:111–121.

7 Adult advanced life support (1993) The Australian Resuscitation Council guidelines. *Med J Aust* **159**:616–621.

8 Otto CW (1993) *Current Concepts in Cardiopulmonary Resuscitation.* 1993 Annual Refresher Course Lectures. Washington DC: American Society of Anesthesiologists.

9 Paradis NA, Martin GB, Rivers EP *et al.* (1990) Coronary perfusion pressure and the return of spontaneous circulation in human cardiopulmonary resuscitation. *J Am Med Assoc* **263**:1106–1113.

10 European Resuscitation Council Basic Life Support Working Group (1993) Guidelines for basic life support. *Br Med J* **306**:1587–1589.

11 European Resuscitation Council Working Party (1993) Adult advanced cardiac life support: the European Resuscitation Council guidelines 1992 (abridged). *Br Med J* **306**:1589–1593.

12 Carden E and Hughes T (1975) An evaluation of manually operated self-inflating resuscitation bags. *Anesth Analg* **54**:133–138.

13 Mills PJ, Baptiste J, Preston J and Barnas GM (1991) Manual resuscitators and spontaneous ventilation – an evaluation. *Crit Care Med* **19**:1425–1431.

14 Elling R and Politis J (1983) An evaluation of emergency medical technicians' ability to use ventilation devices. *Ann Emerg Med* **12**:765–768.

15 Johannigman JA, Branson RD, Davis K *et al.* (1991) Techniques of emergency ventilation: a model to evaluate tidal volume, airway pressure and gastric insufflation. *J Trauma* **31**:93–98.

16 Sack JB, Kesselbrenner MB and Bregman D (1992) Survival from in-hospital cardiac arrest with interposed abdominal counterpulsation during cardiopulmonary resuscitation. *J Am Med Assoc* **267**:379–385.

17 Cohen TJ, Tucker KJ, Lurie KG *et al.* (1992) Active compression–decompression: a new method of cardiopulmonary resuscitation. *J Am Med Assoc* **267**:2916–2923.

18 Robertson C (1993) New standards in emergency cardiac care. *Curr Opinion Anesthesiol* **6**:359–364.

19 Hapnes SA and Robertson C (1992) CPR – Drug delivery routes and systems. *Resuscitation* **24**:137–142.

20 Aitkenhead AR (1991) Drug administration during CPR: which route? *Resuscitation* **22**:191–195.

21 Pedersen A, Jespersen H and Torp-Pedersen C (1991) The place of intracardiac injections in the treatment of cardiac arrest. *Drugs* **42**:915–918.

22 Otto CW and Yakaitis RW (1984) The role of epinephrine in CPR: a reappraisal. *Ann Emerg Med* **13**:840–843.

23 Otto CW and Yakaitis RW (1984) Effects of epinephrine on defibrillation in ischemic ventricular fibrillation. *Am J Emerg Med* **3**:285–291.

24 Bishop RI and Weisfeld TML (1976) Sodium bicarbonate administration during cardiac arrest. Effect on arterial pH, P_{CO_2}, and osmolality. *J Am Med Assoc* **235**:506–509.

25 Grundler WG, Weil MH, Yamaguchi M *et al.* (1984) The paradox of venous acidosis and arterial alkalosis during CPR. *Chest* **86**:282–291.

26 von Planta M and Chamberlain D (1992) Drug treatment of arrhythmias during cardiopulmonary resuscitation. *Resuscitation* **24**:227–232.

27 Waller DG (1991) Treatment and prevention of ventricular fibrillation: are there better agents? *Resuscitation* **22**:159–166.

28 Hallstrom AP, Cobb LA, Yu BH, Weaver WD and Fahrenbruck CE (1991) An antiarrhythmic drug experience in 941 patients resuscitated from an initial cardiac arrest between 1970 and 1985. *Am J Cardiol* **68**:1025–1031.

29 Chamberlain DA (1991) Lignocaine and bretylium as adjuncts to electrical defibrillation. *Resuscitation* **22**:152–157.

30 Sanders AB, Kern KB, Otto CW *et al.* (1989) End-tidal carbon dioxide monitoring during cardiopulmonary resuscitation: a prognostic indicator for survival. *J Am Med Assoc* **262**:1347–1351.

31 Doyal L and Wilsher D (1993) Withholding cardiopulmonary resuscitation: proposals for formal guidelines. *Br Med J* **306**:1593–1596.

32 Florin D (1994) Decisions about cardiopulmonary resuscitation. *Br Med J* **308**:1653.

33 Kerridge IH, Myser C, Mitchell KR and Hamblin J (1994) Guidelines for no-CPR orders. *Med J Aust* **161**:270–272.

34 Tunstall-Pedoe H, Bailey L, Chamberlain DA, Marsden AK, Ward ME and Zideman DA (1992) Survey of 3765 cardiopulmonary resuscitations in British hospitals (the BRESUS study): methods and results. *Br Med J* **304**:1347–1351.

35 Schneider AP, Nelson DJ and Brown DD (1993) In-hospital cardiopulmonary resuscitation: a 30 year review. *J Am Board Fam Pract* **6**:91–101.

36 Martens PR, Mullie A, Buylaert W, Call P and van Hoeyweghen R (1992) Early prediction of non-survival for patients suffering cardiac arrest – a word of caution. The Belgian Cerebral Resuscitation Study Group. *Inten-*

sive Care Med **18**:11–14.

37 So HY, Buckley TA and Oh TE (1994) Factors affecting outcome following cardiopulmonary resuscitation. *Anaesth Intens Care* **22**:647–658.

38 Task Force of Representatives from the European Resuscitation Council, American Heart Association, Heart and Stroke Foundation of Canada, and Australian Resuscitation Council (1992) Recommended guidelines for uniform reporting of data from out-of-hospital cardiac arrest (new abridged version): the 'Utstein style'. *Br Heart J* **67**:325–333.

8 | Cardiac arrhythmias

KD Donovan and BEF Hockings

Cardiac arrhythmias are common in critically ill patients,[1] Whether arrhythmias *per se* increase mortality or are merely markers of illness severity is debatable. Nevertheless, arrhythmias such as ventricular tachycardia (VT), ventricular fibrillation (VF) and complete heart block are life-threatening and require urgent management. Precipitating factors (Table 8.1) should be searched for and corrected. Cardiac status must be evaluated, as arrhythmias are more common in patients with structural heart disease, and are more likely to cause haemodynamic deterioration when cardiac function is poor. Assessment involves a careful history, examination and appropriate investigations.

Basic electrophysiology[2,3]

The phospholipid cell membrane has gates through which ions such as sodium (Na^+), potassium (K^+) and calcium (Ca^{2+}) move, generating electrical potentials. The Na^+–K^+ pump expels intracellular Na^+ against electrical and concentration gradients, and allows K^+ into the cell against its concentration gradient, resulting in high concentrations of K^+ inside and of Na^+ outside the cell. Adjacent cardiac cells are joined

Table 8.1 Arrhythmias in intensive care – some potentially reversible causes

Oxygen delivery (Do_2) decreased

Acidosis, alkalosis

Electrolyte disturbances (e.g. K^+, Mg^{2+} and Ca^{2+})

Drugs (inotropic agents, antiarrhythmic agents, other drugs such as erythromycin or theophylline)

Mechanical stimulation of cardiac chambers (e.g. pacing lead, central venous catheter and pulmonary artery catheter)

Pacemaker malfunction

by low-resistance intercalated discs which permit rapid conduction of electrical impulses between cells. Atria and ventricles hence function as a synchronous, coherent, cellular network.

Action potential

Depolarization (i.e. decrease in electronegativity in a resting cell) occurs when Na^+ and Ca^{++} enter the cell, generating inward ionic currents. Repolarization (i.e. return to resting potential) occurs when K^+ moves out of the cell (and to a lesser extent chloride (Cl^-) moves into the cell), generating outward currents. The cardiac action potential results from structural changes in proteins that control ion fluxes across the membrane.[2]

The interior of a resting cell has a negative potential relative to the outside, usually -50 to -90 mV. A stimulus will reduce (depolarize) the resting membrane potential, and once the threshold potential is reached, an action potential occurs. This is an all-or-none response; larger stimuli will not increase the action potential response. The action potential is conducted throughout all cells to initiate mechanical contraction. There are five phases (Fig. 8.1a):

1 *Phase 0:* Rapid depolarization of the cell membrane occurs. A dramatic influx of Na^+ through open fast channels causes a rapid rise in membrane potential from -80 or -90 mV to $+30$ mV. Action potentials from the sinoatrial (SA) and atrioventricular (AV) nodes and other pacemaker cells have a slow upstroke of phase 0 (Fig. 8.1b), related to slower opening Ca^{2+} channels. Conduction through the AV node is hence delayed. In the SA node, varying rates of Ca^{2+} channel opening help modulate heart rate.
2 *Phase 1:* Early rapid incomplete repolarization of the membrane to approximately 0 mV occurs.
3 *Phase 2:* A slow, prolonged plateau repolarization occurs. Membrane conductance to all ions is low.

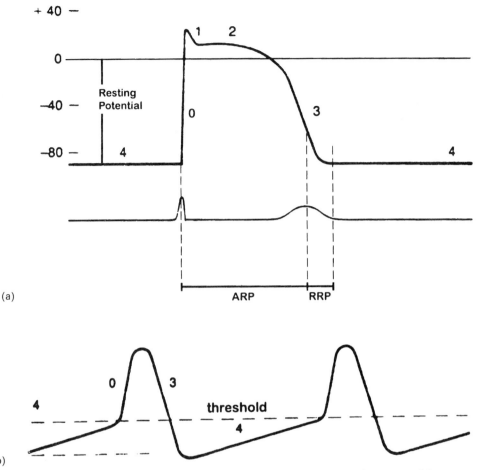

Fig. 8.1 (a) Action potential in a non-pacemaker cell: phases 0–4, membrane potential (− 80 mV), absolute refractory period (ARP) and relative refractory period (RRP). (b) Action potential in a pacemaker cell. The upward slope of phase 4, on reaching threshold potential, results in an action potential.

4 *Phase 3:* Relatively rapid repolarization occurs, with restoration of the resting membrane potential.
5 *Phase 4:* This is a stable electrical state in non-pacemaking cells (Fig. 8.1a). However, in the SA and AV nodes and certain pacemaking cells, resting membrane potential does not remain constant but gradually depolarizes (Fig. 8.1b). The pacemaker cells eventually reach their threshold potential, and action potentials ensue, which are conducted to other cardiac cells.

Electrophysiological properties of cardiac cells

1 *Automaticity:* i.e. ability of pacemaking cells to initiate and maintain a rhythmic beat. A steeper slope of phase 4 has a higher pacemaker discharge rate. The SA node's discharge rate exceeds others, and thus initiates cardiac rhythm. Should the dominant SA node fail, a subsidiary pacemaker will usually provide emergency standby 'escape' rhythm. Automaticity can be altered by autonomic influences and various drugs (e.g. *β*-sympathomimetics increase automaticity).
2 *Excitability:* i.e. ability of a cell to respond to an appropriate stimulus. The threshold for excitation is the stimulus that just provokes an action potential (Fig. 8.1b). Excitability will increase if threshold potential is decreased (e.g. *β*-adrenergic stimulation), and will decrease if threshold potential is increased (e.g. *β*-adrenergic blockade).
3 *Refractoriness:* i.e. a post-excitation period of non-excitability. The absolute refractory period is followed by the relative refractory period when only strong stimuli will provoke an action potential (Fig. 8.1a). The refractory period is proportional to

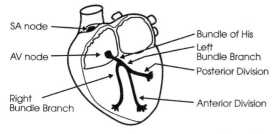

Fig. 8.2 Conduction system of the heart. SA = Sinoatrial; AV = atrioventricular.

Table 8.2 A classification of cardiac arrhythmias

Disorders of impulse formation
Automaticity
  Normal: sinus tachycardia; sinus bradycardia
  Abnormal: accelerated junctional rhythms; accelerated idioventricular rhythms; automatic atrial tachycardias
Triggered activity (early and late afterdepolarizations): long QT syndrome with torsade de pointes; digitalis intoxication
Disorders of impulse conduction
Re-entry: AV nodal re-entry tachycardia; AV re-entry tachycardia, atrial flutter; atrial fibrillation; ventricular fibrillation; ventricular tachycardia (usually)
Block: SA and AV blocks; bundle branch blocks.

AV = Atrioventricular; SA = sinoatrial.

the duration of the previous cycle, shortening with increasing heart rate. It is affected by autonomic stimuli (i.e. sympathetic stimulation shortens, and parasympathetic activity lengthens the AV node refractory period).

4 *Conductivity:* i.e. ability to propagate the excitation process to neighbouring cells. When the first cell in the network is activated, it will conduct an impulse to the next and so on, until the entire atria or ventricles have been stimulated. The specialized conduction system of the heart comprises cells which conduct normal cardiac impulses from the SA node to the rest of the heart via the AV node, the His bundle, right and left bundles and Purkinje fibres (Fig. 8.2). Normally, the only electrical connection between the atrial and ventricular myocardium is the AV nodal conduction system. The speed of conduction (conduction velocity) varies in different conducting tissues, being fastest in the His–Purkinje system and slowest in the AV node.

action potential. These afterdepolarizations may reach threshold potential, and thus initiate and perpetuate a series of action potentials, resulting in tachycardia.

Disorders of impulse conduction

Conduction delay and block of the cardiac impulse can result in either tachyarrhythmias or brady-arrhythmias.

1 *Re-entry:* Occurs when a single impulse activates the same group of cells twice or more. A normal cardiac impulse from the SA node is eventually extinguished when all adjacent cells are refractory (Fig. 8.3). Another sinus impulse will restart the sequence. When unidirectional block is present, a group of depolarized cells may not be refractory, but may have recovered excitability before the initial impulse dies out (Fig. 8.3). These cells may

Classification of cardiac arrhythmias

Arrhythmias may arise from *abnormalities of impulse formation* or *disorders of impulse conduction* (Table 8.2). The classification has limitations, as some combinations of both may be involved.

Disorders of impulse formation

1 *Increased automaticity* may result in a fast discharge rate from the normal pacemaker (e.g. sinus tachycardia). Subsidiary pacemakers provide an 'escape' rhythm when the SA node fails or if AV block occurs. A subsidiary pacemaker may inappropriately speed up and become the dominant pacemaker (e.g. an ectopic atrial tachycardia).

2 *Triggered activity:* Pacemaker activity may be triggered by afterdepolarizations from the previous

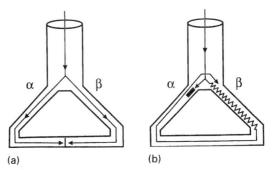

(a)   (b)

Fig. 8.3 Re-entry conduction. (a) Normally, cardiac impulse passes into both limbs of the circuit and is eventually extinguished, as all myocardial cells are refractory. (b) Cardiac impulse to the α-pathway is blocked, but the impulse through the β-pathway is conducted retrogradely up the α-pathway. The impulse may then be conducted down the β-pathway again if cells have recovered their excitability, causing a single ectopic beat or re-entry tachycardia if the impulse is repetitively conducted.

re-excite other cells that have now recovered from the initial depolarization, i.e. re-entry. Re-entry is responsible for most tachyarrhythmias (Table 8.2). Requirements for re-entry are:

(a) block of impulse in one limb of the circuit;
(b) slow conduction in the other limb;
(c) the impulse returns in the opposite direction along the pathway initially blocked, to re-enter and re-excite tissue proximal to the block.

2 *Block:* The cardiac impulse may be conducted at an abnormally slow velocity or blocked (see the section on AV block, below).

Management of the patient with a cardiac arrhythmia

History and physical examination

A careful history is important. Specific questions should confirm or exclude palpitations, syncope, chest pain, shortness of breath, ischaemic heart disease (especially previous myocardial infarction), congestive cardiac failure, valvular heart disease, thyrotoxicosis and diuretic therapy without adequate potassium supplements. A family history is helpful for arrhythmias associated with inherited disorders (e.g. long QT syndrome and hypertrophic obstructive cardiomyopathy).

The physical examination looks for underlying structural heart disease and signs to assist diagnosis, and assesses haemodynamic consequences of the arrhythmia.

Vagal manoeuvres

Vagal manoeuvres may be undertaken during examination. These reflexly increase vagal tone, thereby prolonging AV node conduction and refractoriness. The effect may be:

1 transient slowing of sinus tachycardia as SA nodal discharge rate is slowed;
2 termination of AV nodal re-entry and AV re-entry tachycardias;
3 unmasking (but not reversion) of atrial tachycardia, flutter (Fig. 8.4) and fibrillation.

VT is not affected. Carotid sinus massage is most commonly used; Valsalva manoeuvre or iced water to the face may be useful. Eyeball pressure should be avoided as eye damage may result. Carotid sinus massage is performed with the patient supine, with head extended and turned away from the side to be massaged. After auscultation to exclude carotid bruits, the carotid bifurcation is gently palpated by placing two fingers anterior to the sternocleidomastoid muscle, just below the angle of the jaw. Massage is applied one side at a time, and *never* both sides simultaneously. It is contraindicated in those with known or suspected cerebrovascular disease.

Investigations

A *12-lead electrocardiogram (ECG)* should be recorded with a longer rhythm strip (usually lead II or V1). If P waves are not visible, atrial activity may be recorded using an oesophageal electrode or pacing lead, or via a central venous catheter or the right atrial injectate port of a pulmonary artery catheter, using 20% saline and a bedside monitor.[4]

Holter monitoring requires prolonged (usually 24–72 h), non-invasive, ambulatory ECG monitoring, sometimes combined with exercise testing.

Invasive electrophysiological testing with programmed electrical stimulation attempts to reproduce the spontaneously occurring arrhythmia. It is not superior to Holter monitoring in evaluating drug treatment for ventricular arrhythmias.[5]

Other investigative techniques being studied include signal-averaged ECG, heart rate variability and electrical alternans measurement.[6]

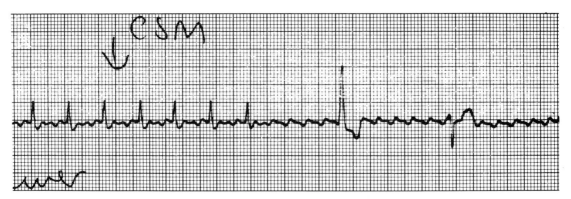

Fig. 8.4 Atrial flutter with 2:1 atrioventricular (AV) block. Carotid sinus massage (CSM) increases AV block and unmasks flutter waves.

Management of specific arrhythmias

Treatment has two aspects: acute termination of the arrhythmia and long-term prophylaxis. The decision whether to treat depends on the rhythm diagnosis, haemodynamic consequences, aetiology of the arrhythmia and the prognosis (e.g. risks of sudden death or long-term complications).

Sinus rhythm

Normal sinus rhythm is arbitrarily defined as cardiac impulse formation initiated in the SA node with a rate of 60–100 beats/min. Sinus arrhythmia with phasic changes in SA node discharge rate usually related to respiration is a normal variant.

ECG

In sinus rhythm the P wave is always upright in aVF and precedes each QRS complex.

Sinus tachycardia

Sinus tachycardia is sinus rhythm at a rate greater than 100 beats/min.

ECG

The ECG is similar to sinus rhythm with normal P waves and QRS complexes at a rate >100/min.

Clinical

Sinus tachycardia is usually a physiological response to exercise, emotion or fever. If inappropriate, search for a cause (e.g. anaemia, heart failure, sepsis and thyrotoxicosis) or consider the possibility of incorrect diagnosis (e.g. atrial flutter with 2:1 AV block).

Treatment

Treat underlying cause.

Sinus bradycardia

Sinus bradycardia is sinus rhythm at a rate <60 beats/min.

ECG

The ECG is similar to sinus rhythm with normal P waves and QRS complexes at <60/min.

Clinical

Sinus bradycardia is often physiological in athletes and during sleep. It may be caused by inferior myocardial infarction, sick sinus syndrome, drugs (e.g. β-adrenergic blockers, calcium-channel blockers or digoxin), jaundice, increased intracranial pressure and hypothyroidism.

Treatment

Treatment with atropine, isoprenaline or pacing is only required when the sinus bradycardia is symptomatic.

Ectopic beats

These are premature impulses originating from the atria, AV junction or ventricles. The coupling interval (time between the ectopic and the preceding beat) is shorter than the cycle duration of the dominant rhythm.

Premature atrial ectopic beats (Fig. 8.5)

This common arrhythmia may occasionally precede atrial fibrillation (AF) or flutter, and can occur in the absence of underlying organic heart disease. Precipitating factors include alcohol, caffeine and smoking.

ECG

Premature atrial ectopics result in an early and abnormal P wave which may be superimposed on the T wave. Due to resetting of the SA node, there is usually an incomplete compensatory pause (i.e. the interval between the normal P–QRS complexes on either side of the atrial ectopic will be less than twice that of the dominant sinus rhythm). Premature atrial ectopics are usually conducted to the ventricles in a normal manner (i.e. PR interval <120 ms) and followed by a narrow QRS complex. Sometimes the atrial ectopic may be delayed or blocked in either the AV node or bundle branches, resulting in prolonged PR interval, a wide QRS due to bundle branch block (usually right), or completely blocked atrial impulse (i.e. no QRS after the P wave).

Treatment

No treatment is usually required.

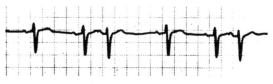

Fig. 8.5 Premature atrial ectopic beats. Note incomplete compensatory pause.

Premature AV junctional ectopic beats

These are recognized by a premature narrow complex QRS without a preceding P wave. The P wave is commonly buried in or follows the QRS complex. No treatment is necessary.

Premature ventricular ectopic beats (VEBs)

These are also known as ventricular premature beats (VPBs) and ventricular premature complexes (VPCs). The ventricle is not activated normally via the rapidly conducting bundle branches, and a wide QRS complex results from slow ventricular conduction.

ECG

There is no preceding P wave, there is a premature wide (>120 ms) QRS and a T wave of opposite polarity to the QRS (Fig. 8.6). Usually the VEB is not conducted retrogradely to the SA node. The SA node is therefore not reset, and there is temporary AV dissociation with a full compensatory pause – the interval between the normal QRS complexes on either side of the ventricular ectopic will usually be twice that of the dominant sinus rhythm. Occasionally, VEBs may not produce any pause, and are said to be interpolated (Fig. 8.7). A VEB following each sinus beat is ventricular bigeminy (Fig. 8.8). Ventricular trigeminy refers to recurring sequences of a VEB followed by two sinus beats. Two VEBS in succession are a couplet (Fig. 8.9), and three, a triplet (Fig. 8.10).

Clinical

VEBs, even when frequent, complex, or in short runs of non-sustained VT, are *not* associated with risk of sudden death in asymptomatic healthy adults.[7] However, in acute myocardial infarction, frequent and complex VEBs often precede VF and sustained VT. In this situation, prophylactic intravenous (IV) lignocaine can no longer be recommended as it may

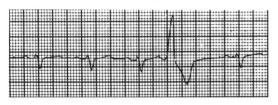

Fig. 8.6 Sinus rhythm with ventricular ectopic beat. Note complete compensatory pause.

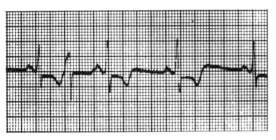

Fig. 8.7 Sinus rhythm with interpolated ventricular ectopic beat. Note absence of any compensatory pause.

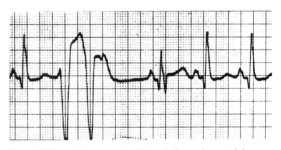

Fig. 8.9 Ventricular couplet. Note independent atrial activity continues during the couplet (see P wave buried in T wave after second ventricular ectopic beat).

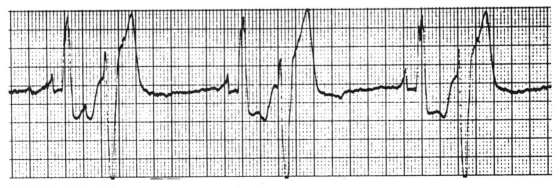

Fig. 8.8 Ventricular bigeminy.

increase total mortality,[8–10] but IV β-adrenergic blockers may improve survival.[10–12] Long-term VEB suppression after acute myocardial infarction with class Ic agents (flecainide and encainide) has increased mortality[13,14] (see Chapter 9). Apart from ischaemic heart disease, VEBs may be associated with cardiomyopathy, valvular disease, myocarditis and non-cardiac precipitating factors (e.g. electrolyte and acid-base disturbances, hypoxia and drugs such as digoxin).

Treatment

Drug treatment of VEBs is rarely indicated and may be dangerous. Adequate potassium and magnesium supplementation is essential. Severely symptomatic patients with frequent complex VPBs may benefit from judicious β-blockade. The underlying cause of VEBs is often more clinically relevant than the arrhythmia.

Parasystole

Ventricular parasystole results from the regular discharge of an automatic focus in the ventricle. The focus is protected from sinus node impulses (entrance block). There is frequently an intermittent exit block from the parasystolic focus, so that the interectopic intervals are always multiples of some common denominator. Variable coupling intervals and fusion beats occur, as the ventricle may sometimes be depolarized partly by atrial impulses via the AV node, and partly by the parasystolic ectopic focus.

Parasystole may also occur in the atria and the AV junction.

Escape rhythms

When the SA node fails to discharge or normal conduction is blocked, other subsidiary latent pacemakers may 'escape' and provide a 'back-up' cardiac rhythm. The escape interval is always greater than the cycle duration of the dominant rhythm. Escape beats usually arise from the AV junction (narrow QRS – escape rate usually 40–60/min; Figs 8.11 and Fig. 8.12) or the ventricles (wide QRS – escape rate usually 20–40/min; see section on third-degree AV block, below).

Treatment

Escape rhythms should not be suppressed with drugs. Treatment is usually unnecessary unless the escape rhythm is so slow that the patient is symptomatic. IV atropine or cardiac pacing is then used.

Supraventricular tachycardias (SVTs: Table 8.3)[15]

SVTs arise from the atria or AV junction and are usually conducted rapidly through the bundle branches (with narrow QRS complexes). Confusion exists regarding the nomenclature of narrow-complex

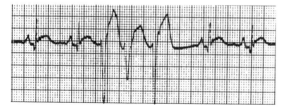

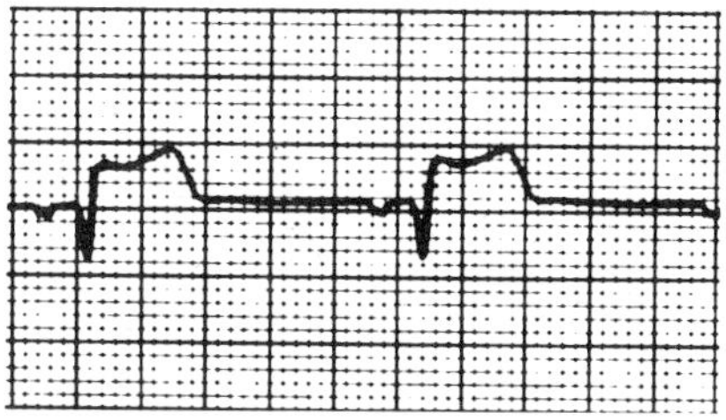

Fig. 8.10 Ventricular triplet.

Fig. 8.12 Rhythm strip (aVF) of junctional rhythm (58/min). Note abnormal inverted P wave preceding each QRS complex, indicating that the junctional focus has also activated the atria retrogradely.

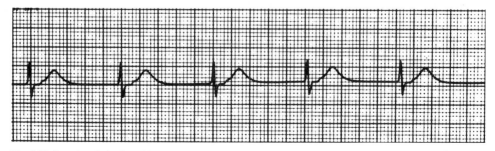

Fig. 8.11 Junctional rhythm (60 beats/min). Note that P wave is probably buried in T wave (see beginning of T-wave upstroke).

Table 8.3 Classification of supraventricular tachycardias

Junctional tachycardias (AV node integral part of arrhythmia circuit)

AV nodal re-entry tachycardia (AVNRT): re-entry within the AV node

AV re-entry tachycardia (AVRT): re-entry via an additional (accessory) AV pathway which connects the atria and ventricles

Accelerated junctional rhythm: increased automaticity of the AV junction resulting in a more rapid (70–120/min) junctional discharge rate

Atrial tachycardias (AV node not an integral part of the arrhythmia circuit)

Atrial flutter: re-entry circuit confined to the atria

Atrial fibrillation: multiple re-entry circuits confined to the atria

Unifocal atrial tachycardia: usually due to increased automaticity, but may occasionally be due to intra-atrial re-entry

Multifocal atrial tachycardia: enhanced automaticity, although triggered activity is also a possible mechanism

Others: For example, sinus node re-entry tachycardia

AV = Atrioventricular.

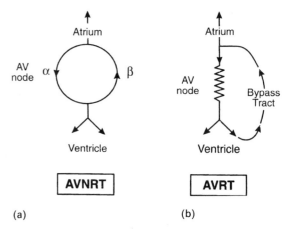

Fig. 8.13 (a) Atrioventricular nodal re-entry tachycardia (AVNRT). Re-entry circuit with dual pathways contained within (or very close to) the atrioventricular (AV) node. (b) Atrioventricular re-entry tachycardia (AVRT). Re-entry circuit involving the AV node and an accessory AV pathway. The impulse usually passes anterogradely through the AV node and retrogradely up the bypass tract.

tachycardias. A useful system classifies SVTs into junctional or atrial.[16]

Junctional tachycardias

The AV node or junction is an integral part of the tachycardia circuit, e.g. AV nodal re-entry tachycardia (AVNRT) and AV re-entry tachycardia (AVRT; see below).

Atrial tachycardias

Atrial tissue only is required for the initiation and maintenance of the tachycardia. The AV node is merely a 'bystander'. Examples include atrial flutter and fibrillation.

At times rhythm diagnosis may not be possible, and a SVT may best be described as a regular narrow complex tachycardia. Vagal manoeuvres or drugs that prolong AV nodal refractoriness (e.g. adenosine) may assist in diagnosis: temporary AV block with unchanged atrial rate indicates a tachycardia of atrial origin, whereas slowing or reversion of the tachycardia suggests a junctional tachycardia.

AV nodal re-entry tachycardia[17]

Re-entry tachycardia is confined to the AV node. Anterograde conduction to the ventricles usually occurs over the slow (α) pathway and retrograde conduction over the fast (β) pathway (Fig. 8.13).

ECG

Regular narrow-complex tachycardia (140–220 beats/min) with abrupt onset and termination. P waves are usually not observed as they are buried in the QRS complexes (Fig. 8.14).

Clinical

AVNRT is common arrhythmia which is usually not associated with structural heart disease. The major symptom is palpitations.

Treatment

Vagal manoeuvres slow conduction through the AV node and may 'break' the tachycardia. If carotid sinus massage fails, adenosine is the drug of choice – IV 6 mg, and if ineffective, 12 mg, to a maximum of 18 mg. Nearly all AVNRTs will revert with adenosine. Verapamil IV 5–10 mg in 1-mg increments may be used if adenosine is unavailable or ineffective, but has a much longer half-life. Cardiac function is depressed and it should be avoided in patients receiving β-adrenergic blockers.

Sotalol, amiodarone and flecainide may also be effective but are rarely used. Rapid atrial pacing will usually terminate AVNRT but is rarely needed. Cardioversion is occasionally necessary when drugs are ineffective or when severe haemodynamic instability is present.

Prevention

Troublesome recurring episodes of AVNRT can be cured by radiofrequency ablation, using a

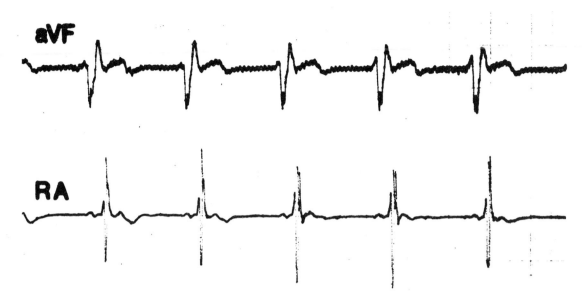

Fig. 8.14 Atrioventricular nodal re-entry tachycardia (AVNRT). Rhythm strip (aVF) shows narrow-complex tachycardia (paper speed 50 mm/s; rate 133/min). There is no recognizable P wave. Intracardiac electrocardiograph from the right atrium (RA) shows that atrial activity occurs immediately after the QRS, indicating that the rhythm is probably AVNRT.

transvenous catheter to interrupt the re-entrant circuit permanently.

AV re-entry tachycardia

The re-entry pathway consists of the AV node and an accessory pathway which bypasses the AV node (Fig. 8.13). The accessory pathway may be evident during sinus rhythm; ECG will show pre-excitation (see Wolff–Parkinson–White (WPW) syndrome, below, under pre-excitation syndrome). However, if the accessory pathway conducts only retrogradely from ventricle to atria, then ECG pre-excitation will be concealed in sinus rhythm.

ECG

The ECG is similar to AVNRT. The length of the re-entry circuit is however greater, and the accessory AV pathway is some distance from the AV node. It therefore takes longer for the impulse to be conducted backwards to the atria, and so the retrograde P wave usually occurs *after* the QRS, sometimes at some distance (Fig. 8.15).

Clinical

AVRT is similar to AVNRT, although antegrade conduction over the accessory pathway may be very rapid with WPW syndrome, should AF occur.

Treatment

Acute treatment is identical to AVNRT, but verapamil should probably be avoided in WPW syndrome, as it may block the AV node, facilitating very rapid conduction to the ventricles via the accessory pathway.

Prevention

Drugs such as sotalol and flecainide may prevent recurrence of the tachycardia. Radiofrequency ablation of the accessory pathway is usually curative.

Accelerated junctional rhythm (accelerated idiojunctional rhythm)

Increased automaticity of the AV junction (above the inherent discharge rate of 40–60/min) is the usual cause of this arrhythmia. The often-used term non-paroxysmal AV junctional tachycardia is cumbersome and misleading; junctional rate is commonly 60–100/min, not strictly a tachycardia. AV dissociation is often present, but there may be synchronization of the two pacemakers – so-called isorhythmic dissociation.

ECG

There are narrow complexes on the ECG at a regular rate (60–130/min; Fig. 8.16), often with independent atrial activity. With isorhythmic dissociation, P wave

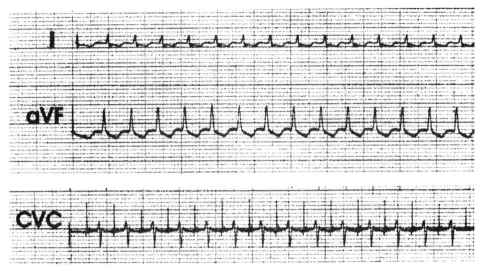

Fig. 8.15 Atrioventricular re-entry tachycardia (AVRT). No P waves are evident in surface leads (I, aVF). The atrial electrogram from the central venous catheter (CVC) demonstrates atrial activity occurring some time after the QRS, suggesting that the rhythm is AVRT.

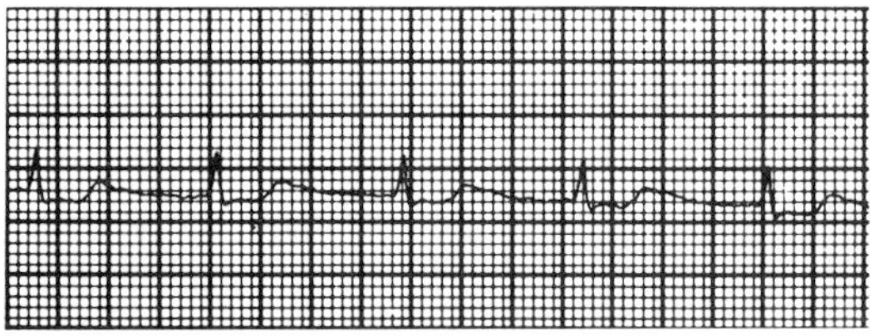

Fig. 8.16 Accelerated junctional rhythm (rate 84/min).

is either fixed relative to the QRS complex (usually just after) or oscillates to and fro across the QRS in a rhythmical manner.

Clinical

It may be observed in normal persons, but is often associated with structural heart disease, especially following inferior myocardial infarction. Digoxin intoxication is another important cause.

Treatment

In most cases, the rhythm is transient and well-tolerated, and no treatment is required. Treatment is otherwise directed towards the underlying cause.

Unifocal atrial tachycardia[15]

This is sometimes called ectopic atrial tachycardia to distinguish it from the atrial tachycardias (referring collectively to unifocal atrial tachycardia, atrial flutter and AF). It is, however, inappropriate to call atrial tachycardia paroxysmal atrial tachycardia. Paroxysmal, by definition, indicates an abrupt onset and termination, which applies less commonly to unifocal atrial tachycardia. Vagal manoeuvres will not terminate the arrhythmia, but AV block may be induced, or increased if already present.

ECG

P-wave morphology is abnormal but monomorphic. Atrial rate is often 130–160/min, and may occasionally exceed 200/min. QRS complexes will usually be narrow (Fig. 8.17). AV block is common (Fig. 8.18).

Clinical

Digitalis intoxication is the most common cause, especially when AV block is present. Other causes include myocardial infarction, chronic lung disease and metabolic disturbances.

Treatment

If applicable, digitalis is stopped and the toxicity treated. Otherwise digoxin may be used to control the ventricular rate. β-Adrenergic blockers or amiodarone are alternatives. Rapid atrial pacing may be ineffective if the arrhythmia is due to increased automaticity, although it may increase AV block, thereby slowing ventricular rate. Synchronized DC shock may be necessary, but is avoided in digitalis intoxication. Low energy levels (e.g. 10 J) should be used initially.

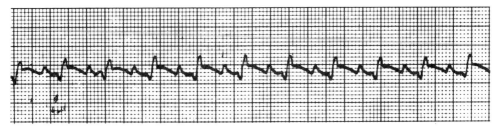

Fig. 8.17 Unifocal atrial tachycardia with 1:1 atrioventricular conduction. (rate about 125/min).

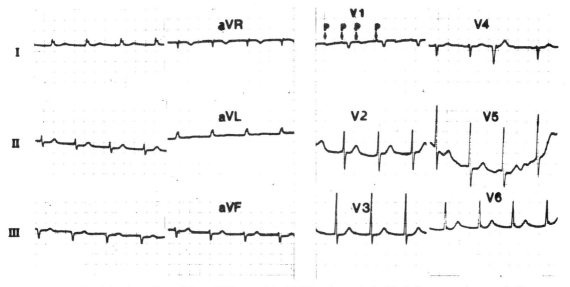

Fig. 8.18 Unifocal atrial tachycardia (atrial rate 185 beats/min) with 2:1 atrioventricular block. P waves are best seen in V1.

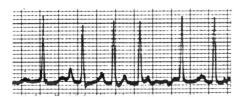

Fig. 8.19 Multifocal atrial tachycardia. Note irregular P waves (atrial rate about 160/min) with differing morphology. Most P waves are conducted to the ventricles.

Multifocal atrial tachycardia[18]

This is an uncommon arrhythmia, also known as chaotic or mixed atrial tachycardia.

ECG

There are irregular atrial rates, usually 100–130/min, with varying P-wave morphology and some degree of AV block (Fig. 8.19). Most P waves are conducted to the ventricles, usually with narrow QRS complexes.

Clinical

Multifocal atrial tachycardia is often misdiagnosed and inappropriately treated as AF. This rhythm occurs most commonly in critically ill elderly patients with chronic lung disease, and is associated with a very high mortality from underlying disease. Theophylline has been implicated as a precipitating cause, and digoxin, rarely.

Treatment

Treatment should correct the underlying cause (e.g. electrolyte and acid–base abnormalities and theophylline toxicity). A spontaneous reversion rate is common, and few patients require antiarrhythmic therapy. β-Blockers are probably more effective than verapamil, but should be avoided in obstructive lung disease. Digoxin is ineffective.

Atrial flutter[19]

Atrial rate during classical atrial flutter is 250–350/min, and in most cases, close to 300/min. Atrial flutter is

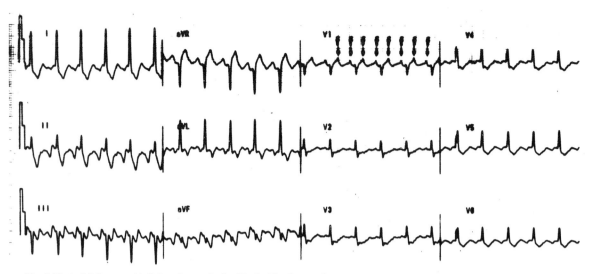

Fig. 8.20 Atrial flutter with 2:1 atrioventricular block. The flutter (f) waves are best seen in V1.

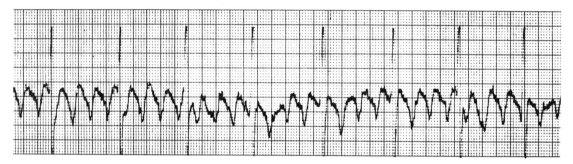

Fig. 8.21 Atrial flutter: typical flutter waves. Atrioventricular (AV) block (4:1) is due to the drug effect on the AV node.

due to a single re-entry circuit lying within the right atrium.

ECG

Atrial flutter waves (characteristic sawtooth appearance with no isoelectric line) are best seen in V1 (Fig. 8.20) or aVF, but leads II and III may also be useful. The flutter waves are usually negative in aVF. Rapid QRS waves may obscure typical flutter waves, and vagal manoeuvres may unmask them (Fig. 8.4). AV conduction block (usually 2:1) is usually present, so that alternate flutter waves are conducted to the ventricles, with a ventricular rate close to 150 beats/min. Treatment with drugs that affect AV node conduction may lead to higher degrees of AV block (Fig. 8.21) and/or variable AV block with irregular QRS duration. Rarely, atrial flutter with 1:1 conduction occurs (Fig. 8.22). This is usually associated with sympathetic overactivity or class 1 antiarrhythmic drugs (which slow atrial discharge rate to 200/min, thereby allowing each atrial impulse to

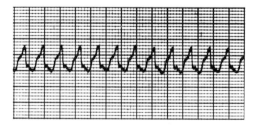

Fig. 8.22 Atrial flutter with 1:1 atrioventricular conduction. Heart rate approaches 300 beats/min.

be conducted). QRS complexes are usually narrow, as conduction through the bundle branches is normal.

Clinical

Atrial flutter is less common than AF. It may occur in ischaemic heart disease, cardiomyopathy, rheumatic heart disease, thyrotoxicosis and after cardiac surgery. Structural heart disease is probably less commonly associated than with AF.

Treatment

No drug will reliably terminate atrial flutter.[19] Synchronized DC cardioversion, often with low energies (25–50 J), is a reliable treatment option. Rapid atrial pacing faster than the flutter rate will terminate classical atrial flutter in most patients. Flecainide and procainamide may occasionally be effective. However, class 1a and 1c drugs may lead to 1:1 AV conduction. Class 1 drugs should probably be avoided unless ventricular response has been slowed with calcium channel or β-adrenergic blocking drugs.

Prevention

Prevention of atrial flutter is often difficult. Drugs used include sotalol and amiodarone at low doses. Class 1c agents (e.g. flecainide) may be used in patients without significant structural heart disease. Occasionally, refractory atrial flutter may be cured by radiofrequency ablation to interrupt the re-entry circuit,[20] but recurrence is high.

Atrial fibrillation[21,22]

AF is the commonest arrhythmia requiring treatment and/or hospital admission. The incidence increases

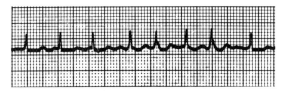

Fig. 8.23 Atrial fibrillation: wavy baseline and irregular QRS complexes.

with age – 5% over 70 years have this arrhythmia. AF is common in congestive cardiac failure (40%), after coronary artery bypass grafting (25–50%),[23] and in critically ill patients (15%).[1] AF is often mistakenly regarded as being relatively benign. Idiopathic or lone AF (i.e. with no structural heart disease or precipitating factor) in someone under 60 years has an excellent prognosis, but AF developing after cardiac surgery is associated with increased stroke, life-threatening arrhythmias and longer ICU and hospital stays.[24]

ECG

Atrial activity is chaotic with rapid (350–600/min) and irregular depolarizations varying in amplitude and morphology (fibrillation waves). Ventricular response is irregularly irregular (Fig. 8.23). Most atrial impulses are not conducted to the ventricles, resulting in an untreated ventricular rate of 100–180/min. (Fig. 8.24). QRS complexes will usually be narrow. When the ventricular rate is very rapid or very slow, ventricular irregularity may be missed (Fig. 8.24).

Clinical

AF is more common in patients with underlying heart disease (particularly those with dilated left atrium) and abnormal atrial electrophysiology. Causes include ischaemic and valvular heart disease, hypertension, cardiac failure, thyrotoxicosis and alcohol abuse. AF may also occur after cardiac surgery and thoracotomy. AF can be chronic, or intermittent with paroxysmal attacks. Chronic AF has a poorer prognosis. AF is associated with:

1 *adverse haemodynamic effects.* Rapid ventricular rate and loss of atrial systole may increase pulmonary capillary wedge pressure, while stroke volume and cardiac output decline;
2 *systemic embolism and stroke.* AF increases the risk of non-haemorrhagic stroke five-fold;

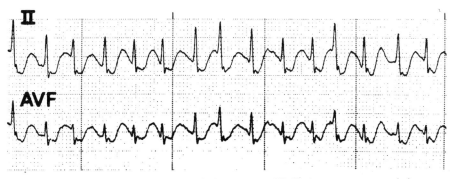

Fig. 8.24 Atrial fibrillation with rapid ventricular response. Fibrillation waves are not obvious. QRS irregularity may be missed as ventricular rate is rapid.

3 *tachycardiomyopathy* – reversible global cardio-myopathy secondary to rapid heart rate.[25]

Treatment

Recent-onset AF (paroxysmal AF)

Spontaneous reversion of AF is common. Treatment may not be necessary, and a reasonable strategy is based on clinical status:

1 haemodynamically unstable with rapid ventricular rate – immediate synchronized DC shock;
2 haemodynamically stable, symptomatic with de-pressed left ventricular function – semi-urgent synchronized DC shock or drug therapy to control ventricular rate until spontaneous reversion occurs (e.g. amiodarone infusion 5–7 mg/kg over 30 min followed by 50 mg/h, or digoxin 15 μg/kg IV over 1 h);
3 haemodynamically stable, symptomatic, normal left ventricular function – control of ventricular response with amiodarone, digoxin, β-adrenergic blockade or verapamil.
4 haemodynamically stable, with minimal or no symptoms – no immediate treatment. Most cases will revert spontaneously within 24 h.[26]

Cardioversion is usually indicated if AF lasts 36–48 h. However, it should probably not be attempted after 48–72 h of onset, until the patient has been anticoagulated for 3 weeks. Stroke rate is 0–1% with anticoagulation, and 3–7% without anticoagulation.[27] Cardioversion is less likely to be successful if AF has been present for over a year, left atrial size is >45 mm, and untreated conditions are present (e.g. thyrotoxicosis, valvular heart disease and heart failure).

Antiarrhythmic drugs can be used after cardioversion to prevent recurrence. Unfortunately most drugs are relatively ineffective and possibly dangerous. About 50% will remain in sinus rhythm 1 year after cardioversion with drugs and 25% without drugs. Quinidine prophylaxis, although more effective than placebo, appears to increase mortality.[28] Sotalol may be safer but may provoke dangerous arrhythmias (e.g. torsade de pointes; see below).[29] Amiodarone has many potential side-effects, but is a reasonable option. Low doses (e.g. 100–200 mg/day) should be used. Class 1c agents (e.g. flecainide) are widely used in patients without structural heart disease. Digoxin does not prevent AF recurrence.[30]

Chronic AF

Treatment aims at ventricular rate control and prevention of embolic stroke.

Digoxin orally remains the drug of choice, but is often ineffective at controlling ventricular rate during exercise. Judicious addition of a small dose of a β-adrenergic blocker or verapamil may be necessary. Rarely, His-bundle ablation with permanent cardiac pacing may be required for severe cases refractory to drug therapy.[31]

Anticoagulation should be considered in all patients.[32,33] Risk of embolic stroke is increased with enlarged left atrium (> 45 mm), congestive cardiac failure or valvular heart disease. Warfarin decreases the incidence from 8% to 3%, although intracranial haemorrhage occurs (0.3%/year). Low-dose warfarin (international normalized ratio 1.5–2.0) is effective with fewer haemorrhagic complications. The risk of intracranial haemorrhage has to increase six-fold to justify withholding warfarin. Patients under 60 years with lone AF have a very low incidence of non-haemorrhagic stroke and aspirin (e.g. 325 mg/day) is recommended. Patients over 75 years, or those with diabetes, hypertension or previous embolic episodes, have a stroke incidence of 10%, and should probably receive warfarin unless haemorrhagic risks are deemed unacceptably high.

Pre-excitation syndrome[3]

Pre-excitation syndromes have an additional or accessory AV pathway. The term WPW syndrome is usually applied when tachyarrhythmias are present.

ECG

During sinus rhythm an atrial impulse will reach the ventricles via both the AV node and the accessory AV pathway. The latter conducts the atrial impulse to the ventricles before the AV node (Fig. 8.13), resulting in ventricular pre-excitation and a short PR interval. On reaching the ventricles, the pre-excitation impulse is not conducted via the specialized conducting system. Hence early ventricular activation will be slow (resulting in a δ wave) until the AV node impulse arrives. Ventricular depolarization by both the accessory pathway and the AV node results in a fusion beat. WPW ECG characteristics are short PR interval, wide QRS, δ wave and T-wave abnormalities (Fig. 8.25). δ-Wave polarity in a 12-lead ECG may help localize the anatomical position of the accessory pathway. Classification into type A (positive complex in V1) and type B (negative complex V1) is not helpful.

Clinical

AVRT or AF (Fig. 8.26) can occur with WPW. During AVRT, the re-entry impulse usually travels down the AV node and back up the accessory pathway; δ waves will not be present. Occasionally, the re-entry impulse may pass in the opposite direction (down the accessory pathway and up the AV node), resulting in a wide QRS complex tachycardia. Treatment is the same as for AVRT (i.e. IV adenosine).

AF is uncommon in WPW, but may be life-threatening.[34] Most impulses are conducted via

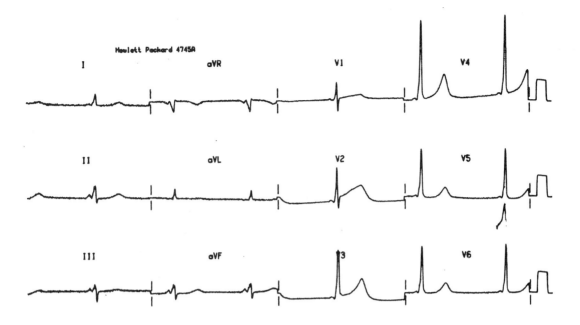

Fig. 8.25 Wolff–Parkinson–White (WPW) syndrome. Note the short PR interval, wide QRS and δ wave.

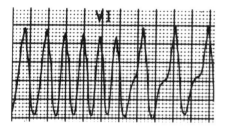

Fig. 8.26 Atrial fibrillation with Wolff–Parkinson–White syndrome. Note the irregular and wide QRS complexes.

the accessory pathway, leading to wide QRS complexes (δ waves). The ECG of WPW with AF usually shows rapid, irregular QRS complexes with variable QRS width (Fig. 8.26). Ventricular response is very rapid, leading to hypotension or cardiogenic shock. The arrhythmia may degenerate to VF.

Treatment usually involves synchronized DC shock. Antiarrhythmic drugs may be used when patients are haemodynamically stable and the ventricular rate is not excessively rapid. Drugs that prolong the refractory period of the accessory pathway are useful (e.g. sotalol, amiodarone, flecainide and procainamide). Drugs which shorten that refractory period (e.g. digoxin) may accelerate ventricular rate and are contraindicated. Verapamil and lignocaine may increase the ventricular rate during AF, and are also best avoided. β-Adrenergic blockers have no effect

on the refractory period of the accessory pathway. Long-term management by radiofrequency ablation of the accessory pathway is effective in selected patients.

Ventricular tachycardia

VT is defined as three or more VEBs at a rate greater than 130/min, and may exceed 300/min. VT lasting over 30 s is considered to be sustained. Non-sustained VT may not cause symptoms, but is associated with increased mortality in certain patients (e.g. after myocardial infarction). VT may be monomorphic (i.e. same QRS morphology; Fig. 8.27) or polymorphic.

Monomorphic VT[3,35]

This is the most common form of VT. It is commonly associated with previous myocardial infarction, and often causes symptoms (e.g. palpitations, shortness of breath, chest pain or syncope). It may result in cardiac arrest, due to the tachycardia itself or degeneration into VF. The most common mechanism is re-entry secondary to inhomogeneous activation of the myocardium and slow conduction through scar tissue from a previous myocardial infarction. AV dissociation (i.e. independent atrial and ventricular activity; Fig. 8.28) is present in about 75% of instances, whereas retrograde ventricle to atrial (VA) conduction occurs in about 25%. AV dissociation is virtually diagnostic for VT during a wide-complex tachycardia,

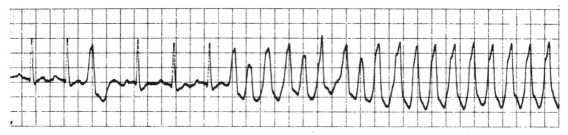

Fig. 8.27 Monomorphic ventricular tachycardia. Sinus rhythm with ventricular ectopic beats (third and seventh beats) of identical morphology are followed by ventricular tachycardia.

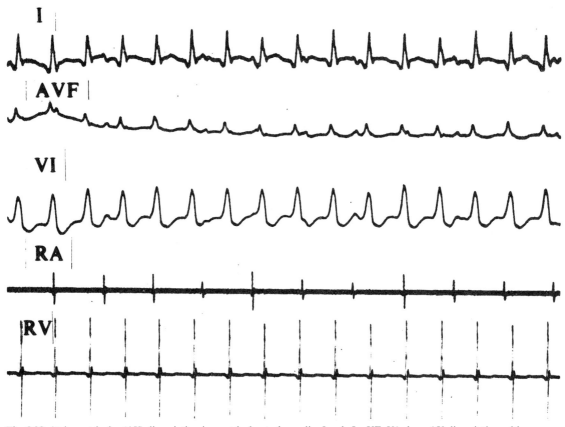

Fig. 8.28 Atrioventricular (AV) dissociation in ventricular tachycardia. Leads I, aVF, V1 show AV dissociation with regular P waves (rate 94/min) unrelated to QRS complexes (135/min). AV dissociation is confirmed by intracardiac electrocardiogram recorded via pacing electrodes. Atrial activity (RA = right atrium) is independent of ventricular activity (RV = right ventricle).

but ECG recognition of independent (and slower) atrial activity is difficult.

VT is the most common cause of a wide-complex tachycardia (QRS $\geqslant$ 120 ms)[35] and any such tachycardia should be considered VT until proven otherwise. Mistakes in diagnosis are common; SVT with aberrant condution is often mistaken for VT.[36]

Inappropriate treatment based on incorrect diagnosis can result in disastrous consequences.[37]

ECG

Older criteria[38] (e.g. QRS $\geqslant$ 140 ms and extreme electrical axis changes) are unhelpful in rhythm

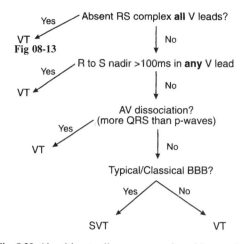

Fig. 8.29 Algorithm to diagnose a regular wide-complex tachycardia. VT = Ventricular tachycardia; AV = atrioventricular; BBB = bundle branch block; SVT = supraventricular tachycardia.

diagnosis. New ECG criteria permit accurate diagnosis in four steps (Fig. 8.29).[39-41]

1 Is a RS complex present in any precordial (V) lead? (QR, QRS, QS, monophasic R and rSR are not considered RS complexes.) If not (Fig. 8.30), the diagnosis is VT.
2 If a RS is present, then measure the duration of the R to S nadir (lowest part of the S wave). If this duration > 100 ms in any V lead (Fig. 8.31), the rhythm is VT.
3 If RS ⩽ 100 ms, then AV dissociation is searched for (more QRS complexes than P waves; Fig. 8.28). Indirect evidence of AV dissociation such as capture or fusion beats may be present. Capture beats occur when atrial impulses via the AV node activate the ventricle before the ventricle can be depolarized from the VT. Even a single capture or fusion beat confirms AV dissociation and VT (Fig. 8.32).
4 If AV dissociation is not present, then decide whether the wide QRS has a right or left bundle branch block (BBB) pattern. If the BBB is typical

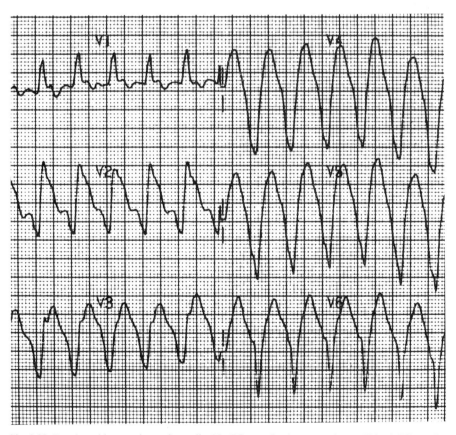

Fig. 8.30 Regular wide-complex tachycardia. No RS complex is present in any V lead. Diagnosis is ventricular tachycardia.

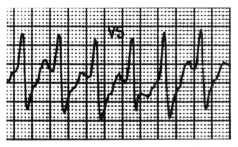

Fig. 8.31 Regular wide-complex tachycardia RS nadir > 100 ms. Diagnosis is ventricular tachycardia.

in both V1 and V6 leads, the rhythm is supraventricular in origin. Typical left BBB pattern requires an rS or QS nadir < 70 ms in V1 and R wave, with no Q wave in V6. Typical right BBB pattern requires an rSR' pattern with R' > r in V1 and R > S in V6 (see the section on bundle branch block, below). If there are any atypical features, the rhythm is considered to be VT (Fig. 8.33).[41]

Termination of a wide-complex tachycardia by IV adenosine strongly suggests the arrhythmia as SVT.[42] Demonstration of AV dissociation by intracardiac ECG from a central venous catheter or a transvenous pacing lead signifies VT.

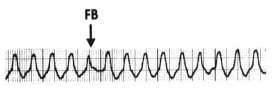

Fig. 8.32 Ventricular tachycardia. Fusion beat (FB) indicates atrioventricular dissociation.

Clinical

The major cause of VT is significant ischaemic heart disease. Other causes include cardiomyopathy, myocarditis and valvular heart disease. Symptoms will depend on the ventricular rate, duration of tachycardia and underlying cardiac function. There are no haemodynamic differences between VT and SVT with aberrant conduction.

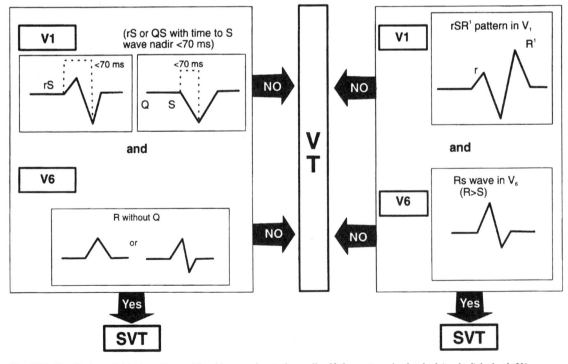

Fig. 8.33 Bundle branch block pattern with wide-complex tachycardia. If the pattern is classical (typical) in both V1 and V6, the diagnosis is supraventricular tachycardia. Otherwise the rhythm is considered ventricular tachycardia. LBBB = Left bundle branch block; RBBB = right bundle branch block; SVT = supraventricular tachycardia.

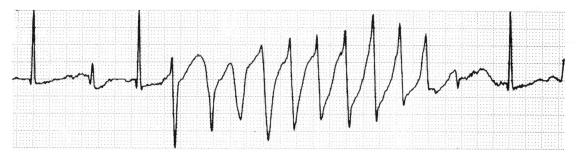

Fig. 8.34 Torsade de pointes. Note prolonged QT$_c$ interval.

Treatment

DC shock is indicated if a patient is haemodynamically unstable. Antiarrhythmic drugs may otherwise be administered (below). No more than two drugs should be used. If ineffective, synchronized DC shock is indicated. Rapid right ventricular pacing may also be effective.

1 *Lignocaine* 1.5–2.0 mg/kg IV over 2–5 min, followed by an infusion of 4 mg/min for 1 h, then 2 mg/min for 2 h, thereafter 1 mg/min remains the traditional drug of choice, despite doubts on its efficacy.
2 *Sotalol* 0.5–1.5 mg/kg IV over 5–20 min is probably more effective than lignocaine.[43]
3 *Procainamide* 6–13 mg/kg IV slowly (< 50 mg/min) has also been shown to be superior to lignocaine.[44]
4 *Amiodarone* 5–7 mg/kg IV over 30 min, followed by an infusion of 50 mg/h may also terminate VT, but often not immediately.

Long-term prevention of VT and sudden death[6] is difficult. Sotalol guided by Holter ECG or electrophysiological testing[29], and empirical (i.e. non-guided) amiodarone[45] are superior to other drugs in preventing arrhythmia recurrences. Empirical β-adrenergic blockers[46] also have a role. Implantable defibrillators can recognize and automatically terminate VT by rapid ventricular pacing or, should this fail, by internal DC cardioversion, and may be life-saving.[6]

Polymorphic VT and torsade de pointes

This arrhythmia has QRS complexes at 200/min or greater, which change in amplitude and direction so that they appear to twist around the baseline (Fig. 8.34). Torsade de pointes has prolonged QT during sinus rhythm, and U waves are often present.

Clinical

The long QT syndrome may be idiopathic (congenital) or acquired. The latter is caused by antiarrhythmic drugs (e.g. quinidine, procainamide, flecainide,[47] sotalol[29] and amiodarone). Bradycardia, hypokalaemia, hypomagnesaemia and other non-antiarrhythmic

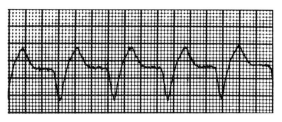

Fig. 8.35 Accelerated idioventricular rhythm (ventricular rate 88/min).

drugs (e.g. tricyclic antidepressants and erythromycin) are also causes.

Treatment

Polymorphic VT associated with a normal QT interval during sinus rhythm (e.g. following acute myocardial infarction) should be treated in the same way as monomorphic VT. However, some conventional antiarrhythmics may increase QT interval (i.e. class 1a, 1c and 3 drugs; see Chapter 9), and should be avoided in torsade de pointes. This is suppressed by IV magnesium[48] 8 mmol IV over 1–2 min followed by 20 mmol over 6 h[49] and/or temporary atrial or ventricular pacing faster than the sinus rate. If pacing is not immediately available, an isoprenaline infusion may be useful.

Accelerated idioventricular rhythm (AIVR)

This is often inappropriately called slow VT. Increased automaticity is probably the mechanism responsible for this relatively benign arrhythmia.

ECG

Wide QRS with a rate of 60–110 beats/min (Fig. 8.35). Sinus rate is often only slightly slower than the arrhythmia, so the dominant rhythm may be intermittent AIVR and sinus rhythm. Fusion beats are therefore common.

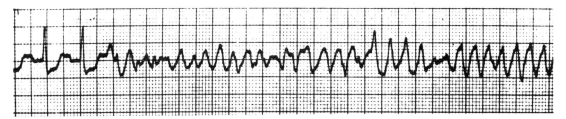

Fig. 8.36 Ventricular fibrillation.

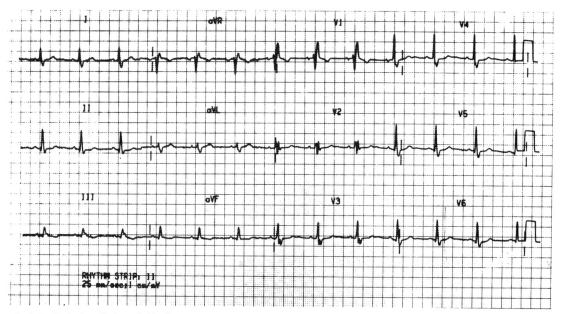

Fig. 8.37 Right bundle branch block.

Clinical

The rhythm is commonly encountered in inferior myocardial infarction. AIVR may be misdiagnosed as VT. Occasionally, AIVR causes haemodynamic deterioration, usually due to loss of atrial systole. Increasing the atrial rate with either atropine or atrial pacing may then be necessary.

Ventricular fibrillation

VF always causes haemodynamic collapse, loss of consciousness and death if not immediately treated. Of patients resuscitated from VF, 20–30% have sustained an acute myocardial infarction, although 75% have coronary artery disease. VF (and VT) unassociated with acute myocardial infarction is likely to be recurrent; 50% die within 3 years.[6]

ECG

The ECG shows irregular waves of varying morphology and amplitude (Fig. 8.36).

Clinical

VF is usually associated with ischaemic heart disease, although other causes include cardiomyopathy, antiarrhythmic drugs, severe hypoxia and non-synchronized DC cardioversion.

Treatment

Immediate non-synchronized DC shock at 200 J, and if ineffective, repeated at 200, 360 and 360 J. (see Chapter 7). Time should not be wasted with basic life support if immediate defibrillation can be delivered. Afterwards, IV lignocaine should be administered, and precipitating factors sought and treated. Bretylium is useful for recurrent VF.

Bundle branch block

Right bundle branch block (RBBB; Fig. 8.37)

In RBBB, activation of the right ventricle is delayed.

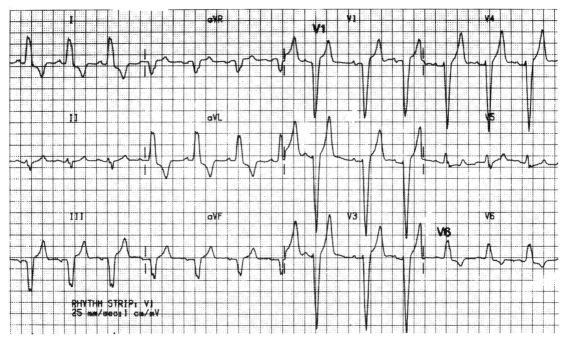

Fig. 8.38 Left bundle branch block.

ECG

The ECG shows wide QRS >120 ms, r(S)R′ in right ventricular leads V1 or V2 (often M-shaped), and a broad S wave in left ventricular leads, especially I and V6. Partial RBBB is identical, except the QRS duration is 110–120 ms.

Clinical

This is a normal variant, but may occur with massive pulmonary embolism, right ventricular hypertrophy, ischaemic heart disease and congenital heart disease. (Note: myocardial infarction can be diagnosed in the presence of RBBB.)

Left bundle branch block (LBBB; Fig. 8.38)

In LBBB, the interventricular septum is activated from right to left (i.e. in the opposite direction to normal).

ECG

Wide QRS (>120 ms), primary and secondary R waves (RR′; often M-shaped in left ventricular leads, especially V6). Q waves are never seen in left ventricular leads (V4–V6). (Note: myocardial infarction usually cannot be diagnosed in the presence of LBBB.) Partial LBBB is similar, except that the QRS duration is 110–120 ms.

Clinical

LBBB is often associated with heart disease such as coronary artery disease, cardiomyopathy or left ventricular hypertrophy.

Hemiblocks

The left branch of the bundle of His conducts impulses to the anterior superior left ventricle via the left anterior division, and to the posterior inferior part of the left ventricle via the posterior inferior division. Block can occur in either division.

Left anterior hemiblock (Fig. 8.39)

Left axis deviation usually (lead I predominantly positive, leads II and III predominantly negative) with initial R wave in inferior leads (II, III, aVF).

Left posterior hemiblock

There is usually right axis deviation (lead I predominantly negative and lead III predominantly positive). Other causes of right axis deviation (e.g. right ventricular hypertrophy) need to be excluded.

Clinical

RBBB with either left anterior hemiblock or left posterior hemiblock indicates an extensive conduction defect and a poor prognosis (high risk of complete heart block), especially in acute myocardial infarction.

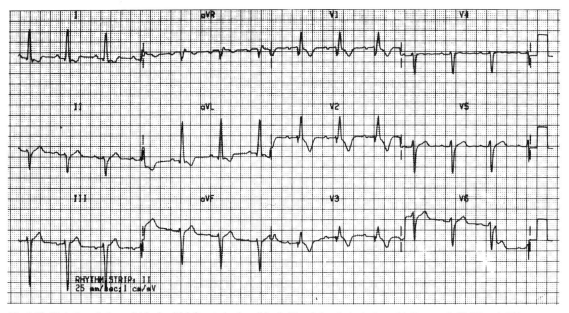

Fig. 8.39 Right bundle branch block with left anterior hemiblock. Note left axis deviation with R waves in II, III and aVF.

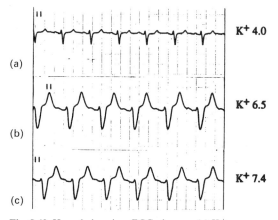

Fig. 8.40 Hyperkalaemia – ECG changes. (a) K⁺ 4.0 mmol/l, normal ECG; (b) K⁺ 6.5 mmol/l, P waves less prominent, widening of QRS and peaked T waves; (c) K⁺ 7.4 mmol/l, P waves obscured, QRS complexes nearly 200 ms.

Hyperkalaemia

A high serum K^+ can produce ECG changes (Fig. 8.40). Early changes consist of tall peaked T waves with reduced P-wave amplitude. Progressive widening of the QRS may be confused with BBB. Cardiac arrest may eventually occur.

Atrioventricular block

AV block is a delay or failure of impulse conduction from the atria to the ventricles. AV block is classified according to whether conduction of atrial impulses is delayed (first-degree), blocked intermittently (second-degree) or blocked completely (third-degree).

First-degree AV block

ECG

PR interval (measured from the onset of the P wave to the onset of the QRS) exceeds 200 ms (Fig. 8.41).

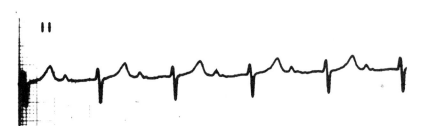

Fig. 8.41 First-degree atrioventricular block. PR interval is 320 ms.

Each P-wave is followed by a QRS. PR intervals may be prolonged to such a degree that the P wave is buried in the previous T wave or even QRS (Fig. 8.42).

Clinical

First-degree AV block is commonly associated with increased vagal tone, and occasionally with drugs (especially digoxin), ischaemic heart disease (particularly inferior myocardial infarction) and rheumatic fever. It usually causes no symptoms and requires no treatment. If associated with digoxin, the drug should be ceased or the dose decreased.

Second-degree AV block

Second-degree AV block is classified into Mobitz types I and II.

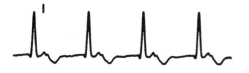

Fig. 8.42 First-degree atrioventricular block. P wave is hidden in initial part of the T wave.

Mobitz type I (Wenckebach)

Delay in AV conduction increases with each atrial impulse until an atrial impulse fails to conduct. This is usually a repetitive pattern.

ECG

There is progressive lengthening of the PR interval over successive cardiac cycles, culminating in a non-conducted P wave, resulting in a missed beat (Fig. 8.43).

Clinical

The condition is generally benign, although it may occur with inferior infarction. Treatment is rarely necessary.

Mobitz type II

There is intermittent failure of conduction of atrial impulses to the ventricles without preceding increases in the PR interval. The ratio of conducted to non-conducted atrial impulses varies, e.g. every second or fourth atrial impulse may be conducted (i.e. 2:1 or 4:1 second-degree AV block).

ECG

PR interval remains constant prior to the blocked P wave (Fig. 8.44). There is always a constant P–QRS

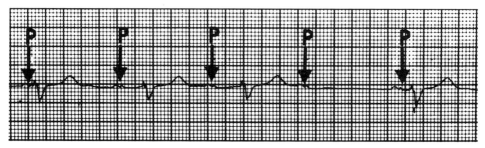

Fig. 8.43 Mobitz type I (Wenckebach) atrioventricular block. PR interval increases until a P wave (see fourth P wave) fails to be conducted.

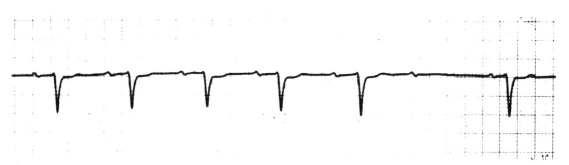

Fig. 8.44 Mobitz type II atrioventricular block. PR interval in sinus rhythm is prolonged in this example.

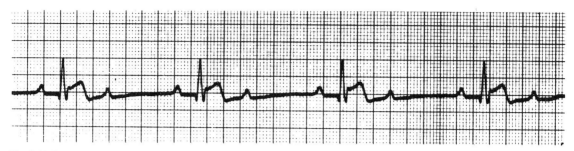

Fig. 8.45 Second-degree (2:1) atrioventricular block. Atrial rate 76/min, ventricular rate 38/min.

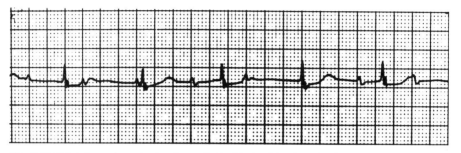

Fig. 8.46 Third-degree (complete) atrioventricular block with a junctional (narrow QRS) escape rhythm. Note independent atrial and ventricular activity (atrial rate 100/min; ventricular rate 68/min).

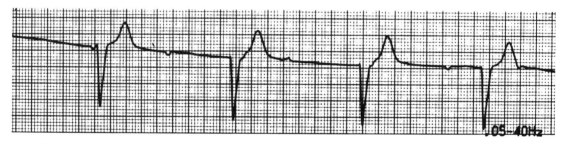

Fig. 8.47 Third-degree (complete) atrioventricular block. Atria and ventricles are dissociated. The ventricular escape pacemaker is discharging at about 38 beats/min.

wave ratio with the P waves two (Fig. 8.45), three (rare) or four times more frequent than QRS waves.

Clinical

It is likely to be associated with structural heart disease. Slower symptomatic ventricular rates may require pacing. The AV block may be intermittent (Fig. 8.44) or persistent (Fig. 8.45).

Third-degree (complete) AV block

This rhythm occurs when no atrial impulses are conducted to the ventricles; atria and the ventricular contraction are dissociated. The SA node usually continues to depolarize the atria, whereas ventricular activation depends on a standby escape pacemaker

located below the block. The escape pacemaker may be close to the His bundle (narrow QRS, stable pacemaker usually 40–60/min; Fig. 8.46), or more distal in ventricular tissue (wide QRS, relatively unstable pacemaker with a rate 20–40/min; Fig. 8.47). Should no ectopic escape pacemaker emerge, ventricular asystole will occur (Fig. 8.48), resulting in a Stokes–Adams attack, or death if the episode is prolonged. Torsade de pointes may also occur associated with the bradycardia.

ECG

The ECG shows normal regular P waves completely dissociated from QRS complexes. The QRS rate is always significantly slower than the P-wave rate and may be very slow at times.

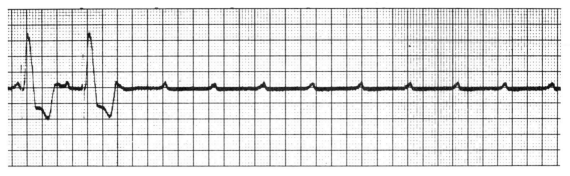

Fig. 8.48 Third-degree (complete) atrioventricular block and ventricular asystole. Failure of ventricular pacing is followed by complete heart block. Sinoatrial node discharge continues (P waves) but no ventricular escape pacemaker emerges.

Clinical

Idiopathic fibrosis of the conduction system is the most common cause. Other causes include myocardial infarction, valvular heart disease, cardiac surgery and a congenital form of complete heart block. Cardiac pacing is usually required to increase heart rate and cardiac output.

Congenital forms often have a relatively fast escape ventricular rate, and patients may remain asymptomatic for many years.

Sinoatrial block

SA block occurs when impulses originating in the SA node are not transmitted to surrounding atrial tissue. Two types are clinically relevant: second-degree SA block and third-degree or complete SA block. As with other bradycardias, escape rhythms may occur.

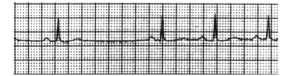

Fig. 8.49 Second-degree sinoatrial (SA) block. Abrupt doubling of heart rate indicates that 2:1 SA block has terminated.

Second-degree SA block

There is intermittent failure of atrial activation, resulting in P-wave intervals which are multiples of the cycle length during sinus rhythm.

ECG

The ECG shows missed PQRS complexes (Fig. 8.49). The PP interval (including the missed PQRS) is two, three, four or more times the length of the normal PP interval.

Third-degree SA block

This is indistinguishable from sinus arrest.

ECG

There are no P waves with an isoelectric line seen on the ECG, until an escape rhythm occurs or sinus rhythm is restored (Fig. 8.50).

Treatment

SA block is often associated with excessive vagal stimulation (e.g. vomiting or inferior myocardial infarction). Both second- and third-degree AV block usually require no treatment unless symptomatic. If cardiac output is inadequate, atropine 0.6 mg IV (repeated if necessary) or atrial pacing may be required.

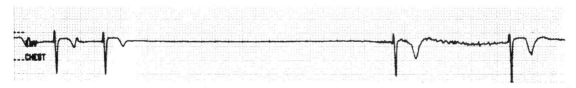

Fig. 8.50 Third-degree sinoatrial (SA) block. Prolonged sinus pause (sinus arrest) in a patient with a grossly prolonged PR interval.

Sick sinus syndrome (SSS)

This consists of a number of sinus node abnormalities including inappropriate sinus bradycardia, SA blocks or sinus arrest. When sinus bradycardia or SA block occurs, junctional escape rhythms are common. There may also be abnormalities of AV conduction. Paroxysms of AF or atrial flutter may alternate with episodes of bradycardia (bradycardia–tachycardia syndrome).

Clinical

The bradycardias associated with SSS may result in syncope or near-syncope. SSS is often not associated with structural heart disease, but may occur with ischaemic and congenital heart disease.

Treatment

Cardiac pacing is usually required to control bradycardic symptoms. Atropine and low-dose isoprenaline may be useful prior to pacing, in the haemodynamically compromised patient. Bradycardia–tachycardia syndrome may require both pacing (for the bradycardia) and antiarrhythmic drugs (for the tachycardia). Anticoagulation needs to be considered if episodes of AF occur.

Hypersensitive carotid sinus syndrome

This syndrome is usually characterized by ventricular asystole associated with SA arrest and atrial asystole. Classification is usually as:

1 *Cardioinhibitory* – ventricular asystole ≥ 3 s with carotid sinus massage. Cardiac pacing will usually prevent the bradycardia.
2 *Vasodepressor* – hypotension prior to a bradycardia. Cardiac pacing may not be useful.

References

1 Artucio H and Pereira M (1990) Cardiac arrhythmias in critically ill patients: epidemiologic study. *Crit Care Med* 18:1383–1388.
2 Katz AM (1993) Cardiac ion channels. *N Engl J Med* 328:1244–1251.
3 Zipes DP (1992) Specific arrhythmias: diagnosis and treatment. In: Braunwald E (ed.) *Heart Disease: A Textbook of Cardiovascular Medicine*. Philadelphia: WB Saunders, pp. 667–718.
4 Donovan KD, Power BM, Hockings BE, Lee KY, Barrowcliffe MB and Lovett M (1993) Usefulness of atrial electrograms recorded via central venous catheters in the diagnosis of complex cardiac arrhythmias. *Crit Care Med* 21: 532–537.
5 Mason JW (1993) A comparison of electrophysiologic testing with Holter monitoring to predict antiarrhythmic drug efficacy for ventricular tachyarrhythmias. *N Engl J Med* 329:445–451.
6 Gilman JK, Jalal S and Naccarelli GV (1994) Predicting and preventing sudden death from cardiac causes. *Circulation* 90:1083–1092.
7 Kennedy HL, Whitlock JA, Sprague MK, Kennedy LJ, Buckingham TA and Goldberg RJ (1985) Long-term follow-up of asymptomatic healthy subjects with frequent and complex ventricular ectopy. *N Engl J Med* 312:193–197.
8 Wesley RC, Rash W and Zimmerman D (1991) Reconsiderations of the routine and preoperational use of lidocaine in the emergent treatment of ventricular arrhythmias. *Crit Care Med* 19:1439–1444.
9 Antman EM and Berlin JA (1992) Declining incidence of ventricular fibrillation in myocardial infarction: implications for the prophylactic use of lignocaine. *Circulation* 86:764–773.
10 Teo KK, Yusuf S and Furberg CD (1993) Effects of prophylactic antiarrhythmic drug therapy in acute myocardial infarction: an overview of results from randomized controlled trials. *J Am Med Assoc* 270:1589–1595.
11 ISIS-1 (First International Study of Infarct Survival) collaborative group (1986) Randomized trial of intravenous atenolol among 16027 cases of suspected acute myocardial infarction ISIS-1. *Lancet* 2:57.
12 Friedman LM, Byington RP, Capone RJ, Furberg CD, Goldstein S and Lichstein E (1986) Writing group for the Beta-Blocker Heart Attack Trial Research Group. Effect of propranolol in patients with myocardial infarction and ventricular arrhythmia. *J Am Coll Cardiol* 7:1–8.
13 The Cardiac Arrhythmia Suppression Trial (CAST) investigators (1989). Preliminary report: effect of encainide and flecainide on mortality in a randomized trial of arrhythmia suppression after myocardial infarction. *N Engl J Med* 321:406–412.
14 The Cardiac Arrhythmia Suppression Trial II investigators (1992) Effect of the antiarrhythmic agent moricizine on survival after myocardial infarction. *N Engl J Med* 327:227–233.
15 Ganz LI and Friedman PL (1995) Supraventricular tachycardia. *N Engl J Med* 332:162–173. 173.
16 Wathen MS, Klein GJ, Yee R and Natale A (1993) Classification and terminology of supraventricular tachycardia. Diagnosis and management of the atrial tachycardias. *Cardiol Clin* 11:109–120.
17 Sung RJ, Lauer MR and Chun H (1994) Atrioventricular node reentry: current concepts and new perspectives. *Pace* 17:1413–1427.
18 Scher DL and Arsura EL (1989) Multifocal atrial tachycardia: mechanisms, clinical correlates and treatment. *Am Heart J* 118:574–580.
19 Olshansky B, Wilber DJ and Hariman RJ (1992) Atrial flutter – update on the mechanism and treatment. *Pace* 15:2308–2335.

20 Haissaguerre M and Saoudi N (1994) Role of catheter ablation for supraventricular tachyarrhythmias with emphasis on atrial flutter and atrial tachycardia. *Curr Opinion Cardiol* **9**:40–52.

21 Pritchett ELC (1992) Management of atrial fibrillation. *N Engl J Med* **326**:1264–1271.

22 Prytowski EN, Benson DW, Fuster V *et al.* (1996) Management of patients with atrial fibrillation. *Circulation* **93**:1262–1277.

23 Cox JL (1993) A perspective of postoperative atrial fibrillation in cardiac operations. *Ann Thorac Surg* **56**:405–409.

24 Creswell LL, Schuessler RB, Rosenbloom M and Cox JL (1993) Hazards of postoperative atrial arrhythmias. *Ann Thorac Surg* **56**:539–549.

25 Grogan M, Smith HC, Gersh BJ and Wood DL (1992) Left ventricular dysfunction due to atrial fibrillation in patients initially believed to have idiopathic dilated cardiomyopathy. *Am J Cardiol* **69**:1570–1573.

26 Donovan KD, Power BM, Hockings EF, Dobb GJ and Lee KY (1995) Intravenous flecainide vs amiodarone for recent-onset atrial fibrillation. *Am J Cardiol* **75**:693–697.

27 Arnold AZ, Mick MJ, Mazurek RP, Loop FD and Trohman RG (1992) Role of prophylactic anticoagulation for direct current cardioversion in patients with atrial fibrillation or atrial flutter. *J Am Coll Cardiol* **19**:851–855.

28 Coplen SE, Antman EM, Berlin JA, Hewitt P and Chalmers TC (1990) Efficacy and safety of quinidine therapy for maintenance of sinus rhythm after cardioversion. *Circulation* **82**:1106–1116.

29 Mason JW (1993) A comparison of seven antiarrhythmic drugs in patients with ventricular tachyarrhythmias. *N Engl J Med* **329**:452–458.

30 Rawles JM, Metcalfe MJ and Jennings K (1990) Time of occurrence, duration and ventricular rate of paroxysmal atrial fibrillation: the effect of digoxin. *Br Heart J* **63**:225–227.

31 Brignole M, Giafranchi L, Menozzi C *et al.* (1994) Influence of atrioventricular junction radiofrequency ablation in patients with chronic atrial fibrillation and flutter on quality of life and cardiac performance. *Am J Cardiol* **74**:242–246.

32 The National Heart, Lung, and Blood Institute working group on atrial fibrillation (1993) Atrial fibrillation: current understandings and research imperatives. *J Am Coll Cardiol* **22**:1830–1834.

33 Laupacis A (1993) Anticoagulants for atrial fibrillation. *Lancet* **342**:1251.

34 Garratt C, Antoniou A, Ward D and Camm AJ (1989) Misuse of verapamil in pre-existent atrial fibrillation. *Lancet* **1**:367–9.

35 Hsia HH and Buxton AF (1993) Work-up and management of patients with sustained and non-sustained monomorphic ventricular tachycardias. *Cardiol Clin* **11**:21–37.

36 Steinman RT, Herrera C, Schuger CD and Lehmann MH (1989) Wide QRS tachycardia in the conscious adult: ventricular tachycardia is the most frequent cause. *J Am Med Assoc* **261**:1013–1016.

37 Stewart RB, Bardy GH and Greene HL (1986) Wide complex tachycardia: misdiagnosis and outcome after emergent therapy. *Ann Intern Med* **104**:766–771.

38 Wellens HJJ, Bär FWHM, Lie KL (1978) The value of the electrocardiogram in the differential diagnosis of a tachycardia with a widened QRS complex. *Am J Med* **64**:27–33.

39 Brugada P, Brugada J, Mont L, Smeets J and Andries EW (1991) A new approach to the differential diagnosis of a regular tachycardia with a wide QRS complex. *Circulation* **83**:1649–1659.

40 Antunes E, Brugada J, Steurer G, Andries A and Brugada P (1994) The differential diagnosis of a regular tachycardia with a wide QRS complex on the 12-lead ECG: ventricular tachycardia, supraventricular tachycardia with aberrant intraventricular conduction, and supraventricular tachycardia with anterograde conduction over an accessory pathway. *Pace* **17**:1515–1524.

41 Griffith MJ, Garratt CJ, Mounsey P and Camm AJ (1994) Ventricular tachycardia as a default diagnosis in broad complex tachycardia. *Lancet* **343**:386–388.

42 Camm AJ and Garratt CJ (1991) Adenosine and supraventricular tachycardia. *N Engl J Med* **325**:1621–1629.

43 Ho DSW, Zecchin RP, Richards DA, Uther JB and Ross DL (1994) Double blind trial of lignocaine versus sotalol for acute termination of spontaneous ventricular tachycardia. *Lancet* **344**:18–23.

44 Gorgels AP, von den Dool A, Hofs A, Smeets JL, Brugada P and Vos MA (1989) Procainamide is superior to lignocaine in terminating sustained ventricular tachycardia. *Circulation* **80** (suppl. II):652.

45 The CASCADE investigators (1993) Randomized antiarrhythmic drug therapy in survivors of cardiac arrest (the CASCADE study). *Am J Cardiol* **72**:280–287.

46 Steinbeck G, Andresen D, Back P *et al.* (1992) A comparison of electrophysiologically guided antiarrhythmic drug therapy with beta-blocker therapy in patients with symptomatic, sustained ventricular tachyarrhythmias. *N Engl J Med* **327**:987–992.

47 Donovan KD, Dobb GJ, Coombs LJ *et al.* (1991) Reversion of recent-onset atrial fibrillation of sinus rhythm by intravenous flecainide. *Am J Cardiol* **67**:137–141.

48 Tzivoni D, Bonai S, Schuger C *et al.* (1988) Treatment of torsade de pointes with magnesium sulphate. *Circulation* **77**:392–397.

49 Arsenian MA (1993) Magnesium and cardiovascular disease. *Prog Cardiovasc Dis* **35**:271–310.

9 Antiarrhythmic drugs

KD Donovan and BEF Hockings

Antiarrhythmic drugs are the mainstay treatment of cardiac arrhythmias. They are given to terminate an arrhythmia, slow arrhythmia-induced tachycardia or prevent arrhythmia recurrences. Benefit is greatest when given to terminate an acute sustained symptomatic tachyarrhythmia (e.g. ventricular tachycardia, VT). However, except for β-blockers after myocardial infarction, antiarrhythmic drugs have not been shown to improve patient survival. Also, benefits of antiarrythmics for long-term treatment of recurrent arrhythmias are unclear. Any potential benefits must be weighed against risks of adverse effects (Table 9.1).[1] Before antiarrhythmic drugs are administered, reversible or precipitating causes of arrhythmias (e.g. electrolyte abnormalities and digoxin or aminophylline toxicity) should be excluded or corrected. Other therapeutic options (e.g. vagal manoeuvres, cardioversion, cardiac pacing, radiofrequency ablation or surgery) should be considered when appropriate.

Classification and mechanisms of drug action

Antiarrhythmic drugs are divided into four classes (Table 9.2),[2-4] according to mechanisms of drug action. This classification is incomplete, as some agents (e.g. adenosine, magnesium and digoxin) are not included. Also, an agent may have more than one antiarrhythmic action (e.g. class III drug amiodarone possesses properties of all four classes).

Adverse effects

Antiarrhythmic drugs have a narrow toxic–therapeutic relationship. Serious side-effects can arise from mildly toxic serum concentrations. Hence drug metabolism and excretion are important in prescribing practice. Dosage regimens and therapeutic concentrations are shown in Table 9.3.[5]

Antiarrhythmic drugs are proarrhythmic, i.e. they can worsen arrhythmias or induce new ones.[6] Malignant ventricular arrhythmias are more likely to be provoked in patients with poor left ventricular (LV) function, pre-existing prolonged QT intervals, or who are receiving digoxin and diuretics.[7] Drug-induced arrhythmias include bradyarrhythmias, atrial flutter with 1:1 atrioventricular (AV) conduction (e.g. quinidine, procainamide and flecainide), torsade de pointes (e.g. quinidine, procainamide and sotalol), and incessant VT (e.g. encainide and flecainide). Most proarrhythmic events occur soon after starting the drug, but late arrhythmias are also a significant problem.[7-9]

Risks of long-term therapy with antiarrhythmic drugs have been underestimated. The cardiac arrhythmia suppression trial (CAST)[9] tested the hypothesis that in survivors of myocardial infarction, suppression of venricular ectopic beats (VEBs) improves survival. However, treatment with flecainide and encainide (which are effective in suppressing VEBs) had a mortality rate 2–3 times that of placebo patients. Most deaths were probably due to drug-induced arrhythmias. This treatment strategy should no longer be followed. An overview of 138 randomized trials (98 000 patients)[10] suggests that in myocardial infarction survivors, class I antiarrhythmic agents may increase mortality; class II agents reduce mortality; amiodarone (a class III agent) may be beneficial;[11] and class IV agents are probably ineffective or harmful.

Class I antiarrhythmic drugs

Most, if not all, class I drugs increase mortality given the appropriate clinical milieu.[12] They are not appropriate first-line treatment for long-term prevention of ventricular arrhythmias.[13]

Table 9.1 Antiarrhythmic drug therapy – benefits and risks

	Comment
Benefits	
Improve survival	β-Blockers (post myocardial infarction) – yes
	All other drugs unproven or may increase mortality
Symptomatic improvement	Acute arrhythmias – yes
	Chronic arrhythmias – probably
Risks – side-effects	
Cardiac	Some agents may increase cardiovascular mortality.
	Most agents are negatively inotropic
	Proarrhythmic effects may worsen existing arrhythmia or
	cause a new arrhythmia; either tachycardia or bradycardia
Non-cardiac	Occasional idiosyncratic reactions such as bone marrow
	depression (tocainide), thrombocytopenia (quinidine)
	Frequently minor and reversible (e.g. nausea and
	diarrhoea)

Table 9.2 Singh and Vaughan-Williams classification of anti-arrhythmic drugs

Class I	Na$^+$ channel blockers – slow rate of rise (V$_{max}$) of phase 0 of the action potential
Class Ia	Action potential duration prolonged (e.g. quinidine, procainamide, disopyramide)
Class Ib	Action potential duration shortened (e.g. lignocaine, tocainide, mexilitine, phenytoin)
Class Ic	Little effect on action potential duration. Conduction slowed with minimal effect on refractoriness (e.g. flecainide, encainide, propafenone)
Class II	β-Adrenergic blockers (e.g. propranolol, timolol, atenolol, metoprolol, esmolol)
Class III	K$^+$ channel blockers. duration of action potential and refractory period) prolonged (e.g. amiodarone, bretylium, sotalol)
Class IV	Ca^{2+} channel blockers (e.g. verapamil, diltiazem)

Class Ia drugs

Quinidine[5]

Quinidine blocks the Na$^+$ channels at fast heart rates, and prolongs repolarization at slower rates.[14] The effective refractory period is prolonged more than action potential duration. It has an anticholinergic effect, and AV node conduction may be enhanced until its direct negative dromotropism becomes effective. Quinidine usually has no effect on sinus rate or PR interval. The ECG may show QRS and QT interval prolongation (QT > 500 ms is usually present in quinidine-induced torsade de pointes). Myocardial contractility and systemic vascular resistance (SVR) are decreased.

Clinical use

Quinidine is effective against atrial and ventricular arrhythmias, but is not usually used because of its side-effects. The drug is never used IV because severe hypotension and myocardial depression may result. Caution should be exercised in prolonged administration. Quinidine effectively maintains sinus rhythm after cardioversion from atrial fibrillation (AF), but total mortality is increased.[15] Quinidine should probably be limited to patients with life-threatening arrhythmias, where it has been 'proven' to be effective by invasive electrophysiological testing. Even then, other drugs may be more effective.

Adverse effects

Severe side-effects necessitate stopping quinidine in 30–40% of patients.[1] Diarrhoea, nausea and vomiting are common. Central nervous system (CNS) toxicity includes tinnitus, visual disturbances, headache and confusion (cinhonism). Allergic reactions include rash, fever, thrombocytopenia and haemolytic anaemia. Cardiac failure may be precipitated in susceptible patients. Quinidine toxicity slows cardiac conduction, causing conduction disturbances, e.g. AV block. Torsade de pointes may occur, usually not associated with toxic concentrations; treatment requires stopping quinidine, avoiding other QT-prolonging drugs and suppression of the polymorphic VT by atrial or ventricular pacing, or IV magnesium.[16]

Quinidine therapy for VEBs is associated with increased mortality.[17] Quinidine may slow the atrial rate in atrial flutter, but AV nodal conduction may be enhanced, causing a potentially life-threatening 1:1 AV conduction and ventricular response of 200/min or greater. If used in atrial flutter or fibrillation, prior slowing of the ventricular response with β-blockers, calcium-channel blockers or digoxin is essential.

Table 9.3 Antiarrhythmic drug dosage and therapeutic plasma concentrations

Drug	Loading dose (IV)	Maintenance dose (IV)	Loading dose (PO)	Maintenance dose (PO)	Elimination route $T^{1/2}$ (major; h)		Therapeutic plasma concentration (mg/l)
Quinidine			300–600 mg q.i.d	500–750 mg b.d.*	Liver	5–9	3–6
Procainamide	6–13 mg/kg at <50 mg/min	2–6 mg/min			Kidneys	3–5	4–10
Disopyramide	1–2 mg/kg (max. 150 mg) over 15–30 min	1 mg/kg per h (max. 800 mg/day)		100–200 mg t.i.d./q.i.d.	Kidneys	8–9	2–5
Lignocaine	1.5–2.0 mg/kg over 2 min	1–4 mg/min			Liver	1–2	1–5
Mexiletine	100–250 mg over 5–10 min	0.5–1.0 mg/min	400–600 mg	200–300 mg t.i.d.	Liver	10–12	0.75–2.0
Phenytoin	15 mg/kg at 100 mg/min		1000 mg	300 mg/day	Liver	18–36	10–20
Flecainide	2 mg/kg (max. 150 mg)			100–200 mg b.d.	Liver	20	0.2–1.0
Propafenone	1–2 mg/kg		600–900 mg	150–300 mg b.d./t.i.d.	Liver	5–8	0.2–3.0
Propanolol	0.5 mg/min max. 0.2 mg/kg			10–200 mg t.i.d./q.i.d.	Liver	2–6	NR
Metoprolol	1–2 mg/min max. dose 15–20 mg			50–100 mg b.d.	Liver	3–4	NR
Esmolol	0.5 mg/kg over 1–2 min	50–300 µg/kg per min			RBC	9 min	NR
Amiodarone	5–7 mg/kg over 30 min then 50 mg/h for 24–48 h		1200 mg/day for 7 days	200–400 mg/day	Liver	50 days	1.0–2.5
Bretylium	5–10 mg/kg at 1–2 mg/kg per min	0.5–2.0 mg/min			Liver	3–6	NR
Sotalol	100 mg over 5–20 min			80–160 mg b.d.	Kidneys	15	1–3
Verapamil	1 mg/min (max. 10–15 mg)	5 µg/kg per min		80–120 mg t.i.d./q.i.d.	Liver	3–8	0.1–0.15
Adenosine	6–18 mg rapid					1–2 s	NR

*Sustained release: IV = intravenous; p.o. = per oral; $T^{1/2}$ half-life; RBC = red blood cell; NR = not relevant.

Drug interactions are common. Serum digoxin concentrations may be increased. Cimetidine and some β-blockers (e.g. propranolol) reduce hepatic flow and may cause toxic plasma quinidine concentrations. Phenytoin and phenobarbitone induce hepatic enzymes, and therefore decrease plasma quinidine concentrations (rate of elimination is increased).

Procainamide[5]

Procainamide has similar electrophysiological and electrocardiographic effects to quinidine. Its major metabolite *N*-acetyl-procainamide has a longer duration of action and different electrophysiological properties to the parent compound. Compared to disopyramide and quinidine, procainamide exerts the least vagolytic effect.

Clinical use

Procainamide can be used to treat both atrial and ventricular arrhythmias. IV procainamide may be more effective than lignocaine for terminating VT.[18] Procainamide is also effective for conversion of AV nodal, AV re-entry tachycardias, and possibly AF.[19] Oral procainamide is not widely used due to its short half-life and side-effect profile.

Adverse effects

A reversible lupus-like syndrome develops in 20–30% of patients receiving procainamide long-term. Other side-effects include gastrointestinal disturbances (less common than with quinidine), CNS manifestations and cardiac depression. As with quinidine, the ventricular response may be accelerated if given for supraventricular tachycardias. QT interval prolongation and torsade de pointes may also occur.

Disopyramide[5,20]

Disopyramide has similar electrophysiological actions to quinidine and procainamide. Anticholinergic effects are greater than quinidine or procainamide.

Clinical use

Disopyramide has a significant negative inotropic effect which limits its usefulness. It has been used to treat both supraventricular and ventricular arrhythmias. Although not a first-line drug, disopyramide terminates AV nodal and AV re-entry tachycardias, and may prevent recurrences. It is as effective as quinidine in preventing recurrence of AF after cardioversion, but again, caution must be exercised in long-term use. Disopyramide should not be used to treat AF or atrial flutter without prior ventricular rate control with β-blockers or verapamil.

Adverse effects

The most common side-effects are anticholinergic (e.g. dry mouth, blurred vision, urinary hesitancy or retention, constipation and closed-angle glaucoma). Proarrhythmic effects include increased ventricular response with atrial flutter or fibrillation, and ventricular tachyarrhythmias, especially prolonged QT-associated torsade de pointes. Disopyramide causes myocardial depression, which is more pronounced in pre-existing cardiac dysfunction. Cardiac failure can be precipitated, with occasionally cardiovascular collapse and cardiogenic shock.[20]

Class Ib drugs

Lignocaine[5,21]

Lignocaine is still considered a first-line drug to treat acute, sustained ventricular tachyarrhythmias. It is ineffective against supraventricular arrhythmias. Lignocaine has no effect on sinoatrial (SA) node automaticity, but depresses automaticity in other pacemaker tissues. Its Na^+ channel-blocking effect is increased in myocardial ischaemia. Normally, lignocaine has little or no effect on conduction. The electrocardiogram (ECG) shows no changes in sinus rate, PR interval, QRS width or QT interval with lignocaine.

Clinical use

Lignocaine is used mainly to treat malignant ventricular tachyarrhythmias, especially in acute myocardial ischaemia. However, lignocaine prophylaxis to prevent ventricular fibrillation (VF) in acute myocardial infarction can no longer be recommended. Lignocaine in this setting increases mortality,[10,21] possibly by inducing asystole despite reducing the incidence of VF.[22] It increases the current required for defibrillation, and may be detrimental during an episode of VF.[21] In the absence of acute ischaemia, its benefit in treating sustained ventricular arrhythmias is unproven;[21,23,24] Sotalol is more effective.[25] Its role in this setting requires further evaluation.

Extensive first-pass hepatic metabolism precludes oral use of lignocaine. IV dose should be reduced by 30–50% in severe liver disease or heart failure. The distribution half-life is about 8 min, and elimination half-life 1.5 h in normal patients (but may be increased >10 h in severe heart failure or shock). An initial bolus of IV lignocaine 1.5–2.0 mg/kg over 1–2 min, followed by an infusion of 4 mg/min for 1 h, then 2 mg/min for 2 h, and thereafter 1–2 mg/min, is recommended. Increasing the maintenance infusion rate without an additional bolus requires about 6 h (4 elimination half-lives) to reach a steady state. If the initial bolus is ineffective, another bolus of 1 mg/kg may be given after 5 min. Another dosage regimen is 1.5–2.0 mg/kg initially, and 0.8 mg/kg at 8-min intervals for three doses (i.e. 3 distribution half-lives), and thereafter 1–2 mg/min by infusion.

Adverse effects

CNS toxicity with high plasma concentrations are the most common (e.g. dizziness, paraesthesia, confusion, and coma and convulsions). Uncommonly, AV block or cardiac depression may occur.[5,26] Cimetidine reduces lignocaine clearance, potentially causing toxic drug concentrations.

Mexiletine[5]

Mexiletine is similar to lignocaine in its electrophysiological, haemodynamic and therapeutic effects. It can be given IV or orally, sometimes in combination with other antiarrhythmics. Clearance is mainly by liver metabolism. It has a narrow toxic–therapeutic ratio. Toxic effects are common; 30–40% of patients have intolerable nausea, vomiting, dizziness, confusion and ataxia. Cardiovascular side-effects (e.g. bradycardia and hypotension) occur mainly after IV use. Like other class I drugs, mexiletine may be proarrhythmic.

Tocainide[5]

Tocainide is a primary amine analogue of lignocaine protected from first-pass hepatic elimination, and is effective orally. Electrophysiological, therapeutic and haemodynamic effects are similar to lignocaine. Tocainide is ineffective for supraventricular arrhythmias. Adverse effects are similar to those of lignocaine. Proarrhythmic effects may occur. Serious effects (e.g. agranulocytosis, thrombocytopenia, and pulmonary fibrosis) prohibit its use except in exceptional circumstances, such as life-threatening ventricular arrhythmias where other agents are ineffective or contraindicated.

Phenytoin[5]

Clinical use

Phenytoin is mainly used to treat seizure disorders. It has limited value as an antiarrhythmic agent, except for arrhythmias caused by digitalis intoxication. Phenytoin abolishes abnormal automaticity caused by delayed afterdepolarizations. Numerous drugs can increase or decrease phenytoin concentrations during chronic administration; frequent monitoring of plasma phenytoin concentration is necessary. Phenytoin may be administered orally or IV. It is very alkalotic and a central vein should be used for IV administration.

Adverse effects

Phenytoin may cause CNS effects (e.g. nystagmus, ataxia and altered consciousness, sometimes progress-ing to coma), related closely to plasma concentrations. It can also exacerbate or provoke arrhythmias, but has minimal haemodynamic effects. Long-term administration can cause megaloblastic anaemia, gingival hyperplasia, peripheral neuropathy and blood sugar disturbances.

Moricizine

Moricizine (ethmozin) is a new oral phenothiazine-derivative antiarrhythmic, not widely available. The CAST II[27] showed that it acutely increased the occurrence of sudden cardiac death. This supports an adverse effect common to all class I (rather than only class Ic) drugs.[12]

Class Ic drugs

Flecainide[5,28]

Flecainide exhibits rate-dependent Na^+ channel blockade, with marked slowing of conduction in all cardiac tissue, and little prolongation of refractoriness. In the CAST,[9] suppression of VEBs after myocardial infarction with flecainide was associated with increased mortality.

Clinical use

Flecainide can be administered IV or orally. It should be avoided in second- (or third-) degree AV block unless a pacemaker is *in situ*. The drug depresses cardiac contractility and is usually contraindicated in patients with abnormal LV function. Flecainide may revert AV nodal and AV re-entry tachycardias, although adenosine or verapamil is more widely used. It may also be useful in supraventricular tachy-arrhythmias, including AF[29,30] and possibly atrial flutter. Although controversial, flecainide may be given in life-threatening VT. If flecainide is deemed necessary for prophylaxis of ventricular arrhythmias, therapy should start with ECG monitoring.

Adverse effects

Proarrhythmic events are common, especially in patients with depressed LV function, and may be life-threatening. Torsade de pointes may occur,[29] even in patients without structural heart disease. Incessant VT may be induced,[28] unresponsive to any therapy, including cardioversion. Although flecainide depresses intracardiac conduction, a paradoxical increase in ventricular rate may occur with atrial flutter or fibrillation.[31] Flecainide's negative inotropic effects can worsen or precipitate heart failure. Flecainide increases the pacing threshold. CNS effects include visual disturbances, dizziness and nausea.

Encainide

The electrophysiological and haemodynamic effects of encainide resemble flecainide. It has, however, a shorter elimination half-life. Adverse effects are also similar.

Propafenone

Propafenone has a similar electrophysiological, haemodynamic and side-effect profile to flecainide and encainide. Use of propafenone should probably be limited, even though it was not included in the CAST.[9]

Class II antiarrhythmic drugs (β-adrenoreceptor blockers)[5]

Various β-blocking drugs have different properties, such as relative cardioselectivity (e.g. atenolol and metoprolol), non-cardioselectivity (e.g. propranolol), intrinsic sympathomimatic activity (mild activation of the β-receptor, e.g. pindolol) and membrane-depressant effects (e.g. propranolol). Such properties may confer advantages under certain circumstances, such as cardioselectivity for a patient with reversible airways disease – cardioselectivity is however lost with higher doses. Antiarrhythmic properties appear to be a class II effect; no specific β-blocker is intrinsically superior.

β-Blockers competitively inhibit catecholamine binding at β-adrenergic receptor sites. Some drugs such as propranolol have a direct membrane-stabilizing or 'quinidine-like' action, but the clinical relevance is negligible, as this effect occurs at doses far greater than those used clinically. The anti-ischaemic properties of β-blockers may have important indirect antiarrhythmic consequences, but overall, β-blockade is the principal antiarrhythmic action. This reduces phase 4 slope of the action potential of pacemaker cells, prolongs their refractoriness and slows conduction in the AV node. Refractoriness and conduction in the His–Purkinje system are unchanged.

Clinical use

β-Blockers are most effective in arrhythmias associated with increased cardiac adrenergic stimulation (e.g. those of thyrotoxicosis, phaeochromocytoma, exercise or emotion).

Supraventricular tachycardias

β-Blockers may terminate supraventricular tachyarrhythmias when the AV node is an intrinsic part of the re-entry arrhythmia circuit (e.g. AV nodal and AV re-entry tachycardias), but adenosine and verapamil are more effective. Atrial flutter and fibrillation do not revert with β-blockade, but the ventricular response will be slowed. Metoprolol may be effective in patients with multifocal atrial tachycardia,[32] although β-blockers should be avoided in patients with reversible airways disease (often associated with this arrhythmia).

Ventricular arrhythmias

β-Blockers are generally ineffective for the emergency treatment of sustained VT. Empirical prophylactic metoprolol administration appears to be as effective in arrhythmia prevention as electrophysiologically guided drug methods,[33] but the role of β-blockade in preventing ventricular tachyarrhythmias long-term awaits further study.

Myocardial infarction

Survival in patients with acute myocardial infarction is probably improved by early IV β-blockade.[34] There may be other benefits such as decreased incidence of VF and relief of chest pain. The ISIS-1[34] regimen used atenolol 5 mg IV over 5 min, repeated 10 min later if heart rate exceeded 60 beats/min. If the heart rate exceeded 40 beats/min 10 min later, oral atenolol 50 mg was administered and continued at 100 mg daily. Long-term β-blockade reduces mortality following myocardial infarction,[10,35] the benefit being greatest in those at highest risk for sudden death. Suppression of ventricular ectopy is, however, not a requisite for benefit. Drugs with intrinsic sympathomimatic activity have not been shown to improve survival after acute myocardial infarction.

Esmolol

Esmolol[36] is an ultrashort-acting (distribution half-life 2 min, elimination half-life 9 min) cardioselective β-blocker which is especially useful for rapid control of ventricular rate in atrial flutter or fibrillation. The short half-life may be particularly useful in critically ill patients. Esmolol permits careful titration of β-blockade. Infusion is initiated with a loading dose of 500 μg/kg over 1 min, followed by a maintenance dose of 50 μg/kg per min for 4 min. If a satisfactory response is not achieved, the loading dose should be repeated and the maintenance dose increased to 100 μg/kg per min and infused for a further 4 min. If no adequate response follows, the procedure may be repeated with 50 μg/kg per min increments in the maintenance infusion, until 300 μg/kg per min is reached. Further increases in infusion rate are unlikely to be successful.

Class III drugs

Class III drugs block potassium channels, thereby prolonging the action potential duration and repolarization.

Amiodarone[5,37,38]

Amiodarone is a potent antiarrhythmic agent with a complex electrophysiological and pharmacological profile. It prolongs action potential duration and increases the refractoriness of all cardiac tissue. Other electrophysiological actions include Na^+ channel blockade (class I), antiadrenergic (class II), calcium-channel blockade (class IV) and antifibrillatory effects. QT prolongation reflects a global prolongation of repolarization and diminished ventricular dispersion, and is closely associated with its antiarrhythmic effects.[38] When given IV, amiodarone has little immediate class III effect; the major action is on the AV node, causing a delay in intranodal conduction and a prolongation of refractoriness.[37] This probably explains why IV amiodarone controls the ventricular rate in recent-onset AF, but is ineffective for termination of this arrhythmia.[30] IV administration causes some cardiac depression, but cardiac index is often unchanged because of its vasodilator properties.

Clinical use

Amiodarone is effective in suppressing both supraventricular and ventricular tachyarrhythmias. It has a long elimination half-life (mean > 50 days). Absorption from oral administration is incomplete, with a delayed onset of action (days to weeks). Loading doses reduce this interval, e.g. 1200 mg/day for 1–2 weeks, reducing to 400–600 mg/day and then 100–400 mg/day after 2–3 months. The dose should probably not be reduced below 400 mg/day with life-threatening ventricular arrhythmias, whereas with more benign arrhythmias such as AF, 100–200 mg/day may suffice. Amiodarone can also be administered IV when rapid loading is required or in an emergency (see above). Commonly used IV doses are 5–7 mg/kg over 30 min, followed by 50 mg/h for several days.

Supraventricular tachycardias

Amiodarone is effective in terminating and suppressing recurrences of AV nodal and AV re-entry tachycardias, although adenosine (for acute reversion) or verapamil (acute termination and long-term prophylaxis) is superior. IV amiodarone does not revert atrial flutter or fibrillation, but the ventricular rate will slow.[30] Administration over a longer time span (days to weeks) may be more effective in reverting recent-onset AF.[39] In preventing recurrence of AF after reversion, amiodarone is comparable in efficacy to quinidine and flecainide.

Ventricular tachyarrhythmias

IV amiodarone may be effective in treating life-threatening ventricular tachyarrhythmias refractory to other drugs,[38] especially in myocardial infarction and poor LV function. However, it is not a first-line drug in the emergency treatment of VT or recurrent VF. Long-term oral amiodarone is useful in controlling symptomatic VT and VF, especially when other conventional antiarrhythmics have failed.[40] The absence of negative inotropism is useful in those with severely depressed LV function, but its many adverse effects limit widespread use. The CASCADE study[41] demonstrated that empirical amiodarone treatment was superior to guided (non-invasive Holter or invasive electrophysiology testing) class I drugs in survivors of VF unassociated with acute myocardial infarction. Amiodarone prevented arrhythmia recurrence and decreased the incidence of sudden death. Thus, amiodarone or sotalol (see below) can be considered as first-line drugs to prevent life-threatening ventricular tachyarrhythmias.

Myocardial infarction

Data are limited at present, but amiodarone may improve survival in patients after myocardial infarction.[10]

Adverse effects

Adverse effects will occur in the majority of patients if they receive amiodarone for long enough. Most are reversible when the drug is discontinued. Adverse effects include:[38]

1 dermatological – photosensitivity, bluish/grey skin discoloration ('slate-blue' skin);
2 eyes – corneal microdeposits (almost 100%) with little or no clinical significance;
3 gastrointestinal disturbances;
4 hypo- and hyperthyroidism;
5 liver dysfunction – asymptomatic increases in liver enzymes are common, and do not require amiodarone cessation unless enzymes are 2–3 times normal – hepatitis is rare;
6 neuropathy, myopathy and cerebellar abnormalities;
7 pulmonary toxicity.

Acute respiratory distress syndrome has been reported in patients undergoing cardiopulmonary bypass surgery.[42] Pulmonary toxicity is the most serious, with a reported incidence of 10% at 3 years.[41] Shortness of breath, cough and fever with pulmonary crepitations are usually present. Chest X-ray shows widespread pulmonary infiltrates. Mortality is 10%. Immediate discontinuation is necessary. Use of steroids is controversial.

Amiodarone interacts with other drugs potentiating warfarin, digoxin and other antiarrhythmic agents. When administered concurrently, doses of these drugs should be reduced accordingly. On the plus side, long-term amiodarone is unlikely to precipitate or worsen heart failure, and proarrhythmias are uncommon.[43]

Bretylium[5,44,45]

Bretylium increases action potential duration and the refractory period of cardiac tissues. It initially causes noradrenaline release, and then produces the equivalent of a sympathectomy, preventing noradrenaline release. Bretylium has an antifibrillatory effect on ventricular muscle, which may be more important than the class III effects in the emergency treatment of malignant ventricular arrhythmias. The initial release of noradrenaline may cause hypertension, which is followed by a fall in blood pressure when adrenergic tone is decreased. Bretylium does not depress myocardial contractility.

Clinical use

Bretylium is a useful adjunctive therapy to DC shock in managing life-threatening ventricular tachyarrhythmias, especially refractory VF. Although it has theoretical advantages over lignocaine, no significant differences were noted between them in managing out-of-hospital VF.[46] The recommended IV dose is 5 mg/kg over 15–20 min, but in a life-threatening emergency, this is often given over 1–2 min, and repeated once or twice if the arrhythmia persists. Maintenance infusion is 0.5–2.0 mg/min. Alternatively, a dose of 5–10 mg/kg may be infused slowly (over 15–30 min) every 6 h.

Adverse effects

The most significant side-effect is orthostatic hypotension. Nausea and vomiting may occur. Parotid pain only occurs with long-term oral therapy, which is never used nowadays.

Sotalol[47]

Sotalol prolongs action potential duration, thereby prolonging the effective refractory period in the atria, ventricles, AV node and accessory AV pathways. It is also a potent non-cardioselective β-adrenergic blocker (class II). Sotalol also has antifibrillatory actions which are superior to those of conventional β-blockers. It can worsen heart failure in patients with depressed LV function. The negative inotropic β-blocking effect is slightly offset by a weak positive inotropism, probably due to prolongation of the action potential (resulting in more time for calcium influx into myocardial cells).[47]

Clinical use

Higher doses of sotalol are required to prolong cardiac repolarization than to cause β-blockade.[47] Sotalol may be administered IV or orally, and is excreted by the kidneys (elimination half-life 15 h). IV dose is 0.5–1.5 mg/kg over 5–20 min. Oral therapy is initiated at 80 mg b.d. and increased to 160 mg b.d., although doses of 320 mg b.d. have been administered.

Supraventricular arrhythmias

Sotalol is effective in AV nodal and AV re-entry tachycardias, although adenosine and verapamil are superior. Long-term sotalol will prevent recurrences of these arrhythmias. Sotalol is probably ineffective for reversion of atrial flutter and fibrillation, but is effective in preventing recurrence of AF after cardioversion. Should AF recur, heart rate is likely to be well-controlled with sotalol.

Ventricular arrhythmias

Sotalol is as safe as, and more effective than, lignocaine to terminate sustained VT,[25] and should be considered a first-line drug. Oral sotalol is more effective than class I drugs for the long-term prevention of VT or VF.[8] Guided (Holter or electrophysiological testing) sotalol[8] or empirical amiodarone[40] (see above) are first-line drugs to prevent recurrences of VT and VF over the long term.

Adverse effects

Side-effects of sotalol are due mainly to β-blockade (e.g. bronchospasm, heart failure or AV conduction problems) and prolongation of QT (e.g. torsade de pointes – similar 2% incidence as quinidine, which may occur early during drug titration or later during long-term treatment).[8]

Class IV antiarrhythmic drugs

Class IV drugs block the slow calcium channels in cardiac tissue. Verapamil and diltiazem have similar electrophysiological effects. Nifedipine does not have any significant electrophysiological actions.

Verapamil[5]

Verapamil depresses the slope of diastolic depolarization in SA node cells, the rate of rise of phase 0 and action potential amplitude in SA and AV nodal cells, and slows conduction and prolongs the refractory period of the AV node.[5] Its main antiarrhythmic actions are associated with prolonged conduction and increased refractory period of the AV node. Refractoriness of atrial cells, ventricular muscle cells and accessory pathways is unchanged. Tachyarrhythmias incorporating the AV node as an integral part of the arrhythmia circuit will often terminate with verapamil. The sinus rate usually does not change significantly, because verapamil-induced peripheral vasodilatation causes reflect sympathetic stimulation of the SA node. Verapamil has marked negative inotropic actions, but cardiac index may not decline because afterload is reduced.

Clinical use

Verapamil may be given IV or orally. After IV administration, prolongation of AV conduction occurs within 1–2 min. The IV dose to treat a supraventricular tachycardia is 1.0 mg/min to a maximum of about 10 mg. Cardiac rhythm and blood pressure should be monitored. IV verapamil should be avoided in patients with poor cardiac function and those receiving β-blockers or disopyramide.

Verapamil will usually terminate AV nodal and AV re-entry tachycardias, although adenosine is probably the drug of choice. Verapamil slows the rapid ventricular response in atrial flutter and fibrillation (an infusion may be required), although termination of the arrhythmia is uncommon. Indeed, verapamil may, through a proarrhythmic effect, prolong episodes of AF.[48] Verapamil may increase the ventricular response in AF associated with the Wolff–Parkinson–White syndrome, and should be avoided in this situation. In general, verapamil should not be given to patients with a wide-complex tachycardia, because haemodynamic collapse may occur if the rhythm is VT.

Adverse effects

Constipation is the most common side-effect. Adverse haemodynamic effects may be counteracted to some extent by IV calcium. IV administration may cause hypotension and extreme bradycardia in patients with poor LV function, or who are receiving other cardiac-depressant drugs. It is contraindicated in patients with sinus node abnormalities, second- or third-degree AV block, VT and AF associated with Wolff–Parkinson–White syndrome. Verapamil increases serum digoxin concentrations.

Diltiazem

Diltiazem has similar electrophysiological effects to verapamil, but less negative inotropic effects.

Other antiarrhythmic drugs

Adenosine[49]

Adenosine stimulates specific A_1 receptors present on the surface of cardiac cells, thereby influencing adenosine-sensitive K^+ channel cyclic adenosine monophosphate production. It slows the sinus rate and prolongs AV node conduction, usually causing transient high-degree AV block. The half-life of adenosine is usually less than 2 s[49,50] as it is taken up by red blood cells and deaminated in the plasma. This ultrashort half-life is a major advantage over other antiarrhythmic drugs. The effects of adenosine can be antagonized by methylxanthines, especially aminophylline. Dipyridamole, an adenosine uptake blocker, potentiates the effect of adenosine.

Clinical use

Adenosine is the drug of choice to terminate AV nodal and AV re-entry tachycardias. Expected reversion rates exceed 90%. Its AV nodal blocking actions may unmask atrial activity (e.g. flutter waves in atrial flutter). Diagnosis of a wide-complex tachycardia may be assisted by the use of adenosine. Supraventricular tachycardias with intraventricular conduction block will terminate with adenosine, whereas few VTs will revert. Adenosine should probably be administered to all patients with a regular wide-complex tachycardia, unless it is considered that the tachycardia is ventricular in origin, or the mechanism is automatic or intra-atrial re-entry. Adenosine will not revert AF. Ventricular rate may transiently increase in AF associated with the Wolff–Parkinson–White syndrome.

Adenosine is given as a rapid bolus through a large peripheral or central vein followed by a saline flush, at intervals less than 60 s. The usual dose is 6 mg, followed by 12 mg if response is ineffective. Another 18 mg can be given if the last dose was well-tolerated.

Adverse effects

Most patients experience transient side-effects such as flushing, shortness of breath and chest discomfort. Adenosine should not be given to asthmatic patients; bronchospasm may result.

Digoxin

Digoxin slows the ventricular response in atrial flutter and fibrillation via an indirect vagal effect. Often other drugs (e.g. β-blockers or verapamil) are also required in patients with chronic AF, because digoxin will not effectively limit the ventricular response during exercise. Digoxin shortens the action potential duration of atrial tissue, and is ineffective for reverting supraventricular tachycardias such as AF, atrial flutter, AV nodal and AV re-entry tachycardias.

Magnesium[51]

Adequate potassium and magnesium repletion is necessary for all cardiac arrhythmias. Magnesium is a necessary co-factor for the membrane enzyme Na^+–K^+ATPase, and lack of magnesium may lead to intracellular K^+ depletion, which cannot be repleted until adequate magnesium has been administered. Magnesium may also have intrinsic antiarrhythmic actions. Torsade de pointes and ventricular arrhythmias associated with digitalis intoxication and possibly multifocal atrial tachycardia may benefit from magnesium therapy. In an emergency, magnesium (8 mmol) can be given as an IV bolus over 1–2 min, followed by 20 mmol over 6 h.[51] Magnesium is probably ineffective to treat sustained monomorphic VT, unless hypomagnesaemia is present.

The LIMIT-II study[52] (1500 patients) showed a significant improvement in survival when magnesium was given to patients with myocardial infarction. A much larger study (58 000 patients,[53] however, did not confirm this benefit, and there were possible adverse effects. At present, magnesium cannot be recommended as standard treatment for patients with acute myocardial infarction.

References

1 Roden DM (1994) Risks and benefits of antiarrhythmic therapy. *N Engl J Med* **331**:785–790.

2 Singh BN and Vaughan-Williams EM (1970) A third class of antiarrhythmic action: effects on atrial and ventricular intracellular potentials and other pharmacological actions on cardiac muscle of MJ 1999 and AH 3474. *Br J Pharmacol* **39**:675–687.

3 Singh BN and Vaughan Williams EM (1972) A fourth class of anti-dysrhythmic action? Effect of verapamil on ouabain toxicity, on atrial and ventricular intracellular potentials and on other features of cardiac function. *Cardiovasc Res* **6**:109–119.

4 Harrison DC (1986) Current classification of antiarrhythmic drugs as a guide to their rational use. *Drugs* **31**:93–95.

5 Zipes DP (1992) Management of cardiac arrhythmias: pharmacological, electrical and surgical techniques. In: Braunwald E (ed.) *Heart Disease: A Text Book of Cardiovascular Medicine.* Philadelphia: WB Saunders, pp. 628–666.

6 Stanton MS, Prystowsky EN, Fineberg NS, Miles WM, Zipes DP and Heger JJ (1989) Arrhythmogenic effects of antiarrhythmic drugs: a study of 506 patients treated for ventricular tachycardia or fibrillation. *J Am Coll Cardiol* **14**:209–215.

7 Minardo JD, Heger JJ, Miles WM *et al.* (1988) Clinical characteristics of patients with ventricular fibrillation during antiarrhythmic drug therapy. *N Engl J Med* **319**:257–262.

8 Mason JW (1993) A comparison of seven antiarrhythmic drugs in patients with ventricular tachyarrhythmias. *N Engl J Med* **329**:452–458.

9 The Cardiac Arrhythmia Suppression Trial (CAST) investigators (1989). Preliminary report: effect of encainide and flecainide on mortality in a randomized trial of arrhythmia suppression after myocardial infarction. *N Engl J Med* **321**:406–412.

10 Teo KK, Yusuf S and Furberg CD (1993) Effects of prophylactic antiarrhythmic drug therapy in acute myocardial infarction: an overview of results from randomized controlled trials. *J Am Med Assoc* **270**:1589–1595.

11 Burkhart F, Pfisterer M, Kiowski W, Follath F, Burckhardt D and Jordi H (1990) Effect of antiarrhythmic therapy on mortality in survivors of myocardial infarction with asymptomatic complex ventricular arrhythmias: BASEL antiarrhythmic study of infarct survival (BASIS). *J Am Coll Cardiol* **16**:1711–1718.

12 Ahmed R and Singh BN (1994) Antiarrhythmic drugs. *Curr Opinion Cardiol* **8**:10–21.

13 Singh BN and Ahmed R (1994) Class III antiarrhythmic drugs. *Curr Opinion Cardiol* **9**:12–22.

14 Hondeghem LM and Snyders DJ (1990) Class III antiarrhythmic agents have a lot of potential but a long way to go. Reduced effectiveness and dangers of reverse use dependence. *Circulation* **81**:686–690.

15 Coplen SE, Antman EM, Berlin JA, Hewitt P and Chalmers TC (1990) Efficacy and safety of quinidine therapy for maintenance of sinus rhythm after cardioversion. *Circulation* **82**:1106–1116.

16 Tzivoni D, Bonai S, Schuger C *et al.* (1988) Treatment of torsade de pointes with magnesium sulphate. *Circulation* **77**:392–397.

17 Morganroth J and Goin JE (1991) Quinidine-related mortality in the short to medium-term treatment of ventricular arrhythmias: a meta-analysis. *Circulation* **84**: 1977–1983.

18 Gorgels APM, Van den Dool A, Hofs A *et al.* (1989) Procainamide is superior to lidocaine in terminating sustained ventricular tachycardia. *Circulation* **80**:652.

19 Fenster PE, Comess KA, Marsh R, Katzenberg C and Hager WD (1983) Conversion of atrial fibrillation to sinus rhythm by acute intravenous procainamide infusion. *Am Heart J* **106**:510–514.

20 Podrid PJ, Schoeneberger A and Lown B (1980) Congestive heart failure caused by oral disopyramide. *N Engl J Med* **302**:614–617.

21 Wesley RC, Resh W and Zimmerman D (1991) Reconsiderations of the routine and preferential use of lidocaine – the emergent treatment of ventricular arrhythmias. *Crit Care Med* **9**:1439–1444.

22 Antman EM and Berlin JA (1992) Declining incidence of ventricular fibrillation in myocardial infarction: implications for the prophylactic use of lignocaine. *Circulation* **86**:764–773.

23 Armengol RE, Groff J, Baerman JM and Swiryn S (1989) Lack of effectiveness of lidocaine for sustained, wide QRS complex tachycardia. *Ann Emerg Med* **18**:254–257.

24 Nasir N, Taylor A, Doyle TK and Pacifico A (1994) Evaluation of intravenous lidocaine for the termination of sustained monomorphic ventricular tachycardia in patients with coronary artery disease with or without healed myocardial infarction. *Am J Cardiol* **74**:1183–1186.

25 Ho DSW, Zecchin RP, Richards DAB, Uther JB and Ross DL (1994) Double-blind trial of lignocaine versus sotalol for acute termination of spontaneous sustained ventricular tachycardia. *Lancet* **344**:18–23.

26 Gottlieb SS and Packer M (1989) Deleterious hemodynamic effects of lidocaine in severe congestive heart failure. *Am Heart J* **118**:611–612.

27 The Cardiac Arrhythmia Suppression Trial II Investigators (1992) Effect of the antiarrhythmic agent moricizine on survival after myocardial infarction. *N Engl J Med* **327**:227–233.

28 Roden DM and Woosley RL (1986) Flecainide. *N Engl J Med* **315**:36–41.

29 Donovan KD, Dobb GJ, Coombs LJ *et al.* (1991) Reversion of recent-onset atrial fibrillation to sinus rhythm by intravenous flecainide. *Am J Cardiol* **75**:693–697.

30 Donovan KD, Power BM, Hockings BEF, Dobb GJ and Lee K-Y (1995) Intravenous flecainide vs amiodarone for recent-onset atrial fibrillation. *Am J Cardiol* (in press).

31 Randozzo DN, Schweitzer P, Stein E, Banas Jr JS and Winters SL (1994) Flecainide induced atrial tachycardia with 1:1 ventricular conduction during exercise testing. *Pace* **17**:1509–1512.

32 Arsura E, Lefkin AS, Scher DL, Solar M and Tessler S (1988) A randomized double-blind placebo-controlled study of verapamil and metoprolol in treatment of multifocal atrial tachycardia. *Am J Med* **85**:519–524.

33 Steinbeck G, Andresen D, Bach P *et al.* (1992) A comparison of electrophysiologically guided antiarrhythmic drug therapy with beta-blocker therapy in patients with symptomatic, sustained ventricular tachyarrhythmias. *N Engl J Med* **327**:987–992.

34 ISIS-1 (First International Study of Infarct Survival) Collaborative Group (1986) Randomized trial of intravenous atenolol among 16 027 cases of suspected acute myocardial infarction. ISIS-1. *Lancet* **2**:57–65.

35 The Norwegian Multicenter Study Group (1981) Timolol-induced reduction in mortality and reinfarction in patients surviving acute myocardial infarction. *N Engl J Med* **304**:801–807.

36 Frishman WH, Murthy S and Strom JA (1988) Ultra-short-acting β-adrenergic blockers. *Med Clin North Am* **72**: 359–371.

37 Singh BN, Venkatesh N, Nademanee K, Josephson MA and Kannan R (1989) The historical development, cellular electrophysiology and pharmacology of amiodarone. *Prog Cardiovasc Dis* **31**:249–280.

38 Gill J, Heel RC and Fitton A. Amiodarone. *Drugs* **43**:69–110.

39 Pilati G, Lenzi T, Trisolino G *et al.* (1991) Amiodarone versus quinidine for the acute conversion of recent-onset atrial fibrillation to sinus rhythm. *Curr Ther Res* **49**:140–146.

40 Weinberg BA, Miles WM, Klein LS and Zipes DP (1993) Five year follow-up of 589 patients treated with amiodarone. *Am Heart J* **125**:109–115.

41 The CASCADE investigators (1993) Randomized antiarrhythmic drug therapy in survivors of cardiac arrest (the CASCADE study). *Am J Cardiol* **72**:280–287.

42 Hohnloser SH, Klingenheben T and Singh BN (1994) Amiodarone-associated proarrhythmic effects: a review with special reference to torsade de pointes tachycardia. *Ann Intern Med* **121**:529–535.

43 Greenspon AJ, Kidwell GA, Hurley W and Mannion J (1991) Amiodarone-related postoperative adult respiratory distress syndrome. *Circulation* **84**:407–415.

44 Anderson JL (1985) Bretylium tosylate: profile of the only available class III antiarrhythmic agent. *Clin Ther* **7**:205–224.

45 Paddu PE, Jouve R, Saadjian A and Torresani J (1986) Experimental and clinical pharmacology of bretylium tosylate in acute myocardial infarction: a 15-year journey. *J Pharmacol* **17**:223–243.

46 Haynes RE, Chinn TL, Copass MK and Cobb LA (1981) Comparison of bretylium tosylate and lidocaine in management of out of hospital ventricular fibrillation: a randomized clinical trial. *Am J Cardiol* **48**:353–356.

47 Hohnloser SH and Woosley RL. Sotalol. *N Engl J Med* **331**:32–38.

48 Shenasa M, Kus T, Fromer M, Le Blanc RA, Duboc M and Nadeau R (1988) Effects of intravenous and oral calcium antagonists (diltiazem and verapamil) on sustenance of atrial fibrillation. *Am J Cardiol* **62**:403–407.

49 Camm AJ and Garratt CJ (1991) Adenosine and supraventricular tachycardia. *N Engl J Med* **325**:1621–1629.

50 Barber MJ (1992) Clinical use of adenosine for arrhythmias. *Cor Art Dis* **3**:1127–1134.

51 Arsenian MA (1993) Magnesium and cardiovascular disease. *Prog Cardiovasc Dis* **35**:271–310.

52 Woods KL, Fletcher S and Roffe C (1992) Intravenous magnesium sulphate in suspected acute myocardial infarction: results of the second Leicester intravenous magnesium intervention trial (LIMIT-II). *Lancet* **339**:1553–1558.

53 ISIS-4 (Fourth International Study of Infarct Survival) Collaborative Group (1995) A randomised trial assessing oral captopril, oral mononitrate and intravenous magnesium sulphate in 58,050 patients with suspected acute myocardial infarction. *Lancet* **345**:669–685.

<table>
</table>

10	**Cardiac pacing**

KD Donovan and BEF Hockings

Cardiac pacing repetitively delivers very low electrical energies to the heart, thus initiating and maintaining cardiac rhythm. ICU physicians should be skilled in the procedure of temporary pacing, and familiar with the principles and devices of permanent pacing. Pacing may be temporary, with an external pulse generator, or permanent, with an implanted pulse generator. It is often associated with the treatment of bradycardia, but rapid atrial or ventricular pacing can be used to terminate certain supraventricular tachycardias (SVTs) and ventricular tachycardias (VTs) respectively.

Cardiac pacing in bradyarrhythmias

Electrode types

Pacing electrodes may be unipolar or bipolar.

Unipolar (Fig. 10.1)

The pacing lead has only one conducting wire and electrode. Electric current returns to the pacemaker via the body fluids. A unipolar lead is rarely used for temporary pacing, as a skin electrode is also needed for the return current pathway, which may cause muscle twitching. Unipolar systems are commonly used for permanent pacing. Over-sensing of electromagnetic interference or skeletal muscle potentials may be a significant problem.[1]

Bipolar (Fig. 10.2)

A bipolar lead has two conducting wires surrounded by a layer of insulation. Electric current travels down one wire to an electrode (usually the distal), passes through cardiac tissue to cause depolarization, and returns to the pacemaker via the second electrode. Inappropriate sensing of electromagnetic interference or myopotentials is uncommon. Bipolar pacing is the method of choice for temporary pacing. Should one limb fail, a bipolar system can be converted to a unipolar system by connecting the other limb tone pacemaker pole (usually positive). The other pole (usually negative) is connected to an electrocardiogram (ECG) skin electrode to complete a unipolar pacing circuit.

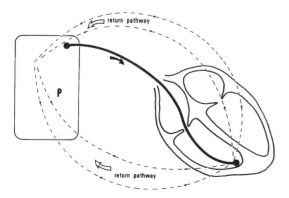

Fig. 10.1 Unipolar pacing lead. P = Pacemaker.

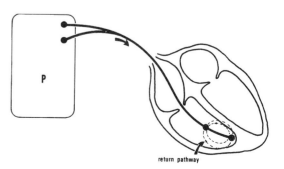

Fig. 10.2 Bipolar pacing lead. P = Pacemaker.

Pacing sites

Transvenous endocardial

The pacing lead is passed via a vein to the endocardial surface of the right atrium (RA), or most commonly, the right ventricle (RV; Fig. 10.1). Rarely, the left atrium (LA) may be paced via the coronary sinus.

Epicardial

This is mainly used in conjunction with cardiac surgery, where the electrodes are attached directly to the epicardial surface of the atrium and/or ventricle.

Transcutaneous (external transthoracic)[2]

Non-invasive transcutaneous cardiac pacing was previously unreliable and uncomfortable. The small-sized electrodes delivered a high current density and produced painful muscle stimulation. Recently, larger electrodes (8 cm diameter) have been developed which are better tolerated by the patient. Transcutaneous pacing devices can sense intrinsic ventricular rhythm and deliver adequate, adjustable current outputs (50–150 mA) and stimuli of long duration (pulse widths 10–40 ms). Some patients will still experience significant pain and may need analgesics. Although transcutaneous pacing can be initiated quickly by personnel unskilled in transvenous pacing, it is only a temporizing measure until the latter can be instituted. Reliable transcutaneous pacing has rendered prophylactic temporary transvenous pacing obsolete in most situations.

Other sites and methods

1 *Transthoracic myocardial puncture*[3] is dangerous and unreliable and should be abandoned in favour of transcutaneous pacing.
2 *Transoesophageal atrial pacing*[4] is safe and effective in refractory atrial flutter,[5] but should probably be replaced by transcutaneous pacing in most situations.

Pacing leads

Temporary pacing

Ventricular pacing

There are basically two types of leads:

1 *Semirigid (5–7 FG):* leads are fairly rigid, but are still flexible enough to be manipulated under fluoroscopic control to the correct position.
2 *Balloon-tipped:*[6] leads float the electrode into the correct position in the RV. If fluoroscopy is unavailable, intracardiac ECG should be monitored to assist with lead placement.

Atrial pacing

Atrial leads have a preformed J tip to hook into the RA appendage, as this usually ensures pacing lead stability with a low pacing threshold and good sensing capacity.

Permanent pacing

Leads for permanent pacing commonly use passive fixation with tines or fins close to the tip to ensure entanglement of the electrode in the trabeculae. Alternatively, active fixation with myocardial penetration by an extendable screw at the electrode tip is used.

Pacemaker modes

The North American Society of Pacing and Electrophysiology/British Pacing and Electrophysiology Group (NASPE/BPEG) code[7] is a generic code used to identify different modes of pacemaker (Table 10.1). The first three positions or letters refer exclusively to antibradycardia functions and describe all available emergency external pacing modes. The fourth and fifth positions describe additional functions which are only available with certain implantable devices. In practice, these letters are not often stated, except for R, which indicates a sensor-driven, rate-responsive pacemaker (see below).

Table 10.1 The pacemaker code NASPE/BPEG[7]

Position	I	II	III	IV	V
Category	Chamber(s) paced	Chamber(s) sensed	Response to sensing	Programmability, rate modulation	Antitachyarrhythmia function(s)
	O = None	O = None	O = None	O = None	O = None
	A = Atrium	A = Atrium	T = Triggered	P = Simple programmable	P = Pacing (antitachyarrhythmia)
	V = Ventricle	V = Ventricle	I = Inhibited	M = Multiprogrammable	S = Shock
	D = Dual	D = Dual	D = Dual		D = Dual
	(A + V)	(A + V)	(T + I)	R = Rate modulation	(P + S)

Positions I–III are used exclusively for antibradyarrhythmia function.

1 *Position I* refers to the chamber(s) paced, e.g. V for ventricle.
2 *Position II* refers to the chamber(s) sensed, e.g. V for ventricle.
3 *Position III* refers to the response to sensing (if any). This may be:
   (a) *I* (inhibition) – a pacemaker's discharge is inhibited (switched off) by a sensed signal, e.g. VVI, where ventricular pacing is inhibited by spontaneous ventricular activity.
   (b) *T* (triggering) – a pacemaker's discharge is triggered by a sensed signal, e.g. VAT, where ventricular pacing is triggered (after a suitable atrioventricular (AV) delay) by sensed P waves.
4 *Position IV* refers to programmability (ability to change *externally* certain parameters of the permanent internal pacemaker) and adaptive rate pacing. Possible descriptions include:
   (a) *P* or simple programmability – an ability to change simple parameters, usually rate and current output.
   (b) *M* or multiprogrammability – a more complex ability to change more parameters.
   (c) *C* or communicating – a telemetry function of the internal pacemaker.
   (d) *R* or rate-adaptive – an ability to vary the pacing rate through sensing one or more biological parameters that reflect the need for changes in cardiac output. This is in effect an artificial sinoatrial (SA) node. Currently available sensors include vibration (to detect physical activity), respiration, Q-T intervals, core temperature, RV oxygen saturation and blood pH.
5 *Position V* refers only to tachyarrhythmic functions:
   (a) *P* or pacing for tachycardias;
   (b) *S* or shock – an ability to deliver a DC shock when a tachycardia (usually VT or ventricular fibrillation, VF) is sensed.
   (c) *D* or dual, offering both pacing and DC shock. It is essential to distinguish clearly between antibradycardia and antitachycardia functions in permanent pacemakers. For example, an implantable defibrillator designated OOOMS will deliver a DC shock for detected VT or VF, whereas a VVIMS unit will, in addition, provide ventricular pacing should this be required. Both may have multiple parameters changed non-invasively.

Specific pacing modes

The three-position code (Fig. 10.3) is adequate to describe emergency temporary pacing and most forms of permanent pacing in the ICU (Table 10.2).

Single chamber pacing

1 *AOO and VOO (asynchronous atrial and ventricular)* pacing: There is no ability to sense cardiac activity (Fig. 10.4). Such pacing is obsolete.
2 *AAI (atrial demand) pacing:* This is indicated for sinus bradycardia provided AV conduction is intact (to maintain AV synchrony).
3 *VVI (ventricular demand) pacing (Fig. 10.5):* This is the most commonly used mode and the mode of choice in life-threatening bradyarrhythmias. Spontaneous cardiac rhythm is sensed, and there is minimal danger of pacemaker-induced ventricular tachyarrhythmia (Fig. 10.6). AV synchrony is, however, lost and there is no 'speed up for need'.

Dual chamber pacing

Two sets of electrodes are required (atrial and ventricular).

1 *DVI (AV sequential) pacing:* Atria and ventricles are paced in sequence (Fig. 10.7). After a stimulus is delivered to the atrium, there is a delay to enable the impulse to be conducted in a normal manner to the ventricles. If AV conduction is successful, the ventricular output of the pacemaker is then inhibited, otherwise the ventricle is paced. The advantage of this mode is that the atria and ventricles usually contract in sequence. To maintain AV synchrony in the absence of atrial sensing, the pacemaker discharge rate must be greater than the spontaneous atrial rate; asynchronous atrial pacing can precipitate atrial fibrillation (AF). Self-inhibition ('cross-talk') can occur, i.e. inappropriate detection of the atrial pacing stimulus by the ventricular channel; if there is no escape rhythm, asystole may result. DVI pacing is indicated when there is impaired AV conduction with an atrial bradycardia. It is of no value when atrial tachyarrhythmias are present.
2 *VDD (atrial synchronous ventricular inhibited) pacing:* This mode paces only the ventricle. Sensing takes place in both atrium and ventricle. A sensed P wave triggers ventricular pacing. VDD pacing is useful when normal sinus rhythm with a high degree of AV block is present.
3 *DDD pacing:* There is pacing and sensing in both chambers (Fig. 10.8). An atrial impulse will trigger a ventricular output and simultaneously inhibit an atrial output. If the impulse is conducted normally to the ventricle, the ventricular output is then inhibited, as with the DVI mode. Upper rate-limiters prevent the pacemaker from following excessive atrial activity with paced ventricular responses. Pacemaker function depends on the underlying cardiac rhythm:
   (a) Atrial bradycardia with intact AV conduction – atrial pacing.
   (b) Normal sinus rhythm with high-degree AV block – tracking of P waves with synchronized ventricular pacing.

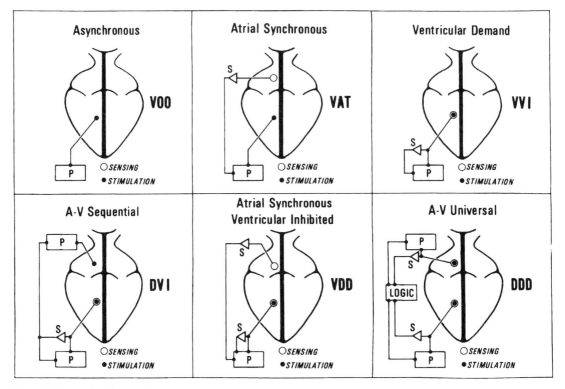

Fig. 10.3 Examples of pacemaker modes and their three-position (letter) codes. A-V = Atrioventricular; P = pacemaker; S = sensing.

(c) Sinus bradycardia with AV block – pacing the atria and ventricles sequentially.

(d) Normal sinus rhythm and AV conduction – inhibition of both atrial and ventricular pacing.

Self-inhibition can be prevented by introducing a ventricular blank (refractory) period coinciding with the atrial pacing stimulus. With DDD and VDD pacing, re-entry pacemaker-mediated 'endless-loop' tachycardias are possible.[8] These are commonly initiated by a ventricular premature beat (Fig. 10.9) conducted retrogradely to the atria, where it is sensed and ventricular pacing is triggered with an endless loop: the circuit's ante-rograde limb is the pacemaker, and the retrograde limb is via the AV node. Conversion to asynchronous (non-sensing) mode or increasing the pacemaker atrial refractory period will prevent endless-loop tachycardia.

4 *DDI pacing:* This has recently been introduced[9] and is available in some external pacemakers. Sensing occurs in both atria and ventricle, but sensed atrial events do not trigger ventricular pacing. This mode therefore prevents endless-loop tachycardias, and is useful in patients with SA node dysfunction and episodes of atrial tachyarrhythmias. During atrial tachyarrhythmias, the DDI pacemaker will simply pace the ventricle at its back-up rate and not track the tachycardia.

Haemodynamics of cardiac pacing

In the normal heart, cardiac output increases three- to fourfold during exercise, due mainly to increased heart rate and increased stroke volume. Synchronized contraction of the atria and ventricles (i.e. AV synchrony) contributes about 20% of cardiac output. Thus AV synchrony and an ability of pacemakers to increase heart rate (i.e. rate-adaptive) are important. Many permanent pacemakers are rate-adaptive. When temporary pacing is used, the arbitrarily set rate of 70–80 min may need to be increased if oxygen delivery is inadequate. For life-threatening bradyarrhythmias, increasing heart rate with VVI mode pacing is the treatment of choice. Permanent VVIR pacing (most commonly using an activity or a respiration sensor) will allow heart rate modulation. However, in ICU, adaptive rate changes may not occur. For example, no activity will be sensed in a patient with septic shock, even when cardiac output is low.

Table 10.2 Pacemaker modes

Code		Common designation	Comment
VOO	Paces the ventricle, no sensing	Fixed rate, asynchronous	Obsolete – except for pacemaker testing
VVI	Paces the ventricle, senses ventricular activity, ventricular activity inhibits the pacemaker	Ventricular demand	Most commonly used in life-threatening bradycardia
AAI	Paces the atrium, senses atrial activity, atrial activity inhibits the pacemaker		Indicated in sinus bradycardia with intact AV conduction
VAT	Paces the ventricle, senses atrial activity, atrial activity triggers ventricular pacing	Atrial synchronized, P-wave triggered	Obsolete – replaced by VDD and DDD
DVI	Paces both atrium and ventricle, senses only ventricular activity, ventricular activity inhibits atrial and ventricular pacing	AV sequential	Commonly used dual chamber pacing mode in ICU
VDD	Paces the ventricle only, senses atrial and ventricular activity	Atrial synchronous, ventricular inhibited	May be useful when normal sinus rhythm is present with a high-degree AV block
DDD	Paces and senses both atrium and ventricle: atrial activity triggers ventricular pacing		Often ideal but more complicated
DDI	Paces and senses both atrium and ventricle. Atrial activity not tracked; thus atrial tachyarrhythmias do not trigger rapid atrial pacing		Useful for sinus bradycardia with AV block and paroxysmal supra-ventricular tachyarrhythmias

AV = Atrioventricular: ICU = intensive care unit.

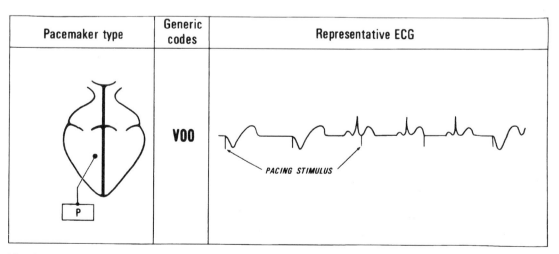

Fig. 10.4 Fixed-rate ventricular pacing VOO. P = Pacemaker.

Pacemaker type	Generic codes	Representative ECG
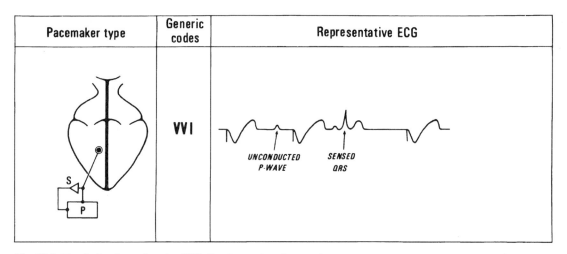	**VVI**	

Fig. 10.5 Ventricular demand pacing VVI. P = Pacemaker; S = sensing.

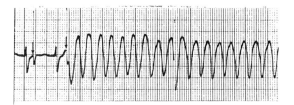

Fig. 10.6 Non-sensing of QRS (see first two beats). Pacing spikes (arrows) fall on the T wave with subsequent pacemaker-induced ventricular tachycardia.

During VVI and VVIR pacing, the atria and ventricles beat independently and AV synchrony is lost. Sometimes, when atria contract against closed AV valves, significant regurgitation of blood into the pulmonary and systemic circulation occurs with serious haemodynamic compromise. This 'pacemaker syndrome'[10] can be eliminated by restoring AV synchrony by atrial pacing or dual chamber pacing.

Physiological pacing means pacing the heart and maintaining synchrony of atrial and ventricular contraction and a heart rate response similar to that of a normal SA node. Emergency and long-term

Pacemaker type	Generic codes	Representative ECG
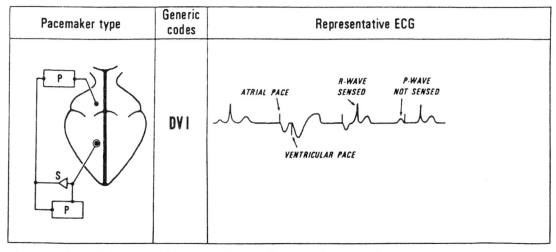	**DVI**	

Fig. 10.7 Atrioventricular sequential demand pacing DVI. P = Pacemaker; S = sensing.

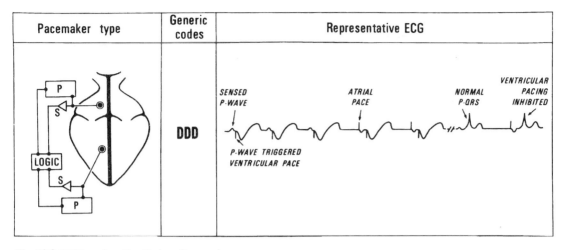

Pacemaker type	Generic codes	Representative ECG
	DDD	

Fig. 10.8 DDD pacing. P = Pacing; S = sensing.

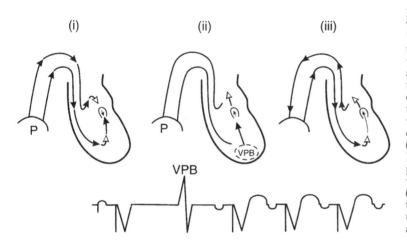

Fig. 10.9 Pacemaker-mediated 'endless-loop' tachycardia. *Note:* (1) Under normal conditions (first beat) there is no conduction from the ventricles to the atria because of atrioventricular block or because the atrial and ventricular impulses collide and extinguish each other in the atrioventricular node. (2) If a ventricular premature beat (VPB) is conducted retrogradely to the atria (second beat) inducing an inverted P wave, this may be sensed by the pacemaker (P) which then triggers a ventricular paced beat (third beat). (3) If the paced ventricular beat is then retrogradely conducted from the ventricle to the atria and sensed, an endless loop may occur (beats 4,5).

haemodynamic effects of physiological pacing are superior to VVI pacing.[11-13] Physiological pacing requires two pacing leads, one each in the RA and RV. AAI and DVI pacing under appropriate conditions provide AV synchrony but not rate adaptation. VDD and DDD pacing will usually ensure AV synchrony and heart rate responsiveness, and thus deliver physiological pacing, provided the SA node is normal.

Dual chamber pacemakers require the AV interval to be set as close as possible to the normal PR interval (140–200 ms). Traditionally, the pacing AV interval is arbitrarily set at about 150–200 ms. If interatrial conduction time (between RA and LA) is significantly prolonged, the LV may contract before or at the same time as the LA, causing a DDD pacemaker syndrome[14] with decreased stroke volume and cardiac output (due to LA contraction against a closed mitral valve). Hence, if there is evidence of inadequate cardiac output or impaired oxygen delivery, the AV interval may need to be increased appropriately, or optimized (e.g. by cardiac output or echocardiography measurements at various AV intervals). Favourable experience with pacing at a *short* AV interval has been reported in patients with severe hypertrophic obstructive cardiomyopathy[15] and severe idiopathic cardiomyopathy.[16,17]

Indications for cardiac pacing in bradyarrhythmias

Temporary pacing

Cardiac pacing is indicated for any sustained symptomatic bradycardia which does not promptly respond to medical treatment. Pacing may also be indicated if a bradycardia predisposes to malignant ventricular arrhythmias. The decision to pace is based on bradycardia associated with haemodynamic deterioration, and not on the specific rhythm disturbance. For example, pacing is indicated in a patient with AF and a ventricular response of 50/min, associated with a blood pressure of 70/40 mmHg (9.3/5.3 kPa), cardiac failure and oliguria. Pacing is not indicated in an asymptomatic, normotensive patient with an inferior infarction, complete heart block and a ventricular rate of 45/min.

Temporary pacing may be indicated prophylactically after cardiac (especially valve) surgery, and occasionally during cardiac catheterization and percutaneous transluminal coronary angioplasty. Asymptomatic patients with bifascicular block do not require prophylactic pacing prior to general anaesthesia, although transcutaneous pacing should be readily available. Patients with second- or third-degree AV block should be paced prior to general anaesthesia and surgery.

The role of temporary pacing in asymptomatic patients with acute myocardial infarction (AMI) is unclear. Many patients will have received thrombolytic agents, and central venous cannulation should be avoided. Prognosis is related to infarct size rather than the degree of AV block. Transcutaneous pacing obviates the need for prophylactic temporary transvenous pacing leads in high-risk patients. Pacing is sometimes required for patients with anterior or inferior myocardial infarction (Table 10.3).

Permanent pacing

Guidelines for permanent pacing have been published.[18] Indications are grouped into three classes:

1 *Class I:* Generally agreed indications, e.g. chronic symptomatic second- or third-degree AV block, SA node dysfunction with syncope or other major symptoms, and recurrent syncope associated with hypersensitive carotid sinus.
2 *Class II:* Controversial, but often used indications, e.g. asymptomatic complete AV block and resistant sinus bradycardia (<40/min) with minimal symptoms.

3 *Class III:* Pacing is not indicated, e.g. first-degree heart block and sinus bradycardia with no symptoms.

Technique of temporary transvenous pacing

Ventricular pacing

A sterile technique is mandatory. In emergencies, transcutaneous pacing is used first while transvenous VVI pacing is being prepared. A bipolar lead introduced under fluoroscopic control is most commonly used. If fluoroscopy is not immediately available, balloon-tipped leads or an atrial J lead may be used. The latter will invariably enter the RV when advanced far enough, to cause ventricular ectopy[19] and establish ventricular pacing. Blind passage of a standard lead, even with use of intracavity ECG monitoring, is unreliable and tedious.

Percutaneous insertion via the right internal jugular vein probably offers least complications with ease of manipulation and stability of the lead. Antecubital veins are associated with lead instability and thrombophlebitis. The femoral vein is best avoided except in patients who have received thrombolytic agents, because of problems with sterility and increased risk of deep vein thrombosis.[20] The pacing lead is introduced using the Seldinger technique and manipulated under fluoroscopic control to the apex of the RV (Fig. 10.10). The lead may occasionally enter the coronary sinus and pace the LA instead of the RV. If this is suspected, the lead is repositioned and checked by lateral chest X-ray or fluoroscopy.

Atrial pacing

Inserting the atrial J lead is similar to that for ventricular pacing. Correct positioning requires experience and should not be undertaken in an emergency. The right atrial appendage is anterior and medial, and the lead tip is advanced anteriorly and to the patient's left, after passing from the superior vena cava to the RA (Fig. 10.10). The correct position can be confirmed by a lateral chest X-ray or fluoroscopy.

Table 10.3 Complete atrioventricular (AV) block in acute myocardial infarction

	Inferior	Anterior
Onset	Slow (usually via Mobitz 1)	Sudden (usually via Mobitz II)
QRS complex	Narrow	Wide
Ventricular rate	>45 beats/min	<45 beats/min (often 20–30 beats/min)
Escape pacemaker	Stable	Unstable
Drug response (e.g. atropine)	Yes	No
Haemodynamic effects	No (usually)	Yes
Permanent pacing	No	Yes (if high-degree AV block persists)
Prognosis	Good	Very poor

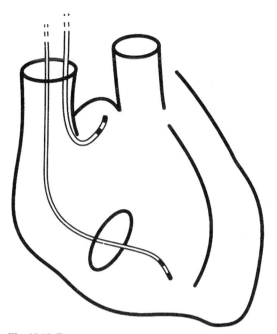

Fig. 10.10 Temporary transvenous pacing leads. Ideally positioned in the right atrium (right atrial appendage) and apex of right ventricle.

Dual chamber pacing

Older dual chamber external pacemakers provide only DVI pacing. Modern external pacemakers are available (*see* Plate 1) which will pace in all modes These units are small and can fit into a small pouch suitable for mobile patients.

Testing the pacing leads

Pacing threshold and sensing can be tested adequately using the external pacemaker. Occasionally, a more sophisticated pacing systems analyser may be required.

Pacing threshold

The lead is attached to the external pulse generator with the distal electrode connected to the negative pacemaker terminal. The cardiac chamber is then paced at 5–10 beats/min faster than patient heart rate, while the pulse generator's output is slowly decreased until consistent capture outside the myocardial refractory period is lost. Threshold testing is always performed at an identical pulse duration, usually 0.5–1.0 ms. Ideally, ventricular pacing threshold should be ≤ 1.0 V and the atrial threshold ≤ 1.5 V. Pacemaker output is usually set at 2–3 times pacing threshold, to allow a reasonable safety margin. After AMI, the amplitude must not be set higher than

necessary, as inadvertent pacing during the vulnerable period of the cardiac cycle may result in VT or VF.

Sensing

A pacemaker senses the potential difference between the two pacing electrodes. The amplitude of the ventricular signal is commonly 5–15 mV and the atrial signal 2–5 mV. Most pacemakers can sense signals as small as 1 mV. Pacing systems analysers can directly measure atrial and ventricular signals, but use of external pulse generators is simpler. The pacing amplitude is set at zero, thereby avoiding potentially dangerous competition between the pacemaker and the spontaneous cardiac rhythm. Pacing rate is then set lower than the spontaneous rate of the tested cardiac chamber, and the pacemaker sensitivity is decreased until there is competition between paced and spontaneous cardiac rhythms. The pacemaker sensitivity is then set at twice that value. This involves reducing the numerical sensitivity value (e.g. changing sensitivity from 2.0 to 1.0 mV will double the sensitivity). This method should not be attempted in completely pacemaker-dependent patients.

Assessment of sensing is important particularly in inferior infarction with RV involvement, when the intracardiac ventricular signal may be very small and not sensed. The resultant competition between pacemaker and spontaneous cardiac rhythm can initiate VT[21] (Fig. 10.6) or VF.[22]

Complications of temporary pacing[23,24]

Temporary transvenous pacemaker insertions should have a very low complication rate. Complications may include:

1 those associated with central venous line insertion. Perforation of the RV can occur, but rarely results in cardiac tamponade;
2 undersensing, with pacemaker-induced arrhythmias; oversensing, with pacemaker inhibition and loss of pacing stimuli; and failure to capture due usually to device defects, unstable lead position, increasing pacing threshold and RV perforation;
3 diaphragmatic pacing which may be associated with RV perforation;
4 thrombus formation, which is uncommon.

Failure to pace

A life-threatening situation may arise if the pacemaker suddenly fails. The following is an approach to such an emergency.

1 The pacemaker output is increased to its maximum setting (usually 20 mA or 10 V).
2 The asynchronous VOO mode is selected to prevent oversensing.

3 All leads and connections are checked. Faulty leads and connections are the most common causes of pacemaker failure.
4 Consideration is given to replacing the pacemaker unit or the batteries.
5 External transcutaneous pacing should be started if available, until a new pacing system can be placed.
6 Cardiopulmonary resuscitation and positive chronotropic drugs such as atropine and isoprenaline may be necessary.

Programmers for permanent implanted pacemakers[25]

A programmable pacemaker can have its mode and parameters reset by signals emitted from an external programmer. Programmability is helpful to assess various pacemaker complications. The pacemaker format best suited to a particular patient's needs may change with time, and programmability enables optimal pacemaker function to be achieved, i.e. 'prescribed'. Simple programmable pacemakers usually allow alteration of pacing rate, output (voltage and pulse width) and sensitivity. Pacing rate changes may be indicated under certain circumstances (e.g. decreased in a stable patient with angina or AMI to reduce myocardial oxygen consumption, or increased in a patient with haemorrhagic shock or cardiac failure). Multiprogrammable (usually dual chamber) pacemakers can adjust other pacing parameters (Table 10.4).

Cardiac pacing in tachyarrhythmias[26–28]

Certain tachyarrhythmias may be treated safely and effectively by rapid pacing and/or premature electrical stimulation. These include:

1 AV nodal re-entry tachycardia (AVNRT);
2 AV re-entry tachycardia (AVRT);
3 atrial flutter;
4 VT.

AVNRT and AVRT rarely require rapid atrial pacing, as treatment with drugs such as adenosine or verapamil is usually successful. Atrial flutter, however, is often resistant to drug therapy, and rapid atrial pacing will usually convert it to sinus rhythm.[24] Dual chamber pacing with a short AV interval can be used to prevent occasional drug-resistant AVNRT or AVRT.[29,30] Rapid continuous atrial pacing can be used to slow ventricular rate during resistant SVTs associated with a rapid ventricular response,[31] by

Table 10.4 Multiprogrammable permanent dual chamber pacemakers

Parameter	Adjustment	Comments
Rate	Increase	Increase cardiac output
	Decrease	Reduce myocardial oxygen consumption
		To assess underlying cardiac rhythm
Output	Increase	Increasing output may result in successful pacing when there is failure to capture
	Decrease	Increases battery life
Sensitivity	Increase	Reducing numerical value increases sensing ability
		May cause oversensing occasionally
	Decrease	Increasing numerical value decreases sensing ability
		Useful in oversensing, e.g. T-wave sensing
Mode	DDD to DDI, DVI	To prevent endless-loop tachycardias in patients with sinus bradycardia and supraventricular tachycardias
	DDD to VVI	Necessary if chronic atrial fibrillation develops
AV Interval	Increase/decrease	To optimize stroke volume and cardiac output
Refractory period (atrial/ventricular)	Increase	To minimize oversensing, e.g. to prevent ventricular sensing in AAI pacing
	Decrease	To optimize sensing under certain circumstances
Hysteresis		To preserve AV synchrony by delaying the onset of VVI pacing until the spontaneous heart rate is significantly less than the back-up ventricular pacing rate
Polarity	Unipolar mode	To improve sensing. Occasionally to allow pacing to continue when fracture of the other conducting wire occurs
	Bipolar	To prevent oversensing, e.g. muscle potentials

AV = Atrioventricular.

Table 10.5 Pacing versus cardioversion for the treatment of tachyarrhythmias

Pacing may assist in rhythm diagnosis
Pacing may be used (cautiously) in digitalis intoxication
Pacing does not require a general anaesthetic
Pacing avoids complications of DC shock, especially myocardial depression
Repeated reversions are easier with pacing
Standby pacing is immediately available should bradycardia or asystole occur after electrical reversion

DC = Direct current.

Table 10.6 Pacing versus drug therapy for the treatment of tachyarrhythmias

Pacing may aid in arrhythmia diagnosis
Pacing avoids drug-induced cardiac depression and other drug side-effects
Pacing can be used when drug therapy has failed
Termination of the tachycardia with pacing is often immediate
Standby pacing is immediately available

Table 10.7 Indications for rapid cardiac pacing in suitable arrhythmias

Failure of drug therapy
Recurrent arrhythmias
Contraindication for cardioversion (e.g. digitalis intoxication)
Aid to arrhythmia diagnosis (e.g. wide-complex tachycardia to differentiate ventricular tachycardia from supraventricular tachycardia)

inducing AF and a high degree of AV block. Sustained VT is responsive to rapid ventricular pacing, but this should not be used for very rapid ventricular rates (e.g. >300/min), or when severe haemodynamic compromise is present and immediate DC cardioversion is indicated. Rapid cardiac pacing may at times have advantages over DC cardioversion (Table 10.5) and drug therapy (Table 10.6), but is of no value in sinus tachycardia, AF and VF (Table 10.7).

Supraventricular tachyarrhythmias

The pacing lead is manipulated to a suitable position in the RA or coronary sinus. Atrial pacing is started at a slow rate (e.g. 60–80/min) and increased slowly to about 10–20% faster than the spontaneous atrial rate. Inadvertent ventricular pacing, especially at rapid rates, must be avoided. The atrium is paced for about 30 s and the pacemaker is then switched off. Normal sinus rhythm should ensue (Fig. 10.11). If not, the pacing lead is manipulated to a different position and/or a faster pacing rate is tried. A more prolonged pacing period may be effective. If sinus rhythm still does not result, AF is deliberately precipitated by rapid atrial pacing at 400–800/min. This is an unstable rhythm which usually reverts spontaneously to normal sinus rhythm. AF persists ccasionally, but the ventricular rate is usually slower and more responsive to drug therapy than that of the SVT.[31]

Ventricular tachycardia

Useful techniques to pace VT include:

1. underdrive ventricular pacing at rates less than that of the tachycardia;
2. overdrive atrial pacing may be useful if there is 1:1 AV conduction;
3. timed ventricular premature beats may be effective but this is complex.
4. Ventricular burst pacing (similar to rapid atrial pacing) is simple and effective. The ventricle is paced at a rate about 120% of the spontaneous VT rate for 5–10 beats. Normal sinus rhythm should ensue (Fig. 10.12). Potential complications include entrainment (Fig. 10.13, i.e. speeding up of VT) and precipitation of VF. Trained personnel, a defibrillator, and resuscitation facilities must be available.

Implantable cardioverter/defibrillator (ICD)[32]

This is an implantable device which can recognize and automatically terminate VT or VF. The ICD may be

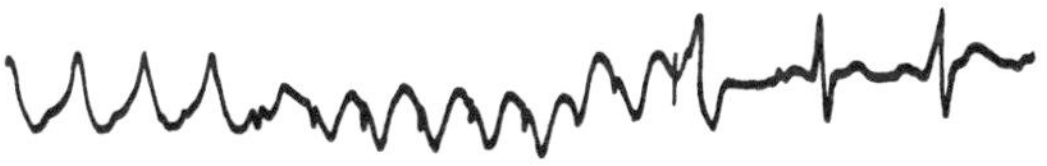

Fig. 10.12 Wide-complex tachycardia. Ventricular burst pacing with ventricular capture results in normal sinus rhythm on cessation of pacing.

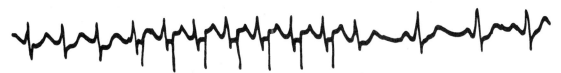

Fig. 10.11 Narrow-complex tachycardia. Rapid atrial pacing with atrial capture results in sinus rhythm on cessation of pacing.

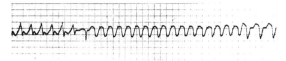

Fig. 10.13 Example of entrainment. Wide-complex tachycardia is followed by ventricular burst pacing. When pacing is discontinued, a wide-complex tachycardia of opposite polarity is precipitated.

indicated for long-term treatment of life-threatening malignant ventricular arrhythmias not associated with recent myocardial infarction. Modern devices are programmable, have multiple function modes, are capable of ventricular pacing and defibrillation, and can store detected arrhythmias which can subsequently be transmitted by telemetry. ICDs can be programmed to function in a sequential manner; rapid ventricular pacing occurs when VT is sensed, and should reversion not occur, low-energy, followed, if necessary, by high-energy shock is discharged. ICD systems with transvenous leads are now available. A single-lead system has recently been introduced[33]. It is generally considered that ICDs decrease the incidence of sudden death in high-risk patients,[34,35] but total mortality remains disturbingly high.

References

1 Levine PA, Caplan CH, Klein MD, Brodsky SJ and Ryan JJ (1982) Myopotential inhibition of unipolar lithium pacemakers. *Chest* **82**:101–103.

2 Kelly JS and Royster RL (1989 Non-invasive transcutaneous cardiac pacing. *Anesth Analg* **69**:229–238.

3 Tintinalli JE and White BC (1981) Transthoracic pacing during CPR. *Ann Emerg Med* **10**:113–116.

4 Barold SS (1990) Transesophageal pacing. *Pace* **13**:1324–1325.

5 Tucker KJ and Wilson C (1993) A comparison of transoesophageal atrial pacing and direct current cardioversion for the termination of atrial flutter: a prospective, randomised clinical trial. *Br Heart J* **69**:530–535.

6 Lang R, David D, Klein HO *et al.* (1981) The use of the balloon-tipped floating catheter in temporary transvenous cardiac pacing. *Pace* **4**:491–496.

7 Bernstein AD, Camm AJ, Fletcher RD *et al.* (1987) The NASPE/BPEG generic pacemaker code for antibradyarrhythmic and adaptive rate pacing and antitachyarrhythmic devices. *Pace* **10**:794–799.

8 Furman S and Fisher JD (1982) Endless-loop tachycardia in an AV universal (DDD) pacemaker. *Pace* **5**:486–489.

9 Irwin M, Harris L, Cameron D, Louis C, Radvanszky E and Goldman B (1994) DDI pacing: indication, expectations and follow-up. *Pace* **17**:274–279.

10 Johnson AD, Laiken SL and Engler RL (1978) Hemodynamic compromise associated with ventriculo-atrial conduction following transvenous pacemaker placement. *Am J Med* **65**:75–81.

11 Wirtzfeld A, Schmidt G, Himmler FC and Stangl K (1987) Physiological pacing: present status and future developments.

12 Kruse I, Arnman K, Conradson TB and Ryden L (1982) A comparison of the acute and long-term hemodynamic effects of ventricular inhibited and atrial synchronous ventricular inhibited pacing. *Circulation* **65**:846–855.

13 Donovan KD, Dobb GJ and Lee KY (1991) The haemodynamic importance of maintaining atrioventricular synchrony during cardiac pacing in critically ill patients. *Crit Care Med* **19**:320–326.

14 Pierantozzi A, Bocconcelli P and Sgarbi E (1994) DDD pacemaker syndrome and atrial conduction time. *Pace* **17**:374–376.

15 Fananapazir L, Cannon RO III, Trilpodi D and Panza JA (1992) Impact of dual-chamber permanent pacing in patients with obstructive hypertrophic cardiomyopathy with symptoms refractory to verapamil and β-adrenergic blocker therapy. *Circulation* **85**:2149–2161.

16 Hochleitner M, Hörtnagl H, Fridrich L and Gschnitzner F (1992) Long-term efficacy of physiologic dual chamber pacing in treatment of end-stage idiopathic dilated cardiomyopathy. *Am J Cardiol* **70**:1320–1325.

17 Auricchio A, Sommariva L, Salo RW, Scafuri A and Chiariello L (1993) Improvement of cardiac function in patients with severe congestive heart failure and coronary artery disease by dual chamber pacing with shortened AV delay. *Pace* **16**:2034–2047.

18 Dreifus LS, Fisch C, Griffen JC, Gillette PC, Mason JW and Parsonnet V (1991) Guidelines for implantation of cardiac pacemaker and antiarrhythmia devices. ACC/AHA task force report. *Circulation* **84**:455–467.

19 Davis MJE (1990) Emergency ventricular pacing using a J-electrode without fluoroscopy. *Med J Aust* **152**:194–195.

20 Pandian NG Kosowsky BD and Gurewich V (1980) Transfemoral temporary pacing and deep vein thrombosis. *Am Heart J* **100**:847–880.

21 Ceuni TA, White RA and Burkart F (1980) Pacemaker-induced ventricular tachycardia in patients with acute inferior myocardial infarction. *Internat J Cardiol* **1**:93–97.

22 Mooss AN, Ross WB and Esterbrooks DJ (1982) Ventricular fibrillation complicating pacemaker insertion in acute myocardial infarction. *Cath Cardiol Diag* **8**:253–259.

23 Austin R, Preis JK, Crampton WS, Beller GA and Martin RP (1983) Analysis of pacemaker function and complications of temporary pacing in the coronary care unit. *Am J Cardiol* **49**:301–306.

24 Donovan KD and Lee KY (1985) Indications for and complications of temporary transvenous cardiac pacing. *Anaesth Intens Care* **13**:63–70.

25 Schoenfeld MH (1993) A primer on pacemaker programmes. *Pace* **16**:2044–2051.

26 Zipes DP (1987) Electrical treatment of tachycardia. *Circulation* **75** (suppl. III):190–193.

27 Fisher JD, Kim SG and Mercando AD (1988) Electrical devices for the treatment of arrhythmias. *Am J Cardiol* **61**:45A–57A.

28 De Belder MA, Malik M, Ward DE and Camm AJ (1990) Pacing modalities for tachycardia termination. *Pace* **13**:231–248.

29 Attuel P, Pellerin D, Mugica J and Coumel PH (1988) DDD pacing: an effective treatment modality for recurrent atrial arrhythmias. *Pace* **11**:1647–1654.

30 Davies CW, Butrous GS, Spurrell RA and Camm AJ (1987) Pacing techniques in the prophylaxis of junctional reentry tachycardia. *Pace* **10**:519–532.

31 Moreira DAR, Shepard RB and Waldo AL (1989) Chronic rapid atrial pacing to maintain atrial fibrillation: use to permit control of ventricular rate in order to treat tachycardia induced cardiomyopathy. *Pace* **10**:519–532.

32 Raitt MH and Bardy GH (1994) Advances in implantable cardioverter-defibrillator therapy. *Curr Opinion Cardiol* **9**:23–29.

33 Bardy GH, Johnson G, Poole JE *et al.* (1993) A simplified, single-lead uinpolar transvenous cardioverson defibrillation system. *Circulation* **88**:543–547.

34 Nisam S, Mower M and Moser S (1991) ICD clinical update: first decade, initial 10 000 patients. *Pace* **14**:255–262.

35 Gilman JK, Jalal S and Naccerelli GV (1994) Predicting and preventing sudden death from cardiac causes. *Circulation* **90**:1083–1092.

11 | Cardioversion and defibrillation

RP Lee

Cardioversion and defibrillation are electrical therapies to treat arrhythmias. Cardioversion refers to the passage of electrical current across the heart, usually synchronized to the electrocardiogram (ECG), to revert organized supraventricular or ventricular arrhythimias. It is applied when tachyarrhythmias are symptomatic or resistant to drug therapy, being most useful for re-entry tachyarrhythmias. Defibrillation refers to the passage of high-dose electrical current to treat ventricular fibrillation (VF). It is the principal therapy for VF. Time from cardiac arrest to defibrillation is the most important determinant of outcome after cardiac arrest[1-4] (see Chapter 7).

General principles[5-7]

The aim of electrical therapy is to provide current through the myocardium to change enough myocardial cells to the same electrical state, for sufficient time to break re-entrant circuits or produce electrical homogeneity. This allows a stable rhythm to be re-established from the sinus node. Animal experiments have shown that the period of homogeneity needs to be 4–12 ms. More organized arrhythmias (e.g. atrial flutter or monomorphic ventricular tachycardia (VT)) require less energy to break the circuit (5–10 J internal, 20–100 J external) compared to disorganized rhythms (e.g. VF, 10–30 J internal, 200–300 J external).

After defibrillation, normal electrical impulse generation is established and myocardial contraction follows. However, contraction may be extremely weak ('stunned'), recovering over minutes to hours, depending on the duration of pre-existing arrhythmia.[8]

Equipment

Electricity was first used in experiments in the 18th century to revive animals. The first human experience of defibrillation was with alternating current (AC), which is more likely to produce arrhythmias and myocardial damage. Modern defibrillators deliver a variable amount of direct current (DC) energy across two electrodes. The output waveform is usually half sinusoidal. Electrodes are placed on the chest, on opposite sides of the heart.

The resultant current through the myocardium to achieve myocardial depolarization is dependent on the energy selected, electrical properties of the conductive medium (e.g. gel or pad), paddle or electrode placement, and resistance to current flow through the chest, i.e. transthoracic impedance (TI), usually 15–150 ohms (Ω) in humans.[9] (Current achieved is a product of energy selected divided by TI.) As little as 4% of the delivered current actually traverses the heart, and 96% takes alternate routes through the chest wall.[10] Total impedance to current flow is dependent on electrode size, coupling material, number and interval of previous shocks, phase of respiration, size of the chest, presence of lung disease and paddle pressure.

Most defibrillators have the capacity to sense the patient's QRST and synchronize events to the ECG. A light on the machine flashes with each QRS, and a spike is shown on the QRS on the oscilloscope. Synchronized cardioversion should be used for all arrhythmias with the exception of VF and polymorphic VT. Synchronization delivers the current during the R wave of the ECG, and not during a vulnerable period just before the T wave, which risks producing VF.

A DC defibrillator usually has a variable transformer, an AC to DC converter, a capacitor to store the energy, and charge and discharge switches to complete the circuit. Defibrillators are available in various configurations for different purposes:

1 Automated external defibrillators (AEDs), which may be manually operated (for medical officer use), semiautomatic (for ambulance officer use) and automatic (for lay operator use).

2 Automatic implanted defibrillators (AIDs) for high-risk patients (see Chapter 8).

A manual AED requires the operator to diagnose the rhythm disturbance, select the charge, charge up the device, and deliver a shock. A semiautomatic AED will diagnose the rhythm; the operator is then able to proceed to shock. Any nurse or ambulance officer, after a short period of training, is able to use the semiautomatic AED. An automatic AED proceeds through all steps automatically, including shocking the patient. It may be used by lay rescuers or relatives of at-risk patients. A potential shortcoming of automatic and semiautomatic AEDs is their inability to detect and respond to fine VF, defined arbitrarily as a deflection smaller than 1 mm on the surface ECG. They are not available for children.

Defibrillators can interface with the patient using:

1 paddles with liquid gel, cream or paste;
2 paddles with disposable impregnated pads;
3 disposable self-adhesive electrode pads;
4 intracardiac or epicardial electrodes;
5 epicardial paddles.

The interface choice is dependent on the setting. Electrolyte-impregnated pads have superseded the use of liquid gel for most external defibrillations, because of ease of use, less risk of electrode–electrode contact, and the chest is not too greasy for external cardiac compression.[11] Gel can smear, creating a low-impedance pathway for current to flow across the skin. Self-adhesive electrode pads are commonly used in semiautomatic or automatic AEDs, and require skin prepping.[12] The optimum electrode size is 13 cm in adults, 8–10 cm in children and 4.5–5.0 cm in infants.[13]

Positioning of the electrodes or paddles can be:

1 transthoracic, either anterior chest-to-apex (usual positioning in emergencies), or anterior-to-posterior chest;
2 epicardial/endocardial (i.e. an AID or use during cardiac surgery);
3 oesphageal (which is being studied).

The electrodes should not be placed over the sternum, vertebral column or scapula. Bone has a high impedance, and will cause current to traverse skin and subcutaneous tissues around the chest.

Maintenance of defibrillators[14]

Defibrillator malfunction in an emergency may lose the opportunity to resuscitate a patient in VF successfully. A high proportion of defibrillators have been reported to have malfunctioned or failed performance standards. The majority of reported malfunctions are due to improper operation or maintenance (including the batteries). Defibrillator function must be regularly checked (e.g. with each change of staff), and a checklist is essential to identify problems. Each check must be recorded. Proper electrical maintenance must also be regularly performed and recorded.

Specific techniques

Cardioversion

Elective cardioversion is used to treat atrial flutter, atrial fibrillation (AF), supraventricular tachycardia and non-pulseless VT, particularly if they are refractory to drug therapy or are associated with angina, heart failure or low cardiac output. If time permits, the patient should be fasted (nil by mouth) for 6 h, and anticoagulation considered. Cardioversion of AF has a thromboembolic risk of 3–7% if anticoagulation is not administered. Anticoagulation should be administered to patients with AF of longer than 48 h duration. It is usually not administered to patients with acute-onset AF after thoracic or cardiac surgery (see Chapter 8). Transoesophageal echocardiographic detection of left atrial thrombus before cardioversion is infrequent in non-valvular AF. However, thromboembolic complications without pre-existing left atrial thrombus suggest that cardioversion may promote new thrombus formation in the atrium.[8]

Serum electrolyte measurements must be checked beforehand, and digoxin toxicity excluded.[15] Informed consent should be obtained. The procedure should be performed with adequate monitoring and resuscitation facilities including suction, oxygen source, emergency pacing, ECG monitoring, non-invasive blood pressure monitoring and pulse oximetry.

A large-bore IV cannula is inserted, and an equipment check is carried out. The patient is pre-oxygenated for 4 min with 100% oxygen, prior to administration of anaesthesia. Benzodiazepines, thiopentone and propofol have been successfully used. Synchronization is checked before charging and then discharging the defibrillator. The amount of energy selected is dependent on the arrhythmia. Energy in the range of 25–50 J terminates most supraventricular arrhythmias other than AF, which requires starting levels in the range of 50–100 J. Patients with stable monomorphic VT require initial levels of 25–50 J. Polymorphic VT, which is more rapid and disorganized, behaves like VF, and the initial shock should therefore be 200 J.

Cardioversion restores sinus rhythm in 70–95% of patients, depending on the type of tachyarrhythmia. Sinus rhythm remains after 12 months in less than one-third to one-half of patients with chronic AF.

Defibrillation

Emergency defibrillation should be used to treat VF or pulseless VT. The interval between collapse and delivery of an effective shock is the strongest determinant of survival. There is no time for preparation beyond diagnosis of the rhythm, charging and discharging the defibrillator. Defibrillation is a priority in cardiac arrest because:

1 most patients will be in VF;
2 electrical defibrillation is the only effective method of terminating VF;
3 prospects of success decline rapidly with time; VF degenerates into asystole;
4 basic life support is a poor substitute for normal cardiac and respiratory function;
5 modern defibrillators have rapid diagnosis and charge times.

The defibrillator should not be in synchronized mode, because there is no organized electrical cardiac activity in VT or VF. The energy level chosen for the initial shock is a compromise between risking myocardial damage from excessive current[16–18] and unsuccessful defibrillation from too low a current.[19] The American Heart Association,[6] Australian Resuscitation Council[20] and the European Resuscitation Council[21] recommend 200 J for the first attempt in adults (2 J/kg in children). Since TI declines with successive shocks, the second attempt may be at 200–300 J. If this fails then another shock at maximum joules (360 J) is administered. The causes of failed defibrillation are listed in Table 11.1. Full cardiopulmonary resuscitation is discussed in Chapter 7.

Impedance may be reduced by strong pressure on the paddles, anteroposterior positioning of the paddles, repetitive shocks and delivery of the shock during expiration.[22,23] Precautions must be taken to avoid the following:

1 discharge over ECG electrodes;
2 discharge over nitroglycerin skin patches – explosions can occur;
3 discharge over an implanted device (e.g. pacemaker box);
4 direct or indirect contact with the patient during discharge;
5 patient contact with metal fixtures.

Complications

Embolic phenomena may occur after cardioversion of AF. The myocardium may be damaged from high-energy shocks. Myocardial necrosis, enzyme changes and ECG changes have been reported. VF can result from a low-energy shock during the vulnerable period. Bradycardias or asystole may follow the electrical shock. Pacemaker malfunction may occur transiently

Table 11.1 Causes of defibrillation failures

Myocardial unresponsiveness
Prolonged VF (declining ECG amplitude due to prolonged VF is strongly associated with decreased survival and stability of rhythm)

Acidosis

Electrolyte imbalance (e.g. hypokalaemia, hypomagnesaemia)

Hypoglycaemia

Digoxin toxicity

Failure to deliver current (suggested by absence of muscle twitch response)
Defibrillator failure

Dead battery

Broken leads

Increased transthoracic impedance
Poor paddle contact or pressure

Failure to use a conductive medium (e.g. gel, cream, pad)

Poor electrode placement (e.g. over bone)

Large chest diameter (e.g. inspiration, obesity)

VF = Ventricular fibrillation; ECG = electrocardiogram.

with loss of capture, or permanently with elevation of threshold. In emergencies, aspiration of gastric contents may be a serious complication if the airway is unprotected. Burns to the chest wall may result from repetitive high-dose shocks or poor paddle contact. Operator injury may occur if there is any electrical contact with the patient.

Special situations

Implantable defibrillators[24]

These devices are becoming common. They are useful for patients with recurrent VF or pulseless VT. The defibrillator is larger than a pacemaker, and is usually implanted in the upper abdomen. It is attached to the heart by suturing defibrillation pads directly on the epicardium or pericardium. A standard pacing wire is inserted into the right ventricle. More recently, a non-thoracotomy approach has been used, placing all leads epicardially via the subclavian vein.

When the device recognizes VT or VF, a shock of 0.5–36 J will be delivered after charging for 20–30 s. Up to seven successive shocks can be delivered during an event. This produces a visible muscle spasm, and a shock can be felt by a person in contact with the patient (although the energy reaching the surface is probably only 2 J from a 30 J shock). If external defibrillation is indicated after the internal unit is disabled, this is best achieved in the usual way, with anteroposterior placement of paddles.

Pacemakers[25]

Patients with pacemakers can be safely defibrillated, but the pacemaker or the junction between the tip of the pacing wire and the myocardium may be damaged. These risks can be minimized by using the lowest effective energy, and by placing the paddles perpendicular to, and far from, the pacemaker sensing dipole and the pacing unit. Pacing threshold is more likely increased by VF of sufficient duration to produce myocardial hypoxaemia.

For patients with a pacemaker in the pectoral region and a lead in the right ventricular apex, an anteroposterior placement of the paddles that encompasses the heart is theoretically safer. Facilities for back-up pacing should be available. After defibrillation, the pacemaker should be checked, as early and late problems with pacemaker function following DC shocks have been reported.

Pregnancy[26]

Defibrillation during pregnancy has been shown to be safe with conventional paddle placement. If possible, fetal ECG should be monitored, although the fetal heart on auscultation before and after cardioversion has been reported to be safe.

The future

Certain developments may lead to safer and more effective electrical therapies for arrhythmias. Current-based defibrillation[27] (in amperes, instead of energy-based in joules) may provide more reliable electrical therapy with less risk of myocardial damage, since the optimum current for most arrhythmias is known (e.g. 30–40 A for VF, 18 A for monomorphic VT, 14 A for atrial flutter and 30 A for AF). The defibrillator determines the TI of the patient by delivering a small preliminary shock. It is then able to compute and deliver a set current.

At present, most defibrillators deliver a damped, sinusoidal waveform single pulse between two electrodes. Research has shown that with internal defibrillation, multiple electrodes to deliver multipulse, multi-pathway biphasic shocks may be more efficacious. This may have application to external defibrillators in the future.[28–30]

References

1 Martin TG, Hawkins NS, Weigel JA *et al.* (1986) Initial treatment of ventricular fibrillation. *Am J Emerg Med* 6:113–119.
2 Cummins R, Ornato J and Thies W (1991) Improving survival from sudden cardiac arrest: the chain of survival concept. *Circulation* 83:1832–1847.
3 Eisenberg MS, Copass MK, Hallstrom AP *et al.* (1980) Treatment of out-of-hospital cardiac arrests with rapid defibrillation by emergency medical technicians. *N Engl J Med* 302:1379–1383.
4 White RD, Vukov LF and Bugliosi TF (1994) Early defibrillation by police: initial experience with measurement of critical time intervals and patient outcome. *Ann Emerg Med* 23:1009–1013.
5 Kerber RE (1993) Electrical treatment of cardiac arrhythmias: defibrillation and cardioversion. *Ann Emerg Med* 22:296–301.
6 Recommendations of the 1992 National Conference (1992) Guidelines for cardiopulmonary resuscitation and emergency cardiac care. *J Am Med Assoc* 268:2211–2213.
7 Bossaert L and Koster R (1992 Defibrillation: methods and strategies. A statement for the Advanced Life Support Working Party of the European Resuscitation Council. *Resuscitation* 24:211–225.
8 Fatkin D, Kuchar DL, Thorburn CW *et al.* (1994) Transoesophageal echocardiography before and during direct current cardioversion of atrial fibrillation: evidence for atrial stunning as a mechanism of thromboembolic complications. *J Am Coll Cardiol* 23:307–316.
9 Kerber RE, Grayzel J, Hoyt R *et al.* (1981) Transthoracic resistance of human defibrillation: influence of body weight, chest size, serial shocks, paddle size and paddle contact pressure. *Circulation* 63:676–682.
10 Lerman BB and Deale OC (1990) Relation between transcardiac and transthoracic current during defibrillation in humans. *Circulation Research* 67:1420–1426.
11 Anon. (1990) Defibrillation: Ensuring its success. Evaluation: Disposable defibrillator pads and electrodes. *Devices* 19:33–56.
12 Stults KR, Brown DD, Cooley F *et al.* (1987) Self-adhesive monitor/defibrillation pads improve prehospital defibrillation success. *Ann Emerg Med* 16:872–877.
13 Dalzell G, Cunningham S, Anderson J *et al.* (1989) Electrode pad size, transthoracic impedance and success of external ventricular defibrillation. *Am J Cardiol* 64:741–744.
14 White RD (1993) Maintenance of defibrillators in a state of readiness. *Annals of Emergency Medicine* 22:302–306.
15 Ditchey RV and Karliner JS (1981) Safety of electrical cardioversion in patients without digitalis toxicity. *Ann Intern Med* 95:676–679.
16 Chun PK, Davia JE and Donohue DJ (1981) ST segment elevation with elective dc cardioversion. *Circulation* 63:220–224.
17 Reiffel JA, Gambino SR, McCarthy DM and Leahey EB Jr (1978) Direct current cardioversion. Effect on creatine kinase, lactic dehydrogenase and myocardial isoenzymes. *J Am Med Assoc* 239:122–124.
18 Dahl CF, Ewy GA, Warner ED *et al.* (1974) Myocardial necrosis from direct current countershock: effect of paddle electrode size and time interval between discharges. *Circulation* 50:956–961.
19 Kerber RE (1986) Energy requirements for defibrillation. *Circulation* 74 (suppl IV):117–119.

20 The Advanced Life Support Committee of the Australian Resuscitation Council (1993) Adult advanced life support. *Med J Aust* **159**:616–621.

21 Advanced Life Support Working Party of the European Resuscitation Council (1992) Guidelines for advanced life support. *Resuscitation* **24**:111–121.

22 Sirna SJ, Ferguson DW, Charbonnier F *et al.* (1988) Factors affecting transthoracic impedance during electrical cardioversion. *Am J Cardiol* **62**:1048–1052.

23 Kerber RE, Jensen SR, Grayzel J *et al.* (1981) Elective cardioversion: influence of paddle electrode location and size on success rates and energy requirements. *N Engl J Med* **305**:658–662.

24 Mirowski M (1985) The automatic implantable defibrillation: an overview. *J Am Coll Cardiol* **6**:461–466.

25 Levine PA, Barold SS, Fletcher RD *et al.* (1983) Adverse acute and chronic effects of electrical defibrillation and cardioversion on impanted unipolar cardiac pacing systems. *J Am Coll Cardiol* **1**:1413–1422.

26 Schroeder JS and Harrison DC (1971) Repeated cardioversion during pregnancy. *Am J Cardiol* **27**:445–446.

27 Lerman BB, Di Marco JP and Haines DE (1988) Current-based versus energy-based ventricular defibrillation: a prospective study. *J Am Coll Cardiol* **12**:1259–1264.

28 Hoch DH, Batsford WP, Greenberg SM *et al.* (1994) Double sequential external shocks for refractory ventriculation fibrillation. *J Am Coll Cardiol* **23**:1141–1145.

29 Swartz JF, Fletcher RD and Karasik PE (1993) Optimization of biphasic waveforms for human non-thoracotomy defibrillation. *Circulation* **88**:2646–2654.

30 Cohen TJ (1993) Innovative emergency defibrillation methods for refractory ventricular fibrillation in a variety of hospital settings. *Am Heart J* **126**:962–968.

12 Inotropic drugs

JA Myburgh and WB Runciman

Circulatory failure[1] may be due to inadequate preload, myocardial failure (systolic $\pm$ diastolic dysfunction),[2,3] or maldistribution (e.g. anaphylaxis and septic shock;[4] see Chapters 13–15 and 61). In a patient with circulatory failure, an initial priority is to achieve an optimal preload using fluid infusons under close haemodynamic monitoring; hypovolaemia *per se* may be associated with some myocardial dysfunction.[5] If circulatory failure persists after optimal volume loading, a positive inotropic agent may be used to increase myocardial contractility.

Inotropic agents

The primary aim of inotropic agents is to increase contractility by increasing the velocity and force of myocardial fibre shortening. There is no ideal inotrope (Table 12.1) available. All agents have other effects on the peripheral vasculature and heart rate.[6] The choice of inotrope will be influenced by the cause of the circulatory failure, haemodynamic status of the patient and mechanism of action of the drug. Interactions between disease states and the pharmacokinetic profiles of the various inotropes are complex. Marked interindividual variability in the response of inotropic agents is well-described.[7] An appropriate inotrope should be selected according to each situation, with careful monitoring of its pharmacodynamic and haemodynamic effects.

As myocardial oxygenation is important, the selected inotrope should not cause tachycardia or arrhythmias, and should raise or maintain diastolic blood pressure, so that coronary perfusion pressure and myocardial oxygen delivery are sustained.[8] This is particularly important in patients with predominantly diastolic failure. The inotrope should be titrated to improve mean arterial pressure (MAP) and cardiac output. This should result in improved tissue perfusion, with reversal of any metabolic acidosis, increased oxygen consumption and an adequate urinary output.[8,9] The dose or agent should

Table 12.1 The ideal inotrope

Increases contractility
  Increases mean arterial pressure
  Increases cardiac output
  Improves tissue hypoxia
Does not increase myocardial oxygen consumption
  There is no resultant tachycardia
  It is non-arrhythmogenic
  Maintains diastolic blood pressure
Does not develop tolerance
Is titratable
  Rapid onset
  Rapid termination of action
Is compatible with other drugs
Is non-toxic
Is cost-effective

be changed if there is no satisfactory response, or if undesirable effects are obtained.[9]

The common, ultimate cellular mechanism of action of inotropic agents involves the release, utilization or sequestration of intracellular calcium (Fig. 12.1). Inotropes can be classified according to whether or not their actions depend on increases in intracellular cyclic adenosine 3',5'-monophosphate (cAMP;[10] Table 12.2).

Catecholamines

These are the most frequently used inotropic agents in the ICU. All act directly on adrenergic receptors.[11] β-Receptor occupancy activates adenyl cyclase to increase the conversion of adenosine triphosphate to cAMP. α_1-Receptor occupancy acts independently of cAMP by activation of phospholipase C, which increases inositol phosphates (IP_3 and IP_4) and diacyl glycerol. These second messengers promote the release of calcium from intracellular stores and increase membrane calcium permeability.[6,11,12] Subsequent

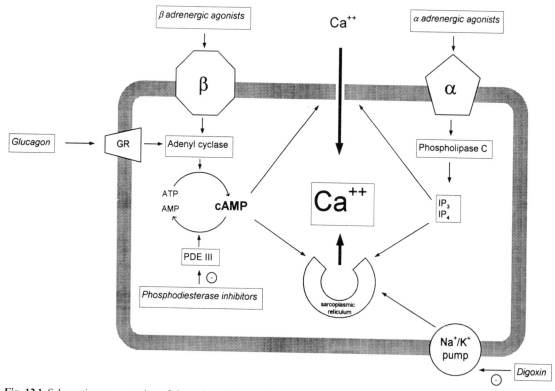

Fig. 12.1 Schematic representation of the action of inotropic agents on intracellular calcium in myocytes. GR = Glucagon receptor; ATP = adenosine triphosphate; AMP = adenosine monophosphate; cAMP = cyclic AMP; PDE III = phosphodiesterase III; IP$_3$ = inositol phosphate 3.

Table 12.2 Classification of inotropic agents

cAMP-dependent	*cAMP-independent*
Catecholamines (β-adrenergic agonists)	*Catecholamines (α-adrenergic agonists)*
Adrenaline	Adrenaline
Noradrenaline	Noradrenaline
Dopamine	Dopamine
Dobutamine	
Dopexamine	*Digoxin*
Isoprenaline	
	Calcium salts
Phosphodiesterase inhibitors	
Amrinone	*Thyroid hormone*
Milrinone	
Enoximone	
Glucagon	

cAMP = Cyclic adenosine monophosphate.

phosphorylation of substrate proteins via protein kinases acts as third messengers to trigger a cascade of events which lead to specific cardiovascular effects.[12] (Table 12.3).

Classification of catecholamines into α- and β-agonists (Table 12.3) is only a crude predictor of likely effects in normal individuals, as the effect of any sympathomimetic amine on any end-organ may be greatly influenced by many local factors acting on both presynaptic terminals and receptors.[7]

Adrenaline, noradrenaline and *dopamine* are catecholamines which occur naturally in humans. Dopamine is the precursor of noradrenaline, and noradrenaline is that of adrenaline. All are predominantly β-agonists at low doses, with increasing α$_1$-effects becoming evident with increasing doses.[11]

Table 12.3 Cardiovascular effects of catecholamines

Agent	β_1 effects	β_2 effects	α_1 effects	α_2 effects
	+ Chronotropy + Dromotropy + Inotropy	+ Inotropy Vasodilatation Bronchodilatation	+ Inotropy Vasoconstriction	+ Inotropy Vasoconstriction
Noradrenaline		β effects predominate at low dose; α effects predominate at high dose		
Adrenaline		β effects predominate at low dose; α effects predominate at high dose		
Dopamine		β effects predominate at low dose; α effects predominate at high dose		
Dobutamine	+	+	(+)	−
Isoprenaline	+	(+)	−	−
Dopexamine	+	+	−	−

+ = Stimulation; (+) = mild effect; − = no effect.

The haemodynamic effects of these three agents vary considerably between individuals, but all tend to increase stroke volume, cardiac output and MAP, with little change in heart rate and a low incidence of dysrhythmias.[7,11]

Noradrenaline is the peripheral sympathetic chemo-transmitter in humans, and thus the agonist which usually acts on β-receptors (augmented by circulating adrenaline at times of stress).[13] There is evidence of markedly depleted stores of noradrenaline and reduced sensitivity and density of β-adrenergic receptors in the failing myocardium (i.e. downregulation). Here, cardiac output is maintained only by increased sympathetic drive. This is well-described in chronic cardiac failure,[2] following cardiopulmonary bypass[14] and in septic shock.[4] Thus α_1- and α_2-adrenergic receptors are important in maintaining inotropy in the ischaemic or failing myocardium.[15] This may explain why increased doses of catecholamines are required to maintain MAP and cardiac output in these patients. The exogenous catecholamine infusions may simply be augmenting endogenous mechanisms which are failing at a number of levels.[11]

Adrenaline and noradrenaline infusions, at rates suggested below, produce blood concentrations similar to those produced endogenously in shock states, whereas dopamine infusions produce much higher concentrations than those naturally encountered.[11] Dopamine may exert much of its effect by being converted to noradrenaline, thus bypassing the rate-limiting (tyrosine hydroxylase) step in catecholamine synthesis.[11,16] At low doses (< 2 μg/kg per min) it may exert vasodilatory effects on specific dopaminergic renal and mesenteric vessel receptors.[17] However, there is little evidence that these effects are important in humans at the doses usually used (100–2000 μg/min). The renal protective effect of low-dose dopamine has been increasingly questioned. Most of the increase in urine flow with dopamine in patients with left ventricular dysfunction is due not to renal vasodilatation, but to inhibition of proximal tubular sodium reabsorption and improvement in MAP and cardiac output.[17,18] Equal or better improvements in these renal parameters have been demonstrated with both noradrenaline[19]

and dobutamine.[20] Distinction between dopamine's predominantly β-effects at low doses and α-effects at higher doses is probably spurious in clinical practice, due to marked interindividual variation and interactions.[7]

Isoprenaline is a synthetic catecholamine. It is predominantly a chronotrope, and tends to produce marked increases in heart rate and cardiac output, without a significant change or a fall in blood pressure, due to predominant β_2-receptor-induced vasodilatation. The positive chronotropic effect is associated with increased myocardial oxygen consumption. Tachycardia and weak activity in maintaining diastolic pressure make this a poor first-line inotrope.[6,11]

Dobutamine is a synthetic derivative of isoprenaline that acts primarily on β_1-receptors in the heart. It exerts a more prominent inotropic than chronotropic action than isoprenaline, and usually increases cardiac output with little change in systemic vascular resistance and moderate increases in heart rate.[6,11]

Dopexamine is a synthetic analogue of dopamine with a similar action and profile, acting primarily at β-receptors. Early reports of improved splanchnic and renal blood flow have not been substantiated and, like dopamine, dopexamine probably exerts most of its effects by increasing MAP and/or cardiac output.[21]

Dosage and administration

All catecholamines have very short biological half-lives (1–2 min), due largely to reuptake into tissues and to degradation by catechol O-methyltransferase in liver and lung. A steady-state plasma concentration is achieved within 5–10 min after the start of a constant infusion. Adrenaline, noradrenaline and isoprenaline all have hydroxyl groups on the β-carbon atom of the side chain, and this is associated with 100-fold greater potency than dopamine or dobutamine, which do not.[11] Adrenaline, noradrenaline and isoprenaline are generally used in adult doses of 1–70 μg/min, and dopamine and dobutamine in doses of 100–2000 μg/min. Doses are frequently referenced to body weight, with ranges prescribed to predict relative predominance of β- or α-effects. This distinction has no clinical use.

Solutions should be titrated against prescribed clinical end-points (e.g. MAP, cardiac output, systemic vascular resistance and oxygen consumption and delivery).

Catecholamines must be administered by continuous infusion, preferably into a large central vein (via a catheter used solely for this purpose) to avoid skin sloughing if extravasation occurs. A recommended concentration protocol for adrenaline, noradrenaline and isoprenaline infusions using drug delivery systems (e.g. infusion pumps) is 6 mg of drug in 100 ml 5% dextrose, where ml/h approximates μg/min. Dopamine and dobutamine infusions may be made up as 400 mg/100 ml and 500 mg/100 ml solutions respectively. These infusions in ml/h approximate μg/kg per min. Heart rate and MAP must be accurately monitored, ideally with an intra-arterial line.

Phosphodiesterase inhibitors

Phosphodiesterase inhibitors are compounds that cause non-receptor-mediated competitive inhibition of phosphodiesterase (PDE) isoenzymes, resulting in increased levels of cAMP (Fig. 12.1).[22,23] Importantly, cAMP also affects diastolic heart function through the regulation of phospholamban, the regulatory subunit of the calcium pump of the sarcoplasmic reticulum.[12] This enhances the rate of calcium re-sequestration and thereby diastolic relaxation. For cardiovascular tissue, inhibition of isoenzyme PDE III is responsible for the therapeutic effects. Cardiac effects are characterized by positive inotropy and improved diastolic relaxation. The latter is termed lusitropy and may be beneficial in patients with reduced ventricular compliance or predominant diastolic failure.[22] These agents also cause potent vasodilatation with reductions in preload and afterload, as well as pulmonary vascular resistance.[24] The term inodilation has been used to describe this dual haemodynamic effect. Myocardial oxygen consumption and heart rate are not significantly increased. Tolerance is not a feature. Thus these agents may have a place in managing patients with β-receptor down-regulation, by causing intrinsic inotropic stimulation and by sensitizing the myocardium to β-agonists.[22] Other speculative actions include inhibition of platelet aggregation and reduction of post ischaemic reperfusion injury.

Titration pharmacokinetics of phosphodiesterase inhibitors are markedly different to the catecholamines. Drug half-lives can be prolonged, and excretion is predominantly renal. Hypotension may result from vasodilatation. Combined use with catecholamines (e.g. adrenaline or noradrenaline) may be necessary and complementary to maintain MAP.[25]

Early phosphodiesterase inhibitors include theophylline and caffeine, but these have serious side-effects at doses required to produce useful positive inotropism. Newer phosphodiesterase inhibitors include the bipyridine derivatives *amrinone* and *milrinone* and the imidazolones *enoximone* and *piroximone*. Their cardiovascular effects are similar. The oral form of amrinone is no longer used clinically, due to a high incidence of thrombocytopenia, and gastrointestinal and neurological side-effects. Milrinone and enoximone are more potent agents, and are currently used in clinical practice, with the latter exhibiting more inotropic effects than vasodilatation. Enoximone is more rapidly metabolized, but the metabolite is active and its cardiovascular effects persist for some hours. There is evidence that prolonged use of these agents is associated with an increased mortality in patients with severe heart failure.[26]

Dosage and administration

Recommended doses based on previous experience have proven to be insufficient.[22] A widely accepted dosage regimen for milrinone is a loading dose of 50 μg/kg together with a maintenance dose of 0.5 μg/kg per min; enoximone 0.5–1.0 mg/kg loading and infusion of 5–10 μg/kg per min. As with catecholamines, patients must be closely monitored and the haemodynamic response evaluated.

Digoxin

Digitalis glycosides have been used to treat heart failure for 200 years and the vagotonic effects used to control the ventricular response in selected supraventricular tachyarrhythmias. The effects of digoxin are largely mediated by an increase in intracellular calcium concentrations produced indirectly by inhibition of the Na^+/K^+ membrane pump, resulting in increased myocardial contraction (Fig. 12.1). Peripheral resistance is also increased, by a direct mechanism and by increased sympathetic activity. The effects on impulse conduction are mediated through change in both vagal and sympathetic tone.[27] Digoxin has a narrow therapeutic index, is highly protein-bound, and is largely excreted unchanged in the urine. Alteration in renal function may prolong the normal half-life of about 35 h to 5 days.[27]

The role of digoxin in acute cardiac failure has become increasingly questioned.[28] It has minimal effect as an inotrope, and evaluation of efficacy is difficult. In the presence of high levels of sympathetic activity, the inotropic effect is negligible, and there is usually a poor response in acute myocardial failure, myocarditis, advanced cardiomyopathy, shock states and cardiac tamponade. Digoxin may actually reduce cardiac output in cardiogenic shock, due to its effect on afterload.[27] The potential for toxicity in the critically ill patient is increased by hypokalaemia, hypomagnesaemia, hypercalcaemia, hypoxia and acidosis. Toxicity is manifested by dysrhythmias that may assume any form, including supraventricular tachyarrhythmias, bradycardia, ventricular ectopy and conduction block at any level.[27,29]

Monitoring digoxin levels in critically ill patients is recommended, although interpretation of results is difficult. A concentration of 1–2 ng/ml represents a reasonable risk/benefit ratio, but concentrations of over 2 ng/ml may be associated with toxicity in some patients. However, correlation between blood concentrations, efficacy and toxic manifestations is poor. Clinical criteria remain the most reliable assessment of toxicity, but except for dysrhythmias, may be difficult to elicit in ICU patients. Commonly used drugs in the ICU, such as amiodarone, calcium-channel blockers and erythromycin, demonstrate adverse drug interactions with digoxin, and may interfere with the radioimmunoassay to reflect apparently increased blood digoxin concentrations.[27–29]

The role of digoxin in the ICU is limited, due to its unpredictable efficacy and toxicity. Careful titration of short-acting inotropes, and use of antiarrhythmic agents (e.g. amiodarone) to control ventricular rate in supraventricular tachycardia, have largely superseded its use. Digoxin should therefore be reserved for patients with symptomatic chronic left ventricular failure with cardiomegaly who are refractory to diuretic and/or vasodilator therapy.

Dosage and administration

In critically ill patients, digoxin must be administered by slow IV injection, as oral bioavailability varies considerably due to altered gastric motility or perfusion. A loading dose (1.0–1.5 mg in three or four divided doses, 4–6 h apart) followed by a maintenance dose (0.125–0.5 mg/day) is a satisfactory regimen.[26] Smaller doses should be used in the elderly, small patients, and those with renal dysfunction, electrolyte and acid–base disturbances and myxoedema.[29] Blood for assay should be taken at least 6 h after an oral dose, and 1 h after an IV dose.

Other inotropic agents

Glucagon

Glucagon is a naturally occurring polypeptide that directly stimulates adenyl cyclase via receptors to increase cAMP concentration in myocardial cells, resulting in positive inotropy without producing myocardial excitability. Large doses are required to achieve this effect which is associated with a high incidence of metabolic side-effects. No definitive cardiovascular role for this agent has been established apart from anecdotal reports of use in severe β-blocker poisoning.

Calcium salts

Although calcium ions are essential in myocardial excitation–contraction coupling, the role of exogenously administered calcium salts for cardiopulmonary resuscitation and in circulatory failure has not been established.[6,30,31] Calcium has deleterious effects in ischaemic areas of the brain and myocardium, and results in an unpredictable and variable effect on cardiac output, MAP and heart rate. These actions are short-acting, lasting for less than 5 min.[31] When administered with β-adrenergic agonists, calcium frequently impairs their cardiovascular actions. Calcium salts may improve haemodynamics following cardiopulmonary bypass, but in general, they should only be used if significant hyperkalaemia, ionized hypocalcaemia or poisoning from calcium-channel blockers are the primary cause of circulatory failure.[6,31]

Thyroid hormone

Thyroid hormone is required for synthesis of contractile proteins and normal myocardial contraction. It is also a regulator of the synthesis of adrenergic receptors. Low levels of thyroid hormone have been demonstrated in brain-dead organ donors and following cardiopulmonary bypass. Preliminary studies suggest that treatment with thyroid hormone in these patients may reduce the need for inotropic agents and vasopressors to achieve satisfactory haemodynamics. Further studies are required in these areas.[6]

Clinical usage of inotropic agents

Cardiopulmonary resuscitation (CPR)

Adrenaline remains the drug of first choice in cardiac arrest, although other strong α-adrenergic catecholamines (e.g. methoxamine, phenylephrine or dopamine) appear equally effective. Efficacy lies fundamentally in α-adrenergic receptor stimulation;[32] pure β-receptor stimulation does not influence outcome and may be deleterious.[32,33] The relative importance of maintaining diastolic pressure and coronary perfusion, diverting blood to essential central organs and increasing venous return, has not been established. Adrenaline is given as IV bolus doses of 1 mg, and infusion rates of 10–100 μg/min. The value of high doses (5–18 mg) is conflicting, but a 5-mg IV dose should be considered if response is lacking, especially if asystole persists.[34–36] (see Chapter 7).

Isoprenaline has previously been recommended for medical pacing for severe bradyarrhythmias that do not respond to atropine. However, the lack of α-activity and increase in myocardial oxygen consumption has raised concerns about its efficacy. Adrenaline is now regarded as the first-line agent in this situation.[36]

Anaphylaxis

Adrenaline is the drug of choice for anaphylactic reactions and for life-threatening bronchospasm, as it blocks mediator release and specifically reverses end-organ effects[37] (see Chapter 58). A dose of 0.3–1.0 mg (0.5 mg is often sufficient) may be injected subcutaneously or intramuscularly. This may be repeated every few minutes, if necessary. If shock compromises muscle blood flow, or as a chosen alternative, an IV infusion of 1–2 mg in 100 ml saline (at a rate up to 100 μg/min) is started with ECG monitoring. A strong slowing pulse indicates a pressor effect, and provides a useful clinical end-point for the rate of infusion.

Weaning from cardiopulmonary bypass

Catecholamine administration is an important treatment for the life-threatening low cardiac output state that may follow cardiopulmonary bypass.[25,38] Numerous combinations of catecholamines have been used successfully, but no significant benefit of one catecholamine (or mixture) over another has been demonstrated. Similarly, the question whether mechanical support devices offer a significant advantage over inotropes remains unanswered. Adrenaline and dopamine, or a mixture of both, increase cardiac output with little increase in heart rate or afterload, and are first-line inotropic drugs during weaning from cardiopulmonary bypass. At higher doses ($>$ 500 μg/min), dopamine has been shown to cause more tachycardia than adrenaline. There is no evidence that these catecholamines cause vasospasm of arterial conduits in clinically used doses.

Dobutamine and isoprenaline may cause significant tachycardia as well as β_2-induced vasodilatation, and cannot be recommended as sole first-line drugs.[38] Phosphodiesterase inhibitors, either as sole agents or in conjunction with adrenaline or noradrenaline, have been used successfully, and may have a role in patients with valve replacement, pulmonary hypertension or preoperative diastolic failure.[39]

Cardiac failure after acute myocardial infarction

Theoretically, a low-dose catecholamine infusion may confer some advantages in cardiogenic shock.[40] Adrenaline, dopamine and dobutamine have been shown to cause satisfactory short-term effects but no increased long-term survival.[41] Isoprenaline is not a first-line drug in this situation, because of its chronotropic effect. Phosphodiesterase inhibitors and β-blockade may have a role in managing acute congestive cardiac failure, especially in patients with diastolic dysfunction[2,3] (see Chapter 6).

Septic shock

The cardiovascular effects of severe sepsis are complex, and range from a hyperdynamic, vasodilated state to one of increasing myocardial failure and paralysis of the peripheral vasculature (vasoplegia).[4] An increasing body of literature supports the use of noradrenaline,

adrenaline or dopamine as first-line agents in septic shock[42–46] to maintain MAP, cardiac output and oxygen delivery. Improved haemodynamic profile results predominantly from increased cardiac output, as systemic vascular resistance is not significantly altered.[44] Thus, these agents should be regarded primarily as inotropes rather than vasoconstrictors in septic shock. Noradrenaline and adrenaline rarely cause tachycardia, whereas dopamine causes an increase in heart rate in about 20% of all patients. All produce a diuresis in 60–80% of previously oliguric, volume-loaded patients, in doses maintaining an adequate MAP.[19,43,46]. Thus, maintenance of a critical renal perfusion pressure appears more important than the specific dopaminergic effect. All three agents will increase oxygen delivery and consumption, but evidence that they improve or prevent pathological oxygen supply dependency is lacking (see Chapters 22 and 61). Use of dobutamine and isoprenaline in septic shock appears to be limited to situations in which first-line catecholamines have not produced an adequate response. Use of phosphodiesterase inhibitors in sepsis has not been established.

References

1 Astiz ME, Rackow EC and Weil MH (1993) Pathophysiology and treatment of circulatory shock. *Crit Care Clin* **9**:183–203.

2 Gaasch WH (1994) Diagnosis and treatment of heart failure based on left ventricular systolic or diastolic dysfunction. *J Am Med Assoc* **271**:1276–1280.

3 Grossman W (1991) Diastolic dysfunction and congestive heart failure. *N Engl J Med* **325**:1557–1564.

4 Parrillo JE (1993) Pathogenetic mechanisms in septic shock. *N Engl J Med* **328**:1471–1477.

5 Rutishauser W and Lerch R (1994) Determinants of cardiac output and their measurement. *Anaesth Pharm Rev* **2**:301–307.

6 Zaloga GP, Prielipp RC, Butterworth JF *et al.* (1993) Pharmacologic cardiovascular support. *Crit Care Clin* **9**:335–362.

7 Runciman WB, Myburgh JA and Upton RN (1990) Pharmacokinetics and pharmacodynamics in the critically ill. In: Dobb GJ (ed.) *Clinical Anaesthesiology. International Practice and Research.* London: Baillière Tindall, pp. 271–303.

8 Linberg DM and Pearl RG (1993) Inotropic therapy in the critically ill. *Int Anesthesiol Clin* **31**:49–71.

9 Stanford GG (1991) Use of inotropic agents in critical illness. *Surg Clin North Am* **71**:683–698.

10 Remme WJ (1993) Congestive heart failure. Drug therapy: central or peripheral approach? *Cardiologia* **38**:51–59.

11 Runciman WB and Morris JL (1993) Adrenoceptor agonists. In: Feldman SA, Paton W and Scurr C (eds) *Mechanism of Drugs in Anaesthesia.* London: Edward Arnold, pp. 262–291.

12 Katz AM (1993) Cardiac ion channels. *N Engl J Med* **328**:1244–1251.

13 Motomura S, Zerkowski H-R, Daul A *et al.* (1990) On the physiologic role of beta-2 adrenoceptors in the human heart: *in vitro* and *in vivo* studies. *Am Heart J* **119**: 608–619.

14 Schwinn DA, Leone BJ, Spahn DR *et al.* (1991) Desensitisation of myocardial β-adrenergic receptors during cardiopulmonary bypass. Evidence of early uncoupling and late downregulation. *Circulation* **84**:2559–2567.

15 Heusch G (1990) α-Adrenergic mechanisms in myocardial ischemia. *Circulation* **81**:1–13.

16 Anderson FL, Port JD, Reid BB *et al.* (1992) Effect of therapeutic dopamine administration on myocardial catecholamine and neuropeptide Y concentrations in the failing ventricles of patients with idiopathic dilated cardiomyopathy. *J Cardiovasc Pharmacol* **20**: 800–806.

17 Duke GJ and Bersten AD (1992) Dopamine and renal salvage in the critically ill. *Anaesth Intens Care* **20**: 277–287.

18 Myles PS, Buckland MR, Schenk NJ *et al.* (1993) Effect of 'renal dose' dopamine on renal function following cardiac surgery. *Anaesth Intens Care* **21**:56–61.

19 Martin C, Eon B, Saux P *et al.* (1990) Renal effects of norepinephrine used to treat septic shock patients. *Crit Care Med* **18**:282–285.

20 Duke GJ, Briedis JH and Weaver RA (1994) Renal support in critically ill patients: low dose dopamine or low dose dobutamine? *Crit Care Med* **22**:1919–1925.

21 Fitton A and Benfield P (1990) Dopexamine hydrochloride. A review of its pharmacodynamic and pharmacokinetic properties and therapeutic potential in acute cardiac insufficiency. *Drugs* **39**:308–330.

22 Kaufman MA and Pargger H (1994) Role of phospho-diesterase inhibitors in acute myocardial contractile failure. *Anaesth Pharmacol Rev* **2**:324–331.

23 Skoyles JR and Sherry KM (1992) Pharmacology, mechanisms of action and uses of selective phospho-diesterase inhibitors. *Br J Anaesth* **68**:293–302.

24 Nolan J, Sanderson A, Taddei F *et al.* (1992) Acute effects of intravenous phosphodiesterase inhibition in chronic heart failure: simultaneous pre- and afterload reduction with a single agent. *Int J Cardiol* **35**:343–349.

25 Butterworth JF (1993) Selecting an inotrope for the cardiac surgery patient. *J Cardiothor Vasc Anesth* **7**:26–32.

26 Packer M, Carver JR, Rodeffer RJ *et al.* (1991) Effect of oral milrinone on mortality in severe chronic heart failure. *N Engl J Med* **325**:1468–1475.

27 Pentel PR and Salerno DM (1990) Cardiac drug toxicity: digitalis glycosides and calcium channel and β-blocking agents. *Med J Aust* **152**:88–95.

28 Ewy GA (1990) Urgent digoxin therapy: a requiem. *J Am Coll Cardiol* **15**:1248–1249.

29 Worfford JL, Hickey AR, Ettinger WH *et al.* (1992) Lack of age related differences in the clinical presentation of digoxin toxicity. *Arch Intern Med* **152**:2261–2264.

30 Erdmann E and Reuschel-Janetschek E (1991) Calcium for resuscitation? *Br J Anaesth* **67**:178–184.

31 Zaloga GP (1992) Hypocalcaemia in critically ill patients. *Crit Care Med* **20**:251–262.

32 Niemann JT (1992) Cardiopulmonary resuscitation. *N Engl J Med* **327**:1075–1080.

33 Lindner KH, Ahnefeld FW, Scheurmann W *et al.* (1990) Epinephrine and norepinephrine in cardiopulmonary resuscitation. Effects on myocardial oxygen delivery and consumption. *Chest* **97**:1458–1462.

34 Brown CG, Martin DR, Pepe PE *et al.* (1992) A comparison of standard-dose and high dose epinephrine in cardiac arrest outside the hospital. *N Engl J Med* **327**:1051–1055.

35 Callaham ME, Madsen CD, Barton CW *et al.* (1992) A randomized clinical trial of high dose epinephrine and norepinephrine vs standard dose epinephrine in prehospital cardiac arrest. *J Am Med Assoc* **268**: 2667–2672.

36 American Heart Association (1992) Adult advanced cardiac life support. *J Am Med Assoc* **268**:2199–2242.

37 Atkinson TP (1992) Anaphylaxis. *Med Clin North Am* **76**:841–855.

38 Hardy JF and Belisle S (1993) Inotropic support of the heart that fails to successfully wean from cardiopulmonary bypass: the Montreal Heart Institute experience. *J Cardiothor Vasc Anesth* **7**:33–39.

39 Tarr TJ, Moore NA, Frazer RS *et al.* (1993) Haemodynamic effects and comparison of enoximone, dobutamine and dopamine following mitral valve surgery. *Eur J Anaesthesiol* **8**:15–24.

40 Califf RM and Bengtson JR (1994) Cardiogenic shock. *N Engl J Med* **330**:1724–1730.

41 Lowenstein E (1993) Clinical markers and clinical consequences of stunned myocardium. *J Card Surg* **8**:232–234.

42 Mackenzie SJ, Kapadia GR, Nimmo IR *et al.* (1991) Adrenalin in treatment of septic shock: effects on haemodynamics and oxygen transport. *Intens Care Med* **17**:36–39.

43 Martin C, Papazian L, Perrin G *et al.* (1993) Norepinephrine or dopamine for treatment of hyper-dynamic septic shock? *Chest* **103**:1826–1831.

44 Moran JL, O'Fathartaigh MS, Peisach AR *et al.* (1993) Epinephrine as an inotropic agent in septic shock: a dose profile analysis. *Crit Care Med* **21**:70–77.

45 Schreuder WO, Schneider AJ, Groeneveld J *et al.* (1989) Effect of dopamine vs norepinephrine on hemodynamics in septic shock. *Chest* **95**:1282–1288.

46 Fukuoka T, Nishimura M, Imanaka H *et al.* (1989) Effects of norepinephrine on renal function in septic patients with normal and elevated serum lactate levels. *Crit Care Med* **17**:1104–1111.

13 | Heart failure

JE Sanderson and RJ Young

Heart failure is a serious public health problem with a prevalence in Europe and the USA of about 0.4–2.0%, and 10% in elderly subjects.[1,2] Before the 1970s, it was regarded as a disorder causing oedema and fluid retention. There was much debate about 'backward' and 'forward' heart failure, and the major treatment was diuretics. Attention in the 1970s and 1980s shifted to peripheral vascular constriction and vasodilator therapy. The past decade has pointed to the pathogenetic importance of neurohormonal mechanisms and new treatments to block these mechanisms.[3]

Heart failure has a high mortality. In the USA, annual mortality of severe cases may exceed 60%;[1,2,4] about a third die within 2 years of diagnosis.[1] Major risk factors are hypertension and coronary artery disease. In Asia, hypertension also appears to be a major risk factor, although coronary artery disease is the major cause in younger men.[5]

Pathophysiology

Performance of the intact ventricle (Fig. 13.1)

The four factors governing performance of the isolated cardiac muscle (preload, afterload, contractility and heart rate) are also used to describe the intact ventricle.[6]

Preload (Fig. 13.2a)

This is the tension placed on resting muscle before the onset of contraction. In the intact heart, ventricular end-diastolic wall stress is equivalent to the preload of isolated muscle, and thus determines the resting lengths of sarcomeres. Increases in preload augment stroke volume (SV), and the relationship between end-diastolic volume (EDV) or pressure (EDP) and SV is called the Frank–Starling mechanism. In heart failure, this ventricular function curve is displaced downwards, so that increasing EDV or EDP have smaller effects on SV. Conversely, a very low filling pressure would lead to a reduced SV. Clinically, preload should thus be maximized, but without reaching a level to cause pulmonary oedema.

Afterload (Fig. 13.2b)

Afterload is the tension, force or stress (force per unit cross-sectional area) acting on the fibres in the ventricle wall after the onset of shortening. Major determinants of afterload are arterial pressure and left ventricular (LV) wall stress itself. Increasing cardiac size increases LV wall stress, as predicted by Laplace's law for a sphere:

$$\text{Circumferential wall stress} = Pr \,/\, 2h$$

where P = intraventricular pressure; r = radius at the endocardial surface; and h = wall thickness. Excessive increases in preload causing ventricular dilatation will also increase afterload. Afterload has a critical role in regulating cardiac output, especially if ventricular function is impaired (Fig. 13.2b). Small increases in afterload will then significantly reduce cardiac output. This is the rationale for using arterial vasodilators in heart failure.

Contractility

Contractility defines the improvement in cardiac function which occurs after stimuli, when preload and afterload remain constant. Inotropic stimuli generally act through altered calcium availability to the myofilaments, or through an alteration in myofilament calcium sensitivity.

Heart rate

At a constant SV, cardiac output is a linear function of heart rate. Thus in acute heart failure, increased heart rate is an important compensatory mechanism.

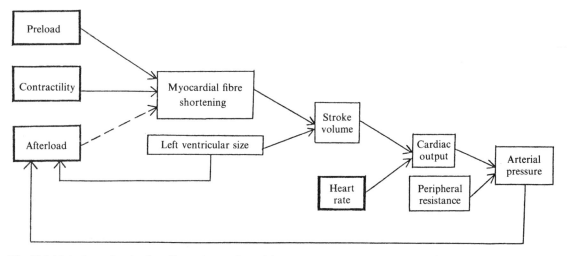

Fig. 13.1 Main determinants of cardiac output and arterial pressure.

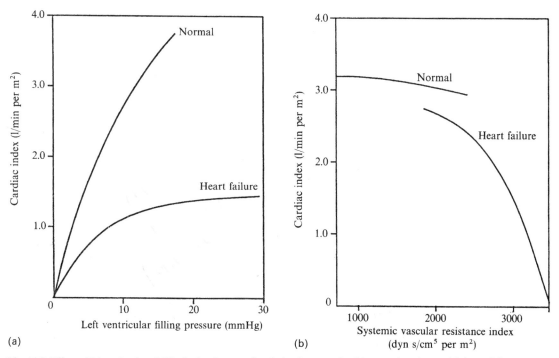

(a)

(b)

Fig. 13.2 Effect of (a) preload and (b) afterload on cardiac index in normal subjects and patients with heart failure.

In chronic heart failure, however, reducing heart rate may be beneficial to improve diastolic filling and function.

Acute and chronic heart failure

The pathophysiology of acute and chronic heart failure is different. In the former, haemodynamics and sympathetic activity are more prominent, while in chronic failure, slow neuroendocrine mechanisms predominate.

Low-output and high-output heart failure

Low-output heart failure occurs when the primary problem is reduced cardiac output. High-output failure is due to excessive vasodilatation or shunting, and may occur in anaemia, hyperthyroidism, arteriovenous fistulae, beriberi, or postpartum.[7] Hyperthyroidism can also *reduce* cardiac output due to myocardial damage and thyrotoxic cardiomyopathy.[8]

Compensatory mechanisms[9]

Myocardial damage initiates important haemodynamic and neurohormonal compensatory mechanisms, which initially provide inotropic support but at a price of increased LV wall stress.

Frank–Starling mechanism

Decreased ventricular emptying during systole increases EDV, and this, via the Frank–Starling mechanism, augments the force and frequency of contraction of the remaining sarcomeres.

Sympathetic nervous system activation

Sympathetic activation occurs early in heart failure, with tachycardia, increased force of contraction and peripheral vasoconstriction.[10]

LV hypertrophy

LV hypertrophy develops because the increase in wall stress induces specific oncogenes.[11] Initially, this helps reduce wall stress but increases LV 'stiffness'.

Renin–angiotensin–aldosterone system (RAAS) activation

Activation of the RAAS increases vasoconstriction (due to angiotensin II) and sodium and water retention. The RAAS is activated more after treatment with diuretics.[12,13]

Sodium and water retention

Sodium and water retention from RAAS activation and renal hypoperfusion results in increased venous return. This improves preload, but also increases LV wall stress (because of ventricular dilatation) and leads to oedema formation.

Atrial natriuretic peptide (ANP) and brain natriuretic peptide (BNP) release

Atrial stretch from increased atrial pressure causes release of ANP and BNP.[14] These inhibit the release and action of noradrenaline,[15] produce vasodilatation and natriuresis, and reduce haemodynamic stress. However, they quickly become depleted.[14]

Endothelin

Endothelin is a potent endothelial-derived venous and arterial vasoconstrictor that may also moderate RAAS, augment inotropy, and stimulate vascular smooth muscle proliferation and cardiac hypertrophy. Levels of endothelin correlate with the degree of heart failure.[16]

A vicious cycle thus exists. Compensatory mechanisms increase afterload and preload, thus increasing cardiac workload and exacerbating the original situation (Fig. 13.3). Further factors contribute to this functional deterioration. Aldosterone and angiotensin II stimulate the generation of fibrous tissue.[17] Cardiotoxic cytokines are released with noradrenaline and angiotensin.[18] Many of these systems also interact – sympathetic activation increases release of renin, and angiotensin enhances the release of noradrenaline and vasopressin.[19] Also, oedema itself increases afterload. Arrhythmias are induced by increased sympathetic activity and RAAS activation.[20] Baroreceptors are reset in heart failure, and this may also promote arrhythmias.[21]

Diastolic heart failure

Impairment of diastolic function is also important in heart failure. In rare cases, diastolic dysfunction may be the main cause of heart failure (e.g. hypertrophic cardiomyopathy, amyloid heart disease and endo-myocardial fibrosis). However, many patients with ischaemic heart disease and hypertension develop myocardial fibrosis in association with hypertrophy, resulting in increased LV wall stiffness and reduced relaxation. This impairs LV filling and raises LV diastolic pressure. Myocardial fibroblasts respond to circulatory aldosterone and tissue angiotensin, which are both increased in heart failure.[17] Impaired diastolic function is a predictor of poor prognosis.[22]

Neural control of cardiac function

The parasympathetic system also has an important role in the immediate control of myocardial function which is less appreciated. Stimulation of the vagus nerve has a negative inotropic action.[23]

Clinical presentation

Main symptoms are breathlessness (due to the high pulmonary venous pressure and changes in muscle mechanics) and fatigue (due to the low cardiac output and poor muscle perfusion). Physical signs are due to:

1 sympathomimetic activation (i.e. tachycardia, cold peripheries and sweating);
2 fluid retention (i.e. raised jugular venous pressure (JVP), oedema, bilateral basal crepitations, ascites and pleural and pericardial effusions);

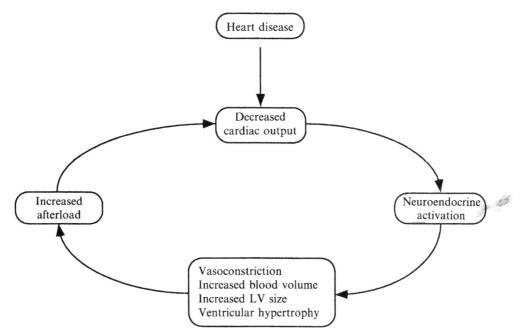

Fig. 13.3 The 'vicious cycle' of heart failure. LV = Left ventricular.

3 signs of myocardial dysfunction (e.g. S3, S4, gallop rhythm and mitral and tricuspid valve regurgitation).

Diagnosis

The diagnosis is frequently obvious, but any part of the heart, including coronary arteries, pericardium, myocardium, valves and endocardium can cause heart failure. Failure can occur with a normal-size heart in mitral stenosis, aortic stenosis, hypertrophic cardiomyopathy and constrictive pericarditis. Pericardial tamponade must always be excluded before starting treatment with diuretics and vasodilators. Causes of sudden deterioration in a patient with well-compensated chronic heart failure include uncontrolled arrhythmias, hypertension, pulmonary emboli, infection and poor compliance or inappropriate drug therapy. Silent myocardial infarctions are important causes of heart failure, especially in diabetics and the elderly.

Investigations

1 *Blood tests* include full blood count, blood urea and serum electrolytes and creatinine. Anaemia and thyrotoxicosis should be excluded.
2 *ECG:* Arrhythmias and recent myocardial infarction should be excluded. Atrial flutter should be considered in any patient with heart failure who has a fixed heart rate of 150 beats/min.

3 *Chest X-ray* is required to assess cardiac size and evidence of pulmonary oedema.
4 *Echocardiography* is a key investigation for all patients. Reversible causes of heart failure, such as valvular or pericardial disease, can be quickly excluded.
5 *Invasive investigations:* are indicated for these reasons:
   (a) Suspected coronary heart disease should be identified, as revascularization by coronary artery bypass grafting may improve LV function in some patients.[24,25]
   (b) Electrophysiological studies (EPS) and radio-frequency ablation are useful for atrial dys-rhythmias that precipitate heart failure or incessant ventricular tachycardia.
   (c) Endomyocardial biopsy is used to identify chronic lymphocytic myocarditis or acute myocarditis that may respond to immuno-suppressive therapy. It can also reveal specific heart muscle diseases, such as amyloidosis or haemochromatosis.[26]
6 *Exercise testing:* Peak oxygen uptake on exercise reflects circulatory status, and is used to assess potential patients for cardiac transplant; values below 14 ml/kg per min suggest transplantation.
7 *Neuroendocrine hormones:* Plasma adrenaline concentrations correlate directly with the severity of LV dysfunction and prognosis.[27] Measurement of BNP may be useful to select post myocardial infarction patients for treatment with angiotensin-converting enzyme (ACE) inhibitors.[28]

8 *Radionucleotide ventriculography (multiple gated acquisition or MUGA scan)* is useful for more accurate assessment of LV ejection fraction.

Management

Emphasis in treating heart failure has shifted from attempts to improve systolic performance to correcting pathophysiological abnormalities of the whole circulation. This latter approach appears to be more effective in improving symptoms and prolonging life.

General measures

Rest is important in acute heart failure, but gentle exercise is beneficial in chronic failure. Weight reduction and a low sodium intake should be encouraged.

Diuretics[29]

Diuretics are effective in relieving breathlessness and oedema, and have a mild vasodilating action. However, they stimulate RAAS and thereby increase afterload. Improved survival in heart failure with diuretics has not been proven. Frusemide is the usual diuretic. If large doses (e.g. over 120 mg/day) are required, addition of a thiazide diuretic achieves synergism. Bendrofluazide 5–10 mg daily is effective. Metolazone is a powerful thiazide useful for severe oedema, but should be used with caution. Hypokalaemia and overdiuresis must be avoided.

ACE inhibitors

ACE inhibitors are a major advance in heart failure treatment. They improve exercise tolerance and symptoms and signs of all grades of failure. The CONSENSUS, SAVE and SOLVD trials[30–33] confirmed that mortality is reduced with their use. ACE inhibitors should be introduced cautiously to patients with severe heart failure, low systolic blood pressure, low serum sodium concentrations (<130 mmol/l) and possible hypovolaemia. They should probably not be given to patients with renal impairment (e.g. serum creatinine >200 mmol/l). Diuretics are stopped for 24 h before starting a low dose (e.g. captopril 6.25 mg or enalapril 2.5 mg). Renal function is checked after 2–3 weeks before increasing the dose. Improved survival is associated with comparably large doses (e.g. captopril 150 mg and enalapril 20 mg daily). Diuretics are commonly used in combination.

Side-effects of ACE inhibitors are as follows:

1 *Hypotension* occurs in about 2.2%, but many can tolerate a systolic blood pressure of 90 mmHg (12 kPa) without obvious symptoms.

2 *Renal dysfunction* occurs in some patients, especially those with atheromatous renal arteries. However, improvement of the circulation may reduce creatinine and urea concentrations. Deteriorating renal function may be due to overdiuresis, and the diuretic dose will need to be reduced if improvement follows ACE inhibitors. Non-steroidal anti-inflammatory drugs (NSAIDs) may also cause renal dysfunction and should be avoided.

3 *Hyperkalaemia* is uncommon.

4 *Cough* is a common side-effect, but also occurs in heart failure because of the raised pulmonary venous pressure.

Hydralazine and nitrates

This vasodilator combination is more effective than placebo,[34] but less than enalapril[35] on mortality. Side-effects are frequent, and the combination is not often used. Hydralazine increases sympathetic activity and RAAS, which may blunt any favourable haemodynamic changes.

Calcium antagonists

Treatment with the calcium anatagonists verapamil, nifedipine and diltiazem increases the risk of worsening heart failure and cardiovascular death.[36] Amlodipine and felodipine are a newer class of calcium antagonists that decrease sympathetic activity. They may have some value in heart failure, but results of trials are still awaited.

Digoxin

There is renewed interest in digoxin, because it may have some important effects other than inotropy.[37] Digoxin is able to reduce sympathetic activity and increase vagal activity, and thus slow heart rate. It has been shown to benefit patients with sinus rhythm heart failure, when given with ACE inhibitors and diuretics.[37] Therefore, digoxin can be added to patients who still have symptoms despite receiving ACE inhibitors and diuretics.

β-Adrenergic blockers[38]

Use of β-blockers in heart failure was controversial, but they have been shown to improve survival in patients with severe heart failure after myocardial infarction. Also, symptomatic improvement and reduced need for cardiac transplantation in dilated cardiomyopathy are possible benefits. Many trials are now assessing β-blockers in a wider group of patients with heart failure, including those with ischaemic heart disease.

Other pharmacological agents

Newer drugs to oppose neurohormonal activation (e.g. endothelin and inhibitors of angiotensin II receptors) are presently undergoing trials. Ventricular arrhythmias are a common cause of death in heart failure, but all antiarrhythmic drugs except amiodarone have a negative inotropic action. Only amiodarone has been assessed in heart failure and it may reduce mortality.[39]

Inotropic drugs seem to have little value in chronic heart failure. Several drugs used to treat chronic failure (e.g. dobutamine, milrinone, enoximone, xamoterol, flosequinan, vesnarinone and a prostaglandin analogue epoprostenol) have been shown to increase mortality.[36]

Surgical treatments

1 Coronary bypass grafting is effective to improve symptoms and prognosis of patients with three-vessel disease and impaired LV function. 'Hibernating' areas of normal myocardium may still be present within ischaemic areas, and overall LV function can improve significantly after reperfusion. Patients are assessed by coronary angiography and nuclear imaging techniques, including positron emission tomography scanning.
2 Cardiac transplantation is effective therapy, with a possible 75% 5-year survival and 55% at 10 years.[40] Absolute contraindications include pulmonary hypertension, interstitial lung disease, recent pulmonary embolism or infarction, active infection, continual alcohol or drug abuse, significant peripheral or cerebral vascular disease, and malignancy.
3 Other surgical procedures such as cardiomyoplasty, implantable ventricular support devices and total artificial hearts are still being evaluated.

Management of acute left ventricular failure

Acute heart failure is a medical emergency requiring urgent treatment. Diagnosis is usually straightforward. Sudden onset of dyspnoea (with or without chest pain or tightness), sweating, tachycardia, cardiac enlargement (not always), S3, S4 or gallop rhythm, and bilateral crepitations or wheezing are usual features. Raised JVP and peripheral oedema may be absent. Differential diagnosis includes exacerbation of airways disease, aortic dissection, pulmonary embolism and acute pericardial tamponade. If possible, echocardiography should be promptly performed. Other investigations required include blood biochemistry, haematology, arterial gases, chest X-ray and electrocardiogram (ECG).

Immediate treatment is as follows:

1 High-flow oxygen is given by facemask.

2 The patient is sat upright. This reduces preload and improves ventilation:perfusion mismatch.[41]
3 Morphine, titrated slowly, is given in 2.5–5.0 mg IV boluses. Its mechanism of action is not clear,[42] but is probably by venodilatation, thereby decreasing LV filling pressure.[43]
4 Frusemide 40–120 mg IV bolus is given. Traditional teaching advocates giving a loop-acting diuretic to reduce LV filling pressure through rapid diuresis and venodilatation.[44] However, frusemide causes an early rise in LV filling pressure and a fall in cardiac output, associated with an increase in systemic vascular resistance.[45–47] These findings suggest potential harm from frusemide administration, particularly in the setting of myocardial ischaemia. None the less, conventional opinion currently supports the use of frusemide for acute LV failure.
5 Vasodilators, nitrates or sodium nitroprusside may improve acute LV failure by reducing LV filling pressure and afterload. Nitrates are more widely used, as (in low doses) they are primarily veno-dilators. (Higher doses of nitrates can cause arterial dilatation, and may be used to reduce systemic arterial pressure.) Nitroprusside produces a more balanced arterial and venous dilatation,[48] but may have a deleterious effect soon after acute myocardial infarction.[49] Nitroglycerin 600 μg can be given sublingually for an acute effect in the emergency room. This should be followed by an infusion, starting at 0.25 μg/kg per min and titrated every 5–10 min against blood pressure. Usual dose range is 0.5–1.5 μg/kg per min. Although special poly-ethylene administration sets are available, standard polyvinyl chloride tubing can be used, since infusion is titrated against clinical effect.[50] Intravenous ACE inhibitors have been used in acute LV failure with good effect,[51,52] but their role is not established.
6 Positive airway pressure (i.e. positive end-expiratory pressure (PEEP) and continuous positive airways pressure (CPAP)) is effective in LV failure.[53] It increases functional residual capacity and lung compliance, reduces work of breathing, and improves ventilation:perfusion mismatch. Extra-vascular lung water is not decreased[54] (see Chapter 26). PEEP may also improve cardiac function in severe LV failure, due to reduced LV afterload associated with increased intrathoracic pressure.[55,56]
7 Inotropes may be required, aiming to improve vital organ perfusion and reduce LV filling pressure without causing significant myocardial oxygen supply : demand imbalance (i.e. avoid tachycardia and increased LV afterload). Catecholamine receptor activity may be abnormal. Myocardial noradrenaline stores may be decreased with 'down-regulation' of β-receptors.[57,58] Dobutamine (1–20 μg/kg per min) is recommended, since it reduces afterload and has little effect on heart rate. However, it may occasionally cause tachycardia, and is often

inadequate in the hypotensive patient. Dopamine (1–20 µg/kg per min) or adrenaline (1–20 µg/min) may provide better pressor effects. Phosphodiesterase inhibitors (e.g. amrinone, milrinone and enoximone) combine positive inotropic and vasodilating properties, and have been shown to have beneficial haemodynamic effects in acute LV failure.[59]

8 Mechanical circulatory assisted device, i.e. intraaortic balloon pump (IABP), may reduce LV work, increase cardiac output and decrease LV filling pressure.[60] However, mortality remains high despite its use. None the less, it provides cardiovascular support to allow time for more definitive therapy (e.g. coronary artery bypass grafting or angioplasty). With this combined therapy, survival from cardiogenic shock complicating myocardial infarction has significantly improved.[61]

9 *Other treatment modalities:* Venesection, while probably effective, risks hypovolaemia and reduced cardiac output. Rotating tourniquets are effective in achieving venous pooling, but can increase systemic vascular resistance and LV diastolic volume, and reduce LV ejection fraction and cardiac output.[62]

References

1 Packer M (1993) How should physicians view heart failure? The philosophical and physiological evolution of three conceptual models of the disease. *Am J Cardiol* **71**:3C–11C.

2 Kannel WB, Ho K and Thom T (1994) Changing epidemiological features of heart failure. *Br Heart J* **72**:3–9.

3 Ho KK, Anderson KM, Kannel WB, Grossman W and Levy D (1993) Survival after the onset of congestive heart failure in Framingham Heart Study subjects. *Circulation* **88**:107–115.

4 Schocker DD, Arrieta MI, Leaverton PE and Ross EA (1992) Prevalence and mortality rate of congestive heart failure in the United States. *J Am Coll Cardiol* **20**:301–306.

5 Sanderson JE, Chan KW and Woo KS. Hypertension is the main cause of heart failure in the Chinese population of Hong Kong – results from a prospective study of 730 patients. *Eur Heart J* **15**:615.

6 Ross JJ (1976) Afterload mismatch and preload reserve: a conceptual framework for the analysis of ventricular function. *Prog Cardiovasc Dis* **18**:255–264.

7 Sanderson JE, Adesanya CO, Anjorin F *et al.* (1979) Postpartum cardiac failure – heart failure due to volume overload? *Am Heart J* **97**:613–621.

8 Kenneth AW (1992) Thyrotoxicosis and the heart. *N Engl J Med* **327**:94–98.

9 Packer M (1992) Pathophysiology of chronic heart failure. *Lancet* **340**:88–92.

10 Leimbach WN, Wallin BG, Victor RG *et al.* (1986) Direct evidence from intraneural recordings for increased central sympathetic outflow in patients with heart failure. *Circulation* **73**:913–919.

11 Morgan HE and Baker KM (1991) Cardiac hypertrophy: mechanical, neural, and endocrine dependence. *Circulation* **83**:13–25.

12 Lindpaintner K and Ganten D (1991) The cardiac renin-angiotensin system: an appraisal of present experimental and clinical evidence. *Circ Res* **68**: 905–921.

13 Anand IS, Ferrari R, Kalra GS, Wahi PL, Poole-Wilson PA and Harris PC (1989) Congestive heart failure: oedema of cardiac origins: studies of body water and sodium, renal function; hemodynamic indexes and plasma hormones in untreated congestive heart failure. *Circulation* **80**:299–305.

14 Wei C-M, Heublein DM, Perrella MA *et al.* (1993) Natriuretic peptide system in human heart failure. *Circulation* **88**:1004–1009.

15 Floras JS (1990) Sympathoinhibitory effects of atrial natriuretic factor in normal humans. *Circulation* **81**:1860–1873.

16 Wei CM, Lerman A, Rodeheffer RJ *et al.* (1994) Endothelin in human congestive heart failure. *Circulation* **89**:1580–1586.

17 Weber KT, Sun Y, Tyagi SC and Cleutjens JPM (1994) Collagen network of the myocardium: function, structural remodelling and regulatory mechanisms. *J Mol Cell Cardiol* **26**:279–292.

18 Levine B, Kalman J, Mayer L *et al.* (1990) Elevated circulating levels of tumour necrosis factor in congestive heart failure. *N Engl J Med* **323**:236–241.

19 Hirsch AT, Dzau VJ and Mager MA (1987) Baroreceptor function in congestive heart failure: effect on neuro-hormonal activation and regional vascular resistance. *Circulation* **75**:36–48.

20 Podrid PJ, Fuchs T and Candinas R (1990) Role of the sympathetic nervous system in the genesis of ventricular arrhythmia. *Circulation* **82**:103–113.

21 Creager MA and Creager SJ (1994) Arterial baroreceptor regulation of blood pressure in patients with congestive heart failure. *J Am Coll Cardiol* **23**:401–405.

22 Yie G-Y, Berk MR, Smith MD, Gurley JC and DeMaria AN (1994) Prognostic value of Doppler transmitral flow patterns in patients with congestive heart failure. *J Am Coll Cardiol* **24**:132–139.

23 Casadei B, Meyer TE, Coats AJS *et al.* (1992) Baroreflex control of stroke volume: an effect mediated by the vagus. *J Physiol* **448**:539–550.

24 Rahimtoola SH (1989) The hibernating myocardium. *Am Heart J* **117**:211–221.

25 Bounous EP, Mark DB, Pollock BG *et al.* (1988) Surgical survival benefits for coronary disease patients with left ventricular dysfunction. *Circulation* **78**:1151–1157.

26 Kasper EK, Agema WRP, Hutchins GM, Deckers JW, Hare JM and Baughman KL (1994) The causes of dilated cardiomyopathy: a clinicopathologic review of 673 consecutive patients. *J Am Coll Cardiol* **23**: 586–590.

27 Cohn JN, Levine TB, Olivari MT *et al.* (1984) Plasma norepinephrine as a guide to prognosis in patients with congestive heart failure. *N Engl J Med* **311**:819–823.

28 Motwani J, McAlpine H, Kennedy N and Struthers A (1993) Plasma brain natriuretic peptide as an indicator for angiotensin-converting-enzyme inhibition after myocardial infarction. *Lancet* **341**:1109–1113.

29 van Swieten PA (1994) Neuroendocrine effects of diuretics in heart failure. *Br Heart J* **72**:51–53.

30 CONSENSUS Trial Study Group (1987) Effects of enalapril on mortality in severe congestive heart failure. Results of the cooperative north Scandinavian enalpril survivel study. *N Engl J Med* **316**:1429–1435.

31 Pfeffer MA, Braunwald E, Moye LA *et al.* for the SAVE investigators (1992) Effect of captopril on mortality and morbidity in patients with left ventricular dysfunction after myocardial infarction. Results of the survival and ventricular enlargement trial. *N Engl J Med* **327**:669–677.

32 The SOLVD investigators (1992) Effect of enalapril on mortality and the development of heart failure in asymptomatic patients with reduced left ventricular ejection fractions. *N Engl J Med* **327**:685–691.

33 The SOLVD investigators (1991) Effect of enalapril on survival in patients with reduced left ventricular ejection fractions and congestive heart failure. *N Engl J Med* **325**:293–302.

34 Cohn JN, Archibald DG, Ziesche S *et al.* (1986) Effect of vasodilator therapy on mortality in chronic congestive heart failure. Results of a Veterans Affairs Administration cooperative study. *N Engl J Med* **314**:1547–1552.

35 Cohn JN, Johnson G, Ziesche S *et al.* (1991) A comparison of enalapril with hydralazine–isosorbide dinitrate in the treatment of chronic congestive heart failure. *N Engl J Med* **325**:303–310.

36 Packer M (1992) Treatment of chronic heart failure. *Lancet* **340**:92–95.

37 Smith TW (1993) Digoxin in heart failure. *N Engl J Med* **329**:51–53.

38 Doughty RN, MacMahon S and Sharpe N (1994) Beta blockers in heart failure: promising or proved? *J Am Coll Cardiol* **23**:814–821.

39 Doval HC, Nul DR, Grancelli HO *et al.* (1994) Randomised trial of low-dose amiodarone in severe congestive heart failure. *Lancet* **344**:493–498.

40 Hunt SA (1993) 24th Bethesda conference: cardiac transplantation. *J Am Coll Cardiol* **22**:1–64.

41 Nunn JF (1993) *Respiratory Physiology*, 4th edn. Oxford: Butterworth-Heinemann.

42 Jaffe JH and Martin WR (1991) Opioid analgesics and antagonists. In: Gilman AG, Rall TW, Nies AS and Taylor P (eds) *Goodman & Gilman's The Pharmacological Basis of Therapeutics,* 8th edn. New York: Maxwell Macmillan, pp. 485–521.

43 Vismara LA, Leamon DM and Zelis R (1976) The effect of morphine on venous tone in patients with acute pulmonary oedema. *Circulation* **54**:335–337.

44 Dikshit K, Vyden JK, Forrester JS, Chatterjee K, Prakash R and Swan HJC (1973) Renal and extrarenal effects of frusemide in congestive heart failure after acute myocardial infarction. *N Engl J Med* **288**: 1087–1090.

45 Francis GS, Siegel RM, Goldsmith SR, Olivari MT, Levine TB and Cohn JN (1985) Acute vasoconstrictor response to intravenous furosemide in patients with chronic congestive heart failure. Activation of the neurohumoral axis. *Ann Intern Med* **103**:1–6.

46 Kraus PA and Lipman J (1990) Acute preload effects of frusemide. *Chest* **98**:124–128.

47 Nelson GIC, Silke B, Ahuja RC, Hussain M and Taylor SH (1983) Haemodynamic advantages of isosorbide dinitrate over frusemide in acute heart failure following myocardial infarction. *Lancet* **i**: 730–733.

48 Francis GS (1991) Vasodilators in the intensive care unit. *Am Heart J* **121**:1875–1878.

49 Cohn JN, Franciosa JA, Francis GS *et al.* (1982) Effect of short-term infusion of sodium nitroprusside on mortality rate in acute myocardial infarction complicated by left ventricular failure. *N Engl J Med* **306**: 1129–1135.

50 Young JB, Pratt CM, Farmer JA *et al.* (1984) Specialized delivery systems for intravenous nitroglycerin; are they necessary in the clinical setting? *Am J Med* **76**:27–37.

51 Ahmad S, Giles TD, Roffidal LE, Haney Y, Given MB and Sander GE (1990) Intravenous captopril in congestive heart failure. *J Clin Pharmacol* **30**:609–614.

52 Tohmo H, Karanko M, Korpilahti K, Scheinin M, Viinamaki O and Neuvonen P (1994) Enalaprilat in acute intractable heart failure after myocardial infarction: a prospective, consecutive sample, before–after trial. *Crit Care Med* **22**:965–973.

53 Bersten AD, Holt AW, Vedig AE, Skowronski GA and Baggoley CJ (1991) Treatment of severe cardiogenic pulmonary oedema with continuous positive airway pressure delivered by face mask. *N Engl J Med* **325**: 1825–1830.

54 Rizk NW and Murray JF (1982) PEEP and pulmonary oedema. *Am J Med* **72**:381–383.

55 Bradley TD, Holloway RM, McLaughlin PR, Ross BL, Walters J and Liu PP (1992) Cardiac output response to continuous positive airway pressure in congestive heart failure. *Am Rev Respir Dis* **145**: 377–382.

56 Buda AJ, Pinsky MR, Ingels NB, Daughters GT, Stinson EB and Alderman EL (1979) Effect of intrathoracic pressure on left ventricular performance. *N Engl J Med* **301**:453–459.

57 Runciman WB (1980) Sympathomimetic amines. *Anaesth Intens Care* **8**:289–309.

58 Fowler MB, Laser JA, Hopkins GL *et al.* (1986) Assessment of the beta-adrenergic receptor pathway in the intact failing human heart: progressive down-regulation and subsensitivity to agonist response. *Circulation* **74**:1290–1302.

59 Chatterjee K, Wolfe CL and DeMarco T (1994) Nonglycoside inotropes in congestive heart failure. Are they beneficial or harmful? *Cardiol Clin* **12**:63–72.

60 Nanas JN and Moulopoulos SD (1994) Counter-pulsation: historical background, technical improvements, hemodynamic and metabolic effects. *Cardiology* **84**:156–167.

61 Mueller HS (1994) Role of intra-aortic counterpulsation in cardiogenic shock and acute myocardial infarction.

Cardiology **84**:168–174.

62 Klein HO, Brodsky E, Ninio R, Kaplinsky E and Di Segni E (1993) The effect of venous occlusion with tourniqets on peripheral blood pooling and ventricular function. *Chest* **103**:521–527.

14 | Circulatory shock

GA Skowronski

Circulatory shock may be defined as a state of cardiovascular dysfunction resulting in a generalized inadequacy of tissue perfusion relative to metabolic requirements. Tissue hypoxia leads to progressive failure of cellular metabolism, eventually resulting in multiple organ dysfunction or death. The term actually encompasses a group of cardiovascular disorders with distinctive aetiologies and pathophysiological patterns. *Hypovolaemic, septic* and *cardiogenic shock* are the most commonly classified and discussed subgroups, but others are also recognized, based on aetiology or characteristic pathophysiological patterns. Examples include anaphylactic, spinal, traumatic, neurogenic and toxic shock.

Aetiology

Hypovolaemic shock is due to inadequate left ventricular preload, which usually requires a relative or absolute reduction in the circulating blood volume by 15–25%,[1] leading to a significant fall in cardiac output. Haemorrhage is the commonest cause, but loss of plasma or protein-free extracellular fluid can also result in hypovolaemic shock. Commonly associated clinical conditions include trauma, burns, severe vomiting, diarrhoea, fistulae and excessive diuresis.

Septic shock (see Chapter 61) may be caused by infections due to Gram-negative or Gram-positive bacteria, fungi (most commonly *Candida* spp.), protozoa (e.g. malaria) or viruses (e.g. dengue fever). A clinically indistinguishable shock state may follow severe non-infective insults such as pancreatitis (see Chapter 85). Toxic shock classically follows localized infection with *Staphylococcus aureus*,[2] but may be produced by severe infection with group A *Streptococcus pyogenes*.[3]

Cardiogenic shock is discussed in Chapter 15. It occurs most commonly as a complication of myocardial infarction, but may arise from myocarditis or tamponade. Neurogenic shock most commonly

results from trauma to the cervical spine, while anaphylactic shock follows exposure to allergens (see Chapters 58 and 69). Different shock states commonly coexist, such as when hypovolaemia complicates septic shock.

Pathogenesis and pathophysiology[4-6]

Cellular changes

Most of the cellular changes and compensatory mechanisms are common to all forms of shock. Ischaemia and impaired tissue perfusion lead to generalized cellular damage, although organs may vary considerably in their ability to withstand ischaemia. Anaerobic cellular metabolism leads to depletion of adenosine triphosphate and failure of the cell membrane sodium–potassium pump.[7] Cell swelling occurs due to sodium and water influx. Anaerobic metabolism also produces a progressively worsening metabolic (lactic) acidosis, and blood lactate levels may be used as a guide to the severity, prognosis and effectiveness of therapy in shock.[8] Mitochondrial calcium loss further impairs the efficiency of oxidation and phosphorylation, and may interfere with other organ-specific functions such as myocardial contractility.[9] Eventually, a large number of cytotoxic, vasodilator, vasoactive and other substances are released into the circulation, resulting in progressive vasodilatation, myocardial depression, increased capillary permeability, and eventually, intravascular coagulation. These substances include histamine, serotonin, kinins, lysosomal enzymes, and endogenous mediators (see below)[10-14]

Organ dysfunction

Heart

Myocardial dysfunction is common in shock. Ischaemic heart disease contributes, especially in cardiogenic shock. In septic and hypovolaemic shock, the effects of several myocardial depressant substances[15] and down-regulation of cardiac β-receptors[16] are more important. Pulmonary hypertension and diastolic dysfunction also contribute to myocardial failure in septic and cardiogenic shock, especially if the acute respiratory distress syndrome (ARDS) is present.[17]

Kidneys

In early shock, the glomerular filtration rate (GFR) is well-preserved by autoregulation, but oliguria nevertheless occurs, due to antidiuretic hormone (ADH) and aldosterone secretion. As GFR falls, oliguria persists or worsens. These changes may be modified by renal trauma, pre-existing renal disease or infection, crush injuries or nephrotoxic drugs such as aminoglycosides. If shock is severe or prolonged, acute renal failure may result. This is initiated by a temporary disorder of glomerular blood flow regulation, and histological phenomena such as the presence of acute tubular necrosis may be of less physiological significance than was once believed[18] (see Chapter 38).

Liver

Both hepatic arterial and portal venous blood flow are reduced in shock. The commonest clinical consequence is the development of intrahepatic cholestasis, especially in relation to septic shock.[19] Profound hypoxia or hypotension may produce more severe liver dysfunction, with marked transaminase rises.[20] Also, the liver's reticuloendothelial function is impaired following shock,[21] but the clinical significance of this is uncertain.

Gastrointestinal tract

Splanchnic blood flow is reduced during shock, and mucosal injury may follow the production of free oxygen radicals after reperfusion. It is proposed that this allows translocation of bacteria and their toxins, which can then pass through the liver because of its reticuloendothelial dysfunction, and hence into the systemic circulation.[22] Evidence for this 'gut hypothesis' is inconclusive. Splanchnic ischaemia is reflected by intramucosal gastric acidosis, which can be detected clinically by gastric tonometry. This has been suggested as a sensitive indicator of tissue hypoxia in shock and a predictor of organ failure.[23]

Lungs

Hyperventilation occurs early in shock due to peripheral chemoreceptor stimulation.[24] Reduced pulmonary blood flow results in increased physiological dead space, which is more than compensated by the increase in respiratory rate and minute volume. Pa_{O_2} is often well-maintained, but advanced shock may result in respiratory failure due to progressive atelectasis, ARDS, respiratory muscle fatigue from respiratory muscle hypoperfusion,[25] or, more rarely, respiratory centre depression due to inadequate cerebral perfusion. Pre-existing lung disease, chest trauma and cardiac failure may contribute.

Brain

Mental state abnormalities are common during shock, and are associated with poor outcome.[26] Respiratory alkalosis, hypoxaemia, electrolyte disturbances and hypoperfusion all contribute, but permanent ischaemic injury is uncommon.

Intermediary metabolism

Hyperglycaemia is mainly due to insulin resistance, to which catecholamines, glucagon and glucocorticoid secretion all contribute. Catecholamines also inhibit insulin release. Catabolism of both fat and carbohydrate is inhibited in shock, and there is increased reliance on skeletal muscle amino acids, especially branched-chain amino acids, as a fuel source. Lactic acid production is increased due to mitochondrial dysfunction and hypoxia.

Oxygen transport

An imbalance between oxygen supply and tissue demands is fundamental to the nature of shock. Under normal circumstances, whole body oxygen consumption (V_{O_2}) is maintained over a wide range of oxygen delivery (D_{O_2}) by varying oxygen extraction (i.e. 'supply-independent' oxygen transport). Once D_{O_2} falls below a critical level, however, V_{O_2} becomes linearly dependent (Fig. 14.1). This supply-dependent

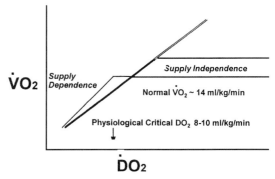

Fig. 14.1 Oxygen consumption (V_{O_2}): supply (V_{O_2}) dependence. The thin line is the physiological relationship and shows critical D_{O_2} and physiological oxygen supply dependence. Pathological supply dependence is shown by the thick line; critical D_{O_2} and V_{O_2} are increased, and the relationship may be linear throughout the clinical range of D_{O_2} (double line).

state defines shock in physiological terms, and measures of the accumulated oxygen debt, such as blood lactate, correlate with morbidity and mortality.[27] In sepsis and ARDS, tissue oxygen extraction efficiency is reduced, and critical D_{O_2} is substantially raised (Fig. 14.1). This $V_{O_2}:D_{O_2}$ relationship may indeed be linear throughout the full range of supply.[28] However, the existence and physiological relevance of 'pathological supply dependence' are questioned[29] (see Chapter 22).

Haemodynamic changes

An increase in heart rate and contractility occurs due to increased sympathetic discharge. This also results in arteriolar and venular vasoconstriction, thus tending to improve cardiac output, venous return and blood pressure. Blood is diverted away from less important areas to vital organs, which initially include the brain, heart, kidneys, liver and respiratory muscles. In cardiogenic and hypovolaemic shock, these mechanisms are insufficient to correct adequately the progressively falling cardiac output, while septic shock is characterized by a generalized failure of systemic arteriolar tone with flow maldistribution at tissue level. Oxygen delivery is reduced despite the hyperdynamic, vasodilated circulation. Pulmonary hypertension is also common in septic shock, and is associated with a poor prognosis.[30]

Mediators

A large number of endogenous substances are triggered by a variety of stimuli, including drugs, infectious agents, tissue injury or ischaemia, haematomas and inflammatory disorders.

Eicosanoids

Eicosanoids are fatty acid metabolites derived from the cell membrane phospholipid component, arachidonic acid. Following release from cell membranes, arachidonic acid is metabolized via one of two main cascading enzyme pathways. The *cyclooxygenase* pathway is responsible for the production of thromboxane and a variety of prostaglandins, which have a diversity of platelet and vasoactive effects. The *lipoxygenase* pathway results in the production of proinflammatory products known as leukotrienes. Platelet-activating factor (PAF) is a related cell membrane phospholipid derivative, though not strictly an arachidonic acid metabolite. All these compounds have variable effects on smooth muscle tone, capillary permeability and neutrophil and platelet activity. Their infusion or inhibition can affect the progress of shock in a number of experimental models,[31] although results of clinical trials have been disappointing.

Endorphins

Endorphins are endogenous opioid peptides derived (along with adrenocorticotrophic hormone, melanocyte-stimulating hormone and enkephalin) from β-lipotropin, which is produced in the anterior pituitary gland in response to systemic stress. Concentrations of endorphins are increased in haemorrhagic and septic shock, and may exacerbate hypotension. Naloxone, an opioid antagonist, can reverse hypotension in animal models, but has not affected outcome in humans.[32]

Cytokines

Cytokines are small proteins produced by macrophages and other immune cells, and are primary mediators of inflammation. They include tumour necrosis factor (TNF; cachectin) and a cascading series of interleukins (IL). Levels of TNF, IL-1 and IL-6 are all elevated in septic shock, and may correlate with mortality,[33] though interventions directed against them have not proven consistently effective in humans.[34]

Complement

Complement comprises a cascading system of plasma proteins which non-specifically assist the immune system in immune cell activation, cytolysis and opsonization (facilitation of bacterial phagocytosis). The cascade is normally activated by antigen–antibody complexes (the classical pathway), but can also be directly activated by bacterial cell membranes and other substances (the alternative pathway). The complement system (particlarly components C3a and C5a) contributes to neutrophil activation, increased capillary permeability and hypotension, particularly in septic and anaphylactic shock.[35]

Nitric oxide

Nitric oxide (previously known as endothelium-derived relaxing factor, EDRF) is synthesized by platelets, nervous and immune systems, and endothelial cells, and is a potent, but extremely evanescent, vasodilator.[36] It is produced from L-arginine by the enzyme nitric oxide synthetase, which is found in constitutive and inducible forms. The latter can be activated by endotoxin, and inhibited by compounds such as *N*-monomethyl-L-arginine (L-NMMA), which may be useful to ameliorate hypotension in septic shock.[37]

Other proposed mediators in shock include bradykinin, free oxygen radicals, neutrophil proteases and endothelins.[38]

Clinical presentation

The terms hypotension and shock are not interchangeable, as either can occur without the other being present. Classical features of hypovolaemic shock include, in addition to hypotension, tachycardia, pallor, sweating, cyanosis, hyperventilation, confusion and oliguria. The presentation of septic shock is much more variable, but fever and vasodilatation with warm extremities may be seen, and confusion may be more prominent, particularly in the elderly. Cardiogenic shock is often complicated by arrhythmias or pulmonary oedema, while pulmonary embolism or pericardial tamponade are characterized by prominent signs of right heart failure. Combinations of shock subtypes may coexist, particularly septic shock combined with hypovolaemia. Additional problems such as respiratory failure may further complicate the clinical picture.

As the blood pressure falls, pulse pressure narrows, and measurement by non-invasive methods may become increasingly difficult and inaccurate.[39] Tachycardia usually precedes hypotension, but may not be present if the patient has pre-existing heart disease or has been taking β-adrenergic blocking drugs.

Management

Shock is a life-threatening and dynamic disorder in which haemodynamic and metabolic variables are continually changing. An urgent and well-organized approach is important, and frequent or even continuous reassessment is required. The diagnostic and therapeutic processes must proceed in parallel, rather than in series.

Ventilation and oxygenation

As with other types of resuscitation, airway and breathing should receive immediate attention. The combination of shock and respiratory failure has an extremely high mortality.[40] Hence, all shocked patients should receive high-flow oxygen by facemask, and intubation and mechanical ventilation should be instituted early if respiration is inadequate. Pneumothorax should be specifically sought and treated in trauma cases.

Volume resuscitation

When gross hypovolaemia is present, insertion of large-bore peripheral intravenous cannulae is more appropriate than urgent central venous catheterization, unless peripheral access is unavailable. Obvious external haemorrhage should be controlled by local pressure, but procedures such as urgent thoracotomy with aortic cross-clamping are probably of little value in the vast majority of cases.[41] The use of a PASG (pneumatic anti-shock garment), MAST (military antishock trousers) suit remains controversial,[42] but may help tamponade intra-abdominal bleeding in some circumstances. When the response to resuscitation suggests ongoing intra-abdominal or intrathoracic bleeding, complex investigations should be kept to a minimum, and every effort should be made to organize urgent definitive surgery.

In septic shock, volume requirements are more variable, and are best guided by haemodynamic monitoring, while volume loading is usually contra-indicated in cardiogenic shock.

Choice of intravenous fluids

As a general rule, the fluid chosen should most closely match the fluid lost. Controversy continues over the relative merits of crystalloids and colloids as plasma expanders.[43,44] Supporters of colloids contend that resuscitation with colloids is more rapid and with fewer adverse effects on the lungs. However, crystalloid users consider that crystalloids are more appropriate, as they equilibrate between intravascular and interstitial fluid spaces, overcoming the main problem in shock (i.e. shrinkage of the entire extracellular compartment). Crystalloids are also cheaper, although 2–4 times the volume may be required to achieve a comparable degree of resuscitation. Colloids present a very small risk of allergic reactions (see Chapter 87). There is, however, no clear evidence to favour either fluid type, especially as regards adverse influence on pulmonary function.[45–47] A mixture of colloids (initially for rapid improvement) and crystalloids is commonly used in practice.[48]

There is some interest in using hypertonic saline solutions (e.g. 3%) for plasma expansion and resuscitation.[46] Plasma volume expansion is thought to be due to an increased osmolality, drawing intracellular fluid into the extracellular spaces. Smaller volumes are required to achieve the same physiological end-points, and improvement may be more sustained if dextran is added.[49] The precise place of hypertonic saline in volume resuscitation is yet to be determined.

Blood should be transfused where significant blood loss has occurred, with the aim of maximizing tissue oxygen delivery by maintaining a haematocrit of at least 0.3 (equivalent to a haemoglobin concentration of about 10 g/dl).[50] The use of oxygen-carrying blood substitutes such as perfluorocarbons[51] and stroma-free haemoglobin is not established.

Monitoring

Heart rate, blood pressure, respiratory rate, urine output, mental state and temperature should all be measured and recorded frequently. A central venous catheter may be used to assess the right ventricular preload, particularly if trends rather than individual readings are observed. However, the central venous pressure (CVP) may be difficult to interpret in patients with lung disease or selective right or left ventricular dysfunction. In more complex cases, and particularly in septic or cardiogenic shock, a pulmonary artery (Swan–Ganz) catheter may be helpful. This allows cardiovascular support to be based on biventricular filling pressures, as well as haemodynamics and oxygen transport. However, in uncomplicated hypovolaemia, pulmonary artery catheterization is uncommonly required, and should never delay urgent investigation or surgery. Neither the CVP nor the pulmonary capillary wedge pressure (PCWP) provides a meaningful measure of the circulating blood volume.[52]

Regular laboratory investigations should include blood gases, electrolyte and acid–base status, renal and liver function, blood glucose, coagulation and routine haematology. Blood lactate monitoring, as a guide to the effectiveness of cardiovascular support, is frequently used, especially in septic shock.[53]

Acid–base and electrolyte therapy

Hypokalaemia, hyponatraemia and metabolic acidosis are characteristic of most shock states, and should be managed conventionally. Hyponatraemia and acidosis will usually respond to cardiovascular optimization with appropriate fluids or inotropes. Bicarbonate administration carries a considerable concurrent sodium load, may worsen intracellular acidosis, tissue oxygen delivery, and hypokalaemia, and does not improve haemodynamics.[54] Hence, only severe and persistent acidosis should be treated in this way.

Inotropic drugs

Failure of the patient to respond to fluid replacement in hypovolaemic shock should prompt a careful search for some other problem (e.g. tension pneumothorax, pericardial tamponade, or continuing bleeding). In septic or cardiogenic shock, use of an inotrope may be indicated, and the choice will depend on the clinical setting. However, differences among these agents are probably of less clinical importance than is commonly asserted, and infusions of adrenaline (1–20 μg/min), noradrenaline (1–20 μg/min), dopamine (1–20 μg/kg per min) and dobutamine (1–20 μg/kg per min) are commonly used.[55] Phosphodiesterase inhibitors, such as milrinone (25 μg/kg bolus, followed by infusion at 0.5 μg/kg per min), may be useful in cardiogenic shock.[56]

Diuretics

Frusemide (10–40 mg) or mannitol (10–20 g) are often given intravenously when oliguria persists despite apparently adequate fluid resuscitation. However,

there is no clear evidence that this improves renal perfusion or can prevent or ameliorate the development of acute renal failure.[57–59] Care must be taken to ensure that a brisk diuresis does not worsen hypovolaemia or hypokalaemia. There is some evidence to suggest that infusion of dopamine at low dosage (2–5 μg/kg per min) may be helpful, but this has never been confirmed in controlled trials.[60,61]

Other treatment

There is no clinical evidence to support the use of corticosteroids in shock, despite theoretical and laboratory-based support for their use.[62] They are contraindicated if concurrent sepsis is present.[63,64]

Naloxone has been used in shock, and anecdotal reports suggest it may temporarily reverse hypotension, possibly by antagonizing central δ-receptors. Currently there is no good evidence that naloxone can improve outcome.[65]

Antibodies against endotoxin, TNF and IL-1 receptors have all had some success experimentally, but there is insufficient evidence to justify routine clinical use.[34,66,67] A number of other agents have potential value in the therapy of shock. Those of note include thyrotropin-releasing hormone (TRH),[68] fibronectin,[69] and various prostaglandins and their inhibitors.[70] All require considerably more study before they can be recommended for clinical use.

Outcome

The prognosis of shock depends on the underlying cause, severity and duration of the shock state, as well as the patient's age and pre-existing illness. Maintenance of a high cardiac output and oxygen delivery are associated with survival.[71] Cardiogenic shock not amenable to surgical intervention carries a mortality of 80%, although an aggressive interventive approach may achieve considerably better results.[72] Septic shock is generally reported to have about 50% mortality, but this is highly dependent on the site and reversibility of the septic focus. The prognosis in hypovolaemic shock is strongly related to the nature of the underlying problem, but with early, aggressive resuscitation and a correctable cause, the outlook is excellent.

References

1 Hardaway RM (1979) Monitoring of the patient in a state of shock. *Surg Gynecol Obstet* **148**:339–345.
2 Reingold AL (1991) Toxic shock syndrome: an update. *Am J Obstet Gynecol* **165**:1236–1239.
3 Wood TF, Potter MA and Jonasson O (1993) Streptococcal toxic shock-like syndrome. The importance of surgical intervention. *Ann Surg* **217**:109–114.

4 George RJD and Tinker J (1983) The pathophysiology of shock. In: Tinker J and Rapin M (eds) *Care of the Critically Ill Patient*. Berlin: Springer-Verlag, pp. 163–187.

5 Skowronski GA (1988) The pathophysiology of shock. *Med J Aust* **148**:576–583.

6 Shoemaker WC (1987) Circulatory mechanisms of shock and their mediators. *Crit Care Med* **15**:787–794.

7 Sayeed MM (1982) Membrane sodium–potassium transport and ancillary phenomenon in circulatory shock. In: Cowley R and Trump B (eds) *Pathophysiology of Shock, Anoxia and Ischaemia*. Baltimore: Williams & Wilkins, pp. 112–132.

8 Vincent JL, Dufaye P, Berre J et al. (1983) Serial lactate determinations during circulatory shock. *Crit Care Med* **11**:449–451.

9 Haugaard N, Haugaard ES, Lee NH and Horn RS (1969) Possible role of mitochondria in the regulation of cardiac contractility. *Fed Proc* **28**:1657–1662.

10 Schayer RW (1962) Evidence that induced histamine is an intrinsic regulator of the microcirculatory system. *Am J Physiol* **202**:66–72.

11 Reichgolt MJ, Forsyth RP and Melman KI (1971) Effects of bradykinin and autonomic nervous system inhibition on systemic and regional hemodynamics in the unanaesthetized rhesus monkey. *Circ Res* **29**:367–374.

12 Fredlund PE, Ockerman PA and Vang JO (1972) Plasma activities of acid hydrolases in experimental oligemic shock in the pig. *Am J Surg* **124**:300–306.

13 Fletcher JR and Romwell PW (1980) The effects of prostacyclin on endotoxin shock and endotoxin induced platelet aggregation in dogs. *Circ Shock* **7**: 299–308.

14 Beutter B and Ceramin A (1986) Cachectin and tumour necrosis factor as two sides of the same biological coin. *Nature* **320**:584–588.

15 Parillo JE, Burche C, Shelhamer JH et al. (1985) A circulating myocardial depressant substance in humans with septic shock. *J Clin Invest* **76**:1539–1553.

16 Romano FD and Jones SB (1986) Characteristics of myocardial β-adrenergic receptors during endotoxicosis in the rat. *Am J Physiol* **251**:R359–R364.

17 Jafri S, Levine S, Field B et al. (1990) Left ventricular diastolic dysfunction in sepsis. *Crit Care Med* **18**: 709–714.

18 Brezis M, Rosen S, Silva P et al. (1984) Renal ischaemia: a new perspective. *Kidney Int* **26**:375–383.

19 Franson T, Hierholzer W and LaBrecque D (1985) Frequency and characteristics of hyperbilirubinemia associated with bacteremia. *Rev Infect Dis* **7**:1–9.

20 Birgens H, Henrickson J, Matzen P et al. (1978) The shock liver: clinical and biochemical findings in patients with centrilobular liver necrosis following cardiogenic shock. *Acta Med Scand* **204**:417–423.

21 Grun M, Brolsch CE and Walter J (1980) Influence of portal hepatic flow on RES function. In: Liehr H and Grun M (eds) *Reticuloendothelial System and Pathogenesis of Liver Disease*. New York: Elsevier/North Holland Biomedical Press, pp. 149–158.

22 Reilly PM and Bulkley GB (1993) Vasoactive mediators and splanchnic perfusion. *Crit Care Med* **21**:S55–S68.

23 Fiddian-Green RG (1993) Associations between intra-mucosal acidosis in the gut and organ failure. *Crit Care Med* **21**:S103–S107.

24 Douglas ME, Downs JB, Dannemiller FJ and Hodges MR (1976) Acute respiratory failure and intravascular coagulation. *Surg Gynecol Obstet* **143**:555–560.

25 Roussos C and Macklem PT (1982) The respiratory muscles. *N Engl J Med* **307**:786–797.

26 Sprung CL, Peduzzi PN, Shatney CH et al. (1990) The impact of encephalopathy on mortality in the sepsis syndrome. *Crit Care Med* **18**:801–806.

27 Durham M, Siegel J and Weirter L (1991) Oxygen debt and metabolic acidemia as quantitative predictors of mortality and the severity of the ischaemic insult in haemorrhagic shock. *Crit Care Med* **19**:231–243.

28 Guttierez G and Pohil RJ (1986) Oxygen consumption is linearly related to oxygen supply in critically ill patients. *J Crit Care* **1**:45–48.

29 Phang PT, Cunningham KF, Ronco JJ, Wiggs BR and Russell JA (1994) Mathematical coupling explains dependence of oxygen consumption on oxygen delivery in ARDS. *Am J Respir Crit Care Med* **150**:318–323.

30 Sibbald WJ, Paterson NAM, Holliday RL, Anderson RA, Lobb TR and Duff JH (1978) Pulmonary hypertension in sepsis. Measurement by pumonary arterial diastolic – pulmonary wedge pressure gradient and the influence of passive and active factors. *Chest* **73**:583–591.

31 Lefer AM (1989) Significance of lipid mediators in shock states. *Circ Shock* **27**:3–12.

32 Hinds CJ (1987) Endogenous opioid peptides in shock. In: Vincent JL and Thijs LG (eds) *Septic Shock: European View. Update in Intensive Care and Emergency Medicine*, volume 4. Berlin: Springer-Verlag, pp. 268–275.

33 Calandra T, Baumgartner JD, Grau G et al. (1990) Prognostic values of tumour necrosis factor/cachectin, interleukin 1, interferon-α and interferon-γ in the serum of patients with septic shock. *J Infect Dis* **161**: 982–987.

34 Natanson C, Hoffman WD, Suffredini AF, Eichacker PQ and Danner RL (1994) Selected treatment strategies for septic shock based on proposed mechanisms of pathogenesis. *Ann Intern Med* **120**:771–783.

35 Slotman G, Burchard K, Williams J et al. (1986) Interaction of prostaglandins, activated complement and granulocytes in clinical sepsis and hypotension. *Surgery* **99**:744–750.

36 Tibballs J (1993) The role of nitric oxide (formerly endothelium-derived relaxing factor – EDRF) in vasodilatation and vasodilator therapy. *Anaesth Intens Care* **21**:759–773.

37 Petras A, Bennett D and Vallance P (1991) Effect of nitric oxide synthase inhibitors on hypotension in patients with septic shock. *Lancet* **338**:1557–1558.

38 Astiz ME, Rackow EC and Weil MH (1993) Pathophysiology and treatment of circulatory shock. *Crit Care Clin* **9**:183–203.

39 Rutten AJ, Ilsley AH, Skowronski GA and Runciman WB (1986) A comparative study of mean arterial blood pressure using automatic oscillometers, arterial cannulation and auscultation. *Anaesth Intens Care* **14**: 58–65.

40 Proctor HJ, Ballantine TVN, Broussard ND *et al.* (1970) An analysis of pulmonary function following penetrating pulmonary injury with recommendations for therapy. *Surgery* **68**:92–98.

41 Moore EE, Moore JB, Galloway AC *et al.* (1979) Post injury thoracotomy in the emergency department. A critical evaluation. *Surgery* **86**:590–597.

42 Mackersie RC, Christensen JM and Lewis R (1984) The prehospital use of external counterpressure: does MAST make a difference? *J Trauma* **24**:882–888.

43 Skillman JJ, Restall DS and Salzman EW (1975) Randomized trial of albumin vs electrolyte solutions during abdominal aortic operations. *Surgery* **78**:291–303.

44 Hauser CJ, Shoemaker WC, Turpin I and Goldberg SJ (1980) Oxygen transport responses to colloids and crystalloids in critically surgical patients. *Surg Gynecol Obstet* **150**:811–816.

45 Ramsay G (1988) Intravenous volume replacement: indications and choices. *Br Med J* **296**:1422–1423.

46 Smith JAR and Norman JN (1982) The fluid of choice for resuscitation of severe shock. *Br J Surg* **69**: 702–705.

47 Moss GS and Gould SA (1988) Plasma expansion: an update. *Am J Surg* **155**:425–434.

48 Haljamae H (1993) Volume substitution in shock. *Acta Anaesthesiol Scand* **98**(suppl):25–28.
volume hypertonic saline solutions. *Crit Care Med* **15**:385.

50 Messner K (1975) Hemodilution. *Surg Clin North Am* **154**:577–586.

51 Mitsuno T, Ohyanagi H and Nasio R (1982) Clinical studies of a perfluorochemical whole blood substitute (Fluosol-DA). *Ann Surg* **195**:60–69.

52 Shippy CR, Appel PL and Shoemaker WC (1984) Reliability of clinical monitoring to assess blood volume in critically ill patients. *Crit Care Med* **12**: 107–112.

53 Vincent J, Roman A, De Backer D and Kahn RJ (1990) Oxygen uptake/supply dependency. *Am Rev Resp Dis* **142**:2–7.

54 Cooper DJ, Walley KR, Wiggs BR and Russell JA (1990) Bicarbonate does not improve hemodynamics in critically ill patients who have lactic acidosis. *Ann Intern Med* **112**: 492–498.

55 Martin C, Papazian L, Perrin G, Saux P and Gouin F (1993) Norepinephrine or dopamine for the treatment of hyperdynamic septic shock? *Chest* **103**:1826–1831.

56 Young RA and Ward A (1988) Milrinone. A preliminary review of its pharmacological properties and therapeutic use. *Drugs* **36**:158–192.

57 Corwin HL and Bonventre JV (1988) Acute renal failure in the intensive care unit. Part 2. *Intens Care Med* **14**: 86–96.

58 Bidani A and Churchill PC (1989) Acute renal failure. *Dis Mon* **35**:63–132.

59 Pass LJ, Eberhart RC, Brown JC *et al.* (1988) The effect of mannitol and dopamine on the renal response to thoracic aortic cross-clamping. *J Thorac Cardiovasc Surg* **95**:608–612.

60 Swygert TH, Roberts LC, Valek TR *et al.* (1991) Effect of intraoperative low-dose dopamine on renal function in liver transplant patients. *Anesthesiology* **75**:571–576.

61 Myles PS, Buckland MR and Schenk NJ (1993) Effect of 'renal-dose' dopamine on renal function following cardiac surgery. *Anaesth Intens Care* **21**:56–61.

62 Oh TE (1985) Corticosteroid agents in intensive care. *Med J Aust* **143**:290–293.

63 Bone RC, Fisher CJ, Clemmer TP *et al.* (1987) A controlled clinical trial of high-dose methylprednisolone in the treatment of severe sepsis and septic shock. *N Engl J Med* **317**:653–658.

64 The Veterans Administration Systemic Sepsis Cooperative Study Group. Effect of high dose glucocorticoid therapy on mortality in patients with clinical signs of systemic sepsis. *N Engl J Med* **317**:659–665.

65 Croeger JS (1986) Opioid antagonists in circulatory shock. *Crit Care Med* **14**:170–171.

66 Cunnion RE (1992) Clinical trials of immunotherapy for sepsis (editorial). *Crit Care Med* **20**:721–723.

67 Beutler B (1993) Endotoxin, tumor necrosis factor, and related mediators: new approaches to shock. *New Horizons* **1**:3–12.

68 Holaday JW and Bernton EW (1984) Protirelin (TRH). A potent neuromodulator with therapeutic potential. *Arch Intern Med* **144**:1138–1140.

69 Mansenberger AR, Doran JE, Treat R *et al.* (1989) The influence of fibronectin administration on the incidence of sepsis and septic mortality in severely injured patients. *Ann Surg* **210**:297–307.

70 Reuhaag A, Michie H, Hanson J *et al.* (1988) Inhibition of cyclo-oxygenase attenuates the metabolic response to endotoxin in humans. *Arch Surg* **123**:162–170.

71 Tuschmidt JA and Mecher CE (1994) Predictors of outcome from critical illness, shock and cardiopulmonary resuscitation. *Crit Care Clin* **10**:179–195.

72 Schreiber TL, Miller DH and Zola B (1989) Management of myocardial infarction shock: current status. *Am Heart J* **117**:435–443.

15 · Cardiogenic shock

GJ Dobb

Shock caused by severe sepsis, burns, pancreatitis or trauma is accompanied by increased plasma cytokine concentrations and impaired myocardial function. Tumour necrosis factor-α has marked negative inotropic effects.[1,2] However, the term cardiogenic shock is reserved for patients with shock primarily caused by heart disease. It is a clinical syndrome defined by:[3]

1 a systolic arterial pressure less than 90 mmHg (23 kPa);
2 evidence of reduced blood flow as shown by:
  (a) urine output less than 20 ml/h;
  (b) impaired mental function; and
  (c) peripheral vasoconstriction with a cold, clammy skin.

Hypotension resulting from pain, vasovagal reaction, serious arrhythmias, drug reaction or hypovolaemia is excluded. In patients with known hypertension, a reduction in the blood pressure of 30 mmHg (4 kPa) is used to define hypotension. Occasionally, urine output or cerebral function is preserved.

Other changes seen in cardiogenic shock include reduced coronary blood flow, myocardial lactate production, abnormally high myocardial oxygen extraction, and an intense neurohumoral stress response. There are large increases in plasma concentrations of adrenaline and noradrenaline, glucose, free fatty acids, cortisol, renin, angiotensin II and glucagon, and decreased concentrations of insulin. Clinical trials using criteria from invasive haemodynamic monitoring to define cardiogenic shock usually require a cardiac index of less than 2.2 l/min per m^2 with a pulmonary artery occluded pressure (PAOP) greater than 15 mmHg (2 kPa). The arteriovenous oxygen difference is usually greater than 55 ml/l.

Aetiology (Table 15.1)

The most common cause of cardiogenic shock is myocardial infarction (MI). Cardiogenic shock is reported to affect 5–20% of those admitted to hospital with an acute infarct, depending on the definition used and the population studied, and is the commonest cause of hospital death. In large randomized trials of thrombolysis for MI, the frequency of cardiogenic shock has been approximately 7%.[4,5] Although thrombolytic treatment has been shown to reduce infarct size and overall mortality, early improvements in left ventricular (LV) function have been less striking. In part, this may be a result of myocardial stunning associated with reperfusion injury.[6] Stunned myocardium has delayed functional recovery so that recovery of systolic function is only modest after 3 days, with further recovery occurring between 3 days and 6 months.

Clinical differentiation between stunning and permanent myocardial injury is impossible, but there

Table 15.1 Causes of cardiogenic shock

Myocardial infarction
  Critical loss of left ventricular muscle mass
  Right ventricular infarction
Myocardial dysfunction after cardiac surgery
Myocardial contusion by direct chest trauma
Reduced systemic flow from left ventricular contraction
  Rupture of the interventricular septum
  Acute mitral regurgitation
  Acute aortic regurgitation
  Left ventricular aneurysm
Obstruction to flow
  Myxoma
  Hypertrophic obstructive cardiomyopathy
  Critical valvular stenosis, aortic or mitral
Cardiomyopathy
Myocarditis
Heart transplant rejection
Poisoning and drug overdose

are clear implications for the duration of ongoing support for patients who have undergone reperfusion treatment and have cardiogenic shock in the absence of a surgically correctable lesion. There is evidence that thrombolyic therapy is ineffective in patients with established cardiogenic shock. Thrombolytics appear dependent on a normal aortic root pressure for their efficacy in coronary reperfusion,[7] and may therefore be more effective when used in conjunction with intra-aortic balloon counterpulsation.[8]

Factors associated with an increased risk of cardiogenic shock from MI are age, diabetes, previous MI, a history of angina or congestive heart failure,[9] and anterior (rather than inferior) infarction. Myocardial dysfunction after cardiac surgery is considered in Chapter 19. Patients with severe cardiomyopathy suitable for heart transplant may need admission to an ICU for assessment and support while awaiting a donor heart.

Pathophysiology

Autopsy studies show that over 40% of functioning myocardium has been lost in patients who die of cardiogenic shock after MI. The effects of recent and old infarction are additive. Extension of the area of infarction during a single hospital admission is common in patients who develop cardiogenic shock.[10] This may represent loss of viability of an ischaemic zone surrounding the initial infarct.

The neurohumoral changes seen in cardiogenic shock (and to a lesser extent after any infarct) cause an increase in heart rate, contractility and blood pressure. In response to a reduced cardiac output, the heart rate and systemic vascular resistance (SVR) increase to try and maintain arterial pressure.[11] The neurohumeral responses and these reflex changes increase myocardial oxygen demand at a time when myocardial perfusion is reduced by hypotension. The result is to jeopardize further ischaemic but potentially viable tissue, and further impair LV function, completing a vicious circle which ends with the patient's death (Fig. 15.1).

In cardiogenic shock caused by septal perforation, ventricular aneurysm or acute valvular regurgitation, there is reduced flow through the systemic circulation because a proportion of the blood ejected from the left ventricle is directed into the right ventricle, the aneurysm, the left atrium or back into the left ventricle.

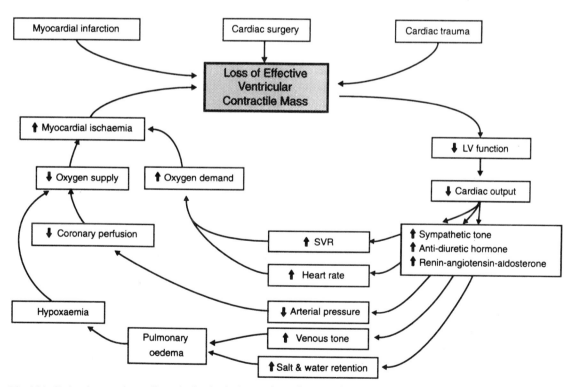

Fig. 15.1 Cycle of events in cardiogenic shock: the haemodynamic events leading to progressive loss of effective ventricular contractile mass and the neurohumeral interactions. LV = Left ventricle; SVR = systemic vascular resistance.

Clinical presentation

The clinical features are in keeping with the definition of cardiogenic shock. Arrhythmias and the extremes of heart rate, cardiac tamponade, pulmonary embolism and other causes of shock must be excluded. Most patients with cardiogenic shock also have pulmonary oedema with raised left ventricular end-diastolic pressure (LVEDP) and PAOP. Pulmonary oedema may cause severe dyspnoea, central cyanosis and crepitations. The diagnosis of pulmonary oedema can be confirmed by an erect chest X-ray.

Less often, cardiogenic shock occurs without the PAOP being elevated in:

1 patients with clinical and radiological evidence of pulmonary oedema, but normal or low PAOP.[12] Causes include diuretic therapy or plasma volume depletion by the fluid lost into the lungs;
2 patients with relative hypovolaemia, i.e. below the level of risk for pulmonary oedema (18–20 mmHg, 2.4–2.7 kPa);
3 patients with significant right ventricular infarction. Hypotension in patients with inferior infarction and the clinical signs of right heart failure should alert one to this possibility,[13,14] although the signs are more specific than sensitive. Right ventricular infarction can also mimic pericardial tamponade or pericardial constriction.

Patients presenting with these three syndromes are a minority of those with cardiogenic shock, but it is important to identify them. They may improve dramatically with plasma volume expansion and deteriorate if diuretics are given inappropriately.

A systolic murmur appearing after MI suggests mitral regurgitation or septal perforation. Clinical distinction between them is difficult. Patients with infarction who respond to volume expansion or who have a mechanical lesion amenable to surgery have potentially reversible cardiogenic shock. All patients with cardiogenic shock who are being actively treated should have an echocardiogram. Echocardiography defines the extent of LV dysfunction, demonstrates lesions of the valves and septum or right ventricular infarction when these are present, and helps exclude other causes of shock including pulmonary embolism, cardiac tamponade or atrial myxoma. Transoesophageal echocardiography is relatively easy in patients needing mechanical ventilation and usually provides clearer images than transthoracic insonation, but is otherwise poorly tolerated by distressed patients. (see Chapter 21).

Shock due solely to extensive LV infarction is usually irreversible. If cardiogenic shock fails to respond to treatment, multiple organ failure, metabolic acidosis, hypothermia and coma may precede death.

Management

The treatment of cardiogenic shock is difficult and the results often disappointing. Efforts have therefore been made to reduce the incidence of cardiogenic shock by techniques that will preserve myocardium during cardiopulmonary bypass[15] and limit the amount damaged by MI. Because of the disappointing results from thrombolysis in cardiogenic shock, alternative methods of revascularization have been investigated. Studies in acute MI suggest improved global LV function in patients treated with angioplasty. Evidence from prospective randomized studies now suggests that coronary angioplasty is the preferred treatment for patients with acute MI complicated by cardiogenic shock.[16] Mortality in a consecutive series of 79 patients with cardiogenic shock treated by primary angioplasty was 44%.[17] In another study mortality was 60% in patients with cardiogenic shock having early revascularization by coronary angioplasty and 19% in those having coronary artery bypass graft surgery,[18] but selection bias makes interpretation of these results difficult. What is clear is that for patients to benefit from active management of acute coronary occlusion, treatment must occur within the first few hours from the onset of symptoms, and preferably within 2–4 h. This is impossible without 24-h availability of cardiac catheterization and surgical expertise.

General supportive measures

These include relief of pain, correction of severe acid–base or electrolyte disturbances and treatment of cardiac arrhythmias. Patients with bradyarrhythmias caused by atrioventricular block or junctional bradycardia may respond dramatically to sequential atrioventricular or atrial pacing[19] (see Chapter 10). Oxygen is given to correct hypoxaemia. If hypoxaemia persists in patients with potentially reversible shock, continuous positive airway pressure (CPAP) or tracheal intubation and mechanical ventilation with positive end-expiratory pressure (PEEP) may be used. The copious frothy sputum of severe pulmonary oedema is controlled by increasing PEEP rather than repeated endotracheal suction. Patients with cardiogenic shock may become profoundly hypotensive when given sedation for intubation.

Monitoring

The principles and methods for monitoring any critically ill patient apply to cardiogenic shock. These should include:

1 measurement of intra-arterial blood pressure;
2 assessment of venous pressures: direct measurement of central venous pressure is more accurate than clinical assessment of the jugular venous pressure,

but only reflects the right ventricular filling pressure. Pulmonary oedema may be diagnosed by hearing widespread crepitations and confirmed by the chest X-ray, but the most accurate assessment of LV filling pressure is gained by measuring the PAOP;

3 assessment of cardiac output: while skin perfusion, hourly urine output and mental state provide clinical guides to cardiac output, changes in cardiac output with time or treatment are best measured directly by the thermodilution method;

4 other investigations:
(a) electrocardiogram and cardiac enzymes to confirm a diagnosis of MI.
(b) blood gases, pH and plasma lactate.
(c) haemoglobin, electrolytes, urea and creatinine.
(d) echocardiography.

Insertion of a pulmonary artery balloon flotation (Swan–Ganz) catheter helps to characterize the haemodynamic problems. Despite suggestions of overuse and a lack of clinical trials to show improved outcome, the pulmonary artery catheter remains the mainstay of bedside monitoring of cardiac function.[20] When cardiogenic shock is caused by septal perforation, blood sampling during insertion of the catheter will show an increase in oxygen saturation between the right atrium and the right ventricle. Patients with severe mitral regurgitation usually have a large V wave on the wedge pressure trace, but this is non-specific; large V waves are also seen in the absence of mitral regurgitation.[21]

Improvement of haemodynamic disturbance

The same principles can be applied in cardiogenic shock from nearly all causes. The overall prognosis should carefully be considered before starting invasive monitoring and aggressive support, especially if presentation is late, there is no access to urgent coronary angiography, the appropriateness of active treatment is limited by coexisting disease, or in patients with large myocardial infarcts without a correctable lesion and those with severe cardiomyopathy.

PAOP <18 mmHg (2.4 kPa)

Plasma volume expansion is the initial treatment. Although a LV filling pressure of 18 mmHg (2.4 kPa) is greater than normal, this is usually the optimum for ventricular performance in patients with recent MI. Blood should be used to correct anaemia, otherwise repeated fluid challenges with 100–200 ml of colloid are used.

In patients with predominant right ventricular infarction, fluid loading may produce a central venous pressure (CVP) of 30 mmHg (4 kPa) or more. Conversely, drugs conventionally used in the treatment of acute MI which reduce preload exacerbate hypoperfusion in these patients.[13]

PAOP > 18 mmHg (2.4 kPa)

This group contains most patients with cardiogenic shock, including those who initially have low PAOPs and remain hypotensive after fluid loading. The treatments available include drugs and mechanical circulatory assistance.

Drug therapy

1 *Catecholamines*, including adrenaline, noradrenaline, isoprenaline, dopamine and dobutamine. The aim of these drugs is to increase arterial pressure and improve coronary perfusion. They do this by varying degrees of increased cardiac contractility and rate (β-adrenergic stimulation) and peripheral vasoconstriction (α-adrenergic effect). The increased arterial pressure is, however, at the expense of increased myocardial oxygen consumption which may endanger additional areas of myocardium. Other side-effects include potentiation of arrhythmias by β-stimulation and a reduction in renal blood flow by α-mediated vasoconstriction.

Dobutamine acts mainly on β_1-adrenergic receptors. In the majority of patients, it has little effect on SVR or heart rate in lower doses. Reduction of venous pressures and SVR may, however, cause hypotension and tachycardia in some patients with shock. The range of infusion rates is 2–40 μg/kg per min. Comparisons in patients with a low cardiac output between dopamine and dobutamine have shown greater haemodynamic benefit from dobutamine,[22] but there is considerable variation between patients. Overall, dobutamine is the preferred sympathomimetic amine in cardiogenic shock unless there is profound hypotension;[23] it augments diastolic coronary blood flow and collateral blood flow to the ischaemic area.

Dopamine at infusion rates of 5–20 μg/kg per min causes increasing β-adrenergic stimulation, and above 20 μg/kg per min α-adrenergic stimulation and vasoconstriction become increasingly prominent. It is useful when hypotension is a predominant feature, though relatively low doses of noradrenaline or adrenaline (1–5 μg/min) are equally effective (see Chapter 12).

When low cardiac output complicates recovery from cardiac surgery, there can be considerable changes in the response to an inotropic drug with time.[24]

2 *Phosphodiesterase inhibitors* (milrinone, amrinone, enoximone) have both inotropic and vasodilator effects. They should be used with extreme caution and close haemodynamic monitoring in patients with cardiogenic shock, and especially when arterial pressure is borderline or low. A need for loading doses and longer half-lives tends to make their use more difficult than catecholamines. When used in conjunction with catecholamines there may be additive arrhythmic effects.

3 *Digoxin* has been used to improve myocardial

contractility but its relatively slow onset of action, long half-life and low therapeutic ratio make it less suitable as an inotropic drug in cardiogenic shock.

4 *Vasodilators* used in cardiogenic shock include sodium nitroprusside, nitroglycerin, isosorbide dinitrate and angiotensin-converting enzyme (ACE) inhibitors. The potential benefits are a reduction in myocardial work and oxygen demand; pooling of blood on the venous side of the circulation with a reduction in atrial pressures to promote clearing of pulmonary oedema; and possibly a redistribution of blood flow within organs and tissues to improve the supply of oxygen and metabolites at cellular level. The greatest danger is a precipitous fall in arterial pressure which reduces coronary perfusion. Invasive haemodynamic monitoring is therefore essential. Vasodilators also tend to increase hypoxaemia by increasing intrapulmonary shunting.

Sodium nitroprusside infusion consistently increases cardiac output in patients with LV failure and shock after MI. An initial dose of $10\,\mu g/min$ should be increased slowly to a maximum of $500\,\mu g/min$, above which cyanide toxicity becomes a hazard of prolonged infusion. Patients with cardiogenic shock are usually quite sensitive to its effects.

Nitroglycerin is predominantly a venodilator when given by infusion. The rapid onset of action is useful in the management of pulmonary oedema. The acute haemodynamic effects of intravenous isosorbide dinitrate in MI[25] are very similar.

Impressive results were reported in a small group of patients with cardiogenic shock given the ACE inhibitor captopril.[26] More often, ACE inhibitors are used to treat residual cardiac failure in patients being weaned off intravenous drugs.

5 *Other drugs:* steroids, glucagon and glucose–insulin–potassium infusions have been used in patients with cardiogenic shock. They are generally considered ineffective.

A combination of catecholamine and vasodilator is often found to produce the best haemodynamic response.

Mechanical circulatory assistance

This should be considered for patients who remain hypotensive and shocked after a short trial of aggressive medical treatment. Factors favouring its use are a potentially reversible cause of cardiogenic shock and shock after cardiac surgery or chest trauma.

Intra-aortic counterpulsation with a balloon pump (IABP) is the method of choice. It increases the chances of successful thrombolysis in cardiogenic shock caused by acute coronary occlusion and assists in stabilizing patients during early coronary angioplasty. The IABP is contraindicated in patients with aortic regurgitation. Percutaneous insertion of the IABP has generally superseded surgical arteriotomy. Using the Seldinger technique to place the introducer in the femoral artery

and inserting the balloon over a flexible-tip J-wire guide under fluoroscopy, an IABP can be inserted quickly and comparatively atraumatically in nearly all patients.[27,28] Potential hazards include limb ischaemia from occlusion of the femoral artery by the balloon catheter or thrombus, aortic dissection, infection and embolization. Peripheral vascular complications are more common in women.[28]

The IABP is synchronized with the patient's ECG. Inflation and deflation are adjusted by inspection of the ECG and arterial pressure wave form. The balloon is inflated during early diastole (on the dicrotic notch of the arterial wave form), thus increasing diastolic pressure and coronary perfusion. The balloon is deflated immediately before ventricular systole, decreasing aortic pressure and so reducing ventricular afterload. The net effect is to increase cardiac output and coronary perfusion, while decreasing myocardial work and oxygen demand (Fig. 15.2).

Other mechanical ventricular assist devices (VAD) have been used in patients with cardiogenic shock which is unresponsive to drugs and IABP.[29] Those available include an implantable turbine pump (Hemopump), centrifugal pumps, various configurations of percutaneous cardiopulmonary support systems, and experimental artificial hearts. Most of the patients treated with VAD have had recent cardiac surgery but other indications have included shock after MI, myocarditis, poisoning and drug overdose, and support while awaiting cardiac transplantation.

Patients with cardiogenic shock after surgery or trauma frequently improve with time and can be weaned off mechanical support. In those with cardiogenic shock after MI, the mechanical support is usually a prelude to coronary angiography and ventriculography to demonstrate lesions correctable by surgery.

Specific treatment

Unless there are contraindications, patients with cardiogenic shock and surgically correctable lesions of the heart valves or intraventricular septum should undergo urgent surgical correction. Systemic blood flow can be improved in patients with acute valvular regurgitation or a ventricular septal defect by afterload reduction with vasodilators and the IABP, but early surgery improves the overall outcome.[30,31] The definitive treatment of an obstructing atrial myxoma is also surgical. Urgent balloon valvuloplasty has been used as an alternative to surgery for cardiogenic shock caused by severe aortic stenosis.[32]

Hypoperfusion in patients with hypertrophic obstructive cardiomyopathy will usually be exacerbated by the measures used to treat other forms of cardiogenic shock (i.e. inotropic drugs and afterload reduction). Plasma volume expansion and intravenous titration of β-adrenergic blocking drugs reduce

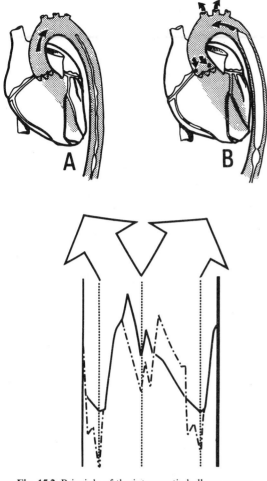

Fig. 15.2 Principle of the intra-aortic balloon pump (IABP). The continuous line is the arterial pressure wave form without circulatory assistance. The dotted line is the arterial pressure with the IABP on. (A) Balloon deflation just before ventricular systole enhances left ventricular ejection by reducing end-diastolic pressure. Peak systolic pressure is reduced. (B) Balloon inflation occurs early in diastole, causing an increase in diastolic pressure and augmenting coronary flow.

ventricular outflow obstruction and improve cardiac output.

Patients remaining dependent on inotropic drugs or mechanical assistance may be considered for heart transplantation. Patients with dilated cardiomyopathy are particularly suitable candidates because they are usually young adults who are otherwise healthy and over 50% die within 2 years of diagnosis, but the option of transplantation should be reviewed in all patients without contraindications. Contraindications to heart transplantation vary between different countries and units. Age over 55–65 years, widespread

vascular disease, high pulmonary vascular resistance, diabetes mellitus, recent pulmonary infarction, active infection and neoplastic disease are common exclusion criteria[33] (see Chapter 94). Cardiogenic shock caused by poor compliance with immunosuppressive treatment in patients with a cardiac transplant can respond rapidly to high-dose intravenous steroids.[34]

Prognosis

The prognosis of cardiogenic shock associated with myocardial infarction is poor. In the absence of a surgically correctable lesion, only about one-third of patients treated actively survive the initial episode, and many of the survivors have continuing angina, congestive heart failure and decreased exercise tolerance.[27] Approximately half the patients with a surgically correctable intracardiac lesion should survive to leave hospital. Right ventricular function usually returns to normal in survivors of cardiogenic shock associated with right ventricular infarction.[14]

The mortality in patients who need maximal therapy and IABP to separate from cardiopulmonary bypass is about 50%.[27] Survival in patients who have required VAD in addition to inotropic drugs and the IABP has been 35–45%. The functional prognosis for these survivors seems reasonably good.[35]

The prognosis after cardiac transplantation is relatively good, with 70–80% surviving 2–4 years (see Chapter 94).

References

1 Giroir BP, Horton JW, White DJ, McIntyre KL and Lin CQ (1994) Inhibition of tumor necrosis factor prevents myocardial dysfunction during burn shock. *Am J Physiol* **167**:H118–H124.

2 Kapadia S, Torre AC, Yokoyama T and Mann DL (1995) Soluble TNF binding proteins modulate the negative inotropic properties of TNF-alpha *in vitro*. *Am J Physiol* **268**:H517–H525.

3 Shaw HJC, Forrester JS, Diamond G, Chatterjee K and Parmley WW (1972) Haemodynamic spectrum of myocardial infarction and cardiogenic shock. *Circulation* **45**:1097–1110.

4 The International Study Group (1990) In hospital mortality and clinical course of 20 891 patients with suspected acute myocardial infarction randomised between alteplase and streptokinase with or without heparin. *Lancet* **336**:71–76.

5 ISIS-3 (Third International Study of Infarct Survival) Collaborative Group (1992) ISIS-3: a randomised comparison of streptokinase vs. tissue plasminogen activator vs anisteplase and of aspirin plus heparin vs aspirin alone among 41 299 cases of suspected acute myocardial infarction. *Lancet* **229**:753–770.

6 Grech ED, Jackson MJ and Ramsdale DR (1995)

Reperfusion injury after acute myocardial infarction. *Br Med J* **301**:477–478.

7 Garbor PJ, Mathieson AL, Ducas J, Patton JN, Geddes JS and Prewitt RM (1995) Thrombolytic therapy in cardiogenic shock: effect of increased aortic pressure and rapid tPa administration. *Can J Cardiol* **11**:30–36.

8 Stomel RJ, Rosak M and Bates ER (1994) Treatment strategies for acute myocardial infarction complicated by cardiogenic shock in a community hospital. *Chest* **105**:997–1002.

9 Leor J, Goldbourt U, Reicher-Reiss H, Kaplinsky E and Behar S (1993) SPRINT study group. Cardiogenic shock complicating acute mycardial infarction in patients without heart failure on admission: incidence, risk factors, and outcome. *Am J Med* **94**:265–273.

10 Alonso DR, Scheidt S, Post M and Killip T (1973) Pathophysiology of cardiogenic shock. *Circulation* **48**:588–596.

11 Forrester JS, Diamond G, Chaterjee K and Swan HJC (1976) Medical therapy of acute myocardial infarction by application of hemodynamic subsets. *N Engl J Med* **295**: 1256–1262.

12 Timmis AD, Fowler MB, Burwood RJ, Gishen P, Vincent R and Chamberlain DA (1981) Pulmonary oedema without critical increase in left atrial pressure in acute myocardial infarction. *Br Med J* **283**:636–638.

13 Isner JM (1988) Right ventricular myocardial infarction. *Journal of the American Medical Association* **259**:712–718.

14 Kinsh JW and Ryan TJ (1994) Right ventricular infarction. *N Engl J Med* **330**:1211–1217.

15 Buckberg GD (1987) Strategies and logic of caridoplegic delivery to prevent, avoid and reverse ischemic and reperfusion damage. *J Thorac Cardiovasc Surg* **93**: 127–139.

16 Landau C, Glamann DB, Willard JE, Hillis LD and Lange RA (1994) Coronary angioplasty in the patient with acute myocardial infarction. *Am J Med* **96**: 536–543.

17 O'Keefe JH, Bailey WL, Rutherford BD and Hartzler CO (1993) Primary angioplasty for acute myocardial infarction in 1000 consecutive patients. Results in an unselected population and high risk subgroups. *Am J Cardiol* **72**:107C–115C.

18 Hochman JS, Boland J, Sleeper LA *et al.* (1995) Current spectrum of cardiogenic shock and effect of early revascularisation on mortality. Results of an international registry. *Circulation* **91**:873–881.

19 Abraham KA, Brown MA and Norris RM (1985) Right ventricular infarction, bradyarrhythmias, and cardiogenic shock: importance of atrial or atrioventricular sequential pacing. *Aust NZ J Med* **15**:52–54.

20 Shephard JN, Brecker SJ and Evans TW (1994) Bedside assessment of myocardial performance in the critically ill. *Intens Care Med* **20**:513–521.

21 Pichard AD, Kay R, Smith H, Rentrop P, Holt J and Gorlin R (1982) Large V waves in the pulmonary artery wedge pressure tracing in the absence of mitral regurgitation. *Am J Cardiol* **50**:1044–1050.

22 Francis GS, Sharma B and Hodges M (1982) Comparative hemodynamic effects of dopamine and dobutamine in patients with acute cardiogenic circulatory collapse. *Am Heart J* **103**:995–1000.

23 Califf RM and Bengtson JR (1994) Cardiogenic shock. *N Engl J Med* **330**:1724–1730.

24 Van Tright P, Spray T, Pasque M *et al.* (1983) The influence of time on the response to dopamine after coronary artery bypass grafting: assessment of left ventricular performance and contractility using pressure/dimension analyses. *Ann Thorac Surg* **35**: 3–11.

25 Cintron GB, Glasser SP, Weston BA, Linares E, Conti CR and participating investigators (1988) Effect of intravenous isosorbide dinitrate versus nitroglycerin on elevated pulmonary arterial wedge pressure during acute myocardial infarction. *Am J Cardiol* **61**:21–25.

26 Lipkin DP, Frenneaux M and Maseri A (1987) Beneficial effect of captopril in cardiogenic shock. *Lancet* **2**:327.

27 Sanfelippo PM, Baker NH, Ewy HG *et al.* (1986) Experience with intra-aortic balloon counterpulsation. *Ann Thorac Surg* **41**:36–39.

28 Sanders KM, Stern TA, O'Gara PT *et al.* (1992) Medical and neuropsychiatric complications associated with use of the intra-aortic balloon pump. *J Intens Care Med* **7**:154–164.

29 Zumbro GL, Kitchens WR, Shearer G, Harville G, Bailey L and Galloway RF (1987) Mechanical assistance for cardiogenic shock following cardiac surgery, myocardial infarction and cardiac transplantation. *Ann Thorac Surg* **44**:11–13.

30 Nishimura RA, Schaff HV, Shub C, Gersh BJ, Edwards WD and Tajik AJ (1983) Papillary muscle rupture complicating acute myocardial infarction: analysis of 17 patients. *Am J Cardiol* **51**:373–377.

31 Miyamoto AT, Lee ME, Kass RM *et al.* (1983) Post myocardial infarction ventricular septal defect. *J Thorac Cardiovasc Surg* **86**:41–46.

32 Moreno PR, Jang IK, Newell JB, Black PC and Palacios IF (1994) The role of percutaneous aortic balloon valvuloplasty in patients with cardiogenic shock and critical aortic stenosis. *J Am Coll Cardiol* **28**: 1076–1078.

33 Perloth MG (1991) Cardiac transplantation: a review for the intensivists. *J Intens Care Med* **6**:47–54.

34 Stevenson LW, Lewis W, Macalpin RN and Clark S (1986) Acute reversible cardiogenic shock: immune-mediated with mild histologic change. *Am Heart J* **111**: 611–613.

35 Pae WE Jr, Pierce WS, Pennock JL, Campbell DB and Waldhaussen JA (1987) Long term results of ventricular assist pumping in post cardiotomy cardiogenic shock. *J Thorac Cardiovasc Surg* **93**:434–441.

16 | Acute hypertension and vasodilators

PT Chui and JM Low

Patients with acute hypertension are at risk of serious cardiovascular, central nervous system and renal complications.[1] A diastolic arterial pressure exceeding 120 mmHg (16 kPa) is considered a hypertensive crisis.[2] However, the rate of rise of the arterial pressure is also important in precipitating a crisis. Hypertensive crises are categorized into emergencies and urgencies (Table 16.1).[3,4] Hypertensive emergencies are accompanied by acute ongoing vascular or target-organ damage. By contrast, patients with hypertensive urgencies have no evidence of progressive vascular or target-organ damage. They may develop hypertensive emergencies if the hypertension remains uncontrolled.

Hypertensive emergencies require immediate treatment to prevent or limit target-organ damage. Traditionally, parenteral agents are used for immediate reduction of arterial pressure. However, oral and sublingual medications have been successfully used recently.[5]

Pathophysiology

Acute hypertension can produce abrupt damage to vessel walls. The brain, heart and kidney receive the greater proportion of cardiac output (CO) and are particularly at risk. Pathogenetic mechanisms of hypertension are complex and inadequately understood. They include:

1 excessive humoral pressor substances (e.g. catecholamines and renin–angiotensin–aldosterone);
2 inadequate secretion of circulating vasodilators (e.g. bradykinin and prostaglandin);
3 neurogenic mechanisms – excessive central nervous system stimulation and increased sympathetic activity;
4 sodium excess and consequent excess in circulating volume;
5 increased vascular reactivity and rigidity;
6 abnormal baroreceptor setting.

Table 16.1 Hypertensive emergencies and urgencies

Hypertensive emergencies
Hypertensive encephalopathy

Accelerated malignant hypertension

Hypertension with acute cardiovascular complications: acute myocardial ischaemia, acute left ventricular failure and acute aortic dissection

Hypertension with acute stroke: intracerebral haemorrhage, subarachnoid haemorrhage and ischaemic stroke

Hypertension with acute renal complications: acute glomerulo-nephritis, collagen vascular disease

Eclampsia and severe pre-eclampsia

Phaeochromocytoma crisis

Hypertensive urgencies
Perioperative hypertension: coronary bypass, carotid endarterectomy, aortic aneurysmectomy

Hypertension associated with catecholamine excess: phaeochromocytoma, withdrawal of antihypertensives, interactions with monoamine oxidase inhibitors, cocaine ingestion

Role of nitric oxide[6,7]

The vascular endothelium releases nitric oxide under basal conditions and in response to stimuli such as sheer stress, platelet-derived factors and acetylcholine.[8] Nitric oxide activates guanylate cyclase in the vascular smooth muscle, with an increase in cyclic guanosine monophosphate which results in smooth muscle relaxation. Nitric oxide is also the common end-product by which the diverse nitro-based vasodilators exert their effects.[9,10] Injection of NG-mono-methyl arginine, which inhibits formation of nitric oxide from L-arginine, causes an immediate and substantial rise in arterial pressure, which can be reversed by L-arginine. Continuous release of nitric oxide from the endothelium probably keeps blood vessels in a dilated state. Defective synthesis of nitric oxide may be implicated in the pathogenesis of hypertension.

Accelerated malignant hypertension

Accelerated hypertension refers to an increase in diastolic arterial pressure exceeding 120 mmHg (16 kPa) accompanied by retinopathy, with flame-shaped haemorrhages and cotton-wool exudates, but without papilloedema (grade III Keith–Wagener retinopathy). Malignant hypertension occurs when accelerated hypertension is also complicated by raised intracranial pressure and papilloedema (grade IV Keith– Wagener retinopathy).

The hallmark of accelerated malignant hypertension is ongoing arteriolar damage with necrotizing arteriolitis, proliferative endarteritis and fibrinoid necrosis. Disruption of the endothelium results in the exposure of the intima-media layers that trigger platelet activation and fibrin deposition. Circulating red cells are damaged, leading to microangiopathic haemolytic anaemia. Consequences of arteriolar damage include loss of autoregulation and impaired organ perfusion. The hypertension in accelerated malignant hypertension is perpetuated by enhanced vascular reactivity, increased levels of vasoconstricting hormones (e.g. angiotensin II, noradrenaline and antidiuretic hormone), and reduced levels of vasodilating substances (e.g. kinins and prostacyclins). However, body sodium and intravascular volume are depleted because of pressure diuresis in the kidneys.

Hypertensive encephalopathy

Hypertensive encephalopathy occurs when acute severe hypertension results in retinal changes (grade III or IV Keith–Wagener retinopathy) and neurological dysfunctions, that are reversible by lowering the arterial pressure. A pathogenic theory is the breakthrough theory.[11] With progressive hypertension, autoregulation of cerebral blood flow is overcome. Breakthrough vasodilatation and hyperaemia result in increased capillary pressure, endothelial damage, capillary transudation and disruption of the blood–brain barrier, eventually leading to cerebral oedema and intracranial hypertension. Fibrinoid necrosis of the arterioles produces multiple thrombi, microinfarcts and petechial haemorrhages.

Target-organ damage and acute hypertension

Acute left ventricular failure, unstable angina, acute myocardial infarction (MI), acute aortic dissection and stroke are often accompanied by acute hypertension. Increased arterial pressure can be both a cause and a consequence of the target-organ disease. Pathogenic factors for the acute hypertension in these conditions remain largely unknown, but probably relate to reflex sympathoadrenal outflow initiated by pain, stress, hypoxaemia, myocardial or cerebral ischaemia.[12]

Management of hypertensive crises

General principles

Complications of acute hypertension require urgent treatment. A full history and clinical examination should aim to determine the precipitating cause of the acute hypertension (Table 16.2), and evidence of ongoing target-organ damage. Symptoms of cardiac and cerebral pathology, previous diagnosis of hypertension and treatment are noted, especially non-prescription drugs, sympathomimetics and anti-depressants. Physical examination should include fundoscopy and full neurological assessment. Investigations include:

1 full blood count;
2 electrolytes, glucose, urea and creatinine;
3 urinanalysis;
4 chest X-ray;
5 electrocardiogram;
6 plasma renin (if renovascular hypertension is suspected);
7 urinary metanephrine, catecholamines and vanillyl-mandellic acid; and plasma catecholamines (if phaeochromocytoma is suspected).

A management programme should be established. Certain conditions require specific treatment (see below). Careful monitoring is needed to avoid hypotensive overshoot, especially in conditions such as stroke. Intravascular volume may be depleted, particularly in patients with excessive circulating catecholamines. Use of drugs with rapid action requires continuous cardiovascular monitoring. Treatment should be implemented with close monitoring of cardiac, renal and neurological functions. The

Table 16.2 Precipitating conditions in hypertensive crises

Chronic essential hypertension

Renal: acute glomerulonephritis, renovascular hypertension

Neurological: stroke, head injuries

Endocrine: phaeochromocytoma, renin-secreting tumour

Drugs: withdrawal of antihypertensives, sympathomimetics, monoamine oxidase inhibitors, antidepressants, oral contraceptives, steroids, ergot alkaloid, cocaine

Pregnancy-induced hypertension

Collagen vascular disease

decision to lower arterial pressure rapidly should not be based on the arterial pressure alone. The aim is to prevent and to reverse target-organ damage. Benefits of treatment must be considered against risks.[13,14]

Antihypertensive therapy

Parenteral and oral antihypertensive drugs with rapid onset of actions are available. Short-acting parenteral drugs allow rapid control and titration of dosage to haemodynamic response.[15] Indeed, infusion by computer control can be used to manage acute hypertension.[16] In hypertensive emergencies, the aim is to reduce mean arterial pressure (MAP) by about 15–25% within 24 h, depending on the clinical condition. Immediate normalization of arterial pressure is not advisable. Overzealous or uncontrolled reduction in arterial pressure may result in stroke, myocardial infarction and acute renal failure. In patients with chronic hypertension, cerebral autoregulation is shifted to the right. They are at risk of cerebral ischaemia when arterial pressure is lowered too abruptly. Following urgent control of arterial pressure, oral medication may be initiated, and the parenteral agents gradually withdrawn. During this unstable phase, the patient is monitored for response as well as side-effects. Vasodilators are also used to treat heart failure and myocardial ischaemia. Those suitable for acute hypertension are discussed below (Table 16.3).

Direct vasodilators

Sodium nitroprusside (SNP)

SNP has a rapid onset and evanescent action, and is excellent for emergency reduction of arterial pressure. It directly dilates both arteriolar and venous smooth muscles, and thus reduces systemic vascular resistance (SVR) and increases venous capacity. CO is maintained or even increased, unless venous return is greatly reduced.

SNP is converted to cyanide in plasma (2%) and in erythrocytes. Only plasma cyanide is available for metabolism. Cyanide is metabolized to thiocyanate by liver rhodanase, a slow rate-limiting process that requires a sulphur group usually from thiosulphate. Thiocyanate is excreted in the urine. Some cyanide combines with vitamin B_{12} to form cyanocobalamin. Cyanide toxicity is increased in renal or hepatic failure, nutritional deficiency, vitamin B_{12} deficiency and prolonged use. SNP is probably inadvisable in pregnancy and prolonged use in paediatrics. Cyanide toxicity produces nausea, vomiting, disorientation, lactic acidosis and arrhythmias, which may be masked by coexisting conditions in critically ill patients. Arterial blood gas, plasma thiocyanate and lactate estimations are indicated in the above risk situations, but are neither specific nor sensitive for cyanide toxicity.[17] Thiocyanate toxicity is less common,

occurring in patients with renal impairment after high-dose SNP infusion. Manifestations include nausea, vomiting, fatigue, delirium, muscle spasm and convulsions.

SNP is the preferred agent in ICU for the management of most hypertensive emergencies, except when there is acute myocardial ischaemia, for which glyceryl trinitrate is indicated. In acute aortic dissection, SNP must be used with concomitant β-adrenergic blockade, to avoid undesirable increase in heart rate, myocardial contractility and CO. SNP is usually used as a (0.01%) solution of 50 mg in 500 ml 5% dextrose. The solution is kept shielded from light and used within 4 h. It should be infused with a syringe or infusion pump. The dose range is 0.3–10 μg/kg per min. To avoid cyanide toxicity, infusion exceeding 2 μg/kg per min should not be used for longer than 3 h.[18] Tachyphylaxis is common, and is probably due to the activation of renin–angiotensin. Rebound hypertension following discontinuation of SNP infusion can be attenuated by β-adrenergic antagonists.

Glyceryl trinitrate/nitroglycerin

Glyceryl trinitrate (GTN) also produces a rapid-onset action. Its major effect is venodilatation rather than arteriodilatation. Arterial, central venous and pulmonary capillary wedge pressures are decreased. Coronary perfusion is increased, even at low-dose infusions. GTN is predominantly metabolized in the liver by glutathione–organic nitrate reductase. This is completed on first pass through the portal circulation, resulting in rapid termination of action. Methaemoglobinaemia is a theoretical toxic hazard.

GTN is particularly suitable for patients with myocardial ischaemia. It is used in ICU to control acute hypertension that is complicated by pulmonary oedema, left ventricular failure and myocardial ischaemia. As with SNP, GTN should be infused with a controllable device, and under continuous arterial monitoring. The dose range is 5–100 μg/min and onset of action is 2–5 min. Polyvinyl chloride absorbs the drug and special polyethylene administration sets are available.

Hydralazine

Hydralazine is a direct arteriodilator with little venodilatation. It reduces the diastolic pressure more than the systolic, and can induce reflex increase in heart rate and CO. Hydralazine is metabolized in the liver by acetylation. The level of hepatic N-acetyl transferase (acetylator status) is genetically determined. Side-effects include reflex tachycardia, headache, nausea, vomiting, flushing and skin rash. A lupus syndrome (10% incidence) can develop in prolonged therapy, renal impairment and 'slow' acetylator phenotypes. Reflex tachycardia (blunted in

Table 16.3 Antihypertensive drugs in hypertensive crises

Drug	Dose	Onset	Special indications	Caution
Sodium nitroprusside	0.25–10 μg/kg per min as IV infusion; maximal dose for 10 min only; limit infusions >2 μg/kg per min for < 3 h only	Immediate	All hypertensive emergencies	Photodegradation; cyanide and thiocyanate toxicity; raised intracranial pressure; rebound hypertension
Glyceryl trinitrate	5–100 μg/min by IV infusion	2–5 min	Acute myocardial ischaemia	Headache; flushing; drug binding to polyvinyl chloride
Diazoxide	50–100 mg by repeated IV boluses; 15–30 mg/min by IV infusion	1–2 min		Hypotension; tachycardia; myocardial ischaemia; hyperglycaemia
Hydralazine	10–20 mg by repeated IV boluses	10 min	Eclampsia	Hypotension; tachycardia; myocardial ischaemia
Phentolamine	5–15 mg IV	1–2 min	Phaeochromocytoma, catecholamine excess	Tachycardia
Trimetaphan	1–4 mg/min by IV infusion	1–5 min	Acute aortic dissection	Mydriasis; dry mouth; ileus; respiratory arrest
Labetalol	20–80 mg by repeated IV boluses every 10 min; or 0.5–4.0 mg/min by IV infusion	5–10 min	Postoperative hypertension	Bronchospasm; heart block
Esmolol	200–500 μg/kg IV, followed by infusion 100–300 μg/kg per min	1–2 min	Aortic dissection	Bronchospasm; bradycardia; heart block
Enalaprilat	0.5–1.0 mg IV, followed by 1–2 mg at 1-h intervals to a maximum dose of 5 mg	15–60 min	Congestive cardiac failure	Renal impairment; renal artery stenosis; pregnancy
Nifedipine	5–20 mg capsules by bite-and-swallow	15–30 min		Hypotension
Captopril	12.5–25 mg sublingually	15–30 min		Renal failure; renal artery stenosis; pregnancy
Clonidine	0.2 mg PO, then 0.1 mg/h to a maximum dose of 0.8 mg			Drowsiness; dry mouth; bradycardia

IV = Intravenous; PO = orally.

patients with chronic heart failure) may precipitate myocardial ischaemia.

Hydralazine is used extensively for hypertension in pre-eclampsia or eclampsia. It can be given in oral or IV form, the latter being more rapid in onset (10–20 min). An oral dose of 75–100 mg is equivalent to an IV dose of 20–25 mg, probably due to first-pass metabolism. The onset and duration of action are affected by the acetylation status. In hypertensive emergencies, IV boluses of 10–20 mg can be repeated if necessary, at about 15-min intervals, to a maximum of 50 mg. It can be given as an infusion of

0.5–1.0 mg/min. Hydralazine can be combined with a central α_2-agonist or a β-blocker to decrease reflex sympathetic outflow.

Diazoxide

Diazoxide is a direct arteriodilator with a rapid onset of action. CO is increased due to decreased SVR and reflex increase in heart rate and contractility. Unwanted effects include salt and water retention and hyperglycaemia. ECG changes contradict its use in MI. A bolus dose of 300 mg IV decreases MAP by about 30%, but effects are unpredictable. It is safer to give the drug by infusion or by repeated, small (25–75 mg) IV boluses. Diazoxide for acute hypertension has been superseded by other agents.

Trimetaphan

Trimetaphan is a ganglionic blocker at both sympathetic and parasympathetic ganglia. At high doses, it also causes direct peripheral vasodilatation and histamine release. Trimetaphan produces both arterio- and venodilatation. CO is decreased because of reduced venous return and myocardial contractility. The effect on heart rate is unpredictable, depending on the extent of parasympathetic blockade. Adverse effects are those of parasympathetic blockade, including dry mucous membrane, mydriasis, paralytic ileus and urinary retention. It can cause respiratory arrest by direct depression on the respiratory centre, in addition to neuromuscular blockade.

Onset of action after trimetaphan is immediate, and the duration is around 10 min, making it suitable for infusion. Following an IV bolus of 3–5 mg, an infusion of 50–100 μg/kg per min may be titrated against arterial pressure. Reflex tachycardia and tachyphylaxis are common. Trimetaphan is reserved for the treatment of acute aortic dissection, often in combination with a β-adrenergic blocker.

Adrenergic antagonists

Current concepts of the peripheral effects of sympathetic stimulation are based on Ahlquist's classification of α- and β-adrenoreceptors. Sympathetic overactivity may be blocked at these receptors.

α-Adrenergic blockers

Prazosin

Prazosin is a competitive postsynaptic α_1-blocker that dilates both arteries and veins. It is available only as an oral drug, rapidly and completely absorbed after administration, with an onset of action around 30 min. It is most effective for acute hypertension associated with increased circulating catecholamines (e.g. sympathomimetics ingestion, cocaine abuse, clonidine withdrawal and monoamine oxidase (MAO)

inhibitors interaction). The dose is 1–2 mg. First dose response, however, is unpredictable and may cause hypotension.

Phentolamine

Phentolamine competitively blocks both postsynaptic (α_1) and presynaptic (α_2) adrenoreceptors, especially the former. It is used in the treatment of hypertensive crises from excessive sympathomimetics, MAO inhibitors and phaeochromocytoma (see below). The onset of action is 1–2 min, and the duration is 3–10 min after 5 mg IV.

β-Adrenergic blockers

Indications of β-adrenergic blockers in ICU include hypertension, myocardial ischaemia and infarction, acute aortic dissection and phaeochromocytoma. Many drugs are available, differing in cardioselectivity (predominant β_1 effects), intrinsic sympathomimetic activity, membrane stabilization, duration of action, hepatic first-pass metabolism and concomitant α-adrenoreceptor blockade. Commonly used parenteral preparations are described below.

Propranolol

Propranolol is non-cardioselective and has extensive first-pass hepatic metabolism. It is suitable for repeated (titrated) injection. Initial dose of 1.0 mg IV can be supplemented by further increments of 0.5 mg up to a total dose of about 10 mg. A history of chronic obstructive airway disease with or without asthma may preclude its use.

Esmolol

Esmolol is an ultrashort-acting β_1-selective adrenergic blocker with an elimination half-life of only 9 min. It is useful in acute settings because of its rapid action and easy reversibility not found in other β-blockers. Esmolol is eminently suitable for IV infusion. An initial dose of 200–500 μg/kg is followed by maintenance infusion at 100–300 μg/kg per min.

Labetalol

Labetalol is a competitive blocker of both β- and α_1-adrenoreceptors. β-Adrenergic blockade predominates during IV administration, being 3–7 times that of α-blockade. The non-selective β-adrenergic blockade prevents reflex increase in heart rate, cardiac output and myocardial oxygen consumption. In acute hypertension, IV labetalol can be given as a single bolus of 1–2 mg/kg over 10 min, repeated mini-boluses of 20 mg followed by 20–80 mg every 10 min, or an incremental infusion of 0.5 mg to 2–4 mg/min. The last method is least likely to cause hypotension and bradycardia.[19] Labetalol should be avoided in patients with bronchial hyperreactivity, advanced atrioventricular block and congestive heart failure.

Calcium-channel antagonists

These drugs specifically block the voltage-operated calcium channels, and inhibit the transmembrane influx of calcium ions into cardiac and vascular smooth muscles. Their antihypertensive effects result from reduction of tension generation during excitation–contraction coupling, and interference with calcium-mediated secretion of catecholamines and aldosterone. They are used to treat angina, heart failure and hypertension. Commonly used drugs are described below.

Verapamil

Verapamil is a papaverine derivative. It is selectively taken up into the atrioventricular node, and is particularly effective for supraventricular tachy-arrhythmias. Verapamil has been used for acute hypertension; however, its usefulness is limited by its negative inotropic effect and interference with atrioventricular conduction. The oral dose is 80–160 mg t.d.s., whilst the IV dose should be limited to 5–10 mg over 20 min.

Nifedipine

Nifedipine is a dihydropyridine derivative. It is a potent arteriodilator that reduces arterial pressure by lowering SVR and can induce reflex tachycardia. In severe hypertension, nifedipine in 5–20 mg doses sublingually, buccally or orally, can produce a prompt and consistent reduction in arterial pressure. Onset of action is slower after oral administration (15–20 min) than after sublingual or buccal administration (5–10 min). The drug is poorly absorbed through the oral mucosa,[20] but absorption is delayed when the whole capsule is swallowed.[21] The 'bite-and-swallow' method is recommended when rapid onset of action is required. Overshoot hypotension with cerebral or myocardial ischaemia can occur, especially in patients who are hypovolaemic, elderly, receiving concomitant antihypertensives, or given repeated doses of nifedipine in less than 1.0 h.[22,23]

Diltiazem

This is a benzothiazepine derivative which has less negative inotropic effect than either nifedipine or verapamil. It is also a lesser vasodilator than nifedipine, although it is useful for supraventricular arrhythmias. The usual dose is 60–90 mg t.d.s.; due to its high first-pass metabolism, the parenteral dose is only 75–150 μg/kg.

Nicardipine

Nicardipine is a new dihydropyridine derivative. It is a pure arteriodilator that increases coronary and cerebral blood flow. It causes minimal myocardial depression, but may induce reflex tachycardia. Unlike nifedipine, it is soluble in water and insensitive to light. Intravenous nicardipine lowers arterial pressure in 5–15 min.[24] In treating acute hypertension, IV infusion of nicardipine has been shown to be similar to SNP, in allowing easy titration to effective doses.[25] Nicardipine can be given by a two-step infusion. A loading infusion of 10–15 mg/h is given until the desired therapeutic response, followed by a maintenance infusion of 2–5 mg/h. Side-effects after IV nicardipine include headache, and nausea and vomiting.

Central α-agonists

These agents stimulate central postsynaptic α_2-receptors in the medullary vasomotor centre. They inhibit peripheral sympathetic outflow and lower arterial pressure by decreasing heart rate, CO, SVR and venous return. Clonidine and methyldopa have been used for acute hypertension. The onset of action of IV methyldopa is delayed by up to 2–4 h, and its effectiveness is also inconsistent.

Clonidine is available both as oral and IV preparations. Systemic absorption after oral clonidine is rapid and complete, producing onset of action after 30–60 min, peak action in 2–4 h, and duration of action of 12–16 h. An initial oral dose of 0.2 mg is followed by 0.1 mg every hour, up to a maximum of 0.6–0.8 mg. Excessive hypotension can occur in elderly patients and in patients given other antihypertensive agents. Sedation is a common side-effect and may interfere with neurological observation. Other side-effects include dry mouth, bradycardia, heart block and postural hypotension. Intravenous clonidine offers no advantage in its onset of action and may produce an initial pressor response.

Angiotensin-converting enzyme inhibitors

These agents competitively inhibit the angiotensin-converting enzyme (ACE), and block the conversion of angiotensin I to angiotensin II. Angiotensin II is 40 times as potent a vasoconstrictor as noradrenaline. ACE inhibitors also block bradykinin kinase and increase the concentration of bradykinin, a potent vasodilator. ACE inhibitors do not induce reflex tachycardia, and this is a distinct advantage over direct arteriodilators.

Captopril

Captopril contains a sulphydryl group that interacts with the Zn^{2+} of the ACE receptor-binding site, with greater affinity than angiotensin I. Captopril is particularly effective in renovascular hypertension. However, it is also effective in anephric patients and in low-renin hypertension, probably the result of local effects on tissue ACE receptor sites in blood vessels. Side-effects may be serious and include agranulocytosis, renal failure and hyperkalaemia. Profound hypotension is a risk, particularly in patients with depleted intravascular volume or taking adrenergic antagonists. Captopril is contraindicated in patients with bilateral renal artery stenosis, or stenosis in a solitary kidney. In acute hypertension, captopril 25 mg can be given sublingually, producing onset of action in 20–30 min, maximum effect around 50 min, and duration of action around 4 h.[26] Captopril is particularly effective in high-renin states, such as malignant hypertension in scleroderma crisis.

Enalapril and enalaprilat

Enalapril was developed to overcome some of the complications of captopril. In enalapril, the sulphydryl group is substituted by phenylanaline. Enalapril is a prodrug, effective by hepatic metabolism to enalaprilat, and producing slower and more controlled action. Enalaprilat is excreted in the kidneys. It is poorly absorbed orally, and is available as an IV preparation. Intravenous enalaprilat is given in 1–5 mg doses. The onset of action is 15 min, and the duration is 6–12 h. Enalaprilat is useful for acute hypertension associated with left ventricular failure or high circulating renin.[27] The hypotensive response is variable, partly dependent on intravascular volume. A lower dose should be used in patients with renal impairment, renovascular hypertension and diuretic therapy. These drugs should be avoided during pregnancy.

Other ACE inhibitors

Lisinipril, a lysine analogue of enalaprilat, does not require metabolic conversion for its activity; however, its clearance is dependent on adequate renal function. Lisinipril is prescribed as a single 5 mg oral dose daily. *Fosinopril*, a new phosphinyl ester prodrug, is rapidly hydrolysed to the active diacid fosinoprilat, which is rapidly cleared by both hepatic and renal routes. Fosinopril can be given as a 10 mg daily oral dose.

Specific hypertensive conditions

Hypertensive encephalopathy[1]

The clinical picture is an insidious onset over 1–3 days of severe generalized headache, nausea and vomiting, apprehension, mental confusion, seizures and focal neurological deficits. Pre-existing essential hypertension is present in about 50% of the patients, and typically, treatment has been inadequate or

discontinued. MAP should be lowered gradually over 2–4 h, but by not more than 25%. The syndrome usually resolves within a few hours following the control of the arterial pressure. The drug of choice is SNP. SNP is a cerebral vasodilator and may induce increase in cerebral blood flow and intracranial pressure, particularly at low doses. However, the fall in arterial pressure will attenuate an increase in intracranial pressure.

Phaeochromocytoma[28]

Tumours of the adrenal medulla secrete catecholamines and produce hypertension that is paroxysmal initially, but later becomes sustained. Most are single benign adrenal tumours, but 10% are bilateral or multiple, and 5–15% are malignant. Common symptoms include hypertension (98%), headache, palpitations, tachycardia, sweating, anxiety and nervousness, nausea and vomiting, and weight loss. Orthostatic hypotension is seen occasionally. Fundoscopic changes are seen in up to 70%. The association with pregnancy carries a 40% mortality. It can be easily confused with eclampsia.

Laboratory confirmation includes spot urinary metanephrine. Urinary catecholamines, and vanillyl-mandelic acid, a metabolite of metanephrine, may be raised. Plasma catecholamines are more sensitive and should be measured whenever possible. Provocative testing of catecholamine secretion (e.g. with histamine, tyramine, or glucagon) is contraindicated. Computed tomography (CT) examination has simplified tumour location, although the limits of detection remain at about 2 cm. For extra-adrenal tumours, combination of CT with radioisotope scanning using meta-iodobenzyl-guanidine (MIBG), an analogue of noradrenaline, has increased both sensitivity and selectivity. Magnetic resonance imaging may help in difficult cases. Selective venous sampling of blood with measurements of plasma catecholamine levels is useful for localization of phaeochromocytoma.

Acute hypertensive crises are managed with phentolamine 2–5 mg IV boluses, repeated at 5-min intervals. Continuous intra-arterial monitoring is necessary. Tumour β-adrenergic stimulation may exhibit excessive vasodilatation, and pressor drugs and IV fluids may be required. Preparation for surgery involves adequate α-adrenergic blockade, using phenoxybenzamine 10 mg b.d.–t.d.s. orally, increasing by 10–20 mg/day, until arterial pressure is controlled (after about a week). Adequate fluid replacement must accompany re-expansion of the contracted intravascular volume. Excessive β-adrenergic effects (e.g. tachycardia, palpitations and angina) can be treated by β-adrenergic antagonists *after* sufficient α-blockade. Postoperative plasma catecholamine concentrations remain elevated for 10–14 days.

Pregnancy-induced hypertension

This is discussed in Chapter 55.

Perioperative hypertension[29]

Major surgical procedures are associated with activation of the sympathetic nervous system and release of stress hormones, as well as inhibition of insulin and atrial natriuretic peptide. The net cardiovascular result is vasoconstriction and increased SVR. The stress response results from anxiety, surgery, general anaesthesia and pain, as well as physiological changes such as volume depletion and hypothermia. Management should consider the aetiological background. Inadequate analgesia, hypothermia, hypoxia or hypercarbia must be corrected before antihypertensive therapy. In addition, attention is paid to preoperative medication and drug-induced hypertension (either cessation of antihypertensives or previous administration of MAO inhibitors). The same principles of general management of acute hypertension should apply.

Drug interaction

Withdrawal of antihypertensive treatment

Abrupt cessation of antihypertensive treatment may result in rebound hypertension. Drugs associated with this discontinuation syndrome include centrally acting drugs (e.g. clonidine, methyldopa and guanabenz), β-adrenergic blockers, guanethidine, bethanidine, reserpine and diuretics. The severity of the rebound response depends on sudden cessation of treatment, combination therapy, pretreatment arterial pressure, renin status, development of renovascular disease and the presence of ischaemic heart disease. The condition should be managed by the same principles and the specific drug therapy is reinstituted.

Interaction with MAO inhibitors

In patients treated with MAO inhibitors, sudden release of catecholamines results from ingestion of tyramine-containing foods with drugs such as pethidine and indirect sympathomimetics. Since the mechanism of hypertension involves adrenergic receptor mediation, this may be best managed by IV α- and β-adrenergic blockers. The acute vasoconstriction of rarely seen ergot poisoning may be treated in similar fashion.

Target-organ diseases

Acute stroke

Acute hypertension is common after acute stroke, particularly in patients with pre-existing chronic hypertension. Arterial pressure, however, will often fall spontaneously within the next day, and to the pre-stroke level after 3–4 days.[30] Continuation of pre-stroke antihypertensive treatment will usually suffice. Extreme caution should be exercised in lowering the arterial pressure in the presence of already impaired cerebral perfusion.[31] New antihypertensives should be withheld until after 24 h of observation, and restricted to patients whose diastolic arterial pressures continue to exceed 130 mmHg (17.3 kPa).[32] During antihypertensive treatment, neurological deterioration may signify cerebral hypoperfusion, and discontinuation of the treatment should be considered. In patients with extensive stroke, intracranial pressure monitoring is advisable. The drug of choice is SNP because its effect can be readily controlled. Labetalol IV is a suitable alternative.

Acute myocardial ischaemia

Acute myocardial ischaemia with or without myocardial infarction is sometimes accompanied by severe hypertension. Myocardial ischaemia is exacerbated because the elevated SVR increases left ventricular wall tension and myocardial oxygen demand. The treatment of choice is IV GTN, as it reduces SVR and improves coronary perfusion. Intravenous labetalol and calcium-channel antagonists are also suitable. SNP is reserved for refractory hypertension.

Acute left ventricular failure

Severely elevated SVR and arterial pressure increase left ventricular workload and can precipitate or aggravate left ventricular failure. Reduction of arterial pressure can restore cardiac compensation without resorting to inotropes. SNP is the agent of choice as it reduces both preload and afterload. SNP should be administered with oxygen, morphine and a loop diuretic. Intravenous GTN is a suitable alternative to SNP. ACE inhibitors such as captopril and enalapril can be used in the acute situation, and they are also required for long-term therapy.

Acute aortic dissection[33,34]

This acutely dangerous situation should be suspected in any patient presenting with severe hypertension and pain in the chest, back or abdomen. Immediate control of cardiac output as well as arterial pressure is required to prevent extension of the dissection. The aim is to decrease the shear forces between the aortic blood flow and the arterial wall, which is related to the index of myocardial contractility $(dP/dT)_{max}$. This can be achieved by the concurrent use of β-adrenergic blockers with SNP or trimetaphan. Intravenous labetalol is also suitable. Systolic arterial pressure should be controlled below 120 mmHg (16 kPa), and in patients with ongoing pain, this can be reduced to 80 mmHg (10.6 kPa) provided urine output is adequate. For aortic dissection distal to the left subclavian artery, antihypertensive treatment is the therapy of choice. For proximal dissection involving the ascending aorta, the patient should proceed to surgery after control of arterial pressure.

Renal failure

Acute hypertension may be caused by renal artery stenosis and renal parenchymal diseases such as glomerulonephritis and vasculitis. Excessive hypertension can also damage the renal parenchyma, and through the renin–angiotensin system, result in further aggravation of the deranged cardiovascular control. There is also impaired secretion of the renal vasodilators, e.g. prostaglandins, renomedullary lipids and the renal kallikrein–bradykinin system. The use of ACE inhibitors may be appropriate in addition to other vasodilators. In chronic hypertensive patients, renal artery stenosis should be excluded by angiography. Transluminal renal artery angioplasty is a possible alternative to surgical endarterectomy.

References

1 Houston MC (1989) Pathophysiology, clinical aspects, and treatment of hypertensive crises. *Prog Cardiovasc Dis* **32**:99–148.

2 Calhoun DA and Oparil S (1990) Treatment of hypertensive crisis. *N Engl J Med* **323**:1177–1183.

3 Gifford RW Jr (1991) Management of hypertensive crises. *J Am Med Assoc* **266**:829–835.
Journal of the American Medical Association **266**:829–835.

4 Kaplan NM (1994) Management of hypertensive emergencies. *Lancet* **344**:1335–1338.

5 Editorial (1991) Hypertensive emergencies. *Lancet* **338**:220–221.

6 Vallance P and Collier J (1994) Biology and clinical relevance of nitric oxide. *Br Med J* **309**:453–457.

7 Kam PCA and Govender G (1994) Nitric oxide: basic science and clinical applications. *Anaesthesia* **49**:515–521.

8 Furchgott RF and Zawadzki JV (1980) The obligatory role of endothelial cells in the relaxation of arterial smooth muscle by acetyl choline. *Nature* **288**:373–376.

9 Katsuki S, Arnold W, Mittal C and Murad F (1977) Stimulation of guanylate cyclase by sodium nitroprusside, nitroglycerin and nitric oxide in various tissue preparations and comparison to the effects of sodium azide and hydroxylamine. *J Cyclic Nucleotide Res* **3**:23–35.

10 Harrison DG and Bates JN (1993) The nitrovasodilators – new ideas about old drugs. *Circulation* **87**:1461–1467.

11 Tamaki K, Sadoshima S, Baumbach GL, Iadecola C, Reis DJ and Heistad DD (1984) Evidence that disruption of the blood brain barrier precedes reduction in cerebral blood flow in hypertensive encephalopathy. *Hypertension* **6**(suppl I):I-75–I-81.

12 Jansen PAF, Thien T, Gribnau FWJ *et al.* (1988) Blood pressure and both venous and urinary catecholamines after cerebral infarction. *Clin Neurol Neurosurg* **90**:41–45.

13 Ferguson RK and Vlasses PH (1989) How urgent is 'urgent' hypertension? *Arch Intern Med* **149**:257–258.

14 Ziegler MG (1992) Advances in the acute therapy of hypertension. *Crit Care Med* **20**:1630–1631.

15 Chun G and Frishman WH (1990) Rapid-acting parenteral antihypertensive agents. *J Clin Pharmacol* **30**:195–209.

16 Chitwood WR Jr, Cosgrove DM III and Lust RM (1992) Multicentre trial of automated nitroprusside infusion for postoperative hypertension. *Ann Thorac Surg* **54**: 517–522.

17 Robin ED and McCauley R (1992) Nitroprusside-related cyanide poisoning: time (long past due) for urgent, effective interventions. *Chest* **102**:1842–1845.

18 Nightingale SI (1991) New labeling for sodium nitroprusside emphasizes risk of cyanide toxicity. *J Am Med Assoc* **265**:847.

19 Cumming AMM, Brown JJ, Lever AF and Robertson JIS (1982) Intravenous labetalol in the treatment of severe hypertension. *Br J Clin Pharmacol* **13**(suppl 1): 93S–96S.

20 McAllister RG Jr (1986) Kinetics and dynamics of nifedipine after oral and sublingual doses. *Am J Med* **81**(suppl 6A):2–5.

21 Stephen JM and Avila JA (1991) Treatment of hypertensive crisis. *N Engl J Med* **324**:993.

22 O'Mailia JJ, Sander GE and Giles TD (1987) Nifedipine associated myocardial ischaemia or infarction in the treatment of hypertensive urgencies. *Ann Intern Med* **107**:185–187.

23 Wachter RM (1987) Symptomatic hypotension induced by nifedipine in the acute treatment of severe hypertension. *Arch Intern Med* **147**:556–558.

24 Ram CV (1991) Management of hypertensive emergencies: changing therapeutic options. *Am Heart J* **122**: 356–363.

25 Halpern NA, Goldberg M, Neely C *et al.* (1992) Postoperative hypertension: a multicenter, prospective, randomized comparison between intravenous nicardipine and sodium nitroprusside. *Crit Care Med* **20**: 1637–1643.

26 Angeli P, Chiesa M, Caregaro L *et al.* (1991) Comparison of sublingual captopril and nifedipine in immediate treatment of hypertensive emergencies. *Arch Intern Med* **151**:678–682.

27 Strauss R, Gavras I, Vlahakos D and Gavras H (1986) Enalaprilat in hypertensive emergencies. *J Clin Pharmacol* **26**:39–43.

28 Karet FE and Brown MJ (1994) Phaeochromocytoma: diagnosis and management. *Postgrad Med J* **70**: 326–328.

29 Leslie JB (1993) Incidence and aetiology of perioperative hypertension. *Acta Anaesthesiol Scand* **37**(suppl) 99):5–9.

30 Carlberg B, Asplund K and Hägg E (1991) Course of blood pressure in different subsets of patients after acute stroke. *Cerebrovasc Dis* **1**:281–287.

31 Phillips SJ (1994) Pathophysiology and management of

hypertension in acute ischaemic stroke. *Hypertension* **23**:131–136.

32 Strandgaard S and Paulson OB (1994) Cerebrovascular consequences of hypertension. *Lancet* **344**:519–521.

33 Asfoura JY and Vidt DG (1991) Acute aortic dissection. *Chest* **99**:724–729.

34 Banning AP, Ruttley MS, Musumeci F and Fraser AG (1995) Acute dissection of the thoracic aorta. *Br Med J* **310**:72–73.

17 Valvular and congenital heart disease

JE Sanderson

Valvular heart disease

Valvular heart disease is still common, although in most developed countries the main cause is no longer rheumatic heart disease but congenital conditions, such as mitral valve prolapse and bicuspid aortic valves.[1] However, in many parts of the world, rheumatic fever and rheumatic heart disease are still major health problems, especially in the young.[2,3] Diseases of heart valves cause stenosis, incompetence or both. The major causes are rheumatic fever, degenerative conditions, congenital and endocarditis.

Rheumatic fever

This acute fibrile illness is due to a cross-reaction following a group A β-haemolytic streptococci pharyngitis, which causes inflammatory lesions involving the joints, heart and subcutaneous tissues. It presents with polyarthritis, carditis, subcutaneous nodules, rash (erythema marginatum) and chorea. Carditis consists of murmurs (most commonly mitral, aortic regurgitation or the mid diastolic Carey Coombs murmur), pericarditis, cardiomegaly or congestive heart failure.[4] Chronic rheumatic heart disease occurs in about 40% of those with apical and basal diastolic murmurs, and 70% with heart failure or pericarditis during the acute attacks. It is still common in the Middle East, India, Africa and South America, and causes between 20–40% of all cardiovascular disease in the Third World.[2] It is rare now in North America, western Europe, Australiasia and parts of Asia.

Mitral stenosis

Rheumatic fever is the main cause; other rare causes are left atrial mxyoma, ball-valve thrombus, calcifica-tion of the annulus or systemic lupus erythematosus. Scarring or fibrosis of the valves, especially at the edges and sometimes involving the subvalvular apparatus, causes narrowing and hence increased left atrial pressure, pulmonary venous hypertension and pulmonary arterial hypertension. Thus the lungs and right ventricle suffer the most burden. Main symptoms are breathlessness on exertion, recurrent bronchitis, fatigue, palpitations due to paroxysmal atrial fibrillation (AF), haemoptysis and stroke. The onset of AF is usually associated with marked symptomatic deterioration and increases significantly the risk for left atrial thrombus formation and embolism.

Classic signs of mitral stenosis are mitral facies (peripheral cyanosis on the cheeks), a small-volume pulse which may be irregular (AF common), right ventricular hypertrophy, a tapping apex due to a palpable first heart sound, a loud first heart sound, and an opening snap with a rumbling diastolic murmur. An opening snap is present if the valve is not calcified and occurs between 0.04 and 0.10 s after S2. An electrocardiogram (ECG) shows a broad P wave in lead 2. Chest X-ray shows an enlarged left atrium and appendage, prominent upper lobe pulmonary veins, but heart size is usually within normal limits. The diagnosis can readily be confirmed by echocardiography, which allows assessment of the valve anatomy, and estimation of valve area and gradient. Severe stenosis is considered to be present if the valve area is < 1 cm^2.

Treatment is the use of β-blockers to slow the heart rate and increase diastolic filling time, diuretics and digoxin if the patient is in AF. Anticoagulation is essential if there is significant mitral stenosis and AF. Mitral balloon valvuloplasty has been shown to be very successful therapy with excellent long-term outcome, and compares well with surgical treatment.[5] The main contraindications to balloon valvuloplasty are significant mitral regurgitation and heavy calcification.

Mitral regurgitation

There is a considerable difference between acute and chronic mitral regurgitation (Table 17.1). In chronic

Table 17.1 Mitral regurgitation

Chronic	*Acute*
Causes	
Mitral valve prolapse	Ruptured chordae
Rheumatic heart disease	Ruptured papillary muscle (MI)
LV dilatation (IHD, cardiomyopathies, etc.)	Perforation of leaflet (IE)
Prosthetic valves	Prosthetic valves
Physiology	
LV volume overload	Sudden pressure overload of LA and
LV dilatation and hypertrophy	pulmonary veins
Increased LA size (mean pressure normal initially because of increased compliance)	No change in LV dimension
Symptoms	
Asymptomatic initially	Severe dyspnoea
Fatigue	
Dyspnoea	
Examination	
Pansystolic apical murmur radiating to axilla/lower sternal edge.	Harsh pansystolic murmur radiating to axilla and back
Third heart sound	Third heart sound
ECG	
LV hypertrophy	No change (or acute MI)
LA hypertrophy	
Chest X-ray	
Increased-size LV	Normal LV and LA dimension
Increased-size LA	Pulmonary oedema
Echocardiography	
Diagnostic	Diagnostic
Treatment	
Vasodilators and ACE inhibitors (reduce afterload)	Preload and afterload reduction and prepare for urgent surgery
Diuretics and digitalis	
Surgery if symptoms and LV size increase (before LV end-systolic diameter >4.5 cm or LV ejection fraction <60%)	

MI = Myocardial infarction; LV = left ventricle/ventricular; IHD = ischaemic heart disease; IE = infective endocarditis; LA = left atrium/atrial; ECG = electrocardiogram; ACE = angiotensin-converting enzyme.

mitral regurgitation there is time for the left ventricle and left atrium to adapt to the increasing regurgitation, leading to their gradual enlargement. In acute mitral regurgitation, the sudden pressure overload of the left atrium and pulmonary veins leads to severe pulmonary oedema. The treatment for acute mitral regurgitation is urgent surgery. The management of chronic mitral regurgitation is more difficult. Initially, medical therapy can be helpful, but the probability of postoperative death or persistent severe heart failure after valve replacement increases abruptly, when the left ventricular (LV) end-systolic diameter exceeds 45 mm on echocardiography, or ejection fraction falls below 60%.[6] In patients without mitral stenosis, mitral valve repair is preferable to replacement, and evidence suggests that preservation of the chordae improves postoperative LV function.[7]

Mitral valve prolapse[8]

This is a common condition affecting 5% of the adult population, more women than men. It has a number of synonyms such as Barlow and click-murmur syndrome. It is due to the myxomatous degeneration of the valve, with redundancy of the leaflets which may affect both the anterior and posterior valves. At the end of diastole, the valve closes normally, but as LV pressure rises during systole, a portion of the valve leaflet prolapses in the left atrium, with associated regurgitation. It is usually mild, but can progress and become more severe, and rarely, the chordae may rupture to produce severe acute regurgitation.

Mitral valve prolapse is usually asymptomatic, but a wide variety of symptoms have been associated, including odd chest pains, palpitations and fatigue.

On examination, typical findings are a mid-systolic click and a late systolic murmur, which are separated from the first heart sound, but usually reaching the second heart sound. The murmur may have a crescendo–decrescendo quality. It is usually louder with the Valsalva manoeuvre and on standing. Echocardiography is diagnostic, and can accurately assess the degree of severity of mitral valve prolapse. In most patients, mitral prolapse is a benign condition with a good prognosis. It poses a risk for infective endocarditis, which then leads to a substantial risk of death and need for mitral valve surgery. There is a very small increased incidence of neurological ischaemic events.[9]

Aortic stenosis

The commonest cause of aortic stenosis is degeneration of a bicuspid aortic valve. Valve stenosis leads to increased LV systolic pressure, LV hypertrophy and reduced LV compliance. The increased LV work may induce subendocardial ischaemia, arrhythmias and sudden death. Main symptoms are angina, syncopy and breathlessness. Typical findings on examination are a slowly rising small-volume pulse which may be associated with a systolic thrill in the carotid, evidence of LV hypertrophy without an enlarged heart, and a harsh ejection systolic murmur radiating into the neck. If the valve is calcified, there is no click and the A2 is soft. An ECG confirms LV hypertrophy. The chest X-ray shows a normal heart size, a poststenotic dilatation in the ascending aorta and presence of calcification. Echocardiography is diagnostic, and allows the measurement of aortic valve area gradient and the degree of aortic incompetence. Medical treatment is not effective. Surgery should be performed even if the patient is asymptomatic, if the gradient is >60 mmHg or the valve area is <0.8 cm^2 as there is an increased risk of sudden death.[10]

Aortic regurgitation

Like mitral regurgitation, the features of chronic and acute aortic regurgitation are different. *Chronic aortic regurgitation* has a number of causes, including rheumatic, connective tissue disorders (e.g. ankylosing spondylitis, Reiter's syndrome and rheumatoid disease), syphilitic aortitis, cystic medial necrosis (Marfan's syndrome), aortic root dilatation due to hypertension and a congenital bicuspid aortic valve. Endocarditis can produce aortic regurgitation in a normal valve. The leak from the aorta increases LV volume, causing LV dilatation and LV hypertrophy. Initially, this is well tolerated but eventually LV function declines.

Main symptoms are fatigue and dyspnoea. Typical findings on examination are a large-volume, bounding, wide pulse pressure which is collapsing in nature. Other classical physical signs include Corrigan's (visible carotoid pulsation) and nailbed capillary pulsation (Quincke's sign) which all reflect the rapid 'run-off'. The heart is usually enlarged with a displaced apex, and there is a high-pitched early diastolic blowing murmur which radiates from the left sternal edge to the apex. There may be a mid-diastolic murmur (Austin Flint) due to the regurgitant aortic jet hitting the anterior mitral valve leaflet. An ECG shows LV hypertrophy, usually with a strain pattern. A chest X-ray shows an enlarged heart with a dilated aorta. Echocardiography is diagnostic and can demonstrate the degree of aortic regurgitation, LV size and function.

The decision to undertake aortic valve replacement in patients with pure aortic regurgitation is difficult. Many patients can survive despite enlarged left ventricles. In general, patients should be advised to have an operation before LV end-systolic dimension exceeds 55 mm or ejection fraction <60%. Medical therapy with vasodilators such as nefedipine or ACE inhibitors can reduce or delay the need for valve replacement.[11] Surgery should not be delayed for too long, otherwise irreversible LV dysfunction ensues.

Acute aortic regurgitation is a severe disease with a high mortality, usually due to endocarditis (*Staphylococcus* or *Pneumococcus*).[12] There is acute LV diastolic pressure and volume overload, which leads to severe pulmonary oedema without LV dilatation. It can be difficult to diagnose clinically, because the early diastolic murmur is very short and soft. An echocardiogram, however, is completely diagnostic, and can demonstrate severe aortic regurgitation, and more importantly, early closure of the mitral valve. The treatment is urgent surgery without delay.

Tricuspid regurgitation

Tricuspid regurgitation is usually secondary to right ventricular (RV) dilatation/hypertrophy because of pulmonary hypertension. However, increasingly, infective endocarditis (usually *Staphylococcus*) in drug addicts is a common cause.[13] The diagnosis is made by the presence of large V waves in the jugular venous pressure, pansystolic murmur at the left sternal edge and echocardiography. Surgery may be necessary if the degree of valvular regurgitation is severe.

Infective endocarditis

This is one of the most important diagnoses not to miss, because, untreated, it is lethal.[14,15] It should be considered in any patient who has a murmur and a fever. Half of all endocarditis is on normal valves when it may follow a more acute course. Endocarditis on a prosthetic valve may occur early or late after implantation and has a high mortality; usually the prosthetic valve needs to be replaced. Clinical features of chronic endocarditis may be misleading, and often the symptoms are vague ill health, weight loss, malaise with night sweats and mild fever, and many patients are assumed to have influenza. In more chronic cases, there may be nail and conjunctival splinter haemorrhages, clubbing, splenomegaly and anaemia. Regurgitant murmurs (aortic, mitral or tricuspid) are usually present, and heart failure is a bad prognostic sign. Emboli may occur causing strokes. Mycotic aneurysms are frequently lethal.

The most important investigation is blood cultures (three sets) which should be taken preferably at different times and from different sites. Echocardiography may show vegetations, but only if they are > 3 mm, but will confirm the degree of regurgitation.[15] Echocardiography alone cannot be relied on to diagnose infective endocarditis. *Streptococcus bovis* is an unusual cause of endocarditis, and is associated with colonic carcinoma which may be occult.

Treatment for infective endocarditis should be prolonged antibiotic therapy (usually 4–6 weeks). If blind therapy is required, a combination of benzylpenicillin (1 g 4-hourly IV) is used, gentamicin 80 mg 12-hourly IV and flucloxacillin 2 g 6-hourly IV. Increasingly, surgical intervention is used and this improves outcome[16,17] (see Chapter 18).

Congenital heart disease in adults

The number of adults with congenital heart disease is steadily increasing, and includes not only patients with congenital heart disease who have survived into adulthood, but an increasing number of patients who have had cardiac surgery. The commonest congenital conditions found in adults are ostium secondum atrial septal defects, pulmonary valve stenosis, patent ductus arteriosus, uncomplicated congenitally corrected transposition of the great arteries, small perimembranous ventricular septal defects and Fallot's tetralogy.

Ostium secondum atrial septal defect

This is the commonest congenital cardiac abnormality in adults. It is often unrecognized because symptoms may be absent and the physical signs are subtle. Older patients may develop AF and cardiac failure. Paradoxical emboli through the defect are rare. Examination typically shows a pulmonary ejection systolic murmur with a wide and fixed second heart sound. ECG usually shows a right bundle branch block (and a left axis deviation with a primum defect). Chest X-ray will show pulmonary plethora. Echocardiography, especially transoesophageal echocardiography, can demonstrate the defect and give an estimate of the pulmonary artery pressure. There is an increased risk of developing Eisenmenger's syndrome but no risk of endocarditis. Many patients can live to a good age but overall life expectancy is not normal. Surgical closure is usually recommended if the size of the shunt is > 1.5:1.0, although this has recently been challenged.[18]

Patent ductus arteriosus (PDA)

This congenital abnormality is often asymptomatic and survival is usual. At about the age of 20, the risk of infective endocarditis increases, and at the age of about 30, patients with sizeable left-to-right shunts will begin to develop cardiac failure. Patients with significant shunts should have the PDA closed by surgery, or increasingly, by transcatheter using an umbrella device.[19]

Ventricular septal defects (VSD)

These are very common at birth but are seldom found in adults. The occasional adult will survive with a persistent small perimembranous VSD which is a risk for endocarditis.

Fallot's tetralogy

This is the cyanotic malformation most frequently associated with survival to adulthood. In these patients, the pulmonary stenosis is usually sufficient to prevent excessive pulmonary blood flow, but not too severe to cause large degrees of shunting from the right to the left ventricle. An increasing number of patients who have had complete repair are surviving into adulthood, and overall outcome is excellent.[20] The 30-year actuarial survival rate is 90% of the expected, and late health status is very good.

Non-cardiac surgery in adults with congenital heart disease

Cyanotic congenital heart disease

These patients have an increased risk of acute cholecystitis caused by calcium bilirubinate stones, and cholecystectomy is a procedure to be anticipated. Blood taken for phlebotomy can be stored for transfusion later. Oxygen inhalation appears to be desirable. Care must be taken with all IV lines, infusions and drugs, so that air is not introduced because of the risk of systemic embolism. If patients with Fallot's tetralogy have a sudden fall in blood pressure because of a fall in systemic resistance, intense cyanosis and occasionally death may occur. Conversely, a sudden rise in systemic resistance may severely depress systemic blood flow. Prophylaxis is required for infective endocarditis. Cyanotic patients with elevated fixed pulmonary vascular resistance (Eisenmenger's syndrome) are not able to respond rapidly to haemodynamic changes. In these patients, a sudden fall or rise in systemic vascular resistance can be very dangerous.

Ostium secondum atrial septal defect

In asymptomatic adults with this malformation and with normal pulmonary artery pressure, there is little risk during non-cardiac surgery. However, a rise in peripheral vascular resistance will increase left-to-right shunting; with hypotension, right-to-left shunting may occur. Systemic paradoxical emboli from leg veins can occur and early mobilization is recommended.

Congenital complete heart block

If the QRS is narrow and the subsidiary pacemaker is reliable with a reasonable ventricular rate, then temporary RV pacing is not required. However, all vagotonic stimuli should be minimized. If the QRS complex is wide and there is a relatively slow ventricular response, a temporary pacemaker should be inserted preoperatively.

References

1 Hall RJ and Julian DG (1989) *Diseases of the Cardiac Valves.* New York: Churchill Livingstone.

2 Sanderson JE and Woo KS (1994) Rheumatic fever and rheumatic heart disease – declining but not gone. *Int J Cardiol* **43**:231–232.

3 Eisenberg MJ (1993) Rheumatic heart disease in the developing world: prevalence, prevention, and control. *Eur Heart J* **14**:122–128.

4 Barlow JB (1992) Aspects of active rheumatic carditis. *Aust NZ J Med* **22**:592–600.

5 Reyes VP, Raju BS, Wynne J *et al.* Percutaneous balloon valvuloplasty compared with open surgical commissurotomy for mitral stenosis. *N Engl Med J Med* **331**:961–967.

6 Wisenbaugh T, Skudicky D and Sareli P (1994) Prediction of outcome after valve replacement for rheumatic mitral regurgitation in the era of chordal preservation. *Circulation* **89**:191–197.

7 Straub U, Feindt P, Huwer H *et al.* (1994) Mitral valve replacement with preservation of the subvalvular structures where possible: an echocardiographic and clinical comparison with laser where preservation was not possible. *Thorac Cardiovasc Surg* **42**:2–8.

8 Devereux RB (1995) Recent developments in the diagnosis and management of mitral valve prolapse. *Curr Opinion Cardiol* **10**:107–116.

9 Frary W, Devereux RB, Kramer-Fox R *et al.* (1994) Clinical and health-care cost consequences of infective endocarditis in mitral valve prolapse. *Am J Cardiol* **73**:263–267.

10 Davies SW, Gershlick AH and Balcon R (1991) The progression of valvular aortic stenosis in a long term retrospective study. *Eur Heart J* **12**:10–14.

11 Scognamiglio R, Rahimtoola SH, Fasoli G, Nishi S and Volta SD (1994) Nifedipine in asymptomatic patients with severe aortic regurgitation and normal left ventricular function. *N Engl J Med* **331**:689–694.

12 Benolti JR (1987) Acute aortic insufficiency. In: Dalen JE and Alpert JS (eds). *Valvular Heart Disease,* 2nd edn. Boston: Little, Brown, pp. 319–352.

13 Robbins MJ, Sveiro R, Fishman WH and Strom JA (1986) Right sided valvular endocarditis: etiology, diagnosis and approach to therapy. *Am Heart J* **109**:558–566.

14 Korzeniowski OM and Kaye D (1992) Infective endocarditis. In: Braunwald E (ed.) *Heart Disease.* Philadelphia: Saunders, pp. 1078–1105.

15 Durack DT, Lukes AS and Bright DK (1994) New criteria for diagnosis of infective endocarditis: utilization of specific echocardiographic findings. *Am J Med* **96**: 200–209.

16 Verheul HA, Vanderbrink RBA, Vanvreeland T, Moulijn AC, Duren DR and Dunning AJ (1993) Effects of changes in management of active infective endocarditis on outcome in a 25-year period. *Am J Cardiol* **72**: 682–687.

17 Watanabe G, Haverich A, Speier R, Dresler C and Borst HG (1994) Surgical treatment of active infective endocarditis with paravalvular involvement. *J Thorac Cardiovasc Surg* **107**:171–177.

18 Ward C (1994) Secundum atrial septal defect: routine surgical treatment is not of proven benefit. *Br Heart J* **71**:219–223.

19 Schenck MH, O'Laughlin MP, Rokey R, Ludomirsky A and Mullins CE (1993) Transcatheter occlusion of patient ductus arteriosus in adults. *Am J Cardiol* **72**:591–595.

20 Murphy JG, Gersh BJ, Mair DD *et al.* (1993) Long term outcome in patients undergoing surgical repair of tetralogy of Fallot. *N Engl Engl J Med* **329**:593–599.

18 • Infective endocarditis

BL Lloyd

Infective endocarditis (IE) is infection by any microorganism located on the lining (endocardium) of the heart. Although the heart valves are most commonly affected, the disease may involve the endocardium elsewhere in the heart (e.g. in association with ventricular and atrial septal defects and ventricular aneurysms). Infection may occur in endocardium outside the heart such as with coarctation and patent ductus arteriosus. In contrast with IE, non-infective forms may occur in rheumatic fever, in systemic lupus erythematosus (SLE; Libman–Sacks disease), leukaemia, and rarely, in terminal cachectic states. While differentiation between acute and subacute endocarditis has diminished in favour, it remains a useful clinical classification in many patients.

Acute endocarditis

This is caused by virulent pathogenic microorganisms (*Staphylococcus aureus, Streptococcus pneumoniae, β*-haemolytic streptococcus and *Neisseria gonorrhoeae*) and often affects normal valves. Inadequate host defences may be a causative/predisposing factor. The clinical course is usually short, more complicated and associated with a high mortality rate. Treatment needs to be early and aggressive.

Subacute endocarditis

This is caused by organisms regarded as commensals which are of lesser pathogenicity (e.g. *Staphylococcus epidermidis* or *Streptococcus viridans*), and tends to occur with pre-existing valvular disease and runs a more chronic course with a lower mortality.

Aetiology[1–5]

Transient or persisting bacteraemia by any organism in a subject 'at risk' may induce endocarditis. With more virulent organisms, infection may occur in the absence of valvular or endocardial disease.

Cardiac/endocardial abnormality

While the disease is most commonly associated with turbulent blood flow caused by abnormalities of the aortic and/or mitral valves, a change in flow dynamics by other cardiac lesions may also predispose to the infection. Rheumatic and degenerative valvular disease has been a common underlying cause of IE, but mitral valve prolapse and prosthetic valves are increasingly recognized now. Common congenital heart conditions involved are aortic stenosis, bicuspid aortic valve, patent ductus arteriosus, ventricular septal defect and tetralogy of Fallot – the most common cyanotic form of congenital heart disease. Infection involving the right heart is uncommon except in drug addicts.

Acute infection may occur in a normal heart during massive bacteraemia such as in 'mainlining' drug addicts or when bacteraemia with a virulent organism (e.g. *Staphylococcus aureus*) is present.

Infection may also occur in the presence of, and associated with, foreign bodies such as prosthetic valves, pacemaker electrodes, indwelling catheters such as central venous and parenteral nutrition lines and haemodialysis shunts. In ICU patients, right-sided IE may develop as a consequence of invasive lines such as Swan–Ganz catheters.[6]

Nosocomial or hospital-acquired infection may occur in 13–29% of cases of IE. Of 30 cases recently reviewed,[7] *S. aureus* occurred in 57% of cases, *Enterococcus faecalis* in 10% and fungi in 10%. Examination of source of infection revealed that 8 patients had a central venous catheter, 2 a peripheral venous catheter, 1 a pacemaker, 2 had cardiac catheterization and 3 had had prior recent cardiac surgery. Mortality was 40% compared with 18% in community-acquired infection.[7]

Table 18.1 Infecting organisms in adults with infective endocarditis (%)

Organism	<60 years	>60 years	Addict v	Early post prosthetic valve	Late post prosthetic valve
Streptococci	50–70	30	6–12	5–10	25–30
Enterococci	10	15	8	<1	5–10
Staphylococci	25	45	60	45–50	30–40
S. aureus	(90)	(65)	(99)	(45–50)	(30)
S. epidermidis	(10)	(35)	(1)	(50–55)	(70)
Gram-negative bacilli	<1	5	10	20	10–12
Fungi	<1		5	10–12	5–8
Diphtheroids	<1		2	5–10	4–5
Polymicrobial			5	1–5	1–5
Culture-negative	5–10	5	4–10	5–10	5–10
Other	<1			8	8

Modified from Ref. 9.

Infecting organism

The relative frequency of various microorganisms infecting the heart has changed over the last 20–30 years.[8] Table 18.1 shows the variety of infecting organisms in younger and older adult patients, drug addicts and in those with prosthetic heart valves. There has been a decline in frequency of *Streptococcus viridans* and culture-negative episodes, and a significant increase in *Staphylococcus aureus* and coagulase-negative staphylococci.[8,9]

Non-bacterial causes of endocarditis may occur, including fungi (e.g. *Candida*), rickettsia (e.g. Q fever), psitticosis, *Mycoplasma* species, *Brucella* species, *Chlamydia* species, *Legionella* species, *Histoplasma capsulatum* and *Aspergillus* species.

A portal of entry of the infecting organism such as dental therapy[1] or genitourinary instrumentation[3] may be evident. However, in a significant proportion of cases (40–60%), a direct causal relationship may not be evident.

Host factors

Various disease states and drug usage may predispose to the development of endocarditis (e.g. collagen disorders, diabetes mellitus, immunosuppressant drugs and chemotherapy).

Incidence

The incidence of endocarditis is difficult to establish, but it has been estimated[10] that in UK, about 20 cases/million population per year occur, many of whom are older than 65 years. It was estimated that 20% of these patients would die.

Clinical manifestations

Classical diagnostic features involve a heart murmur, septicaemia and embolism. The clinical features are often insidious, and the diagnosis should be considered in any patient with a cardiac murmur who shows signs of infection, or develops an unexplained fever. With septicaemia involving more virulent organisms (e.g. *S. aureus*), endocarditis should be suspected despite the absence of a murmur in the early stages, since in many patients it will develop later. The clinical features of IE have changed considerably over recent decades and the previous 'classical' features are frequently not present. The diagnosis ought to be considered[4,5,9,11–13] in patients with unexplained anaemia, glomerulonephritis, stroke, valvular heart disease with rapidly progressive symptoms, poorly controlled congestive heart failure, peripheral embolism, multiple pulmonary emboli, and saccular aneurysms; and in the postoperative cardiac patient and the elderly patient with general symptoms of malaise, weight loss and fever, especially a few weeks or months after a diagnostic or manipulative procedure (e.g. sigmoidoscopy or dilatation and curettage).

Presenting symptoms

Presenting symptoms are generally non-specific constitutional symptoms, most commonly fever, chills, weakness, dyspnoea, sweats, malaise and cough.[13] Less frequent symptoms include skin lesions, stroke, nausea, vomiting, headache, chest pain, oedema, myalgia, arthralgia and arthritis, and abdominal and low back pain.

Physical findings

Heart murmur is present in 90% of patients,[13] but may not be detectable at the initial examination or may develop some time later, particularly with acute or right-sided endocarditis. Murmurs will not be present with mural endocarditis (e.g. aneurysm). 'Changing murmurs', particularly systolic, may occur in a variety of conditions, and are of little diagnostic support except where new or worsening regurgitant

Table 18.2 Physical signs of infective endocarditis[13]

	Percentage of patients
Heart murmur	90
Fever	77
Embolic phenomena	50
Skin manifestations	50
Splenomegaly	28
Septic complications	19
Myotic aneurysms	18
Glomerulonephritis	15
Finger clubbing	12
Retinal lesions	9

murmurs develop (indicating valve destruction). Other common physical findings are shown in Table 18.2. Skin manifestations include petechiae and splinter haemorrhages, both commonly found in a general hospital population, and are therefore non-specific. More specific signs are Osler's nodes and Janeway lesions, but in recent years these are rarely seen. Osler's nodes are smaller, nodular red to purple tender lesions on the pulp spaces of the terminal phalanges or, less frequently, on the feet. Janeway lesions are small (1–4 cm), flat, erythematous, non-tender macules on the thenar and hypothenar eminences of the hands and soles of the feet.

Complications

More common complications include the following:

1 *Cardiac* – including congestive heart failure, arrhythmias, development of atrioventricular block, valve destruction and perforation, myocardial and aortic ring abscess, purulent pericarditis, fistulae (ventriculoatrial, aortopulmonary, aorto–right atrial), aneurysms, obstruction to valvular or coronary flow by vegetation, myocardial infarction and myocarditis.
2 *Embolic phenomena* – occur in up to 50% of patients. Common sites involved are coronary, cerebral, splenic and renal arteries, often associated with organ infarction. Mycotic aneurysms may occur and, occasionally, with rupture of the involved vessel. Fungal endocarditis often results in large vegetations which, on fragmentation, may cause major artery obstruction.
3 *Renal* – including renal infarction, haematuria, glomerulonephritis and abscess formation.
4 *Neurological* – including cerebrovascular accidents arising secondary to embolism or mycotic aneurysm, cerebral abscess, toxic and psychiatric states, meningoencephalitis, cranial nerve lesions, dyskinesia and spinal cord or peripheral nerve involvement.

A majority of emboli occur prior to treatment, within 48 h of treatment initiation or where infection is uncontrolled. Risk of embolization is highest in patients with left-sided IE and with vegetations greater than 10 mm. Rarely, embolization may occur up to months later following successful treatment.

In a recent series of 300 episodes of endocarditis in 287 patients,[14] a total of 386 complications occurred in 74% of the patients. Cardiac complications were the most common, but fatality rates were higher with neurological and septic complications, which were the leading cause of death.

Diagnosis

Since the presenting symptoms and clinical findings are usually non-specific, and classic features of fever, heart murmur embolism and anaemia are not uniformly present, the diagnosis is often difficult. Similar vague constitutional symptoms and findings may be present in various malignancies, viral illnesses, arthritis and anaemias of other causes, and with atrial myxoma.

Blood cultures

In suspected IE, the most important laboratory finding is isolation of the infecting microorganism from at least two blood cultures. Despite absence of murmur, IE should be suspected where blood cultures are positive and no other source of infection is evident. In approximately 90–95% of patients the infecting organism will be isolated from appropriately collected blood specimens. Cultures are more likely to be negative where there has been prior administration of antibiotics, and with organisms requiring special culture techniques (e.g. anaerobic, L forms, *Brucella* and streptococcal variants).[11] Negative cultures are also frequently observed with right-sided and mural IE, in uraemia and some chronic forms of endocarditis, and with non-bacterial causes (Q fever, psitticosis, fungal and viral infections).

Three sets of blood specimens obtained at least 3–4 h apart from different venepuncture sites, and over a 24–48 h period, are generally considered adequate for detection of bacteraemia in most patients,[11] but occasionally more specimens are necessary (especially if antibiotics have been given). Collection of arterial blood does not usually provide additional diagnostic information and is indicated. It is imperative that aerobic and anaerobic culture media be used. If a patient had been commenced on an antibiotic, use of antibiotic absorption or neutralization media should be considered. Where cultures are negative after several days, or in patients where multiple organisms are suspected (e.g. drug addicts and the immunocompromised), then culture bottles ought to remain incubated for up to 3 weeks and several repeat specimens collected.

Table 18.3 Laboratory findings in infective endocarditis

Positive blood cultures	90% of patients
Positive serology	Variable frequency
Normochromic, normocytic anaemia	50–80%
Elevated white cell count	75%
Elevated ESR	90%
Anaemia	50–80%
Rheumatoid factor present	35–50%
C-reactive protein elevation	Frequency uncertain

ESR = Erythrocyte sedimentation rate.

Serology

In some patients a positive serological diagnosis may establish the organism, e.g. Q fever, *Brucella, Candida, Myocoplasma, Chlamydia, Legionella, Histoplasma* and *Aspergillus.*

Other laboratory findings

Other finding are frequently present, but are non-specific (Table 18.3).

Urinalysis

Urine may show haematuria, red blood cell casts and proteinuria.

Echocardiography – Doppler examination (see below)

Management

The difficulties in diagnosis and management of IE usually warrant early and close collaboration and consultation with a cardiologist, infectious diseases/ microbiology consultant and, where necessary, a cardiac surgeon.

Confirmation of diagnosis

In suspected subacute bacterial endocarditis without prior antibiotic treatment (and positive cultures are likely), it is usually reasonable to delay treatment for 1–2 days until the organism is isolated. With acute endocarditis, blood cultures should be drawn over 1–2 h and any potential source (e.g. infected tooth or urine) be swabbed and/or cultured, and treatment initiated usually without further delay, in view of the poor prognosis and the rapid deterioration which may occur.

Antibiotics

Bactericidal antibiotics are generally used and need to be given in adequate dosage and duration, usually by the IV route. Where combinations of antibiotics are used they should be synergistic. Efficacy against the organism must be evaluated by *in vitro* sensitivity tests, and minimum inhibitory or bactericidal concentrations should be determined (see Chapter 64). IV administration is usually intermittent. Complications must be minimized by selection of lower-toxicity antibiotics, constant monitoring of serum drug concentrations and monitoring renal function. Doses may require adjustment in very obese or lean patients, or with altered renal function.

Antibiotic treatment is discussed in detail elsewhere,[4,5,9,15] both for native and prosthetic valve involvement, and requires individualization dependent upon the particular organism and its likely or proven sensitivities, the clinical course and complications. Selection of antibiotics ought to be in collaboration with an infectious disease consultant, but Tables 18.4–18.8 show general guidelines for adults. Dosages may need to be adjusted for patient size. Cephalosporins should be avoided with known penicillin hypersensitivity.

If a patient is penicillin-sensitive, an attempt at desensitization is too time-consuming and impracticable in endocarditis. Usually, other antibiotics can be used in place of penicillin, e.g. cephalosporins, lincomycin, clindamycin, fucidin, co-trimoxazole and vancomycin. The duration of antibiotic treatment is related to the antibiotic used and the organism's sensitivity; average duration is 4–6 weeks. There is a high tendency for relapse in patients treated for less than 3 weeks.

Table 18.4 General guidelines for therapy for endocarditis in adults due to penicillin-susceptible *Streptococcus viridans* and *S. bovis* (MIC ≤ 0.1 µg/ml)[15]

Antibiotic	Adult dose and route	Duration (weeks)
Aqueous crystalline penicillin G	10–20 million U/24 h IV either continuously or in six equally divided doses	4
Aqueous crystalline penicillin G	10–20 million U/24 h IV either continuously or in six equally divided doses	
with streptomycin	7.5 mg/kg IM (not to exceed 500 mg) every 12 h	2
or gentamicin	1 mg/kg IM or IV (not to exceed 80 mg) every 8 h	2–4

MIC = Minimum inhibitory concentration; IV = intravenous; IM = intramuscular

Table 18.5 General guidelines for therapy for endocarditis in adults due to penicillin-susceptible *Streptococcus viridans* and *S. bovis* (MIC 0.1 µg/ml) in patients allergic to penicillin[15]

Antibiotic	Adult dose and route	Duration (weeks)
Cephalothin	2 g IV every 4 h	4
or		
Cefazolin	1 g IM or IV every 8 h	4
or		
Vancomycin	30 mg/kg per 24 h IV in two or four equally divided doses, not to exceed 2 g/24 h unless serum concentrations are monitored	4

MIC = Minimum inhibitory concentration; IV = intravenous; IM = intramuscular

Table 18.6 General guidelines for therapy for endocarditis due to strains of *Streptococcus viridans* and *S. bovis* relatively resistant to penicillin G (MIC >0.1 µg/ml and <0.5 µg/ml)[15]

Antibiotic	Adult dose and route	Duration (weeks)
Aqueous crystalline penicillin G	20 million U/24 h IV either continuously or in six equally divided doses.	4
with		
Streptomycin	7.5 mg/kg IM (not to exceed 500 mg) every 12 h	2
or		
Gentamicin	1 mg/kg IM or IV (not to exceed 80 mg) every 8 h	2

MIC = Minimum inhibitory concentration; IV = intravenous; IM = intramuscular

Table 18.7 Therapy for endocarditis due to *Staphylococcus* in the absence of prosthetic material[15]

Antibiotic	Adult dose and route	Duration
	Methicillin-susceptible staphylococci	
Non-penicillin-allergic patients		
Nafcillin	2 g IV every 4 h	4–6 weeks
or		
Oxacillin	2 g IV every 4 h	4–6 weeks
With optional addition of gentamicin	1 mg/kg IM or IV (<80 mg) every 8 h	3–5 days
Penicillin-allergic patients		
Cephalothin	2 g IV every 4 h	4–6 weeks
or		
Cefazolin	2 g IV every 8 h	4–6 weeks
With optional addition of gentamicin	1 mg/kg IM or IV (not to exceed 80 mg)	3–5 days
or		
Vancomycin	30 mg/kg per 24 h IV in two or four equally divided doses (<2 g/24 h unless serum levels are monitored)	4–6 weeks
	Methicillin-resistant staphylococci	
Vancomycin	30 mg/kg per 24 h IV in two or four equally divided doses (<2 g/24 h unless serum levels are monitored)	4–6 weeks

IV = intravenous; IM = intramuscular

Monitoring

Clinical

Patients should be carefully observed for the development of congestive cardiac failure, which is associated with increased mortality,[16] and for worsening regurgitation. The presence of moderate or severe congestive heart failure requires urgent and aggressive medical therapy in an ICU or cardiac care unit with digoxin, diuretic and vasodilators, and usually measurement of left ventricular filling pressures via a pulmonary artery catheter.[6]

After control or stabilization of failure, or with clinically deteriorating haemodynamics, the patient

Table 18.8 Treatment of staphylococcal endocarditis in the presence of a prosthetic valve or other prosthetic material[15]

Antibiotic	Adult dose and route	Duration
	Methicillin-resistant staphylococci	
Vancomycin	30 mg/kg per 24 h IV in two or four equally divided doses	6 weeks
with	(<2 g/24 h unless serum levels are monitored)	
Rifampin	300 mg PO every 8 h	6 weeks
plus		
Gentamicin	1.0 mg/kg IM or IV (not to exceed 80 mg) every 8 h	2 weeks
	Methicillin-susceptible staphylococci	
Nafcillin or oxacillin	2 g IV every 4 h	⩾6 weeks
with		
Rifampin	300 mg PO every 8 h	⩾6 weeks
plus		
Gentamicin	1.0 mg/kg IM or IV (not to exceed 80 mg) every 8 h	2 weeks

IV = Intravenous; PO = orally; IM = intramuscular.

should be considered for corrective cardiac surgery. This may be assessed using non-invasive echo Doppler techniques or possibly cardiac catheterization, depending upon the patient's condition, valve affected and age.

Patients with mild congestive heart failure should be similarly treated, except that if failure is easily controlled, then a decision regarding surgery can often be delayed for 4–6 weeks.[16]

Electrocardiogram

Electrocardiogram evidence of new conduction defects often indicates abscess or aneurysm formation, and further investigations and possible surgical intervention need to be considered.

Echocardiography–Doppler ultrasound

Echocardiography has now assumed a major role in the diagnosis and assessment of infective endocarditis[17,19] (see Chapter 21). Valvular vegetation can be detected in 35–100% of patients, depending upon the series studied, the likelihood of active disease and its severity, and the technique used. In patients with clinical disease, two-dimensional echocardiography by the transthoracic route will detect vegetations in 38–100% of patients, the average being around 50%.[17] The sensitivity is higher with two-dimensional views than with M-mode studies. However, technical limitations and inadequate views, particularly in the sicker ICU patients, may result in inadequate studies in 20–30% of patients.

Transoesophageal echocardiography has allowed higher resolution and less frequent inadequate studies. By this route, detection of vegetations in definite cases frequently approaches 100%.[17] If a vegetation is not seen, alternative causes of an infective site ought to

be sought. 'False positive' vegetations may be reported with old healed vegetations, the redundancy of mitral valve prolapse, in thickened rheumatic valves, thrombus attached to a valve, and with some tumours.

Transoesophageal echocardiography is the preferred approach for assessment of possible vegetations on a prosthetic valve, but differentiation of vegetation from thrombus and pannus ingrowth may be indistinguishable and, frequently, echoreflectance makes visualization suboptimal.

Echocardiography also uniquely allows assessment of the infective process and haemodynamic complications. Infective processes of particular importance are fenestration or torn leaflet margins and valve disruption, chordal rupture and second valve infection (e.g. mitral valve aneurysm with aortic valve endocarditis). Extension of infection into perivalvular tissue or interventricular septum are detectable, as are infective pericarditis and fistulae. With prosthetic valves, necrosis and abscess formation in the annulus and valve disturbances can be detected.

Doppler ultrasound examination is useful in the detection of valvular regurgitation when often not clinically apparent, assessing the severity of a valvular regurgitation or stenosis, and in the detection of other abnormalities or shunts which develop as a complication of the infective procedure (e.g. aortic to right ventricular shunt). The extent of haemodynamic deterioration can be serially monitored, such as worsening aortic, mitral and tricuspid regurgitation.

Prognostic significance can be attached to the presence of vegetation. Patients with clinical evidence of IE and vegetations detected at echocardiography are at least twice as likely to have complications as patients without vegetations. If the vegetation size is greater than 10 mm, then congestive cardiac failure, embolic events, need for surgical intervention and death are more frequent.[18]

Table 18.9 Recommendations for prophylaxis in prevention of endocarditis in adults in Australia[23]

Low-risk patients (without prosthetic valves or prior infective endocarditis)
For dental procedures, oral surgery, or upper respiratory tract surgery:
1 If not receiving long-term penicillin: amoxycillin 3 g, 1 h before procedure
2 If having general anaesthetic (amoxy)ampicillin 1 g IV just before the procedure commences (or IM 30 min prior), followed by 500 mg IV, IM or orally, 6 h later
3 If hypersensitive to penicillin or receiving long-term penicillin: clindamycin 600 mg orally, 1–2 h before the procedure, followed by 300 mg orally, 6 h later
   or
   vancomycin 1 g IV slowly (at least over 1 h), the infusion ending just before the procedure commences

High-risk patients (with prosthetic valves or prior endocarditis)
For dental procedures, oral surgery or upper respiratory tract surgery, gastrointestinal or genitourinary procedures
1 (Amoxy)ampicillin 1 g IV just prior to the procedure (or IM 30 min prior to the procedure) followed by 500 mg IV, IM or orally 6 h later,
   plus
   gentamicin 1.5mg/kg IV just before the procedure commences (or IM 30 min before procedure commences)
2 If hypersensitive to penicillin:
   vancomycin 1 g IV slowly (at least over 1 h), the infusion ending just before the procedure commences.
   followed by:
   gentamicin 1.5 mg/kg IV just before the procedure commences.
For special situations such as renal failure, specific known infections, prolonged labour, specialist consultation may be indicated

IV = Intravenous; IM = intramuscular.

Table 18.10 Recommendations for prophylaxis in prevention of endocarditis in adults in the UK[24,25]

1 *Dental extractions, scaling or periodontal surgery under local or no anaesthesia*
   (a) Not allergic to penicillin and not given penicillin more than once in the previous month; 3 g amoxycillin orally taken under supervision 1 h prior to the procedure
   (b) If allergic to penicillin: 600 mg clindamycin orally taken under supervision 1 h before the procedure.

2 *Dental extractions, scaling or periodontal surgery under general anaesthesia*
   (c) Not allergic to penicillin and not given penicillin more than once in the previous month: amoxycillin IV or IM 1 g at the time of induction *plus* 500 mg orally 6 h later
   or
   3 g amoxycillin orally 4 h before anaesthesia, followed by a further 3 g orally as soon as possible after the operation
   or
   Amoxycillin 3 g together with probenicid 1 g orally 4 h before operation
Special-risk patients who should be referred to hospital:
   (i) Patients with prosthetic valves who are able to have a general anaesthetic.

Table 18.10 *Continued*
   (ii) Patients who are to have a general anaesthetic *and* who are allergic to pencillin or who have had pencillin more than once in the previous month.
   (iii) Patients who have had a previous attack of endocarditis.

Recommendations for these patients are:
   (d) If not allergic to penicillin and who have not had penicillin more than once in the previous month:
   1 g amoxycillin IV or 1 g amoxycillin in 2.5 ml 1% lignocaine hydrochlode IM
   plus
   120 mg gentamicin IV or IM at induction, then 500 mg amoxycillin orally 6 h later.
   (e) If allergic to penicillin or who have had penicillin more than once in the previous month:
   (i) vancomycin 1 g by slow IV infusion over at least 100 min
   followed by
   gentamicin 120 mg IV at induction or 15 min before the surgical procedure
   or
   (ii) teicoplanin 400 mg IV
   plus
   gentamicin 120 mg IV at induction or 15 min before the surgical procedure
   or
   (iii) clindamycin 300 mg by IV infusion over at least 10 min at induction or 15 min before the surgical procedure, followed by 150 mg orally or 150 mg by IV infusion over at least 10 min, 6 h later

3 *Surgery or instrumentation of upper-respiratory tract*
Recommended cover is for 1 (a) to 2 (e)(iii), but postoperative antibiotics may have to be given IM or IV if swallowing is painful.

4 *Genitourinary surgery or instrumentation*
For patients with sterile urine, the suggested cover is directed against faecal streptococci and is as for 2(d), 2(e)(i), or 2(e)(ii) above, but clindamycin regimens are not suitable for this purpose. If the urine is infected, prophylaxis should also cover the pathogens involved

5 *Obstetric and gynaecological procedures*
Cover is suggested for patients with prosthetic valves or patients who have had a previous attack of endocarditis and is as for 2(d), 2 (e)(i) or 2(e)(ii) above because of the risk from faecal streptococci. Clindamycin regimens are not suitable for this purpose

6 *Gastrointestinal procedures*
Cover is suggested for patients with prosthetic valves or patients who have had a previous attack of endocarditis and is as for 2 (d), 2 (e)(i), or 2 (e)(ii) above because of the risk from faecal streptococci. Clindamycin regimens are not suitable for this purpose.

IV = Intravenous; IM = intramuscular.

Antibiotic therapy

Efficacy against the infecting organism must be evaluated as discussed above.

Surgery

Indications for valve surgery in IE[4,5,16,19,20] include congestive cardiac failure, significant structural

Table 18.11 Recommendations for the prophylaxis of endocarditis in adults in the USA[22]

Indication	Regimen
Standard regimen For dental procedures; oral or upper respiratory tract surgery; minor GI or GU tract procedures	Amoxycillin, 3.0 g orally 1 h before, then 1.5 g 6 h later
Special regimens Oral regimen for penicillin-allergic patients (oral and respiratory tract only)	Clindamycin, 300 mg orally 1 h before, then 150 mg 6 h later
Parenteral regimen for high-risk patients; also for GI or GU tract procedures	Ampicillin, 2.0 g IM or IV, plus gentamicin 1.5 mg/kg IM or IV, 0.5 h before, followed by amoxicillin 1.5 g PO 6 h after initial dose; alternatively, the parenteral regimen may be repeated 8 h after initial dose.
Parenteral regimen for penicillin-allergic patients	Vancomycin 1.0 g IV slowly over 1 h, starting 1 h before; add gentamicin 1.5 mg/kg IM or IV if GI or GU tract is involved
Cardiac surgery including implantation of prosthetic valves	Cefazolin, 2.0 g IV at induction of anaesthesia, repeated 8 and 16 h later† or vancomycin, 1.0 g IV slowly over 1 h, starting at induction, then 0.5 g IV 12 h later†‡

*These regimens are empirical suggestions; no regimen has been proved effective for the prevention of endocarditis, and prevention failures may occur with any regimen. These regimens are not intended to cover all clinical situations; practitioners should use their own judgement on safety and cost–benefit issues in each individual case. One or two additional doses may be given if the period of risk for bacteraemia is prolonged.
†Gentamicin, 1.5 mg/kg IV, may be given with each dose if postoperative Gram-negative infections have occurred with significant frequency at the hospital.
‡This regimen is recommended for units where *Staphylococcus epidermidis* prosthetic valve infection is a problem.
GI = gastrointestinal; GU = genitourinary.

damage of a valve (especially aortic with severe regurgitation), or with other catastrophes (e.g. ruptured sinus of Valsalva, and perivalvular and myocardial abscess). Early surgery is often required for certain infections, including *Staphylococcus, Serratia*, Gram-negative bacterial and fungal infection. Other possible indications include very large mobile vegetations and recurrent septic emboli despite adequate antibiotic therapy, failure of response of the infective process despite appropriate antibiotic therapy, relapse or recurrent endocarditis.

Where IE occurs early after prosthetic valve insertion, replacement may be necessary if signs of infection fail to resolve or decompensation occurs.

Prognosis

Prognosis in IE clearly depends upon underlying valvular disease, presence of decompensation, organism involved and delay in diagnosis or adequate treatment. Case fatality rates range from 14% with no or mild heart failure, to 100% with severe congestive heart failure when treated medically, compared with 6% and 33% respectively when treated surgically.[16] Cure rates are highest for native valve endocarditis with streptococci (90%) or enterococci (75–90%) compared with staphylococci, where mortality may be 30–40%. Mortality is higher with left-sided infection compared with right-sided infection and in patients with prosthetic valve endocarditis.

Prophylaxis

It is accepted practice that patients considered at risk of endocarditis should be administered antibiotics prophylactically prior to procedures known to result in bacteraemia, such as dental therapy, operations in the upper respiratory tract, and surgery or instrumentation of the genitourinary or gastrointestinal tract. There have been no controlled clinical trials on prophylaxis, and many treatment regimens have been recommended, partly influenced by ease of administration, need for fasting, etc. It is clear that in addition to the procedure being performed, the species of microorganism present in the particular community or hospital environment and the immediate past history of the patient direct the type of antibiotic that would provide the most extensive cover. The recommendations are empirical and often vary between countries. Recommendations in Australia, USA and the UK are presented in Tables 18.9–18.11. Details on procedures requiring or not requiring prophylaxis, special risk groups, adjustment for anticoagulation and general anaesthesia are discussed elsewhere.[21,22]

References

1 Baylis SR, Clarke C, Oakly CM, Somerville W and Whitfield AGW (1983) The teeth and infective endocarditis. *Br Heart J* **50**:506–512.

2 Baylis SR, Clarke C, Oakly CM *et al.* (1983) The microbiology and pathogenesis of infective endocarditis. *Br Heart J* **50**:513–519.

3 Baylis SR, Clarke C, Oakly CM *et al.* (1983) The bowel, the genito-urinary tract and infective endocarditis. *Br Heart J* **51**:339–345.

4 Molavi A (1993) Endocarditis: recognition, management, and prophylaxis. In: Frankl WS and Brest AN (eds) *Valvular Heart Disease: Comprehensive Evaluation and Treatment. Cardiovascular Clinics.* Philadelphia: FA Davis, pp. 139–174.

5 Mehra A and Rahimtoola SH (1994) Infective endocarditis. In: Zaibag MA and Duran CMG (eds) *Valvular Heart Disease.* New York: Marcel Dekker.

6 Rowley KM, Clubb KS, Smith GJW and Cabin HS (1984) Right-sided infective endocarditis as a consequence of flow-directed pulmonary artery catheterisation. *N Engl J Med* **311**:1152–1156.

7 Chen SCA, Dwyer DE and Sorrell TC (1992) A comparison of hospital and community acquired infective endocarditis. *Am J Cardiol* **70**:1449–1452.

8 McCartney AC (1992) Changing trends in infective endocarditis. *J Clin Pathol* **45**:945–948.

9 Korzeniowski OM and Kaye D (1992) Infective endocarditis. In: Braunwald E (ed.) *Heart Disease, A Textbook of Cardiovascular Medicine,* 4th edn. Philadelphia: WB Saunders, pp. 1078–1105.

10 Young SE (1987) Aetiology and epidemiology of infective endocarditis in England and Wales. *J Antimicrob Chemother* **20**(Suppl A):7–15.

11 Gregoratos G and Karliner JS (1979) Infective endocarditis: diagnosis and management. *Med Clin North Am* **63**:173–199.

12 Editorial (1984) Infective endocarditis. *Lancet* i:6034.

13 Pelletier LL and Petersdorf RG (1977) Infective endocarditis: a review of 125 cases from the University of Washington Hospitals 1963–72. *Medicine* **56**:287–313.

14 MansurAJ, Grinberg M, da Luz PL and Bellotti G (1992) The complications of infective endocarditis. A reappraisal in the 1980s. *Arch Intern Med* **152**:2428–2432.

15 Bisno AL, Dismukes WE, Durack DT *et al.* (1989) Antimicrobial treatment of infective endocarditis due to viridans streptococci, enterococci, and staphylococci. *J Am Med Assoc* **261**:1471–1477.

16 Rahimtoola SH (1983) Valvular heart disease: a perspective. *J Am Coll Cardiol* **1**:199–215.

17 Yvorchuk KJ and Chan K-L (1994) Application of transthoracic and transesophageal echocardiography in the diagnosis and management of infective endocarditis. *J Am Soc Echocardiogr* **14**:294–308.

18 Aragam J R and Weymouth AE (1994) Echocardiographic findings in infective endocarditis. In: Weymouth AE (ed.) *Principles and Practice of Echocardiology,* 2nd edn. Philadelphia: Lea & Febiger, pp. 1178–1197.

19 Alsip SG, Blackstone EH, Kirklin JW and Cobbs CG (1985) Indications for cardiac surgery in patients with active endocarditis. *Am J Med* **78**:13843.

20 Karp RB (1987) Role of surgery in infective endocarditis. *Cardiovasc Clin* **17**:141–162.

21 Dajani AS, Bisno AL, Chung KJ *et al.* (1990) Prevention of bacterial endocarditis. *J Am Med Assoc* **264**:2919–2922.

22 Durack DT (1994) Prophylaxis of infective endocarditis. In: Mandell G (ed.) *Principles and Practice of Infectious Diseases.* New York: Churchill Livingstone, pp.793–799.

23 Victorian Medical Postgraduate Foundation (1994) *Antibiotic Guidelines of the Victorian Drug Usage Advisory Committee,* 8th edn. Australia.

24 Simmons NA, Ball AP, Cawson RA (1992) Antibiotic practice and infective endocarditis. *Lancet* **229**:1292–1293.

25 Simmons NA (1993) Recommendations for endocarditis prophylaxis. *J Antimicrob Chemother* **31**:437–438. **31**:437–438.

19 Postoperative cardiac intensive care

RP Lee and JM Branch

Postoperative cardiac intensive care involves managing the patient with cardiac disease after non-cardiac or cardiac surgery. The principles in each setting are similar, although cardiac function should be improved by surgical correction of the underlying cardiac defect. It is important to understand the cardiac condition, the patient's functional status, stresses produced by procedures, and basic principles of cardiac physiology and energy balance.

Physiology

Factors which determine cardiac function and vital organ blood flow are shown in Figure 19.1. Central to adequate cardiovascular function is stroke volume, which is determined by interdependent preload, afterload and contractility.

Preload

Preload is defined as the initial fibre length of a muscle before contraction. Clinically, this is interpreted as left ventricular end-diastolic volume (LVEDV). It is an important determinant of stroke volume; the Frank–Starling law of the heart states that the energy of contraction is proportional to the length of the muscle fibres before contraction.[1] This is now suggested to be a linear relationship[2] (Fig. 19.2). It is misguided to use pressure, whether left ventricular end-diastolic pressure (LVEDP), left atrial (LA) pressure or pulmonary capillary wedge pressure (PCWP) as an indicator of preload.[3] This assumes that increases in transmural pressure result in proportional increases in ventricular volume (or ventricular compliance remains constant). In fact, the relationship between ventricular volume and pressure is non-linear, and may be shifted by events (Fig. 19.3). Compliance increases with nitroglycerin, relief of ischaemia or hypoxia or dilated cardiomyopathy, and decreases with overload, right ventricular (RV) distension, catecholamines, hypoxia and ischaemia.[4] Hence, increased LVEDP (and pulmonary oedema) may indicate ischaemia, rather than increased preload (Fig. 19.4).

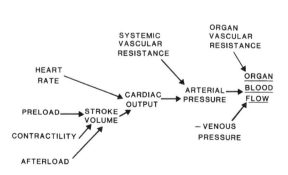

Fig. 19.1 Determinants of cardiac output and organ blood flow.

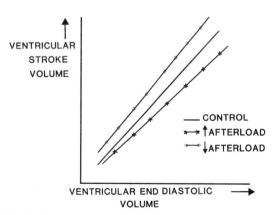

Fig. 19.2 Relationship between left ventricular end-diastolic volume and stroke volume.

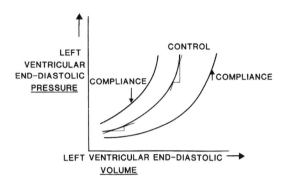

Fig. 19.3 Left ventricular compliance. Normal increased and decreased compliance curves are shown.

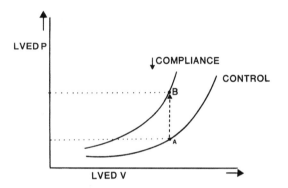

Fig. 19.4 Left ventricular end-diastolic pressure (LVEDP) and preload (LVEDV). Decreased compliance (A→B) leads to increased LVEDP for the same preload, and may precipitate pulmonary oedema. LVEDV = Left ventricular end-diastolic volume.

Afterload

Afterload is defined as the load on a muscle after the commencement of contraction, and best equates with systolic myocardial wall tension. It is not synonymous with systemic vascular resistance (SVR).[5] From Laplace's law, the tension (T) is given by the relationship:

$$T = \frac{Ptm \times R}{2H}$$

where Ptm = ventricular transmural pressure, R = ventricular radius, H = ventricular wall thickness. Hence factors which increase left ventricular (LV) afterload include:

1 increased ventricular radius;
2 increased intracavity pressure;

3 increased aortic impedance/SVR;
4 negative intrathoracic pressure.

Conversely, factors which decrease LV afterload include:

1 increased wall thickness;
2 positive intrathoracic pressure;
3 decreased intracavity pressure;
4 decreased aortic impedance/SVR.

As afterload rises, the speed of muscle fibre shortening and external work performed fall (Fig. 19.5). In the clinical setting, increased afterload, particularly in the failing heart, produces a decrease in cardiac output (Fig. 19.6).

Contractility

Contractility is the inherent property of the ventricle to perform external work, independent of afterload

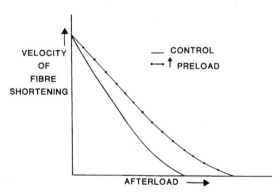

Fig. 19.5 Increased afterload and velocity of fibre shortening. Velocity of fibre shortening falls with increasing afterload, in control fibre and fibre with increased preload.

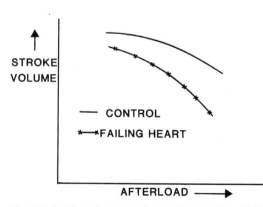

Fig. 19.6 Stroke volume and afterload in normal and failing heart.

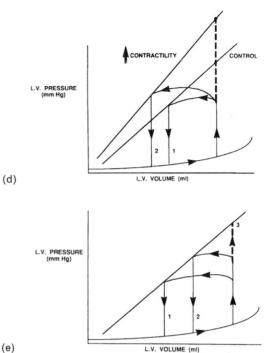

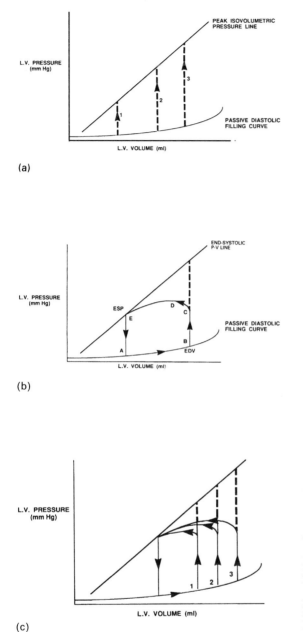

Fig. 19.7 (a) Isovolumetric pressure–volume relation. In the isolated heart preparation, if ejection is prevented and the diastolic volume is increased, the peak pressure developed by contractions (beat 1–3) is increased, and describes a line – the peak isovolumetric pressure line. LV = Left ventricular. (b) Pressure–volume loop of an ejecting left ventricle. The end-systolic pressure (ESP) point lies on or close to the peak isovolumetric pressure line. A–B = ventricular filling; B–C = isovolumetric ventricular contraction; C = aortic valve opens; C–D = rapid ejection; D–E = reduced ejection; E = aortic valve closes; E–A = isovolumetric ventricular relaxation. EDV = End-diastolic volume. (c) Diagrammatic pressure–volume loop, showing the effects of progressively increasing end-diastolic volume beats 2 and 3). At equivalent end-systolic pressure (ESP) the stroke volume increases. (d) Pressure–volume loops, showing the effect of increasing contractility. Note the increased peak systolic pressure and stroke volume. (e) Pressure–volume loops, showing the effect of increasing end-systolic pressure by increasing mean arterial pressure or aortic impedance (beat 1–2). Note the reduction in stroke volume. Beat 3 represents an isovolumetric contraction.

and preload. It cannot be measured directly. Contractility is increased by catecholamines, calcium, relief of ischaemia and digoxin, and decreased by hypoxia, ischaemia and drugs (e.g. thiopentone, β-adrenergic blockers, calcium-channel blockers or sedatives).

Myocardial performance is best understood by the construction of the pressure–volume ($P–V$) loop

relationship for the whole cardiac cycle. It allows stroke work to be measured, and ventricular stiffness and contractility to be assessed. The four phases of the cardiac cycle and the effects of changes in preload, afterload and contractility[6,7] are seen (Fig. 19.7a–e). The slope of the end-systolic P–V line may be used to represent contractility.

Myocardial oxygen supply and demand[8]

Anatomy

The myocardium is supplied by the left and right coronary arteries (LCA, RCA). The LCA divides into left anterior descending and circumflex coronary arteries, and supplies the anterior and lateral aspects of the LV, plus the right bundle branch, anterior fascicle of the left bundle branch, and the anterior two-thirds of the interventricular septum. Flow in the LCA occurs predominantly during diastole (Fig. 19.8). The RCA gives off branches to the right atrium (RA), RV, diaphragmatic and posterior walls of the LV, and the lower third of the septum. A branch of the RCA supplies the sinoatrial (SA) node in 55% of humans and the atrioventricular (AV) node in 90%. Flow in the RCA occurs throughout the cardiac cycle. Although flow through the LCA is several times that of the RCA, territorial dominance of flow is ascribed according to which artery supplies the posterior descending artery.

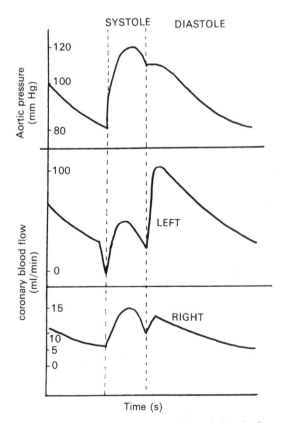

Fig. 19.8 Diagrammatic representation of blood flow during systole and diastole in the right and left coronary arteries.

Regulation of coronary artery flow

Oxygen extraction from coronary artery blood is normally 60–70%. Increased extraction cannot compensate for changing myocardial oxygen demand, which may increase fourfold. Hence, increased myocardial blood supply in response to stress is essential. Since LV perfusion essentially occurs during diastole (Fig. 19.8), diastolic conditions are paramount. As flow is pressure gradient divided by resistance, LCA or coronary blood flow (CBF) is expressed by the equation:

$$CBF\,(LCA) = \frac{(Aortic\ diastolic\ pressure - LVEDP)}{Coronary\ artery\ resistance}$$

As oxygen supply is the product of blood flow and oxygen content, supply to LV is thus decreased by:

1 anaemia or hypoxia;
2 increased heart rate (decreased diastolic time);
3 decreased diastolic aortic pressure;
4 coronary artery disease;
5 raised LVEDP.

Oxygen demand is dependent on heart rate, afterload and contractility. LV oxygen demand is increased by:

1 increased heart rate;
2 increased contractility;
3 increased afterload or wall tension (e.g. increased ventricular pressure, radius, aortic impedance, SVR and aortic stenosis).

It is a conventional belief that perioperative myocardial ischaemia is due to increased demand associated with tachycardia and hypertension or hypotension, but recent work suggests that coronary vasoconstriction and thrombotic occlusion impairing supply may also contribute.[9] The resultant imbalance between supply and demand leads to myocardial ischaemia evidenced by increased ventricular stiffness, wall motion abnormalities and increased LVEDP.[10] Angina, electrocardiogram (ECG) changes and decreased ventricular ejection fraction may follow, and lead to heart failure and shock (see Chapter 13). Thus, general principles of managing ischaemic heart disease patients are to maintain coronary blood flow, avoid rapid increases in oxygen consumption, maintain preload and avoid increases in afterload.

Specific cardiac disorders

Coronary artery disease (CAD)

CAD impairs myocardial oxygen supply. A high risk of perioperative infarction is associated with diseases of LCA or equivalent (i.e. left anterior descending plus circumflex arteries). Diffuse disease or ventricular hypertrophy makes myocardial protection with cardioplegia during cardiac surgery difficult, and may lead to postoperative complications, including low-output state and arrhythmias. In chronic obstruction from atherosclerosis, normally small intramural collateral vessels open to supply potentially ischaemic areas. Coronary artery steal, or diversion of blood from areas dependent on collateral flow, can occur (e.g. distal vasodilatation of the normal coronary artery may divert blood flow from the ischaemia-prone area). This may be provoked by agents such as sodium nitroprusside or isoflurane.

Mitral stenosis (MS)

Symptoms present early and progress slowly. Decompensation to acute pulmonary oedema may be precipitated by pregnancy, infection or paroxysmal atrial fibrillation (AF). There is a fixed stroke volume. Hence decreases in heart rate or SVR may lead to hypotension. AF or increases in heart rate will lead to impaired LV filling. Increased LA pressure leads eventually to pulmonary congestion. In the late stage, RV failure ensues, with further reduction of forward flow and distortion of LV (by the bulging RV). Valve replacement leads to greatly increased LV filling, and perhaps, ventricular distension, with ensuing increase in LV afterload.

Mitral regurgitation (MR)

MR leads to LV volume overload. Acute regurgitation associated with acute myocardial infarction (AMI) leads to acutely impaired LV function, pulmonary oedema and shock. Chronic MR allows time for compensation by LV hypertrophy/dilatation and LA dilatation. Most patients are in AF. A fall in heart rate may lead to increased LV volume, regurgitation and LA pressure, with ensuing pulmonary oedema. Increased SVR may lead to increased regurgitation, with similar consequences. Myocardial contractility is impaired due to the chronic LV overload, and the patient is thus sensitive to myocardial depressants. Vasodilator therapy and use of the intra-aortic balloon pump (IABP) improve cardiac output. Valve replacement may precipitate LV failure in the presence of high SVR.

Aortic regurgitation (AR)

AR leads to LV volume overload and dilatation. Bradycardia may lead to increase LV distension and failure. Vasodilators will decrease regurgitation, and increase forward flow and cardiac output. Vasoconstrictors will, conversely, worsen cardiac function and failure. There is impaired contractility, with chronic volume overload and increased sensitivity to myocardial depressants. IABP is contraindicated

in AR because regurgitation is enhanced, leading to acute heart failure.[11]

Aortic stenosis (AS)

AS causes pressure overload on LV. Compensatory hypertrophy to reduce wall tension follows. This leads to decreased LV compliance, and requires a high LVEDP (and LA pressure) for filling. Up to 40% of cardiac output is due to atrial contraction in AS. Sinus rhythm with 'atrial kick' is important for LV filling. Gross imbalance between oxygen supply and demand is due to the increased demand of the pressure load on LV and decreased supply from a relatively low aortic pressure, increased systolic time and LVEDP, and impaired perfusion of the thickened wall. These patients are at risk of sudden death. Prognosis is poor without valve replacement if symptoms develop. It is important to maintain sinus rhythm and aortic diastolic pressure, and avoid myocardial depression and vasodilatation.

Secondary cardiomyopathy

This may develop secondary to any condition of pressure or volume overload. Compensatory hypertrophy mechanisms eventually cause degenerative changes in cardiac muscle. There is a decreased exercise capacity and an inability to respond to postoperative stresses by increasing cardiac output.

Other organ dysfunction

Cardiac or related diseases and/or complications of treatment may impair function of other organ systems.

1 *Kidneys:* Renal vascular disease, heart failure, low cardiac output, diuretic use and diabetes may lead to impaired renal function.
2 *Liver:* Congestion from heart failure may impair hepatic metabolism of drugs and production of coagulation factors.
3 *Brain:* Diffuse vascular disease involving extra-/intracranial vessels increases the risk of neurological damage during surgery.
4 *Lungs:* Pulmonary hypertension and varying degrees of pulmonary oedema are common.
5 *Blood:* Polycythaemia is common in congenital heart disease.
6 *Nutrition:* Cardiac cachexia with impaired vital capacity and wound healing is seen in end-stage heart disease, due to decreased calorie intake, anorexia, malabsorption and increased metabolic needs.[12]

Preoperative assessment

Many cardiac patients are asymptomatic, and ischaemia is often silent. Some patient groups (e.g. those for vascular surgery) should be investigated to determine their cardiac risk, even if symptoms are absent. Mainstays of risk stratification for myocardial ischaemia are the history and examination. The preoperative assessment involves the following:

History

Details of cardiac disease, past history and medications are sought. Exertional tolerance points to the patient's functional reserve and response to stress.

Examination

Cardiorespiratory signs and variables are recorded, including pulse quality and rhythm, cyanosis, capillary filling, carotid bruits, ascites, oedema, elevated jugular venous pressure, hepatomegaly, murmurs, extra heart sounds and respiratory effort.

Investigations

Basic baseline investigations include full blood count, serum urea, creatinine and electrolytes, coagulation studies, ECG and chest X-ray. A normal ECG does not exclude CAD, but suggests that a cardiac event is less likely.[13] More complex investigations are:

Holter monitoring

From the preoperative to the postoperative period, Holter monitoring has been shown to predict and strongly correlate with adverse cardiac events.[14]

Exercise ECG

This determines heart rate, blood pressure and level of exertion when ischaemia and arrhythmias are detected. It helps CAD detection and risk stratification. Severe CAD is suggested by:

1 ST depression over 2 mm;
2 early ECG changes and angina;
3 ECG changes without increased heart rate or blood pressure;
4 hypotension.

Radionuclide tests

Thallium scanning

Thallium scanning shows myocardial uptake and, hence, perfusion abnormalities. This can be combined with dipyridamole, which dilates coronary arteries and induces a steal to reveal myocardium supplied by stenotic arteries.[15,16] Dipyridamole–thallium scintigraphy has been used in risk assessment of vascular patients, but a recent study found that age and history of cardiac disease were better predictors of cardiac risk before abdominal aortic surgery.[17]

Technetium blood pool scanning

Technetium blood pool scanning, gated to the ECG, allows assessment of both regional and global ventricular functions.[18]

Echocardiography

Echocardiography shows valve areas and abnormalities, chamber size and thickness and ventricular function[19] (see Chapter 21).

Cardiac catheterization

This shows the location and severity of coronary artery lesions, collateral flow, distal vessel disease, ventricular function, valve function, pressure gradients, vascular pressures, cardiac output and shunts (see Chapter 20). The need for invasive investigation and monitoring perioperatively is indicated by:

1 a history of myocardial infarction, episodes of chronic cardiac failure, dyspnoea at rest, paroxysmal nocturnal dyspnoea and angina;
2 signs of cardiac failure;
3 ischaemic ST–T wave abnormalities on the ECG;
4 ejection fraction less than 40% on echocardiography, gated heart pool scan or angiography;
5 LVEDP at rest greater than 15 mmHg (2.5 kPa);
6 cardiac index less than 2.2 l/min per m².

Medications

Medications may complicate the postoperative course:

1 Aspirin increases bleeding time for up to 7 days.
2 Digoxin effects should be assessed by ECG and serum concentration.
3 β-Adrenergic blockers should be continued; systolic blood pressure and heart rate are better controlled perioperatively, and the incidence of infarction and arrhythmia is reduced.
4 Antihypertensives should be continued to the time of the surgery.
5 Diuretics may be associated with electrolyte abnormalities and hypovolaemia.

Management of the cardiac patient after non-cardiac surgery

Incidence and risk factors

From the Framingham study, the chance of developing cardiovascular disease by 65 years was 37% for men and 22% for women. Patients with cardiovascular disease are at risk from postoperative cardiac complications, including AMI, arrhythmias, cardiac failure and death. The perioperative infarction rate in 1962 was 6.1% (mortality 58%) in those with previous AMI, and 0.7% (mortality 19%) in those with no previous AMI. The reinfarction rate remained unchanged to the late 1970s[20,21] (Table 19.1). Since then, better invasive monitoring and management may have improved the reinfarction rate (Table 19.1).[22] Recently, the Perioperative Ischemia Research Group reported 5% in-hospital mortality and 23% mortality at 2 years in high-risk patients.[23]

Patients with peripheral vascular disease have a high incidence of associated CAD, even though they may be asymptomatic. They should undergo stress testing by either exercise ECG or dipyrimadole–thallium scintigraphy. AMI is a common late problem, accounting for 50% of late deaths. Mortality in these patients may be reduced, if they undergo coronary artery bypass grafting before their peripheral vascular surgery. Suggested risk factors for AMI are hypertensive disease, major blood pressure changes during surgery, heart failure and emergency surgery.

An index of cardiac risk for non-cardiac surgical procedures was proposed by Goldman *et al.*[24] (Table 19.2). Patients were classified into risk groups I–IV, according to points scored for nine adverse risk factors; higher scores correspond to higher complication rates (Table 19.3). Preoperative predictors of cardiac risk reported by the Perioperative Ischemia Research Group included ECG evidence of LV hypertrophy, hypertension, diabetes, definite CAD and digoxin use. Patients with four predictors had a 77% incidence of postoperative myocardial ischaemia.[23] During surgery, 70% of new regional wall motion abnormalities (reflecting ischaemia) develop under stable haemodynamic conditions, and are probably caused by changes in coronary blood flow induced by spasm, steal, increased viscosity, or increased coagulability.

Preoperative guidelines

1 Patients with suspected cardiac disease should not undergo elective surgery without a complete assessment. Risk stratification and preoperative intervention are essential.[25] With emergency surgery, the risks of delaying surgery must be weighed against those of proceeding.
2 Elective surgery should not proceed if AMI has occurred within 6 months, as mortality is much higher.[26]
3 Anaesthetic technique appears to make a significant difference only in ophthalmological and urological surgery; regional techniques are associated with lower cardiac morbidity.
4 Patients with valve lesions or congenital defects require perioperative antibiotic cover.[27] (see Chapter 18).
5 Extreme caution must be taken to avoid IV entry of air bubbles into patients with septal defects.

Table 19.2 Goldman's risk factors and weighting

	Points
S3 gallop, raised JVP	11
AMI episode <6 months	10
Non-sinus rhythmn	7
>5 ventricular ectopic beats/min	7
Age >70 years	5
Aortic stenosis	3
Operation: emergency, thoracic, aortic	3
Poor condition: P_{O_2} <60 mmHg (8.0 kPa)	3
P_{CO_2} >50 mmHg (6.7 kPa)	

JVP = Jugular venous pressure; AMI = acute myocardial infarction; P_{O_2} = partial pressure of oxygen; P_{CO_2} = partial pressure of carbon dioxide.

Table 19.3 Risk of complications for Goldman scores

Class	Points	Complications (%)		
		Nil/minor	Serious	Cardiac deaths
I	0–5	99	0.7	0.2
II	6–12	93	5	2
III	13–25	86	11	2
IV	>25	77	22	56

Table 19.1 Myocardial reinfarction rate

			Reinfarction rate		
Reference	Year	Patient numbers	Previous infarct <3 months	<4–6 months	>6 months
Tarhan *et al.*[20]	1972	32 877	37%	16%	3%
Steen *et al.*[21]	1978	73 321	27%	11%	6%
Rao *et al.*[22]	1973–76	364	36%	26%	
	1977–82	733	5.7%	2.3%	

6 Patients with valvular heart disease, especially severe MS or symptomatic AS, may warrant valve replacement before undertaking major surgery, and should be assessed accordingly.

7 Cardiac pacing should be instituted preoperatively in patients with complete heart block. Those with bifascicular block do not require prophylactic pacing.

8 If surgery is unavoidable, and CAD is severe or AMI is recent, other less invasive surgical options should be considered as well as balloon or laser angioplasty.

Postoperative management

Ideally, high-risk patients should be monitored in ICU for at least 3 days.[22] The postoperative period is the time of greatest stress and risk of ischaemia. Potential stresses are associated with the end of anaesthesia and transfer to the ICU, and a smooth transition is important. Oxygen and adequate analgesia are given, with continuous monitoring of ECG and Sao_2 by pulse oximeter. Postoperative myocardial ischaemia is difficult to diagnose, and many episodes are silent. Unexplained hypotension, arrhythmia or pulmonary oedema may indicate AMI. Twelve-lead ECG and cardiac enzymes should be checked in at-risk patients.

Ventilation

Mechanical ventilation should be continued until the patient is warm, well-oxygenated, haemodynamically stable and able to protect the airway. Shivering increases myocardial oxygen demand and is reduced by morphine.[28]

Circulation

Blood pressure and heart rate should be maintained within 10% of the patient's normal level. Fluid shifts and continued blood loss are the main causes of haemodynamic disturbance in this period. Volume replacement is guided by regular assessments of pulse, blood pressure, central venous pressure (CVP) and chest X-ray. In the unstable patient, PCWP monitoring is useful. Perioperative problems include:

1 *Hypertension* (mean arterial pressure (MAP) > 100 mmHg or 13.3 kPa) – urinary retention, pain, hypoxia and hypercarbia are excluded. Vasodilators by infusion (e.g. nitroprusside or nitroglycerin) are next considered.

2 *Hypotension* (MAP < 70 mmHg or 9.3 kPa) – complications (e.g. pneumothorax, tamponade and ischaemia) are excluded. Preload is optimized and inotrope support is considered.
Tachycardia (> 100 beats/min) – pain, hypovolaemia, hypoxia, hypercarbia are considered.

3 *ST depression with hypertension* – analgesia, nitroglycerin and vasodilators are considered.

4 *ST depression with tachycardia* – analgesia and β-adrenergic blockers are considered.

5 *ST depression with increased PCWP* – nitroglycerin, vasodilators and diuretics are considered.

6 *ST depression with hypotension* – volume infusion and inotropes/vasopressors are considered.

Fluid therapy

This is dependent on anticipated and observed losses (revealed and concealed) of blood and fluids. It is guided by strict fluid balance, haemodynamic variables and clinical assessment.

Basic monitoring

1 *ECG* – to detect rhythm disturbances and ST- and T-wave changes (leads II and V5). More sophisticated monitoring has not been proven to be superior to standard two-lead Holter monitoring.[29]

2 *Arterial line* – to monitor blood pressure continuously. MAP provides the most reliable measure, aiming to maintain MAP > 70 mmHg (9.3 kPa) and within 10% of resting normal. Before initiating treatment, it is wise to measure blood pressure in the other arm, particularly in patients with peripheral vascular disease.

3 *Temperature core (rectal or nasal) and skin* – to quantify hypothermia, detect fever and reflect peripheral perfusion.

4 *Fluid balance* – to track measurable losses.

5 *Urine output* (normally > 0.5 ml/kg per h) – to reflect vital organ perfusion (except when mannitol or frusemide has been given) and track fluid balance.

6 *CVP* – in patients with normal ventricular function and pulmonary circulation, changes in CVP follow changes in LVEDP. Trends in CVP provide an additional monitor of cardiac function and fluid therapy.

7 *PCWP* – provides an early sign of myocardial ischaemia and guides fluid therapy in cardiac dysfunction.

Investigations

Routine tests on arrival in ICU include arterial blood gases, full blood count, serum electrolytes and creatinine, coagulation studies and chest X-ray.

Management of the cardiac patient after cardiac surgery

In-hospital mortality ranges from being negligible for repair of atrial septal defect and coronary artery bypass grafting, to appreciable with complex procedures (e.g. repair of Fallot's tetralogy). In adults, factors which influence the postoperative course are:

Preoperative factors

The preoperative symptomatic state affects the probability of postoperative mortality.[30] This is assessed by the preoperative examination, as detailed above.

Surgical procedure

Postoperative cardiac performance is dependent on the surgical result (e.g. adequacy of revascularization or valve repair). Surgical trauma may give rise to postoperative problems (e.g. cannulation for bypass causing RA irritation, dissection of aorta or shedding of atheroma from the aorta; and resection or stitching of the conducting pathways leading to conduction abnormalities).

Myocardial protection[31]

Cross-clamping of the aorta facilitates surgery, but produces immediate global myocardial ischaemia. Current techniques of myocardial protection use systemic and topical hypothermia, and infusion of cold cardioplegia solutions containing potassium, magnesium, bicarbonate and dextrose with or without blood into the coronary arteries, to produce chemical asystole, and rapidly to minimize energy needs and reperfusion damage. Newer techniques include the following:

1 addition of calcium-channel blockers;
2 addition of substrates such as aspartate or glutamate;
3 addition of adenosine-regulating agents;[32]
4 use of warm blood cardioplegia before the removal of the cross-clamp;[33]
5 retrograde cardioplegia via the coronary sinus.[34]

Complications of cardioplegia include complete heart block secondary to potassium overload and, rarely, infusion of contaminated fluid. Diffuse CAD, myocardial hypertrophy and decreased myocardial reserves shorten the usual 20-min period of protection between doses. If the cardioplegia solution cannot be efficiently infused into the coronary arteries (e.g. due to diffuse disease or previous grafting), it should be administered retrogradely via the coronary sinus.[34]

Anaesthetic technique[35]

Cardiopulmonary bypass (CPB)

Although CPB has been an important advance, it may produce some damaging effects which continue into the postoperative state. Exposure of blood to non-endothelial surfaces and shear stresses from suctioning, pumping, acceleration and deceleration, may cause the following:

1 clotting, leading to depletion of platelets and fibrinogen – the patient is hence fully heparinized before CPB;
2 trauma to red blood cells, producing haemoglobinaemia and haemoglobinuria;
3 a diffuse inflammatory reaction via activation of leukocytes and the complement system;
4 microembolism of air and formed elements to cerebral or coronary circulation, particularly during heart manipulation, transport and posturing. This may lead to focal neurological deficits and myocardial dysfunction.

Presently, most defects become significant only if complicated by other problems (e.g. poor haemostasis, prolonged bypass greater than 150 min or a difficult repeat operation).

Postoperative complications (see below)

Postoperative management

Transfer to the ICU postoperatively is a particularly dangerous period. It is imperative that mechanical ventilation and ECG and blood pressure monitoring are maintained, and sedation, inotropes and vasodilators continued by pump infusion. The pacemaker box should easily be visualized. On arrival in ICU a complete handover is given.

Ventilation

Routine cases may be extubated early (i.e. after 2–6 h).[36] Sicker or more complex cases should be ventilated overnight, until cardiovascular support has been weaned. Extubation or resumption of spontaneous ventilation provides new stresses to the myocardium, including increased work of breathing[37] and increased LV afterload by the generation of negative intrathoracic pressure.[38] Positive end-expiratory pressure (PEEP) in the failing heart may aid cardiac output by reducing LVEDP, ventricular size and LV afterload. Removal of PEEP in patients with severe LV dysfunction may precipitate cardiac failure.[39] Extubation is indicated by an alert, cooperative patient, able to protect the airway, with stable cardiovascular and respiratory systems and without excessive bleeding. Respiratory and central stimulants (e.g. naloxone) may provoke massive sympathetic stimulation, and should be avoided. Postextubation basal atelectasis and sputum retention are common, and may be reduced by intermittent mask continuous positive airways pressure (CPAP).[40]

Circulation

In the immediate postoperative period, continuing diuresis, rewarming vasodilatation and some blood loss require volume expansion. This is achieved with autologous blood, pump blood and plasma expanders. Haemoglobin is maintained over 10 g/dl in most patients, although young and otherwise healthy patients tolerate a concentration around 8 g/dl. Free water and sodium are restricted, as total body water and sodium have been expanded during CPB. Mobilization of this fluid usually occurs at postoperative day 2–3. Occasionally, diuretics may be required. Myocardial function after CPB is impaired functionally and metabolically. The nadir appears to be at about 4 h. The heart may be at risk of ischaemia despite revascularization.

Electrolytes

Requirements for potassium and magnesium may be large, depending on the amount of cardioplegia given, preoperative state and postoperative diuresis. If the serum potassium immediately after CPB is normal, then 5 mmol/h KCl is required until the diuresis settles. $MgSO_4$ 20–40 mmol is given in the first postoperative 24 h. If ventricular ectopic beats or tachycardia occur, extra KCl and $MgSO_4$ may be indicated. Metabolic acidosis may persist postoperatively due to poor tissue perfusion. Essentially, management involves improving cardiac output (see below).

Monitoring

Simple operations (e.g. valvotomy, atrial septal defect repair or coronary artery bypass grafting with a good LV) require basic clinical monitoring as for all cardiac patients, continued for the period of haemodynamic instability (24–48 h). If complications supervene, a LA line or Swan–Ganz catheter may be placed. However, morbidity from complex invasive techniques (e.g. Swan–Ganz catheterization and prolonged tracheal intubation) may be worse than that from surgery itself. More complex cases (e.g. infarct ventricular septal defect or a 'sick mitral') require more invasive monitoring.

Special considerations

There may be discrepancies between mean aortic and radial artery blood pressure (of 10–30 mmHg or 1.3–3.9 kPa) in the immediate post CPB period (up to 60 min).[41] If suspected, femoral artery pressure recordings should be performed. LA pressure monitoring is performed intraoperatively if haemodynamic instability is encountered. PCWP monitoring is started preoperatively before complex operations in sick patients, and may be needed postoperatively if a low-output state develops.

Aspirin is useful in improving long-term graft patency. If 100 mg is given within 1 postoperative day, saphenous grafts have a 90% patency at 4 months versus 68% in controls.[42] Anticoagulation is required after valve surgery. Agents used and duration of treatment will depend on the type and postition of the valve. In general, patients with mechanical valves will need long-term warfarin, whereas those with tissue valves will require warfarin for 8–12 weeks, followed by aspirin.

Specific problems after cardiac surgery

Problems arising in this setting must be treated rapidly before a vicious cycle leads to irreversible problems.[43]

Bleeding[42]

Bleeding is minimized by careful haemostasis, autologous blood transfusion, cessation of drugs which may increase bleeding, and use of haemostasis-enhancing drugs (e.g. desmopressin (DDAVP) or aprotinin). Continuing major postoperative blood loss may be due to:

1 difficult surgery (e.g. 're-do' operation) or poor surgical haemostasis. Common sites of surgical bleeding are graft anastomoses, sternal wire insertion and internal mammary artery pedicle;
2 reinfusion of retrieved pump blood containing heparin;
3 pre-existing liver disease secondary to heart failure;
4 preoperative therapy with aspirin,[44] non-steroidal anti-inflammatory drug or warfarin;
5 CPB-generated platelet and clotting factor problems due to activation of complement and kallikreins by the plastic surfaces. Prophylactic use of aprotinin and ε-aminocaproic acid have been shown to reduce blood loss and transfusion rate in high-risk patients.[42]

If bleeding occurs, treatment includes:

1 protamine for reversal of heparin, guided by activated clotting time or activated partial thromboplastin time;
2 fresh frozen plasma guided by coagulation studies, to replace consumed clotting factors;
3 platelet infusion to replace platelets consumed on CPB or to provide active platelets to a patient with recent aspirin treatment;
4 DDAVP 0.3 µg/kg over 30 min (to mobilize von Willebrand's factor from endothelial cells) may improve platelet function post CPB;[45]
5 reoperation if bleeding continues at over 200 ml/h for 3 h, or over 400 ml in 1 h.

Low-output state

Low cardiac output state is obvious with hypotension, but other symptoms may be more subtle. Most patients are pale and cool in the periphery after hypothermic CPB, but low cardiac output is suggested by persistent metabolic acidosis, obtundation, high core temperature, oliguria and tachycardia. Causes include:

1 preoperative (e.g. cardiomyopathy);
2 intraoperative (e.g. poor revascularization and myocardial protection);
3 postoperative (e.g. hypovolaemia, tamponade, reaction to protamine,[46] hypoxia and ischaemia).

Tamponade and LV dysfunction may be difficult to differentiate, as both may be associated with increased jugular venous pressure and CVP, and hypotension. Echocardiography or Swan–Ganz catheterization may aid diagnosis, but the chest needs to be reopened to exclude tamponade if hypotension is progressive. If there is evidence of new ischaemia after coronary artery bypass grafting associated with circulatory instability, chest reopening and inspection of the grafts may be necessary.

Treatment of hypotension includes:

1 treating the reversible cause (e.g. tamponade, kinked graft);
2 volume restoration;
3 treating arrhythmias (see below);
4 vasodilators – patients with low cardiac output, high SVR and normal or slightly low blood pressure may respond to vasodilatation with an increase in cardiac output. Choice of vasodilators is between nitroprusside and nitroglycerin.[47] Theoretically, nitroprusside may produce a coronary steal in the presence of incomplete revascularization. However, trials with nitroglycerin during CPB have failed to show a benefit,[48] due perhaps to tolerance. Nitrates increase venous capacitance, decrease SVR and increase coronary vascular diameter without increasing 'steal'. Tolerance develops rapidly, due perhaps to depletion of sulphydryl groups in vascular smooth muscle or decreased sensitivity of guanylyl cyclase.[49] Tolerance is less likely with the use of nitroprusside, because it acts by directly increasing nitric oxide.
5 inotropic agents are used in patients unresponsive to volume loading. Effects are often unpredictable.[50,51] Choice of inotrope depends on the degree of myocardial dysfunction, state of circulation and local experience (see Chapter 12).
   (a) *Dopamine* experimentally produces selective splanchnic vasodilatation at 0.5–3 µg/kg per min, even in the presence of vasopressor infusion.[52] With high doses, peripheral vasoconstriction and increased pulmonary artery pressures develop. Dopamine is known to be diuretic and natriuretic but has not been shown to be renal-protective[53,54] in this setting.
   (b) *Dobutamine* is useful (up to 10 µg/kg per min) for mild hypotension associated with increased SVR. With increasing doses, tachycardia and decreased SVR are seen. It results in better myocardial flow and haemodynamics than dopamine, in low to moderate doses.[55] Dobutamine may have a special place in AR as it increases cardiac output directly without increasing SVR or LVEDP.
   (c) *Adrenaline* is useful for more severe hypotension. Treatment aims to balance the increased myocardial oxygen consumption by a greater increase in perfusion pressure. It produces β_1 and β_2 stimulation, with increasing α stimulation as the dose is increased.
   (d) *Noradrenaline* is used for temporary treatment of severe resistant hypotension, while awaiting reoperation or insertion of IABP. It increases SVR by a strong α effect and some β effect.
   (e) *Milirone/amrinone:* these bipyridine derivatives are phosphodiesterase inhibitors, and are primarily vasodilators with a mild and variable inotropic effect. They have a long half-life and are not recommended for sole treatment of acute heart failure. They may be useful adjuncts to other measures.
6 IABP is considered in patients who are difficult to wean from CPB or who require continued high-dose inotropic agents. It is the only technique to increase perfusion pressure and decrease LV afterload, and is useful for the temporary dysfunction seen post CPB.[56]
7 Mechanical ventilation is continued throughout this period because raised intrathoracic pressure may assist the failing LV by decreasing LVEDV and afterload.[39] Also, re-operation may be necessary, and spontaneous breathing will use a large percentage of cardiac output in shock.[37]
8 Calcium produces temporary haemodynamc improvement (increased MAP and cardiac index) and sustained increased SVR after CBP. Infusion beyond this period adds no advantage.[57]

Hypertension

This is often seen postoperatively in patients with essential hypertension and good LV function. It manifests during rewarming as resistance to vasodilators, often with tachycardia, and may provoke myocardial ischaemia. Pain, hypoxia, hypercarbia or β-adrenergic blocker withdrawal should be excluded. Treatment includes analgesia, increasing vasodilator dose and infusion of β-adrenergic blockers.

Arrhythmias

Arrhythmias should be promptly treated. Causes such as electrolyte abnormalities, hypoxia, hypercarbia, tamponade and hypotension should be sought and treated.

1 Bradycardias are preferably treated with AV sequential pacing. IV bolus atropine and isoprenaline infusion are temporary measures.

2 Atrial tachyarrhythmias may require cardioversion; otherwise digoxin, short-acting β-blockers, amiodarone or verapamil are used. AF is common after the second day (due to atrial distension or irritation from the venous bypass cannula site) requiring digoxin, sotalol or amiodarone, depending on other presenting medical problems.

3 Ventricular ectopic beats are treated more aggressively in the immediate post-bypass period with lignocaine (whilst checking potassium and magnesium levels).

4 Pulseless ventricular tachycardia or fibrillation requires urgent defibrillation.

Hypoxia

Oxygen by mask, physiotherapy and intermittent facemask continuous positive airways pressure breathing is important after extubation. Respiratory failure may develop in patients with pre-existing chronic lung disease, tobacco abuse and general debility from heart failure. Surgical factors such as phrenic nerve palsy and left lower lobe atelectasis during left internal mammary artery harvest are compounded by postoperative pain and sputum retention.

Hypothermia

Patients are often cooled to 25–30°C and then rewarmed on CPB. After CPB, recooling will occur from surgical exposure and perfusion of cold fat layers. This hypothermia may lead to hypertension, myocardial irritability, shivering and increased oxygen reqirements. Rewarming should be accomplished in ICU by the use of warmed IV fluids, humidified ventilation and blankets. Shivering should be suppressed with narcotics and sedatives, but short-acting non-depolarizing muscle relaxants may also be required, if shivering is extreme.

Renal failure

Polyuria usually follows CPB (see above). Renal disease may be secondary to pre-existing conditions, haemolysis, hypoperfusion, renal vasoconstriction, long CPB and nephrotoxic drug use. It should be suspected if there is no postoperative diuresis. Intravascular haemolysis is suspected if the urine is opalescent pink without intact red cells. (Haematuria appears cloudy pink due to intact red cells.) Treatment is along the conventional lines.

Neurological deficits[58,59]

Postoperative obtundation, focal deficits and confusion may occur. Macroemboli from the surgical field cause most neurological complications. The periods of highest risk are during aortic cannulation, onset of bypass and weaning from bypass. Risk factors include atherosclerosis of the ascending aorta, advanced age, cerebrovascular disease, previous neurological event, duration of surgery, diabetes and low cardiac output state. Long-term problems are rare. Investigations include computed tomography scan and Doppler studies. Treatment may include heparinization, but is usually expectant and supportive.

Other non-cardiac problems[60]

Cardiac surgery may be associated with wound infections, gastrointestinal tract haemorrhage and ischaemia, jaundice, cholecystitis, pancreatitis and type II lactic acidosis with use of adrenaline.

References

1 O'Rourke M (1984) Starling's law of the heart: an appraisal 70 years on. *Aust NZ J Med* **14**:879–887.

2 Glower DD, Spratt JJ, Snow ND *et al.* (1985) Linearity of the Frank–Starling relationship in the intact heart: the concept of preload recruitable stroke work. *Circulation* **71**:994–1009.

3 Hansen RM, Viquerat CE and Mathay M (1986) Poor correlation between pulmonary arterial wedge pressure and left ventricular end-diastolic volume after coronary bypass graft surgery. *Anesthesiology* **64**:764–770.

4 Groenberg MA (1988) Ischaemia-induced diastolic dysfunction: new observations, new questions (editorial). *J Am Coll Cardiol* **13**:1071–1072.

5 Lang RM, Borrow KM, Neumann A and Janzen D (1986) Systemic vascular resistance: an unreliable index of left ventricular afterload. *Circulation* **74**:1114–1123.

6 Katz AM (1988) Influence of altered intropy and lusitropy on ventricular pressure–volume loops. *J Am Coll Cardiol* **11**:438–445.

7 Foex P and Leone BJ (1994) Pressure–volume loops: a dynamic approach to the assessment of ventricular function. *J Cardiothorac Vasc Anaesth* **8**:84–96.

8 Goldberg AH and Warltier DC (1990) The coronary circulation: implications for anesthesiologists. *Sem Anaesth* **9**:232–244.

9 Nugent M (1992) Anesthesia and myocardial ischemia: the gains of the past have largely come from control of myocardial oxygen demand; the breakthroughs of the future will involve optimising myocardial oxygen supply. *Anesth Analg* **75**:1–3.

10 Nesto RW and Kowalchuk GJ (1987) The ischemic cascade: temporal sequence of haemodynamic, electro-cardiographic and symptomatic expressions of ischemia. *Am J Cardiol* **57**:23C–30C.

11 Maccioli GA, Lucas WJ and Norfleet EA (1988) The intra-aortic balloon pump: a review. *J Cardiothorac Anaesth* **3**:365–373.

12 Ansari A (1987) Syndromes of cardiac cachexia and the cachectic heart: current perspective. *Prog Cardiovasc Dis* **30**:45–60.

13 Donovan K and Hockings B (1994) Perioperative management of ischaemic heart disease in non-cardiac

surgical patients. In: Keneally J (ed.) *Australian Anaesthesia*. Melbourne: Australian and New Zealand College of Anaesthetists, pp. 75–88.

14 Morgans DT, Browner WS, Hollenberg M *et al.* (1990) Association of perioperative myocardial ischemia with cardiac morbidity and mortality in men undergoing non-cardiac surgery. *N Engl J Med* **323**:1781–1788.

15 Iskandrian AS, Heo J, Askenase A, Segal BL and Auerbach N (1988) Dipyridamole cardiac imaging. *Am Heart J* **115**:432–443.

16 Brown KA (1991) Prognostic value of thallium-201 myocardial perfusion imaging. A diagnostic tool comes of age. *Circulation* **83**:363–381.

17 Baron J, Murdler O, Bertrand M *et al.* (1994) Dipyrimidole-thallium scintigraphy and gated radionuclide angiography to assess cardiac risk before abdominal aortic surgery. *N Engl J Med* **330**:663–669.

18 Iskandrian AS, Heo J and Mostel E (1987) The role of radionuclide cardiac imaging in coronary artery bypass surgery. *Am Heart J* **113**:163–169.

19 Cahalan MK, Litt L, Botvinick EH and Schiller NB (1987) Advances in non-invasive cardiovascular imaging: Implications for the anesthesiologist. *Anesthesiology* **66**:356–372.

20 Tarhan S, Moffitt EA, Taylor WF and Giuliani ER (1972) Myocardial infarction after general anaesthesia. *J Am Heart Med Assoc* **220**:1451–1454.

21 Steen PA, Tinker JH and Tarhan S (1978) Myocardial reinfarction after anesthesia and surgery. *J Am Med Assoc* **239**:2566–2570.

22 Rao TLK, Jacobs KH and El-Etr AA (1983) Reinfarction following anesthesia in patients with myocardial infarction. *Anesthesiology* **59**:499–505.

23 Hollenberg M, Mangano DT, Browner WS *et al.* (1992) Predictors of postoperative myocardia ischemia in patients undergoing noncardiac surgery. *J Am Med Assoc* **268**:205–209 (editorial 252–253).

24 Goldman L, Caldera DL and Nussbaum SR (1977) Multifactoral index of cardiac risk in noncardiac surgical procedures. *N Engl J Med* **297**:845–850.

25 Weitz HH (1993) Cardiac risk stratification prior to vascular surgery. *Med Clin North Am* **77**:377–395.

26 Rivers SP, Scher LA, Gupta SK and Veith FJ (1990) Safety of peripheral vascular surgery after recent acute myocardial infarction. *J Vasc Surg* **11**:70–74.

27 Oakley CM (1987) Controversies in the prophylaxis of endocarditis: a cardiological view. *J Antimicrobial Chemoth* **20**(suppl. A):99–104.

28 Eisenberg MJ, Sondon MJ, Leung JM *et al.* (1992) Monitoring for myocardial ischemia during noncardiac surgery. *J Am Med Assoc* **268**:210–216.

29 Rodriguez JL, Weissman C, Damask MC, Askanazi J, Hyman AI and Kinney JM (1983) Morphine and post-operative rewarming in critically ill patients. *Circulation* **68**:1238–1246.

30 Rutherford JD and Braunwald E (1988) Selection of patients for the surgical treatment of coronary artery disease. *Quart J Med* **67**:369–385.

31 Hearse DJ (1988) The protection of the ischaemic

myocardium surgical success v clinical failure? *Prog Cardiovasc Dis* **30**:381–402.

32 Van Belle H (1993) Nucleoside transport inhibition: a therapeutic approach to cardioprotection via adenosine. *Cardiovasc Res* **27**:68–76.

33 Guyton RA (1993) Warm blood cardioplegia: benefits and risks. *Ann Thorac Surg* **55**:1071–1072.

34 Menasche P and Piwnica A (1991) Cardioplegia by way of the coronary sinus for valvular and coronary surgery. *J Am Coll Cardiol* **18**:628–636.

35 Hall RI (1993) Anaesthesia for coronary artery surgery – a plea for a goal-directed approach. *Can J Anaesth* **40**:1178–1194.

36 Williams BT and Jindane A (1994) New trends in the postoperative management of cardiac surgical patients: review. *J Cardiovasc Surg* **35**:161–163.

37 Ward ME and Roussos C (1985) The respiratory muscles in shock: service or disservice? *Intens Crit Care Digest* **4**:3–5.

38 Hausknecht MJ, Brin KP, Weisfeldt ML, Permutt S and Yin FCP (1988) Effects of left ventricular loading by negative intrathoracic pressure in dogs. *Circ Res* **62**:620–631.

39 Mathru M (1984) Editorial. Mechanical breath. Nonpharmacologic support for a failing heart? *Chest* **85**:1.

40 Ricksten S, Bengtsson A, Soderberg C, Thorden M and Kvist H (1986) Effects of periodic positive airway pressure by mask on post-operative pulmonary function. *Chest* **89**:774–780.

41 Mohr R, Lavee J and Goor DA (1987) Inaccuracy of radial artery pressure measurement after cardiac operations. *J Thorac Cardiovasc Surg* **94**:286–290.

42 Kondo NI, Maddi R, Ewenstein BM *et al.* (1994) Anticoagulation and haemostasis in cardiac surgical patients. *J Cardiac Surg* **9**:440–442.

43 Cutfield G, Harrison GA and Junius F (1993) Practical crisis. Management in the perioperative care of cardiac surgical patients. *Clin Anaesthesiol* **7**:423–469.

44 Levy JH (1994) Aspirin and bleeding after coronary artery bypass grafting. *Anaesth Analg* **79**:1–3.

45 Salzman EW, Weinstein MJ, Weintraub RM *et al.* (1986) Treatment with desmopressin acetate to reduce blood loss after cardiac surgery. *N Engl J Med* **314**:1402–1405.

46 Lowenstein E and Zapol WM (1990) Protamine reactions, explosive mediator release and pulmonary vasoconstriction. *Anesthesiology* **73**:573–575.

47 Cont CR (1991) Why use a nitrate in 1990? *Eur Heart J* **12**(suppl A):2–4.

48 Gallagher JD, Moore RA, Jose AB, Botros SB and Clark DL (1986) Prophylactic nitroglycerin infusions during coronary bypass surgery. *Anesthesiology* **64**:785–789.

49 Abrams J (1991) Chemical aspects of nitrate tolerance. *Eur Heart J* **12**(suppl E):42–52.

50 Di Sesa VJ (1987) The rational selection of inotropic drugs in cardiac surgery. *J Cardiac Surg* **2**:385–406.

51 Leir CV (1986) Cardiotonic drugs. A clinical survey. In: Leir CV (ed.) *Basic and Clinical Cardiology*, vol. 7. New

York:Marcel Dekker, pp. 49–84.

52 Schaer GL, Fink MP and Parrilio JE (1985) Norepinephrine alone versus norepinephrine plus low-dose dopamine: enhanced renal blood flow with combination pressor therapy. *Crit Care Med* **13**:495–496.

53 Duke GJ and Bersten AD (1992) Dopamine and renal salvage in the critically ill patient. *Anaesth Intens Care* **20**:277–302.

54 Szeric HM (1991) Renal-dose dopamine: fact or fiction? *Ann Intern Med* **115**:153–154.

55 Fowler MB, Alderman EL, Osterle SN *et al.* (1984) Dobutamine and dopamine after cardiac surgery: greater augmentation of myocardial blood flow with dobutamine. *Circulation* **70**:103.

56 Swanton RH (1984) Editorial. Who requires balloon pumping? *Intens Care Med* **10**:271–273.

57 Shapira N, Schaff HV, White RD and Pluth JR (1984) Haemodynamic effects of calcium chloride injection following cardiopulmonary bypass: response to bolus injection and continuous infusion. *Ann Thorac Surg* **37**:133–140.

58 Shaw PJ, Bates D, Cartlidge NEF *et al.* (1987) Long-term intellectual dysfunction folllowing coronary artery bypass graft surgery: a six month follow-up study. *Quart J Med* **62**:259–268.

59 Nussmeier NA (1994) Neuropsychiatric complications of cardiac surgery. *J Cardiothorac Vasc Anaesth* **8**:13–18.

60 Alfieri A and Kotler MN (1990) Noncardiac complications of open-heart surgery. *Am Heart J* **119**:149–158.

20 | Cardiac investigations and interventions

JE Sanderson

Contemporary cardiovascular physicians have a wide array of investigative tools to study myocardial anatomy, physiology and pathology. Diagnosis still begins with a careful, thorough history and examination followed by a resting 12-lead electrocardiogram (ECG). A diagnostic hypothesis is made which can then be confirmed or refuted by a variety of laboratory tests. These include blood tests (cardiac enzymes), chest X-ray, cardiac catheterization with coronary angiography, echocardiography (including intravascular ultrasound of coronary arteries, ventricles and aorta), exercise testing, 24-h ambulatory (Holter) monitoring, electrophysiological studies, nuclear cardiology, computed tomography (CT) and magnetic resonance imaging (MRI) scanning, myocardial biopsy, and more recently, the tools of molecular biology. Each one of these subjects is a major area of research and study. ECGs will not be discussed in detail. Routine 12-lead ECGs are essential for the accurate diagnosis of arrhythmias and helpful in the diagnosis of chest pain, but have limited usefulness in most other circumstances. Echocardiography is discussed in Chapter 21.

Exercise testing[1]

Exercise testing is designed either to provoke a symptom (usually chest pain or breathlessness) or a specific ECG abnormality (i.e. ST segment depression or arrhythmia), and to determine the workload which is achieved at the time of maximum effort. The ECG is the most widely used method of assessment, though increasingly nuclear cardiology (i.e. myocardial perfusion scanning) and echocardiography are used for additional information. The main indications for exercise testing are:[1]

1 Ischaemic heart disease – for diagnosis, risk stratification, assessment of symptoms and exercise capacity during regular follow-up, and screening asymptomatic men in specific professions (e.g. pilots);
2 post acute myocardial infarction – for risk stratification and assessment of exercise capacity;
3 assessment of patients post angioplasty or bypass grafting;
4 heart failure – to assess exercise capacity, especially with a view for cardiac transplantation;
5 arrhythmias – assessment of exercise-induced arrhythmias and associated symptoms.

Although ST segment depression on ECG is the most frequently used index of ischaemia, it does not occur in all patients with proven coronary artery disease (CAD), and conversely develops in some patients who have normal coronary arteries. Downsloping or planar ST depression are more reliable indicators; upsloping ST depression is not an indicator of ischaemia. The sensitivity and specificity of ST segment depression for the presence of CAD depend importantly on the prevalence, or pretest likelihood, of CAD in the patient population (Bayes theorem).[2] In a review of 24 074 subjects who had both coronary angiography and exercise testing, mean sensitivity was 68% (range 23–100%), and mean specificity was 77% (range 17–100%).[3] If the pretest likelihood of CAD is high (e.g. middle-aged, or older men with a history of angina and risk factors) most positive tests will be truly positive. In a population with low prevalence (e.g. younger women with non-specific chest pain) there may be many false positives. Exercise testing to detect CAD in young or middle-aged asymptomatic subjects without risk factors is not useful, since the pretest likelihood of CAD is very low, and a normal or abnormal exercise ECG result is difficult to interpret. Exercise testing is best used for assessing patients with symptoms of angina to determine whether they need further investigation.

Protocols[4]

The Bruce protocol is the most commonly used; it starts at 1.7 mph and 10% incline, increasing by 0.8

mph and 2% every 3 min. This is a fast protocol producing large increases in workload. The modified Bruce protocol has two 3-min warm-up stages at 1.7 mph and 0.5% incline, and is suitable for post myocardial infarction and older subjects. Other protocols are occasionally used for specific reasons (e.g. heart failure patients) such as the Naughton protocol.[5] In certain circumstances, maximum oxygen uptake is measured and this is especially useful for assessing patients for cardiac transplantation (consider if peak $V_{O_2} < 15$ ml/min per kg).[6] Post myocardial infarction exercise testing can be carried out safely at 7–10 days. The prognosis of patients post myocardial infarction depends primarily on left ventricular function, and thus low exercise capacity and failure of systolic blood pressure to rise above 30 mmHg (4 kPa) identify a high-risk group.[7] The diagnostic accuracy of exercise testing is improved when combined with nuclear perfusion techniques (see below).

Ambulatory 24-h (Holter) monitoring[8]

Holter monitoring is now a standard tool for:

1 diagnosing arrhythmias:
2 assessing antiarrhythmic therapy;
3 assessing pacemakers, or implanted defibrillators (ICD);
4 detecting ischaemia.

Modern systems record at least two simultaneous ECG channels with a third channel devoted to timing pulses and/or a patient-activated event marker. Most recorders use a magnetic tape, but solid-state systems are now available. Usually a 24–48-h period is recorded. Intermittent recorders are also available; these can be activated by the patient at the time of an arrhythmia, and are useful for assessing infrequent arrhythmias. Another variety allows long-term recordings with retention of the previous 30 s before a selected event. Analysis is usually automatic, with recordings being played back between 60 and 240 times the recording speed; areas of interest are usually reviewed by a technician before printing. Holter monitoring is a valuable tool to diagnose symptoms which occurred during the recording period. Frequently, arrhythmias can be excluded as a cause of the symptoms. Conversely, serious asymptomatic arrhythmias may be detected in patients with repetitive unexplained syncope. Holter recordings are also used extensively for the investigation of silent ischaemia, and have contributed to the concept of the total ischaemic burden.[9] Painless ischaemia is now considered to have the same pathophysiological significance as painful ischaemia.[10] Ambulatory ECG

monitoring has demonstrated that many arrhythmias occur frequently in the normal population and are not pathological, e.g. supraventricular ectopic beats, isolated infrequent ventricular ectopic beats, first-degree heart block, Wenckebach atrioventricular (AV) block, sinus arrhythmia and brief episodes of atrial fibrillation (3–4 beats).[11,12] Minor arrhythmias are especially common in elderly patients.[11,12]

Nuclear cardiology[13]

Nuclear cardiology is useful for non-invasive assessment of myocardial perfusion and left ventricular function. The techniques and isotopes used include:

1 myocardial perfusion imaging: thallium 201 (a potassium analogue), technetium 99m Sesta MIBI (isonitrile derivative), and positron emission tomography (PET) using rubidium 82, which is also a potassium analogue;[14]
2 ventricular function: first-pass radionucleotide ventriculography or gated blood pool radionuclear ventriculography (multiple gated acquisition; MUGA), which can provide an accurate measurement of ventricular volumes and ejection fraction.[15]

Nuclear cardiography is also used, less frequently, for:

1 myocardial necrosis imaging – using [111]IM antimyosin antibody imaging and ^{99m}Tc-Sm-pyrophosphate for diagnosis of a myocardial infarction, which appears as a 'hot spot';[16]
2 myocardium metabolism with PET scanning (using a variety of positron emitters to assess carbohydrate, amino acid or fatty acid metabolism);[17]
3 imaging of cardiac sympathetic nerves and adrenergic receptors using an analogue of noradrenaline.[18]

Nuclear myocardial imaging for myocardial perfusion is usually combined with exercise testing, with the isotope injected at maximum exercise or ischaemia. Thallium and MIBI scans considerably improve the specificity and sensitivity of exercise tests. Multiple views are taken using single-photon emission computed tomography (SPECT) imaging. A three-dimensional view can be reconstructed, and the exact site and size of ischaemic or infarcted areas can be seen. These nuclear techniques are especially useful in patients with abnormal resting ECGs in whom exercise-induced ST segment changes are difficult to interpret, and for detecting hibernating myocardium in patients with ischaemic cardiomyopathy who may benefit from revascularization. Myocardial perfusion scanning in patients who are unable to exercise can be carried out using a pharmacological stress such as

IV dipyridamole,[19] adenosine or dobutamine,[20] all of which increase heart rate, myocardial oxygen consumption, and induce ischaemia in patients with significant CAD.

Cardiac catheterization and coronary angiography

The major advances in imaging technology, especially echocardiography, have reduced the requirement for cardiac catheterization in patients with valvular heart disease. The main indications for cardiac catheterization are:

1. coronary arteriography and other forms of angiography;
2. measurement of intracardiac pressure, oxygen saturation and cardiac output in patients with valvular heart disease or shunts;
3. intervention procedures, e.g. percutaneous transluminal coronary angioplasty (PTCA), atherectomy, valvuloplasty (especially of the mitral valve), and various paediatric interventional procedures such as placing of patent ductus arteriosus (PDA) occluder;
4. cardiac biopsy to diagnose acute or chronic lymphocytic myocarditis and some forms of cardiomyopathy.

Techniques of cardiac catheterization in the cardiac laboratory[21]

Catheterization is usually performed via the right femoral vein and artery. In other situations, right heart catheterization can be done via the cubital, subclavian or internal jugular vein. Left heart catheterization is occasionally done via a brachial arteriotomy. However, the Seldinger percutaneous technique has proved to be quick and efficient. After inserting local anaesthetic and making a small skin incision the artery or vein is punctured with a Seldinger-type needle below the inguinal ligament. A guide wire is inserted through the needle which is then removed. An introducer-sheath is inserted over the guide wire. The guide wire and introducer are removed leaving only the sheath in place. A sheath with a haemostatic valve and a side port are generally used, and this allows rapid and frequent catheter changes without patient discomfort. A catheter is usually inserted into the right or left heart via long guide wires. At the end of the procedure, haemostasis is achieved by a firm pressure on the groin for 10–15 min. Overnight bedrest is usually recommended, but increasingly, outpatient day-care catheterization is being performed without any increase in complications.

Pressures are recorded in the right atrium, right ventricle, pulmonary artery, pulmonary capillary wedge pressure (PCWP), aorta, and left ventricle.

Valve stenosis is assessed by the pressure gradient, and if cardiac output is measured, valve area can be calculated using the Gorlin formula.[21] Mitral regurgitation is assessed by the presence of a systolic wave in the PCWP trace and by left ventricular angiography. Aortic regurgitation is assessed by aortic angiography, but this is not particularly accurate and only allows regurgitation to be categorized into mild, moderate or severe. Assessment of shunts is made by taking multiple samples for oxygen saturation. The ratio of pulmonary to systemic flow is estimated by:

$$\frac{\text{Pulmonary flow}}{\text{Systemic flow}} =$$

$$\frac{\text{Aortic saturation} - \text{mixed venous saturation (SVC)}}{\text{Pulmonary venous saturation} - \text{PA saturation}}$$

where SVC = superior vena cava and PA = pulmonary artery. (Pulmonary venous saturation is usually taken as 98% unless it is directly obtained.)

In general, pulmonary systemic flow ratios < 2:1 are haemodynamically insignificant. In the cardiac catheterization laboratory, cardiac output is usually assessed using the thermodilution technique or direct Fick method (using oxygen consumption). Left atrial pressure can be measured directly via a transeptal technique. Previously, this was done infrequently, but now it is done more commonly as part of the technique for mitral balloon valvuloplasty.

Coronary angiography

Although angiography is the gold standard for establishing the presence, site and severity of CAD, it has some limitations. Conventionally, the degree of obstruction is estimated as a percentage reduction of luminal diameter, but there is significant interobserver variability and a significant underestimation of degree of atherosclerosis compared to postmortem studies. Anatomical information can be improved by measurement of flow using Doppler-tipped guide wires[22] and intravascular ultrasound.[23] Coronary angiography is, and should be, very safe. In most laboratories, mortality is less than 0.2% and the risk of a major adverse event (stroke, myocardial infarction or major bleeding) is less than 0.5%.[24] The main indications for coronary angiography are listed in Table 20.1.[25] It is occasionally justified in asymptomatic individuals if there is evidence of high risk on non-invasive testing, and in subjects whose occupations involve the safety of other individuals (e.g. pilots or bus drivers). Coronary angiography is often done in patients with atypical chest pain of uncertain origin, to exclude significant CAD, especially if there have been multiple hospital admissions.

Table 20.1 Main indications for coronary angiography

Symptomatic angina pectoris unresponsive to medical, surgical or PTCA treatment

Unstable angina

Angina associated with other evidence of high risk (e.g. strongly positive exercise ECG testing)

Major vascular surgery (e.g. repair of aortic aneurysms) if angina pectoris is present

Post-resuscitation from cardiac arrest (sudden death syndrome) in the absence of acute myocardial infarction

Patients over 35 years in whom valve surgery is being considered[25]

PTCA = Percutaneous transluminal coronary angioplasty; ECG = electrocardiogram.

Percutaneous transluminal coronary angioplasty (PTCA)

Increasingly cardiac catheterization techniques are used for treating as well as diagnosing cardiovascular lesions, and this new application is known as *interventional cardiology*. In 1979 Gruentzig *et al.* used a balloon-tipped catheter to dilate a coronary artery stenosis.[26] Since then there have been major advances in techniques and adjuvant therapy. The current technique uses specialized guide wires (0.3–0.5 mm diameter) which are steerable, and can be manipulated across a stenosis located anywhere in the coronary tree. The guide wire acts as a railroad-track for the passage of the dilatation catheters. These have very low profiles and can tolerate high inflation pressures (up to 20 atm). After dilatation, the balloon is withdrawn and the result is confirmed by repeat angiography, or by measurement of the translesional pressure gradient. The dilated segment is then observed for 5–10 min to document stability. Other techniques may be utilized, including rotational or directional atherectomy to remove atheromatous plaque.[27] Coronary artery stenting is used increasingly *de novo*[28] and to deal with complications such as coronary artery dissection and abrupt closure. The re-stenosis rate is lower after stent placement compared to PTCA only.[29] The success of PTCA is partly dependent on the type of lesion: high success is associated with a discreet, concentric, easily accessible, smooth stenosis, with little or no calcification in a non-angulated segment.[30] Age less than 65 years, male gender, single-vessel disease, a single lesion and good ventricular function also favour a successful outcome. Diffuse lesions with excessive tortuosity or angulation, side or branch lesions and other stenoses of the same vessel, are associated with a poor outcome. Increasingly, multivessel PTCA is being undertaken in an attempt to produce complete revascularization. Initially, PTCA was indicated only for patients with chronic stable angina, but now it is used increasingly in patients with more unstable patterns and in patients with acute myocardial infarction as an alternative to thrombolysis.[31,32] Saphenous vein and internal mammary artery grafts can also be dilated. Complications of PTCA are:[32]

1 risks associated with cardiac catheterization (e.g. arrhythmias, embolization and arterial vascular injury);
2 abrupt vessel closure due to extensive dissection in conjunction with local vasospasm or thrombus formation, which occurs in approximately 4% of patients undergoing dilatation of long eccentric or curved stenotic segments. Perfusion or shunt catheters can be placed across the occluded segment to perfuse the distal bed;[33]
3 restenosis is a major disadvantage and occurs up to 40% of patients.[32] Many therapies, including antiplatelets agents, anticoagulants and angiotensin-converting enzyme inhibitors have been tried, but failed to decrease the incidence. Of various mechanical procedures, only stenting has been shown to lower the rate of restenosis.[29] Molecular biology techniques using oligonucleotides and other molecular inhibitors to stop smooth muscle cell growth are presently under trial.[34]

Mitral balloon valvuloplasty[35]

Percutaneous transeptal mitral commissurotomy (PTMC) has emerged as a very successful technique for the treatment of rheumatic mitral stenosis (providing no or only mild mitral regurgitation and no calcification). The results are comparable to surgery. Aortic balloon valvuloplasty provides only a temporary improvement in the aortic valve area, but may be of some value in patients with poor left ventricular function, advanced age or other medical problems, to allow improvement prior to aortic valve replacement.

Electrophysiological studies (EPS)[36]

The development of radiofrequency ablation (RFA) has given considerable impetus to the investigation of cardiac arrhythmias by cardiac catheterization. RFA of either accessory pathways or of atrioventricular pathways has revolutionized the treatment of supraventricular tachycardias, producing permanent cure in nearly 90%.[37] RFA delivers heat through a purpose-built steerable catheter with a large surface-area distal electrode, producing a small lesion about 5 mm diameter. The heat desiccates and destroys the conducting pathways, which are the basis of the re-entry mechanism causing the tachycardia. It does not cause pain, and therefore can be carried out under local anaesthesia. Success rates are uniformly high (85–99%) and serious complications are very rare. A wide range of tachycardias can be treated, including atrial nodal re-entry tachycardias, atrioventricular re-entry tachycardias (of the Wolff–Parkinson–White type),[38] re-entry ventricular tachycardias and atrial flutter. Patients with symptomatic tachycardias not readily controlled by medical drug therapy should be considered for EPS and ablation therapy. For patients with Wolff–Parkinson–White syndrome and atrial fibrillation, ablation of the accessory pathway is the treatment of choice, as this gives a complete cure and removes the risk of very fast ventricular rates and ventricular fibrillation during atrial fibrillation.[27,28]

Cardiac MRI[39]

Development of ECG-gated angiographic sequences has facilitated the rapid acquisition of excellent images of vascular structures, including the heart. MRI has several advantages, including safety and, except in a few circumstances, contrast agents are not required. Angiographic-type pictures can be produced (magnetic resonance angiography or MRA). The main indications for MRI are:

1 *Aortic disease* – now the investigation of choice for the definition of thoracic as well as abdominal aortic disease, particularly aortic dissection and aortic aneurysms. Coexisting aortic valve regurgitation, ventricular function, and valve morphology can also be assessed.
2 *Pericardial disease* – MRI is useful for the assessment of loculated pericardial effusions or constrictive pericarditis not adequately demonstrated by echocardiography.
3 *CAD* – as well as assessing left and right ventricular function, MRI can differentiate between infarcted and ischaemic myocardium, measure the size of myocardial infarctions and provide information on myocardial perfusion.
4 *Congenital heart disease* – MRI is the best non-invasive method for demonstrating the pulmonary artery and aortic arch disease associated with congenital heart disease. Atrial and ventricular defects can be well-visualized, and MRI is excellent for detecting sinus venosus defects and partial anomalous pulmonary venous drainage.
5 *Assessment of valve disease* – MRA is a sensitive method for detecting valve regurgitation, especially paraprosthetic regurgitation, and a semiquantitative assessment of the severity can be made.
6 *Evaluation of coronary bypass graft patency* – MRI or MRAs are likely to become major investigative tools for cardiovascular diseases.

References

1 Froelicher VF (1987) *Exercise and the Heart: Clinical Concepts,* 2nd edn. Chicago: Yearbook Medical Publishers.
2 Patterson RE and Horowitz SF (1989) Importance of epidemiology and biostatistics in deciding clinical strategies for using diagnostic tests: a simplified approach using examples from coronary artery disease. *J Am Coll Cardiol* **13**:1653–1665.
3 Gianrossi R, Detrano R, Mulvihill D *et al.* (1989) Exercise-induced ST depression in the diagnosis of coronary artery disease. A meta-analysis. *Circulation* **80**:87–98.
4 Ellestad MH (1986) *Stress Testing. Principles and Practice,* 3rd edn. Philadelphia: FA Davies.
5 Chaitman B. Exercise stress testing. In: Braunwald E (ed.) *Heart Disease,* 4th edn. Philadelphia: W B Saunders, pp. 163–164.
6 Mancini DM, Eisen H, Kussmaul W *et al.* (1991) Value of peak exercise oxygen consumption for optimal timing of cardiac transplantation in ambulatory patients with heart failure. *Circulation* **83**:778–786.
7 Moss AJ, Bigger JT and Odoroff CL (1987) Postinfartion risk stratification. *Prog Cardiovasc Dis* **29**:389–412.
8 ACC/AHA Task Force Report (1989) Guidelines for ambulatory electrocardiography. *J Am Coll Cardiol* **13**:249–258.
9 Deanfied JE, Maseri A, Selwyn AP *et al.* (1983) Myocardial ischaemia during daily life in patients with stable angina: its relation to symptoms and heart rate changes. *Lancet* **2**:753–758.
10 Yeung AC, Barry V, Orav J *et al.* (1991) Effects of asymptomatic ischemia on long-term prognosis in chronic stable coronary disease. *Circulation* **83**:1598–1604.
11 Bjerregaard P (1982) Premature beats in healthy subjects 40–79 years of age. *Eur Heart J* **3**:493–503.
12 Bjerregaard P (1983) Mean 24-hour heart rate, minimal heart rate and pauses in healthy subjects 40–79 years of age. *Eur Heart J* **4**:44–51.
13 Zaret B, Wackers FJ Th and Soufer R (1992) Nuclear cardiology. In: Braunwald E (ed.) *Heart Disease,* 4th edn. Philadelphia: W B Saunders, pp. 276–311.
14 Kotler TS and Diamond GA (1990) Exercise thallium-201 scintigraphy in the diagnosis and prognosis of coronary artery disease. *Ann Intern Med* **113**:684–702.
15 Links JM, Becker LC, Shindledecker JG *et al.* Measurement of absolute left ventricular volume from gated blood pool studies. *Circulation* **65**:82–87.
16 Johnson LL, Seldin DW, Becker LC *et al.* (1989) Antimyosin imaging in acute transmural myocardial infarctions. Results of a multicenter clinical trial. *J Am Coll Cardiol* **13**:27–35.
17 Brunken RC and Schelbert HR (1989) Positron emission (1994) Dipyridamole is superior to dobutamine for *Br Heart J* **71**:129–134.
18 Dae MW, O Connell JW, Botunick EH *et al.* (1989) Scintigraphic assessment of regional cardiac adrenergic innervation. *Circulation* **79**:634–644.
19 Kumar EB, Steel SA, Howey S, Caplin JL and Aber CP

(1994) Dipyradomole is superior to dobutamine for thallium stress imaging: a randomized cross-over study. *British Heart Journal* **71**:129–134.

20 Mairesse GH, Marwizk TH, Vanoverschelde JLJ *et al.* (1994) How accurate is dobutamine. Stress electrocardiography for detection of coronary artery disease. *J Am Coll Cardiol* **24**:920–927.

21 Grossman W and Baim DS (1991) *Cardiac Catheterisation, Angiography, and Intervention,* 4th edn. Philadelphia: Lea & Febiger.

22 Doucette JW, Corl PD, Payne HM *et al.* (1992) Validation of a Doppler guide wire for intravascular measurement of coronary artery flow velocity. *Circulation* **85**:1899–1911.

23 York PG, Mullen WL and Fitgerald PJ (1994) Intravascular ultrasound: an inside view. *Br Heart J* **72**:97–98.

24 de Bono D (1993) Complications of diagnostic cardiac catheterisation results from 34 041 patients in the United Kingdom confidential enquiry into cardiac catheter complications. *Br Heart J* **70**:297–300.

25 ACC/AHA Task Force Report (1987) Guidelines for coronary angiography. *Circulation* **76**:963A–977A.

26 Gruentzig AR, Serring A and Siegerthaler WE (1979) Nonoperative dilation of coronary-artery stenosis: percutaneous transluminal coronary angioplasty. *N Engl J Med* **301**:61–68.

27 Holmes DR, Topol EJ, Adelman AG, Cohen EA and Califf RM (1994) Randomized trials of directional coronary arterectomy: implications for clinical practice and future investigation. *J Am Coll Cardiol* **24**:431–439.

28 Vogel JHK (1994) Stents: a time for clinical judgement (editorial). *J Am Coll Cardiol* **24**:1213.

29 Fishman DL, Leon MB, Baim DS *et al.* (1994) A randomized comparison of coronary stent placement and balloon angioplasty in the treatment of coronary artery disease. *N Engl J Med* **331**:496–501.

30 Ellis SG, Vandormael MG, Cowley MJ *et al.* and the Multivessel Angioplasty Prognosis Study group (1990) Coronary morphologic and clinical determinants of procedural outcome with angioplasty for multivessel coronary disease. *Circulation* **82**:1193–1202.

31 Grines CL, Browne KF, Marco J *et al.* A comparison of immediate angioplasty with thrombocytic therapy for acute myocardial infarction. *N Engl J Med* **328**:673–679.

32 Landau C, Lange RA and Hillis D (1994) Percutaneous transluminal coronary angioplasty. *N Engl J Med* **330**:981–993.

33 de Feyter PJ, van den Brand M, Laarman GL, van Domburg R, Serruys PW and Suryapranata H (1991) Acute coronary occlusion during and after percutaneous transluminal coronary angioplasty: frequency, prediction, clinical course, management and followup. *Circulation* **83**:927–986.

34 Muller DWM (1994) Gene therapy for cardiovascular disease (editorial). *Br Heart J* **72**:309–312.

35 Inoue K (1991) Percutaneous transvenous mitral commissurotomy using the Inoue balloon. *Eur Heart J* **12**(suppl B):99–108.

36 ACCAHA Task Force Report (1989) Guidelines for clinical electrophysiological studies. *J Am Coll Cardiol* **14**:1827–1842.

37 ACC Position Statement (1994) Catheter ablation for cardiac arrhythmias: clinical applications, personnel and facilities. *J Am Coll Cardiol* **24**:828–833.

38 Jackman WM, Wang Y, Friday KJ *et al.* (1991) Catheter ablation of accessory atrioventricular pathways (Wolff–Parkinson–White syndrome) by radio-frequency current. *N Engl J Med* **324**:1605–1611.

39 Higgins CB and Caputop GR (1993) Role of MR imaging in acquired and congenital cardiovascular disease. *Am J Roentgenol* **161**:13–22.

Echocardiography in intensive care

RJ Young and JE Sanderson

Echocardiography uses ultrasound to examine the heart and great vessels. The first ultrasound imaging device was developed in 1952[1] but the first large clinical series of investigations was reported in 1967.[2] Echocardiography has since become an invaluable aid to cardiac diagnosis and treatment. Its advantages in intensive care include its portability, ease of performance and non-invasive nature. In recent years, its applications and utility have been further expanded by the advent of Doppler and transoesophageal echocardiographic techniques.

Physical principles

Ultrasound waves are produced by a piezoelectric element which acts as both transmitter and receiver. When the ultrasound beam strikes a tissue interface it is either reflected or refracted, depending on the relative acoustic impedance of the tissues (a function of the tissue density). Thus, by considering the magnitude of the reflected ultrasound and its transit time, one can derive information on the distance to the tissue interface and the relative densities of the tissues.[3]

Modalities of echocardiography

M-mode and two-dimensional echocardiography

Echo-derived information can be presented in a number of ways. M-mode records a one-dimensional view of the heart, with distance from the transducer on the y axis and time on the x axis. Whilst the resultant image lacks spatial orientation, it has excellent temporal resolution, allowing precise measurements of amplitude and rate of motion of cardiac structures. It is used in conjunction with two-dimensional echo which permits targeting of the ultrasound beam through structures of interest[4] (Fig. 21.1). Measurements of left ventricular (LV) wall

thickness and cavity size, valve leaflet excursion and aortic root and left atrial dimensions can be taken from the M-mode trace.

In two-dimensional echocardiography, the ultrasound beam moves continually in an arc so that a pie-shaped slice of the heart is examined. This provides

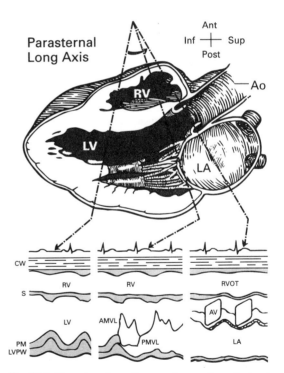

Fig. 21.1 M-mode echocardiogram. Images from the level of the papillary muscles, through the mitral valve apparatus and the aortic root. CW = chest wall; RV = right ventricle; S = septum; LV = left ventricle; PM = papillary muscle; LVPW = left ventricular posterior wall; AMVL = anterior mitral valve leaflet; PMVL = posterior mitral valve leaflet; RVOT = right ventricular outflow tract; AV = aortic valve; LA = left atrium; AO = aorta.

excellent spatial resolution with a continuous, two-dimensional image of cardiac structures in real time.[5] Multiple transducer positions are used to image the heart. Commonly used views are shown in Plate 2.

Doppler echocardiography

Doppler echocardiography uses ultrasound not to generate images, but to measure blood flow velocity.[3] If an ultrasound beam is directed at a moving object (e.g. red cells) then the frequency of the reflected sound will be different from that of the transmitted sound. The difference between the two frequencies is termed the *Doppler shift*, from which it is possible to calculate the speed and direction of blood flow. Different modalities of Doppler are available:

Continuous-wave (CW) Doppler

This uses two transducers, one continuously transmitting and the other continuously receiving. Thus it measures velocity of all blood in the path of the beam and can measure high-velocity blood flow.

Pulsed-wave (PW) Doppler

This uses only one transducer, which transmits a burst of ultrasound, and then acts as a receiver for a specified period. Thus it will only receive ultrasound reflected by a target area. Its range can be set, and one can therefore interrogate a specific area of the heart. However, the velocity of flow measured is limited by the pulse repetition frequency, and so CW Doppler is more commonly used for recording high-velocity flow (e.g. through a stenotic valve).

Colour Doppler

Colour Doppler uses PW with many hundreds of tiny sample regions. The blood flow in each of these regions is analysed separately, and the information is displayed on a colour scale superimposed on a two-dimensional echo sector. By convention, flow towards the transducer is depicted as red, and flow away as blue. Thus blood flow direction, velocity and pattern are displayed in real time, enabling detection of valvular regurgitation, turbulence, septal defects, etc.

Doppler echocardiography for haemodynamic assessment

Haemodynamic assessment by Doppler echo was first described in 1976,[6] and is now a powerful, non-invasive method used for a wide range of cardiac conditions. In some cases it obviates the need for cardiac catheterization[7-9] or invasive monitoring.[10] Examples of its use are:

Pressure gradients

By utilizing the simplified Bernoulli equation, one can calculate the pressure gradient across a stenotic orifice,

$$\Delta P = 4V^2$$

where ΔP is the pressure gradient and V is the blood velocity across the orifice.

Doppler-derived pressure gradient and cardiac catheter findings correlate well in aortic stenosis,[11] mitral stenosis,[6] and pulmonary stenosis.[12] This same technique can be applied to tricuspid regurgitant jets to estimate pulmonary artery systolic pressure.[13]

Stenotic valve areas

Stenotic valve areas are determined by the continuity principle or, in mitral valve stenosis, by consideration of the pressure half-time (the time in diastole for the pressure across the mitral valve to fall by half). Correlation between Doppler and cardiac catheter findings is acceptable.[14,15]

Cardiac output

Blood flow through cardiac structures or great vessels can be calculated using PW Doppler by multiplying the velocity of blood flow by the cross-sectional area of the relevant structure. Since blood flow is pulsatile, the integral of velocity versus time during a cardiac cycle (*time–velocity integral*) is used to calculate stroke volume. Cardiac output has been measured at multiple sites, with the most accurate at the LV outflow tract.[7] Reasonable correlation with thermodilution cardiac output has been reported.[16] Transoesophageal echocardiography can be used to measure cardiac output at the pulmonary artery[17] or LV outflow tract, with close correlation between the latter and thermodilution measurements.[18,19]

Left ventricular contractility

This is difficult to quantify clinically. Ejection fraction (measured by radionuclide scan or estimated by echocardiography) has been traditionally used. However, this is dependent on both preload and afterload. CW Doppler measurement of peak blood flow acceleration in the ascending aorta has been proposed as a good measure of LV contractility, since it is relatively independent of the ventricular load conditions.[20,21] Its use is limited, however, by its dependence on heart rate and systolic load.[7] In mitral regurgitation, the rate of increase in velocity of the regurgitant jet measured by CW Doppler can be used to calculate the maximal rate of pressure rise (dp/dt_{max}) of the LV.[22] Maximal dp/dt in animal models is a good index of contractility.[23]

Diastolic function

It is now clear that diastolic dysfunction is important in the pathogenesis of heart failure. Diastolic function of the LV can be accurately assessed by Doppler analysis of flow across the mitral valve, with normal and abnormal flow patterns well-described.[24,25]

Left atrial pressure

Left atrial pressure can be estimated by Doppler analysis of mitral blood flow[26] or, more accurately, by analysis of pulmonary venous flow.[27]

Transoesophageal echocardiography

Transoesophageal echocardiography (TOE) uses an ultrasound probe attached to the end of a flexible endoscope, which is introduced into the oesophagus. This provides a number of advantages over trans-thoracic echocardiography (TTE), particularly in the intensive care setting:[28,29]

1 TOE, being close to the heart, allows high-quality imaging of the heart and mediastinum without interference from lungs, ribs, fat and superficial obstructions (e.g. dressings), which commonly makes TTE inadequate in the critically ill.
2 TOE provides particularly good views of native and prosthetic valves, cardiac septa, and thoracic aorta.
3 The position of the probe is relatively stable, allowing serial measurements to be made.
4 TOE does not interfere with most surgical procedures, and so can be used for perioperative monitoring.[30]

Early TOE probes had a single, fixed transducer to image in only one plane.[31] Newer biplanar probes have two transducers at right angles (Fig. 21.2). Omniplanar probes are now available, in which the angle of the transducer can be varied to scan in all planes without manipulation of the endoscope tip.[32] TOE provides diagnostic imaging and, by incorporating Doppler technology, allows serial semi-invasive determination of the wide range of haemodynamic variables described above. The safety and use of TOE in critically ill patients have been well-demonstrated.[33–35] Specific indications for the use of TOE in the ICU are shown in Table 21.1 and are discussed further below. It is likely to be used more routinely for investigation and monitoring in the ICU.

Intravascular ultrasound

Ultrasound probes have now been miniaturized to 3F–5F size allowing placement in, and imaging of, peripheral and coronary vessels. This technology is still in its relative infancy, but provides tomographic images of the vessel lumen and vascular pathology (e.g. atheromatous plaques, thrombi and dissections). In addition, catheters are available which combine therapeutic devices, such as angioplasty balloons or atherectomy tools, with intravascular ultrasound probes.[36]

Contrast echocardiography

Ultrasound is extremely sensitive to intravascular gas bubbles. Intravenous injection of almost any liquid produces microbubbles which are revealed as a cluster of echoes on the echocardiogram. This has been used as a sensitive technique for detecting right-to-left shunts. The most commonly used contrast medium is simple agitated saline. The microbubbles lack intravascular stability, are filtered by pulmonary capillaries, and are thus useful only for right heart investigations. However, new commercial agents contain smaller, more uniform and stable bubbles, which are capable of crossing the pulmonary circulation.[37] This allows new applications such as analysis of myocardial contrast enhancement to assess myocardial perfusion,[38] and improved Doppler analysis of left heart blood flow and coronary artery flow.[39]

Indications for echocardiography in intensive care

Echocardiography may be useful to assess haemodynamic function in certain situations in the ICU, as discussed below.

Unexplained shock

Echocardiography is very useful to differentiate causes of shock. TOE, in particular, may have its greatest clinical impact in the diagnosis of shock states.[29]

Hypovolaemia

Echocardiography allows reasonably accurate assessment of LV volume, with good correlation between measurement of LV cross-sectional area and radionuclide estimates of LV volume.[40] The stable position of the TOE probe promotes its use for continuous monitoring of LV volume. TOE also allows Doppler analysis of pulmonary venous flow for estimation of left atrial (LA) pressure.[27]

Cardiogenic shock

This is recognized as a reduction in ejection fraction (which is accurately reflected by fractional area change measured by two-dimensional echocardiography[40]) with or without regional wall motion abnormalities. Using TOE, the pulmonary venous flow pattern will show predominantly diastolic flow as evidence of

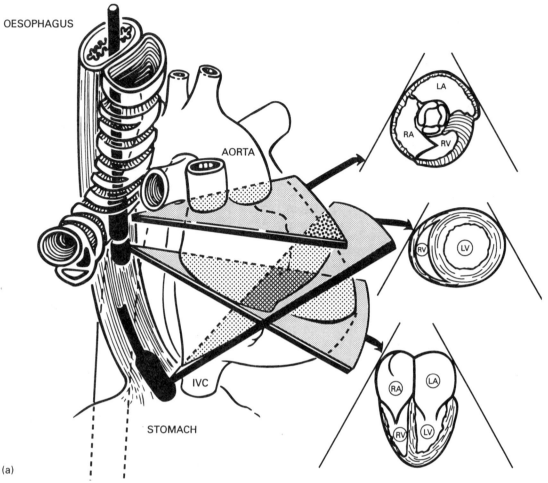

Fig 21.2 Biplanar transoesophageal echocardiogram views. (a) Short axis and (b) long axis. IVC = inferior vena cava; LA = left atrium; RA = right atrium; RV = right ventricle; LV = left ventricle; RPA = right pulmonary artery; SVC = superior vena cava; Ao = aorta; LAA = left atrial appendage.

elevated LA pressure. In shock secondary to right ventricular (RV) infarction, there will be RV dilatation, RV anterior wall hypokinesis, paradoxical septal motion and small LV dimensions.

Cardiac tamponade

Characteristic echocardiographic features of tamponade are initially late diastolic and early systolic collapse of the right atrial (RA) free wall, followed by early diastolic collapse of the right ventricle as cardiac output falls, prior to the development of systemic hypotension. These findings are sensitive and specific for the diagnosis of tamponade.[41]

Aortic dissection

See below.

Assessment of left ventricular function

As discussed above, echocardiography can be used to assess regional ventricular wall function and global systolic function, and, by utilizing Doppler analysis of pulmonary venous flow, for estimation of LA pressure. Thus, it is indicated for diagnosis of pulmonary oedema, investigation of unexplained low cardiac output states and for monitoring myocardial function.

Assessment of myocardial ischaemia and infarction

Diagnosis of ischaemia

The echocardiographic feature of ischaemic myocardium is decreased regional myocardial systolic motion and thickening – the so-called regional wall

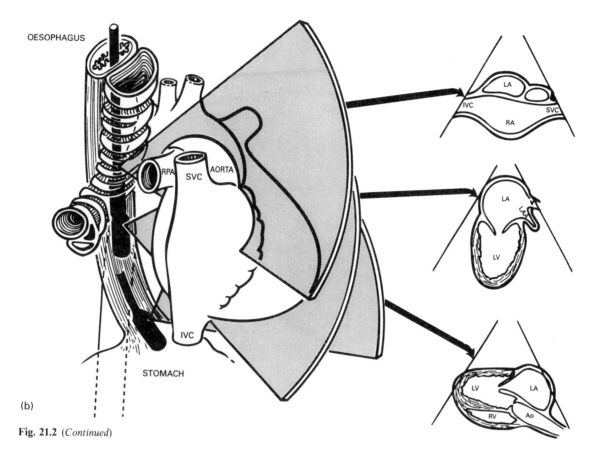

Fig. 21.2 (*Continued*)

Table 21.1 Specific indications for use of transoesophageal echocardiography in intensive care

Inadequate images with transthoracic echocardiography
Suspected aortic dissection
Suspected endocarditis
Evaluation of prosthetic valve function
Suspected massive pulmonary embolism with haemodynamic compromise
Systemic arterial embolism
Suspected thoracic aortic trauma
Monitoring of haemodynamic status

motion abnormality (RWMA). This is a sensitive indicator, and occurs within seconds of onset of regional ischaemia, preceding any ECG changes.[42] TOE monitoring for RWMA has been extensively used intraoperatively,[43,44] but its application to intensive care monitoring is difficult, as it requires continuous monitoring of the TOE image by a skilled operator.

Stress echocardiography, using pacing,[45] dobuta-mine,[46] or dipyridamole,[47] can be used to detect ischaemic myocardium. Further future applications include contrast echocardiography to assess myocardial perfusion[38] and, with TOE, visualization of the proximal coronary arteries and analysis of flow in the left anterior descending artery.[48]

Localization of infarction

Echocardiography can be used to estimate infarct size and location with reasonable accuracy, although this may be less reliable with non-transmural infarction.[3]

Complications of myocardial infarction

Ventricular septal rupture and mitral regurgitation complicating myocardial infarction may both present with cardiovascular collapse and a pansystolic murmur. Echocardiography, using colour and PW Doppler, can readily differentiate between these two conditions, and can quantify the left-to-right shunt of a septal defect.[49] Echocardiography can also diagnose other complications, including LV thrombus, LV aneurysm and pericardial effusion.

Assess complications of cardiac surgery

Haemodynamic instability in the early postoperative phase following cardiac surgery is common, and the cause is often difficult to determine. Adequate imaging by TTE is often impossible due to dressings, drains, wounds, etc., whereas TOE provides good images. Problems readily diagnosed by TOE include pericardial tamponade, myocardial dysfunction, prosthetic valve dysfunction, periprosthetic regurgitation and perioperative infarction.[28]

Suspected valvular heart disease

Echocardiography is the investigation of choice to evaluate valvular heart disease, since it can provide anatomical and quantitative haemodynamic information, enabling an accurate assessment of valvular dysfunction. However, imaging and accuracy of TTE are often inadequate in critically ill patients. In addition, when evaluating prosthetic valves, TTE is limited by attenuation and acoustic shadowing by the prosthetic material. In contrast, TOE provides an unobstructed view of the left atrium, mitral valve and annulus, right atrium, aortic root and ascending aorta.[50,51]

Suspected aortic dissection

Studies have compared available diagnostic techniques for aortic dissection, including aortography, CT scanning, magnetic resonance imaging (MRI) and TOE.[52-54] Sensitivity for TOE is 97-100%, which is matched only by MRI (sensitivity 98-100%) and is superior to aortography, the traditional gold standard. The specificity of TOE (68-97%) is lower than that for MRI (97-100%). However, these studies used monoplanar TOE, which has limitations in visualizing the entire thoracic aorta. Newer biplanar and omniplanar TOE are able to delineate the entire thoracic aorta, and should thus improve diagnostic accuracy,[55] particularly when coupled with Doppler analysis of aortic blood flow.[56] TOE provides a rapid, safe, semi-invasive and highly sensitive technique to diagnose aortic dissection, and is currently probably the method of choice.

Suspected endocarditis

TTE has been used to assess patients suspected of having endocarditis. However, its sensitivity is only about 40-70%. In contrast, TOE has been shown to be highly sensitive (about 90%) and specific.[57-60] TOE is also sensitive to detect complications of endocarditis, e.g. abscesses, fistulae and valve leaflet diverticula or perforation. Most studies to date have used monoplanar TOE. Biplanar and omniplanar TOE can be expected to improve diagnostic accuracy. However, TOE cannot confirm or exclude endocarditis with 100% accuracy, and diagnosis remains dependent on microbiological investigations (see Chapter 18).

Suspected pulmonary embolism

Echocardiography may show changes of increased RV afterload as indirect evidence of pulmonary embolism (PE) when the emboli are large enough to cause obstruction of more than 25% of the pulmonary arterial tree.[61] In addition, TOE enables imaging of the central pulmonary arteries and thus direct visualization of intraluminal thrombus.[62-64] The sensitivity and specificity of TOE for PE has not been determined. Sensitivity is probably low for small emboli but highest for large, haemodynamically significant emboli, which are more likely to be centrally located. The advantage of TOE is that it can be rapidly performed at the bedside (cf. pulmonary angiography or radionuclide scanning), allowing thrombolysis to be commenced with minimal delay. Thus, TOE should be considered early for haemodynamically compromised patients suspected to have PE (see Chapter 30).

Systemic embolism

A number of cardiac and aortic features are associated with systemic arterial emboli. These include LA thrombus, LA spontaneous echo contrast, patent foramen ovale, atrial septal aneurysm and aortic atheroma. TOE has a far higher sensitivity for these findings than TTE.[64,65] In fact, the significance of thoracic aortic atheroma as a source of systemic embolism has only been recognized since the advent of TOE, as only TOE can adequately visualize this region. Thus, all patients with unexplained cerebral or systemic emboli should have TOE performed as part of their diagnostic work-up.

Thoracic trauma

Blunt or penetrating chest trauma may result in injury to cardiac structures or great vessels, which can be difficult to diagnose clinically. The optimal approach for diagnosing myocardial contusion remains controversial (see Chapter 68).[66] Echocardiography is useful for rapid, non-invasive detection of myocardial contusion, pericardial effusion and valvular disruption. TTE may provide limited views in these cases, because of chest wall injuries, dressings and other obstructions. TOE reliably provides good images and should be performed when TTE images are inadequate. With this approach, echocardiography has been reported to be the most sensitive technique to detect myocardial contusion (cf. cardiac enzymes and electrocardiogram).[67] TOE has also been shown to be superior to aortography in evaluating traumatic aortic injury.[68]

Echocardiography has been proposed for all patients with chest trauma.[69] However, as significant cardiac events are few in patients with cardiac contusion who are haemodynamically stable, its use as a universal screening examination is not warranted. It is indicated in patients who are haemodynamically unstable, or who have clinical evidence of cardiac injury. TOE is the preferred technique, and is certainly indicated if TTE is inadequate or if thoracic aortic injury is suspected.

Miscellaneous

TOE has been used during cardiopulmonary resuscitation (CPR) since it readily provides high-quality, continuous imaging without interrupting resuscitation. It has assisted research into the physiology of CPR as well as assessment of new CPR techniques, and may find a role to monitor resuscitation efforts and to diagnose the cause of cardiac arrest.[70]

An automated border detection system is now available (Acoustic Quantification, Hewlett Packard, Andover, Massachusetts) which processes echocardiographic information into a video format. This enables myocardial boundaries to be plotted accurately and automatically and thus continuous quantification of ventricular dimensions, including end-diastolic and -systolic areas, fractional area change (as an index of ejection fraction) and rate of change.[71] Thus TOE may develop as a monitor of cardiovascular function, possibly supplanting the pulmonary artery catheter.

References

1 Wild JJ and Reid JM (1952) Application of echo ranging techniques to the determination of structure of biological tissues. *Science* **115**:226–230.

2 Ebina T, Oka S, Tanaka M, Kosaka S and Terasawa Y (1967) The ultrasono-tomography of the heart and great vessels in living human subjects by means of the ultrasonic reflection technique. *Jap Heart J* **8**:331–333.

3 Feigenbaum H (1986) *Echocardiography*, 4th edn. Philadelphia: Lea & Febiger.

4 Louie EK and Konstadt SK (1992) Doppler echocardiography: diagnostic applications in the intensive care unit. In: Hall JB, Schmidt GA and Wood LDH (eds) *Principles of Critical Care*. New York: McGraw-Hill, pp. 272–291.

5 Weyman AE (1994) *Cross-sectional Echocardiography*. Philadelphia: Lea & Febiger.

6 Holen J, Aaslid R, Landmark K and Simonsen S (1976) Determination of pressure gradient in mitral stenosis with a noninvasive ultrasound Doppler technique. *Acta Med Scand* **199**:455–460.

7 Nishimura RA and Tajik AJ (1994) Quantitative hemodynamics by Doppler echocardiography: a non-invasive alternative to cardiac catheterisation. *Prog Cardiovasc Dis* **36**:309–342.

8 Kotler MN, Jacobs LE, Podolsky LA and Meyerowitz CB (1993) Echo-Doppler in valvular heart disease. *Cardiovasc Clin* **23**:77–103.

9 Reeder GS, Currie PJ, Hagler DJ, Tajik AJ and Seward JB (1986) Use of Doppler techniques (continuous wave, pulsed wave and color flow imaging) in the noninvasive

10 Harrington GR and Hnatiuk OW (1993) Noninvasive monitoring. *Am J Med* **95**:221–228.

11 Currie PJ, Seward JB, Reeder GS *et al.* (1985) Continuous wave Doppler echocardiographic assessment of severity of calcific aortic stenosis: a simultaneous Doppler-catheter correlative study in 100 adult patients. *Circulation* **71**:1162–1169.

12 Currie PJ, Hagler DJ, Seward JB *et al.* (1986) Instantaneous pressure gradient: a simultaneous Doppler and dual catheter correlative study. *J Am Coll Cardiol* **7**:800–806.

13 Yock PG and Popp RL (1984) Noninvasive estimation of right ventricular systolic pressure by Doppler ultrasound in patients with tricuspid regurgitation. *Circulation* **70**:657–662.

14 Smith MD, Widenbaugh T, Grayburn PA, Gurley JC, Spain MG and DeMaria AN (1991) Value and limitations of Doppler pressure half-time in quantifying mitral stenosis: a comparison with micromanometer catheter recordings. *Am Heart J* **21**:480–488.

15 Nakatani S, Masuyama T, Kodama K, Kitabatake A, Fujii K and Kamada T (1988) Value and limitations of Doppler echocardiography in the quantification of stenotic mitral valve area: comparison of pressure half-time and the continuity equation methods. *Circulation* **77**:78–85.

16 Kuecherer HF and Foster E (1993) Hemodynamics by transesophageal echocardiography. *Cardiol Clin* **11**: 475–487.

17 Muhiudeen IA, Kuecherer HF, Lee E *et al.* (1991) Intraoperative assessment of cardiac output by transesophageal pulsed Doppler echocardiography. *Anesthesiology* **74**:9–14.

18 Katz WE, Gasior TA, Quinlan JJ and Gorscan J (1993) Transgastric continuous-wave Doppler to determine cardiac output. *Am J Cardiol* **71**:853–857.

19 Stoddard MF, Prince CR, Ammash N, Goad JL and Vogel RL (1993) Pulsed Doppler transesophageal echocardiographic determination of cardiac output in human beings: comparison with thermodilution technique. *Am Heart J* **126**:956–962.

20 Bennett ED, Barclay SA, Davis AL, Mannering D and Mehta N (1984) Ascending aortic blood velocity and acceleration using Doppler ultrasound in the assessment of left ventricular function. *Cardiovasc Res* **18**: 632–638.

21 Sabbah HN, Khaja F, Brymer JF *et al.* (1986) Noninvasive evaluation of left ventricular performance based on peak aortic blood acceleration measured with a continuous wave Doppler velocity meter. *Circulation* **74**:323–329.

22 Bargiggia GS, Bertucci C, Recusani F *et al.* (1989) A new method for estimating left ventricular dP/dt by continuous wave Doppler echocardiography: validation studies at cardiac catherization. *Circulation* **80**: 1287–1292.

23 Guyton AC (1991) *Textbook of Medical Physiology*, 8th edn. Philadelphia: WB Saunders.

24 Nishimura RA, Housmans PR, Hatle LK and Tajik AJ (1989) Assessment of diastolic function of the heart: background and current applications of Doppler echocardiography. Part I. Physiology and pathophysiologic features. *Mayo Clin Proc* **64**:71–81.

25 Nishimura RA, Abel MD, Hatle LK and Tajik AJ (1989) Assessment of diastolic function of the heart: background and current applications of Doppler echocardiography. Part II. Clinical studies. *Mayo Clin Proc* **64**:181–204.

26 Störk TV, Müller RM, Piske GJ, Ewert CO, Wienhold S and Hochrein H (1990) Noninvasive determination of pulmonary artery wedge pressure: comparative analysis of pulsed Doppler echocardiography and right heart catheterization. *Crit Care Med* **18**:1158–1163.

27 Kuecherer HF, Muhiudeen IA, Kusumoto FM *et al.* (1990) Estimation of mean left atrial pressure from transesophageal pulsed Doppler echocardiography of pulmonary venous flow. *Circulation* **82**:1127–1139.

28 Foster E and Schiller NB (1993) Transesophageal echocardiography in the critical care patient. *Cardiol Clin* **11**:489–503.

29 Oh JK and Freeman WK (1994) Transesophageal echocardiography in critically ill patients. In: Freeman WK, Seward JB, Khandheria BK and Tajik AJ (eds) *Transesophageal Echocardiography*. Boston: Little, Brown, pp. 549–575.

30 Sutton DC and Cahalan MK (1993) Intraoperative assessment of left ventricular function with transesophageal echocardiography. *Cardiol Clin* **11**:389–398.

31 Seward JB, Khanderia BK, Oh JK *et al.* Transesophageal echocardiography: technique, anatomic correlations, implementation, and clinical applications. *Mayo Clin Proc* **63**:649–680.

32 Pandian NG, Hsu T-L, Schwartz SL *et al.* (1992) Multiplane transesophageal echocardiography. Imaging planes, echocardiographic anatomy, and clinical experience with a prototype phased array omniplane probe. *Echocardiography* **9**:649–666.

33 Pearson AC, Castello R and Labovitz AJ (1990) Safety and utility of transesophageal echocardiography in the critically ill patient. *Am Heart J* **119**:1083–1089.

34 Oh JK, Seward JB, Khanderia BK *et al.* (1990) Transesophageal echocardiography in critically ill patients. *Am J Cardiol* **66**:1492–1495.

35 Hwang JJ, Shyu KG, Chen JJ, Tseng YZ, Kuan P and Lien WP (1993) Usefulness of transesophageal echocardiography in the treatment of critically ill patients. *Chest* **104**:861–86.

36 Higano ST and Nishimura RA (1994) Intravascular ultrasonography. *Curr Probl Cardiol* **1**:1–55.

37 Redberg RF (1994) Coronary flow by transesophageal Doppler echocardiography: do saccharide-based contrast agents sweeten the pot? *J Am Coll Cardiol* **23**:191–193.

38 DeMaria A, Dittrich H, Kwan O and Kimura B (1993) Myocardial opacification produced by peripheral venous injection of a new ultrasonic contrast agent. *Circulation* **88**(suppl 1):1–401.

39 Iliceto S, Caiati C, Aragona P, Verde R, Schlief R and Rizzon P (1994) Improved Doppler signal intensity in coronary arteries after peripheral injection of a lung crossing contrast agent (SHU 508A). *J Am Coll Cardiol* **23**:184–190.

40 Clements FM, Harpole DH, Quill T, Jones RH and McCann RL (1990) Estimation of left ventricular volume and ejection fraction by two dimensional transoesophageal echocardiography: comparison of short axis imaging and simultaneous radionuclide angiography. *Br J Anaesth* **64**:331–336.

41 Singh S, Wann LS, Schuchard GH *et al.* (1984) Right ventricular and right atrial collapse in patients with cardiac tamponade – a combined echocardiographic and hemodynamic study. *Circulation* **70**:966.

42 Alam M, Khaja F, Brymer J *et al.* (1986) Echocardiographic evaluation of left ventricular function during coronary artery angioplasty. *Am J Cardiol* **57**:20–25.

43 Freeman WK, O'Leary PW, Abel MD, Losasso TJ and Muzzi DA (1994) Intraoperative applications of transesophageal echocardiography. In: Freeman WK, Seward JB, Khandheria BK, Tajik AJ (eds). *Transesophageal Echocardiography*. Boston: Little, Brown, pp. 501–548.

44 Sutton DC and Cahalan MK (1993) Intraoperative assessment of left ventricular function with transesophageal echocardiography. *Cardiol Clin* **11**:389–398.

45 Lambertz H, Kreis A, Trumper H *et al.* (1990) Simultaneous transesophageal atrial pacing and transesophageal two-dimensional echocardiography. *J Am Coll Cardiol* **16**:1143.

46 Pierard LA, De Landsheere C, Berthe C *et al.* (1990) Identification of viable myocardium by echocardiography during dobutamine infusion in patients with myocardial infarction after thrombolytic therapy: comparison with positron emission tomography. *J Am Coll Cardiol* **15**:1031.

47 Picano E, Severi S, Michelassi C *et al.* (1989) Prognostic importance of dipyridamole-echocardiography test in coronary artery disease. *Circulation* **80**:450–457.

48 Iliceto S, Marangelli V, Memmola C *et al.* (1991) Transesophageal Doppler echocardiography evaluation of coronary blood flow velocity in baseline conditions and during dipyridamole-induced coronary vasodilation. *Circulation* **83**:61–69.

49 Topaz O and Taylor AL (1992) Interventricular septal rupture complicating acute myocardial infarct: from pathophysiologic features to the role of invasive and noninvasive diagnostic modalities in current management. *Am J Med* **93**:683–688.

50 Khanderia BK (1993) Transesophageal echocardiography in the evaluation of prosthetic valves. *Cardiol Clin* **11**:427–436.

51 Karalis DG, Ross JJ, Brown BM and Chandrasekaran K (1993) Transesophageal echocardiography in valvular heart disease. *Cardiovasc Clin* **23**:105–123.

52 Nienaber CA, von Kodolitsch Y, Nicolas V *et al.* (1993) The diagnosis of thoracic aortic dissection by noninvasive imaging procedures. *N Engl J Med* **328**:1–9.

53 Nienaber CA, Spielman RP, von Kodolitsch Y *et al.* Diagnosis of thoracic aortic dissection. Magnetic

resonance imaging versus transesophageal echocardiography. *Circulation* **85**:434–447.

54 Erbel R, Engberding R, Daniel W, Roelandt J, Visser C, Rennollet H and the European Study Group for Echocardiography (1989) Echocardiography in diagnosis of aortic dissection. *Lancet* **1**:457–461.

55 Khanderia BK (1993) Aortic dissection. The last frontier. *Circulation* **87**:1765–1768.

56 Erbel R (1993) Role of transesophageal echocardiography if dissection of the aorta and evaluation of degenerative aortic disease. *Cardiol Clin* **11**:461–473.

57 Shapiro SM, Young E, De Guzman S *et al.* (1994) Transesophageal echocardiography in diagnosis of infective endocarditis. *Chest* **105**:377–382.

58 Birmingham GD, Rahko PS and Ballantyne F (1992) transesophageal echocardiography. *Am Heart J* **125**:774–781.

59 Daniel W, Mugge A, Martin R *et al.* (1991) Improvement in the diagnosis of abscesses associated with endocarditis by transesophageal echocardiography. *N Engl J Med* **324**:795.

60 Shively BK (1993) Transesophageal echocardiography in endocarditis. *Cardiol Clin* **11**:437–446.

61 Wolfe MW, Skibo LK and Goldhaber SZ (1993) Pulmonary embolic disease: diagnosis, pathophysiologic aspects and treatment with thrombolytic therapy. *Curr Prob Cardiol* **18**:587–633.

62 Rittoo D and Sutherland GR (1993) Acute pulmonary artery thromboembolism treated with thrombolysis: diagnostic and monitoring uses of transoesophageal echocardiography. *Br Heart J* **69**:457–459.

63 Rittoo D, Sutherland GR, Samuel L, Flapan AD and

Shaw TRD (1993) Role of transesophageal echocardiography in diagnosis and management of central pulmonary artery thromboembolism. *Am J Cardiol* **71**:1115–1119.

64 Kronzon I and Tunick PA (1993) Transesophageal echocardiography as a tool in the evaluation of patients with embolic disorders. *Prog Cardiovasc Dis* **36**:39–60.

65 Dressler FA and Labovitz AJ (1993) Systemic arterial emboli and cardiac masses. Assessment with transesophageal echocardiography. *Cardiol Clin* **11**:447–460.

66 Brader AH (1993) Chest trauma. In: Kravis TC, Warner CG and Jacobs LM (eds) *Emergency Medicine*, 3rd edn. New York: Raven Press, pp. 1181–1193.

67 Karalis DG, Victor MF, Davis GA *et al.* (1994) The role of echocardiography in blunt chest trauma: a transthoracic and transesophageal echocardiographic study. *J Trauma* **36**:53–58.

68 Kearney PA, Smith DW, Johnson SB, Barker DE, Smith MB and Sapin PM (1993) Use of transesophageal echocardiography in the evaluation of traumatic aortic injury. *J Trauma* **34**:696–703.

69 Clements F (1993) The role of transesophageal echocardiography in patients with cardiac trauma. *Anesth Analg* **77**:1089–1090.

70 Redberg RF, Tucker K and Schiller NB (1993) Transesophageal echocardiography during cardiopulmonary resuscitation. *Cardiol Clin* **11**:529–535.

71 Cahalan MK, Ionescu P, Melton HE, Adler S, Kee LL and Schiller NB (1993). Automated real-time analysis of intraoperative transesophageal echocardiograms. *Anesthesiology* **78**:477–485.

Part III

Respiratory failure

22 · Oxygen therapy

TE Oh

Oxygen is required in aerobic metabolic pathways to produce biological energy from food fuels. With inadequate oxygenation, anaerobic metabolism leads to decreased biological energy and harmful lactic and metabolic acidosis. Oxygen therapy is thus indicated whenever tissue oxygenation is impaired, in order to allow essential metabolic reactions to occur, and to prevent complications attributed to hypoxaemia.[1,2]

The common clinical indications are:

1 cardiac and respiratory arrest;
2 respiratory failure:
  (a) type I: hypoxaemia without CO_2 retention (e.g. asthma, pneumonia, pulmonary oedema and pulmonary embolism);
  (b) type II: hypoxaemia with CO_2 retention (e.g. chronic bronchitis, chest injuries, unconscious drug overdose, postoperative hypoxaemia and neuromuscular disease);
3 cardiac failure or myocardial infarction;
4 shock of any cause;
5 increased metabolic demands (e.g. burns, multiple injuries and severe infections);
6 postoperative states;
7 carbon monoxide poisoning.

Arterial oxygen tension (Pao_2)

Tissue oxygenation depends upon oxygen delivery and extraction. It is difficult to suggest a 'safe' Pao_2 value above which tissue hypoxia does not occur. Pao_2 does not reflect tissue oxygenation, and oxygen extraction mechanisms vary between organs. In general, supplementary oxygen is required when Pao_2 is 60 mmHg (8.0 kPa) or less, and profound hypoxaemia is present and death is imminent when Pao_2 is less than 30 mmHg (4.0 kPa). The clinical significance of common Pao_2 and saturation (Sao_2) values are listed (Table 22.1; see Chapter 98).

Table 22.1 Clinical significance of some Pao_2 and Sao_2 values

Pao_2 mmHg	(kPa)	Sao_2(%)	Clinical significance
150	(20.0)	99	Inspired air at sea level
97	(12.9)	97	Young normal man
80	(10.6)	95	Young normal man asleep
			Old normal man awake
			Inspired air at 5700 m (19 000 ft)
70	(9.3)	93	Lower limit of normal
60	(8.0)	90	Respiratory failure, mild
			Shoulder of oxygen dissociation curve
50	(6.7)	85	Respiratory failure: admit to hospital
40	(5.3)	75	Venous blood, normal
			Arterial, severe respiratory failure
			Acclimatized man at rest at 2700 m (9000 ft)
30	(4.0)	60	Unconscious if not acclimatized
26	(3.5)	50	P_{50} or 50% saturation
20	(2.7)	36	Acclimatized mountaineer exercising at 5700 m (19 000 ft)
			Hypoxic death

Oxygen dissociation curve

Tissue oxygenation depends partly on the oxygen dissociation curve. A shift of the curve to the right (Table 22.2; Fig. 22.1) favours haemoglobin (Hb) unloading of oxygen, and thus oxygen delivery to the tissues. Conversely, a shift to the left (Table 22.2) increases the affinity of Hb for oxygen with reduced tissue oxygenation.

Oxygen delivery and consumption

Oxygen delivery (Do_2) to the cells is represented by the oxygen cascade (Table 22.3). Supply of oxygen is dependent upon the Hb, Sao_2, and cardiac output (Q).

Table 22.2 Factors influencing the position of the oxygen dissociation curve

Factors increasing P_{50} (curve shifts to right)	Factors decreasing P_{50} (curve shifts to left)
Hyperthermia	Hypothermia
Decreased pH (acidaemia)	Increased pH (alkalaemia)
Increased P_{CO_2} (Bohr effect)	Decreased P_{CO_2}
Increased 2,3-DPG	Decreased 2,3-DPG
	Fetal haemoglobin
	Carboxyhaemoglobin
	Methaemoglobin

$P_{50} = Pa_{O_2}$ at 50% saturation; 2,3-DPG = 2,3-diphosphoglycerate.

Table 22.3 Oxygen cascade: pressure gradients for oxygen transfer from inspired gas to tissue cells

	mmHg	*(kPa)*
Inspired air	150	(20.0)
Alveolar	103	(13.7)
Arterial	100	(13.3)
Capillary	51	(6.8)
Tissue	20	(2.7)
Mitochondrial	1–20	(0.13–1.3)

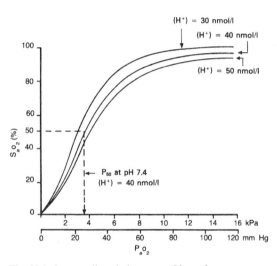

Fig. 22.1 Oxygen dissociation curve. Normal curve at 40 nmol/l H^+) and shifts to left and right. P_{50} = Tension at 50% saturation.

$\dot{D}o_2$ (or oxygen flux) denotes the total amount of oxygen delivered to the body per minute and is given by the equation:

$$\dot{D}o_2 = 1.39 \times Hb \text{ in g/dl} \times \frac{Sa_{O_2}}{100} \times \frac{\dot{Q}}{100} \text{ in ml/min}$$

$$= 1000 \text{ ml/min}.$$

(1.39 = oxygen-carrying capacity of Hb in ml/g Hb.) The amount of oxygen carried dissolved in blood is negligible.

Hence $\dot{D}o_2$ for a normal adult is approximately 1000 ml/min or 14 ml/kg per min. However, not all of this amount is available for cellular utilization. Oxygen diffuses from tissue capillaries to mitochondria in cells. Mean tissue Po_2 varies from organ to organ, and is higher near capillaries.[3] Although mitochondria in tissue cells may operate at a low Pa_{O_2}

of 8–40 mmHg (1.06–5.32 kPa), diffusion requires a capillary–tissue cell gradient. Thus tissue extraction of oxygen from blood is generally limited, and mitochondrial function jeopardized, at a Pa_{O_2} of less than 30 mmHg (4.0 kPa) or a Sa_{O_2} of 30%. The available oxygen per minute is therefore less than the supply (by about 250–300 ml/min) and is approximately 700 ml in a normal man.

Normal oxygen consumption ($\dot{V}o_2$) at rest is about 200–250 ml/min. The oxygen reserve (availability minus consumption) in a normal man at rest is thus about 450–500 ml/min. Some factors in the sick person increase oxygen consumption greatly, e.g. fever, sepsis, shivering, restlessness and hypercatabolism. When other associated factors concomitantly reduce oxygen supply and availability, oxygen reserve may be reduced to critical levels. A minimal $\dot{D}o_2$ compatible with survial at rest appears to be about 400 ml/min. Thus the use of supplemental oxygen to relieve hypoxaemia must be considered with measures to:

1 reduce excessive oxygen requirements (e.g. by cooling, paralysis and mechanical ventilation);
2 increase $\dot{D}o_2$ (by correcting anaemia, low cardiac output and adverse factors which shift the dissociation curve to the left).

Oxygen therapy apparatus and devices (Table 22.4)[1,2,4]

The basic requirements of apparatus or devices for oxygen therapy are:

1 control of fractional inspired oxygen concentration (Fi_{O_2});
2 prevention of excessive CO_2 accumulation;
3 minimal resistance to breathing;
4 efficient and economical use of oxygen;
5 acceptance by patients.

Anaesthetic circuits and resuscitator bags are used to preoxygenate patients prior to endotracheal intubation. Oxygen administration is thus achieved largely by facemasks or nasal catheters. It is important

Table 22.4 Apparatus/devices for oxygen therapy

Apparatus/device	Oxygen flow (l/min)	Concentration (%)
Nasal catheters	2–6	25–40
Semi-rigid mask (e.g. MC, Edinburgh, Hudson, Harris)	4–15	35–70
Venturi-type mask		
Individual concentration masks		24, 28, 35
Interchangeable entrainment discs	6–12	40, 50, 60
Soft plastic masks (e.g. Pneumask, Polymask, Oxyaire)	4–15	40–80
Ventilators	Varying	21–100
Anaesthetic circuits	Varying	21–100
CPAP circuits	Varying	21–100
Plastic head hood	4–8	30–50
Oxygen tent/cot	7–10	60–80
Incubator	3–8	Up to 40%

CPAP = Continuous positive airways pressure.

to know if the Fio_2 delivered by the apparatus will vary with the patient's ventilation. Apart from low-flow breathing circuits, some manual resuscitator bags and ventilators (see Chapter 27), no device will deliver 100% oxygen, unless the oxygen is supplied at a rate greater than peak inspiratory flow rate (PIFR). PIFR in adults is about 25–35 l/min at rest, increasing markedly to over 60 l/min in dyspnoeic states. The apparatus and devices for oxygen therapy are classified below.

Fixed performance systems (Fio_2 is independent of patient factors)

High-flow Venturi-type masks[5]

Oxygen flow entrains air by the Venturi principle to deliver a fixed Fio_2. Venturi masks may individually offer separate oxygen concentrations, e.g. 24%, 28%, 35%, 40%. Others use a facemask with a short 'elephant trunk' hose attached to an interchangeable entrainment disc to allow a range of concentrations. The oxygen flow rate is set at 6–8 l/min depending on the Fio_2 chosen, entraining room air to give a resultant total flow rate of 40–60 l/min. Since room air is entrained, the use of a humidifier is not essential. The high-flow system also eliminates rebreathing and the need for a tight fit to the face. However, these masks may not deliver the intended Fio_2 if severe dyspnoea is present.[6,7] The large PIFR in such patients may exhaust the reservoir in smaller-volume masks, leading to a lower, fluctuant Fio_2.[7] This is overcome by increasing the oxygen flow rate to 12–14 l/min (to give total inspired gas flows over 60 l/min).

Low-flow breathing circuits

These include anaesthetic circuits and circuits to deliver continuous positive airway pressure (CPAP) or spontaneous positive end-expiratory pressure (PEEP;[8] see Chapter 26) These circuits incorporate a reservoir bag to deliver an Fio_2 set by the fresh gas mixture, via an endotracheal tube or tight facemask.

Variable performance systems (Fio_2 depends upon oxygen flow, device factors and patient factors)

No-capacity system

These include nasal catheters at low flow rates (less than 2 l/min). Hence there is insufficient oxygen storage in the airway during the expiratory pause to affect the next inspiration significantly. Fio_2 then depends upon the added oxygen flow rate and the peak inspiratory flow rate. In order to maintain the same Fio_2, the added oxygen flow rate will need to be altered with each change in peak inspiratory flow.

Small-capacity system

Nasal catheters at high flow

Significant oxygen storage occurs during the expiratory pause, and varies with the length of the pause. With the breath-to-breath variation of PIFR, Fio_2 thus varies with ventilation. The high flow rates may cause discomfort and drying of nasal mucosa. However, nasal catheters are cheap and easy to use, and the patient is able to eat or drink with them *in situ*. CO_2 rebreathing does not occur.

Simple, semi-rigid plastic masks (e.g. MC, Edinburgh, Harris, Hudson)

Since some CO_2 rebreathing occurs, especially at low flows, the oxygen flow rate should be set at 4 l/min or greater. Fio_2 varies with patient ventilation and the oxygen flow rate (Table 22.5). A maximum concentration of only 60–70% oxygen is achieved by these

Table 22.5 Approximate oxygen concentrations related to flow rates of semi-rigid masks

Oxygen flow rate (l/min)	Approximate $F_{i}O_2$
4	0.35
6	0.50
8	0.55
10	0.60
12	0.65
15	0.70

masks. Large discrepancies between the delivered $F_{i}O_2$ and that received by the patient (i.e. intratracheal $F_{i}O_2$) occur with increasing rate and depth of breathing (i.e. increased PIFR).[9,10]

Tracheostomy masks

These are small, plastic masks placed over the tracheostomy tube or stoma. The patient will inspire less oxygen than delivered, as dilution by room air occurs. Otherwise, they perform similarly to simple facemasks.

T-piece circuit

A T-piece is a simple, large-bore, non-rebreathing circuit attached directly to an endotracheal or tracheostomy tube. Humidified oxygen is delivered through one limb of the T, and expired gas leaves via the other limb. The T-piece can be a fixed performance device if the fresh gas flow rate and the circuit volume are higher than the patient's PIFR.

Face tent

This is a large, semi-rigid plastic half-mask which wraps around the chin and cheeks. The oxygen mixture is delivered from the bottom of the mask, and gases are exhaled through the open, upper part. It is used to provide added humidification from a heated humidifier. Otherwise it has no advantages over the simple facemask.

Large-capacity system

Significant oxygen and CO_2 storage (i.e. rebreathing) occurs in these devices.

Soft plastic masks, e.g. Pneumask, Polymask, Oxyaire

These masks have an added reservoir bag and thus a large effective dead space. $F_{i}O_2$ greater than semi-rigid masks is possible, but considerable CO_2 rebreathing occurs if the oxygen supply fails or is reduced. They are potentially dangerous in patients without

cardiopulmonary reserve, and should be used with high oxygen flow rates. Rebreathing can be eliminated, and delivered $F_{i}O_2$ increased further, if unidirectional valves are added, but asphyxia may occur in the unconscious patient if a valve becomes faulty.

Oxygen headbox, tents, cots and incubators (see below)

Positive-pressure devices

CPAP maintains a continuous positive airway pressure throughout the spontaneous breathing cycle. Oxygenation is improved mainly as a result of increased functional residual capacity. Lung compliance and work of breathing may also be improved. CPAP can be applied via an endotracheal tube, mask or special nasal prongs. With the latter two methods, gastric distension should be avoided, commonly with nasogatric tube drainage. Other CPAP modifications such as airway pressure release ventilation (APRV) and bi-positive airway pressure (BIPAP) can also be applied (see Chapter 26).

Non-invasive positive-pressure ventilation can be delivered using face or nasal masks. This may be able to provide oxygenation and ventilatory support in some patients without endotracheal intubation.

Other methods of oxygenation

Extracorporeal membrane oxygenation has no benefits over ventilation modes. An intravascular blood gas exchanger (IVOX, an elongated membrane oxygenator to lie within the venae cavae)[11] has been designed, but requires proper clinical evaluation.

Paediatric oxygen therapy

The PIFR of children, because of their smaller size, approximately more closely with the flow rate of oxygen delivery devices. Hence, higher $F_{i}O_2$ is achieved. However, it is difficult to retain nasal catheters and masks on children. A single nasal catheter, placed at the level of the uvula and taped to the face, is well-tolerated and is useful in infants and small children.[1]

Oxygen headbox or hood

Oxygen is delivered into a box encasing the child's head and neck. The $F_{i}O_2$ depends on the fresh gas flow, size of box, leak around the neck, head position and how often the box is removed. It is a useful method in infants and small children, but high flow rates should be supplied, and monitoring of oxygen concentration near the face is essential.

Incubator

Incubators provide oxygen as well as a neutral thermal environment. Patient access and recovery of oxygen concentration after opening the incubator are problems. The use of a headbox inside an incubator is common to give a more stable oxygen environment.

Oxygen cot/tent

Oxygen cots or tents may be used to nurse larger children. Access, long recovery time for oxygen concentration and the diffculty to achieve Fio_2 above 0.4 are problems.

Hazards of oxygen therapy[12]

CO_2 narcosis

When high Fio_2 is administered to patients dependent on a hypoxic (chemoreceptor) drive, e.g. those with acute exacerbation of chronic bronchitis, severe respiratory depression may occur, with loss of consciousness. If this oxygen-induced CO_2 narcosis is suspected, oxygen should not be withdrawn suddenly, as dangerous hypoxaemia will result. Such patients should be encouraged to breathe, or if unconscious, should immediately be ventilated.

Oxygen toxicity

Neurological effects (Paul Bert effects)

Idiopathic epilepsy occurs with exposure to oxygen at more than 3 atm absolute.

Lung toxicity

Pulmonary toxicity following exposure to high Fio_2 is a recognized clinical problem, but knowledge of the disorder remains limited. Progressive decrease in lung compliance occurs, associated with the development of haemorrhagic interstitial and intra-alveolar oedema and, ultimately, fibrosis. The exact mechanism of the toxic effects of oxygen on the lung remains unknown, but it is believed that oxygen directly affects lung tissue. A biochemical pathogenesis of toxic oxygen free radicals (reactive oxygen species) causing lung tissue injury is suggested.[13] Normally protective antioxidants in respiratory tract lining fluids (e.g. mucin, uric acid, ascorbic acid, reduced glutathione, superoxide dismutase and 'sacrificial' proteins) are depleted by a large or prolonged oxidative challenge. Additional indirect factors that have been suggested include increased sympathetic activity, reduced surfactant activity and absorption collapse. Dif-ferentiation of oxygen toxicity from other conditions of lung damage (e.g. acute respiratory distress syndrome, ARDS) is extremely difficult, and the damage may be a common response to different types of injury.

It is generally agreed that oxygen pulmonary toxicity is dependent upon the duration of exposure and the concentration. However, precise details about 'safe' periods of exposure and 'safe' concentrations are unknown. Individual susceptibility to oxygen damage may vary. Even when using high Fio_2, pulmonary toxicity does not always occur.[14] Damage in healthy lungs can occur, but whether the response is similar in lungs with pre-existing disease remains unclear. In general, clinical signs of toxicity (e.g. dyspnoea, substernal pain, deteriorating gas exchange and X-ray changes) are not usually detected with using oxygen less than 50%,[15] or 100% for short periods less than 24 h.

Bronchopulmonary dysplasia,[16] a paediatric chronic lung disease originating in the neonatal period, has similar abnormalities. This is seen when the immature lung is ventilated with high Fio_2. Pathogenetic contributions of immaturity, oxygen toxicity and ventilatory pressure are unknown. Barotrauma may be the major predisposing factor, but oxygen may accelerate the pathological process.

Retrolental fibroplasia[17]

Blindness occurs in premature babies under 1200 g weight (about 28 weeks) exposed to high oxygen concentrations, and relates to Pao_2 and retinal immaturity. Oxygen appears to stimulate immature retinal vessels to spasm and proliferate, resulting in obliteration, haemorrhage, fibrosis, retinal detachment and blindness. Fio_2 should be restricted to keep Pao_2 between 60 and 80 mmHg (6.6–10.6 kPa). Oxygen therapy must be closely monitored.

Barotrauma[18]

Alveolar rupture with interstitial and mediastinal emphysema is a disastrous consequence when oxygen flow is inadvertently delivered at wall outlet or cylinder pressure, directly to the patient's airway.

Clinical application of oxygen

Oxygen is a drug and has to be used correctly. It is usually given as a temporary measure to relieve hypoxaemia, but does not replace definitive treatment of the underlying condition. Oxygen therapy must be assessed by indices of oxygenation (e.g. pulse oximetry Spo_2 arterial blood gases, mixed venous Po_2, and shunt equations; see Chapter 98). Pao_2 must always be related to Fio_2 and the ventilation pattern; a quoted Pao_2 value by itself is meaningless. Oxygen therapy must be continuous. Intermittent oxygen is harmful, as Pao_2 falls (possibly profoundly) when oxygen is withheld.

Oxygen will correct hypoxaemia from hypoventilation or ventilation:perfusion mismatch. Hypoxaemia due to right-to-left shunting (e.g. severe pneumonia, pulmonary embolism and ARDS) is less responsive, and will usually perisist despite 100% oxygen, if the shunt fraction exceeds 20–25%. The lowest Fio_2 to provide adequate oxygenation should be given. However, in profound life-threatening hypoxaemia, high (even 100%) concentrations should never be withheld.

Mild hypoxaemia

Nasal catheters at 2–4 l/min or a simple mask at 4 l/min are suitable.

Moderate hypoxaemia with normal or low $Paco_2$ (type I respiratory failure)

A simple mask is used with a flow rate of 4–15 l/min according to the Pao_2 and patient requirements. Extremely dyspnoeic patients with large PIFR will require oxygen delivered at as high a flow as possible. The standard oxygen flowmeter has a maximum flow rate of only 15 l/min, and may not deliver adequate inspired oxygen. Special high-flow flowmeters or linked dual flowmeters can be used. Oxygen must never be rationed ('asphyxia therapy') in acute asthma[19] and shock.

Hypoxaemia with increased $Paco_2$ (type II respiratory failure)

Hypoventilatory causes (e.g. central depression, neuromuscular dysfunction, head injury and chest wall abnormalities)

A high Fio_2 by simple facemask may be sufficient. Endotracheal intubation may be indicated to protect the airway, and mechanical ventilation is instituted if ventilatory efforts are inadequate. Restricting oxygen to these patients is illogical and dangerous.

Chronic obstructive airways disease

Controlled oxygen therapy with a Venturi-type mask is used. A concentration of 24% is started, and blood gases are measured after 30–60 min. If $Paco_2$ increases less than 10 mmHg (1.3 kPa) and is below 75 mmHg (10 kPa), Fio_2 is increased to 0.28. Since these patients lie on the steep part of the oxygen dissociation curve, a small rise in Pao_2 will result in a relatively large increase in oxygen available to tissues. Fio_2 may be increased further in the same way if hypoxaemia persists. Nasal catheters at low flows may be used but are not ideal. At higher flows, controlled oxygen therapy cannot be achieved with nasal catheters. The concept of limiting Fio_2 for fear of depressing the hypoxic drive to breathe is based on little scientific evidence. In many patients, the danger of hypercarbia is overstressed, and severe hypoxaemia is undertreated.[4,20]

Profound hypoxaemia

Mechanical ventilatory support is indicated. CPAP by mask, or non-invasive pressure ventilation, may be tried initially in awake patients to avoid intubation. PEEP may be used to help reduce Fio_2. (see Chapter 26).

'Supranormal' oxygen supply

In normal humans and animals, $\dot{V}o_2$ remains relatively constant over a wide range of $\dot{D}o_2$. This $\dot{V}o_2$ autoregulation is due to increased oxygen extraction as $\dot{D}o_2$ decreases. However, if $\dot{D}o_2$ decreases below a critical $\dot{D}o_2$ of 5–10 ml/kg per min, $\dot{V}o_2$ then becomes dependent on $\dot{D}o_2$, denoting inadequate oxygen supply to tissues (Fig. 22.2). Some workers have reported that critical $\dot{D}o_2$ is increased in sepsis and ARDS (to 16–22 ml/kg per min) due to impaired oxygen extraction and increased $\dot{V}o_2$ (Fig. 22.2).[21,22] Thus, some workers advocate using 'supranormal' $\dot{D}o_2$ and haemodynamic values (Table 22.6) by increasing Fio_2 haemoglobin and cardiac output, to achieve adequate tissue oxygenation in these patients. Using this objective, lower mortality figures were reported.[23–25] However, this 'pathological supply dependency' concept is not universally accepted. In earlier studies, $\dot{V}o_2$ was calculated rather than measured, and a resultant $\dot{V}o_2/\dot{D}o_2$ relationship was possible from mathematical coupling.[26–28] Data from too few patients were often pooled, and the calorigenic effect of inotropes used was ignored.[29] Evidence of a pathological critical $\dot{D}o_2$

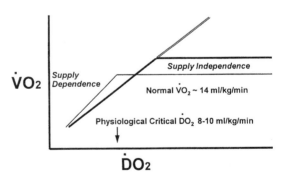

Fig. 22.2. Oxygen consumption ($\dot{V}o_2$) supply ($\dot{D}o_2$) dependency. The thin line is the physiological relationship and shows critical $\dot{D}o_2$ and physiological oxygen supply dependence. Pathological supply dependence is shown by the thick line; critical $\dot{D}o_2$ and $\dot{V}o_2$ are increased, and the relationship may be linear throughout the clinical range of $\dot{D}o_2$ (double line).

Table 22.6 'Supranormal' oxygen delivery end-points

Variable	End-point	(Normal values)
Cardiac index	>4.5 l/min per m^2	(2.5–3.5)
Oxygen delivery index	>650 ml/min per m^2	(400–700)
Systemic vascular resistance	>800 dyn s/cm^5	(770–1500)
Oxygen consumption index	>170 ml/min per m^2	(130–150)
Pulmonary occlusion pressure	>18 mmHg	(15)

with its plateau (Fig. 22.2) has never been demonstrated clinically. More recent studies have not shown a pathological $\dot{V}o_2/\dot{D}o_2$ relationship nor better patient outcome with 'supra-normal' therapy.[26,27,30–32] Therefore, while it is worthwhile improving $\dot{D}o_2$ in critically ill patients, the intensivist should not aggressively apply supranormal end-points to all patients, as attempting this objective may be detrimental.[32]

Hyperbaric oxygen therapy

Hyperbaric oxygen (HBO) therapy delivers 100% oxygen at a pressure above atmospheric, in a pressurized multi- or one-person chamber. Oxygen inhaled at pressure dissolves in plasma, e.g. Pao_2 approaches 1500 mmHg (200 kPa) at 2 atm absolute. Increases in oxygen tensions of tissues vary widely, depending on local perfusion and metabolic conditions. HBO therapy is the treatment for decompression sickness or 'bends'. It has been used in the treatment of carbon monoxide poisoning,[33,34] burns,[35] gas gangrene,[36–38] osteomyelitis, osteoradionecrosis, crush injuries and ischaemic skin grafts. While favourable clinical results have been claimed for each of these conditions, no proper trials have demonstrated benefits of HBO therapy over conventional treatment.[33,38] Complications of HBO therapy include barotrauma to ears, sinuses and lung, oxygen toxicity, grand mal fits, and changes in visual acuity. Patient selection for HBO therapy is probably important.[34]

References

1 Oh TE and Duncan AW (1988) Oxygen therapy. *Med J Aust* **149**:141–166.

2 Leigh JM (1984) Oxygen therapy: physiological principles, monitoring and administration technique. *Crit Care Int* **3**:4–7.

3 Nunn J F (1987) *Applied Respiratory, Physiology,* 3rd edn. London: Butterworths, p. 201.

4 Leach RM and Bateman NT (1993) Acute oxygen therapy. *Br J Hosp Med* **49**:637–644.

5 Goddard JM (1985) Concentrations of oxygen delivered by air entrainment oxygen masks. *Ann Roy Coll Surg Engl* **67**:366–367.

6 Editorial (1982) Oxygen behind the mask. *Lancet* **2**:1197–1198.

7 Campbell EJM (1982) How to use the venturi mask. *Lancet* **2**:1206.

8 Duncan AW, Oh TE and Hillman DR (1986) PEEP and CPAP. *Anaesth Intens Care* **14**:236–250.

9 Wexler HR, Levy H, Cooper JD and Aberman A (1975). Measurement of intratracheal oxygen concentrations during face mask administration of oxygen. *Can Anaesth Soc J* **22**:417–431.

10 Goldstein RS, Young J and Rebuck AS (1982) Effect of breathing pattern on oxygen concentration received from standard face masks. *Lancet* **2**:1188–1190.

11 Mortenson JD (1991) Augmentation of blood gas transfer by means of an intravascular blood gas exchanger (IVOX). In: Marini JJ and Roussos C (eds) *Ventilatory Failure.* Berlin: Springer-Verlag, pp. 318–346.

12 Coates JE (1993) *Lung Function. Assessment and Application in Medicine,* 5th edn. London: Blackwell Scientific Publications, pp. 629–633.

13 Cross CE, van der Vliet A, O'Neill CAO and Eiserich JP (1994) Reactive oxygen species and the lung. *Lancet* **344**:930–933.

14 Gibbs PS, Moorthy SS and Losasso AM (1976) Sustained high inspired Pao_2 without toxic sequelae. *Anesth Analg* **55**:588–589.

15 Klein J (1990) Normobaric pulmonary oxygen toxicity. *Anesth Analg* **70**:195–207.

16 Martin R, Bruce M and Fanaroff A (1989) Bronchopulmonary dysplasia. In: Nussbaum E (ed.) *Pediatric Intensive Care.* New York: Futura, pp. 469–481.

17 Phelps DL (1992) Retinopathy of prematurity. *N Engl J Med* **326**:1078–1080.

18 Newton NI (1991) Supplementart oxygen – potential for disaster. *Anaesthesia* **46**:905–906.

19 Elder AT, Crompton GK (1985) Misleading guidelines on oxygen treatment in asthma. *Br Med J* **291**:823.

20 Schmidt GA and Hall JB. Acute on chronic respiratory failure. Assessment and management of patients with COPD in the emergency setting. *J Am Med Assoc* **261**:3444–3453.

21 Mohensifar Z, Goldbach P, Tashkin DP *et al.* (1983) Relationship between O_2 delivery and O_2 consumption in the adult respiratory distress syndrome. *Chest* **84**:267–271.

22 Danek SJ, Lynch JP, Weg JG and Dantzker DR (1980) The dependence of oxygen uptake on oxygen

delivery in the adult respiratory distress syndrome. *Am Rev Resp Dis* **122**:387–395.

23 Shoemaker WC, Appel PL and Kram HB (1993) Hemodynamic and oxygen transport responses in survivors and nonsurvivors of high-risk surgery. *Crit Care Med* **21**:977–990.

24 Edwards JD, Brown GCS and Nightingale P (1989) Use of survivors' cardiorespiratory values as therapeutic goals in septic shock. *Crit Care Med* **17**:1098–1103.

25 Tuschmidt J, Fired J, Astiz M and Rackow E (1992) Elevation of cardiac output and oxygen delivery improves outcome in septic shock. *Chest* **102**:216–220.

26 Ronco JJ, Phang PT, Walley KR, Wiggs B, Fenwick JC and Russell JA (1991) Oxygen consumption is independent of changes in oxygen delivery in severe adult respiratory distress syndrome. *Am Rev Respir Dis* **143**:1267–1273. methods. *Intens Care Med* **20**:12–18.

27 Wysocki M, Bebes M, Roupie E and Brun-Buisson C (1992) Modification of oxygen extraction ratio by change in oxygen transport in septic shock. *Chest* **102**:221–226.

28 Hanique G, Dugernier T, Laterre PF, Dougnac A, Roeseler J and Reynaert MS (1994) Significance of pathologic oxygen supply dependency in critically ill patients: comparison between measured and calculated methods. *Intensive Care Medicine* **20**:12–18.

29 Bhatt SB, Hutchinson RC, Tomlinson B and Oh TE (1992) Effect of dobutamine infusion on oxygen supply and uptake in healthy volunteers. *Br J Anaesth* **69**:298–303.

30 Vermeij CG, Feenstra BWA, Adrichem WJ and Bruning HA (1991) Independent oxygen uptake and oxygen delivery in septic and postoperative patients. *Chest* **99**:1438–1443.

31 Ronco JJ, Fenwick JC, Wiggs BR, Phang PT, Russell JA and Tweeddale MG (1993) Oxygen consumption is independent of increases in oxygen delivery in septic patients who have normal or increased plasma lactate. *Am Rev Respir Dis* **147**:25–31.

32 Hayes MA, Timmins AC, Yau EH, Palazzo M, Hinds CJ and Watson D (1994) Elevation of systematic oxygen delivery in the treatment of critically ill patients. *N Engl J Med* **330**:1717–1722.

33 Tibbles PM and Perrotta PL (1994) Treatment of carbon monoxide poisoning: a critical review of human outcome studies comparing normobaric oxygen with hyperbaric oxygen. *Ann Emerg Med* **24**:269–276.

34 Gorman DF and Runciman WB (1991) Carbon dioxide poisoning. *Anaesth Intens Care* **19**:506–511.

35 Cianci P and Sato R (1994) Adjunctive hyperbaric oxygen therapy in the treatment of thermal burns: a review. *Burns* **20**:5–14.

36 Thom S (1993) A role for hyperbaric oxygen in clostridial myonecrosis. *Clin Infect Dis* **17**:238.

37 Brown DR, Davis NL, Lepawsky M, Cunningham J and Kortbeek J (1994) A multicenter review of the treatment of major truncal necrotizing infections with and without hyperbaric oxygen therapy. *Am J Surg* **167**:485–489.

38 Heimbach D (1993) Use of hyperbaric oxygen. *Clin Infect Dis* **17**:239–240.

23 ◈ Airway management

KK Young and TE Oh

Management of the obstructed upper airway is a frequent ICU emergency (see Chapter 25). Death and brain injury attributable to inability to intubate and/or ventilate contribute significantly to medicolegal litigation.[1] A difficult airway has been described as one in which a conventionally trained anaesthesiologist experiences difficulty with mask ventilation, tracheal intubation or both.[2] Difficult intubations may be expected in 1–3% of patients presenting for general anaesthesia, and this incidence would generally apply to ICU patients. Airway management consists of techniques which clear the obstructed airway or bypass the obstruction, assist or replace spontaneous ventilation, permit tracheal suctioning and protect the lungs from soiling.

Airway management technique

Airway management can be considered under non-invasive or invasive manoeuvres with respect to instrumentation above or below the glottis (Table 23.1). Established airway management techniques include bag-and-mask ventilation and blind nasal plus direct laryngoscopic intubation. Alternative techniques for difficult intubation have been developed in recent years (particularly using the fibreoptic bronchoscope). Management of failed intubation and ventilation by various techniques (e.g. jet ventilation, cricothyroidotomy and laryngeal mask airway) is now well-described.[3] Procedures for acute upper airway obstruction are described in Chapter 25, but basic management choices are:

1 surgical versus non-surgical initial approach to intubation;
2 awake intubation under local anaesthesia versus intubation after induction of general anaesthesia;
3 preservation of spontaneous ventilation versus ablation of spontaneous ventilation.

The choice of technique will depend on each situation, which is an interaction of patient factors with the clinician's experience (Table 23.2). Other factors include availability of back-up help, levels of training and supervision, and accessibility of equipment. A portable airway box with equipment for difficult airway management (Table 23.3)[4–10] is recommended for an ICU.

The difficult airway

Causes and factors

Difficulties in tracheal intubation or maintaining a patent airway may be encountered in patients with:

1 variants from normal anatomy (in subjects who otherwise appear normal);
2 a short neck, especially if obese or muscular;
3 limited neck and jaw movements (e.g. as a result of trismus, osteoarthritis, ankylosing spondylitis, rheumatoid arthritis and perioral scarring);
4 protruding teeth, a small mouth, a long high curved palate, or a receding lower jaw;
5 space-occupying lesions of the oropharynx and larynx;
6 congenital conditions with any of the above features (e.g. Marfan's syndrome and cystic hygroma).

Experience and training

About 85% of difficult intubations can be managed sucessfully by experienced clinicians with an introducer.[11] The experience of the operator is probably the most important factor determining success or (disastrous) failure. Experience implies greater manual skills, better anticipation of problems and preformulation of strategies, and familiarity with many techniques. Thus training of intensivists must

Table 23.1 Characteristics of airway management techniques

Technique	Experience required	Time	Airway protected	Use in failed intubation/ventilation
Non-invasive				
Bag-and-mask	+	seconds	−	
Laryngeal mask airway (LMA)	−	<1 min	−	+
Combitube	−	<1 min	+	+
Invasive				
Endotracheal intubation				
Direct laryngoscopy	+	variable	+	
Bronchoscopic	+	minutes	+	
Retrograde	−	minutes	+	
Jet ventilation	−	<1 min	−	
Cricothyroidotomy				
Percutaneous	−	variable	±	+
Surgical	+	minutes	+	+
Tracheostomy				
Percutaneous	+	minutes	+	
Surgical	+	minutes	+	+

Table 23.2 Application of airway management techniques

	Difficult direct laryngoscopic intubation +	Difficult mask ventilation
Awake	Fibreoptic bronchoscopic intubation Blind nasal intubation Retrograde intubation Laryngeal mask airway	Transtracheal jet ventilation Percutaneous cricothyroidotomy* Surgical tracheostomy*
Anaesthetized/Coma		
Empty stomach	Bag-and-mask ventilation Direct laryngoscopic intubation 　Different blade 　Bougie/stylet 　Lighted stylet Blind nasal intubation Laryngeal mask airway Fibreoptic bronchoscopic intubation	Laryngeal mask airway Transtracheal jet ventilation Rigid ventilating bronchoscope Percutaneous cricothyroidotomy Surgical tracheostomy
Full stomach	Bag-and-mask with cricoid pressure Combitube	Percutaneous cricothyroidotomy Surgical tracheostomy Combitube

Examples of common alternatives are given. The technique(s) chosen will depend on the clinician.
* Under local anaesthesia.

specifically include airway management skills (e.g. fibreoptic, blind nasal and retrograde intubation, and use of techniques such as percutaneous tracheostomy, cricothyroidotomy and transtracheal jet ventilation).

Supervision and assistance

Airway emergencies are situations when the patient's condition may rapidly deteriorate. If the situation allows, the patient should be moved to the best location for emergency airway interventions. Help must be summoned. Anaesthetists can assist in gaining IV access, administering drugs, setting up equipment

and managing the airway. Surgeons (gowned and standing by) can help to provide a surgical airway or perform rigid bronchoscopy to remove foreign bodies.

Anticipated versus unanticipated difficulty

Acute upper airway obstruction from a foreign body, trauma, oedema or infection is immediately apparent. If the patient has survived the journey to hospital, there will be time to provide supplemental oxygen and plan a strategy in most circumstances. Problems and catastrophes arise when the difficult airway is unanticipated, such as failure to intubate

Table 23.3 Suggested contents of a portable kit for difficult airway management

Masks
Face and nasal masks
Patil endoscopic mask[4] for oral endoscopic intubation
Airways
Oropharyngeal airways
Nasopharyngeal airways
Airway intubator[4] guide for oral endoscopic intubation
Rigid laryngoscope with a variety of designs and sizes[5]
Short handle or variable angle (Patil-Syracuse) laryngoscope
or Kessel or polio blades
Curved blades: Macintosh, Bizarri-Guiffrida
Straight blades: Miller
Tubular blade
Bent blade: Belscope[6]
Fibreoptic stylet laryngoscope or Bullard laryngoscope[7]
Endotracheal tubes of assorted size
Murphy tubes
Microlaryngoscopy tubes
Endotracheal tube stylets
Gum elastic bougie (Eschmann stylet)[8]
Malleable stylet
Tube changer/hollow tube changer (jet stylet)[9]
Lighted stylet
Fibreoptic intubation equipment
Fibreoptic endoscopes, adult and paediatric-sized
Device for emergency non-surgical airway ventilation
Transtracheal jet ventilation
Laryngeal mask airway
Combitube
Emergency surgical airway access
Percutaneous cricothyroidotomy[2]
Exhaled carbon dioxide monitor
Capnometer
Capnograph
Chemical indicator[10]
High-pressure oxygen source should be available at the airway management location
Regulated central wall O_2 pressure (Sanders-type injector)
Unregulated central wall O_2 pressure
Regulated O_2 tank pressure
Anaesthesia machine fresh gas outlet and O_2 flush valve

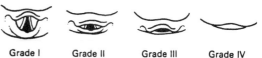

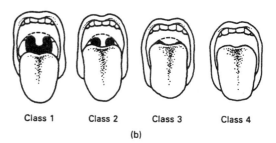

Fig. 23.1 (a) Cormack and Lehane and (b) Mallampatti visual airway classifications. From Yentis *et al.*,[67] with permission.

or mask ventilate a patient who has been given an IV hypnotic and muscle relaxant.[12]

Grading or predicting a difficult airway

Difficulty of intubation can be anticipated or predicted by the following (although many such predicted difficult patients can present with no problems):

1 anatomical or pathological features of difficult intubation (see above);
2 Cormack and Lehane classification of grade III and IV difficult intubation (Fig. 23.1)[13]
   (a) grade I – complete glottis is visible;
   (b) grade II – anterior glottis is not visible;
   (c) grade III – epiglottis but not glottis is visible;
   (d) grade IV – epiglottis is not visible.
3 Mallampatti classification of visualizing the oropharyngeal structures (Fig. 23.1)[14]
   (a) class 1 – visible soft palate, uvula, fauces and pillars
   (b) class 2 – visible soft palate, uvula and fauces;
   (c) class 3 – visible soft palate and base of uvula;
   (d) class 4 – soft palate is not visible.
4 degree of atlanto-occipital extension less than the normal 15°.[15]
5 thyromental distance with neck extended less than 6.5 cm.

Failed intubation algorithm

A preformulated plan in the event of failed intubation is essential. Failed intubation drills have been described.[15,16] The American Society of Anesthesiologists algorithm can be recommended (Fig. 23.2).[3] If the initial attempt at intubation fails, repeated attempts should be avoided unless a more experienced person takes over, or a helpful manoeuvre has been quickly carried out (e.g. repositioning, externally applied laryngeal pressure or change of laryngoscpe blade). Hypoxia will quickly result if the patient is inadequately ventilated between attempts. In addition, the oedema and bleeding caused will impair mask ventilation and the use of alternative techniques such as fibreoptic intubation.[12]

Clearing the airway

Suctioning

The airway may be obstructed by food, vomitus, blood or sputum. Suctioning may be attempted; the

Difficult airway algorithm

1 Assess the likelihood and clinical impact of basic management problems:

    (a) Difficult intubation
    (b) Difficult ventilation
    (c) Difficulty with patient cooperation or consent

2 Consider the relative merits and feasibility of basic management choices:

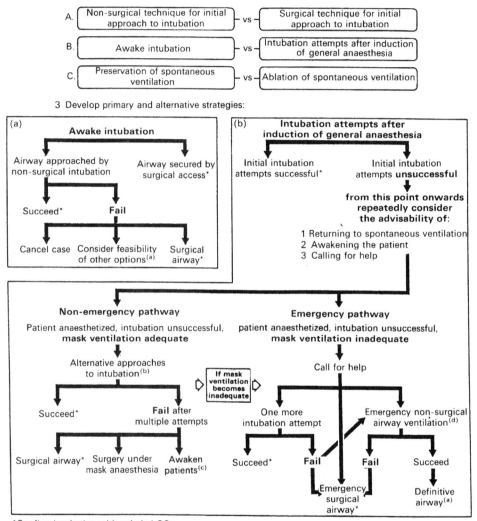

3 Develop primary and alternative strategies:

*Confirm intubation with exhaled CO_2.

(a) Other options include (but are not limited to): surgery under mask anaesthesia, surgery under local anaesthesia infiltration or regional nerve blockade, or intubation attempts after induction of general anaesthesia.

(b) Alternative approaches to difficult intubation include (but are not limited to): use of different laryngoscope blades, blind oral or nasal intubation, fibreoptic intubation, intubating stylet or tube changer, light wand, retograde intubation and surgical airway access.

(c) See awake intubation

(d) Options for emergency non-surgical airway ventilation include (but are not limited to): transtracheal jet ventilation, laryngeal mask ventilation, or oesophageal–tracheal combitube ventilation.

(e) Options for establishing a definite airway include (but are not limited to): returning to awake state with spontaneous ventilation, tracheotomy or endotracheal intubation.

Fig. 23.2 Difficult airway algorithm. From American Society of Anesthesiologists.[68] Reproduced with permission from *Anesthesiology* 1993, **78**:597–602, published by JB Lippincott Co, PA.

suction apparatus should be able to generate at least 300 mmHg (40 kPa) and 30 l/min.[17] For a given negative pressure source, the air flow will increase with the size of the suction catheter. Potential complications of suctioning include laryngospasm, vagal stimulation producing bradycardia and hypotension, mucosal injury and bleeding.[18]

Heimlich manoeuvre

Foreign body upper airway obstruction is a leading cause of death at home in young children, and is also common in the elderly. The obstruction may be infraglottic in up to two-thirds of cases.[19] In the standing or sitting conscious victim, the rescuer should attempt the Heimlich manoeuvre, i.e. application of a thrusting pressure from behind, with the arms encircling the upper abdomen (see Chapter 25). For pregnant or very obese patients, the rescuer's arms should encircle the chest instead, and a fist is placed over the mid-sternum. The unconscious victim is placed supine, and the rescuer kneels astride the patient's thighs and places the heel of one hand on the abdomen between the xiphoid process and navel, with the other hand on top of the first. The rescuer then pushes the abdomen with a quick upward thrust. Back blows are currently not recommended.[20] The Heimlich manoeuvre is used in children, but in infants back blows and chest thrusts are still recommended.[21]

Non-invasive ventilation

Bag-mask ventilation

Mask ventilation is a basic skill of airway management that nevertheless requires experience to master. The bag may be a self-inflating resuscitator or that attached to an anaesthetic circuit. Some resuscitator bags cannot deliver adequate concentrations of oxygen without a reservoir bag in series. Resuscitators with a 'soft feel' on inflation can help the operator to assess the patient's lung compliance. Ventilation with positive end-expiratory pressure (PEEP) may ameliorate airway obstruction due to laryngospasm. Many designs of facemask are available, including the anatomical mask, Trimar mask, Ambu transparent mask and Laerdal mask. The Rendell–Baker–Soucek mask is commonly used in paediatric patients.[5]

Complications of mask ventilation include the following:

1 *Inadequate ventilation:* The seal of the mask against the face may be inadequate. A beard may be covered with a large adhesive plastic dressing with a hole cut out for the mouth, or smeared with petroleum jelly or water-based lubricant. Edentulous patients may be ventilated with a Flotex multifitting mask which is fitted under the chin.[5] Two operators, one to hold the mask and the other to inflate the bag,

are recommended if a mask–face leak is excessive (see Chapter 7).

2 *Gastric insufflation* increases the risk of vomiting and aspiration. Severe distension may cause cardiovascular compromise. Cricoid pressure, first described to prevent passive regurgitation of gastric contents during induction of general anaesthesia,[22] is also effective in preventing gastric gas insufflation during mask ventilation in adults[23] and children.[24]

3 *Pulmonary aspiration:* In the emergency situation where the stomach may not be empty, mask ventilation with cricoid pressure is a temporizing measure until the airway can be secured. Passage of a nasogastric tube to aspirate gastric contents may be reasonable if time permits. However, complete emptying of gastric contents cannot be guaranteed (indeed, large food particles cannot be removed), and vomiting may be induced.

4 *Worsening upper airway foreign body obstruction –* by further impaction.

Oropharyngeal airways

Airways are adjuncts to mask ventilation. In the unconscious patient, functional obstruction may occur due to loss of pharyngeal tone and inspiratory airway narrowing at the levels of the soft palate, epiglottis and base of tongue.[25] Oropharyngeal airways may establish an adequate airway when proper head positioning is insufficient. They may be made of plastic, rubber or metal. The following sizes (length measured from flange to tip) are recommended: large adult: 100 mm (Guedel size 5); medium-sized adult: 90 mm (Guedel size 4); small adult; 80 mm (Guedel size 3).[26] It is inserted with the concavity facing the palate and then rotated 180° into the proper position as it is advanced.[27] Complications of airways include mucosal trauma and worsening of obstruction by pressing the epiglottis against the laryngeal outlet or displacing the tongue more posteriorly.

The nasopharyngeal airway is a soft rubber or plastic tube inserted into the nostril and advanced along the floor of the nose into the posterior pharynx. It is better tolerated by the semiconscious patient than the oropharyngeal airway. Complications include epistaxis and blood aspiration, laryngospasm and advancement into the oesophagus.[27]

Laryngeal mask airway (LMA)[28]

The LMA (Intravent International SA, Henley-on-Thames, UK) is a relatively recent reusable device designed as an intermediate between facemask ventilation and endotracheal intubation.[29] It consists of a silicone rubber tube connected to a distal elliptical spoon-shaped mask with an inflatable rim, which is positioned blindly into the pharynx to form a

Table 23.4 Applications of the laryngeal mask airway (LMA)

Anaesthetized/unconscious patient
Spontaneous ventilation

Positive-pressure ventilation

Guide for bougie for blind intubation with and without removal of the LMA in adults and children[31-33]

Guide for blind intubation by passage of endotracheal tube into shaft of LMA in adults and children[34,35]

Guide for fibreoptic bronchoscopic intubation[36]

In-hospital resuscitation[37]

Out-of-hospital resuscitation[38]

Awake patient
Management of failed fibreoptic intubation[39]

Aid to intubation[40]

Guide for diagnostic bronchoscopy[41]

low-pressure seal against the laryngeal inlet. There are five sizes for use in children and adults. LMAs are widely used in elective general anaesthesia, enabling spontaneous breathing and limited postitive-pressure ventilation. Positive-pressure ventilation must allow for 13–17% leak and increasing risk of gastric insufflation with increasing ventilation pressure.[30] LMAs have also been used for airway management in many emergency situations (Table 23.4)[31-41]

An LMA is prepared for insertion by deflating and smoothing out the cuffed rim to be wrinkle-free, and the posterior surface is lubricated with water-soluble jelly. The patient is positioned as for endotracheal intubation, with slight flexion of the neck and extension of the atlanto-occipital joint ('sniffing the morning air' position). The LMA is inserted with the tip of the cuff continuously applied to the hard palate, and with the right index finger guiding the tube to the back of the tongue until a firm resistance is encountered. The cuff is then inflated with 5–40 ml of air (depending on size used) before attachment of the breathing circuit.

Contraindications for using an LMA are inability to open the mouth adequately, pharyngeal pathology, airway obstruction at or below the larynx, low pulmonary compliance or high airway resistance, inadequate depth of anaesthesia, increased risk of regurgitation and one-lung ventilation. Complications include aspiration, gastric insufflation, partial airway obstruction, coughing, laryngospasm, post-extubation stridor and kinking of the shaft of the LMA. Nitrous oxide diffuses into and overinflates the cuff, which may cause displacement or obstruction.

Combitube (oesophageal–tracheal double-lumen airway)

The oesophageal–tracheal combitube (Sheridan Catheter, NY, USA) is a double-lumen tube that is blindly inserted up to the indicated markings. The oesophageal lumen has a stopper at the distal end and side perforations at the pharyngeal level while the tracheal lumen has a hole at the distal end. It has two cuffs, a distal one and a proximal pharyngeal balloon. The patient is ventilated through the oesophageal lumen initially as the combitube usually enters the oesophagus, with the distal cuff sealing the oesophagus and the proximal balloon, sealing the pharynx. Gas exits the perforations and enters the pharynx and larynx. In the event of failure of ventilation, the tracheal lumen is ventilated and the distal cuff now seals the trachea.[42] The combitube is very similar to the pharyngotracheal lumen airway, and evolved from earlier designs of the oesophageal obturator airway and oesophageal gastric tube airway. Positive-pressure ventilation compares favourably with endotracheal intubation. However, its role in resuscitation and management of the difficult airway is yet to be established.[43]

Invasive ventilation

Endotracheal intubation

The 'gold standard' of airway management is endotracheal intubation. It allows for spontaneous and positive-pressure ventilation, with good (though not absolute) protection from aspiration. Indications for tracheal intubation are:[27]

1 acute airway obstruction;
2 facilitation of tracheal suctioning;
3 protection of the airway in those without protective reflexes;
4 respiratory failure requiring ventilatory support and high inspired concentrations of oxygen.

Intubation techniques

Direct laryngoscopy

A detailed description of the technique of direct laryngoscopic intubation is beyond the scope of this chapter and may be found in textbooks of anaesthesia.[44,45] The route may be orotracheal or nasotracheal, in which case the tip may need to be directed with a Magill forceps to enter the glottis. Advantages of nasotracheal intubation include greater patient comfort and better tolerance, better tube fixation (especially in infants and children), and avoidance of tube occlusion from biting. Disadvantages of nasotracheal intubation include a requirement for a smaller tube (thus increasing airway resistance, risk of obstruction and difficulty of tracheal suctioning) and possible epistaxis, submucosal dissection and sinusitis.

The size of tracheal tubes is described by the internal

diameter in millimetres, and in the absence of obstruction, 8.0–9.0 mm in adult males and 7.0–8.0 mm in adult females are generally used. A great variety of tubes are available, the most common being a disposable Murphy type made of polyvinyl chloride with a high-volume/low-pressure cuff. Special-purpose tubes include double-lumen tubes for lung isolation, spiral embedded tubes and laser-resistant tubes. Tubes that may be useful for narrowed airways include paediatric-sized and microlaryngoscopy tracheal (MLT) tubes.[5]

Blind nasal intubation

This was used during the early days of general anaesthesia.[46] It is still a useful technique today, usually using general anaesthesia and spontaneous ventilation. In the emergency situation, blind nasal intubation can be performed with local anaesthesia. Possible indications for this technique include inability to open the mouth (e.g. mandibular fracture or temporomandibular joint pathology), cervical spine injury and faciomaxillary surgery. Absolute contraindications include bleeding disorders, nasal airway obstruction or distortion, fractured base of skull and sinusitis. The technique requires proficiency; other techniques (below) are usually preferred in difficult intubations.

Retrograde intubation

This is a technique where a wire or catheter is inserted into the cricothyroid membrane and brought up through the mouth or nose. An endotracheal tube is then threaded through it and blindly advanced through the glottis, after which the guide is removed by pulling it through the endotracheal tube.[47,48] The equipment can be assembled from readily available materials (e.g. epidural needle and catheter, IV cannulae and J wire) or available as a commercial kit.[45] As an invasive and blind technique it is less attractive than fibreoptic intubation, but is an alternative if the skill and equipment for the latter are not available.

Stylet guide

Direct laryngoscopic intubation can be difficult if the glottis cannot be visualized, even if there is no obstruction. The 'anterior larynx' can be intubated if a guide is first blindly advanced in the midline and directed anteriorly; the endotracheal tube is then railroaded over the guide. Clinical signs of tracheal placement include coughing, a resistance felt before the guide is fully advanced (due to the carina or bronchus), and a sensation of clicks from the tracheal rings. A number of guides are available, including the gum elastic bougie, tube changer and hollow tube changer. The hollow tube changer can be attached to

a side-stream capnometer, so confirming correct placement. The lighted stylet has a light at the distal end which results in a characteristic midline transillumination appearance when the light enters the larynx.[49] The Belscope (Avulunga, NSW, Australia) and Bullard (Circon ACMI, CT, USA) laryngoscopes may allow visualization of the larynx in this situation.[50]

Fibreoptic bronchoscopic intubation

This technique offers advantages of direct visualization, intubating an awake patient, use of the sitting position if required, diagnosing (and treating) upper airway obstruction,[51] not needing to move the neck, and administering supplemental oxygen during the procedure. However, experience and skill are necessary, especially for dealing with acute upper airway obstruction. Awake intubation also requires a cooperative patient, and this excludes combative and paediatric patients. Fibreoptic intubation may also be performed in anaesthetized patients, using a mouth mask for nasal intubation[52] or a modified facemask with diaphragm[4] for oral intubation. The technique may also be used in emergencies.[53] Nasal intubation is usually performed through the endotracheal tube placed in the nasopharynx, with the tip just above the glottis. The fibreoptic bronchoscope is advanced into the trachea and the tube is railroaded down. A check of correct placement is made before the scope is removed. Fibreoptic intubation orally is more difficult, as there is no guide to keep the scope in the midline. A number of oral airways are available to assist oral fibreoptic intubation.[5,54] The most common cause of failure is obstructed vision from blood or secretions.

Confirmation of tracheal tube placement

Confirming correct intratracheal tube placement is essential. After direct visualization, the most reliable method is measurement of the expired CO_2 with a capnograph. A false-positive may occur with the few breaths after oesophageal intubation (i.e. detectable P_{ECO_2}), if gastric insufflation from mask ventilation has occurred. A false-negative (decreased P_{ECO_2}) may occur with severe hypotension and low cardiac output states. Other clinical signs such as visualization of condensed water vapour, chest wall movement, auscultation of breath sounds and auscultation over the stomach are not reliable.

Complications of endotracheal intubation

These may be classified into those occurring during intubation (e.g. trauma, cardiovascular response to laryngoscopy and intubation, hypoxaemia, aspiration and oesophageal intubation), while the tube is in place (e.g. blockage, dislodgement, damage to larynx and complications of mechanical ventilation), and following extubation (e.g. aspiration and airway obstruction).

Jet ventilation[55,56]

Techniques

Transtracheal jet ventilation (TTJV)

TTJV via a percutaneous cricothyroid catheter has been proposed as a first-line technique in the 'can't intubate, can't ventilate' scenario. The maximum attainable pressure with a self-inflating resuscitation bag is 1–2 psi (6.9–13.8 kPa), requiring a 2.5 mm catheter for adequate positive pressure ventilation.[56] A high-pressure (up to 50 psi or 344 kPa) oxygen source is required for adequate ventilation through a 14–16 FG IV cannula. Ventilation occurs from bulk flow through the catheter plus air entrainment. The method of ventilation is usually manually regulated breaths (with a jet injector or anaesthesia machine flush button). The optimum rate and inspiratory: expiratory ratio is unknown. In upper airway obstruction, prolonged inspiratory time increases the risk of dynamic hyperinflation, haemodynamic compromise and barotrauma (i.e. pneumothorax and pneumomediastinum). It may be prudent to limit respiratory rate to that which will maintain adequate oxygenation, often <30/min, and accepting hypercapnia until a definitive airway is established.

Intratracheal jet ventilation

This may be achieved through a hollow jet stylet[57] or bronchoscope.[58]

High-pressure oxygen sources

The source of high-pressure oxygen may be wall outlet, tank pressure or the anaesthesia machine flush button. Wall outlet pressures should be regulated to minimize the risk of barotrauma, especially in paediatric patients. The pressure from the flush button may be inadequate in those anaesthesia machines not fitted with a check valve downstream from the vaporizers.[59]

Complications of jet ventilation

Complications are due to insertion of the IV cannula (e.g. bleeding and oesophageal perforation), ventilation (e.g. hyperinflation, barotrauma), catheter displacement (i.e. subcutaneous emphysema) and failure to protect the airway (i.e. aspiration). Relative contraindications of using jet ventilation include pathology which precludes palpation of the laryngeal anatomy, bleeding disorder and full stomach.

Surgical airways

Cricothyroidotomy

Cricothyroidotomy is an optional airway intervention in emergencies. There exist many descriptions of the technique with minor variations.[2,26,60] The simplest describes a horizontal incision over and through the cricothyroid membrane and (with the space held wide open by the scalpel handle) insertion of a small tracheostomy tube or a paediatric endotracheal tube (Fig. 23.3).[26] Commercial cricothyroidotomy sets using the Seldinger technique are available.[2] Minitracheostomy is the insertion of a small 4-mm non-cuffed tracheostomy tube (e.g. Portex Mini Trach) through the cricothyroid membrane, mainly to facilitate suctioning in patients with poor cough ability. Cricothyroidotomy or minitracheostomy are now less preferred techniques than percutaneous tracheostomy (below) in many ICUs.

Tracheostomy

The indications for tracheostomy include bypass of obstruction, access for tracheal toilet, provision for prolonged ventilatory support and protection of the airways from aspiration. Surgical tracheostomies are increasingly being replaced in the ICU by percutaneous

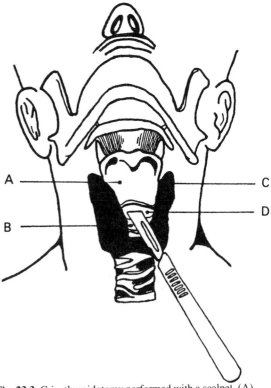

Fig. 23.3 Cricothyroidotomy performed with a scalpel. (A) Thyroid cartilage; (B) cricoid cartilage; (C) thyroid gland; (D) cricothyroid membrane, easily palpable subcutaneously.

tracheostomies performed by intensivists.[61] The endotracheal tube is first withdrawn so that its cuff lies just above the vocal cords. Under sterile conditions, a Seldinger wire is placed in the trachea through the membrane between the cricoid and the first cartilage or between the first and second cartilages. After making an adequate skin incision and using blunt dissection with forceps, a series of dilatation bougies are railroaded over the wire. A tracheostomy tube is then inserted into the trachea and the endotracheal tube removed. Complications of tracheostomy are given in Table 23.5.

Local anaesthesia

Instrumentation of the upper airway in the awake patient will require local anaesthesia to increase patient comfort, improve cooperation and chance of success, attenuate the cardiovascular response and reduce the risk of laryngospasm. There is a trend from nerve blocks (of the internal branch of the superior laryngeal nerve and the glossopharyngeal nerve) to topical administration of local anaesthetics (Table 23.6). The most commonly used local anaesthetic is lignocaine. Cocaine has been a popular choice for its vasoconstrictor properties, but it is toxic and its supply is regulated. Systemic absorption of topically applied lignocaine (maximum dose 3 mg/kg) is variable, and the clinician should be alert for signs and symptoms of toxicity.

Table 23.5 Complications of tracheostomy

Immediate
Procedural complications such as haemorrhage, surgical emphysema, pneumothorax, air embolism and cricoid cartilage damage

Accidental disconnection

Misplacement in pretracheal tissues or right main bronchus

Compression of tube by cuff herniation

Occlusion of the tip against the carina or tracheal wall

Delayed
Blockage with secretions

Infection of the tracheostome or the tracheobronchial tree

Distension of trachea with high-pressure cuffs, proceeding to ulceration and possible rupture

Mucosal ulceration caused by the tip

Deep erosion leading to bleeding from the innominate artery or development of a tracheo-oesophageal fistula

Late
Granulomata of the trachea

Persistent sinus at tracheostomy site

Tracheomalacia and tracheal dilatation

Tracheal stenosis

References

1 Benumof JL (1991) Management of the difficult adult airway. *Anesthesiology* **75**:1087–1110.
2 Bainton CR (1994) Cricothyrotomy. In: Bainton CR (ed.) *International Anesthesiology Clinics: New Concepts in Airway Management*, vol. 32. Boston: Little, Brown, pp. 95–108.
3 Task Force on Guidelines for Management of the Difficult Airway (1993) Practice guidelines for management of the difficult airway. *Anesthesiology* **78**:597–602.
4 Patil V, Stehling LC, Zauder HL and Koch JP (1982) Mechanical aids for fibreoptic endoscopy (letter). *Anesthesiology* **57**:69–70.
5 Dorsch JA and Dorsch SE (1994) *Understanding*

Table 23.6 Local anaesthesia of the upper airway in adults

Technique	Drug dosage
Nerve block[62]	
Internal branch of superior laryngeal nerve	Lignocaine 1% (2 ml/side)
Glossopharyngeal nerve	Lignocaine 1% (3 ml/side)
Topical anaesthesia of the tongue and oropharynx	
Gargle	Lignocaine viscous 4% (5 ml)
Spray	Lignocaine 10% (5–10 sprays = 50–100 mg)
Topical anaesthesia of the nasal mucosa	
Cocaine spray or paste[63]	Cocaine 4% (0.5 ml)
Gel[64]	Lignocaine 2% gel (5 ml)
Lignocaine spray[64]	Lignocaine 10% (10 sprays = 100 mg)
Lignocaine + phenylephrine spray[63]	Lignocaine 3% + phenylephrine 0.25% (0.5 ml)
Topical anaesthesia of glottis and trachea	
Spray-as-you-go through bronchoscope[65]	Lignocaine 1–4% (3 mg/kg)
Cricothyroid membrane puncture[65]	Lignocaine 2% (5 ml)
Nebulized[66]	Lignocaine 4% (4 ml) ± phenylephrine 1% (1 ml)

Anesthesia Equipment, 3rd edn. Baltimore: Williams & Wilkins.

6 Bellhouse CP (1988) An angulated laryngoscope for routine and difficult tracheal intubation. *Anesthesiology* **69**:126–129.

7 Cooper SD, Benumof JL and Ozaki GT (1994) Evaluation of the Bullard laryngoscope using the new intubating stylet: comparison with conventional laryngoscopy. *Anesth Analg* **79**:965–970.

8 McCarroll SM, Lamont BJ, Buckland MR and Yates APB (1988) The gum-elastic bougie: old but still useful (letter). *Anesthesiology* **68**:643–644.

9 Bedger RC and Chang JL (1987) A jet-stylet endotracheal catheter for difficult airway management. *Anesthesiology* **66**:221–223.

10 Bogdonoff DL and Stone DJ (1992) Emergency management of the airway outside the operating room. *Can J Anaesth* **39**:1069–1089.

11 Latto IP (1985) Management of difficult intubation. In: Latto IP and Rosen M (eds) *Difficulties in Tracheal Intubation.* London: Ballliere Tindall, pp. 99–141.

12 Benumof JL (1994) Management of the difficult airway: the ASA algorithm. American Society of Anesthesiologists: 45th Annual Refresher Course Lectures, Oct 15–19. San Francisco: American Society of Anesthesiologists.

13 Cormack RS and Lehane J (1984) Difficult tracheal intubation in obstetrics. *Anaesthesia* **39**:1105–1111.

14 Mallampati SR, Gugino LD, Desai SP and Freiberger D (1985) A clinical sign to predict difficult tracheal intubation: a prospective study. *Can J Anaesth* **32**:429–434.

15 Tunstall ME (1976) Failed intubation drill. *Anaesthesia* **31**:850.

16 Roberts TJ (1983) *Fundamentals of Tracheal Intubation.* New York: Grune & Stratton.

17 Safar P and Bircher NG (1988) *Cardiopulmonary Cerebral Resuscitation,* 3rd edn. Philadelphia: WB Saunders Co.

18 Daya M, Mariani R and Fernandes C (1992) Basic life support. In: Dailey RH, Simon B, Young GP and Stewart RD (eds) *The Airway: Emergency Management.* St Louis: Mosby Year Book, pp. 39–61.

19 Cox GR and Shepherd SM (1992) Acute upper airway obstruction and mediastinal disorders. In: Schwartz GR, Cayten CG, Mangelsen MA, Mayer TA and Hanke BK (eds) *Principles and Practice of Emergency Medicine.* Philadelphia: Lea & Febiger, pp. 500–512.

20 Emergency Cardiac Care Committee and Subcommittees, American Heart Association (1992) Guidelines for cardiopulmonary resuscitation and emergency cardiac care, II: adult basic life support. *J Am Med Assoc* **268**:2184–2198.

21 Emergency Cardiac Care Committee and Subcommittees, American Heart Association (1992) Guidelines for cardiopulmonary resuscitation and emergency cardiac care, V: pediatric basic life support. *J Am Med Assoc* **268**:2251–2261.

22 Sellick BA (1961) Cricoid pressure to control regurgitation of stomach contents during induction of anaesthesia. *Lancet* **2**:404–406.

23 Petito SP and Russell WJ (1988) The prevention of gastric insufflation: a neglected benefit of cricoid pressure. *Anaesth Intens Care* **16**:139–143.

24 Moynihan RJ, Brock-Utne JG, Archer JH, Feld LH and Kreitzman TR (1993) The effect of cricoid pressure on preventing gastric insufflation in infants and children. *Anesthesiology* **78**:652–656.

25 Shorten GD, Opie NJ, Graziotti P, Morris I and Khangure M (1994) Assessment of upper airway anatomy in awake, sedated, and anaesthetised patients using magnetic resonance imaging. *Anaesth Intens Care* **22**:165–169.

26 Albarran-Sotelo R, Anderson M, Atkins JM *et al.* (1990) *Textbook of Advanced Cardiac Life Support,* 2nd edn. Dallas: American Heart Association.

27 Kaur S, Heard SO and Welch GW (1991) Airway management and endotracheal intubation. In: Rippe JM, Irwin RS, Alpert JS and Fink MP (eds) *Intensive Care* airway management. *Br J Anaesth* **55**:801–805.

28 Pennant JH and White PF (1993) The laryngeal mask airway: its uses in anesthesiology. *Anesthesiology* **79**:44–163.

29 Brain AIJ (1983) The laryngeal mask: a new concept in airway management. *British Journal of Anaesthesia* **55**:801–805.

30 Devitt JH, Wenstone R, Noel AG and O'Donnell MP (1994) The laryngeal mask airway and positive-pressure ventilation. *Anesthesiology* **80**:550–555.

31 Allison A and McCrory J (1990) Tracheal placement of a gum elastic bougie using the laryngeal mask airway (letter). *Anaesthesia* **45**:419–420.

32 Brimacombe J and Johns K (1991) Modified intravent LMA (letter). *Anaesth Intens Care* **19**:607.

33 Chadd GD, Crane DL, Phillips RM and Tunell WP (1992) Extubation and reintubation guided by the laryngeal mask airway in a child with the Pierre–Robin syndrome. *Anesthesiology* **76**:640–641.

34 Heath ML and Allagain J (1991) Intubation through the laryngeal mask: a technique for unexpected difficult intubation. *Anaesthesia* **46**:545–548.

35 White AP and Billingham IM (1992) Laryngeal mask guided tracheal intubation in paediatric anaesthesia (letter). *Paed Anaesth* **2**:265.

36 McNamee CJ, Meyns B and Pagliero KM (1991) Flexible bronchoscopy via the laryngeal mask: a new technique. *Thorax* **46**:141–142.

37 Bogetz MS (1994) The laryngeal mask airway – role in managing the difficult airway. In: Bainton CR (ed.) *International Anesthesiology Clinics: New Concepts in Airway Management,* vol. 32, Boston: Little, Brown, pp. 109–117.

38 Pennant JH and Walker MB (1992) Comparison of the endotracheal tube and laryngeal mask in airway management by paramedical personnel. *Anesth Analg* **74**:531–534.

39 Williams PJ and Bailey PM (1993) Management of failed oral fibreoptic intubation with laryngeal mask airway insertion under topical anaesthesia (letter). *Can J Anaesth* **40**:287.

40 Asai T (1992) Use of the laryngeal mask for tracheal intubation in patients at risk of aspiration of gastric

contents. *Anesthesiology* **77**:1029–1030.

41 Brimacombe J, Newell S, Swainston R and Thompson J (1992) A potential new technique for awake fibreoptic bronchoscopy – use of the laryngeal mask airway. *Med J Aust* **156**:876–877.

42 Frass M, Frenzer R, Rauscha F, Weber H, Pacher R and Leithner C (1986) Evaluation of esophageal tracheal combitube in cardiopulmonary resuscitation. *Crit Care Med* **15**:609–611.

43 Pepe PE, Zachariah BS and Chandra NC (1993) Invasive airway techniques in resuscitation. *Ann Emerg Med* **22**:393–403.

44 Otto CW (1989) Tracheal intubation. In: Nunn JF, Utting JE and Brown BR (eds) *General Anaesthesia*. London: Butterworths, pp. 512–539.

45 Stone DJ and Gal TJ (1994) Airway management. In: Miller RD (ed.) *Anesthesia*. New York: Churchill Livingstone, pp. 1403–1435.

46 Magill I (1930) Technique in endotracheal anaesthesia. *Br Med J* **2**:817.

47 Purcell T (1992) Retrograde tracheal intubation. In: Dailey RH, Simon B, Young GP and Stewart RD (eds) *The Airway: Emergency Management*. St Louis: Mosby Year Book, pp. 135–143.

48 McNamara RM (1987) Retrograde intubation of the trachea. *Ann Emerg Med* **16**:680–682.

49 Stewart R (1992) Lighted stylet. In: Dailey RH, Simon B, Young GP and Stewart RD (eds) *The Airway: Emergency Management*. St Louis: Mosby Year Book, pp. 115–121.

50 Good ML (1994) Airway gadgets. American Society of Anesthesiologists: 45th Annual Refresher Course Lectures, Oct 15–19. San Francisco: American Society of Anesthesiologists.

51 Giudice JC, Komansky H, Gordon R and Kaufman JL (1981) Acute upper airway obstruction – fibreoptic bronchoscopy in diagnosis and therapy. *Crit Care Med* **9**:878–879.

52 Nagaro T, Hamami G, Takasaki Y and Arai T (1993) Ventilation via a mouth mask facilitates fibreoptic nasal tracheal intubation in anesthetized patients (letter). *Anesthesiology* **78**:603–604.

53 Afilalo M, Guttman A, Stern E *et al.* (1993) Fibreoptic intubation in the emergency department: a case series. *J Emerg Med* **11**:387–391.

54 Rogers SN and Benumof JL (1983) New and easy techniques for fibreoptic endoscopy-aided tracheal intubation. *Anesthesiology* **59**:569–572.

55 Benumof JL and Scheller MS (1989) The importance of transtracheal jet ventilation in the management of the difficult airway. *Anesthesiology* **71**:769–778.

56 Neff CC, Pfister RC and Van Sonnenberg E (1983) Percutaneous transtracheal ventilation: experimental and practical aspects. *J Trauma* **23**:84–90.

57 Gaughan SD, Benumof JL and Ozaki GT (1992) Quantification of the jet junction of a jet stylet. *Anesth Analg* **74**:580–585.

58 Satyanarayana T, Capan L, Ramanathan S, Chalon J and Turndorf H (1980) Bronchofiberscopic jet ventilation. *Anesth Analg* **59**:350–354.

59 Gaughan SD, Benumof JL and Ozaki GT (1993) Can an anesthesia machine flush valve provide for effective jet ventilation? *Anesth Analg* **76**:800–808.

60 Kress TD and Balasubramaniam S (1982) Crico-thyroidotomy. *Ann Emerg Med* **11**:197–201.

61 Silva WE and Hughes J (1991) Tracheotomy. In: Rippe JM, Irwin RS, Alpert JS and Fink MP (eds) *Intensive Care Medicine*. Boston: Little, Brown, pp. 169–182.

62 Murrin KR (1985) Awake intubation. In: Latto IP and Rosen M (eds) *Difficulties in Tracheal Intubation*. London: Ballière Tindall, pp. 90–98.

63 Gross JB, Hartigan M and Schaffer DW (1984) A suitable substitute for 4% cocaine before blind nasotracheal intubation: 3% lidocaine–0.25% phenylephrine nasal spray. *Anesth Analg* **63**:915–918.

64 Zainudin BMZ, Rafia MH and Sufarlan AW (1993) Topical nasal anaesthesia for fibreoptic bronchoscopy: lignocaine spray or gel? *Sing Med J* **34**:148–149.

65 Webb AR, Fernando SSD, Dalton HR, Arrowsmith JE, Woodhead MA and Cummin ARC (1990) Local anaesthesia for fibreoptic bronchoscopy: transcricoid injection or the 'spray as you go' technique? *Thorax* **45**:474–477.

66 Bourke DL, Katz J and Tonneson A (1985) Nebulized anesthesia for awake endotracheal intubation. *Anesthesiology* **63**:690–692.

67 Yentis SM, Hirsch NP and Smith GB (1993) *Anaesthesia A to Z*. Oxford: Butterworth-Heinemann.

68 American Society of Anesthesiologists (1993) Practice guidelines for management of the difficult airway. *Anesthesiology* **78**:602.

24 · Acute respiratory failure in chronic obstructive airways disease

DV Tuxen

The terms chronic obstructive airways/pulmonary disease (COAD, COPD) apply to patients with reduced expiratory airflow due to chronic bronchitis and/or emphysema. Respiratory reserve is reduced, and superimposed acute respiratory failure (ARF) has significant morbidity and mortality. COAD affects about 5% of the population, and is the only major cause of death increasing in prevalence.[1] However, most precipitating factors of ARF are reversible, and aggressive management is frequently justified.[2]

Precipitants of acute respiratory failure

.A wide variety of factors may precipitate ARF in COAD patients.

Airway infection

Acute bronchitis without pneumonia is the most common precipitant, accounting for 50% of presentations requiring conventional mechanical ventilation (CMV).[3] *Streptococcus pneumoniae* and *Haemophilus influenzae* are isolated in 80% of exacerbations,[4] but *S. viridans*,[5] *Moraxella* (previously *Branhamella*) *catarrhalis*,[6] *Mycoplasma pneumoniae*,[7] and *Pseudomonas aeruginosa* may be found. Viruses are isolated in 20–30% of exacerbations,[7] including rhinovirus, influenza and parainfluenza, corona, adenovirus, and respiratory syncytial virus. Whether these organisms are pathogens or colonizers is often unclear.

Pneumonia

Pneumonia accounts for 20% of presentations requiring CMV,[3] and is most commonly caused by *S. pneumoniae* and *H. influenzae* but *Mycoplasma*, *Legionella*, enteric Gram-negatives and viruses are occasional causes.

Sputum retention

Sputum retention may complicate COAD following elective or emergency surgery, trauma (particularly chest trauma) or any illness reducing conscious state. The primary problem is failure of coughing to remove the increased respiratory secretions in COAD.

Left ventricular (LV) failure

This may result from ischaemic heart disease,[8] fluid overload or biventricular failure secondary to cor pulmonale. Pulmonary congestion can be difficult to diagnose because of the abnormal breath sounds and chest X-ray appearance commonly present in COAD. Lungs affected with COAD are very sensitive to LV failure and ARF may be precipitated even without pulmonary oedema on chest X-ray.

Pulmonary embolism

Pulmonary embolism is not a common cause of ARF in COAD, although it is found in 20–50% of autopsies of COAD patients.[9,10] It causes hypoxia and dyspnoea, but haemoptysis and pleuritic pain are less frequent in patients with COAD.[11]

Pneumothoraces and bullae

Although the risk of pneumothorax is increased in COAD, it occurrs in only 0.3% of COAD patients regularly attending hospital.[12] Large bullae may expand within the lung and precipitate ARF similar to pneumothorax. Subpleural bullae must not be mistaken for pneumothoraces, as placement of an intercostal catheter in a bullus may cause a bronchopleural fistula.

Uncontrolled oxygen administration

This may precipitate acute hypercarbia in a small proportion of patients with more severe COAD, especially those with chronic hypercarbia. Removal of the hypoxic drive to respiration is only a partial explanation. Major factors appear to be dissociation of CO_2 from haemoglobin by O_2 (Haldane effect) and worsening of V/Q mismatch.[13] The latter is probably due to reduced hypoxic vasoconstriction in areas of shunt, allowing more CO_2-rich venous blood into the arterial circulation.

Sedation

Sedation can readily precipitate hypoventilation in severe COAD with resulting hypercarbia and hypoxia. Respiratory failure may persist because of concurrent sputum retention.

Other factors

Non-compliance with medication and bronchospasm may also precipitate ARF. Asthma may cause or coexist with COAD; COAD may cause increased bronchial reactivity in some patients. Coincidental conditions such as aspiration, pleural effusion, upper airway obstruction, myopathy, poor nutrition and mineral deficiency may all precipitate or contribute to ARF.

End-stage lung disease

COAD is progressive (Fig. 24.1) and may ultimately lead to disability and death.[14] End-stage patients present with apparent ARF from absent or trivial precipitating factors. Careful assessment will determine decisions regarding extent of therapy.

Pathophysiology

Reduced expiratory airflow in COAD is due to increased airway resistance and reduced lung elastic recoil (which drives expiratory airflow). Airway resistance is increased by mucosal oedema and hypertrophy, secretions, bronchospasm, airway tortuosity and turbulence, and loss of lung parenchymal elastic tissues supporting small airways. Reduced lung elastic recoil pressure results from loss of lung elastin and alveolar surface tension from alveolar wall destruction.[15] Forced expiration increases alveolar driving pressure, but also causes dynamic airway compression, resulting in no flow improvement. Airflow limitation results in dyspnoea, prolonged expiration, pulmonary hyperinflation and increased work of breathing.

Pulmonary capillary bed loss from alveolar destruction and pulmonary artery (PA) vasoconstriction from hypoxia lead to pulmonary hypertension, secondary vascular changes and, ultimately, cor pulmonale. Increased hypoxia during ARF increases PA pressure[16] and may precipitate acute right heart failure. The combination of airway obstruction, parenchymal disease and pulmonary circulatory disturbance leads to extensive V/Q mismatching. The resultant hypoxaemia may cause secondary polycythaemia and worsen pulmonary hypertension. Shunting also causes arterial hypercarbia, which is normally corrected by increasing minute ventilation. Increased dead space also increases ventilatory requirements for normocarbia and the work of breathing. Since expiration is always incomplete, there is permanent dynamic hyperinflation of the lung (see

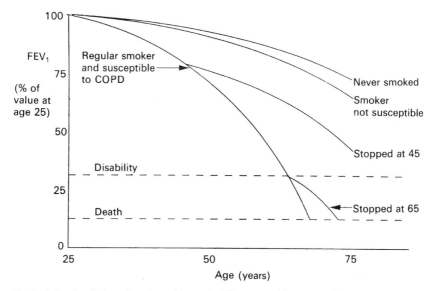

Fig. 24.1 Decline in lung function with age in different smoking categories.
FEV_1 = Forced expiratory volume in 1 s; COPD = chronic obstructive pulmonary disease.

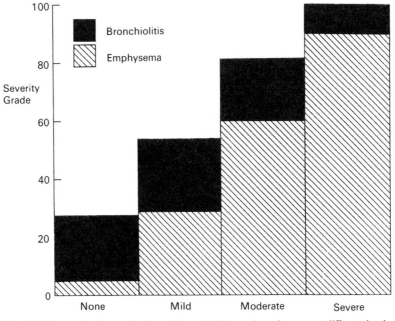

Fig. 24.2 Proportional contributions of bronchiolitis and emphysema at different levels of severity of lung disease

Chapter 32). As lung volume is increased, the respiratory muscles become less efficient, because of shortened fibre length and mechanical disadvantage. When muscle capacity fails to meet increased ventilatory requirements, hypercarbia ensues. Chronic hypercarbia is uncommon in COAD, tends to occur late, and is associated with renal acid–base compensation. It is usually seen in COAD with $FEV_1 < 1.0$ l[17] and is associated with polycythaemia, cor pulmonale and worsening hypercarbia with uncontrolled O_2 administration.

Chronic bronchitis or emphysema

The value of specifying these two diagnoses is uncertain, as they usually coexist, and the principles of management are similar. Indeed, major pathophysiological processes are present to varying degrees in each patient with COAD.[18] Also, pathological components depend more on the stage of the disease than the inherent susceptibility of the patient.[14] Early/mild COAD tends to be dominated by bronchiolitis, with minimal emphysema (Fig. 24.2), whereas the reverse is true with severe COAD. However, recognition that COAD is dominated by one of these patterns is helpful with regard to clinical pattern and prognosis.

Simple chronic bronchitis is common in regular smokers, and is characterized by chronic productive cough without airflow limitation. Only about 15% of regular smokers will develop COAD, possibly because of genetic predisposition.[14] Patients with COAD

dominated by chronic bronchitis have chronic cough, large sputum production, wheeze, fluctuating dyspnoea, and V/Q mismatch. They are thus more prone to hypercarbia, secondary polycythaemia, pulmonary hypertension, cyanosis and cor pulmonale (hence the label 'blue bloaters'). Infection-induced exacerbations present earlier in the course of the disease, which is characterized by exacerbations and remissions.

Patients whose COAD is dominated by emphysema have a more constant level of dyspnoea, with less cough, sputum and wheeze. The pulmonary parenchyma is primarily affected, with alveolar wall loss. V/Q relationships are better preserved than in chronic bronchitis. With less shunting, increased respiratory effort in response to increased ventilatory requirements can nomalize blood gases (hence the label 'pink puffers'). The course is characterized by gradually increasing dyspnoea. Thus patients with emphysema presenting with ARF are often closer to end-stage lung disease than those with chronic bronchitis.

Clinical features

ARF in COAD can present with two distinct clinical patterns.[19]

Increasing dyspnoea ('can't breathe' pattern)

This is the more common presentation, and results from precipitating factors which primarily impair airflow or gas exchange without impairing respiratory drive. There is inability to achieve adequate ventilation despite a maximum ventilatory effort. Dyspnoea, increased sputum production, cough, tachypnoea, use of accessory respiratory muscles and pursed lip breathing are present. Cyanosis and pulmonary hyperinflation may be evident. Rhonchi and expiratory wheeze are usually audible. A loud pulmonary component of the second heart sound, right ventricular (RV) heave, elevated jugular venous pressure and peripheral oedema indicate pulmonary hypertension and cor pulmonale. In severe cases, right heart failure is accompanied by tricuspid incompetence. Signs of consolidation may be present.

Respiratory muscle fatigue is accompanied by a fall in minute ventilation and a further rise in Pa_{CO_2}. As fatigue progresses, abnormal breathing patterns may emerge – abdominal/ribcage breathing (respiratory alternans) or abdominal indrawing during inspiration (abdominal paradox).[20,21] Features of CO_2 retention may become evident (i.e. obtundation, warm dilated periphery, bounding pulse and sweating). Fatigue, abnormal breathing patterns and increasing hypercarbia herald impending respiratory collapse.

Decreasing dyspnoea ('won't breathe' pattern)

This occurs from precipitating factors which primarily impair respiratory drive. It must be differentiated from the advanced stages of the 'can't breathe' pattern. The primary problem is increasing hypercarbia and respiratory acidosis with no increase in dyspnoea. However, sputum retention and V/Q mismatch usually contribute to the hypercarbia. Dominant features are a depressed conscious state and the blood gas abnormalities – increased Pa_{CO_2}, acidaemia and a small decrease in Pa_{O_2}. As respiratory failure worsens, cyanosis, sputum retention, decreasing consciousness, and signs of hypercarbia become apparent.

Diagnosis and assessment

Diagnosis of COAD

The diagnosis of COAD is based on:

1 history of smoking and/or other causative factors;
2 chronic cough and sputum production;
3 long-standing dyspnoea with or without wheeze;
4 lung function tests demonstrating largely irreversible airflow obstruction (see Chapter 97):
   (a) *Spirometry* shows a reduced FEV_1 vital capacity (VC) ratio and minimal response to bronchodilators. VC is initially normal, and decreases later in the disease but less than FEV_1.
   (b) *Flow–volume graphs* demonstrate reduced expiratory flow rates at various lung volumes.
   (c) *Lung volumes* show elevated total lung volume, functional residual capacity and residual volume.

(d) *Carbon monoxide uptake* reflects alveolar surface area; reduction approximates the degree of emphysema. It may be normal or near normal in pure chronic bronchitis.

Assessment of respiratory failure

Arterial blood gases (ABGs)

Chronic hypercarbia is recognized by a bicarbonate concentration > 30 mmol/l and a base excess > 4 mmol/l. Renal compensation to return pH to normal will increase serum bicarbonate by approximately 4 mmol/l for each 10 mmHg (1.33 kPa) of chronic P_{CO_2} rise above 40 mmHg (5.3 kPa). An acute increase in Pa_{CO_2} with a decreased arterial pH indicates that compensatory mechanisms are exhausted.

Spirometry

Spirometry or peak expiratory flow should be performed if possible. It will indicate severity of illness and deterioration, and provide a baseline measurement for subsequent assessments.

Chest X-ray

Chest X-ray is mandatory to diagnose or exclude pneumothorax, collapse, pneumonia or LV failure. It will commonly show hyperinflated lung fields, flattened diaphragms and a paucity of lung markings. Pulmonary hypertension is manifested by enlarged proximal and attenuated distal vascular markings, and by RV and right atrial enlargement. Lung bullae may be evident.

Electrocardiogram (ECG)

ECG is commonly normal but may show right atrial or ventricular hypertrophy and right ventricular (RV) strain. These changes may be chronic or acute. The ECG may also show coexistent ischaemic heart disease.

Sputum microscopy and culture

Sputum samples in COAD will usually culture the causative organism and provide a guide to antibiotic therapy.

Full blood count

Polycythaemia may be present. An elevated white cell count may occur with steroid therapy or infection (indicated by a 'left shift' in neutrophils).

Theophylline assays

Serum theophylline concentrations should be performed on patients receiving theophylline derivatives.

Differential diagnosis

It is important to diagnose or exclude the less common causes of ARF in COAD which require specific therapy.

1 *Left ventricular failure:* Minor degrees of pulmonary oedema and pulmonary venous congestion may precipitate ARF in a severely compromised lung without clinical or radiological features of pulmonary oedema. Comparison with previous films is important. A trial of diuretics may be indicated.
2 *Pulmonary embolism:* Pulmonary embolism should be suspected in any unexplained deterioration.
3 *Pneumothorax.*
4 *Upper airway obstruction:* Unrecognized upper airway obstruction from any cause may precipitate ARF in patients with COAD. Unexplained deterioration, stridor or voice alteration may provide clues.

Management

Oxygen therapy

Most COAD patients will not develop CO_2 retention with oxygen administration, but this is more common in those with severe COAD who present with ARF.[22–24] While high levels of O_2 should be avoided, reversal of hypoxia is important, and O_2 should not be withheld in the presence of hypercarbia nor withdrawn if it worsens. Oxygen given by low-flow intranasal cannulae or 24–35% Venturi mask[22] should be titrated to achieve a saturation (Sao_2) 90–92%. Increases in $Paco_2$ are most common in patients with initial $Pao_2 > 50$ mmHg (6.7 kPa) and pH < 7.35.[22] If the rise in $Paco_2$ is excessive (> 10 mmHg or 1.33 kPa), O_2 delivery should be reduced, titrating Sao_2 to 2–3% below the previous value, and ABGs repeated. If no $Paco_2$ rise occurs, a higher Sao_2 may be targeted with repeat blood gases. Inadequate reversal of hypoxia (e.g. $Sao_2 < 85\%$) is suggestive of a larger shunt (e.g. from pneumonia, pulmonary oedema, embolus or pneumothorax). Investigation of this should commence and a higher O_2 delivery system should be used (see Chapter 22).

Bronchodilators

Bronchodilators are routinely given in all exacerbations of COAD because a small reversible component of airflow obstruction is common, and bronchodilators improve mucociliary clearance of secretions.[25]

1 Anticholinergic agents should be used routinely in COAD with ARF,[14,18] as they have a similar or greater bronchodilator action than β-agonists[26–28] with fewer side-effects and no tachyphylaxis. Ipratropium bromide 0.5 mg in 2 ml is nebulized initially 2-hourly, then every 4–6 h.

2 β-Agonists may cause tachycardia, tremor, mild reductions in potassium and Pao_2 (due to pulmonary vasodilatation),[29] and tachyphylaxis. Nebulized β-agonists (e.g. salbutamol, terbutaline or fenoterol) given 2–4 hourly should be used routinely in combination with ipratropium. This combination is more effective than either agent alone.[27] Parenteral β-agonists are rarely indicated and not recommended for routine use.

3 Aminophylline is a less potent bronchodilator in COAD. Reports of benefits are conflicting.[30,31] The clinical importance of other effects of theophylline (e.g. mild respiratory stimulant and improved diaphragm contractility and mucociliary transport) is unestablished.[32–36] Aminophylline (loading dose 5.6 mg/kg IV over 30 min followed by an infusion of 0.5 mg/kg per h) is commonly given. Serum theophylline levels must be monitored regularly, targeting the low therapeutic range (55–85 μmol/l).[37] The high therapeutic range (85–110 μmol/l) thought necessary for diaphragm contractility and respiratory stimulation effects has little additional benefit and significantly more side-effects.[37]

Steroids

Only 10–20% of patients with stable COAD respond to steroids,[18] but short-term administration improves airflow obstruction in exacerbations[38] and ventilated patients.[39] Steroids should be given, except in cases of bacterial pneumonia. Doses similar to those for acute asthma should be used.

Antibiotics

Antibiotics have an accepted role in the treatment of infection-induced exacerbations of COAD.[40] Amoxycillin is a suitable first-line agent against *Haemophilus influenzae* and *Streptococcus pneumoniae* for outpatient exacerbations.[40] Serious exacerbations requiring hospital admission require newer agents such as ciprofloxacin[41] or a third-generation cephalosporin.[40] Antibiotics for pneumonia are discussed in Chapters 33 and 64.

Secretion clearance

Clearance of lower respiratory secretions is of crucial importance. Chest physiotherapy is discussed in Chapter 4. The benefits of nebulized mucolytic agents (e.g. acetylcysteine) are unproven. Fibreoptic bronchoscopy is indicated if a sputum plug is suspected to cause lobar consolidation, and for bronchoalveolar lavage. Although effective in clearing sputum, it is labour-intensive and poorly tolerated by a patient with ARF. A minitracheostomy tube (4.0 mm Portex Mini-Trach) inserted through the cricothyroid membrane allows suctioning using a fine-bore catheter, but is relatively ineffective at removing tenacious secretions and may partially occlude the airway.

Other measures

Diuretics and digoxin are beneficial if LV failure is present. Even if LV failure is minimal, a trial of diuresis is worthwhile in patients refractory to usual treatment. Digoxin improves LV function in patients with cor pulmonale[42] (but not RV function if the primary problem is increased afterload).[43] Diuretics will reduce fluid overload in cor pulmonale, but if pulmonary hypertension is severe, a decrease in RV filling pressure may result in a low-output state. Pulmonary vasodilators may ameliorate pulmonary hypertension in stable COAD,[44] but outcome is not improved.[45] Although unproven, they have a rational basis in ARF, as pulmonary hypertension is associated with a poor prognosis. Calcium-channel blockers appear to be most promising.[44]

Hypophosphataemia,[46] hypomagnesaemia,[47] hypocalcaemia,[48] and hypokalaemia may impair respiratory muscle function, and must be corrected. Adequate nutrition is important. Excessive carbohydrate calories should be avoided, as this increases CO_2 production.

Respiratory stimulants have not been shown to improve short-term or long-term outcome, and are not generally recommended. Doxapram may have limited application in the 'won't breathe' group. Opioid or benzodiazepine-induced respiratory depression is best managed with their antagonists naloxone or flumazenil.

Mechanical ventilatory support

Justification of ventilation

Mechanical ventilatory support may be withheld in end-stage lung disease, when low survival, poor quality of life or permanent ventilator dependence is likely. Lifestyle[3] and dyspnoea[49] categories may be the most useful factors when deciding to withhold ventilation. Lifestyle categories 3 (housebound and at least partly dependent) and 4 (bed- or chair-bound) indicate both a poor outcome (Fig. 24.3)[3] and a quality of life that may not justify aggressive treatment. Withholding ventilation should be based on the patient fulfilling these criteria:

1 known severe COAD which has failed to respond to adequate therapy;
2 severe limitation by dyspnoea with a poor quality of life;
3 no identifiable reversible factors (e.g. pneumonia, sputum retention or LV failure).

If in doubt, a trial of CMV is undertaken and subsequently withdrawn if unsuccessful. Most COAD patients who present with ARF do not have end-stage disease. Although their immediate problems may be life-threatening, their short-term outcome is sufficiently good to justify full active treatment.

Indications for mechanical ventilation

Hypercarbia or acidosis alone are not indications for CMV, as they can be sustained for some time without respiratory collapse. As with acute asthma, institution of CMV is based on a number of criteria:

1 clinical appearance of fatigue and impending respiratory collapse;
2 increasing $Paco_2$ unrelated to O_2 administration, despite adequate conservative treatment;
3 deteriorating conscious state due to fatigue or hypercarbia or both;
4 hypoxia refractory to high levels of inspired O_2;
5 deterioration due to failure of sputum clearance;
6 respiratory arrest

Non-invasive ventilatory assistance (NIVA)

NIVA may be continuous positive airways pressure (CPAP) alone or in combination with pressure- or volume-supported inspiration. This may be delivered by a ventilator or a specific device (e.g. BiPAP, Respironics, USA) to an occlusive nasal or facemask.

CPAP alone can reduce the work of breathing in COAD during weaning[50] and during sleep.[51] However, pressure support or volume-controlled NIVA offers greater support, and has become the preferred option. Improvements in Pao_2, $Paco_2$ and a reduced requirement for intubated CMV have been reported.[52–54] NIVA may also be tried when CMV is considered inappropriate. Pressure support levels of 10–20 cm $H_2O \pm 3$–7 cm H_2O CPAP are common settings.

CMV

Goals of CMV in COAD are first to support ventilation while reversible components improve, second, to allow respiratory muscle to rest and recover but without wasting; and third, to minimize dynamic hyperinflation. These are accomplished by using low tidal volumes, low minute ventilation and long expiratory times in synchronized intermittent mandatory ventilation mode. Tidal volumes of 8–10 ml/kg are recommended.[55,56] Although controversial, use of a high inspiratory flow rate results in a short inspiratory time, and hence a longer expiratory time for a given ventilatory rate. It has been shown to reduce dynamic hyperinflation and alveolar pressure,[55] and improve gas exchange.[57] Minute ventilation $\leqslant 115$ ml/kg is a guideline.[55] If a higher minute ventilation is required for excessive hypercapnic acidosis, the degree of dynamic hyperinflation and its effects should be determined beforehand. If excessive dynamic hyperinflation causes circulatory compromise or presents a barotrauma risk, minute ventilation should not be increased. Hypercapnic acidosis is accepted, and spontaneous ventilation (which increases dynamic hyperinflation) is discouraged by heavy sedation. Muscle relaxants should be avoided unless essential. Positive end-expiratory pressure (PEEP) increases pulmonary hyperinflation, and should not be applied during controlled ventilation.[58] If dynamic hyperinflation is not excessive, spontaneous ventilation should be encouraged. Flow-by, pressure support and low-level CPAP may reduce the work of spontaneous breathing and promote a better ventilatory pattern. A CPAP level approximately equal to that of intrinsic PEEP is most commonly recommended.[59] These strategies must be used cautiously, as each can increase dynamic hyperinflation; flow-by increases resistance through the expiratory valve, pressure support increases tidal volume and may increase inspiratory time, and CPAP increases functional residual capacity.

Weaning

Weaning a patient with a severe COAD from ventilatory support can be difficult and prolonged. Various proposed weaning criteria have a limited predictive value (see Chapter 26).

Techniques fall into three major categories:

1 *Reduce work of spontaneous breathing:* This may be achieved by various combinations of pressure support, flow-by and CPAP while the SIMV rate is being reduced. These promote a better breathing pattern with less fatigue during weaning, but whether they shorten weaning-to-extubation time remains to be established. Work imposed by the breathing system can be significant.[60]
2 *Muscle rest and training:* This is achieved by protocols of rest periods and supported ventilation. Periods of low-level support or complete spontaneous breathing (usually during the day) are often

alternated with periods of high-level support (usually at night).[51] Muscle training by added loads to breathing has been used with some success in stable COAD, but is not generally used during weaning.

3 *Reduce ventilatory requirement:* A low-glucose, high-fat diet to reduce CO_2 production can assist weaning. Increasing serum bicarbonate from 25 to 35 mmol/l increases the $Paco_2$ required to normalize pH from 42 to 58 mmHg (5.6 to 7.7 kPa), and will reduce ventilatory requirement by 30%. This is an adaptive process to assist weaning when ventilatory capacity is reduced. Bicarbonate may be given if serum bicarbonate is not already increased by renal compensation or diuretics.

Failed weaning

If weaning is unsuccessful, continued prolonged ventilation (i.e. over weeks) has been reported to result in successful weaning in a third to half of patients.[61,62] Home ventilation (continuous or intermittent and by nose/facemask or tracheostomy) may be an option[63,64] for patients who are relatively independent (e.g. continent and able to feed, dress and transfer). Lung transplantation is used in various terminal lung conditions including COAD, with 60–70% 2-year survival;[65] however, it is not indicated for failed weaning. Withdrawal of support may be a preferable alternative for a patient with end-stage disease and a poor quality of life.

Outcome

Patients with COAD have a reduced life expectancy compared with an age-matched general population

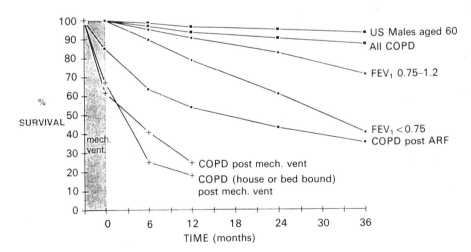

Fig. 24.3 Survival curves for various patient groups with chronic obstructive pulmonary disease (COPD) (Approximations only, based on Menzies *et al.*[3] and Hudson.[66])
FEV_1 = Forced expiratory volume in 1 s; mech, vent. = mechanical ventilation;
ARF = acute respiratory failure.

group. This life expectancy decreases in proportion with severity of COAD as assessed by FEV_1 (Fig. 24.3). An episode of ARF further decreases survival (Fig. 24.3). ARF precipitated by bronchitis only has a better outcome[2] than ARF from serious causes such as pneumonia, LV failure and pulmonary embolus.[66] Although the majority of patients do not require CMV, an episode of ventilation further decreases survival probability (Fig. 24.3). None the less, short-term survival in ventilated patients is still good; hospital survival can be as high as 80%,[67] but 2- and 3-year survival is significantly lower (Fig. 24.3).[68,69] Severity of ARF and the severity of underlying COAD based on FEV_1, lifestyle score and dyspnoea score are also predictors of outcome.[3,66]

References

1 Higgins MW (1989) Chronic airways disease in the United States: trends and determinants. *Chest* **96**:328S–29S.

2 Martin TR, Lewis SW and Albert RK (1982) The prognosis of patients with chronic obstructive pulmonary disease after hospitalization for acute respiratory failure. *Chest* **82**:310–314.

3 Menzies R, Gibbons W and Goldberg P (1989) Determinants of weaning and survival among patients with COPD who require mechanical ventilation for acute respiratory failure. *Chest* **95**:398–405.

4 Schreiner A, Bjerkestrand G, Digranes A *et al.* (1978) Bacteriologic findings in the transtracheal aspirate from patients with acute exacerbations of chronic bronchitis. *Infection* **6**:54–56.

5 Irwin RS, Erickson AD, Pratter MR *et al.* (1982) Prediction of tracheobronchial colonization in current cigarette smokers with chronic obstructive bronchitis. *J Infect Dis* **145**:234–241.

6 Christensen JJ, Gadeberg O and Bruvn B. (1986) *Branhamela catarrhalis*: significance in pulmonary infections and bacteriological features. *Acta Pathol Microbiol Immunol Scand* **94**:89–95.

7 Smith CB, Golden CA, Kanner RE and Renzetti Jr AD (1980) Association of viral and *Mycoplasma pneumoniae* infections with acute respiratory illness in patients with chronic obstructive pulmonary disease. *Am Rev Respir Dis* **121**:225–232.

8 Steele P, Ellis JH, Vandyke D, Sutton F, Creagh E and Davies H (1975) Left ventricular ejection fraction in severe chronic obstructive airways disease. *Am J Med* **59**:21–28.

9 Moser KM, Lemoine JR, Nachtwey FJ and Spragg RG (1981) Deep venous thrombosis and pulmonary embolism. *J Am Med Assoc* **246**:1422–1424.

10 Baum GL and Fisher FD (1960) The relationship of fatal pulmonary insufficiency with cor pulmonale, rightsided mural thrombi and pulmonary emboli: a preliminary report. *Am J Med Sci* **240**:609–612.

11 Sharma GVRK and Sasahara AA (1975) Diagnosis of pulmonary embolism in patients with chronic obstructive pulmonary disease. *J Chronic Dis* **28**:253–257.

12 Dines DE, Clagett OT and Payne WS (1970) Spontaneous pneumothorax in emphysema. *Mayo Clin Proc* **45**:481–487.

13 Aubier M, Murciano D, Fournier M, Milic-Emili J, Pariente R and Derenne JP (1980) Central respiratory drive in acute respiratory failure of patients with chronic obstructive pulmonary disease. *Am Rev Respir Dis* **122**:191–199.

14 Petty TL (1993) Early identification and intervention in chronic obstructive pulmonary disease. In: Hoffman P (ed.) *Lung and Respiration*. Frankfurt: pmi, pp. 2–3.

15 West JB (1987) *Pulmonary Pathophysiology – The Essentials*, 3rd edn. Sydney: Williams & Wilkins.

16 Weitzenblum E, Loiseau A, Hirth C, Mirhom R and Rasaholin-Janahary J (1979) Course of pulmonary hemodynamics in patients with chronic obstructive pulmonary disease. *Chest* **75**:656–662.

17 Burrows B, Strauss RH and Niden AH (1965) Chronic obstructive lung disease: 3. Interrelationships of pulmonary function data. *Am Rev Respir Dis* **91**:861–888.

18 Canadian Thoracic Society Workshop Group (1992). Guidelines for the assessment and management of chronic obstructive pulmonary disease. *Can Med Assoc J* **147**:420–428.

19 Fahey PJ and Hyde RW (1983) 'Won't breathe' versus 'can't breathe'. Detection of depressed ventilatory drive in patients with obstructive pulmonary disease. *Chest* **84**:19–25.

20 Roussos C, Fixley M, Gross D and Macklem PJ (1979) Fatigue of inspiratory muscles and their synergic behavior. *J Appl Physiol* **46**:897–904.

21 Cohen C, Zagelbaum G, Gross D, Roussos C and Macklem PT (1982) Clinical manifestations of inspiratory muscle fatigue. *Am J Med* **73**:308–316.

22 Bone RC, Pierce AK and Johnson RL (1978) Controlled oxygen administration in acute respiratory failure in chronic obstructive pulmonary disease. *Am J Med* **65**:896–902.

23 Aubier M, Murciano D, Milic-Emili *et al.* (1980) Effects of the administration of O_2 on ventilation and blood gases in patients with chronic obstructive pulmonary disease during acute respiratory failure. *Am Rev Respir Dis* **122**:747–754.

24 Degaute OP, Domenigretti J, Naeije R, Vincent JL, Treyvaud D and Perret C (1981) Oxygen delivery in acute exacerbation of chronic obstructive pulmonary disease. Effects of controlled oxygen therapy. *Am Rev Respir Dis* **124**:26–30.

25 Mossberg B, Strandberg K, Philipson K and Camner P (1976) Tracheobronchial clearance and beta-adrenoceptor stimulation in patients with chronic bronchitis. *Scand Respir Dis* **57**:281–289.

26 Braun SR, McKenzie WN, Copeland C, Knight L and Ellersieck M (1989) A comparison of effect of ipratropium and albuterol (salbutamol) in chronic obstructive airway disease. *Arch Intern Med* **149**:544–547.

27 Bone R, COMBIVENT inhalation aerosol study group (1994) In chronic obstructive pulmonary disease,

a combination of ipratropium and albuterol is more effective than either agent alone. An 85 day multicenter trial. *Chest* **105**:1411–1419.

28 Karpel JP (1991) Bronchodilator responses to anticholinergic and beta-adrenergic agents in acute and stable COPD. *Chest* **99**:871–876.

29 Gross NJ and Bankwala Z (1987) Effects of an anticholinergic bronchodilator on arterial blood gases of hypoxemic patients with chronic obstructive pulmonary disease: comparison with a beta-adrenergic agent. *Am Rev Respir Dis* **136**:1091–1094.

30 Rice KL, Leatherman JW, Duane PG *et al.* (1987) Aminophylline for acute exacerbations of chronic obstructive pulmonary disease. *Ann Intern Med* **107**:305–309.

31 Guyatt GH, Townsend M, Pugsley SO *et al.* (1987) Bronchodilators in chronic air-flow limitation. Effects on airway function, exercise capacity, and quality of life. *Am Rev Respir Dis* **135**:1069–1074.

32 Murciano D, Aubier M, Lecocguic Y and Pariente R (1984) Effects of theophylline on diaphragm strength and fatigue in patients with severe chronic pulmonary disease. *N Engl J Med* **311**:349–352.

33 Berry RB, Desa MM, Branum JP and Light RW (1991) Effect of theophylline on sleep and sleep-disordered breathing in patients with chronic obstructive pulmonary disease. *Am Rev Respir Dis* **143**:245–250.

34 Wanner A (1985) Effects of methylxanthines on airway muciciliary function. *Am J Med* **79**:16–21.

35 Matthay RA, Berger RH, Davies R, Loke A, Gottschalk A and Zaret BL (1982) Improvement in cardiac performance by oral long-acting theophylline in chronic obstructive pulmonary disease. *Am Heart J* **104**:1022–1026

36 Pauwels RA (1989) New aspects of the therapeutic potential of theophylline in asthma. *J Allergy Clin Immunol* **83**:548–553.

37 Rogers RM, Owens GR and Pennock BE (1985) The pendulum swings again: toward a rational use of theophylline. *Chest* **87**:280–282.

38 Albert RK, Martin TR and Lewis SW (1980) Controlled clinical trial of methylprednisolone in patients with chronic bronchitis and acute respiratory insufficiency. *Ann Intern Med* **92**:753–758.

39 Rubini S, Rampulla C and Nava S (1994) Acute effect of corticosteroids on respiratory mechanics in mechanically ventilated patients with chronic airflow obstruction and acute respiratory failure. *Am J Respir Crit Care Med* **149**:306–310.

40 Hosker H, Cooke NJ and Hawkey P (1994) Antibiotics in chronic obstructive pulmonary disease. *Br Med J* **308**:871–872.

41 Basran GS, Joseph J, Abbas AM, Hughes C and Tillotson GS (1990) Treatment of acute exacerbations of chronic obstructive airways disease – a comparison of amoxycillin and cyprofloxacin. *J Antimicrob Chemoth* **26**(suppl F):19–24.

42 Mathur PN, Pugsley SO, Powles ACP *et al.* (1980) Effect of digitalis on left ventricular function in chronic cor pulmonale. *Am Rev Respir Dis* **121**:163.

43 Green LH and Smith TW (1977) The use of digitalis in patients with pulmonary disease. *Ann Intern Med* **87**:459–465.

44 Sajkov D, McEvoy RD, Cowie RJ *et al.* (1993) Felodipine improves pulmonary hemodynamics in chronic obstructive pulmonary disease. *Chest* **103**:1354–1361.

45 Salvaterra CG and Rubin LJ (1994) Investigation and management of pulmonary hypertension in chronic obstructive pulmonary disease. *Am Rev Respir Dis* **148**:1414–1417.

46 Aubier M, Murciano D, Lecocguic Y *et al.* (1985) Effect of hypophosphatemia on diaphragmatic contractility in patients with acute respiratory failure. *N Engl J Med* **313**:420–424.

47 Dhingra S, Solven F, Wilson A and McCarthy DS (1984) Hypomagnesemia and respiratory muscle power. *Am Rev Respir Dis* **129**:497–498.

48 Aubier M, Viires N, Piquet J *et al.*(1985) Effects of hypocalcemia on diaphragmatic strength generation. *J Appl Physiol* **58**:2054–2061.

49 Ferris B (1978) Epidemiology standardization project. *Am Rev Respir Dis* **118**(suppl):1–120.

50 Petrov BJ, Legare M, Goldberg P, Milic-Emili J and Gottfried SB (1990) Continuous positive airways pressure reduces work of breathing and dyspnea during weaning from mechanical ventilation in severe chronic obstructive pulmonary disease. *Am Rev Respir Dis* **141**:281–289.

51 Mezzanotte WS, Tangel DJ, Fox AM, Ballard RD and White DP (1994) Nocturnal nasal continuous positive airways pressure in patients with chronic obstructive pulmonary disease. Influence on waking respiratory muscle function. *Chest* **106**:1100–1108.

52 Brochard L, Isabey D, Piquet J, Amaro D, Mancebo J and Messadi AA (1990) Reversal of acute exacerbations of chronic obstructive lung disease by inspiratory assistance with a face mask. *N Engl J Med* **323**:1523–1529.

53. Fernandez M, Blanch Ll, Valles J, Baigorri F and Artigas A (1993) Pressure support ventilation via face mask in acute respiratory failure in hypercapnic COPD patients. *Intens Care Med* **19**:456–461.

54 Vitacca M, Rubini F, Foglio K, Scalvini S, Nava S and Ambrosino N (1993) Non-invasive modalities of acute exacerbations in COLD patients. *Intens Care Med* **19**:450–455.

55 Tuxen DV and Lane S (1987) The effects of ventilatory pattern on hyperinflation, airway pressures, and circulation in mechanical ventilation of patients with severe airflow obstruction. *Am Rev Respir Dis* **136**:872–879.

56 Curtis JR and Hudson LD (1994) Emergent assessment and management of acute respiratory failure in COPD. *Clin Chest Med Respir Emergencies II* **15**:481–500.

57 Connors AF, McCaffree DR and Gray BA (1981) Effect of inspiratory flow rate on gas exchange during mechanical ventilation. *Am Rev Respir Dis* **124**:537–543.

58 Tuxen DV (1989) Detrimental effects of positive end-expiratory pressure during controlled mechanical

ventilation of patients with severe airflow obstruction. *Am Rev Respir Dis* **140**:5–9.

59 Biagorri F, De Monte A, Blanch L *et al.* (1994) Hemodynamic response to external counterbalancing of auto-positive end-expiratory pressure in mechanically ventilated patients with chronic obstructive pulmonary disease. *Crit Care Med* **22**:1782–1791.

60 Oh TE, Lin ES and Bhatt S (1991) Inspiratory work imposed by demand valve ventilator circuits. *Anaesth Intens Care* **19**:187–191.

61 Indihar FJ (1991) A 10-year report of patients in a prolonged respiratory care unit. *Minnesota Med* **74**:23–27.

62 Scheinhorn DJ, Artinian BM and Catline JL (1994) Weaning from mechanical ventilation. The experience of a regional weaning center, *Chest* **105**:534–539.

63 Sadoul P and Cardinaud JP (1986) L'expérience francaise de l'assistance respiratoire à domicile des insuffisants respiratories graves. *Bull Eur Physiopathol Respir* **22**:15–65.

64 Leger P, Bedicam JM, Cornette A *et al.* 1994) Nasal intermittent positive pressure ventilation. Long-term follow-up in patients with severe chronic respiratory insufficiency. *Chest* **105**:100–105.

65 Patterson GA, Maurer JR, Williamsx TJ *et al.* (1991) Comparison of outcomes of double and single lung transplantation for obstructive lung disease. *J Thorac Cardiovasc Surg* **101**:623–632.

66 Hudson LF (1989) Survival data in patients with acute and chronic lung disease requiring mechanical ventilation. *Am Rev Respir Dis* **140**:S19–S24.

67 Petty TL (1984) Acute respiratory failure in chronic obstructive pulmonary disease. In: Shoemaker W, Thompson W and Holbrook P (eds) *Textbook of Critical Care*. Sydney: W. B. Saunders, pp. 264–272.

68 Burk RH and George RB (1972) Acute respiratory failure in chronic obstructive pulmonary disease (immediate and long-term prognosis). *Arch Intern Med* **132**:865–868.

69 Admandsson T and Kilburn KH (1974) Survival after respiratory failure (145 patients observed 5 to 8.5 years). *Ann Intern Med* **80**:54–59.

25   Acute upper airway obstruction

GM Joynt

Acute upper airway obstruction is a life-threatening emergency, resulting from a wide range of patho-physiological processes. Rapid assessment and establishment of a patent airway are vital, often in the absence of a specific diagnosis. As no single treatment modality is universally applicable, the ICU physician must be capable of instituting a variety of airway management techniques.

Anatomy and pathophysiology

The upper airway begins at the nose and mouth, and ends at the carina.[1] Obstruction is likely to occur at sites of anatomical narrowing, such as the hypopharynx at the base of the tongue, and the false and true vocal cords at the laryngeal opening. Sites of airway obstruction are classified as supraglottic (above the true cords), intraglottic (involving the true vocal cords) or infraglottic (below the true cords and above the carina).[1]

The upper airway can also be divided into intrathoracic and extrathoracic portions, which behave differently during inspiration and expiration. The intrathoracic airway dilates during inspiration, i.e. 'pulled outwards' by negative intrapleural pressure. Positive intrapleural pressure during expiration causes compression and narrowing. Conversely the compliant extrathoracic airway, unexposed to intra-pleural pressure, collapses during inspiration, and expands during expiration.[1] Better assessment of clinical signs, radiographs and flow–volume loops can be made if this phenomenon is remembered.[2,3]

Aetiology

Acute upper airway obstruction may result from functional or mechanical causes (Table 25.1). Functional causes involve central nervous system and neuro-muscular dysfunction. Mechanical causes may occur within the lumen, in the wall or extrinsic to the airway.

Table 25.1 Clinical conditions associated with acute upper airway obstruction

Functional causes
Central nervous system depression[28]
    Head injury, cerebrovascular accident, cardiorespiratory arrest, shock, hypoxia, drug overdose, metabolic encepha-lopathies.
Peripheral nervous system and neuromuscular abnormalities
    Recurrent laryngeal nerve palsy (postoperative, inflam-matory or tumour infiltration),[1,2] obstructive sleep apnoea,[51] laryngospasm,[2] myasthenia gravis, Guillain–Barré polyneuritis, hypocalcaemic vocal cord spasm.

Mechanical causes
Foreign body aspiration[5,27]
Infections
    Epiglottitis,[11] retropharyngeal cellulitis or abscess,[32] Ludwig's angina,[35] diphtheria and tetanus,[32] bacterial tracheitis,[52] laryngotracheobronchitis[53]
Laryngeal oedema
    Allergic laryngeal oedema[42] and hereditary angioneurotic oedema[54]
Haemorrhage and haematoma
    Postoperative, anticoagulation therapy[33]
Trauma
Burns[36]
Neoplasm[3]
    Pharyngeal, laryngeal and tracheobronchial carcinoma, vocal cord polyposis
Congenital[2]
    Vascular rings, laryngeal webs, laryngocele
Miscellaneous
    Cricoarytenoid arthritis,[55] achalasia of the oesophagus,[56] hysterical stridor,[57] myxoedema[58]

Clinical presentation

Signs of sudden complete upper airway obstruction are obvious.[3] The victim cannot breathe, speak or cough, and may hold the throat between the thumb and index finger – the universal choking sign.[4] Agitation, panic and vigorous breathing efforts are rapidly followed by cyanosis. Respiratory efforts diminish as consciousness is lost, and death results within 2–5 min if obstruction is not relieved.[1,5]

Signs of partial airway obstruction include choking, drooling, gagging, coughing, inspiratory stridor with noisy respiration and dysphonia.[6] Paradoxical chest wall movements and intercostal and supraclavicular retractions may be marked. Powerful inspiratory efforts may produce dermal ecchymoses and subcutaneous emphysema. Respiratory decompensation may be rapid in onset, and progress to complete obstruction. Lethargy, diminishing respiratory efforts and loss of consciousness are late signs of hypoxaemia and hypercarbia. Bradycardia and hypotension herald impending cardiac arrest.

Special evaluation or investigations

If the patient remains stable, specific diagnostic evaluation may be undertaken, provided airway management facilities are immediately available.[1]

Laryngoscopy and bronchoscopy

Indirect laryngoscopy in a stable, cooperative patient is useful to diagnose foreign bodies, retropharyngeal or laryngeal masses and other glottic pathology.[1,7]

Assessment with a flexible fibreoptic bronchoscope or laryngoscope[8,9] enables direct visualization of upper airway anatomy and function. The procedure can be performed in the Emergency Department without transporting the patient and risking complete obstruction. It can be applied to an awake, spontaneously breathing patient and, with care, should not worsen the obstruction. Definitive airway control by intubation can usually be achieved at the end, by railroading an endotracheal tube into the

trachea. Disadvantages are the need for a skilled operator and a cooperative patient, and a poor visual field if blood and secretions are copious.[10]

Direct laryngoscopy will enable forceps removal of foreign bodies and suctioning of blood, vomitus and secretions. Endotracheal intubation can rapidly be achieved under direct vision. Disadvantages are the need for good local analgesia (often difficult in the emergency setting) or general anaesthesia. It can be traumatic, and may worsen soft-tissue bleeding and oedema.

Radiographic imaging

Anterior–posterior and lateral plain neck X-rays are useful to detect radiopaque foreign bodies, retropharyngeal masses and epiglottitis. The lateral view is obtained in inspiration with the neck fully extended.[1] Swelling of the epiglottis and supraglottic tissues, and ballooning of the hypopharynx, are classical signs of epiglottitis, but are not always present.[11] A computed tomography (CT) scan can assess the thyroid, cricoid and arytenoid cartilages and the airway lumen in stable patients.[12,13] Although magnetic resonance imaging (MRI) has been used to image the upper airway, its use in airway obstruction is unproven.[14]

Gas flow measurement

Flow–volume loop measurement reveals characteristic patterns corresponding to different types and position of pathological lesions (Fig. 25.1).[2,15]

Management

Algorithms to manage partial and complete upper airway obstruction are shown in Figures 25.2 and 25.3.

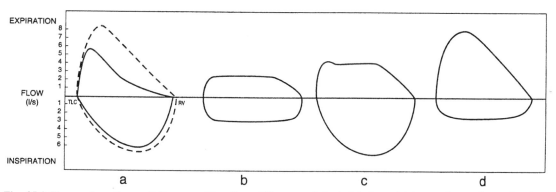

Fig. 25.1 Flow–volume loops. Patterns resulting from different pathological lesions: (a) lower airway obstruction (e.g. chronic obstructive pulmonary disease or asthma), the dashed line represents the normal pattern; (b) fixed, non-variable obstruction (e.g. fibrous ring in trachea); (c) variable obstruction, intrathoracic (e.g. tumour in the lower trachea); (d) variable obstruction, extrathoracic (e.g. vocal cord tumour or paralysis).

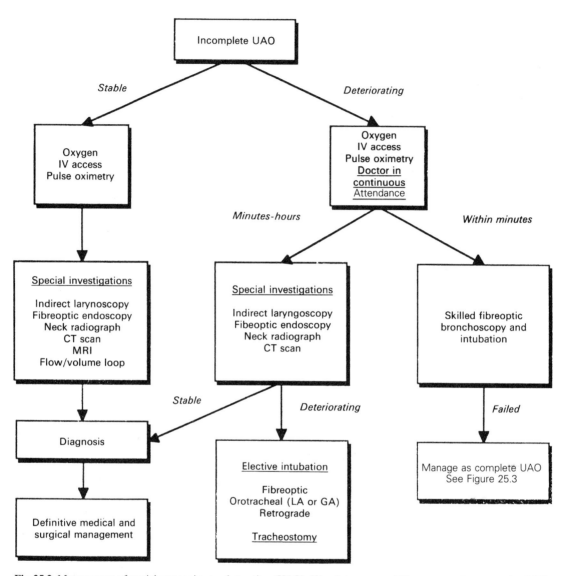

Fig 25.2 Management of partial upper airway obstruction (UAO). IV = Intravenous; CT = computed tomography; MRI = magnetic resonance imaging; LA = local anaesthesia; GA = general anaesthesia).

Improvisation may be required for certain difficult problems. The most appropriate technique should be one in which the clinician has the greatest skill and experience.[7] Special considerations in patients with suspected cervical spine instability are discussed in Chapter 69.

Important general measures

1 Supplemental oxygen (100%) is immediately administered.

2 All equipment for definitive airway control must be available and ready for use. This includes good suction, a choice of laryngoscope blades, a range of endotracheal tube sizes, fibreoptic bronchoscope or laryngoscope, drugs and surgical airway devices (i.e. cricothyroidotomy and tracheostomy sets and transtracheal jet ventilation injectors).

3 Intravenous access must be readily secured.

4 Continuous monitoring of vital signs and pulse oximetry is started.

5 Transport of the patient before securing the airway

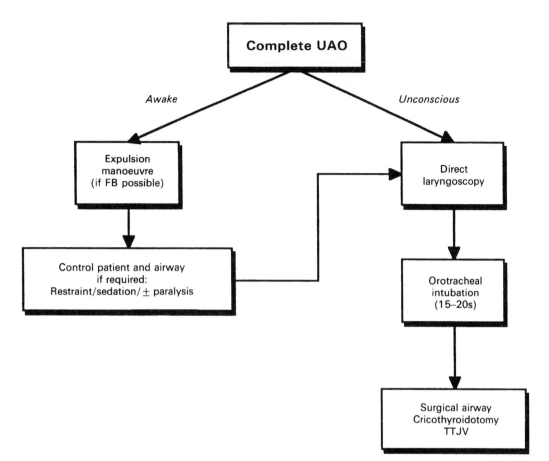

Fig. 25.3 Management of complete upper airway obstruction (UAO). Attempts at orotracheal intubation should not take longer than 10–20 s. FB = Foreign body; TTJV = transtracheal jet ventilation.

must be carefully considered. It is difficult to provide safe conditions during transport or in radiology suites.[7,16]

Principles of airway management techniques[6]

The unconscious patient

If the upper airway is obstructed by the tongue in an unconscious patient, airway patency is achieved by using standard airway manoeuvres[5] and oropharyngeal or nasopharyngeal airways. Direct laryngoscopy allows evaluation of any supraglottic obstruction, and endotracheal intubation can proceed.

Endotracheal intubation

1 *Awake fibreoptic intubation* in a spontaneously breathing patient is recommended.[8,9] The following points are important in acute upper airway obstruction:

(a) The procedure is clearly explained to the patient.

(b) Good local anaesthesia is important. Rapid transcricoid injection of 2–3 ml lignocaine 2% followed by either sprayed or nebulized lignocaine 4% to the nares, posterior pharynx and base of tongue is effective.[9,17,18] Superior laryngeal and glossopharyngeal nerve block techniques[19,20] will improve analgesia but are not essential.

(c) Topical phenylephrine (0.25–0.50%) or cocaine (2 ml 5% solution) vasoconstricts mucosal vasculature and can reduce nasopharyngeal bleeding.[17]

(d) Failure is most commonly due to excessive secretions and bleeding.[9] Additional suction catheters may help.[10]

(e) The suction port of the fibrescope can be used to insufflate 100% oxygen. This provides supplemental oxygen and clears the fibrescope tip of secretions.[8]

(f) The procedure will take 2–10 min or even

longer.[8,9] Urgency of the case must be assessed beforehand with this time frame in mind. An alternative technique should be initiated if there are any delays or if intubation fails after a reasonable time.

2 *Retrograde tracheal intubation* is a less invasive alternative to cricothyroidotomy in proximal obstructions.[21] A J-tip guide wire is introduced percutaneously through the cricothyroid membrane, and advanced through the retropharynx. The tip is retrieved from the oral cavity, and the wire is used to guide an oral endotracheal tube past the obstruction and into the trachea. The procedure is relatively simple and safe.

3 *Blind nasotracheal intubation* is a less useful technique now that fibreoptic laryngoscopes are available.

4 *Direct laryngoscopic intubation under general anaesthesia* requires a skilled operator (see below).

Once endotracheal intubation is safely accomplished, tracheostomy can be performed if considered necessary. Secure fixation of the endotracheal tube is mandatory. The patient's upper limbs may need to be restrained to avoid self-extubation.

Surgical airways (see Chapter 23)

A surgical airway is indicated when endotracheal intubation is not possible, or when an unstable cervical spine is threatened by available airway techniques[22] (see Chapter 69). It is the last line of defence against hypoxia.

1 *Percutaneous transtracheal jet ventilation,*[22,23] using a large-bore intravenous catheter inserted through the cricothyroid membrane, is a simple, effective and relatively safe technique. It is quicker than cricothyroidotomy or tracheostomy. Ventilation through the cannula with a standard manual resuscitator bag is inadequate, and a jet ventilation system is necessary. Expiratory gases must be able to escape via the glottis. Appropriate chest movements during expiration must be noted. The consequence of expiratory obstruction is severe and potentially fatal barotrauma. In cases of complete upper airway obstruction, the technique must not be used.

2 *Cricothyroidotomy,*[24,25] by surgery or percutaneously, is another reliable, safe, and relatively easy way of providing an emergency airway. It is the method of choice if severe to complete upper airway obstruction exists. A tube with internal diameter of 2.5 and 3.0 mm will allow adequate gas flow for bag ventilation and spontaneous breathing respectively, provided supplemental oxygen is used.[23] Since the diameter of the cricothyroid space is 9 by 30 mm, tubes of 8.5 mm outer diameter or less should avoid laryngeal and vocal cord damage. Commercially available percutaneous tracheostomy sets that meet the above requirements are available. Complications such as subglottic stenosis (1.6%), thyroid fracture, haemorrhage and pneumothorax are acceptably low.[24,25]

3 *Tracheostomy* in the emergency setting is rarely required, although surgical tracheostomy under local anaesthesia may be a correct technique under certain controlled conditions. There are reports of percutaneous tracheostomy procedures in urgent cases,[26] but cricothyroidotomy remains the method of choice in an emergency.

Common clinical conditions

Foreign body obstruction

Foreign body obstruction is the most common cause of acute airway obstruction. The elderly, especially those in institutions, are at risk, and dentures, alcohol and depressant drugs are high-risk factors.[5] Fatal food asphyxiation ('café coronary') has an incidence of 0.66 per 100 000 population.[27] The diagnosis should be considered in any acute respiratory arrest where the victim cannot be ventilated.[28]

Expulsion of the foreign body can be attempted with the Heimlich manoeuvre.[4] From behind, the rescuer encircles the arms around the victim, placing the thumb of one fist between the umbilicus and xiphisternum. The fist is gripped by the other hand, and an inward, upward thrust is applied. Chest thrusts and other variations for use in infants, pregnancy and obesity have been described.[28,29] The technique is not without controversy. Unwanted effects such as vomiting, aspiration, fractured ribs, barotrauma and ruptured organs have been reported.[5,30,31] The finger sweep, although recommended, may cause further foreign body impaction.[5] If these fail, management immediately proceeds as shown in Fig. 25.3.

Extrinsic airway compression

Extrinsic space-occupying lesions can cause upper airway obstruction. Compression from haematomas may be associated with trauma, neck surgery, central venous catheterization, anticoagulants and coagulapathies.[7,13,32–34] Haematomas following surgery should immediately be evacuated by removing skin and subcutaneous sutures. If this fails, an artificial airway must be secured. In patients with coagulation abnormalities, intubation is preferred over a surgical airway. Most haematomas secondary to coagulopathy do not require surgical intervention, and resolve spontaneously with conservative therapy (i.e. vitamin K and blood component therapy).

Partial airway obstruction caused by retropharyngeal abscesses[32] is best managed by drainage under local anaesthesia. Gentle fibreoptic examination and intubation or direct laryngoscopy and intubation in the lateral, head-down position is favoured by some.[7] Risks are related to inadvertent rupture of the abscess, with subsequent flooding of the airway. Ludwig's angina is a mixed infection of the floor of the mouth. An inflammatory mass develops in the space between the tongue and the muscles and fascia of the anterior neck.[35] The supraglottic airway is compressed and becomes narrowed. Direct laryngoscopy is difficult, as the tongue cannot be anteriorly displaced. Awake fibreoptic bronchoscopy or a surgical airway are management options.[7,32]

Intrinsic airway compression

Inhalational injury

Patients with facial burns or inhalation injuries develop progressive supraglottic oedema, usually within 24 h.[36] Such patients require early tracheal intubation, even prophylactically (see Chapter 72). Assessment of the injury and tracheal intubation can be achieved under general anaesthesia (see below). Intubation by fibreoptic laryngoscopy or tracheostomy under local anaesthesia is usually a better alternative.

Adult epiglottitis[11,37,38]

Epiglottitis is an uncommon but increasingly recognized infectious disease in adults. It involves the epiglottis and supraglottic larynx, causing swelling with consequent airway obstruction. *Haemophilus influenzae*, and *H. parainfluenzae*, *Streptococcus pneumoniae*, haemolytic steptococci, and *Staphylococcus aureus* are common causative organisms. Mortality is high in adults (6–7%), due to misdiagnosis and inappropriate treatment.[11,38] Clinical features are summarized in Table 25.2. The diagnosis is confirmed by gentle indirect laryngoscopy, lateral neck X-ray or fibreoptic laryngoscopy.

Airway management is controversial. Some recommend securing a definitive airway on presentation,[38] while others suggest close observation in ICU.[37] However, there are numerous reports of sudden obstruction and death with the latter approach.[11,39] Tracheal intubation and tracheostomy are acceptable techniques, but tracheal intubation may result in better long-term outcome.[40] Patient positioning is important, and changing from a sitting to supine position may induce complete obstruction. In more

Table 25.2 Features suggestive of adult epiglottitis

Sudden onset of sore throat
Throat pain greater than suggested by clinical findings
Dysphagia
Voice changes – usually muffling
Stridor
Respiratory distress
Systemic toxaemia
Pain on laryngeal palpation

Adapted from Baxter and Dunn.[11]

stable patients, awake fibreoptic intubation is possible if a skilled operator is available.[7,11] Endotracheal intubation under general anaesthesia using a gaseous induction is frequently recommended. Obstruction can occur, and this procedure must only be undertaken by a skilled anaesthetist in the operating room, with a surgeon scrubbed and ready to perform an emergency trachestomy. Rapid-sequence induction using muscle relaxants is dangerous. Tracheostomy under local anaesthesia is a safe alternative.[7,11]

Medical management consists of appropriate antibiotics and supportive care. Cefuroxime 1.5 g IV 8-hourly[11] or ampicillin 1–2 g IV 6-hourly *plus* chloramphenicol 50 mg/kg per day are empiric regimens.[32,35] Cultures of epiglottal swabs and blood should be undertaken. Supportive care includes adequate sedation and tracheobronchial toilet. Abscesses should be surgically drained. There is no firm evidence for the use of steroids.

Allergic manifestations

Allergic responses involving the upper airway may be localized or part of a systemic anaphylactic reaction.[1,41] Angioedema of the lips, supraglottis, glottis and infraglottis results in airway obstruction.[1,35] The systemic reaction consists of variable combinations of urticaria (79%), bronchospasm (70%), shock, cardiovascular collapse and abdominal pain.[42] Common causative agents are Hymenoptera stings, shellfish ingestion and drugs.[35,42] Angiotensin-converting enzyme (ACE) inhibitor-related angioedema is becoming more common.[43] Treatment consists of immediately ensuring an adequate airway (Fig. 25.2), and administration of oxygen, adrenaline and steroids (see Chapter 58). As it is likely to recur, the patient should be fully investigated.[44]

Hereditary angioneurotic oedema (Quincke's disease) is a rare, inherited disorder of the complement system, caused by functionless or low levels of C_1 esterase inhibitor.[45,46] Angioedema involving skin and subcutaneous tissue occurs in various locations, particularly the upper airway. Precipitating causes include stress, pregnancy, physical exertion and localized trauma (e.g. dental or maxillofacial surgery and laryngoscopy). Management consists of establishing a secure airway (Fig. 25.2) and infusion of fresh frozen plasma to replenish the esterase inhibitor. C_1 esterase inhibitor concentrate is the treatment of choice if available. A poor response to adrenaline, antihistamines and steroids can be expected.[45,46] Danazol, C_1 esterase inhibitor, antifibrinolytic agents (e.g. tranexamic acid) and fresh frozen plasma (2–4 units) can be used prophylactically if time permits.[46]

Post-extubation laryngeal oedema

Laryngeal oedema following extubation is much more common in children (see Chapter 102). It is often associated with airway manipulation and traumatic and prolonged tracheal intubation. Treatment in adults is conservative, with close observation and humidified oxygen therapy. Steroids and nebulized plain adrenaline (1–2 ml 1:1000 solution diluted with 2 ml saline) or racemic adrenaline (0.25–0.5 ml of 2.25% solution) have been used.

Upper airway obstruction in children

This is discussed in Chapter 102.

Postobstruction pulmonary oedema

Postobstruction pulmonary oedema occurs in up to 11% of cases.[47] This appears to be related to the markedly decreased intrathoracic pressure caused by forced inspiration against a closed upper airway, resulting in transudation of fluid from pulmonary capillaries to the interstitium. In addition, increased venous return may increase pulmonary blood flow, further worsening oedema.[48,49] Hypoxia and the hyperadrenergic stress state may also affect capillary hydrostatic pressure. The oedema usually occurs within minutes after the relief of the obstruction, but may be delayed up to 2.5 h.[48] Management includes maintenance of airway patency, oxygen therapy, diuretics, morphine, fluid restriction and continuous positive airways pressure application.[49] Ventilation with positive end-expiratory pressure may be necessary in severe cases. Pulmonary capillary wedge pressure is usually normal and pulmonary artery catheterization should be reserved only for complicated cases.[50]

References

1 Cox GR and Shepherd SM (1992) Acute upper airway obstruction and mediastinal disorders. In: Schwartz GR (ed.) *Emergency Medicine*. Philadelphia: Lea & Febiger, pp. 500–512.

2 Miller RD (1988) Obstructing lesions of the larynx and trachea: clinical and pathophysiological aspects. In: Fishman AP (ed.) *Pulmonary Diseases and Disorders*. New York: McGraw-Hill, pp. 1173–1187.

3 Dailey RH (1983) Acute upper airway obstruction. *Emerg Med Clin North Am* **1**:261–277.

4 Heimlich HJ (1975) A life saving maneuver to prevent food-choking. *J Am Med Assoc* **234**:398–401.

5 Daya M, Mariani R and Fernandes C (1992) Basic life support. In: Dailey RH, Simon B, Young GP and Stewart RD (eds) *The Airway: Emergency Management*. St Louis: Mosby Year Book, pp. 39–61.

6 Dailey RH and Pace S (1992) Autraumatic upper airway obstruction. In: Dailey RH, Simon B, Young GP and Stewart RD (eds). *The Airway: Emergency Management*. St Louis: Mosby Year Book, pp. 309–319.

7 Bogdonoff DL and Stone DJ (1992) Emergency management of the airway outside the emergency room. *Can J Anaesth* **39**:1069–1089.

8 Milnek EJ, Clinton JE, Plummer D and Ruiz E (1990) Fiberoptic intubation in the emergency department. *Ann Emerg Med* **19**:359–362.

9 Afilalo M, Guttman A, Stern E *et al.* (1993) Fiberoptic intubation in the emergency department: a case series. *J Emerg Med* **11**:387–391.

10 Telford RJ and Liban JB (1991) Awake fiberoptic intubation. *British Journal Hospital Medicine* **46**:182–184.

11 Baxter FJ and Dunn GL (1988) Acute epiglottitis in adults. *Can J Anaesth* **35**:428–435.

12 Angood PB, Attia EL, Brown RA and Mulder DS (1986) Extrinsic civilian trauma to the larynx and cervical trachea – important predictors of long term morbidity. *J Trauma* **26**:869–873.

13 Grillo HC, Mathisen DJ and Wain JC (1992) Management of tumours of the trachea. *Oncology* **6**:61–67.

14 Schneider M, Probst R and Wey W (1989) Magnetic resonance imaging – a useful tool for airway measurement. *Acta Anaesthesiol Scand* **33**:429–431.

15 Miller RD and Hyatt RE (1973) Evaluation of obstructing lesions of the trachea and larynx by flow volume loops. *Am Rev Respir Dis* **108**:475–481.

16 Warner JA and Finlay WEI (1985) Fulminating epiglottitis in adults. *Anaesthesia* **40**:348–352.

17 Bourke DL, Katz J and Tonneson A (1985) Nebulized anesthesia for awake endotracheal intubation. *Anesthesiology* **6**:690–692.

18 Webb AR, Fernando SS, Dalton HR, Arrowsmith JE, Woodhead MA and Cummin AR (1990) Local anaesthesia for fiberoptic bronchoscopy: transcricoid injection or the spray as you go technique. *Thorax* **45**:474–477.

19 Gotta AW and Sullivan CA (1984) Superior laryngeal nerve block: an aid to intubating the patient with fractured mandible. *J Trauma* **24**:83–85.

20 Benumof JL (1991) Management of the difficult airway. *Anesthesiology* **75**:1087–1110.

21 McNamara RM (1987) Retrograde intubation of the trachea. *Ann Emerg Med* **16**:680–682.

22 Benumof JL and Scheller MS (1989) The importance of transtracheal jet ventilation in the management of the difficult airway. *Anesthesiology* **71**:769–778.

23 Neff CC, Pfister RC and Van Sonnenberg E (1983) Percutaneous transtracheal ventilation: experimental and practical aspects. *J Trauma* **23**:84–90.

24 Salvino CK, Dries D, Gamelli R, Murphy-Macabobby M and Marshall W (1993) Emergency cricothyroidotomy in trauma victims. *J Trauma* **34**:503–505.

25 Kress TD and Balasubramaniam S (1982) Cricothyroidotomy. *Ann Emerg Med* **11**:197–201.

26 Griggs WM, Myburgh JA and Worthley LIG (1991) Urgent airway access – an indication for percutaneous tracheostomy? *Anaesth Intens Care* **19**:586–587.

27 Mittleman RE and Wetli CV (1982) The fatal cafe coronary: foreign body airway obstruction. *J Am Med Assoc* **247**:1285–1288.

28 Finucane BT and Santora AH (1988) *Principles of Airway Management*. Philadelphia: FA Davis.

29 American Heart Association (1987) *Heartsaver Manual*. Dallas: American Heart Association.

30 Orlowsky JP (1987) Vomiting as a complication of the Heimlich maneuver. *J Am Med Assoc* **258**:512–513.

31 Dupre MW, Silva E and Brotman S (1993) Traumatic rupture of the stomach secondary to Heimlich maneuver. *Am J Emerg Med* **11**:611–612.

32 Boster RS and Martinez SA (1982) Acute upper airway obstruction in the adult. *Postgrad Med* **72**:50–57.

33 Duong TC, Burtch GD and Shatney CH (1986) Upper-airway obstruction as a complication of oral anti-coagulation therapy. *Crit Care Med* **14**:830–831.

34 O'Hara JF, Brand MI and Boutros AR (1994) Acute airway obstruction following placement of a subclavian Hickman catheter. *Can J Anaesth* **41**:241–243.

35 Jacobson S (1989) Upper airway obstruction. *Emerg Med Clin North Am* **7**:205–217.

36 Gough D and Young G (1992) Airway burns and toxic gas inhalation. In: Dailey RH, Simon B, Young GP and Stewart RD (eds) *The Airway: Emergency Management*. St Louis: Mosby Year Book, pp. 297–307.

37 Walker PJ, Dwyer DE and Curotta JH (1988) Adult epiglottis. *Med J Aust* **248**:309–310.

38 Mayo-Smith MF, Hirsch PJ, Wodzinski SF and Schiffman FJ (1986) Acute epiglottitis in adults: an eight-year experience in the state of Rhode Island. *N Engl J Med* **314**:1133–1139.

39 Mayo-Smith M (1993) Fatal respiratory arrest in adult epiglottitis in the intensive care unit. *Chest* **104**:964–965.

40 Schloss MD, Gold JA, Rosales JK and Baxter JD (1983) Acute epiglottitis: current management. *Laryngoscope* **93**:489–493.

41 Fisher MM and More DG (1981) The epidemiology and clinical features of anaphylactic reactions in anaesthesia. *Anaesth Intens Care* **9**:226–234.

42 Corren J and Schocket AL (1990) Anaphylaxis: a preventable emergency. *Postgrad Med* **87**:167–178.

43 Pigman EC and Scott JL (1993) Angioedema in the emergency department: the impact of angiotensin-converting enzyme inhibitors. *Am J Emerg Med* **11**:350–354.

44 Fisher M and Baldo BA (1994) Anaphylaxis during anaesthesia: current aspects of diagnosis and prevention. *Eur J Anaesth* **11**:263–284.

45 Evans TC and Roberge RJ (1987) Quincke's disease of the uvula. *Am J Emerg Med* **5**:211–216.

46 Poppers PJ (1987) Anaesthetic implications of hereditary angioneurotic oedema. *Can J Anaesth* **34**:76–78.

47 Tami TA, Chu F, Wildes TO and Kaplan M (1986) Pulmonary edema and acute upper airway obstruction. *Laryngoscope* **96**:506–509.

48 Willms D and Shure D (1988) Pulmonary edema due to upper airway obstruction in adults. *Chest* **94**:1090–1092.

49 Wiesel S, Gutman JB and Kleiman SJ. Adult epiglottitis and postobstructive pulmonary edema in a patient with severe coronary artery disease. *J Clin Anesth* **5**:158–162.

50 Younker D, Meadors C and Coveler L (1989) Postobstruction pulmonary edema. *Chest* **95**:687–689.

51 Anonsen C (1990) Laryngeal obstruction and obstructive sleep apnea syndrome. *Laryngoscope* **100**:775–778.

52 Campbell TM, Paris PM and Stewart RD (1988) Tracheitis: the other cause of upper airway obstruction. *Ann Emerg Med* **66**:119–121.

53 Deeb ZE and Einhorn KH (1990) Infectious adult croup. *Laryngoscope* **100**:455–457.

54 Frank MM, Gelfand JA and Atkinson JP (1976) Hereditary angioedema: the clinical syndrome and management. *Ann Intern Med* **84**:580–593.

55 Leicht MJ, Harrington TM and Davis DE (1987) Cricoarytenoid arthritis: a cause of laryngeal obstruction. *Ann Emerg Med* **16**:885–888.

56 Dominguez F, Hernandez-Ranz F, Boixeda D and Valdazo P (1987) Acute upper-airway obstruction in achalasia of the oesophagus. *Am J Gastroenterol* **4**:362–364.

57 Snyder HS and Weiss E (1989) Hysterical stridor: a benign cause of upper airway obstruction. *Ann Emerg Med* **18**:991–994.

58 Stahl N and Leiberman A (1988) Acute upper airway obstruction due to myxedema and upper airway abnormalities. *J Laryngol Otol* **102**:733–734.

IKS Tan and TE Oh

Respiratory support forms a major part of an ICU workload. It is uncommonly required in isolation from other problems which may have their own adverse effects on respiratory function. A wide diversity of conditions may affect alveolar gas exchange and ventilation, resulting in two types of respiratory failure: oxygenation failure and ventilatory failure. Management of respiratory failure thus involves first, diagnosis and treatment of the underlying pathology; second, respiratory support, i.e. oxygen therapy (see Chapter 22) and ventilatory support;[1] and third supportive care of other organ systems. Ventilatory support includes continuous positive airway pressure (CPAP) breathing and mechanical ventilation.

Indications

The classical indication for ventilatory support is reversible acute respiratory failure. Most conditions requiring ventilatory support are clear and many often present together (Table 26.1). However, reversibility of the respiratory failure and the appropriateness of ventilatory support are sometimes debatable. Intensivists should justify instituting mechanical ventilation, especially long-term, in patients with little chance of meaningful survival.

When ventilatory support is indicated, timing is important. Indices of gas exchange and work of breathing are guides. These include Sao_2 less than 90% despite supplemental oxygen, progressive hypercarbia and acidosis, fatigue, distress, tachypnoea of more than 35 breaths/min, and decreasing conscious level. Although specific guidelines have been proposed (Table 26.2),[2] initiating ventilatory support remains a clinical decision. The trend of values together with the clinical situation will decide the timing and need for intervention.[3] Hypoxic ward patients (e.g. acute asthmatics) who are likely to require mechanical ventilation should be admitted early to the ICU. The response time of a general ward to worsening hypoxia is too slow to avert a cardiac arrest.[4]

Table 26.1 Clinical applications of mechanical ventilatory support

To maintain gas exchange and reduce work of breathing in respiratory failure
    Pulmonary causes: airway disease, airspace filling, interstitial disease, vascular disease; disorders of the pleura/mediastinum.
    Extrapulmonary causes: disorders of the musculoskeletal system; neurological disorders, including the use of muscle relaxants; all forms of shock
Control of carbon dioxide elimination
    Intracranial hypertension
    Raised pulmonary vascular resistance
    Situations with increased carbon dioxide production.
Reduction of cardiac work in cardiac failure
'Prophylactic' ventilation for patients at high risk of respiratory failure or inability to maintain an adequate work of breathing or cardiac work, e.g. after major surgery, unstable patients, severe sepsis.

Initial management

An alternative means of ventilation (e.g. resuscitator bag; see Chapter 27) must be available. Preparations must be made to deal with the immediate complications of tracheal intubation and ventilation. Initial ventilator settings should aim to achieve adequate oxygenation, with a fractional inspired oxygen concentration (Fio_2) and positive end-expiratory pressure (PEEP) titrated to maintain Sao_2 of at least 90%. Volume-controlled ventilation (VCV; see below) with tidal volume 8–10 ml/kg, at a rate of 12/min, with an inspiratory flow rate of 50–100 l/min or an inspiratory to expiratory time ratio (I:E) of 1:3, and an end-expiratory pause of 10%, is satisfactory. These settings should be adjusted according to the initial response to ventilatory support,[1] and altered to the needs of specific patients and pathologies.

Table 26.2 Traditional criteria for instituting mechanical ventilation

Parameter	Ventilation indicated	Normal range
Mechanics:		
Respiratory rate (breath/min)	>35	10–20
Tidal volume (ml/kg body weight)	<5	5–7
Vital capacity (ml/kg body weight)	<15	65–75
Maximum inspiratory force (cm H_2O)	<25	75–100
Oxygenation		
Pao_2 (mmHg)	<60 Fio_2 0.6)	75–100 (air)
$P(A-aDo_2)$ (mmHg)	>350	25–65 (Fio_2 1.0)
Ventilation		
$Paco_2$ (mmHg)	>60	35–45
$V_D:V_T$ ratio	>0.6	0.3

PEEP and CPAP[5]

PEEP and CPAP do not provide ventilation but are used in spontaneous breathing and with other modes of ventilation to improve oxygenation. PEEP is an airway pressure above atmosphere (i.e. positive) at the end of a ventilator cycle, during which spontaneous breathing is absent. CPAP refers to a positive airway pressure maintained *throughout spontaneous breathing*. By definition, CPAP is not provided if the spontaneous breathing circuit allows airway pressure to become negative on inspiration. Instead, the term *spontaneous PEEP* (sPEEP) can be used for this situation. CPAP is more efficacious than sPEEP. Both PEEP and CPAP act by similar physiological mechanisms, and are applied for similar indications, using similar devices (see Chapter 27). When spontaneous and mechanical breaths are superimposed on PEEP or CPAP, various terms are used according to the ventilatory mode (e.g. intermittent mandatory ventilation (IMV) with CPAP, see below).

PEEP is indicated when a Fio_2 of 0.5 fails to maintain Sao_2 over 90%. PEEP/CPAP increases functional residual capacity (FRC) through alveolar recruitment and prevention of alveolar derecruitment. Lung water also redistributes from the alveolar to perivascular interstitial space. Both these mechanisms improve Pao_2 by improving ventilation–perfusion mismatch. Recruitment of atelectatic areas also leads to less ventilator-induced lung injury from shear forces.[6]

Both PEEP and CPAP can also reduce the work of breathing. Airway resistance and lung compliance may improve with the improvement of functional residual capacity (FRC). In the setting of flow limitation with dynamic hyperinflation (e.g. acute asthma), PEEP will decrease the difference between airway pressure and intrinsic or auto-PEEP (the positive *alveolar* pressure at end-expiration); thus less patient effort is required to initiate inspiration.[7] CPAP and sPEEP may also have a prophylactic role, enabling some patients with moderate respiratory dysfunction to avoid endotracheal intubation and/or mechanical ventilation.[8] A usual range of PEEP or CPAP is 5–15 cm H_2O (0.5–1.5 kPa). The optimal level is disputed, but is one that optimizes oxygen delivery and keeps lung units open (as recognized by an increase in lung compliance). High levels reduce cardiac output and oxygen delivery (even though Pao_2 may be increased). The risk of barotrauma associated with hyperinflation and high intrathoracic pressures is increased. Hyperinflation also increases work of breathing and reduces the efficiency of inspiratory muscles, but in general, PEEP levels less than intrinsic PEEP will not aggravate hyperinflation.[9] Although the best PEEP may be the least PEEP,[10] low levels less than the opening pressure (inflection point) of the pressure–volume curve can cause progressive lung injury.[6]

Modes of ventilation

Different modes of mechanical ventilation were devised to offer improved oxygenation with fewer adverse effects on respiratory mechanics.[8] Minimizing airway pressure has become an important ventilatory strategy. Some mixed spontaneous and mechanical breathing modes were introduced for weaning, but are now used as primary ventilatory modes. The advantage and usefulness of any particular mode will depend on how well it meets the aims of ventilatory support, which may vary between patients and with time in a given patient. Clinically important modes of ventilation are as follows

Conventional mechanical ventilation

Conventional mechanical ventilation (CMV), otherwise called intermittent positive-pressure ventilation (IPPV), provides all ventilatory support mechanically. Sedation, often with muscle relaxants, is usually necessary. It is used when controlled hyperventilation or when minimal work of breathing is required. Common indications are for patients with increased intracranial pressure or with such poor cardiorespiratory reserve that agitation and spontaneous breathing will compromise gas exchange and cardiac function. Optimal choice of tidal volume, rate, inspiratory time, inspiratory flow waveform, end-inspiratory pause and I:E ratio can help minimize adverse physiological side-effects and patient discomfort. The use of traditional large tidal volumes (10–15 ml/kg) will reduce physiological shunt in normal lungs, but may increase the incidence of complications in patients with diseased lungs. High flow rates promote gas maldistribution, but low flow rates lead to longer inspiratory times and increased patient discomfort.

The inspiratory flow waveform does not affect gas exchange. Traditional CMV is *volume-controlled* ventilation, i.e. delivery of preset volumes using a constant flow waveform; airway pressures rise with worsening lung impedance. Whenever possible, peak airway pressures should be kept below 35 cm H_2O (3.5 kPa) to reduce the risk of complications. An alternative strategy is *pressure-controlled* (or pressure-limited) ventilation. Preset pressures are delivered using a decelerating flow waveform and time-cycling, but volumes may vary with lung mechanics. Airway pressures remain constant. Pressure-controlled ventilation appears to reduce peak airway pressure and improve thoracic compliance,[11,12] but the relationship between ventilation and other preset variables is not straightforward or intuitive.[13] For example, increasing the rate in pressure-controlled ventilation may *decrease* minute ventilation.[14] Close monitoring of pressures and volumes is essential. Comparisons are volume- and pressure-controlled ventilation are few, with inconsistent findings. Both strategies are also applicable to mechanical breaths which are triggered by the patient (see below). Other parameters of CMV are discussed elsewhere and in Chapter 27.

Assist-control ventilation (triggering)

Assist-ventilation or triggering is a mode whereby a spontaneous breath by the patient opens a demand valve and triggers a full mechanical breath. Triggering may be operated by airway pressure or flow changes produced by the patient's breath. Flow triggering entails less imposed work of breathing.[15] For safety reasons, most ventilators offer only an assist-control ventilation (ACV) mode whereby triggering initiates delivery of the preset mechanical breath, and a back-up frequency of mechanical breaths starts if no patient effort occurs. Until recently, ACV was volume-controlled, but ventilators are now available with a pressure-controlled ACV mode. Triggering aims to synchronize patient and ventilator, so as to reduce work of breathing,[16] dyspnoea and the need for sedation. However, hyperventilation is a problem with ACV, and patient–ventilator dysynchrony can still occur. Work of breathing performed by the patient is considerable.[17] ACV is uncommonly used other than in weaning or recovery from respiratory failure secondary to central depression.

Synchronized intermittent mandatory ventilation

Currently, ventilators generally provide IMV mode in its synchronized form, SIMV. SIMV allows unassisted spontaneous breathing along with trig-gered mandatory mechanical breaths. A preset back-up rate is available, and the mechanical breaths may be volume-controlled or pressure-controlled. SIMV is accepted as a primary mode of ventilation in patients with inadequate respiratory effort but is generally used more during the weaning process. PEEP or CPAP or both can be applied to SIMV.

Pressure support ventilation

In pressure support ventilation (PSV; also called inspiratory pressure support), the ventilator applies a preset pressure when triggered. Flow, instead of time, determines inspiratory to expiratory cycling. The patient controls the inspiratory time duration, flow and breathing rate. Multiple patient and ventilator factors alter tidal volume. PSV improves synchrony and comfort.[18] The preset pressure level determines the level of ventilatory support. A level of 5–20 cm H_2O (0.5–2.0 kPa) is usually used. High levels of PSV when used as the primary mode of ventilation provide ventilatory support equal to volume-controlled CMV.[19] A PSV level of 20 cm H_2O (2 kPa) decreases inspiratory work of breathing and abolishes the fatigue pattern of diaphragmatic electromyographic activity.[20] PSV combined with SIMV makes available back-up mandatory breaths. PSV is being increasingly used as a primary ventilatory mode. PEEP can be added.

Volume support ventilation (or, more correctly, volume-assured pressure support ventilation) is a new mode available in the Servo 300 ventilator (Siemens-Elema AB, Solna, Sweden). It gives the lowest PSV level necessary to deliver preset volumes to the spontaneously breathing patient, based on pressure and volume calculations of the previous breath and preset values.

Proportional assist ventilation (PAV)[21] is a new mode in which the ventilator applies an airway pressure in proportion to the patient's inspiratory effort (similar to the operation of power steering in a motor car). The patient has better control of overall ventilation, but must be able to increase the respiratory effort – questionable in those with severe muscle fatigue.

Inverse ratio ventilation

Inverse ratio ventilation (IRV)[22] involves setting an I:E ratio of more than 1:1. This recruits collapsed alveoli and allows alveolar units with slow time constants to fill, improving distribution of ventilation and ventilation–perfusion matching. The short expiratory time creates an intrinsic PEEP which prevents alveolar derecruitment. Mechanical breaths are usually pressure-controlled (PC-IRV). IRV requires sedation and paralysis. Adverse effects result from the increase in intrathoracic pressure.

Mandatory minute volume ventilation

In mandatory minute volume (MMV) ventilation the ventilator delivers breaths when spontaneous breathing generates less than the preset minute volume. Thus a constant minute volume is maintained, even in the presence of varying spontaneous ventilation. Unfortunately, many critically ill patients have rapid shallow breathing which is ineffectual in eliminating CO_2 but contributes to the minute volume monitored. Few ventilators offer MMV; if available, success will depend largely on the ventilator design.

Pressure release ventilation

Airway pressure release ventilation (APRV)

In APRV, the ventilator applies CPAP and intermittently releases the airway pressure to a lower level using a time-controlled release valve. High CPAP and lung volume are re-established when the release valve is closed. The APRV pressure versus time profile is the inverse of that for IMV. Gas exchange, and thus ventilator support, is provided by the lung deflation, which is superimposed on spontaneous CPAP breathing. Peak airway pressures never exceed the high CPAP level. The high CPAP, release airway pressure and rate are preset.

Biphasic positive airway pressure (BIPAP)

BIPAP is a confusing term but is essentially similar to APRV. One version[23] allows spontaneous breathing at two airway pressures, with synchronization during cycling between the pressures. Better coordination between spontaneous and pressure release breaths may result. PSV can be added to augment spontaneous breathing. BIPAP can be applied with a mask, which is a useful strategy in some patients, to avoid tracheal intubation or in the immediate postextubation period. BIPAP and APRV appear useful for patients with mild to moderate ventilatory failure, but further clinical assessment is required.

Independent lung ventilation

Independent lung ventilation (ILV) separates ventilation to each lung using double-lumen tracheal tubes. Different parameters and, indeed, different modes can be applied for each lung, and synchronization is not necessarily required. ILV may be useful in unilateral lung disease, e.g. unilateral trauma, bronchopleural fistula, pulmonary haemorrhage or infection.

High-frequency ventilation

High-frequency ventilation[8,24] consists of high-frequency positive pressure ventilation (HFPPV at a rate of 1–2 Hz or 60–120/min), high-frequency oscillation (HFO, at 3–20 Hz or 180–12 000/min), and high-frequency jet ventilation (HFJV). HFJV is the most widely used form in clinical practice today. High-pressure gas (30–300 kPa) is delivered into the airway via a small-bore catheter or a special endotracheal tube with a jet delivery tube in its wall. Ventilation frequencies range between 1 and 5 Hz (60–300/min) and expired minute volumes may be between 10 and 50 l/min. Entrainment of gases is often used but a closed system is also possible. HFJV offers advantages in the management of massive air leaks and disrupted airways. Its superiority over other ventilatory modes in managing severe acute respiratory failure remains unproven. Inadequate humidification of inspiratory gases is a problem.[25] Other disadvantages are increased risk of barotrauma and tracheal mucosal injury when the jet impinges directly on the tracheal wall.

Non-invasion ventilation

Non-invasive ventilation refers to mechanical ventilatory support applied without the use of an artificial airway. Positive-pressure ventilation is delivered using face or nasal masks. Less commonly, negative-pressure ventilation is delivered using a variety of devices. Intermittent nocturnal positive-pressure non-invasive ventilation has improved symptoms and gas exchange in some chronic disorders such as neuromuscular disorders, thoracic cage abnormalities and sleep apnoea. Non-invasive ventilation can reduce the need for endotracheal intubation, length of hospitalization, and mortality rate in selected patients with respiratory failure.[26,27] It may also be useful to avert reintubation following extubation.

Other methods of ventilatory support and gas exchange

These include low-frequency modes, perfluorocarbon-associated ventilatory support (see section on liquid ventilation, below),[28] intratracheal pulmonary ventilation,[29] and the use of inhaled nitric oxide.[30] Extracorporeal membrane oxygenation has no benefits over ventilation modes. A modified technique (extracorporeal CO_2 removal with low-frequency IPPV and PEEP) has been used in adult respiratory distress syndrome,[31] but does not improve survival[32] (see Chapter 29). An intravascular blood gas exchanger (IVOX, an elongated membrane oxygenator to lie within the venae cavae)[33] has been designed. Proper clinical evaluation is needed.

Management of ventilatory support

Management of ventilatory support aims to optimize gas exchange, lessen work of breathing and avoid complications, while maintaining optimal conditions for lung recovery.

Optimal gas exchange

Oxygenation is the first priority of ventilatory support. Ventilator controls influencing oxygenation are Fio_2 (which affects alveolar Po_2) and ventilator-generated pressures (which affect the alveolar–arterial Po_2 difference). Fio_2 and the pattern and levels of airway pressure should be titrated against changes in patient oxygenation. Hypoxaemia during mechanical ventilation requires immediate management, and causes should be promptly determined (Table 26.3). The Fio_2 should be increased to 1.0, equipment and tracheal tube checked, and a physical examination performed. If a cause is not apparent, chest X-rays are required.

CO_2 elimination requires increased minute ventilation. Complications from excessive ventilation can be life-threatening, while hypercarbia is usually safe. The technique of 'permissive hypercarbia' uses hypoventilation to avoid the side-effects of mechanical ventilation.[34,35] This technique cannot be used in situations in which hypercarbia is dangerous (e.g. patients with intracranial hypertension).

Work of breathing

Spontaneous breathing can still occur during mechanical ventilation, with considerable work being performed.[36] It is crucial to minimize work of breathing during ventilatory support.[37] This may be done by reducing ventilatory demand (e.g. eliminating hypoxia, acidosis, anxiety and other stimulants of excessive breathing), by improving lung compliance and resistance, and by minimizing imposed work. Such work of breathing is imposed by the ventilator (e.g. inappropriate settings, patient dysynchrony and ventilator design), and humidifiers, circuits and tracheal tubes.[38–40] The correct choice of ventilator and circuit and optimal setting of ventilatory variables will minimize the work of breathing.

It is important to improve respiratory muscle capacity and efficiency. This may be done by positioning the patient, reducing dynamic hyperinflation and replenishing energy supplies (i.e. adequate perfusion, nutrition and electrolytes) to the respiratory muscles. Reducing the work of breathing also diverts oxygen delivery to other vital tissue beds.

Minimizing complications

Ventilatory support is a dynamic process requiring trained personnel and continuous monitoring. A 1:1 nurse:patient ratio is essential. The patient's airway (i.e. patency, and presence of leaks and secretions), breathing (i.e. rate, depth, bilateral movements, synchronization with the ventilator and oxygenation) and circulatory status (pulse, blood pressure and urine output) must be monitored. Ventilatory equipment must be regularly checked, including Fio_2, ventilator settings, humidifier, breathing circuit, tracheal tube and its cuff pressure. Airway temperature should be monitored. Ventilator alarms can be disabled temporarily but never switched off.

Serial investigations of respiratory function are obtained as indicated. This includes arterial blood gases, oxygen delivery, oxygen consumption and regional oxygenation indices such as gastric intra-mucosal pH.[41] Continuous pulse oximetry is indicated, if not mandatory. It is important to monitor tidal volume in pressure-preset modes (Table 26.4), and airway pressures in volume preset modes (Table 26.5). End-inspiratory volume[35] and intrinsic PEEP monitoring are useful in patients with airflow limitation. Delineation of pressure–volume curves will aid ventilatory management.[42]

The spontaneous breathing pattern and the integrity of the central respiratory drive should be

Table 26.3 Common causes of hypoxaemia during mechanical ventilation

Inadequate Fio_2
Incorrect settings
Circuit leak
Contaminated gas supply

Hypoventilation
Incorrect settings
Inadequate patient effort
Tracheal tube malposition

Ventilation–perfusion mismatch
Endobronchial intubation
Pneumothorax
Pulmonary pathology

Table 26.4 Low tidal volumes in pressure preset modes

Patient factors
Asynchronous breathing

Decreased compliance
 Development of pneumothorax
 Pulmonary pathology

Increased airway resistance/airway obstruction
 Bronchospasm
 Aspiration/secretions
 Allergic reaction to drugs/transfusion

Equipment causes
Ventilator settings
 Inadequate preset pressure
 I:E ratio > 2:1
 Frequency > 20 breath/min

Other equipment
 Gas leak
 Endotracheal tube malposition

assessed regularly.[43] It may also be useful to monitor patient work of breathing.[44] Pulmonary structure may be evaluated with serial chest X-rays; bronchoscopy may be indicated for microbiological sampling[45] or evaluation of pulmonary lesions.

With the use of sedation and paralysis, nursing care of the comatose patient is obligatory. Patient communication is vital. A ventilated patient should be spoken to as if fully alert. A brief explanation must be given before performing any procedure. Patient anxiety and pain must be managed with appropriate sedation and analgesia. Support of other organ systems is essential. This includes stress ulcer prophylaxis, deep vein thrombosis prophylaxis, oral hygiene and metabolic support.

Mechanical ventilation is supportive therapy, and the patient's prognosis depends on the underlying disease and severity of illness.[46] However, complications resulting from mechanical ventilation can affect outcome, and their risks must be minimized. Table 26.6 lists some adverse effects of mechanical ventilation. Equipment-related complications underscore the need for experienced personnel and close monitoring.

Cardiovascular complications[47]

Positive-pressure ventilation increases mean intrathoracic pressure. This reduces systemic venous return and cardiac output. Raised intrathoracic pressure also reduces left ventricular (LV) preload by decreasing LV compliance. The reduction in cardiac output may result in acute hypotension in situations of hypovolaemia and reduced vascular tone (e.g. in sepsis, anaphylaxis and neurogenic shock). Blood volume must be adequately replaced and inotropes should be considered.

Mechanical ventilation of a diseased lung may reduce pulmonary vascular resistance, by attenuating hypoxic pulmonary vasoconstriction and by returning the diseased lung to a normal FRC; collapsed extra-alveolar vessels are reopened. Conversely, overdistension of the lung increases pulmonary vascular resistance due to compression of alveolar vessels.

LV afterload, being dependent on the transmural LV systolic pressure, will be reduced by a rise in intrathoracic pressure (assuming maintenance of systolic arterial pressure). The reduction in LV end-diastolic volume from reduced systemic venous return also reduces LV afterload. Reduced LV afterload partly explains the beneficial action of CPAP in heart failure. This effect also explains the acute LV failure which can occur during weaning in patients with poor LV function.

Lung complications

Positive-pressure ventilation can produce varied unfavourable pulmonary effects such as maldistribution of gas, progressive atelectasis, hyperinflation, ventilation–perfusion mismatch, decreased compliance,

Table 26.5 High airway pressures in volume-preset modes

Patient factors
Asynchronous breathing

Low compliance
  Endobronchial intubation
  Pulmonary pathology
  Pneumothorax
  Ascites

Increased airway resistance/airway obstruction
  Bronchospasm
  Aspiration/secretions
  Allergic reactions

Equipment causes
Ventilator settings
  Excessive flow/volume settings

Other equipment
  Obstruction to flow in circuit, tracheal tube, PEEP valve
  Endotracheal tube malposition

PEEP = Positive end-expiratory pressure.

Table 26.6 Complications associated with mechanical ventilation

Equipment	Malfunction
	Contamination
	Incorrectly used
	Wrong settings
Patient	
Cardiovascular	Decreased cardiac output
Respiratory	Lung injury, imposed work, oxygen toxicity
Neuromuscular	Decreased cerebral perfusion, sedation and paralysis
Psychiatric	Psychosis, suffering, pain
Splanchnic	Decreased splanchnic and renal perfusions, gastrointestinal distension, bleeding
Infection	Loss of host defences, transmission of pathogens
Airway management	Damage to teeth, trachea, vocal cords (see Chapter 23)

reduction in surfactant, increased work of breathing, increased extravascular lung water and decreased bronchial circulation.

Ventilator-induced lung injury[48] includes pulmonary air leaks, pulmonary microvascular leaks with oedema,[49] and pulmonary fibrosis. Ventilation with large lung volumes as well as at low lung volumes may induce lung injury.[50] Preventive strategies include permissive hypercapnia, the use of PEEP to recruit lung volume and reduce shear stress, and ensuring that maximum transalveolar pressures do not exceed 35 cm H_2O (3.5 kPa).[51] Use of high Fio_2 levels and inadequate heating and humidification of inspired gases may lead to airway and lung injury (see Chapter 28). Other complications result from devices and apparatus (e.g. tracheal tube, mask or tracheostomy).

Neuropsychiatric complications

Raised intrathoracic pressure increases intracranial pressure and reduces cardiac output, both reducing cerebral perfusion pressure. Sedation, with or without paralysis, can lead to atelectasis, muscle atrophy, secretion retention and hypotension. However, intubation and ventilation are distressing to the patient. Inadequate sedation will produce restlessness; self-extubation may result in fatality. Sensory overload can cause 'ICU psychosis'.

Infectious complications

Intubation and ventilation bypass natural defences with non-sterile equipment. Many ICU personnel deal with each ventilated patient, and movement between patients transfers microorganisms. Endogenous sources of infection quickly develop with critical illness, and enter the lung by aspiration or translocation from the gut. Nosocomial pneumonia occurs in 30% of ventilated patients and increases mortality two-fold.[52] Prevention includes treatment of the underlying disease, measures to improve host defences, use of the upright position,[53] stress ulcer prophylaxis with sucralfate,[54] infection control measures, hand-washing, proper disinfection of equipment and selective decontamination of the gut (see Chapter 62).

Weaning from ventilatory support

Weaning is the process of gradual discontinuation of ventilatory support. Complications increase with duration of ventilatory support, but premature weaning leads to cardiopulmonary deterioration. Weaning is indicated when the underlying problem has resolved, and the patient can reassume the work of breathing and maintain good gas exchange. This implies an intact central drive, haemodynamic stability, recovery of respiratory muscle weakness and fatigue (with no residual paralysis or effects of sedation) and no major organ dysfunction. Nutritional support (including provision of minerals and vitamins) is important in restoring energy stores to respiratory muscles.

Reported bedside predictors of successful weaning[55] include standard weaning criteria (the opposite of Table 26.2),[56] work of breathing,[56] oxygen cost of breathing,[57,58] mouth occlusion pressure (inspiratory airway pressure at 0.1 s), and an index of compliance, rate, oxygenation and pressure (CROP).[55] However, a simple rate (breath/min)/tidal volume (l) ratio, within a minute after disconnection from the ventilator is more reliable.[55] A ratio over 100 depicts rapid shallow breathing and has a negative (failure) predictive value of 95% (Table 26.7). The inspiratory pressure (P_1)/maximal inspiratory pressure (P_1max) ratio also reasonably separates weaning success and failure.[59] A value > 0.3 has a negative predictive value of 72% (Table 26.7).[59] Combined use of rate/tidal volume ratio and P_1/P_1 max ratio can provide higher accuracy (Table 26.7).[59] Neural networks theoretically outperform traditional statistical predictive models and are under investigation.[60] None the less, the judgement of an experienced clinician is probably the most reliable predictor of weaning outcome.

T-piece weaning has been the traditional weaning technique. However, use of SIMV or PSV in weaning prevents the drastic increase in work of breathing during T-piece sessions.[61] PSV may shorten the duration of weaning and improve weaning success, compared to the T-piece and SIMV.[62] Combined SIMV and PSV are commonly used. Low PEEP/CPAP levels may be useful, and low levels of PSV can be used

Table 26.7 Predictors of weaning outcome – rate, tidal volume and inspiratory pressure indices of respiratory muscle fatigue[58]

Index	Sensitivity	Specificity	Positive predictive value	Negative predictive value
f/V_T (100/min)	0.94	0.73	0.79	0.92
P_1/P_1max (0.3)	0.75	0.67	0.71	0.72
f/V_T and P_1/P_1max	0.81	0.93	0.93	0.83

f = Rate; V_r = tidal volume; P_1 = inspiratory pressure; P_1max = maximal inspiratory pressure.

to overcome imposed work of breathing.[63] The progress and psychological state of the patient must be followed closely. Fatigue of the respiratory muscles and excessive anxiety must be avoided. In prolonged weaning, reinstituting ventilatory support overnight will allow adequate rest. The final stage before extubation is usually PSV ± CPAP or CPAP breathing. Extubation is performed when airway patency and protection are assured (i.e. reflexes are present) and the patient can cough up secretions.

Liquid ventilation

Perfluoration is capable of holding high concentrations of oxygen and carbon dioxide. Gas ventilation of perfluorocarbon-filled lung was originally reported in animal models of respiratory failure and isolated premature babies with infant respiratory distress syndrome.[28,64] Concurrent use with extracorporeal membrane oxygenation (ECMO), i.e. partial liquid ventilation (PLV) in adults, children and neonates has recently been reported.[65;66] In patients who do not respond following mechanical ventilation and ECMO support, perfluorocarbon is gradually instilled into the lungs via the endotracheal tube until a meniscus is seen within the endotracheal tube. Gas ventilation is continued with ECMO. Extra doses of perfluorocarbon are given daily and following tracheal suctioning. PLV appears to improve gas exchange and lung compliance by increased alveolar recruitment (due to perfluorocarbon's high density and low surface tension), and better ventilation:perfusion matching (due to increased redistribution of pulmonary blood flow to non-dependent lung zones). This is an exciting new unconventional technique which requires proper scientific validation.

References

1 Slutsky AS (1993) ACCP consensus conference: mechanical ventilation. *Chest* **104**:1833–1859.
2 Pontoppidan H, Laver MB and Geffin B (1970) Acute respiratory failure in the surgical patient. *Adv Surg* **4**:163–254.
3 Schuster DP (1990) A physiological approach to initiating, maintaining, and withdrawing mechanical ventilatory support during acute respiratory failure. *Am J Med* **88**:268–278.
4 Franklin C and Matthew J (1994) Developing strategies to prevent cardiac arrest: analysing responses of physicians and nurses in the hours before the event. *Crit Care Med* **22**:224–230.
5 Duncan AW, Oh TE and Hillman DR (1986) PEEP and CPAP. *Anaesth Intens Care* **14**:236–250.
6 Muncedere JG, Mullen JBM, Gan K and Slutsky AS (1994) Tidal ventilation at low airway pressures can augment lung injury. *Am J Respir Crit Care Med* **149**:1327–1334.

7 Petrof BJ, Legare M, Goldberg P, Milic-Emili J and Gottfried SB (1990) Continuous positive airway pressure reduces work of breathing and dyspnea during weaning from mechanical ventilation in severe chronic obstructive pulmonary disease. *Am Rev Respir Dis* **141**:281–289.
8 Lin ES and Oh TE (1990) Which mode of ventilation? In Dobb G (ed.) *Intensive Care: Developments and Controversies. Bailliere's Clinical Anaesthesiology.* London: WB Saunders, pp. 441–473.
9 Tan IKS, Bhatt SB, Tam YH and Oh TE (1993) Effects of PEEP on dynamic hyperinflation in patients with airflow limitation. *Br J Anaesth* **70**:267–272.
10 Carroll GC, Tuman KJ, Braverman B, Logas WG, Wool and N, Ivankovich AD (1988) Minimal positive end-expiratory pressure (PEEP) may be 'best PEEP'. *Chest* **93**:1020–1025.
11 Rappaport SH, Shpiner R, Yoshihara G, Wright J, Chang P and Abraham E (1994) Ramdomized prospective trial of pressure-limited versus volume-controlled ventilation in severe respiratory failure. *Crit Care Med* **22**:22–32.
12 Lessard MR, Guerot E, Lorino H, Lemaire F and Brochard L (1994) Effects of pressure-controlled ventilation with different I:E ratios versus volume-controlled ventilation on respiratory mechanics, gas exchange, and hemodynamics in patients with adult respiratory distress syndrome. *Anesthesiology* **80**:983–991.
13 Marini JJ (1991) Controlled ventilation: targets, hazards and options. In: Marini JJ and Roussos C (eds). *Ventilatory Failure.* Berlin: Springer-Verlag, pp. 269–292.
14 Nahum A, Burke WC, Ravenscraft SA *et al.* (1992) Lung mechanics and gas exchange during pressure-control ventilation in dogs: augmentation of CO_2 elimination by an intratracheal catheter. *Am Rev Respir Dis* **146**:965–973.
15 Sassoon CSH, Lodia R, Rheeman CH, Kuei JH, Light RW and Mahutte CK (1992) Inspiratory muscle work of breathing during flow-by, demand-flow, and continuous-flow systems in patients with chronic obstructive pulmonary disease. *Am Rev Respir Dis* **145**:1219–1222.
16 Stock MC (1994) Timing is everything – or is it? *Crit Care Med* **22**:730–731.
17 Marini JJ, Capps JS and Culver BH (1985) The inspiratory work of breathing during assisted mechanical ventilation. *Chest* **87**:612–618.
18 MacIntyre NR, Nishimura M, Usada Y, Takioka H, Takezawa J and Shimida Y (1990) The Nagoya conference on system design and patient–ventilator interactions during pressure support ventilation. *Chest* **97**:1463–1466.
19 MacIntyre NR (1986) Respiratory function during pressure support ventilation. *Chest* **89**:677–683.
20 Brochard L, Harf A, Lorino H and Lemaire F (1989) Inspiratory pressure support prevents diaphragmatic fatigue during weaning from mechanical ventilation. *Am Rev Respir Dis* **139**:513–521.
21 Younes M (1992) Proportional assist ventilation, a new approach to ventilatory support: theory. *American Rev Respir Dis* **145**:114–120.

22 Marcy TW and Marini JJ (1991) Inverse ratio ventilation in ARDS. *Chest* **100**:494–504.

23 Hormann C, Baum M, Putenen C, Mitz NJ and Benzer H (1994) Biphasic positive airway pressure (BIPAP) – a new mode of ventilatory support. *Eur J Anaesthesiol* **11**:37–42.

24 Froese AB and Bryan AC (1987) High frequency ventilation. *Am Rev Respir Dis* **135**:1363–1372.

25 Kan AF, Gin T, Lin ES and Oh TE (1990) Factors influencing humidification in high frequency jet ventilation. *Crit Care Med* **18**:537–539.

26 Brochard L, Mancebo J, Wysocki M *et al.* (1995) Noninvasive ventilation for acute exacerbations of chronic obstructive pulmonary disease. *New Engl J Med* **333**:817– 822.

27 Bersten AD, Holt AW, Vedig AE, Skowronski GA and Baggoley CJ (1991) Treatment of severe cardiogenic pulmonary edema with continuous positive airway pressure delivered by face mask. *N Engl J Med* **325**:1825–1830.

28 Leach CL, Fuhrman BP, Morin FM *et al.* (1993) Perfluorocarbon-associated gas exchange (partial liquid ventilation) in respiratory distress syndrome: a prospective randomized study. *Crit Care Med* **21**:1270–1278.

29 Muller EE, Kolobow T, Mandava S *et al.* (1993) How to ventilate lungs as small as 12.5% of normal: the new technique of intratracheal pulmonary ventilation. *Pediatr Res* **34**:606–610.

30 Roissant R, Falke KJ, Keitel N *et al.* (1993) Inhaled nitric oxide for the adult respiratory distress syndrome. *N Engl J Med* **328**:399–405.

31 Gattinoni L, Agostini A, Pesenti A *et al.* (1980) Treatment of acute respiratory failure with low frequency positive pressure ventilation and extracorporeal removal of CO_2. *Lancet* **2**:292–295.

32 Morris AH, Wallace CJ, Menlove RL *et al.* (1994) Randomized trial of pressure-controlled inverse ratio ventilation and extracorporeal CO_2 removal for adult respiratory distress syndrome. *Am J Respir Crit Care Med* **149**:295–305.

33 Mortenson JD (1991) Augmentation of blood gas transfer by means of an intravascular blood gas exchanger (IVOX). In: Marini JJ and Roussos C (eds) *Ventilatory Failure*. Berlin: Springer-Verlag, pp. 318–346.

34 Hickling KG, Henderson SJ and Jackson R (1990) Low mortality associated with low volume pressure limited ventilation with permissive hypercapnia in severe adult respiratory distress syndrome. *Intens Care Med* **16**:372–377.

35 Tuxen DV, Williams TJ, Scheinkestel CD, Czarny D and Bowes G (1992) Use of a measurement of pulmonary hyperinflation to control the level of mechanical ventilation in patients with acute severe asthma. *Am Rev Respir Dis* **146**:1136–1142.

36 Marini JJ, Smith TC and Lamb VJ (1988) External work output and force generation during synchronized intermittent mechanical ventilation. *Am Rev Respir* **138**:1169–1179.

37 Marini JJ (1990) Strategies to minimize breathing effort during mechanical ventilation. *Crit Care Clin* **6**:635–661.

38 Oh TE, Lin ES and Bhatt S (1991) Inspiratory work imposed by demand valve ventilator circuits. *Anaesth Intens Care* **19**:187–191.

39 Oh TE, Lin ES and Bhatt SB (1991) Resistance of humidifiers and inspiratory work imposed by a ventilator–humidifier circuit. *Br J Anaesth* **56**:258–263.

40 Bersten AD, Rutten AJ, Vedig AE and Skowronski GA (1989) Additional work of breathing imposed by endotracheal tubes, breathing circuits, and intensive care ventilators. *Crit Care Med* **17**:671–677.

41 Mohsenifar Z, Hay A, Hay J, Lewis MI and Koerner SK (1993) Gastric intramural pH as a predictor of success or failure in weaning patients from mechanical ventilation. *Ann Intern Med* **119**:794–798.

42 Fernandez R, Blanch L and Artigas A (1993) Inflation pressure–volume curves of the total respiratory system determined without any instrumentation other than the mechanical ventilator. *Int Care Med* **19**:33–38.

43 Kelley BJ and Matthay MA (1993) Prevalence and ventilator dependent patients. *Crit Care Med* **22**:515–525.

44 Banner MJ, Jaeger MJ and Kirby RR (1994) Components of the work of breathing and implications for monitoring ventilator dependent patients. *Critical Care Medicine* **22**:515–525.

45 Torres A, el Ebiary M, Padro L *et al.* (1994) Validation of different techniques for the diagnosis of ventilator-associated pneumonia. Comparison with immediate post-mortem biopsy. *Am J Respir Crit Care Med* **149**:324–331.

46 Jimenez P, Torres A, Roca J, Cobos A and Rodriguez-Roisin R (1994) Arterial oxygenation does not predict the outcome of patients with acute respiratory failure needing mechanical ventilation. *Eur Respir J* **7**:730–735.

47 Pinsky MR (1990) The effect of mechanical ventilation on the cardiovascular system. *Crit Care Clin* **6**:663–678.

48 Parker JC, Hernandez LA and Peevy KJ (1993) Mechanisms of ventilator-induced lung injury. *Crit Care Med* **21**:131–143.

49 West JB and Mathieu-Costello O (1992) Stress failure of pulmonary capillaries: role in lung and heart disease. *Lancet* **340**:956–961.

50 Dreyfuss D and Saumon G (1994) Should the lung be rested or recruited? The Charybdis and Scylla of ventilator management. *Am J Respir Crit Care Med* **149**:1066–1068.

51 Tsuno K, Miura K, Takeya M, Kolobow T and Morioka T (1991) Histopathological pulmonary changes from mechanical ventilation at high peak airway pressures. *Am Res Respir Dis* **143**:1115–1120.

52 Fagon JY, Chastre J, Hance AJ, Montravers P, Novara A and Gilbert C (1993) Nosocomial pneumonia in ventilated patients: a cohort study evaluating attributable mortality and hospital stay. *Am J Med* **94**:281–288.

53 Torres A, Serra-Batlles J, Ros E *et al.* (1992) Pulmonary aspiration of gastric contents in patients receiving mechanical ventilation: the effect of body position. *Ann Intern Med* **116**:540–543.

54 Prod'hom G, Leuenberger P, Koerfer J *et al.* (1944) Nosocomial pneumonia in mechanically ventilated patients receiving antacids, ranitidine, or sucralfate as prophylaxis for stress ulcer. A randomized controlled trial. *Ann Intern Med* **120**:653–662.

55 Yang KL and Tobin MJ (1991) A prospective study predicting the outcome of trials of weaning from mechanical ventilation. *N Engl J Med* **324**:1445–1450.

56 Fiastro LF, Habib MP, Shon BY and Campbell SC (1988) Comparison of standard weaning parameters and the mechanical work of breathing in mechanically ventilated patients. *Chest* **94**:232–238.

57 Shikora SA, Bistrian B, Borlase BC, Blackburn GL, Stone MD and Benotti PN (1990) Work of breathing: reliable predictor of weaning and extubation. *Crit Care Med* **18**:157–162.

58 Oh TE, Bhatt S, Lin ES, Hutchinson RC and Low JM (1993) Plasma catecholamines and oxygen consumption during weaning from mechanical ventilation. *Intens Care Med* **17**:199–203.

59 Yang KL (1993) Inspiratory pressure/maximal inspiratory pressure ratio: a predictive index of weaning outcome. *Intens Care Med* **19**:204–208.

60 Ashutosh K, Lee H, Mohan CK, Ranka S, Mehrota K and Alexander C (1992) Prediction criteria for successful weaning from respiratory support: statistical and connectionist models. *Crit Care Med* **20**:1295–1301.

61 Sassoon CSH, Light RW, Lodia R, Sieck GC and Mahutte CK (1991) Pressure–time product during continuous positive airway pressure, pressure support ventilation, and T-piece during weaning from mechanical ventilation. *Am Rev Respir Dis* **143**:469–475.

62 Brochard L, Rauss A, Benito S *et al.* (1994) Comparison of three methods of gradual withdrawal from ventilatory support during weaning from mechanical ventilation. *Am J Resp Crit Care Med* **150**:896–903.

63 Brochard L, Rua F, Lorino H, Lemaire F and Harf A (1991). Inspiratory pressure support compensates for the additional work of breathing caused by the endotracheal tube. *Anesthesiology* **75**:739–745.

64 Hirsch RB, Tooley R, Parent AC, Johnson K and Bartlett RH (1995) Improvement of gas exchange, pulmonary function, and lung injury with partial liquid ventilation. A study model in a setting of severe respiratory failure. *Chest* **108**:500–508.

65 Hirschl RB, Pranikoff T, Wise C *et al.* (1996) Initial experience with partial liquid ventilation in adult patients with the acute respiratory distress syndrome. *J Am Med Assoc* **275**:383–389.

66 Hirsch RB, Pranikoff T, Gauger P, Schriner RJ, Dechert R and Bartlett RH (1995) Liquid ventilation in adults, children, and full-term neonates. *Lancet* **346**:1201–1202.

27 Ventilators and resuscitators

AD Bersten and TE Oh

This chapter complements Chapter 26. Ventilators are mechanical devices used to replace or assist spontaneous ventilation. They include conventional positive-pressure machines, negative-pressure devices (e.g. cuirass and iron lung), and devices applied via a nose or facemask, or oral prosthesis for non-invasive ventilation.

Ideal requirements

Patient size

An ideal ventilator should be able to ventilate all sizes of patients from neonates to adults. Dedicated neonatal ventilators evolved from simple T-piece, continuous-flow occlusion devices, but some modern neonatal/paediatric ventilators are more similar to adult ventilators in complexity and versatility.

Versatility of operation

Delivery of an accurate fractional inspired oxygen concentration (Fio_2 from 0.21 to 1.0) and a preset volume, despite changes in respiratory system characteristics, should be expected. Conventional mechanical ventilation (CMV), assist-control ventilation (ACV), synchronized intermittent mandatory ventilation (SIMV), pressure support ventilation (PSV), positive end-expiratory ventilation (PEEP) and continuous positive airway pressure (CPAP) are essential ventilatory modes for a modern ICU ventilator.[1] A range of ventilatory settings should be available, e.g. for inspiratory flow, volume, pressure, time and inspiratory:expiratory (I:E) ratio, although data on optimal ventilatory patterns are generally lacking.

Unimpeded spontaneous respiration

The circuit should have minimal resistance to spontaneous and assisted breathing. Circuit-imposed work of breathing is minimized if fresh gas flow and demand valve respond rapidly to patient-initiated breaths.[2,3]

Monitoring and alarm functions

These requirements are mandatory and complementary, and may include automatic responses to detected abnormalities (e.g. back-up CMV following apnoea and opening of high-pressure relief valves to prevent barotrauma). Continuous monitoring of airway pressures and expired volumes and a disconnect alarm are essential features (Table 27.1).[3] Additional monitoring of respiratory mechanics and metabolic parameters may be desirable.

Effective humidification of inspired gas (see Chapter 28)

Nebulization of drugs

The ventilator should be able to deliver therapeutic aerosols in-line and automatically discount excess gas flow to avoid hyperinflation and barotrauma. Partitioning of aerosolization to inspiration is useful.

Maintenance and reliability

Cleaning and maintenance should be simple, with easy access to parts requiring sterilization. A ventilator should also be reliable, robust and easy to use.

Classification of ventilators[4-6]

Classifying ventilators allows better understanding of functional characteristics of ventilators, enabling a particular ventilator to be used to its full potential.

Mapleson flow or pressure generator[6]

This most commonly used classification considers inspiratory and expiratory flow with their methods of

Table 27.1 Proposed monitoring and alarm requirements for ICU ventilators*

Variable	Critical care	Transport
Pressure		
P_{pk}	Essential	Essential
P_{plat}	Essential	Optional
P_{mean}	Essential	Optional
$PEEP_e$	Essential	Essential
$PEEP_i$	Recommended	Optional
Volume		
V_T expired machine	Essential	Recommended
V_E machine	Essential	Optional
V_T expired spontaneous	Essential	Recommended
V_E spontaneous	Essential	Optional
Timing		
Flow mechanical	Recommended	Optional
Flow spontaneous	Optional	Optional
I:E ratio	Essential	Recommended
Rate: mechanical	Essential	Recommended
Rate: spontaneous	Essential	Recommended
Gas concentration†	Essential	Optional
Alarms‡		
Power failure	Essential	Essential
Apnoea	Essential	Essential
Loss of gas delivery	Essential	Essential
Excess gas delivery	Essential	Essential
Exhale valve failure	Essential	Essential
Timing failure	Essential	Essential
Circuit leak	Essential	Essential
Circuit partially occluded	Essential	Essential
Blender failure	Essential	Essential
Heater/humidifier failure	Essential	Essential
Loss of or excess PEEP	Essential	Essential
Autocycling	Essential	Essential

*Modified from American Association for Respiratory Care[3].
†Equals FiO_2 when the inspiratory flow rate is met.
‡Currently most modern ventilators achieve most of these aims through electrical, pneumatic and circuit pressure monitoring with alarm limits.
P_{pk} = Peak airway pressure; P_{plat} = plateau airway pressure; P_{mean} = mean airway pressure. $PEEP_e$ = extrinsic positive end-expiratory pressure (PEEP): $PEEP_i$ = intrinsic PEEP; V_T = tidal volume; V_E minute volume; I:E = inspiratory :expiratory.

cycling, although clinical usefulness involves mainly inspiratory flow and inspiratory to expiratory cycling (Table 27.2). A flow generator uses a high generating pressure to produce an inspiratory flow unaffected by patient lung changes. The flow pattern may be constant or non-constant. A pressure generator has a lower generating pressure to produce an inspiratory flow that can be influenced by lung changes. Flow pattern may vary, but the pressure waveform remains unchanged, and may be constant or non-constant. Both flow and pressure generators are subdivided into methods of cycling.

Although this classification divides ventilators according to the generating pressure produced to drive gas into the lungs, it is actually a spectrum, with transition from one group to the other at some intermediate point. A ventilator behaves like a flow generator when the generating pressure is high enough to disregard patient impedance. A pressure generator may become a flow generator if its generating pressure is increased to exceed alveolar pressure by 10 times. Modern ICU ventilators use piped gas sources and are electrically controlled, and can act as flow or pressure generators.

Chatburn classification[4]

The ability of modern ventilators to produce varied patterns of ventilation has outgrown Mapleson's and other conventional classifications.[5,6] Chatburn's classification uses a framework of power source, drive mechanism, control mechanism, and output (Table 27.3).[4] A ventilator's functional characteristics are basically described by the control mechanism and output headings, but as much detail of the ventilator in other headings can be added as desired.

Control mechanism

Consideration of the control mechanism is based on the interrelationship of force generated by ventilator and/or respiratory muscles (measured as pressure), gas displacement (measured as volume), and the rate of displacement (i.e. flow), expressed as the equation of motion for the respiratory system:

$$Pressure = volume/system\ compliance + (system\ resistance \times flow)$$

where pressure, volume or flow can vary (i.e. variables) and compliance and resistance are constant (i.e. parameters). The control mechanism is described under three subheadings.

Variable and waveform control

If any one of the variables and its resultant waveform can be preset (i.e. pressure, volume or flow control), it becomes the independent variable, making the other two dependent variables. If no variable can be predetermined, the ventilator is a time-controller.

Table 27.2 Mapleson's flow/pressure generator classification[6]

Generating pressure	Cycling
Flow generator (constant or non-constant flow)	Time Pressure Volume
Pressure generator (constant or non-constant pressure)	Time Pressure Volume Flow

Table 27.3 Classification of ventilators and their modes

Power input
Pneumatic
Electrical | Mains
| Battery

Drive mechanism
External compressor
Internal compressor | Compressed gas
| Electric motor
| Direct
| Rotating crank and piston
| Rack and pinion
Output control valves | Pneumatic
| Diaphragm
| Poppit valve
| Electromagnetic
| Poppit valve
| Proportional valve

Control mechanism
Control circuit | Mechanical
| Pneumatic
| Fluidic
| Electric
| Electronic
Control variables and | Pressure
waveform | Flow
| Volume
| Time
Phase variables | Trigger
| Limit
| Cycle
| Baseline

Conditional variables

Output
Pressure waveform | Rectangular
| Sinusoidal
| Exponential rise
| Oscillating
Volume waveform | Ramp
| Sinusoidal
Flow waveform | Rectangular
| Ramp
| Ascending
| Descending
| Sinusoidal

Alarm systems
Input alarms
Control and circuit alarms
Output alarms

Modified from Chatburn[4].

1 *Pressure control:* the ventilator applies a positive or negative pressure with a set waveform. The flow and volume achieved will depend upon the compliance, resistance and the pressure waveform chosen.

2 *Flow control:* the ventilator delivers a set flow rate and pattern, independent of the patient's respiratory mechanics. Hence resultant volume is also constant. The pressure will depend upon the flow rate and pattern, volume or inspiratory time and respiratory system mechanics.

3 *Volume control:* Volume remains constant, but specific measurement of volume separates volume controllers from flow controllers.

4 *Time control:* When both pressure and volume waveforms are not predetermined, only inspiratory and expiratory times are controlled.

Phase variables (Table 27.4)

This subheading provides details on a particular variable to start, sustain and end each phase of the ventilation cycle.

1 *Trigger variable:* During purely mandatory ventilation, time is used to initiate each breath. With other modes, the ventilator uses one variable (e.g. a fall in airway pressure) to initiate the breath. Breaths may be assisted (i.e. a breath initiation results in a mandatory breath) or supported (i.e. a breath initiation results in partial ventilatory support). The change in the variable required to trigger inspiration is influenced by the sensitivity setting. Over-sensitive settings (e.g. $> -0.5\,cm\,H_2O$ or $0.05\,kPa$ in pressure triggering) will lead to autocycling. Pressure may be sensed at the ventilator (which underestimates effort) or at the Y-piece (which delays sensing by the transducer sited in the ventilator), with no real benefit of one over the other.[7] In flow triggering, loss of a basal flow is sensed as a breath trigger. For a given time delay, flow triggering offers no advantages over pressure triggering, but proper setting of flow sensitivities can reduce inspiratory work.[8]

2 *Limit variable:* Flow, volume or pressure may be set to remain constant or reach a maximum. This variable may be the same as, or unrelated to, the variable that terminates inspiration (e.g. a preset inspiratory pressure is achieved in PSV, but other variables – usually flow – terminate inspiration).

3 *Cycle variable:* A measured (feedback) variable is used to end inspiration. During CMV, most modern ventilators deliver a constant flow pattern which is terminated after a set inspiratory time. As volume is not measured, this should not be classified as volume-cycled.

4 *Baseline variable* is the variable that is controlled during expiration, and pressure control is the most practical and common.

Conditional variables

Some ventilators are capable of offering different patterns of pressure, volume and flow prior to each

Table 27.4 Phasic classification of ventilatory modes

Mode	Trigger	Limit	Cycle	Variable
Mandatory				
CMV	Time	Flow	Volume*	
PCV	Time	Pressure	Time	
IMV†	Time	Flow	Volume*	
PIMV†	Time	Pressure	Time	
APRV‡	Time	Pressure	Time	
Assisted§				
ACV	Patient**	Flow	Volume*	Patient effort/time
PACV	Patient**	Pressure	Time	Patient effort/time
SIMV†	Patient**	Flow	Volume*	Patient effort/time
PSIMV†	Patient**	Pressure	Time	Patient effort/time
APRV‡	Patient**	Pressure	Time	Patient effort/time
Supported				
PSV	Patient**	Pressure	Flow††	
PAV	Patient**	Volume or flow	Volume or flow	
VS	Patient**	Volume	Flow	Volume
VAPS	Patient	Pressure	Flow	Volume
Spontaneous				
CPAP	Patient**	Pressure	Pressure	

Modified from American Association for Respiratory Care[3].
*Inspiratory time may also act as a cycling from inspiration to expiration ± pause.
†Allows additional spontaneous (CPAP) breaths.
‡Spontaneous (CPAP) breaths may occur during both inspiratory and expiratory times.
§Usually includes a preset back-up mandatory mode.
**May be sensed as a change in pressure or flow.
††Inspiration ceases when the inspiratory flow rate decreases below a set rate (often <25% initial flow rate).
CMV = Conventional mechanical ventilation; PCV = pressure-controlled ventilation; IMV = intermittent mandatory ventilation; PIMV = pressure IMV; APRV = airway pressure release ventilation; ACV = assist control ventilation; PACV = pressure ACV; SIMV = synchronized IMV; PSIMV = pressure SIMV; PSV = pressure support ventilation; PAV = proportional assist ventilation; VS = volume support; VAPS = volume-assured pressure support; CPAP = continuous positive airway pressure.

breath, decided by what conditional variables are met. For example, in SIMV, sensed patient effort and an open spontaneous phase ('window') will allow a spontaneous breath; otherwise a mandatory breath is delivered.

Ventilatory modes of ventilators (Fig. 27.1)

Conventional mechanical ventilation

CMV is a time-preset pattern of inspiratory flow at a given rate that delivers a set tidal volume. Patient-initiated breaths are not possible. It is the most basic pattern of positive-pressure respiration, completely taking over ventilation in the apnoeic patient. When a time-preset pattern of inspiratory pressure is delivered, the term pressure-controlled ventilation (PCV) is used.

Assist-control ventilation

During ACV, in addition to a preset background rate of CMV breaths, a patient inspiratory effort initiates a standard CMV breath. Advantages proposed are

reduced respiratory work and sedation requirements. However, respiratory muscles continue to contract during assisted breaths,[9] and work performed by the patient is still significant.[10] When the breath is pressure-limited, the term pressure assist/control ventilation (PACV) is applicable.

Intermittent mandatory ventilation (IMV, SIMV)

IMV was introduced over 20 years ago[11] to aid weaning from CMV, by allowing the patient to take unimpeded breaths while still receiving a background of controlled breaths. Proposed advantages include a reduction in sedation, lower mean intrathoracic pressure with less barotrauma,[12] less haemodynamic depression, improved intrapulmonary gas distribution, continued exercise of respiratory muscles, and faster weaning. SIMV is a modification designed to avoid breath-stacking, in which the ventilator partitions the inspiratory time into patient-initiated and true spontaneous breaths. Neither IMV nor SIMV has been clearly shown to achieve easier weaning than T-piece trials,[13] perhaps due to the inspiratory workload imposed by the circuit.[14,15] Also, SIMV

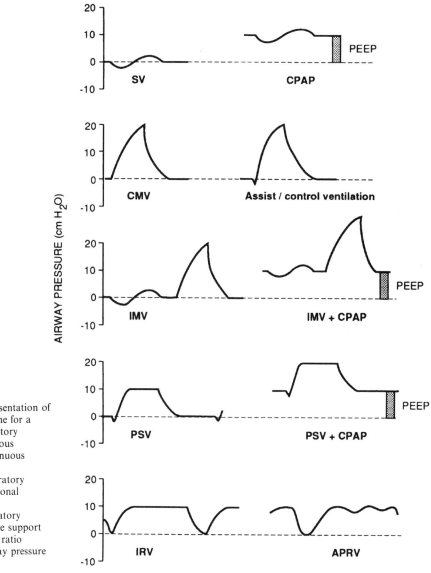

AIRWAY PRESSURE (cm H₂O)

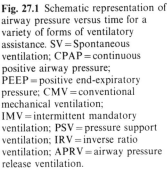

Fig. 27.1 Schematic representation of airway pressure versus time for a variety of forms of ventilatory assistance. SV = Spontaneous ventilation; CPAP = continuous positive airway pressure; PEEP = positive end-expiratory pressure; CMV = conventional mechanical ventilation; IMV = intermittent mandatory ventilation; PSV = pressure support ventilation; IRV = inverse ratio ventilation; APRV = airway pressure release ventilation.

breaths often fail to unload the respiratory muscles, and they impose the same work as intercurrent spontaneous breaths.[16] Use of paediatric circuit tubing, however, has been shown to reduce circuit-imposed work.[17] When the breath is pressure-limited, the correct nomenclature is PIMV or PSIMV.

Pressure support ventilation

During PSV, each patient-triggered breath is supported by gas flow to reach a preset pressure. Inspiration is usually terminated when the inspiratory gas flow falls to 25% of the initial flow rate or less than 5 l/min. PSV may help unload respiratory muscles,[18] and offset the work imposed by the circuit.[19,20] The PSV level to overcome apparatus work will depend upon the disease state, endotracheal tube size, ventilator and inspiratory flow rate, but is usually 5–10 cm H_2O (0.05–0.10 kPa).[20,21] PSV has advantages during weaning over SIMV or T-piece techniques.[13] Disadvantages of PSV are tidal volume and hence, minute volume will vary, excessively large tidal volumes may be delivered, and the high initial flow and termination algorithm may be unsuitable for severe airflow obstruction (although newer ventilators allow adjustment of the initial flow rate or pressure slope). When the limit variable is volume instead of pressure, the correct terminology is volume support (VS; see below).

Proportional assist ventilation (PAV)

PAV is similar to PSV, but inspiratory pressure is applied in proportion to the patient's inspired effort, as determined by inspiratory volume and flow. PAV will be more responsive to patient demand than PSV, but is unsuitable for apnoeic or bradypnoeic patients. It is not available in present commercial ventilators and data are limited.[22]

Volume-assured pressure support (VAPS)

VAPS is a mode of adaptive PSV, where breath-to-breath logic achieves a preset tidal volume, if that is not being achieved with the level of PSV chosen.[23] Similar concepts are encompassed with VS, a mode of assisted, spontaneous ventilation where the tidal volume is preset, and pressure-regulated volume control (PRVC) where tidal volume and respiratory rate are preset and achieved at a minimum constant pressure by a decelerating flow pattern.

Positive end-expiratory pressure and continuous positive airway pressure

PEEP and CPAP are elevations in baseline pressure during mechanical ventilation and spontaneous breathing respectively. Both aim to increase lung volume and oxygenation. In patients with dynamic hyperinflation and auto-PEEP (intrinsic PEEP), an applied PEEP (extrinsic PEEP) may reduce respiratory work during spontaneous or patient-initiated breaths.[24,25] This is apparently due to a reduction in threshold work, as lung compliance and airway resistance are unaffected.[25,26] PEEP is applied by placing an expiratory resistance, e.g. a constriction, a spring-loaded valve, a weighted valve, an underwater column, a Venturi valve, an electronically controlled scissor valve or a pressure-actuated solenoid valve, in the expiratory part of the breathing circuit (Fig. 27.2). A threshold resistor mechanism (i.e. presents minimal resistance to flow above its opening pressure) is preferred to minimize expiratory work and avoid barotrauma during coughing or straining.

A CPAP circuit may use a demand valve or continuous fresh gas flow. Respiratory work is imposed by the circuit design and demand valve. Older ventilators imposed respiratory work similar to normal work of breathing,[14,15] but most modern ventilators impose relatively low work through better demand valves and use of flow triggering.[15,27] A 'flow-by' function in the 7200a (Puritan-Bennett, USA) which uses two different systems (i.e. a demand valve system and a valveless continuous flow system), controlled by a microprocessor, can also reduce CPAP inspiratory work.[27,28]

Airway pressure-release ventilation (APRV)

APRV is similar to a bi-level CPAP, with intermittent decreases in airway pressure augmenting alveolar ventilation in addition to spontaneous breaths at either CPAP level. APRV without spontaneous breathing has a similar profile to pressure-controlled inverse-ratio ventilation (PCIRV), and is similarly intended to limit peak airway pressure and barotrauma. However, no real advantages over conventional ventilation have been demonstrated.[29,30]

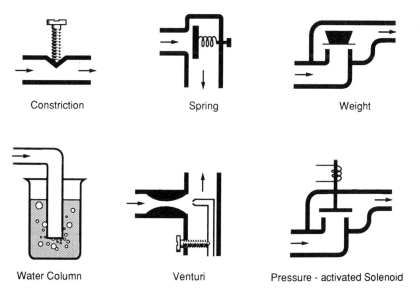

Constriction   Spring   Weight

Water Column   Venturi   Pressure - activated Solenoid

Fig. 27.2 Positive end-expiratory pressure valves.

Non-invasive ventilation (NIV)

Many modes of ventilation may be applied non-invasively via a nasal or facemask or an oral prosthesis. These techniques are commonly employed for obstructive sleep apnoea (nasal CPAP) and nocturnal home ventilation (CMV, ACV, PSV and bipositive airway pressure (BIPAP)),[31,32] but there is growing interest in their use in ICU. Mask CPAP, CMV and PSV have been used with some success in patients with acute pulmonary oedema and acute respiratory failure.[33-35] These ventilatory modes can generally be provided using standard ventilators. BIPAP is a device that provides both inspiratory and expiratory positive airway pressure. Although inspiration is usually patient-triggered, an inspiratory fraction or minimum rate can be preset. The inability to achieve high Fio_2 reduces its usefulness.

High-frequency ventilation (HFV)

HFV[36] encompasses techniques where small tidal volumes (1–3 ml/kg are administered at high respiratory rates (100–3000/min). HFV is provided by purpose-designed ventilators that do not fit into conventional classification systems. Hazards include inadequate humidification and gas trapping in patients with airflow limitation. High-frequency jet ventilation (HFJV) utilizes dry gas from a high-pressure source delivered into an intratracheal catheter. Benefit over conventional ventilation in patients with acute lung injury has not been shown. High-frequency oscillation (HFO) uses oscillatory flow within the airway to provide active inspiration and expiration at rates of 3–20 Hz. HFO offers benefits over conventional ventilation in neonates and children with respective infant and acute respiratory distress syndromes.[37-39]

Other ventilatory features

Inspiratory:expiratory ratio

Most ventilators allow control over the I:E ratio and the inspiratory time. An I:E ratio of 1:2 and inspiratory time of 0.8–1.2 s is commonly used. Shortening the inspiratory time and the I:E ratio (usually by increasing inspiratory flow rate) may be desirable in severe airflow obstruction, as this will increase expiratory time and alleviates gas trapping.[40] Conversely, lengthening inspiratory time and I:E ratio elevates mean airway pressure, and may be used to improve oxygenation. When the I:E ratio is greater than 1:1, this is termed inverse ratio ventilation (IRV), and may be applied as a pressure (PCIRV) or volume-controlled mode (VCIRV) with a decelerating flow pattern. The prolonged inspiratory time may also allow recruitment of alveoli with long time constants. However, IRV is often poorly tolerated, and may lead to gas trapping and auto-PEEP. There are no convincing data on the superiority of IRV over conventional ventilation.[41-43]

Inspiratory flow pattern

Many ventilators offer the choice of square, decelerating and sine-wave inspiratory flow patterns. However, when the I:E ratio and tidal volume are taken into account, these are essentially the same.[36] If VCIRV is used, it is usually delivered with a decelerating flow pattern.

Inspiratory pause

An end-inspiratory pause may improve oxygenation through prolonging inspiratory time, but has no advantage for a given mean airway pressure and inspiratory time. An inspiratory pause also allows measurement of the plateau pressure (P_{plat}) and a calculation of:

1 Static respiratory system compliance (C_{rs}) as:

$$C_{rs} = \text{tidal volume} / (P_{plat} - \text{PEEP})$$

The pause should be sufficiently long (1–2 s) to allow the respiratory system to reach elastic equilibrium. Otherwise, PEEP in the equation should be the sum of extrinsic and auto-PEEP. Failure to account for auto-PEEP may underestimate C_{rs} by 50%.[44] The respiratory muscles must be relaxed, and the compliance of the delivery hoses and humidifier discounted.

2 An approximate respiratory system resistance (R_{rs}) as

$$R_{rs} = P_{pk} - P_{plat} / \text{constant inspiratory flow}$$

where P_{pk} = peak airway pressure. Either R_{rs} or, more simply, the resistive pressure $P_{pk} - P_{plat}$ (providing inspiratory flow is constant),[45] may then be used to trend changes in lung-resistive properties, such as the effect of bronchodilator therapy.

Auto-PEEP

Dynamic hyperinflation results in auto-PEEP, and is most commonly measured by end-expiratory port occlusion.[46,47] Identifying end-expiration may be difficult. Hence end-expiratory hold techniques incorporated into the ventilator are desirable.

Sigh

Most ventilators are able to provide a 'sigh' breath intermittently, often twice the set tidal volume. Designed to prevent atelectasis, sighs fell out of general use when large tidal volume ventilation was shown to result in lower physiological shunts.[48,49]

However, due to concerns regarding lung stretch and barotrauma, small tidal volumes and lower transpulmonary pressures are now recommended.[36] As the occasional sigh prevents atelectasis and fall in lung compliance through the release of pulmonary surfactant,[49,50] this ventilatory option needs to be reassessed. Sighs may also be used for intermittent hyperinflation during closed suctioning techniques.

Monitoring

Nearly all modern ventilators measure pressure, flow and volume variables, and use them as high-pressure and disconnect alarms. In particular, peak, plateau and mean airway pressure, respiratory rate, expired tidal and minute volume are usually measured. These parameters can be used to calculate static and dynamic respiratory mechanics, after adjustments for the compliance of the ventilator circuit (usually 3–4 ml/cm H_2O of the distending pressure, i.e. P_{plat} – PEEP). Although the accuracy of these measures has been questioned,[51] they none the less provide useful information. Other desirable ventilator-derived parameters include static and dynamic pressure–volume curves,[52] absolute lung volume, volume of gas above the lung elastic equilibrium point, and measures of respiratory strength and endurance. Continuous measurement of first, metabolic indices such as oxygen consumption, carbon dioxide production, and respiratory quotient; second, pulse oximetry; and third, arterial blood gases are becoming available. Their integration into the ventilator may allow servo-control of ventilatory parameters.

Portable transport ventilators

Safe, reliable portable ventilators are required to transport critically ill patients from accident sites, between hospitals and within the hospital. Airway pressure, PEEP, disconnection or apnoea and gas supply must be monitored in the same manner as within the ICU. The ventilator must be able to deliver 100% oxygen and have controls to set tidal volume and respiratory rate.[53] Commonly, the I:E ratio is fixed, and a choice of 100% oxygen or 50–60% oxygen from air entrainment is available. The airmix mode is more likely to hyperventilate at low inspiratory pressures, and hypoventilate at high inspiratory pressures.[54] Some basic modes of assisted ventilation, such as IMV/SIMV and PSV, are desirable. IMV and PEEP can be provided using local modifications, but are available in a number of ventilators. Equipment for emergency airway access, a manual resuscitator and portable oxygen and suction must also accompany the ventilator.

Resuscitators

Manual resuscitators

Resuscitators may be gas-powered or manual. The latter is used in ICU for preoxygenating and manually inflating patients' lungs. Manual resuscitators have a self-inflating bag and a non-rebreathing valve. The double-ended bag is held inflated in the resting state by thick foam rubber lining (Ambu bag, Ambu International, Denmark) or the silicone bag material (Laerdal bag, Asmund Laerdal, Norway). The gas inlet at one end allows entry of air. Oxygen can be added through a nipple. Inflation (bag squeezing) forces a flap to close the gas inlet and expel gas in the bag through a non-return valve at the other end, which is attached to a mask or endotracheal tube. A reservoir bag can usually be attached to the gas inlet to give higher Fio_2. The non-rebreathing valve separates fresh gas from expired gas by means of a spring-loaded disc (Ruben and Ambu), labial flaps (Ambu E and E2), mushroom valve (Ambu Mk 3), or duck-bill valve (Laerdal).[55,56] Most valves have an inflation over-pressure blow-off facility.

Function

When applying manual lung inflations, Fio_2 in the range 0.3–0.9 and 0.3–1.0 with a reservoir bag attached can be achieved with 3–15 l/min of oxygen flow. Higher Fio_2 is delivered if high oxygen flows, large tidal volumes and slower rates are used.[55] Disadvantages and hazards of manual resuscitators are the following:

1 Valves may stick, especially when wet. This may result in ambient air being inspired during spontaneous breathing (e.g. Ambu E2), or in high inflating pressures if the valve is jammed in the inspiratory position (e.g. Ruben and Ambu Mk 3).
2 Lower tidal volumes may be delivered with the Ambu E valve, if small volumes at slow rates are inflated. Some gas bypasses the lungs (forward leak) during inflation.
3 The 'feel' of the lungs is lost with bags of thick walls.
4 The operator must use both hands to inflate the bag. If a face mask is attached, the mask is held by a second attendant (see Chapter 7).
5 The dead space of the resuscitators is excessive for children and neonates.
6 Incorrect assembly of the valve components and attachment of the wrong valve port to the bag will result in serious malfunction. Some resuscitators have different-sized ports to eliminate this potential hazard.

References

1 Kacmarek RM (1992) Essential gas delivery features of mechanical ventilators. *Respir Care* **37**:1045–1055.

2 Oh TE, Lin ES and Bhatt S (1991) Inspiratory work imposed by demand valve ventilator circuits. *Anaesth Intens Care* **19**:187–191.

3 American Association for Respiratory Care (1992) Consensus statement on the essentials of mechanical ventilators – 1992. *Respir Care* **37**:1000–1008.

4 Chatburn RL (1992) Classification of mechanical ventilators. *Respir Care* **37**:1009–1025.

5 Oh TE (1990) Ventilators. In: Oh TE (ed.) *Intensive Care Manual*, 3rd edn. Sydney: Butterworths, pp. 162–168.

6 Mushin WW, Rendell-Baker L, Thompson PW and Mapleson WW (1980) *Automatic Ventilation of the Lungs*. Oxford: Blackwell Scientific.

7 Sassoon CSH (1992) Mechanical ventilator design and function: the trigger variable. *Respir Care* **37**:1056–1069.

8 Sassoon CSH, Lodia R, Rheeman CH *et al.* (1992) Inspiratory muscle work of breathing during flow-by, demand-flow and continuous-flow systems in patients with chronic obstructive pulmonary disease. *Am Rev Respir Dis* **145**:1219–1222.

9 Flick GR, Bellamy PE and Simmons DH (1989) Diaphragmatic contraction during assisted mechanical ventilation. *Chest* **96**:130–135.

10 Marini JJ, Rodriguez M and Lamb V (1986) The inspiratory workload of patient-initiated mechanical ventilation. *Am Rev Respir Dis* **134**:902–909.

11 Downs JB, Klein EF, DeSautels D *et al.* (1973) Intermittent mkandatory ventilation: a new approach to weaning patients from mechanical ventilators. *Chest* **64**:331–335.

12 Mathru M, Rao TLK and Venus B (1993) Ventilator induced barotrauma in controlled mechanical ventilation versus intermittent mandatory ventilation. *Crit Care Med* **11**:359–361.

13 Brochard L, Rauss A, Benito S *et al.* (1994) Comparison of three methods of gradual withdrawal from ventilatory support during weaning from mechanical ventilation. *Am J Respir Crit Care Med* **150**:896–903.

14 Gibney RTN, Wilson RS and Pontoppidan H (1982) Comparison of work of breathing on high gas flow and demand valve continuous positive airway pressure systems. *Chest* **82**:692–695.

15 Bersten AD, Rutten AJ, Vedig AE *et al.* (1989) Additional work of breathing imposed by endotracheal tubes, breathing circuits, and intensive care ventilators. *Crit Care Med* **17**:671–677.

16 Imsand C, Feihl F, Perret C *et al.* (1994) Regulation of inspiratory neuromuscular output during synchronized intermittent mechanical ventilation. *Anesthesiology* **80**:13–22.

17 Martin LD, Rafferty JF, Watsel RC and Gioia FR (1989) Inspiratory work during synchronized intermittent mandatory ventilation and pressure support ventilation. *Anesthesiology* **71**:977–981.

18 Brochard L, Harf A, Lorino H *et al.* (1989) Inspiratory pressure support prevents diaphragmatic fatigue during weaning from mechanical ventilation. *Am Rev Respir Dis* **139**:513–521.

19 Fiastro JF, Habib MP and Quan SF (1988) Pressure support compensation for inspiratory work due to endotracheal tubes and demand continuous positive airway pressure. *Chest* **93**:499–505.

20 Brochard L, Rua F, Lorino H *et al.* (1991) Inspiratory pressure support compensates for the additional work of breathing caused by the endotracheal tube. *Anesthesiology* **75**:739–745.

21 Bersten AD, Rutten AJ and Vedig AE (1993) Efficacy of pressure support in compensating for apparatus work. *Anaesth Intens Care* **21**:67–71.

22 Younes M, Puddy A, Roberts D *et al.* (1992) Proportional assist ventilation: Results of an initial clinical trial. *Am Rev Respir Dis* **145**:121–129.

23 MacIntyre NR, Gropper C and Westfall T (1994) Combining pressure-limiting and volume-cycling features in a patient-interactive mechanical breath. *Crit Care Med* **221**:353–357.

24 Smith TC and Marini JJ (1988) Impact of PEEP on lung mechanics and work of breathing in severe airflow obstruction. *J Appl Physiol* **651**:1488–1499.

25 Petrof BJ, Legare M, Goldberg P *et al.* (1990) Continuous positive airway pressure reduces work of breathing and dyspnea during weaning from mechanical ventilation in severe chronic obstructive pulmonary disease. *Am Rev Respir Dis* **1411**:281–289.

26 Shade E, Kawagoe Y, Brower R *et al.* (1994) Effects of hyperinflation and CPAP on work of breathing and respiratory failure in dogs. *J Appl Physiol* **771**:819–827.

27 Sassoon CSH, Lodia R, Rheeman CH *et al.* (1992) Inspiratory muscle work of breathing during flow-by, demand-flow, and continuous-flow systems in patients with chronic obstructive pulmonary disease. *Am Rev Respir Dis* **1451**:1219–1222.

28 Saito S, Tokioka H and Kosaka F (1990) Efficacy of flow-by during continuous positive airway pressure ventilation. *Crit Care Med* **181**:654–656.

29 Rasanen J, Cane RD, Downs JB *et al.* (1991) Airway pressure release ventilation during acute lung injury: A prospective multicentre trial. *Crit Care Med* **191**:1234–1241.

30 Calzia E, Lindner KH, Witt S *et al.* (1994) Pressure–time product and work of breathing during biphasic continuous positive airway pressure and assisted spontaneous breathing. *Am J Respir Crit Care Med* **1501**:904–910.

31 Ellis ER, Bye PT, Brudere JW *et al.* (1987) Treatment of respiratory failure during sleep in patients with neuromuscular disease: positive-pressure ventilation through a nose mask. *Am Rev Respir Dis* **1351**:148–152.

32 Hill NS, Eveloff SE, Carlisle CC *et al.* (1992) Efficacy of nocturnal nasal ventilation in patients with restrictive thoracic disease. *Am Rev Respir Dis* **1451**:365–371.

33 Bersten AD, Holt AW, Vedig AE *et al.* (1991) Treatment of severe cardiogenic pulmonary edema with continuous positive airway pressure delivered by face mask. *N Engl J Med* **3251**:1825–1830.

34 Meduri G, Cohosceti C, Menashe P *et al.* (1989) Non-invasive face mask ventilation in patients with acute respiratory failure. *Chest* **951**:865–870.

35 Fernandez R, Blanch Ll, Valles J *et al.* (1993) Pressure support ventilation via face mask in acute respiratory failure in hypercapnic COPD patients. *Intens Care Med* **191**:456–461.

36 Slutsky AS (1993) Mechanical ventilation. *Chest* **1041**:1833–1859.

37 Clark GH, Gerstmann DR, Null DM *et al.* (1992) Prospective randomized comparison of high frequency oscillation and conventional ventilation in respiratory distress syndrome. *Pediatrics* **891**:5–12.

38 HiFO study group (1993) Randomized study of high-frequency oscillatory ventilation in infants with severe respiratory distress syndrome. *J Pediatr* **122**:609–619.

39 Arnbold JH, Hanson JH, Toro-Figuero LO *et al.* (1994) Prospective, randomized comparison of high-frequency oscillatory ventilation and conventional mechanical ventilation in pediatric respiratory failure. *Crit Care Med* **22**:1530–1539.

40 Tuxen DV and Lane S (1987) The effects of ventilatory pattern on hyperinflation, airway pressures, and circulation in mechanical ventilation of patients with severe airflow obstruction. *Am Rev Respr Dis* **136**:872–879.

41 Shanholtz C and Brower R (1994) Should inverse ratio ventilation be used in adult respiratory distress syndrome? *Am J Respir Crit Care Med* **149**:1354–1358.

42 Lessard MR, Guerot E, Lorino H *et al.* (1994) Effects of pressure-controlled ventilation with different I:E rarios versus volume-controlled ventilation on respiratory mechanics, gas exchange, and hemocynamics in patient with adult respiratory distress syndrome. *Anesthesiology* **80**:983–991.

43 Morris AH, Wallace CJ, Menlove RL *et al.* (1994) Randomized clinical trial of pressure-controlled inverse ratio ventilation and extracorporeal CO_2 removal for adult respiratory distress syndrome. *Am J Respir Crit Care Med* **149**:295–305.

44 Rossi A, Gottfried SB, Zocchi L *et al.* (1985) Measurement of static compliance of the total respiratory system in patients with acute respiratory failure during mechanical ventilation. *Am Rev Respir Dis* **131**:672–677.

45 Manthous CA, Hall JB, Schmidt GA *et al.* (1993) Metered-dose inhaler versus nebulized albuterol in mechanically ventilated patients. *Am Rev Respir Dis* **148**:1567–1570.

46 Pepe PE and Marini JJ (1982) Occult positive end-expiratory presssure in mechanically ventilated patients with airflow obstruction: the auto-PEEP effect. *Am Rev Respir Dis* **126**:166–170.

47 Iotti G and Braschi A (1990) Respiratory mechanics in chronic obstructive pulmonary disease. In: Vincent JL (ed.) *Update in Intensive Care and Emergency Medicine,* vol. 10. Berlin: Springer-Verlag, pp. 223–230.

48 Hedley-White J, Laver MB and Bendixen HH (1964) Effect of changes in tidal ventilation on physiologic shunt. *Am J Physiol* **206**:891–897.

49 Mead J and Collier C (1959) Relation of volume history of lungs to respiratory mechanics in anesthetized dogs. *J Appl Physiol* **14**:669–678.

50 Nicholas TE, Power JHT and Barr HA (1982) The pulmonary consequences of a deep breath. *Respir Physiol* **49**:315–324.

51 Chartrand D, Dionne B, Jodoin C *et al.* (1993) Measurement of respiratory mechanics using the Puritan-Bennett 7200a ventilator. *Can J Anaesth* **40**:1076–1083.

52 Ranieri VM, Giuliani R, Fiore T *et al.* (1994) Volume–pressure curve of the respiratory system predicts effect of PEEP in ARDS: 'Occlusion' versus 'constant flow' technique. *Am J Respir Crit Care Med* **149**:19–27.

53 AARC clinicai practice guidelines (1993) Transport of the mechanically ventilated patient. *Respir Care* **38**:1169–1178.

54 Heinrichs W, Mertzluft F and Dick W (1989) Accuracy of delivered versus preset minute ventilation of portable emergency ventilators. *Crit Care Med* **17**:682–685.

55 Davey A, Moyle JTB and Ward CS (1992) *Ward's Anaesthetic Equipment,* 3rd edn. London: WB Saunders, pp. 188–194.

56 Dorsch JA and Dorsch SE (1984) *Understanding Anesthesia Equipment,* 2nd edn. Baltimore: Williams & Wilkins, pp. 198–209.

28 Humidification and inhalation therapy

AD Bersten and TE Oh

The upper airway normally warms, moistens and filters inspired gas. When these functions are impaired by disease factors, or when the nasopharynx is bypassed by endotracheal intubation, artificial humidification of inspired gases must be provided.

Physical principles

Humidity, the amount of water vapour in a gas, may be expressed as:

1 *Absolute humidity* (AH) – the total mass of water vapour in a given volume of gas at a given temperature (g/m³).
2 *Relative humidity* (RH) – the actual mass of water vapour (per volume of gas) as a percentage of the mass of saturated water vapour, at a given temperature. Saturated water vapour exerts a saturated vapour pressure (SVP). As the SVP has an exponential relation with temperature (Table 28.1), addition of further water vapour to the gas can only occur with a rise in temperature.
3 *Partial pressure*

Table 28.1 Relationship of temperature and saturated vapour pressure

Temperature (°C)	Saturated vapour pressure		Absolute humidity (g/m³)
	mmHg	(kPa)	
0	4.6	(0.6)	4.8
10	9.2	(1.2)	9.3
20	17.5	(2.3)	17.1
30	31.3	(4.2)	30.4
34	39.9	(5.3)	37.5
37	47.1	(6.3)	43.4
40	55.3	(7.4)	51.7
46	78.0	(10.4)	68.7

Physiology

Clearance of surface liquids and particles from the lung depends on beating cilia, airway mucus and transepithelial water flux. Airway mucus is derived from secretions from goblet cells, submucosal glands and Clara cells, and from capillary transudate. Conducting airways are lined with pseudostratified, ciliated columnar epithelium and numerous fluid-secreting glands. As the airway descends, the epithelium becomes stratified, and then cuboidal and partially ciliated, with very few secretory glands at the terminal airways. The cilia beat in a watery (sol) layer over which is a viscous mucus layer (gel), and move a superficial layer of mucus from deep within the lung toward the glottis (at a rate of 10 mm/min at 37°C and 100% RH). Both cilia function and mucus composition depend on temperature and adequate humidification.

The large surface area of the nasal mucosa with its extensive vascular network humidifies and warms inhaled gas more effectively than mouth-breathing. Heating and humidification of dry gas are progressive down the airway, with an isothermic boundary (i.e. 100% RH at 37°C or AH of 43 g/m³) just below the carina.[1] Under resting conditions, approximately 250 ml of water and 1.5 kJ (350 kcal) of energy is lost from the respiratory tract in a day. A proportion (10–25%) is returned to the mucosa during expiration due to condensation.

The minimal moisture level to maintain ciliary function and mucus clearance is uncertain. Although reproducing an isothermic boundary at the carina may be ideal, it does not seem essential in all situations. Mucus flow is markedly reduced when RH at 37°C falls below 75% (AH of 32 g/m³), and ceases when RH is 50% (AH of 22 g/m³).[2] This suggests that an AH exceeding 33 g/m³ is needed to maintain normal function. At this AH level, inspired gas temperature does not appear to be important unless excessive.[3] Mucociliary function is also impaired by upper respiratory tract infection, chronic bronchitis, cystic fibrosis, bronchiectasis, immotile cilia syndrome (including Kartagener's syndrome), dehydration hyperventilation, general anaesthetics, opioids, atropine and exposure to noxious gases. High fractional inspired oxygen concentrations (Fio_2) may lead to acute tracheobronchitis, with depressed tracheal mucus velocity within 3 h.[4] Inhaled β_2-adrenergic agonists increase mucociliary clearance by augmenting ciliary beat frequency, and mucus and water secretion.[5]

Clinical applications of humidification

Tracheal intubation

The need for humidification in endotracheal intubation and tracheostomy is unquestioned. As the upper airway is bypassed, RH of inspired gas falls below 50% with adverse effects including:[6]

1 increased mucus viscosity;
2 depressed ciliary function;
3 cytological damage to the tracheobronchial epithelium, including mucosal ulceration, tracheal inflammation and necrotizing tracheobronchitis,[7]
4 microatelectasis from obstruction of small airways;
5 airway obstruction due to tenacious or inspissated sputum.

Metaplasia of the tracheal epithelium occurs over weeks to months in patients with a permanent tracheostomy. These patients do not usually require humidified gas, suggesting that humidification occurs lower down the respiratory tree. None the less, humidification of inspired gas may be needed during an acute respiratory tract infection.

Heat exchange

The respiratory tract is an important avenue to adjust body temperature by heat exchange. Humidification of gases reduces the fall in body temperature associated with anaesthesia and surgery.[6] In this setting, active humidifiers are of no benefit over heat and moisture exchangers (HMEs).[8] Excessive heat from humidification may produce mucosal damage, hyperthermia and overhumidification.[9] However, if water content is not excessive, mucociliary clearance is unaffected up to temperatures of $42°C$.[3] Overhumidification may increase secretions and impair mucociliary clearance and surfactant activity, resulting in atelectasis.[9]

Ideal humidification

The basic requirements of a humidifier should include the following features:[10]

1 The inspired gas is delivered into the trachea at $32–36°C$ with a water content of $30–43$ g/m^3.
2 The set temperature remains constant and does not fluctuate.
3 Humidification and temperature remain unaffected by a large range of fresh gas flows, especially high flows.
4 The device is simple to use and to service.
5 Humidification can be provided for air, oxygen or any mixture of inspired gas, including anaesthetic agents.
6 The humidifier can be used with spontaneous or controlled ventilation.
7 There are safety mechanisms, with alarms, against overheating, overhydration and electrocution.
8 The resistance, compliance and dead-space characteristics do not adversely affect spontaneous breathing modes.
9 The sterility of the inspired gas is not compromised.

Methods and devices

Water bath humidifiers

Inspired gas is passed over or through a water reservoir to achieve humidification. Their efficiency is dependent on ambient temperature and the surface area available for gas vaporization.

Cold water humidifiers

These units are simple and inexpensive, but are inefficient, with a water content of around 9 g/m^3 (i.e. about 50% RH at ambient temperatures). They are also a potential source of microbiological contamination. Routine use of cold-water humidifiers to deliver oxygen with simple facemasks is unnecessary.

Hot water humidifiers (Figs 28.1 and 28.2)

Inspired gas is passed over (i.e. blow-by humidifier, e.g. Fisher-Paykel, Fisher and Paykel Medical, New Zealand) or through (i.e. bubble or cascade humidifier, e.g. Bennett Cascade, Bennett Medical Equipment, USA) a heated water reservoir. Gas leaving the reservoir contains a high water content, often more than 43 g/m^3. The water bath temperature is thermostatically controlled (e.g. at $45–60°C$) to allow cooling along the hose for an inspired RH of 100% at $37°C$. A heated wire may be sited in the delivery hose to maintain preset gas temperature and humidity (e.g. Fisher-Paykel humidifier). It is commonly believed that hot-water humidifiers do not produce aerosols, but micro-droplets (mostly less than 5 μm diameter) have been reported with bubble humidifiers,[11] and this may be a potential source of infection.

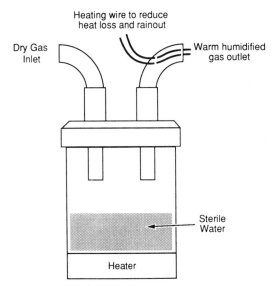

Fig. 28.1 Hot water 'blow-by' humidifier.

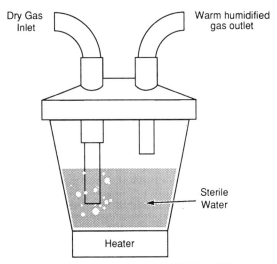

Fig. 28.2 Hot water 'cascade' or 'bubble' humidifer.

Fisher-Paykel humidifier

This is a commonly used blow-by humidifier. Older models (series 328) used an aluminium scroll lined with absorbent paper to increase the vaporizing surface area (713 cm^2 in the reusable unit and 213 cm^2 in the disposable model).[12] Reservoir temperature is variable for flows 3–25 l/min. The delivery hose is heated by an insulated heating wire to achieve a manual preset inspired temperature. An additional servo-control unit is available, while more recent models have a dual servo unit which combines this function in the heater base. Audible alarms indicate disconnection and variations over 2°C from the set delivery temperature. The heater base is protected from overheating by a thermostat set at 47°C. If this fails, another safety thermostat operates at 70°C. The heated wire avoids or minimizes 'rainout', which is a problem in recent models (series 600 and 700). These models are used with a disposable humidification chamber that is filled manually with water or by a gravity-feed set. Although absorbent paper scrolls are no longer used in these models, the smaller water volume and larger base plate temperature allow RH greater than 95% at 37°C over a wide range of gas flows. To minimize rainout, the chamber outlet can be set at a temperature below the delivery hose outlet temperature – 2°C is usually adequate and does not compromise RH. Temperature alarms are fixed at 41°C and 29.5°C, with a back-up safety set at 66°C for the delivery chamber.

Heat and moisture exchangers

Modern HMEs are popular ICU humidifiers due to their simplicity and increased efficiency. They all work on the basic principle of heat and moisture conservation during expiration, allowing inspired gas to be heated and humidified. Most HMEs are hygroscopic, and adsorb moisture on to a foam or paper-like material that is chemically coated (often calcium chloride or lithium chloride). However, large pore-size hygroscopic HMEs are less efficient filters than hydrophobic HMEs (e.g. Pall BB50T, Pall Biomedical, USA). The Pall HME was initially designed as a breathing filter, and consists of a pleated, water-repellent ceramic membrane. This membrane has low thermal conductivity, and the large temperature gradient between inspiration and expiration increases its condenser efficiency. Many HMEs combine humidification with filtration, but some only act as humidifiers.

Modern HMEs are light with a small dead space, but are varied in their level of humidification. As HME efficiency decreases with time[13] and increasing tidal volume,[14] direct comparisons of units are not always possible. None the less, hydrophobic filters (e.g. Pall or Filtra-therm, Intersurgical, UK) are generally less efficient humidifiers (i.e. AH 20–25 g/m^3) than hygroscopic or hygroscopic/ hydrophobic filters (i.e. AH around 30 g/m^3).[13–17] The latter HMEs may be suitable for long-term mechanical ventilation in selected patients,[18] particularly as the majority of reported HME complications (e.g. thick secretions and endotracheal tube occlusion) occurred with units of lower humidification levels.[19–21] Nevertheless, HMEs cannot match the humidification offered by hot-water humidifiers, which remain the 'gold standard', particularly if secretions are thick or bloody, humidification is necessary for more than 4 days,[22] or if used in children and neonates. HME units should be changed daily.

Complications of humidification

Inadequate humidification

An AH exceeding 30 g/m^3 is recommended in respiratory care.[22] Inadequate humidification is usually only a problem with HMEs. With hot-water humidifiers, however, efficiency is reduced by increasing gas flow rates and rainout. A decrease of about 1°C occurs for each 10 cm of tubing beyond the end of the delivery hose (i.e. the Y-connector and right-angled connector), and should be catered for. Inadequate humidification in high-frequency ventilation can be overcome by using superheated humidification of the entrained gas with a temperature thermistor built into the endotracheal tube.[23]

Overhumidification

Overheating malfunction of hot-water humidifiers may cause a rise in core temperature, water intoxication, impaired mucociliary clearance and airway burns.[9]

Imposed work of breathing

The work of breathing imposed by a humidifier is an important additional respiratory load in ICU patients. This imposed work increases with increasing inspiratory flows for both hot-water humidifiers and HMEs[24–26] The progressive increase in water content of HMEs is also associated with increased resistance.[25] The Fisher-Paykel humidifier imposes relatively low work compared to the Bennett cascade.[24] Most HMEs also impose little work at low inspiratory flows,[25,26] but a pressure differential up to 5 cm H_2O (0.5 kPa) is not uncommon at flows of 60 l/min.

Infection

Current evidence argues against humidifiers as important factors in nosocomial respiratory tract infection. Although water reservoirs represent a good culture medium for bacteria such as *Pseudomonas* species, it is rare to culture bacteria from humidifiers. Any such positive finding is usually preceded by colonization of the circuit by the patient's own flora within the first 24 h of use.[27,28] This self-colonization is hence unlikely to be clinically significant. Indeed, the incidence of nosocomial pneumonia is reported to be higher (due to outside contamination) if the circuit is changed too frequently (every 24 h[29] or 48 h[28]

Many HMEs are also effective bacterial filters, with efficiencies usually greater than 99.9977%[14], i.e. less than 23 out of 1 million bacteria will pass through – filters that can exclude all virus particles are not currently available. It thus seems rational to minimize contamination of circuits by placing a filter at the patient end. Fresh circuits and filters should be used for each new patient. Filtration of inspired gases is unnecessary with heated humidifiers, as inspired gas does not recirculate in ICU ventilators. The incidence of nosocomial pneumonia is not altered whether heated humidifiers or HMEs are used.[19] Consequently, humidification capacity is more important than filtration characteristics when choosing an HME for ICU use.

Electrical hazards (see Chapter 74)

Inhalation therapy

Therapeutic aerosols are particles suspended in gas that are inhaled and deposited within the respiratory tract. Numerous factors, including particle size, inertia and physical nature, gravity, volume and pattern of ventilation, temperature and humidity, airway geometry, lung disease and the delivery system alter aerosol deposition. In general, particles of diameter 40 μm deposit in the upper airway, 8–15 μm deposit in bronchi and bronchioles, 3–5 μm deposit in peripheral conducting airways and 0.8–3.0 μm settle in lung parenchyma. Optimal particle size will depend on the clinical indication and agent used (e.g. β_2-adrenergic agonists, anticholinergics, corticosteroids, antibiotics, anti-virals, surfactant therapy, sputum induction and water). Obviously, if an HME with filtration characteristics is being used, the aerosol needs to be delivered proximal to the filter.

Aerosol delivery

Although therapeutic aerosols are usually produced by nebulizers in intensive care patients, metered dose inhalers (MDIs) and dry particle inhalers (DPIs) are also available. MDIs suspend micronized crystals of drug in a propellant gas under high pressure, allowing a relatively fixed volume (i.e. dose) to be delivered with each actuation (e.g. 90 μg for salbutamol and 18 μg for ipratropium).[30] A holding chamber improves their efficacy in drug delivery to intubated or unintubated patients,[31] which may equal[32] or better that of nebulizers.[31] None the less, under some circumstances, MDIs with a chamber may be ineffective.[33] Consequently, nebulized delivery of drugs remains the standard technique in ventilated patients.

Nebulizers

The most common nebulizers are sidestream nebulizers. These use an extrinsic gas flow through a narrow orifice, to create a pressure gradient that draws the drug mixture from a liquid reservoir (i.e. Bernoulli's principle; Fig 28.3). The gas is then directed at a baffle to reduce the mean particle size. This extrinsic gas

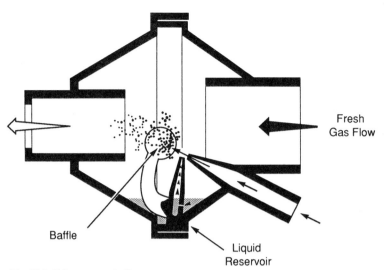

Fig. 28.3 Sidestream nebulizer.

flow (at 3–10 l/min) often adds to the inspiratory flow, and may increase patient tidal volume. However, many modern ventilators will compensate for this in delivering the preset tidal volume.

Mainstream nebulizers employ inspiratory gas flow to actuate nebulization. These are commonly large-volume water nebulizers that entrain air to achieve fresh gas flow rates of 20–30 l/min. They are used to deliver drugs such as bronchodilators, and Fio_2 is usually titratable (e.g. Puritan All Purpose, Puritan-Bennett, CA, USA).

Ultrasonic nebulizers use high-frequency sound waves (typically 1 MHz) to create an aerosol above a liquid reservoir, to produce small uniform droplets (<5 μm) and a high mist density (i.e. 100–200 g/m^3). Disadvantages of ultrasonic nebulizers are the risk of infection, overhydration, and increased airway resistance.

Clinical applications of inhalation therapy

Humidification

Humidifiers produce gas with a water content dictated by temperature and water vapour pressure, whereas nebulizers produce gas with a water content determined by the aerosol content. The latter can provide water to the respiratory tract, particularly if the water reservoir is heated to increase mist density. However, the risk of infection is increased, as droplets can carry bacteria to the alveoli. Consequently, only sterile water should be used to fill the reservoir, and all units should be regularly changed and sterilized. Acetylcysteine has been used as a mucolytic, but may cause bronchospasm. Benefits are not supported by clinical data.[30]

Bronchodilator therapy

Nebulized bronchodilator therapy is extremely common in ventilated patients, but the optimal mode and dosing are unclear. Greater aerosol delivery is associated with low respiratory rates, low inspiratory flows, high inspiratory times and larger nebulizer volumes, but there is marked variation between nebulizers.[34,35] The proportion of actuated drug reaching the lung is small (1–6%) with significant amounts being deposited on the endotracheal tube.[36,37] Given the above variables, choice of drug dose and mode of delivery will depend on patient response and side-effects. Response can be judged clinically, and by changes in peak-to-plateau airway pressure gradient, calculated airways resistance, and auto-PEEP. Numerous studies show effective bronchodilatation with β_2-agonists in ventilated patients, but it is uncertain whether additional nebulized ipratropium or steroids are useful.[30] Although entrainment of nebulized drug in a high-gas-flow CPAP circuit can be expected to reduce drug delivery, good bronchodilator response with salbutamol has been reported in this setting.[38]

Delivery of antibiotics and antiviral agents

Aerosolized antibiotics have generally not been used, as they may not be distributed to consolidated lung. Their use as prophylaxis against nosocomial pneumonia is reported to result in reduced bacterial colonization with no change in outcome, but with emergence of resistant bacteria.[39] In contrast, aerosolized tobramycin reduces the density of *Pseudomonas aeruginosa*, and is associated with improvements in vital capacity and FEV_1 in cystic fibrosis patients.[40] Aerosolized pentamidine for *Pneumocystis carinii* pneumonia and amphotericin B for fungal infection have been proposed, but require proper evaluation.[30] Aerosolized ribavarin is effective for respiratory syncytial virus infection, resulting in a shorter period of ventilation and hospitalization.[41] However, ribavarin deposition in the circuit may cause valve malfunction, and concerns of teratogenicity in health care personnel have dictated its use with care.[41]

Sputum induction

Nebulized 3% saline is effective in sputum induction for diagnosing *P. carinii* pneumonia in patients with the acquired immunodeficiency syndrome, thereby often obviating the need for bronchoscopy.[42] This technique may not be suitable in other immuno-suppressed patients, as the sputum load of *P. carinii* may not be as dense (see Chapter 33).

Surfactant therapy

Surfactant preparations have been delivered by instillation and as an aerosol in neonates with respiratory distress syndrome, and in adults with the acute respiratory distress syndrome. Aerosolized surfactant achieves a more uniform distribution and avoids problems of instilling liquid into injured lungs. However, large amounts are needed for lung deposition, and preferential distribution occurs to less damaged lung areas that receive better ventilation.[43]

References

1 Hedley RM and Allt-Graham J (1994) Heat and moisture exchangers and breathing filters. *Br J Anaesth* **73**:227–236.

2 Forbes AR (1973) Humidification and mucus flow in the intubated trachea. *Br J Anaesth* **45**:874–878.

3 Forbes AR (1974) Temperature, humidity and mucus flow in the intubated trachea. Br J Anaesth **46**:29–34.

4 Sackner MA, Landa J, Hirsch J et al. (1975) Pulmonary effects of oxygen breathing: a six-hour study in normal man. *Ann Intern Med* **82**:40–43.

5 LaFortuna CL and Fazio F (1985) Acute effect of inhaled salbutamol on mucociliary clearance in health and chronic bronchitis. *Respiration* **45**:111–113.

6 Chalon J, Patel C, Ali M et al. (1974) Humidity and the anesthetized patient. *Anesthesiology* **50**:195–198.

7 Circeo LE, Heard SO, Griffiths E et al. (1991) Overwhelming necrotizing tracheobronchitis due to inadequate humidification during high-frequency jet venilation. *Chest* **100**:268–269.

8 Linko K, Honkavaara P and Niemenen MT (1984) Heated humidification after major abdominal surgery. *Eur J Anaesthesiol* **1**:285–291.

9 Shelley MP, Lloyd GM and Park GR (1988) A review of the mechanisms and methods of humidification of inspired gases. *Intens Care Med* **14**:1–9.

10 Chamney AR (1969) Humidification requirements and techniques. *Anaesthesia* **24**:602–617.

11 Rhame FS, Streifel A, McComb C et al. (1986) Bubbling humidifiers produce microaerosols which can carry bacteria. *Infection Control* **7**:403–407.

12 Russell WJ (1983) *Equipment for Anaesthesia and Intensive Care.* Adelaide: Russell, pp. 140–146.

13 Jackson C and Webb AR (1992) An evaluation of the heat and moisture exchange performance of four ventilator circuit filters. *Intens Care Med* **18**:264–268.

14 Mebius C (1992) Heat and moisture exchangers with bacterial filters: a laboratory evaluation. *Acta Anaesthesiol Scand* **36**:572–576.

15 Martin C, Papazian L, Perrin G et al. (1992) Performance evaluation of three vaporizing humidifiers and two heat and moisture exchangers in patients with minute volumes > 10 l/min. *Chest* **102**:1347–1350.

16 Shelley M, Bethune DW and Latimer RD (1986) A comparison of five heat and moisture exchangers. *Anaesthesia* **41**:527–532.

17 Sottiaux T, Mignolet G, Damas P et al. (1993) Comparative evaluation of three heat and moisture exchangers during short-term postoperative mechanical ventilation. *Chest* **104**:220–224.

18 Branson RD, Davis K, Campbell RS et al. (1993) Humidification in the intensive care unit: prospective study of a new protocol utilizing heated humidification and a hygroscopic condenser humidifier. *Chest* **104**:1800–1805.

19 Misset B, Escudier B, Rivara D et al. (1991) Heat and moisture exchanger vs heated humidifier during long-term mechanical ventilation: a prospective randomized study. *Chest* **100**:160–163.

20 Martin C, Perrin G, Gevaudan MJ et al. (1990) Heat and moisture exchangers and vaporizing humidifiers in the intensive care unit. *Chest* **97**:144–149.

21 Cohen IL, Weinberg PF, Fein IA et al. (1988) Endotracheal tube occlusion associated with the use of heat and moisture exchangers in the intensive care unit. *Crit Care Med* **16**:277–279.

22 AARC clinical practice guideline (1992) Humidification during mechanical ventilation. *Respir Care* **37**:887–890.

23 Gluck E, Heard S, Patel C et al. (1993) Use of high frequency ventilation in patients with ARDS: a preliminary report. *Chest* **103**:1413–1420.

24 Oh TE, Lin ES and Bhatt S (1991) Resistance of humidifiers, and inspiratory work imposed by a ventilator-humidifier circuit. *Br J Anaesth* **66**:258–263.

25. Ploysongsang Y, Branson R, Rashkin MC et al. (1988) Pressure flow characteristics of commonly used heat–moisture exchangers. *Am Rev Respir Dis* **138**:675–678.

26 Nishimura M, Nishijima MK, Okada T et al. (1990) Comparison of flow-resistive work load due to humidifying devices. *Chest* **97**:600–604.

27 Craven DE, Goularte TA and Make BJ (1984) Contaminated condensate in mechanical ventilator circuits: a risk factor for nosocomial pneumonia. *Am Rev Respir Dis* **129**:625–628.

28 Dreyfuss D, Djedaini K, Weber P *et al.* (1991) Prospective study of nosocomial pneumonia and of patient and circuit colonisation during mechanical ventilation with circuit changes every 48 hours versus no change. *Am Rev Respir Dis* **143**:738–743.

29 Craven DE, Connolly MG, Lichtenberg DA *et al.* (1982) Contamination of mechanical ventilators with tubing changes every 24 or 48 hours. *N Engl J Med* **306**:1505–1509.

30 Manthous CA and Hall JB (1994) Administration of therapeutic aerosols to mechanically ventilated patients. *Chest* **106**:560–571.

31 Fuller HD, Dolovich MB, Posmituck G *et al.* (1990) Pressurized aerosol versus jet aerosol delivery to mechanically ventilated patients: comparison of dose to the lungs. *Am Rev Respir Dis* **141**:440–444.

32 Gay PC, Patel HG, Nelson SB *et al.* (1991) Metered dose inhalers for bronchodilator delivery in intubated, mechanically ventilated patients. *Chest* **99**:66–71.

33 Manthous CA, Hall JB, Schmidt GA *et al.* (1993) Metered-dose inhaler versus nebulized albuterol in mechanically ventilated patients. *Am Rev Respir Dis* **148**:1567–1570.

34 O'Riordan TG, Greco MJ, Perry RJ *et al.* (1992) Nebulizer function during mechanical ventilation. *Am Rev Respir Dis* **145**:1117–1122.

35 O'Doherty MJ, Thomas SHL, Page CJ *et al.* (1992) Delivery of a nebulized aerosol to a lung model during mechanical ventilation: effect of ventilator settings and nebulizer type, position and volume of fill. *Am Rev Respir Dis* **146**:383–388.

36 Thomas SHL, O'Doherty MJ, Fidler HM *et al.* (1993) Pulmonary deposition of a nebulised aerosol during mechanical ventilation. *Thorax* **48**:154–159.

37 Newhouse MT and Fuller HD (1993) Rose is a rose is a rose? Aerosol therapy in ventilated patients: nebulizers versus metered dose inhalers – a continuing controversy. *Am Rev Respir Dis* **148**:1444–1446.

38 Parkes SN and Bersten AD (1993). Bronchodilator response is maintained when nebulised salbutamol is administered concurrently with continuous positive airway pressure (CPAP) by face mask. *Anaesth Intens Care* **21**:715 (abstract).

39 Lode H, Hoffken G, Kemmerich B *et al.* (1992) Systemic and endotracheal antibiotic prophylaxis of nosocomial pneumonia in ICU. *Intens Care Med* **18**:S24–S27.

40 Ramsey BW, Dorkin HL, Eisenberg JD *et al.* (1993) Efficacy of aerosolized tobramycin in patients with cystic fibrosis. *N Engl J Med* **328**:1740–1746.

41 Committee on infectious diseases (1993) Use of ribavarin in the treatment of respiratory syncytial virus infection. *Pediatrics* **92**:501–504.

42 Bigby TD, Margolskee D, Curtis JL *et al.* (1986) The usefulness of induced sputum in the diagnosis of *Pneumocystis carinii* pneumonia in patients with the acquired immunodeficiency syndrome. *Am Rev Respir Dis* **133**:515–518.

43 Lewis JF and Jobe AH (1993) Surfactant and the adult respiratory distress syndrome. *Am Rev Respir Dis* **147**:218–233.

29 · Acute respiratory distress syndrome ARDS

J Takala

Acute respiratory distress syndrome (ARDS), the most severe type of acute respiratory failure, was first described in the late 1960s.[1] The clinical picture at the onset of the syndrome is characterized by refractory hypoxaemia and non-cardiogenic pulmonary oedema. ARDS may develop as the complication of any event which acutely and severely deranges the homeostasis of the patient.[2,3] Typical examples of these triggering events include severe and prolonged hypovolaemic shock, multiple injury, sepsis with or without shock, pneumonia, peritonitis, aspiration and acute pancreatitis (Table 29.1). Indeed, older terms for ARDS often referred to the triggering cause (e.g. shock lung, perfusion lung and pancreatitis lung). Recently, an American–European consensus conference on ARDS has recommended that the original term *acute* rather than *adult* respiratory distress syndrome should be used, since ARDS is not limited to adults.[3]

It is now evident that ARDS is the most severe manifestation of a spectrum of *acute lung injury* that results from inflammation, endothelial injury and increased microvascular permeability. The definition of when acute lung injury becomes ARDS is arbitrary, since the severity of the disease process is dynamic.[3,4] A practical outline for the diagnostic criteria is shown in Table 29.2.

Incidence and aetiology

The reported incidence of ARDS varies widely due to the variability of the definitions and diagnostic criteria. True incidence is not known but is probably around 1.5–4.0 cases/100 000 inhabitants per year in the developed countries.[3,5]

Various aetiologies of acute lung injury and ARDS have been listed in Table 29.1. All these aetiologies will eventually lead to clinically similar responses and injury of both the endothelium and the epithelium of the lung. Nevertheless, it is conceptually useful to consider two separate main mechanisms of injury: a

Table 29.1 Typical clinical conditions that trigger acute respiratory distress syndrome

Direct lung injury
Aspiration
Near-drowning
Smoke or toxic chemical inhalation
Pulmonary contusion
Pneumonia

Indirect (inflammatory)) lung injury
Severe or prolonged shock of any cause
Sepsis
Pancreatitis
Massive transfusion
Fat embolism
Cardiopulmonary bypass

Table 29.2 Practical diagnostic criteria for acute lung injury and acute respiratory distress syndrome (ARDS)

Acute lung injury
Timing: Acute onset

Oxygenation: $Pao_2/Fio_2 < 300$ mmHg (despite normal $Paco_2$ and regardless of PEEP)*

Chest X-ray: Bilateral diffuse infiltrates

Cardiac: No apparent cardiogenic cause (pulmonary capillary wedge pressure $\leqslant 18$ mmHg or 2.4 kPa if measured, or no clinical evidence of left atrial hypertension)

Risk factor: Known triggering event or risk factor

ARDS – same as above except:
Oxygenation: $Pao_2/Fio_2 < 200$ mmHg (despite normal $Paco_2$ and regardless of PEEP)*

*The Pao_2/Fio_2 criterion is arbitrary.[3]
PEEP = Positive end-expiratory pressure.

direct insult on the lung and the effects of systemic inflammatory response on the lung.

Pathophysiology and pathogenesis

The early stage of ARDS is characterized by alveolar oedema resulting from the endothelial injury and increased microvascular permeability. Aerated lung volume is markedly reduced: less than one-half of the total lung volume may be aerated.[6,7] Destruction of the epithelial cells and leakage of protein into the alveoli reduce the action of surfactant. Gas exchange abnormalities precede the impairment of the mechanical properties of the lung. The lung injury is not homogeneous: while the dependent lung regions tend to be collapsed or consolidated, the non-dependent parts of the lung may be normally or excessively inflated.[6]

The early stage of ARDS is followed by proliferation of alveolar epithelial type II cells. In the interstitium, collagen formation and fibroblast activity are increased.[8] The compliance of the lung decreases substantially, and the resistance of both the airways and the lung tissue increases.

Arterial hypoxaemia due to increased venous admixture is the principal gas exchange abnormality early in ARDS. The increased venous admixture is largely due to increased shunt, although reduced ventilation/perfusion also contributes.[9,10] Later on, the elimination of CO_2 is also impaired due to an increased physiological dead space to tidal volume ratio (V_D/V_T).[9,10]

When acute lung injury is caused by an inflammatory response, the mechanisms and sequence of events are not well-understood. Neutrophils, macrophages and lymphocytes are involved in the cell-mediated inflammatory response.[11] Cell adhesion, chemotaxis/chemokinesis and activation and release of mediators by the cells (e.g. cytokines, proteases, oxidants, lipid mediators) are evidently important in the pathogenesis of tissue damage.[12-15] Other important components of the inflammatory response in acute lung injury and ARDS include activation of the complement cascade and alterations in the coagulation and fibrinolysis. The relative importance of the various components of inflammation is not known.[12] There may also be several alternative chains of events in the pathogenesis of tissue damage.[3] Furthermore, some of the biochemical and immunological observations may represent mere epiphenomena.

Clinical presentation

The clinical signs and symptoms develop acutely, usually within 12–72 h following a triggering event known to be associated with the development of ARDS (Table 29.1). When ARDS develops in patients who are already on mechanical ventilation, the clinical signs and symptoms may be more subtle. The early clinical presentation is dominated by severe respiratory distress, severe hypoxaemia despite normal or low arterial Pa_{CO_2}, bilateral diffuse infiltrates in the chest X-ray and pulmonary oedema without an evident cardiogenic cause. It is important to recognize that simple hydrostatic pulmonary oedema (e.g. due to volume overload) may coexist with or precede the development of acute lung injury.[3]

The severity of hypoxaemia may rapidly fluctuate during the early phase of ARDS, because of changes in regional ventilation/perfusion and alveolar oedema. Since true shunt is the main cause of hypoxaemia, all factors that reduce the mixed venous saturation (i.e. increased oxygen consumption, decreased cardiac output and decreased haemoglobin) will markedly worsen the arterial hypoxaemia. The mechanical properties of the respiratory system are usually relatively well-preserved in the first days of ARDS, but deteriorate rapidly thereafter.[16] Markedly reduced compliance, increased venous admixture and increased dead space/tidal volume are characteristic in established ARDS, usually within approximately 1 week from the onset of the symptoms.[9,17,18] Pulmonary barotrauma, secondary (nosocomial) infections and dysfunction of other organ systems are common in established ARDS[19,20] (see Chapter 85).

From the second week on, recovery from ARDS may gradually start, though individual variability is extremely wide. Death in non-survivors usually occurs within 2–4 weeks, and the leading causes of death are infection and multiple organ failure.[19,20] The survivors may need prolonged weaning from mechanical ventilation due to the impaired gas exchange and respiratory mechanics, and rehabilitation due to a prolonged septic illness and general functional deterioration.

Management

Mechanical ventilatory support

Mechanical ventilation is the basic life-saving supportive therapeutic modality in ARDS. It allows time for the lungs to heal from the primary insult, and has largely eliminated deaths in acute hypoxaemia in the early phase of ARDS. Despite this, mechanical ventilation may also markedly worsen the lung injury, reduce the cardiac output and alter its distribution, and thereby indirectly contribute to the development of organ dysfunction and later death in ARDS.[3,21-23] The main goal of mechanical ventilatory support should be to maintain gas exchange and sufficient tissue oxygenation. Simultaneously, the adverse effects of mechanical ventilation on haemodynamics, lung overdistension and oxygen toxicity should be avoided or minimized.

Table 29.3 Components of systemic oxygen delivery (Do_2)

Arterial oxygen content (Cao_2 ml/l)
= 1.34 × Hb (g/l) X arterial oxygen saturation (Sao_2) + dissolved oxygen [= 0.23 × Po_2 (kPa)]
Cardiac output (Q l/min)
Do_2 (ml/min) = Q × Cao_2

Several different modes of positive-pressure ventilation are capable of supporting oxygenation and alveolar ventilation in ARDS[24–29] (see Chapter 26). None of the ventilatory modes have been shown superior to others in ARDS.[3] Accumulating data from experimental models and clinical studies strongly suggests that avoiding overinflation and high alveolar pressures should be one of the main goals in acute lung injury. Furthermore, prevention of repeated collapse and reinflation of lung units by use of sufficient positive end-expiratory pressure (PEEP) may help to prevent further lung damage.[21]

Oxygenation

Arterial oxygenation can be improved by increasing the fraction of inspired oxygen (Fio_2) and by increasing the mean airway pressure by the use of PEEP or prolonged inspiration time. Since oxygen delivery to the tissues is the product of blood flow and arterial oxygen content (Table 29.3), arterial oxygenation alone cannot be used as a guide to ensure adequate oxygen availability to the tissues. While increasing intrathoracic pressure usually improves arterial oxygenation, cardiac output is reduced in most cases, and oxygen delivery may actually decrease, and the risk for barotrauma increase. High Fio_2 ($\geqslant 0.6$) may be toxic and worsen the lung injury.

It is therefore advisable to target for a reasonable arterial oxygenation: an arterial Pao_2 of $\geqslant 60$ mmHg (8 kPa) and an arterial oxygen saturation of $\geqslant 90\%$ is acceptable. If these goals cannot be achieved with a PEEP of 10–15 cm H_2O (0.10–0.15 kPa), the risks of high levels of PEEP and Fio_2 and their net effect on oxygen delivery against accepting a slightly lower level of Pao_2 should be carefully considered.

In the presence of large shunt in ARDS, a reduction of mixed venous oxygenation due to a decrease in cardiac output or haemoglobin, or an increase in metabolic rate, will have a major impact on arterial oxygenation.[30] Accordingly, increasing haemoglobin and reducing unnecessary metabolic demand (e.g. by sedation) will also help to optimize arterial oxygenation.

Ventilation and CO_2 elimination

The factors contributing to the arterial CO_2 level can be described using the Bohr equation:

$$\text{Arterial } Paco_2 \text{ (kPa)} = \frac{0.115 \times Vco_2}{VE \times (1 - V_D/V_T)}$$

where Vco_2 is CO_2 production (ml/min STPD), VE is minute ventilation (l/min BTPS), and V_D/V_T is the physiological dead space to tidal volume ratio.

V_D/V_T may be markedly increased in ARDS, and the metabolic production of CO_2 is also commonly increased[17]. In order to maintain a normal $Paco_2$, an unreasonably high minute ventilation with large tidal volumes and/or high frequency would be required.[27] This increases the risk of overinflation and barotrauma (see below). It is therefore advisable to allow the $Paco_2$ to rise in order to reduce the ventilatory demand (i.e. permissive hypercapnia).[27,31] If the $Paco_2$ is allowed to rise slowly and renal and circulatory functions are normal, metabolic compensation will help to maintain a normal pH despite a substantially increased $Paco_2$. Depending on the lung mechanics and the level of PEEP, tidal volumes of 5–9 ml/kg body weight will usually allow acceptable alveolar ventilation without excessively high inflation pressures.

Mechanics and ventilator settings

The main effect of acute lung injury on respiratory mechanics is a substantial reduction of compliance.[6,7,16,18] Therefore, more inflation pressure is required to obtain a given tidal volume. Lung injury is inhomogeneous, and compliance in various parts of the lung varies from near normal to markedly reduced.[6,7] The less injured areas with higher compliance will receive more of the tidal volume during inflation, and there is a substantial risk of overdistension and further injury. During expiration, parts of the lung may tend to collapse, and this can be prevented by the cautious use of PEEP.[6,7,32]

The *alveolar pressure* during inflation should be limited to 30–35 cm H_2O (0.30–0.35 kPa). Peak inspiratory pressure depends markedly on the inspiratory flow and the resistance of the ventilator tubing, intubation tube and airway resistance, and is a poor indicator of alveolar pressure.[18,32,33] If an inspiratory pause is used, the *plateau pressure* is a much better indicator of alveolar pressure. The mean alveolar pressure at end-inspiration will be best obtained by occluding the airway at end-inspiration and recording the *static pressure* after 2–5 s of occlusion. This option is available in many modern ventilators. Peak alveolar pressure is always somewhat higher than the static pressure obtained after occlusion. Spontaneous breathing or efforts to breathe may lower the apparent inspiratory pressure, but large transpulmonary pressures may still be present.

When adjusting the ventilator to obtain the desired goals of gas exchange, the pressure during inspiratory pause or end-inspiratory occlusion should be limited to 30–35 cm H_2O (0.30–0.35 kPa). Whenever PEEP is adjusted, the inspiratory pause or occlusion pressure should be checked, and tidal volume readjusted, if necessary.

Estimation of the static compliance (C_{st}) is useful in tuning the ventilator:[6,7,18,32-34]

$$C_{st} = \text{Tidal volume}/(Pi_{st} - \text{PEEP}_{tot})$$

where Pi_{st} is the static pressure after end-inspiratory occlusion (or pause pressure, if inspiratory occlusion is not available), and PEEP_{tot} is the total PEEP, obtained after end-expiratory occlusion.

An increase in C_{st} following a change in PEEP or tidal volume suggests either recruitment of new lung units (e.g. after increased PEEP) or reduction of overdistension (e.g. after reducing the tidal volume or PEEP). Conversely, a decrease in C_{st} in response to a change in the ventilator settings suggests over-distension (e.g. after increasing tidal volume or PEEP), or closure of lung units (e.g. after reduction of PEEP or tidal volume). No change in C_{st} suggests that the lungs operate in the linear part of the pressure–volume relationship, and the risk of overdistension is minimized. The practical goals in setting the ventilator have been summarized in Table 29.4.

Management of oxygen transport and fluid therapy

Oxygen delivery to the tissues should be supported by maintaining adequate cardiac output and blood haemoglobin (120–130 g/l) in addition to optimum ventilator settings. Cardiac performance can be improved by adjusting the preload and afterload,

Table 29.4 Practical goals in setting the ventilator in acute respiratory distress syndrome

Mechanics
Keep static inspiratory or plateau pressure ⩽ 30–35 cm H_2O by adjusting PEEP and tidal volume

Oxygenation
Adjust Fio_2 (⩽ 0.60 if possible) and PEEP to obtain acceptable arterial oxygenation. Pao_2 around 60 mmHg (8 kPa) and Sao_2 90% is sufficient

Evaluate the net effect of ventilator settings on oxygen delivery. High PEEP and large tidal volumes may markedly reduce Do_2 despite improved arterial oxygenation.

Ventilation
Tidal volume of 5–9 ml/kg body weight; adjust to limit the inspiratory pressure (see Mechanics above)

Allow hypercapnia, if necessary, to limit the inspiratory pressures and ventilatory demand (NB: 'permissive hypercapnia' may worsen cerebral oedema and have adverse haemodynamic effects)

PEEP = Positive end-expiratory pressure.

according to measurements of cardiac output and pulmonary capillary wedge pressure (PCWP).[35] When adjusting the PCWP, the minimum level judged adequate should be targeted in order to avoid increasing the pulmonary oedema (see below). Inotropic agents (e.g. dobutamine) can be used to increase contractility. Systemic vasodilator agents should be administered with caution, since they may dramatically increase venous admixture and worsen the mismatch between ventilation and perfusion. Monitoring mixed venous oxygen saturation (aim for > 65%), blood levels of lactate, and possibly gastric mucosal pH, will help to maintain adequate oxygen transport to the tissues.

Since the main physiological reason for the pulmonary oedema in ARDS is increased capillary permeability, both haemodynamic and fluid management should attempt to minimize the capillary hydrostatic pressure without compromising the cardiac output.[3,36] Due to the increased pulmonary vascular resistance in ARDS, the pulmonary capillary hydrostatic pressure is often substantially higher than the PCWP. When a marked gradient between the pulmonary arterial diastolic pressure (PAPd) and the PCWP exists, the pulmonary capillary pressure is closer to the PAPd. Provided that sufficient preload can be maintained, attempting a negative fluid balance in the acute phase of ARDS seems advisable.[37]

Positioning and physiotherapy

Frequent changes of posture, removal of secretions and physiotherapy are important. Airway suctioning should be done with caution to avoid severe hypoxaemia. PEEP, if used, must be maintained at all times. Turning the patient prone may sometimes dramatically improve arterial oxygenation, especially in the early phase of ARDS.[38]

Nutrition support

Most of the patients with ARDS are hypermetabolic throughout the disease. Nutrition support, using the enteral route when possible, should be started early in order to reduce wasting. Energy intake should be aimed to meet the expenditure and protein intake should be around 1.2–1.5 g/kg per day. Nutrient intakes grossly exceeding the energy expenditure should be avoided.[39]

Other therapeutic considerations

1 *Infection control* by appropriate microbiological monitoring and specific antibiotic therapy is important, since infections are a major source of morbidity and mortality in ARDS. Prophylactic use of antibiotics is not indicated.

2 *Extracorporeal lung assistance (ECLA)* has been used by several centres in the treatment of ARDS. At present, controlled clinical studies have demonstrated similar outcome with ECLA as with conventional treatment.[40]

3 *Corticosteroids* have been suggested to reduce lung inflammation in ARDS. There are no data from controlled clinical studies to support this. In contrast, non-specific inhibition of the inflammatory response may be counterproductive.

4 *Miscellaneous experimental agents*, including inhibitors of the prostaglandin system, free radical scavengers, vasodilators, surfactant and various immunotherapies, are under investigation.

Nitric oxide (NO)

NO is involved in a wide variety of physiological and pathological processes.[41–43] NO is synthesized via the L-arginine NO pathway from the amino acid L-arginine, by a family of enzymes, the NO synthases. Under physiological conditions, NO regulates blood pressure and regional perfusion by maintaining basic vasodilatory tone.[41] It acts as a neurotransmitter in the central and peripheral nervous systems; NO-dependent mechanisms contribute to neurogenic vasodilatation. Macrophages can produce large quantities of NO in various host defence responses, and platelet aggregation and leukocyte adhesion are partly controlled by NO. Cytokines induce NO production in the endothelium and vascular smooth muscle.[44]

Normal vasoregulation is controlled by a calcium-dependent *constitutive* NO synthase, located in the endothelium.[41] Several stimuli (e.g. acetylcholine, adenosine diphosphate, bradykinin and shear stress) can increase NO production by the constitutive NO synthase in the endothelium. The NO diffuses into the vascular smooth muscle, and stimulates soluble guanylate cyclase, thus increasing production of cyclic guanosine monophosphate (GMP). Cyclic GMP is the second messenger that brings about vascular smooth-muscle relaxation. NO is produced continuously by the endothelium in order to fine-tune vascular tone. Vasodilatory effects of compounds like acetylcholine or bradykinin depend on the endothelium-derived NO. In contrast, enothelium-independent vasodilators sodium nitroprusside and nitroglycerin release NO to activate guanylate cyclase directly.[41]

A calcium-independent *inducible* isoform of NO synthase can also produce large amounts of NO both in the endothelium and in the vascular smooth muscle.[41–44] Once induced, continuous production of NO will result in a sustained relaxation of vascular smooth muscle. This relaxation can be very resistant to vasopressors, and is believed to contribute to the hypotension in septic shock.[41,44–46] Preliminary studies suggest that NO inhibition may reduce vasopressor needs in septic shock,[45,46] but the safety and efficacy of NO inhibition in septic shock remain undocumented.[44] Selective inhibition of inducible NO synthase, while preserving the activity of constitutive NO synthase, may be a future therapeutic strategy.

The use of NO in acute lung injury and severe pulmonary hypertension is based on the rationale that inhaled NO will directly reach the target tissue.[41–43,47] Since inhaled NO will preferentially reach well-ventilated alveoli, the local vasodilatation (and possibly also bronchodilatation) will result in improved ventilation/perfusion matching and reduced pulmonary hypertension without systemic vasodilatation. In contrast, systemically administered vasodilators dilate pulmonary vasculature non-selectively, and thereby worsen ventilation/perfusion mismatch. Long-term and toxic effects of inhaled NO are currently not known. NO reacts readily with oxygen, and increases the concentration of toxic NO_2. The delivery of NO in clinical experiments requires careful safety considerations.[42] Only 50–80% of patients with ARDS will have a favourable gas exchange response to inhaled NO, and the clinical relevance of this improvement is currently not known. At present, its use should be regarded as experimental.

Outcome

Mortality in ARDS is approximately 50–60%, although the figures may vary substantially depending on the definition of ARDS and the patient categories. Early deaths in hypoxaemia are extremely rare. ARDS patients who die later in the course of the disease, usually die *with* hypoxaemia, not *of* it. The main causes of mortality are sepsis and multiple organ failure.[48–51] Those patients who survive recover to achieve a good functional status, though some pulmonary dysfunction and slightly reduced quality of life is common after 1 year of discharge from the hospital.[51,52]

References

1 Ashbaugh DG, Bigelow DB, Petty TL and Levine BE (1967) Acute respiratory distress in adults. *Lancet* ii: 319–323.

2 Petty TL (1982) Adult respiratory distress syndrome: definition and historical perspective. *Clin Chest Med* 3:3–7.

3 Bernard GR, Artigas A, Brigham KL *et al.* (1994) Report of the American–European consensus conference on ARDS: definitions, mechanisms, relevant outcomes and clinical trial coordination. *Intens Care Med* 20:225–232.

4 Murray JF, Matthay MA, Luce JM and Flick MR (1988) An expanded definition of the adult respiratory distress syndrome. *Am Rev Respir Dis* 138:720–723.

5 Villar J and Slutsky AS (1989) The incidence of the

adult respiratory distress syndrome. *Am Rev Respir Dis* **140**: 814–816.

6 Gattinoni L, Pesenti A, Bombino M *et al.* (1988) Relationships between lung computed tomographic density, gas exchange, and PEEP in acute respiratory failure. *Anesthesiology* **69**:824–832.

7 Pelosi P, D'Andrea L, Vitale G, Pesenti A and Gattinoni L (1994) Vertical gradient of regional lung inflation in adult respiratory distress syndrome. *Am J Respir Crit Care Med* **149**:8–13.

8 Wiener-Kronish JP, Gropper MA and Matthay MA (1990) The adult respiratory distress syndrome: definition and prognosis, pathogenesis and treatment. *Br J Anaesth* **65**:107–129.

9 Lamy M, Fallat RJ, Koeniger E *et al.* (1976) Pathologic features and mechanisms of hypoxemia in adult respiratory distress syndrome. *Am Rev Respir Dis* **114**:267–284.

10 Dantzker DR, Brook CJ, Dehart P, Lynch JP and Weg JG (1979) Ventilation–perfusion distributions in the adult respiratory distress syndrome. *Am Rev Respir Dis* **120**:1039–1052.

11 Repin JE and Beehler CJ (1991) Neutrophils and adult respiratory distress syndrome: two interlocking perspectives in 1991. *Am Rev Respir Dis* **144**:251–252.

12 St. John RC and Dorinsky PM (1993) Immunologic therapy for ARDS, septic shock, and multiple-organ failure. *Chest* **103**:932–943.

13 Bunnell E and Pacht ER (1993) Oxidized glutathione is increased in the alveolar fluid of patients with the adult respiratory distress syndrome. *Am Rev Respir Dis* **148**:1174–1178.

14 Laurent T, Markert M, von Fliedner V *et al.* (1994) CD11b/CD18 expression, adherence, and chemotaxis of granulocytes in adult respiratory distress syndrome. *Am J Respir Crit Care Med* **149**:1534–1538.

15 Tran van Nhieu J, Misset B, Lebargy F, Carlet J and Bernaudin J-F (1993) Expression of tumor necrosis factor-α gene in alveolar macrophages from patients with the adult respiratory distress syndrome. *Am Rev Respir Dis* **147**:1585–1589.

16 Matamis D, Lemaire F, Harf A, Brun-Buisson C, Ansquer JC and Atlan G (1984) Total respiratory pressure–volume curves in the adult respiratory distress syndrome. *Chest* **86**:58-66.

17 Kiiski R and Takala J (1994) Hypermetabolism and efficiency of CO_2 removal in acute respiratory failure. *Chest* **105**:1198–1203.

18 Ranieri M, Giuliani R, Fiore T, Dambrosio M and Milic-Emili J (1994) Volume-pressure curve of the respiratory system predicts effects of PEEP in ARDS: 'occlusion' versus 'constant flow' technique. *Am J Respir Crit Care Med* **149**:19–27.

19 Sloane PJ, Gee MH, Gottlieb JE *et al.* (1992) A multicenter registry of patients with acute respiratory distress syndrome. *Am Rev Respir Dis* **146**:419–426.

20 Suchyta MR, Clemmer TP, Elliott CG, Orme JF and Waver LK (1992) The adult respiratory distress syndrome, a report of survival and modifying factors. *Chest* **101**:1074–1079.

21 Muscedre JG, Mullen JBM, Gan K and Slutsky AS (1994) Tidal ventilation at low airway pressures can augment lung injury. *Am J Respir Crit Care Med* **149**:1327–1334.

22 Rouby JJ, Lherm T, Martin de Lassale E *et al.* (1993) Histologic aspects of pulmonary barotrauma in critically ill patients with acute respiratory failure. *Intens Care Med* **19**:383–389.

23 Dreyfuss D and Saumon G (1994) Should the lung be rested or recruited? The charybdis and scylla of ventilator management (editorial). *Am J Respir Crit Care Med* **149**:1066–1068.

24 Kiiski R, Takala J, Kari A and Milic-Emili J (1992) Effect of tidal volume on gas exchange and oxygen transport in the adult respiratory distress syndrome. *Am Rev Respir Dis* **146**:1131–1135.

25 Sydow M, Burchardi H, Ephraim E, Zielmann S and Crozier TA (1994) Long-term effects of two different ventilatory modes on oxygenation in acute lung injury. *Am J Respir Crit Care Med* **149**:1550–1556.

26 Leatherman JW, Lari RL, Iber C and Ney AL (1991) Tidal volume reduction in ARDS. Effect on cardiac output and arterial oxygenation. *Chest* **99**:1227–12231.

27 Hickling KG, Henderson SJ and Jackson R (1990) Low mortality associated with low volume pressure limited ventilation with permissive hypercapnia in severe adult respiratory distress syndrome. *Intens Care Med* **16**:372–377.

28 Shanholtz C and Brower R (1994) Should inverse ratio ventilation be used in adult respiratory distress syndrome? *Am Rev Respir Dis* **149**:1354–1358.

29 Marini JJ and Kelsen SG (1992) Re-targeting ventilatory objectives in adult respiratory distress syndrome (Editorial). *Am Rev Respir Dis* **146**:2–3.

30 Marshall BE, Hanson CW, Frasch F and Marshall C (1994) Role of hypoxic pulmonary vasoconstriction in pulmonary gas exchange and blood flow distribution. *Intens Care Med* **20**:379–389.

31 Bidani A, Tzouanakis AE, Cardenas VJ and Zwischenberger JB (1994) Permissive hypercapnia in acute respiratory failure. *J Am Med Assoc* **272**:957–962.

32 Valta P, Takala J, Eissa NT and Milic-Emili J (1993) Does alveolar recruitment occur with positive end-expiratory pressure in adult respiratory distress syndrome patients? *J Crit Care* **8**:34–42.

33 Gattinoni L, Pesenti A, Caspani ML *et al.* (1984) The role of total static lung compliance in the management of severe ARDS unresponsive to conventional treatment. *Intens Care Med* **10**:121–126.

34 Brunet F, Mira J-P, Belghith M *et al.* (1994) Extracorporeal carbon dioxide removal technique improves oxygenation without causing overinflation. *Am J Respir Crit Care Med* **149**:1557–1562.

35 Shephard JN, Brecker SJ and Evans TW (1994) Bedside assessment of myocardial performance in the critically ill. *Intens Care Med* **20**:513–521.

36 Harris TR, Bernard GR, Brigham KL *et al.* (1990) Lung microvascular transport properties measured by multiple indicator dilution methods in patients with adult respiratory distress syndrome. A comparison between patients reversing respiratory failure and those failing to reverse. *Am Rev Respir Dis* **141**:272–280.

37 Schuller D, Mitchell JP, Calandrino FS and Schuster DP (1991) Fluid balance during pulmonary edema. Is fluid gain a marker or a cause of poor outcome? *Chest* **100**:1068–1075.

38 Lamm WJE, Graham MM and Albert RK (1994) Mechanism by which the prone position improves oxygenation in acute lung injury. *Am J Respir Crit Care Med* **150**:184–193.

39 Takala J (1993) Nutrition and metabolism in acute respiratory failure. In: Wilmore DW and Carpentier YA

(eds) *Update in Intensive Care and Emergency Medicine 17. Metabolic Support of the Critically Ill Patient*. Berlin: Springer-Verlag, pp. 390–406.

40 Morris AH, Wallace CJ, Menlove RL *et al.* (1994) Randomized clinical trial of pressure-controlled inverse ratio ventilation and extracorporeal CO_2 removal for adult respiratory distress syndrome. *Am J Respir Crit Care Med* **149**:295–305.

41 Moncada S and Higgs A (1993) The L-arginine–nitric oxide pathway. *N Engl J Med* **329**:2002–2012.

42 Zapol WM, Rimar S, Gillis N, Marletta M and Bosken CH (1994) Nitric oxide and the lung. *Am J Respir Crit Care Med* **149**:1375–1380.

43 Hognan M, Frostell CG, Hedenstrom H and Hedenstierna G (1993) Inhalation of nitric oxide modulates adult human bronchial tone. *Am Rev Respir Dis* **148**:1474–1478.

44 Natanson C, Hoffman WD, Suffredinl AF, Eichacker PQ and Danner RL (1994) Selected treatment strategies for septic shock based on proposed mechanisms of pathogenesis. *Ann Intern Med* **120**:771–883.

45 Lorente JA, Landin L and Esteban A (1994) Role of nitric oxide in the regulation of vascular tone in septic shock. In: Vincent J-L (ed.) *Yearbook of Intensive Care and Emergency Medicine*. Berlin: Springer-Verlag, pp. 75–89.

46 Petros A, Lamb G, Leone A, Moncada S, Bennett D and Vallance P (1994) Effects of a nitric synthase inhibitor in humans with septic shock. *Cardiovasc Res* **28**:34–39.

47 Rossaint R, Falke KJ, López F, Slama K, Pison U and Zapol WM (1993) Inhaled nitric oxide for the adult respiratory distress syndrome. *N Engl J Med* **328**:399–405.

48 Suchyta MR, Clemmer TP, Orme JF, Morris AH and Elliott CG (1991) Increased survival of ARDS patients with severe hypoxemia (ECMO criteria). *Chest* **99**: 951–955.

49 Fowler AA, Hamman RF, Zerbe GO, Benson KN and Hyers TM (1985) Adult respiratory distress syndrome. Prognosis after onset. *Am Rev Respir Dis* **132**:472–478.

50 Bone RC, Balk R, Slotman G *et al.* (1992) Adult respiratory distress syndrome. Sequence and importance of development of multiple organ failure. *Chest* **101**:320–326.

51 McHugh LG, Milberg JA, Whitcomb ME, Shoene RB, Maunder RJ and Hudson LD (1994) Recovery of function in survivors of the acute respiratory distress syndrome. *Am J Respir Crit Care Med* **150**:90–94.

52 Elliott CG, Morris AH and Cengiz M (1981) Pulmonary function and exercise gas exchange in survivors of adult respiratory distress syndrome. *Am Rev Respir Dis* **123**:492–495.

30 | Pulmonary embolism

RC Freebairn and TE Oh

Pulmonary embolism (PE) is a complication of deep vein thrombosis (DVT), and is a frequent cause of morbidity and mortality in postoperative and medical patients. Its incidence is estimated to be as high as 630 000 cases annually in the USA.[1] Mortality has been directly attributed to PE in 15% of cases at autopsy. Thus, prophylactic measures against DVT and early diagnosis and treatment of PE are important, especially in critically ill patients.

Aetiology

Most pulmonary emboli result from asymptomatic thromboses in deep veins of the lower limbs, pelvis and inferior vena cava (i.e. proximal DVT), and less frequently from thromboses in the upper limbs, right atrium or ventricle. Thrombosis limited to calf veins (i.e. distal DVT) seldom results in clinically obvious PE.[2]

Predisposing factors for thrombosis involve one or more components of Virchow's triad: stasis of blood flow; damage to vessels; or alterations in coagulation mechanism (Table 30.1). Venous stasis, while augmenting thrombus formation, is insufficient on its own to induce DVT.[3] Increased coagulation results from a lowered clotting threshold or a more rapidly progressive clotting process, once activated. Clot formation involves platelet aggregation and the coagulation cascade (see Chapter 89). Venous thrombi consist of mainly fibrin and red blood cells with relatively few platelets.[4] As vessel walls are often normal, platelet activation plays a minimal role in venous thrombosis.

Risk factors for DVT and PE are multiple and additive. Over 50% of DVT patients were immobilized within the previous 3 months; two-thirds of the immobilizations were less than 2 weeks.[5] Surgery is another major contributor to thromboembolic disease (Table 30.2).[6,7] Thrombotic complications are common in catheterized veins, often associated with catheter-related sepsis.[8] Activated protein C resistance

Table 30.1 Pathophysiological basis of thromboembolic disease[3]

Changes in platelet function
Thrombocytosis
  Reactive
  Pathological
Cytokine activation
Catecholamine activation
Fibrinogenaemia
Increased factor VIII-related antigen

Decreased fibrinolytic activity
Postoperatively
Decreased α_2-antiplasmin levels
Decreased α_1 levels

Decreased natural anticoagulant activity
Antithrombin III
Protein C
α_2-Macroglobulin

Increased procoagulant activity
Fibrinogen
Factor VIII coagulant
Increased factor VIII-related antigen
Interleukin-6

Stasis
Low cardiac output
Arterial or venous occlusion

Vessel wall
Trauma
Toxin

has a high incidence amongst patients with a history of DVT.[9]

Clinical presentation

PE has diverse non-specific presentations, depending on the severity and multiplicity of the embolic

Table 30.2 Risk factors for thromboembolic disease[5-10]

Prolonged immobilization

Age

Surgical
General surgery
Orthopaedic surgery
Surgery of legs and pelvis
Arthroscopy
Valve incompetence of leg veins
Spinal cord injuries
Local trauma
Burns
Electric shock

Coagulation abnormalities
Polycythaemia
Platelet abnormalities
Antithrombin III deficiency
Protein C and S deficiencies
Inherited abnormalities of fibrinogen and plasminogen
Previous venous thrombosis

Medical conditions
Congestive cardiac failure
Myocardial infarction
Cerebrovascular accidents
Obesity
Infection
Malignancy, especially pancreas, lung, stomach, genito-
    urinary tract or breast
Smoking
Oral contraceptive/oestrogen therapy
Pregnancy
Advanced age
Vasculitis
Shock syndromes
Dysproteinaemias
Hyperlipidaemia
Inflammatory bowel disorders
Paroxysmal nocturnal haemaglobinuria
Behçet's syndrome
Sickle-cell anaemia

episode. Symptoms and signs may be masked by or mistaken for manifestations of coexistent diseases. Small heraldic emboli commonly precede a major embolus by days or weeks, and 90% of deaths follow a second embolic attack.[10]

Symptoms

In nearly all patients with acute PE, dyspnoea (73%), tachypnoea (66%) or pleuritic pain (66%) is present.[11] Non-productive cough occurs in 37%. Classic symptoms of pleuritic pain and haemoptysis (13%) are not early symptoms, and are present only if infarction has occurred (10%). Syncope occurs more commonly (17%) in massive embolus than with minor emboli (4%).[11]

Physical signs

There may be minimal clinical signs which are usually non-specific, including:

Respiratory

Tachypnoea with shallow breaths (>20/min) is common (70%). Cyanosis (1%) is usually restricted to cases of massive embolism. A pleural effusion and friction rub (3%) may be found with pulmonary infarction.[11] Wheezing (5%) and rales may also be manifestations of coexisting cardiopulmonary disease.[12]

Cardiovascular

Tachycardia (>100 beats/min) may relate to the site of the obstruction. Onset of bradycardia is an ominous sign. Accentuation of the pulmonary valve closure sound and widened splitting of the second heart sound may reflect a rise in pulmonary artery (PA) pressure. Mean PA pressure is elevated by 5 mmHg (0.67 kPa) when more than 50% of the pulmonary vasculature is acutely obstructed. A palpable right ventricular heave and audible S3 and S4 gallop heart sounds occur in 4% of presentations, and are associated with extensive embolism.[11] Elevated jugular venous pressure and prominent A waves may be seen. Systemic hypotension and shock occur in the presence of massive embolization;[12] a small sharp peripheral pulse may be palpated.

Pulmonary hypertension

Recurrent PE or an underlying cardiopulmonary disease can lead to exacerbation of pulmonary hypertension. Massive PE increases right ventricular afterload, enlarges the right ventricle and deviates the septum to the left, decreasing left ventricular volume and compliance.[13,14] Cardiac output and coronary blood flow, especially to the right heart, are diminished. Resultant ischaemia decreases the contractility of the right heart, developing a cycle of cardiac decompensation. Neurogenic and humoral influences may result in catastrophic pulmonary hypertension, with occlusion of as little as 30% of the pulmonary vascular bed.[15] Once mean PA pressure exceeds 40 mmHg (5.3 kPa), haemodynamic collapse occurs. With right ventricular hypertrophy, higher PA pressures can be generated.[15]

Lower limbs

Clinical evidence of DVT may be present, but is found in only about 30% of patients with PE. The 'normal' leg may give rise to emboli, with DVT found in 36% of contralateral limbs on investigation.[16]

Other signs

Sweating (11%) and fever >38.5°C (7%) are present infrequently.[11] Many signs are transient and persist for only a few hours after the acute embolization, perhaps signifying early lysis and fragmentation with more distal distribution of the embolus.

Differential diagnosis

Differential diagnosis includes myocardial infarction, acute left ventricular failure, aspiration pneumonitis, pleural effusion, acute pneumonia, fat embolism, pneumothorax and dissecting aortic aneurysm.

Investigations

Objective diagnostic tests are essential, as clinical examination and routine tests (e.g. chest X-ray) are neither specific nor sensitive to diagnose PE. The choice and order of investigations are dependent upon the availability of equipment and expertise. Investigations include those to diagnose DVT as well as PE.

Diagnosis of DVT

Evidence of DVT may help diagnose PE, if specialized facilities to confirm PE (see below) are unavailable. The presence of DVT necessitates antithrombolic treatment and consideration of thrombolysis. Investigation of the lower extremities for DVT previously included radioisotope-labelled fibrinogen scanning, but this blood product carries infection and radiation risks and is not clinically useful. Currently used tests are:

1 *Ultrasonography*
   (a) *Doppler ultrasonography* detects flow changes in veins, but is notoriously unreliable in detecting proximal vein thrombi in asymptomatic patients.[13,15] A negative finding does not exclude a DVT.[17]
   (b) *B-mode ultrasonography* is easy to perform, non-invasive and readily available. The vessel compressibility is the criterion for diagnosis. Occasionally, clot may be visualized. In symptomatic patients it is highly accurate, simple and reproducible.[18] Limiting examination to the common femoral and popliteal vessels appears to be adequate.[2]
2 *Impedance plethysmography*: This is a non-invasive technique sensitive for proximal, but not distal DVT. Electrical impedance is measured distally, during inflation and deflation of a mid-thigh pneumatic cuff. It has low specificity and sensitivity.[19] Diagnostic reliability is markedly increased with serial measurements over 10–14 days.[20]
3 *Contrast venography*: Venography is the most accurate diagnostic technique,[21] but visualization of external and common iliac veins is inadequate. A negative venogram cannot exclude DVT with utmost certainty, as embolism may arise from other than the lower extremities. It is invasive and expensive, and complications include pain, hypersensitivity, phlebitis and a low incidence of DVT itself.
4 *Magnetic resonance imaging (MRI)*: MRI using gradient-recalled echo acquisition is sensitive and specific in detecting DVT.[22] With an accuracy of 96%, it may be superior to contrast venography or ultrasound in pelvic thrombosis detection, but the difficulties of MRI in the critically ill preclude its routine use.[22,23]

Diagnosis of PE

Diagnostic investigations include routine laboratory and bedside tests, although these are non-specific. Patients with DVT frequently have PE that are not clinically apparent.[24]

Blood

White cell count may be elevated (>15 × 10⁹ cells/l). Increased serum lactic dehydrogenase, transaminase enzymes and bilirubin levels lack enough specificity to be useful in the acute situation. D-Dimer concentrations are a non-specific but sensitive indicator of PE; concentrations below 500 μg/l virtually exclude the diagnosis.[25] Elevated plasma activator inhibitor levels and immunoglobulin E levels may be predictive of DVT, but are not routinely available.[26,27]

Chest X-ray

In PE, 16% of chest films are normal, and any changes are neither specific nor diagnostic.[11] Comparison with previous films may be helpful. Localized infiltrates, consolidation and atelectasis occur in two-thirds, and a pleural effusion in half of the patients.[28] The classic 'plump' pulmonary arteries with peripheral pruning (Westermark sign) are relatively rare and non-specific.[11] This, along with an elevated diaphragm, is more commonly associated with massive embolus and elevated PA pressures.[28,29]

Electrocardiograph

A normal electrocardiogram (ECG) is found in 30% of cases.[12] Non-specific S-T depression and T-wave inversion in anterior leads are the commonest findings (49%), reflecting right heart strain. The classic pattern of a deep S wave in lead I, and a Q wave and inverted T wave in lead III (i.e. $S_1Q_3T_3$ pattern) is not frequently seen.[30] Left axis deviation occurs more frequently than right axis. P pulmonale, right bundle branch block and atrial arrhythmias are also occasionally present, and persistent if embolization is massive. The ECG is useful in excluding acute myocardial infarction or other primary cardiac abnormalities.

Arterial blood gases

Hypoxaemia is frequently present, but an arterial Po_2 over 80 mmHg (10.6 kPa) occurs in a quarter of PE patients.[12] Recording the inspired oxygen concentration during arterial blood sampling allows calculation of the arterial–alveolar gradient (i.e. $Pao_2 - Pao_2$). Even this may be normal.[31] Tachypnoea may result in hypocarbia. Metabolic acidosis may be present if shock follows a large embolus.

Ventilation/perfusion lung scans

A perfusion lung scan (using IV technetium 99m-labelled albumin) is a sensitive non-invasive test which should be performed whenever PE is suspected. Perfusion defects may be classified as single or multiple, and as subsegmental, segmental or lobar. Current ventilation scans involve inhalation of ^{133}Xe or ^{127}Xe, radioactive ^{81m}Kr or radioactive ^{99m}Tc or ultrafine distribution of carbon laced with ^{99m}Tc.[32,33] Combining ventilation and perfusion scans markedly improves specificity.[33] Defects may mismatch (i.e. normal ventilation in zone of perfusion defect) or match (when the ventilation defect corresponds with the perfusion defect). The probability of PE is classified as high, low or intermediate (Table 30.3).[5] The presence of pre-existing cardiopulmonary disease reduces the diagnostic power of $\dot{V}/\dot{Q}$ scans.[34] For example, up to 60% of lung scans of patients with chronic respiratory disease but without PE can be classified as intermediate probability. The diagnostic strength is increased by clinical assessment and stratification according to pre-existing disease.[35,36] Mean resolution of PE is only 7.4% in the first 24 h, suggesting that a scan performed within this period is likely to show a defect.[37]

Pulmonary angiography

This specific 'gold standard' diagnostic test is unfortunately invasive, with an associated mortality and morbidity. However, risks are sufficiently low to justify use in an appropriate setting.[38] A positive angiogram shows consistent defects in multiple films or sharp cut-offs in vessels over 2.5 mm diameter. Massive PE produces significant filling defects or obstruction in two or more lobar arteries. Indications for pulmonary angiography include the above considerations with $\dot{V}/\dot{Q}$ scans, confirmation of PE in a patient at increased risk of bleeding from anticoagulants, and massive PE to decide the choice of thrombolytic, embolectomy or vena caval inter-

Table 30.3 Interpretation of ventilation/perfusion scans[5]

Probability of PE	Findings
None	Normal perfusion
Very low	Three or fewer small (<25% segment) $\dot{Q}$ defects with normal CXR findings
Low	Non-segmental $\dot{Q}$ defects One-moderate (>25%, <75% segment) with normal CXR findings Any $\dot{Q}$ defect with larger CXR abnormality Three or 4 large (>75% segment) or moderate $\dot{Q}$ defects matched, CXR findings normal or smaller More than three small $\dot{Q}$ defects, normal CXR findings
Intermediate	All not defined in very low, low or high group
High	Two or more large $\dot{Q}$ defects without $\dot{V}$ or CXR matches Two or more moderate $\dot{Q}$ defects with $\dot{Q}$ or CXR matches Four or more moderate $\dot{Q}$ defects with $\dot{V}$ or CXR abnormality

Notes

1 A normal perfusion scan rules out significant PE
2 A high-probability V/Q scan with significant risk factors reliably establishes the diagnosis of PE
3 A low-probability V/Q scan with a high clinical index of suspicion warrants further investigation
4 A high-probability V/Q scan with normal non-invasive tests for deep venous thrombosis and low risk factors should also be confirmed by pulmonary angiography or other confimatory test

PE = pulmonary embolism; $\dot{Q}$ = perfusion; CXR = chest X-ray; $\dot{V}$ = ventilation.

ruption therapy (Fig. 30.1). The pulmonary angiogram catheter may be left *in situ* for measurements of pulmonary artery (PA) pressures, direct infusion of thrombolytic drugs and repeat angiography. Digital subtraction angiography, cineangiography, and balloon occlusion angiography may augment diagnostic accuracy in difficult cases.[10] Full resuscitation facilities should readily be available during radiographic procedures as contrast media can cause catastrophic vasodilatation.

Echocardiography

Transthoracic and transoesophageal echocardiography (TOE) have been used clinically, and transvenous echocardiography used experimentally, in the detection and evaluation of PE.[13,39] The echocardiographic characteristics are listed in Table 30.4. Intraluminal thrombus is occasionally seen. Central pulmonary artery thrombus can be detected by TOE. Echocardiography is useful as a bedside diagnostic modality in ICU.[7,13]

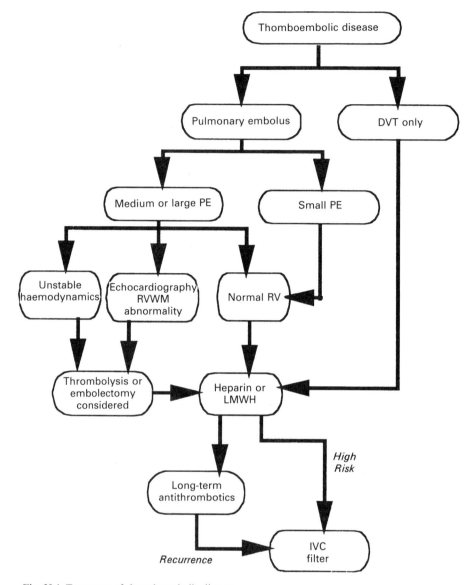

Fig. 30.1 Treatment of thromboembolic disease

Management

General measures

General measures in the acute situation include oxygen therapy, haemodynamic support and treating shock in massive PE. Cardiopulmonary resuscitation is undertaken in acute cardiovascular collapse.

Oxygen therapy

Oxygen is given initially by mask. High flows must be used because air entrainment during marked hyperventilation results in a lower than expected

inspired oxygen concentration (see Chapter 22). Intubation and mechanical ventilation may be necessary.

Haemodynamic support

It is imperative to maintain right heart filling pressures. Leg elevation will increase venous return by autotransfusion, and assist right heart filling pressures (Starling effect). Overfilling the right ventricle in the presence of pulmonary hypertension may be detrimental.[13,14] PA catheter placement, although not essential, will enable monitoring of

Table 30.4 Echocardiographic changes in pulmonary embolism[13]

Decreased mitral valve opening
Thromboemboli in right heart or pulmonary artery
Right ventricular dilatation
Right ventricular hypokinesis
Abnormal septal position/paradoxical systolic movement
Reduced left ventricular size
Increase right/left ventricular diameter ratio
Pulmonary artery dilatation
Tricuspid or pulmonary valve insufficiency jets

Table 30.5 Antithrombotic treatment for pulmonary embolism (PE) or deep venous thrombosis (DVT)[10,44]

Antithrombotic treatment of PE should be the same as for DVT

Subcutaneous or IV heparin titrated to APPT of 1.5–2.0 times normal; standard doses of LMWH can be used

Warfarin may be started simultaneously with heparin only in *stable* patients
    Loading dose is 25–30 mg over 36 h
    Maintenance is about 5 mg/day, titrated against regular prothrombin time estimations ($\times 2$ control) or INR 2–3

Heparin therapy should be continued to day 6 if INR is therapeutic (or day 8 in massive PE)

Oral warfarin therapy should continue for 3 months with repeated monitoring

Patients with ongoing risk factors or recurrent emboli should be treated indefinitely

IV = intravenous; APPT = activated partial prothrombin time; LMWH = low-molecular-weight heparin; INR = international normalized ratio.

responses to fluids, and vasoactive and thrombolytic agents. Fluid infusion and inotropes may help to maintain systemic and pulmonary circulations. Dobutamine, adrenaline, noradrenaline and amrinone all have benefits if titrated appropriately to clinical effects.[15,40,41] Isoprenaline, a potent inotrope and pulmonary vasodilator, is arrhythmogenic and a systemic vasodilator, and is detrimental.[15] Nitroprusside reduces right ventricular coronary perfusion.[15] Extracorporeal oxygenation and circulatory assistance has been used to support the circulation until thrombolytic therapy or embolectomy can be undertaken.

Definitive therapy for DVT and PE

Definitive treatment is directed towards the prevention of new thrombus formation, thrombolysis, blocking migration of emboli and emboli removal (Fig. 30.1).

Heparin therapy (Table 30.5)[43]

Heparin enhances the inhibitory effect of antithrombin III on thrombin and factor Xa (see Chapter 89). Heparin anticoagulation by infusion is safe and more efficacious than intermittent IV bolus doses for preventing new thrombus formation. Treating proximal DVT with subcutaneous heparin is as safe as, and possibly more effective than, continuous IV therapy.[42] An initial 15 000–20 000 unit bolus, followed by an infusion of 1000–1500 units/h, is advocated. Platelet-released serotonin and histamine exacerbation of pulmonary hypertension associated with PE may be antagonized by heparin.

The paradoxical heparin-induced thrombotic thrombocytopenia syndromes may result from heparin usage (see Chapter 89). In severe cases, heparin should be discontinued, and an alternative treatment of oral anticoagulants combined with ancrod or lomoparan commenced.[45,46]

Low-molecular-weight heparins (LMWH)

LMWH are derivatives of unfractionated heparin, with mean molecular weights of 4–7 kDa. Compared with subcutaneous standard heparin, LMWH have a longer anti-Xa anticoagulant effect. When used subcutaneously, they compare favourably with IV standard heparin in the treatment of thromboembolism;[47] mortality and recurrence of DVT have been reduced. Associated bleeding occurs in high-risk groups, and is unrelated to activated partial prothrombin time (APPT) or anticoagulant dose.[47] The fixed dosing regimens based on body mass, with reduced dosing frequency and need for monitoring, have advantages over standard heparin regimens.

Warfarin therapy (Table 30.5)

Warfarin and other coumarin derivatives inhibit synthesis of vitamin K-dependent clotting factors (factors II, VII, IX and X) and reduce antithrombotic protein C levels. Thus a hypercoagulable state may exist during the early stages of warfarin therapy, before all vitamin K-dependent factors with longer half-lives (II, IX and X) are inhibited. Hence, heparin therapy must continue for 5 more days after the start of warfarin, even though the prothrombin time may reflect a therapeutic international normalized ratio (INR) after 2–3 days.

Haemorrhage is the important side-effect of warfarin anticoagulation. Age and interaction with other drugs (e.g. salicylates, phenothiazines and phenylbutazone) increase the risk of bleeding. Warfarin-induced haemorrhage may occur into kidneys, gastrointestinal tract, lungs, subdural or subarachnoid space, skin, mucous membranes and muscles. Bleeding into the retroperitoneal space is often insidious. Contraindications to anticoagulation are given in Table 30.6.

Vitamin K reverses warfarin's effects but disturbs the control of prothrombin time for 2–3 weeks

Table 30.6 Contraindications to anticoagulant and thrombolytic therapy

Anticoagulant therapy	Thrombolytic therapy
Peptic ulceration	Neurosurgery <6 months
Hiatus hernia	Major GI bleed <6 months
Hepatic disease	Severe hepatic insufficiency
Steatorrhoea	History of CVA/TIA
Uncontrolled hypertension	Uncontrolled hypertension
Retinopathy	Ophthalmic surgery within 6 weeks
Infective endocarditis	Infective endocarditis
Uraemia	Renal insufficiency
Alcoholism	Alcoholism
Pregnancy	Pregnancy/ <10 days postpartum
Recent surgery and trauma	Recent surgery and trauma (<2 months)
Cerebral haemorrhage	Cerebral haemorrhage/tumour/ abscess
Haemostatic defect	Haemostatic defect
Poor patient compliance	Incompressible venous puncture <48 h
	CPR for >1 min, less than 2 weeks previously

GI = Gastrointestinal; CVA = cerebrovascular accident; TIA = transient ischaemic attack; CPR = cardiopulmonary resuscitation

Table 30.7 Recommended thrombolytic regimens[7]

Drug	Loading dose	Maintenance
Streptokinase	250 000 U IV over 30 min	100 000 U/h IV over 24 h
Urokinase	900 U/kg IV over 10 min	900 U/kg/h for 24 h
rTPA	100 mg over 2 h	Nil

rTPA = Recombinant tissue plasma activator.

following recommencement of warfarin. A 1 mg dose may shorten the prothrombin time sufficiently with minimal interference with later anticoagulation. Complete reversal of anticoagulation requires doses of up to 50 mg. If anticoagulation is to be interrupted for elective surgery, withholding warfarin for about 3–4 days beforehand is best. Acute reversal of warfarin therapy is promptly achieved by administration of fresh frozen plasma and factor concentrates.

Thrombolytic therapy

Streptokinase, urokinase and recombinant tissue plasminogen activator (rTPA) accelerate clot lysis in the treatment of PE. However, with all three agents, despite consistent and more rapid resolution of radiographic and haemodynamic parameters, no reduction in morbidity or mortality has been demonstrated.[48–50] Bleeding complications are more frequent and important in patients on thrombolysis. None the less, thrombolytic therapy restricted to massive PE with haemodynamic compromise or severe pulmonary hypertension may improve outcome.[15,48–51] Successful direct intraembolic thrombolysis, avoiding systemic anticoagulation in selected patients, has been reported.[52] Further trials are pending.

Thrombolytic therapy for DVT is equally controversial. Current recommendations are for use in proximal occlusive DVT associated with significant swelling, if there are no contraindications.[7] These circumstances rarely exist in critically ill patients.

Recommended regimens are listed in Table 30.7.[7] Streptokinase, despite its potential pyrogenic and antigenic properties, is commonly used. It has a molecular weight of 43 kDa, and is rapidly bound to the patient's previously generated circulating antibodies. Thus the dose must be sufficiently large to provide a free excess for fibrinolytic activity. There is a significant risk of anaphylaxis, and resuscitation facilities should be immediately available. Urokinase is non-antigenic and may be used repeatedly, but remains very expensive. Therapy with rTPA is more rapid and safer than urokinase.[51]

Coagulation monitoring is not mandatory during thrombolytic therapy.[7] Heparin is recommended after the thrombolytic therapy is complete. The main disadvantages of thrombolytic therapy are bleeding and allergic reactions; contraindications of use are listed in Table 30.6. Intramuscular injections must be avoided (as with heparin therapy) and venepuncture minimized and restricted to sites where digital compression is possible. If complications occur, the thrombolytic infusion must be stopped. Fresh frozen plasma is infused to replenish depleted coagulation factors. ε-Aminocaproic acid (amicar, 5–8 g) or aprotinin (trasylol, 500 000 units) has been used to antagonize streptokinase fibrinolytic action more rapidly.

Inferior vena cava (IVC) filter

Mechanical barriers against migration of emboli in the IVC should be considered, if another PE may prove fatal. Indications are:[53–55]

1 recurrent PE despite adequate anticoagulation;
2 inability to tolerate anticoagulation;
3 a large, free-floating thrombus in the ileofemoral veins;
4 immediately following pulmonary embolectomy.

IVC filters can be placed surgically or transvenously, and are effective in preventing recurrent pulmonary emboli.[54] There is no ideal filter, and none is distinctly superior.[7] Heparin should be started 12 h after placement of filter in those without contraindications. Morbidity associated with placement or subsequent migration reduces their suitability for more widespread or prophylactic use (Table 30.8).

Embolectomy

Most patients with massive PE respond well to conservative therapy and surgical embolectomy is rarely indicated. Mortality with embolectomy approaches 40%.[56] Specific criteria for pulmonary embolectomy are difficult to derive. Haemodynamic improvement following streptokinase therapy is similar to that of pulmonary embolectomy with cardiopulmonary bypass, but surgical treatment of massive pulmonary embolus may produce a better outcome than medical treatment.[53]

Pulmonary embolectomy is an acceptable procedure if thrombolytic therapy is contraindicated or unsuccessful, and there is persistent hypotension, oliguria, hypoxia and metabolic acidosis, with radiological confirmation of greater than 50% occlusion of the pulmonary arterial tree. This may be attempted by open thoracotomy or by special transvenous catheters.[57] Recent thrombosis formation, if demonstrated by venography, warrants consideration for venous thrombectomy.

Prophylaxis against DVT and PE

Prevention of PE is largely the prevention of DVT. Measures to reduce risks in critically ill patients, particularly those with protracted immobilization, are frequently neglected[58] (Table 30.9). Perioperative low-dose heparin (5000 units SC twice daily) offers significant protection against both DVT and PE, and with early mobilization exercises, is recommended for all patients at risk.[10,59] LMWH is more effective with a similar risk of bleeding.[60] Prolonged anticoagulation with oral agents is useful in patients at high risk of

Table 30.8 Complications of inferior vena cava (IVC) filters

	Incidence
Fatal	0.12%
Migration	0.04%
Misplacement	0.04%
Cardiac arrest	0.04%
Non-fatal	
Technical difficulty	4.3%
Insertion-site DVT	2.0%
Migration complications	53%
IVC wall erosion	14–24%
IVC obstruction	5–18%

DVT = Deep venous thrombosis.

Table 30.9 Recommended deep venous thrombosis/pulmonary embolism prophylaxis[7,10,13]

Group	Risk factors	Prophylaxis
General surgery		
Low risk	Age < 40 years Minor surgery	Early ambulation
Moderate risk		GCES, LDH, LMWH or IPC
High risk	Age > 40 years Major surgery and one other risk factor	LDH (8-hourly) or LMWH If haemotoma or bleeding then IPC or dextran
Very high risk	Multiple risk factors	LDH/LMWH and IPC and perioperative warfarin
Orthopaedic		
Low/moderate risk	Total hip replacement Hip fractures Knee replacement	LDH, warfarin or LMWH Warfarin or LMWH IPC
High risk	Multiple risk factors	IVC filter
Neurosurgery	Intracranial operation	IPC ± GCES
Spinal injury	With paralysis	Adjusted-dose heparin or LMWH Alternatives: IPC or warfarin
Multi-trauma	Varied	IPC, warfarin or LMWH whenever possible
Myocardial infarction	All patients	LDH; full anticoagulation may be used. LMWH, IPC, GCES may be useful
Ischaemic stroke	Lower-limb paralysis	LDH or LMWH

GCES = Graduated compression elastic stockings; LDH = low-dose heparin; LMWH = low-molecular-weight heparin; IPC = intermittent pneumatic compression; IVC = inferior vena cava.

recurrent emboli. If anticoagulant therapy or prophylaxis is contraindicated (e.g. in neurosurgical, ophthalmic or orthopaedic joint replacement procedures), intermittent pneumatic compression of the legs should be employed early in the immobilization period. This is continued until fully ambulatory or another prophylaxis is started.[61] Graduated elastic stockings donned preoperatively improve venous return from lower extremities and augment other measures.

Dihydroergotamine increases tone of capacitance vessels. The combination with subcutaneous LMWH improves effectiveness.[62] Alteration of vascular responses in myocardial and peripheral ischaemia remains a concern. Aspirin is a controversial but probably underutilized adjunct to thromboprophylaxis.[63] Very-low-dose warfarin is effective prophylaxis against thromboembolus in certain groups with malignancy.[64] Recombinant hirudin, a promising antithrombotic with little effect on haemostasis, is undergoing evaluation.[65] Other agents being investigated are activated protein C, D-phenylalanyl-L-arginyl-chlormethylketone and defibrotide.[66-68] Other modalities tried with some success include antiplatelet agents or dipryidamole, and dextran infusions.[69]

Prognosis

The mortality of in-hospital DVT is 5% but increases with age.[70] Following PE, initial mortality is 2.5%, mostly due to recurrent PE. The greatest risk occurs in the initial period following clot migration to the pulmonary vascular bed.[1] The 1-year mortality following PE is 24%, with most patients dying from their underlying disease.[71] With continued anticoagulation, the long-term prognosis from PE itself is excellent; haemodynamic problems resolve with clot lysis.[1] Pulmonary hypertension follows only multiple emboli or underlying disease.

Other pulmonary embolic pathologies

PA obstruction may result from embolization with bone marrow, fat, tumour (choriocarcinoma and renal vein tumours), air and amniotic fluid (see Chapter 31). General principles of resuscitation are applied.

Air embolism may result from the aspiration of air into large open veins at operation, or after inadvertent disconnection of large-bore central venous catheters. Therapeutic manoeuvres include compresssion or occlusion of the air source, immediate positioning to left lateral with head-down tilt, and placement of a central venous line for aspiration of air from the right atrium, ventricle or pulmonary artery. Anticoagulation may be required to prevent thrombus forming around residual intracardiopulmonary air collections. Associated acute pulmonary hypertension may facilitate paradoxical embolus across a patent foramen ovale.

Amniotic fluid embolism often results in catastrophic cardiovascular collapse with an acute bleeding diathesis and anaphylactic shock. A central venous catheter is placed to aspirate intracardiac amniotic fluid to confirm the diagnosis and monitor the cardiovascular status. Cardiopulmonary resuscitation, fresh blood, coagulation factors and fibrinolytic inhibitors may be required (see Chapter 56). Major air and amniotic fluid embolization is associated with a high mortality.

References

1 Alpert JS and Dalen JE (1994) Epidemiology and natural history of venous thromboembolism. *Prog Cardiovasc Dis* **36**:417–422.

2 Cogo A, Lensing AWA, Prandoni P and Hirsh J (1993) Distribution of thrombosis inpatients with symptomatic deep vein thrombosis. *Arch Intern Med* **153**:2777–2780.

3 Gibbs NM (1994) Postoperative hypercoagulability: mechanisms and clinical implications. In: Keneally J (ed.) *Australasian Anaesthesia 1994*. Melbourne: Australia and New Zealand College of Anaesthetists, pp. 89–96.

4 Handlin RI (1987) Bleeding and thrombosis. In: Wilson JD, Braunwald E, Isselbacher KJ *et al.* (eds) *Harrisons Principles of Internal Medicine*, 12th edn. New York: McGraw Hill, pp. 343-353.

5 A Collaborative Study by the PIOPED Investigators (1990) Value of the ventilation/perfusion scan in acute pulmonary embolism – results of the prospective investigation of pulmonary embolsim diagnosis (PIOPED). *J Am Med Assoc* **263**:2753–2759.

6 Bick RL (1994) Hypercoagulability and thrombosis. *Med Clin North Am* **78**:635–665.

7 Tapson VF and Fulkerson WJ (1994) Pulmonary embolism in the intensive care unit. *J Intens Care Med* **9**:119–131.

8 Raad II, Luna M, Khalil SM, Costerton JW, Lam C and Bodey GP (1994) The relationship between the thrombotic and infectious complications of central venous catheters. *J Am Med Assoc* **271**:1014–1016.

9 Svensson PJ and Dahlbäck B (1994) Resistance to activated protein C as a basis for venous thrombosis. *N Engl J Med* **330**:517–522.

10 Stein P (1994) Acute pulmonary embolism. *Disease-a-month* **40**:467–523.

11 Stein PD, Terrin ML, Hales CA *et al.* (1991) Clinical laboratory roentgenographic and electrocardiographic findings in patients with acute pulmonary embolism and no pre-existing cardiac or pulmonary disease. *Chest* **100**:598–603.

12 Stein PD, Willis PW III and DeMets DL (1981) History and physical examination in acute pulmonary embolism in patients without pre-existing cardiac or pulmonary disease. *Am J Cardiol* **47**:218–223.

13 Wolfe MW, Skibo LK and Goldhaber SZ (1993) Pulmonary embolic disease: diagnosis, pathophysiological aspects, and treatment with thrombolytic agents. *Curr Probl Cardiol* **10**:587–633.

14 Belenkie I, Dani R, Smith ER and Tyberg JV (1989) Effects of volume loading during experimental actue pulmonary embolism. *Circulation* **80**:178–188.

15 Dries DJ and Mathru M (1992) Cardiovascular performance in embolism. *Anesthesiol Clin North Am* **10**:755–780.

16 Lohr JM, Hasselfeld KA, Byrne MP, Deshmukh RM and Cranley JJ (1994) Does the asymptomatic limb harbor deep venous thrombosis? *Am J Surg* **168**:184–187.

17 Davidson BL, Elliot CG, Lensing AWA *et al.* (1992) Low accuracy of color Doppler ultrasound in the detection of proximal leg vein thrombosis in asymptomatic high risk patients. *Ann Intern Med* **117**:735–738.

18 Lensing AWA, Prandoni P, Brandjes D *et al.* (1989) Detection of deep vein thrombosis by real time B-mode ultrasonography. *N Engl J Med* **320**:342–345.

19 Anderson DR, Lensing AWA, Wells PS *et al.* (1993) Limitations of impedance plethysmography in the diagnosis of clinically suspected deep-vein thrombosis. *Ann Intern Med* **118**:25–30.

20 Huisman MV, Buller HR and ten Cate JW (1986) Serial impedance plethysmography for suspected deep vein thrombosis in outpatients. *N Engl J Med* **314**:823–828.

21 Rabinov K and Paulin S (1972) Roentgen diagnosis of venous thrombosis of the leg. *Arch Surg* **104**:134–144.

22 Spritzer CE, Norconk JJ, Sostman HD and Coleman RE (1993) Detection of deep vein thrombosis by magnetic resonance imaging. *Chest* **103**:54–60.

23 Evans AJ, Tapson VF, Sostman HD *et al.* (1992) The diagnosis of deep vein thrombosis: a prospective comparison of venography and magnetic resonance imaging. *Chest* **102**:120S.

24 Moser KM, Fedullo PF, Littlejohn JK and Crawford R (1994) Frequent asymptomatic pulmonary embolism in patients with deep venous thrombosis. *J Am Med Assoc* **271**:223–225.

25 Bounameaux H, Cirafici P, De Moerloose P *et al.* (1991) Measurement of D-dimer in plasma as a diagnostic aid in suspected pulmonary embolism. *Lancet* **337**:196–200.

26 Wickham NWR, Bradshaw A, Evans J, Bevan DH and Mansi J (1994) Endothelial function and malignant coagulopathy. Vascular endothelium response to stress. NATO/ASI Symposium Plenum Press.

27 Takekawa H, Miyamoto K, Yamguchi E, Muankata M and Kawakami Y (1993) Acute rise in serum immunoglobulin E concentration in pulmonary thrombolembolism. *Chest* **104**:61–64.

28 Stein PD, Willis PW III, DeMets DL *et al.* (1987) Plain chest roentgenogram in patients with acute pulmonary embolism and no preexisting cardiac or pulmonary disease. *Am J Noninvas Cardiol* **1**:171–176.

29 Stein PD, Athanasoulis C, Greenspan RH *et al.* (1992) Relation of plain chest radiographic findings to pulmonary artery pressure and arterial blood oxygen levels in patients with acute pulmonary embolism. *Am J Cardiol* **69**:394–396.

30 Stein PD, Dalen JE, McIntyre KM *et al.* (1975) The electrocardiogram in acute pulmonary embolism. *Prog Cardiovasc Dis* **17**:247–257.

31 Overton TD and Bocka JJ (1988) The alveolar–arterial gradient in patients with documented pulmonary emboli. *Arch Intern Med* **148**:1617–1619.

32 Fawdry RM and Gruenewald SM (1988) Initial experience with technegas: a new ventilation agent. *Aust Radiol* **32**:232–238.

33 Stein PD and Gottschalk A (1994) Critical review of ventilation/perfusion lung scans in acute pulmonary embolism. *Prog Cardiovasc Dis* **37**:13–24.

34 Lesser BA, Leeper KV, Stein PD *et al.* (1992) The diagnosis of pulmonary embolism in patients with chronic obstructive airways disease. *Chest* **102**:17–22.

35 Stein PD, Gottschalk A, Henry JW and Shivkumar K (1993) Stratification of patients according to prior cardiopulmonary disease and probability assessment based on the number of mismatched segmental equivalent perfusion defects. *Chest* **104**:1461–1467.

36 Stein PD, Henry JW and Gottschalk A (1993) The addition of clinical assessment to stratification according to prior cardiopulmonary disease further optimises the interpretation of ventilation/perfusion lung scans in pulmonary embolism. *Chest* **104**:1472–1476.

37 Urokinase Pulmonary Embolism Trial (1973) Perfusion scanning. *Circulation* **47** (suppl):II46–50.

38 Stein PD, Athanasoulis C, Alavi A *et al.* (1992) Complications and validity of pulmonary angiography in acute pulmonary embolism. *Circulation* **85**:462–468.

39 Tapson VF, Davidson CJ, Gurbel PA, Sheikh KH, Kisslo KB and Stack RS (1991) Rapid and accurate diagnosis of pulmonary emboli in a canine model using intravascular ultrasound imaging. *Chest* **100**:1410–14113.

40 Wolfe MW, Saad RM and Spence TH (1992) Hemodynamic effects of amrinone in a canine model of massive pulmonary embolism. *Chest* **102**:274–278.

41 Hirsch LJ, Rooney MW, Wat SS, Kleinmann B and Mathru M (1991) Norepinephrine and phenylephrine effects on right ventricular function in experimental canine pulmonary embolism. *Chest* **100**:796–801.

42 Holmes DW, Bura A, Mazzolai L, Büller HR and Ten Cate JW (1982) Subcutaneous heparin compared with continuous intravenous heparin administration in the initial treatment of deep vein thrombosis. *Ann Intern Med* **116**:279–284.

43 Hull RD, Raskob GE, Hirsh J *et al.* (1986) Continuous intravenous heparin compared with intermittent subcutaneous heparin in the initial treatment of proximal vein thrombosis. *N Engl J Med* **315**:1109–1114.

44 Hyers TM, Hull RD and Weg JD (1992) Anti-thrombotic therapy for venous thromboembolic disease. *Chest* **102** (suppl):408S–425S.

45 Demers C, Ginsberg JS, Brill-Edwards P *et al.* (1991) Rapid anticoagulation using ancrod for heparin induced thrombocytopenia. *Blood* **78**:2194–2197.

46 Ortel TL, Gockerman JP, Califf RM *et al.* (1992) Parenteral anticoagulation with the heparinoid lomoparan (Org 10172) in patients with heparin induced thrombocytopenia and thrombosis. *Thromb Haemos*

67:292–296.

47 Hull RD, Raskob GE, Pineo GF *et al.* (1992) Subcutaneous low-molecular-weight heparin compared with continuous intravenous heparin in the treatment of proximal deep vein thrombosis. *N Engl J Med* **326**:975–982.

48 Anderson DR and Levine MN (1992) Thrombolytic therapy for the treatment of acute pulmonary embolism. *Can Med Assoc J* **146**:1317–1324.

49 A Collaborative Study by the PIOPED Investigators (1990) Tissue plasminogen activator for the treatment of acute pulmonary embolism. *Chest* **97**:528–533.

50 Goldhaber SZ (1992) Evolving concepts in thrombolytic therapy for pulmonary embolism. *Chest* **101** (suppl):183S–185S.

51 Goldhaber SZ, Heit J, Sharma GVRK *et al.* (1988) Randomised controlled trial of recombinant tissue plasminogen activator versus urokinase in the treatment of acute pulmonary embolism. *Lancet* **2**:293–298.

52 Tapson VF, Davidson CJ, Bauman R *et al.* (1992) Rapid thrombolysis of massive pulmonary emboli without systemic fibrinogenolysis: intraembolic infusion of thrombolytic therapy. *Am Rev Respir Dis* **145**:A719.

53 Gulba DC, Schmid C, Borst H-G, Lichtien P, Dietz R and Luft FC (1994) Medical compared with surgical treatment for massive pulmonary embolism. *Lancet* **343**:576–577.

54 Becker DM, Philbrick JT and Selby JB (1992) Inferior vena cava filters. Indications, safety, effectiveness. *Arch Intern Med* **152**:1985–1994.

55 Alexander JJ, Yuhas JP and Piotrowski JJ (1994) Is the increasing use of prophylactic percutaneous IVC filters justified? *Am J Surg* **168**:102–106.

56 Meyer G, Tamisier D, Sors H *et al.* (1991) Pulmonary embolectomy: a 20 year experience at one center. *Ann Thorac Surg* **51**:232–236.

57 Timsit J-F, Reynaud P, Meyer G and Sors H (1991) Pulmonary embolectomy by catheter device in massive pulmonary embolectomy. *Chest* **100**:655–658.

58 Keane MG, Ingenito EP and Goldhaber SZ (1994) Utilization of venous thromboembolism prophylaxis in the medical intensive care unit. *Chest* **106**:13-22.

59 Collins R, Scrimgeour A, Yusuf S and Peto R (1988) Reduction in fatal pulmonary embolism and venous thrombosis by perioperative administration of sub-cutaneous heparin. *N Engl J Med* **318**:1162–1173.

60 Nurmohamed MT, Rosendaal FR, Bller HR *et al.* (1992) Low-molecular weight heparin versus standard heparin in general and orthopaedic surgery: a meta-analysis. *Lancet* **340**;152–156.

61 Skillman JJ, Collins REC, Coe NP *et al.* (1978) Prevention of deep vein thrombosis in neurosurgical patients: a controlled randomized trial of external pneumatic compression boots. *Surgery* **83**:354–358.

62 The Multicenter Trial Committee (1984) Dihydroergotamine–heparin prophylaxis of postoperative deep vein thrombosis. *J Am Med Assoc* **251**:2960–2966.

63 Antiplatelet Trialist Collaboration (1994) Collaborative overview of randomised trials of antiplatelet therapy – III: Reduction in venous thrombosis and pulmonary embolism by antiplatelet prophylaxis among surgical and medical patients. *Br Med J* **308**:235–246.

64 Levine M, Hirsch J, Gent M *et al.* (1994) Double-blind randomised trial of very-low-dose warfarin for prevention of thromboembolism in stage IV breast cancer. *Lancet* **343**:886–889.

65 Bichler J and Fritz H (1991) Hirudin. A new therapeutic tool? *Ann Hematol* **63**:67–76.

66 Gruber A, Griffin JH, Harker AL and Hanson R (1989) Inhibition of platelet dependent thrombus formation by human activated protein C in a primate model. *Blood* **73**:639–642.

67 Hanson SR and Harker AL (1988) Interruption of acute platelet dependent thrombosis by the synthetic antithrombin D-phenylalanyl-L-arginyl chlormethyl ketone. *Proc Nat Acad Sci* **85**:3184–3188.

68 Pescador R, Porta R, Mantovani M and Prino G (1991) Cardioprotective effects of deofibrotide: a mini review. *Sem Thromb Hemos* **17**(suppl 1):96–100.

69 Harris WH, Salzman EW, Desanctis RW and Coutts RD (1972) Prevention of venous thromboembolism following total hip replacement. Warfarin vs dextran 40. *J Am Med Assoc* **220**:1319–1322.

70 Anderson FA, Wheeler HB, Goldberg RJ *et al.* (1991) A population based perspective of the incidence and case fatality rates of deep vein thrombosis and pulmonary embolism. *Arch Intern Med* **151**:933–938.

71 Carson JL, Kelley MA, Duff A *et al.* (1992) The clinical course of pulmonary embolism. *N Engl J Med* **326**:1240–1245.

31 Fat embolism syndrome

RC Freebairn and TE Oh

The fat embolism syndrome is an infrequent but potentially lethal complication of trauma, orthopaedic surgery and other disorders (Table 31.1), characterized by the triad of respiratory failure, confusion and petechial haemorrhage.[1,2-14] Intravascular fat emboli are found in 90% of skeletal trauma victims, but only 3.5–5.0% develop the syndrome.[15-18] The incidence of the fat embolism syndrome is 0.25–29% depending on diagnostic criteria and population groups.[18] It is more frequent in the second and third decade of life, but can occur in the elderly and in neonates.[17,19]

Aetiology and pathogenesis

The aetiology remains controversial. There is no doubt about the relationship with fractures and trauma. However, the concentration of fat microemboli within the pulmonary and systemic vasculature appears unrelated to the severity of the disorder.[20] Only few patients with fat embolism develop the syndrome, which appears to require three components: first, a source of circulating fat; second, embolization of fat globules to pulmonary capillaries; and third, other precipitating factors which activate the fat emboli to develop the syndrome.

There are two major theories on the pathogenesis of the fat embolism syndrome.

Mechanical theory

This proposes that mechanical obstruction in pulmonary capillaries results from fat emboli (>8–20 μm) from the marrow or adipose tissue. Some fat particles pass through to the systemic circulation, via intracardiac or pulmonary routes, to embolize in the renal, cerebral, skin or retinal capillaries. The presence of a patent foramen ovale (in 25% of population) and the fluidity of fat globules encourage systemic spread.

Table 31.1 Conditions associated with the fat embolism syndrome[8-19]

Orthopaedic trauma	Liposuction
Pancreatitis	Sickle-cell disease
Diabetes mellitus	Fatty liver of pregnancy
Cardiac massage	Renal transplant
Parenteral nutrition	Animal bites
Systemic lupus erythematosus	Bone marrow transplants
Chemotherapy	

Physicochemical theory

This may be a toxic or obstructive mechanism. The toxic proposal maintains that free fatty acids (FFA) released at the time of trauma, or during the breakdown of fat in the lung, directly affect pneumocytes, resulting in an inflammatory response – acute respiratory distress syndrome (ARDS). FFA may originate from lipid stores mobilized by circulating catecholamines.[21] The obstructive theory proposes that a chemical event at the trauma site releases mediators that affect the solubility of circulating lipids, resulting in coalescence and subsequent embolization. Normal chylomicrons may coalesce into fat globules of 10–40 μm, large enough to occlude pulmonary capillaries.[21] Calcium-dependent C-reactive protein and adrenal hormones are postulated to precipitate the coalescence.[22]

Circulating fat may originate from:

1 *Bone marrow*: Fractures, particularly of the pelvis or long bones, cause fat and marrow to enter the venous system through ruptured medullary sinuses. Haematomas, movement and reaming may further increase intramedullary pressure and facilitate fat entry.[18] Closed fractures have a higher incidence of the syndrome. Tourniquets placed proximal to the fracture site may delay the passage of fat centrally.

2 *Adipose tissues*: Massive trauma (e.g. from high-velocity projectiles and explosion), liposuction and

extensive burns, may disrupt adipose tissue, causing entry of fat globules into the venous circulation.[8,18]

3 *Circulating fat* is usually emulsified in the form of neutral triglycerides bound to albumin or low-density lipoproteins. In the microscopic (1 μm) chylomicron form, they are stable and a major energy source. Following trauma or other stress, increased mobilization of depot fat may overwhelm fat transport mechanisms, causing chylomicrons to become unstable and coalesce into larger (20 μm) particles.[21]

Pathophysiology

The major pathophysiological effect is occlusion of small vessels in the lung by fat emboli. This obstruction is aggravated by the adherence of platelets and fibrin to emboli, forming a plug. The neutral fat is hydrolysed by lung lipase, producing toxic FFA. Severe inflammatory changes produce endothelial damage, inactivate lung surfactant and increase capillary permeability. These events commonly induce acute lung injury or ARDS. The time for the conversion of embolized fat to FFA equates to the 24–48 h latency period between the onset of injury and symptoms of vasculitis and pneumonitis.[23] Catastrophic cor pulmonale can result if adequate pulmonary vasodilatation does not occur.[18,24] Other humoral changes are implicated in the pulmonary pathology. Large numbers of platelets are sequestered and broken down, with release of serotonin and 5-hydroxytryptamine. Endogenous vasopressors are released from the injury site, while histamine is released from the lung parenchyma. These combine to induce pulmonary vasospasm, bronchospasm and vascular endothelial injury.[21] Hypoxia results from shunting, ventilation:perfusion mismatch, diffusion impairment, increased dead space:tidal volume ratio, congestive atelectasis and decreased compliance.

The pathophysiology of cerebral manifestations remains unclear. Large fat emboli may increase right atrial pressures and thus induce foramen ovale patency. These paradoxical emboli are thought to underlie the neurological manifestations.[25] Cerebral oedema may be a major contributor to decreased consciousness.[26]

Skin and renal petechiae result from microinfarction, capillary distension and increased endothelial fragility. Thrombocytopenia is not an important factor. The upper body distribution is presumed to reflect the buoyancy of fat in blood.[18]

Clinical presentation

Presentation usually occurs 24–72 h following the initial insult. The classic syndrome involves pulmonary, cerebral and cutaneous manifestations.

Pulmonary

Tachypnoea, dyspnoea and cyanosis are common, and are often accompanied by tachycardia and pyrexia. Respiratory distress is the most common presenting feature, followed by neurological deterioration.[27] Auscultation reveals crackles and wheezes, with an occasional friction rub.

Cerebral

Headache, irritability and delirium are common, with stupor, coma and convulsions in severe cases. Retinal signs are exudates, oedematous patches, 'cotton-wool' spots, perivascular or petechial haemorrhages and intravascular fat globules.[21] Focal neurological signs are rare, and usually suggest another diagnosis (e.g. expanding subdural haematoma).

Cutaneous

By 72 h, 40–50% of patients develop a petechial rash in non-dependent parts of the body, classically the chest, axillae and conjunctiva, which often pass unnoticed.[21,28]

Acute fulminant fat embolism syndrome is rare. It develops within minutes to hours of injury, with profound hypoxaemia and hypotension, and carries a high mortality.[29]

Diagnosis

The syndrome has no pathognomonic sign or symptom. Diagnosis is made on clinical grounds. Differential diagnosis includes pulmonary thromboembolism, air embolism, cardiac or pulmonary contusion, septic shock, fluid overload, intracranial injury, aspiration pneumonitis, ARDS and transfusion reaction. Proposed diagnostic criteria lack specificity (Table 31.2)[30] or require full validation (Table 31.3).[31] Metabolic and drug-induced delirium should be excluded. Investigations include the following list, but no single test has the specificity or sensitivity to be diagnostic. Repeated clinical assessments with arterial blood-gas analyses are important for early diagnosis and treatment.[32]

Investigations

Arterial blood gases

Arterial blood gases will show hypoxaemia and respiratory alkalosis from hyperventilation. Increased shunt (alveolar–arterial oxygen gradient and the shunt equation; see Chapter 97) is a common and early change.[23]

Electrocardiograph

The electrocardiogram (ECG) may be normal, or show sinus tachycardia or right heart strain. Non-specific T-wave changes secondary to hypoxia may be present.

Imaging investigations

The chest X-ray may be normal. In severe cases, progressive diffuse bilateral interstitial and alveolar infiltrates produce a classical 'snowstorm' pattern. Complete opacification may occur in conjunction with decreased compliance and progressive hypoxaemia, producing a condition indistinguishable from ARDS. Chest ventilation:perfusion scans demonstrate reduced perfusion and ventilation, more frequently in the upper zones (in contrast to pulmonary embolus).[33] A computed tomography scan may exclude other intracranial disorders in the differential diagnosis.

Echocardiography

Transoesophageal echocardiography (TEE) may be useful to detect fat embolism in at-risk patients early after orthopaedic surgery,[25] but the benefits of routine intraoperative use have not been established.

Pulmonary artery cytology

Aspiration of blood through a pulmonary artery flotation catheter for cytological examination of fat globules has been advocated.[34]

Bronchoscopy

In patients with the fat embolism syndrome, 31–82% of cells obtained from bronchopulmonary lavage are positive for fat globules, compared with 2% of cells in patients without the syndrome.[34] This finding remains controversial,[31] but the technique in high-risk groups may allow early detection in asymptomatic patients.

Haematological and coagulation profile

Increased fibrin degradation products, thrombocytopenia and coagulation abnormalities may be detected during the acute phase. Fibrinogen decreases initially, but rebound hyperfibrinogenaemia occurs within 5 days.[18] Bleeding problems are infrequently seen. Red cell loss from intra-alveolar haemorrhage and mild haemolysis results in a decreased haemoglobin concentration.[18]

Urine examination

The presence of fat in the urine is neither sensitive nor specific enough to aid diagnosis.[23,25]

Table 31.2 Fat embolism syndrome: Gurd and Wilson's diagnostic criteria[30] (one major, four minor criteria and fat macroglobulinaemia are required for diagnosis)

Major
Petechial rash
Respiratory symptoms, signs and radiographic changes
Cerebral signs unrelated to head injury or other conditions

Minor
Tachycardia
Pyrexia
Retinal changes (fat or petechiae)
Renal changes
Jaundice

Laboratory
Acute fall in haemoglobin
Sudden thrombocytopenia
High erythrocyte sedimentation rate
Fat macroglobulinaemia (>8 μm)

Table 31.3 Fat embolism syndrome diagnostic criteria Vedrienne et al.[31]

Signs	Absent (0 point)	Present	
		Mild (1 point)	Severe (2 points)
Pulmonary infiltrates	0	Moderate or localized	Diffuse
Neurological EEG	0	Disturbance of consciousness or typical EEG changes	Disturbance of consciousness *and* typical EEG changes
Petechiae	0	Moderate	Diffuse
Platelet count	$>200\,000/mm^3$	$200\,000–100\,000/mm^3$	$<100\,000/mm^3$
Retinal changes	0	Haemorrhage or retinal emboli	Haemorrhage *and* retinal emboli
Cholesterol (mmol/l)	>3.5	<3.5	Phospholipids <1.9
Fracture (long bone/pelvis)	0	1	$2+$

EEG = Electroencephalogram.

Serum investigations

Hypocalcaemia is common but rarely poses problems. Serum triglyceride and lipid concentrations bear no relationship to the fat embolism syndrome. Serum lipase concentration increases after bone trauma, but does not correlate well with the syndrome.[21]

Intraoperative detection

Microemboli of fat and marrow can be reflected by changes in pulmonary artery pressure, but not by capnography or systemic and right atrial pressures.[36]

Management

The fat embolism syndrome is a self-limiting disease, and therapy is mainly supportive. Numerous pharmacological therapies (see below) have been advocated, but there is no conclusive evidence to recommend any agent for routine use. Immobilization of the fracture is essential, as movement precipitates intravascular entry of fat.[37] Early internal fixation of fractures produces smaller quantities of intraoperative emboli[25] and a decreased incidence of the syndrome, compared with delayed fixation.[38-48] Surgical embolectomy is usually not practical, as the emboli are mostly minute.[18]

Supportive treatment

Early attention to assessment and treatment of airway, ventilation and circulation problems is crucial. Continuous pulse oximetry monitoring will help clinical assessment. Oxygen by facemask corrects mild hypoxaemia. Mask continuous positive airways pressure (CPAP) and, if necessary, non-invasive ventilation, may avoid endotracheal intubation and ventilation. Full mechanical ventilation should be instituted if Sao_2 cannot be maintained above 90%, or if severe respiratory distress, hypercarbia or exhaustion is present.[41] Optimal oxygen delivery with the lowest possible inspired oxygen (Fio_2) is the aim.[18,41] Application of positive end-expiratory (PEEP) may decrease shunt fractions and reduce Fio_2 requirements. However, cardiac output may fall, and right-to-left shunt through a patent foramen ovale may increase, thus decreasing oxygen delivery.[42] An adequate cardiac output must be maintained with replacement of fluid or blood and infusion of inotropes. Blood and fluid loss at the fracture site is often underestimated.[18] Central venous and pulmonary artery catheters will aid fluid therapy (see Chapter 29).

Pharmacological therapies

Corticosteroids have been advocated to reduce the incidence and severity of hypoxaemia in fat embolism.[35,43] Recommendations for their use have traditionally followed those for ARDS.[18] However, steroids do not affect the haemodynamic or prostanoid response in fat embolism,[44] and the outcomes of those given steroids or supportive therapy only are no different.[45]

Albumin reduces pulmonary injury in animal models of the fat embolism syndrome, as albumin–FFA complexes are non-toxic.[46] However, no large clinical trials have been performed.

Ethanol is a lipase inhibitor and emulsifying agent, and theoretically may be beneficial. Intoxicated patients are noted to develop the fat embolism syndrome less frequently.[47] However, blood alcohol and circulating FFA concentrations and the development of the fat embolism syndrome have no relationship. Ethanol use is not recommended.[21]

Aprotinin attenuated the decrease in platelets following orthopaedic surgery, but did not affect subsequent hypoxaemia.[48] Its use is unclear.

Dextran, *aspirin* and *heparin* may exacerbate bleeding. No clinical benefit has been conclusively demonstrated with any of these agents.[18,23]

Outcome

The fat embolism syndrome results in considerable morbidity and a mortality of 10–20%.[23] Death is usually from respiratory failure, but other causes such as renal failure, cerebral haemorrhage and cardiac conduction system insults have been described[49,50]. Survivors usually have an excellent prognosis. Mortality and morbidity may be reduced by early diagnosis and prophylactic administration of oxygen to at-risk patients.[32]

References

1 Peltier LF (1984) Fat embolism – an appraisal of the problem. *Clin Orthop* **187**:3–17.

2 Gossling HR and Pelligrine Jr VD (1982) Fat embolism syndrome – a review of the pathophysiology and physiological basis of treatment. *Clin Orthop* **165**:68—82.

3 Guardia SN, Bilbao JM, Murray D *et al.* (1989) Fat embolism in acute pancreatitis. *Arch Pathol Lab Med* **113**:503–506.

4 Cuppage FE (1963) Fat embolism in diabetes mellitus. *Am J Clin Pathol* **40**:270–275.

5 Jackson C and Greendyke RM (1965) Pulmonary and cerebral fat embolism after closed cardiac massage. *Surg Gynecol Obstet* **120**:25–27.

6 Kitchell CC and Balogh K (1986) Pulmonary lipid emboli in association with long term hyperalimentation. *Human Pathol* **17**:83–85.

7 Katz DA, Ben-Ezra J, Factor SM, Horoupian DS and Goldfischer S (1983) Fatal pulmonary and cerebral fat embolism in systemic lupus erythematosus. *J Am Med Assoc* **250**:2666–2669.

8 Boezaart AP, Clinton CW, Braun S, Oettle C and Lee NP (1990) Fulminant adult respiratory distress syndrome after suction lipectomy. *S Afr Med J* **78**:693–695.

9 Shapiro MP and Hayes JA (1984) Fat embolism in sickle cell disease. *Arch Intern Med* **144**:181–182.

10 Jones MB (1993) Pulmonary fat emboli associated with acute fatty liver of pregnancy. *Am J Gastroenterol* **88**:791–792.

11 Jones JP, Engleman EP and Najaran JS (1965) Systemic fat embolism after renal homotransplantation and treatment with corticosteroid. *N Engl J Med* **273**:1453–1458.

12 Bloch B (1976) Fatal fat embolism following severe donkey bites. *J Forens Sci Soc* **16**:231–233.

13 Lipton JH, Russell JA, Burgess KR and Hwang WS (1987) Fat embolization and pulmonary infiltrates after bone marrow transplantation. *Med Pediatr Oncol* **15**:24–27.

14 Menendez LR, Bacon W, Kempf RA and Moore TM (1990) Fat embolism syndrome complicating intraarterial chemotherapy with cis-platinum. *Clin Orthopaed Rel Res* **254**:294–297.

15 Benatar SR, Fergusson AD and Goldschmidt RB (1972) Fat embolism – some clinical observations and a review of the controversial aspects. *Quart J Med* **41**:85–98.

16 ten Duis HT, Nijsten MWN, Klasen JH and Binnedijk B (1988) Fat embolism in patients with an isolated fracture of the skeletal shaft. *J Trauma* **28**:383–390.

17 Moore P, James O and Saltos N (1981) Fat embolism syndrome: incidence, significance and early features. *Aust NZ J Surg* **51**:546–551.

18 Capan LM, Miller SM and Patel KP (1993) Fat embolism. *Anaesthesiol Clin North Am* **11**:25–54.

19 Puntis JL and Rushton DI (1991) Pulmonary intra-vascular lipid in neonatal necropsy specimens. *Arch Dis Child* **66**:26–28.

20 Gitin TA, Seidel T, Cera PJ, Glidewell OJ and Smith JL (1993) Pulmonary microvascular fat: the significance? *Crit Care Med* **21**:673–677.

21 Levy D (1990) The fat embolism syndrome: a review. *Clin Orthopaed* **261**:281–286.

22 Hulman G (1988) Pathogenesis of nontraumatic fat embolism. *Lancet* **1**:13667.

23 Fabian TC (1993) Unravelling the fat embolism syndrome. *N Engl J Med* **329**:961–963.

24 Reid CBA and Hill DA (1992) Acute cor pulmonale and death due to massive fat embolim. *Aust NZ J Surg* **62**:320–322.

25 Pell ACH, Christie J, Keating JF and Sutherland GR (1993) The detection of fat embolism by transoesophageal echocardiography during reamed intramedullary nailing. A study of 24 patients with femoral and tibial features. *J Bone Joint Surg* **75**:921–925.

26 Meeke RI, Fitzpatrick GJ and Phelan DM (1987) Cerebral oedema and the fat embolism syndrome. *Intens Care Med* **13**:291–297.

27 Jacobson DM, Terence CF and Reinmuth OM (1986) The neurologic manifestations of fat embolism. *Neurology* **36**:847–851.

28 Fabian TC, Hoots AV, Stanford DS, Patterson CR and Mangiante EC (1990) Fat embolism syndrome: prospective evaluation in 92 fracture patients. *Crit Care Med* **18**:42–46.

29 Hagley SR (1983) The fulminant fat embolism syndrome. *Anaesth Intens Care* **11**:162–166.

30 Gurd AR and Wilson RI (1974) Fat embolism syndrome. *J Bone Joint Surg* **58**:408–416.

31 Vedrienne JM, Guillaume C and Gagnieu MC (1992) Bronchoalveolar lavage in trauma patients for diagnosis of fat embolism syndrome. *Chest* **102**:1323–1327.

32 Peltier LF (1988) Fat embolism. A perspective. *Clin Orthopaed* **232**:263–270.

33 Skarzynski JJ, Slavin JD, Spencer RP and Karimeddini MK (1986) Matching ventilation/perfusion images in fat embolization. *Clin Nucl Med* **11**:40–41.

34 Chastre J, Fagon J-Y, Soler P *et al.* (1990) Broncho-alveolar lavage for rapid diagnosis of the fat embolus syndrome in trauma patients. *Ann Intern Med* **113**:583–588.

35 Schonfeld SA, Polysongsans Y, Dilisio R *et al.* (1983) Fat embolism prophylaxis with corticosteroids. *Ann Intern Med* **99**:438–443.

36 Byrick RB, Kay CJ and Mullen JB (1989) Capnography is not as sensitive as pulmonary artery pressure monitoring in detecting marrow microembolism. *Anesth Analg* **68**:94–100.

37 Tachakra SS, Potts D and Idowu A (1990) Early operative fracture management of patients with multiple injuries *Br J Surg* **77**:1194.

38 Behrman SW, Fabian TC, Kudsk KA and Taylor JC (1990) Improved outcome with femur fractures: early vs delayed fixation. *J Trauma* **30**:792–798.

39 Bone LB, Johnson KD, Weigelt J and Scheinberg R (1989) Early versus delayed stabilization of femoral fractures: a prospective randomized study. *J Bone Surg* **71**:336–340.

40 Svenningsen S, Nesse O, Finsen V, Hole A and Benum P (1987) Prevention of fat embolism syndrome in patients with femoral fractures – immediate or delayed operative fixation. *Ann Chirurg Gynaecolog* **76**:163–166.

41 Slutsky AS (1994) Consensus conference on mechanical ventilation – January 28–30 1993 at Northbrook, Illinois, USA. Part I. Consensus conference on mechanical ventilation. *Intens Care Med* **20**:64–79.

42 Elliot CG (1992) Pulmonary physiology during pulmonary embolism. *Chest* **101**:163S–171S.

43 Kallenbach J, Lewis M, Zaltzman M, Feldman C, Orford A and Zwi S. 'Low-dose' corticosteroid prophylaxis against fat embolism. *J Trauma* **27**:1173–1176.

44 Byrick RJ, Mullen JB, Wong PY, Kay JC, Wigglesworth D and Doran RJ (1991) Prostanoid production and pulmonary hypertension after fat embolism are not modified by methylprenisolone. *Can J Anaesth* **38**:660–667.

45 Worthley LIG and Fisher M McD (1979) The fat embolism syndrome treated with oxygen, diuretics, sodium restriction and spontaneous ventilation. *Anaesth Intens Care* **7**:136–142.

46 Agantis N, Gyras M, Tserkezoglou N *et al.* (1988) Therapeutic effect of bovine albumin in the experimental fat embolism syndrome. *Respiration* **53**:50–57.

47 Myers R and Taljaard JJF (1977) Blood alcohol and fat embolism syndrome. *J Bone Joint Surg* **59**:878–880.

48 Sari A, Migauchi Y, Yamashito S *et al.* (1986) The magnitude of hypoxemia in elderly patients with fractures of the femoral neck. *Anesth Analg* **65**:892–894.

49 Schwartz DA, Finkelstein SD and Lumb GD (1988) Fat embolism to the cardiac conduction system associated with sudden death. *Hum Pathol* **19**:116–119.

50 Weisz GM and Steiner E (1971) The causes of death in fat embolism. *Chest* **59**:511–516.

32 Acute severe asthma

DV Tuxen and TE Oh

Acute severe asthma is a medical emergency requiring prompt careful assessment and management. Its prevalence has risen from 4% prior to 1960 to 10% today, affecting 8% of adults and 15–20% of children.[1] There is geographical variation (e.g. it is common in New Zealand and uncommon in Asia). Life-threatening episodes affect 0.5% of asthmatic patients per year,[2] and mortality ranges from 0.4 to 6 per 100 000 population, depending on the age and population group.[3]

Aetiology

The pathogenesis is incompletely understood, but immunological mechanisms are important. Airways are hyperreactive to allergens (e.g. housemite and pollen), non-specific precipitating factors (e.g. cold air, exercise, atmospheric and industrial irritants, viral infection) and drugs affecting chemical airway control (e.g. aspirin and β-adrenergic blockers). No precipitant can be identified in over 30% of patients.[4]

Clinical presentation

Emergency presentation commonly arises from two clinical backgrounds, described below. Both clinical patterns have been associated with the need for mechanical ventilation and with mortality.[5]

Acute severe asthma

This is more common and arises in patients (more frequently females) with poorly controlled asthma[6] and persistent airflow obstruction. Symptoms of asthma may be minimal, because of underperception of breathlessness,[7] denial and behaviour modification. Hence, late presentation, underestimation of severity and undertreatment are common.[5] Severe attacks may develop over hours to days, and presentation follows a prolonged exacerbation or recurrent episodes.[6]

Predominant airway pathology is chronic inflammatory changes, including oedema, hypertrophy and mucus plugging. Large doses of inhaled β-agonists have often been used, but with limited response. Improvement usually requires steroids and may be slow. Respiratory fatigue and need for ventilatory support may arise before clinical improvement occurs.

Hyperacute fulminating asthma

This occurs in younger patients (more commonly male) with relatively normal lung function but high bronchial reactivity.[6,8,9] Previous episodes of severe asthma or evidence of bronchial reactivity may be present, such as diurnal variation of symptoms or exercise-induced asthma. However, life-threatening asthma may arise de novo. The attack is usually rapid and may lead to severe respiratory insufficiency within hours – and occasionally within minutes – of onset. Response to aggressive treatment is usually prompt, and may avert respiratory support or shorten its duration.

Clinical features and assessment of severity

The clinical features of asthma are well-known, but the assessment of severity is more difficult. Underestimation of asthma severity is a risk factor for mortality.[10]

Airflow obstruction

Although expiratory wheeze is the hallmark of asthma, the loudness of wheezing is a poor guide to the severity of airway obstruction.[11] Very soft breath sounds on auscultation or especially a 'silent chest' may indicate grossly inadequate airflow ('locked lung syndrome'). Airflow obstruction results in pulmonary hyperinflation (see below).

Ventilation–perfusion (*V*/*Q*) mismatch

Hypoxaemia and increased minute ventilation are invariably present due to increased *V*/*Q* mismatch, which is roughly proportional to the severity of airflow obstruction. Hypoxaemia and central cyanosis refractory to supplemental oxygen may occur with severe asthma. Cyanosis may be clinically detected with as little as 1.5 g/dl deoxyhaemoglobin (*P*aO_2 of approximately 60 mmHg or 8.0 kPa),[12] but it is a late sign. Thus hypoxaemia must be averted with high-flow oxygen therapy, and tracked using pulse oximetry or arterial blood gases.

Tachycardia and arrhythmias may be present, often associated with stress, increased work of breathing, sympathomimetic drugs and electrolyte disturbances. Nevertheless, severe hypoxaemia is a cause of tachycardia of over 130 beats/min.[13]

Increased minute ventilation requirement primarily results in tachypnoea because of a limited capacity to increase tidal volume. As asthma worsens, ventilation requirement increases and tidal volume falls, causing increasing tachypnoea. Lessening tachypnoea without improvement in airflow obstruction indicates fatigue and impending respiratory collapse.

Increased work of breathing

Increased work of breathing due to airflow obstruction and the mechanical disadvantage of hyperinflation results in an increased requirement for respiratory muscle force generation and the use of accessory respiratory muscles.[10] This in turn results in dyspnoea[7] and, as airflow obstruction worsens, respiratory distress. Assessment of respiratory distress by both the patient and experienced doctor[14] can indicate the severity of asthma. However, some patients have minimal symptoms despite severe airflow obstruction, and individual patient assessments may also be inaccurate. Increased work of breathing is also accompanied by assumption of an upright posture, sweating and inability to speak – all valuable indicators of asthma severity.

The increased negative intrathoracic pressure generated during inspiration is also responsible for pulsus paradoxus. Pulsus paradoxus is an exaggeration of the normal slight fall in blood pressure and pulse volume on inspiration. A difference in systolic blood pressure between inspiration and expiration >10 mmHg (1.3 kPa) indicates severe asthma.[15] However, the degree of pulsus paradoxus does not necessarily correlate with the severity of asthma, as it is also dependent on the capacity of the inspiratory muscles to generate negative intrathoracic pressure. If the inspiratory muscles are weak, or if their force generation is impaired by hyperinflation and fatigue, then pulsus paradoxus may be small or even diminish, as airflow obstruction becomes more severe.

Ventilatory failure

When ventilation required for normocarbia cannot be achieved, ventilatory failure ensues, manifested by a rising *P*aCO_2, marked distress, restlessness and anxiety. As higher levels of *P*aCO_2 are reached, flushing, further sweating and bounding pulse occur. When accompanied by exhaustion, obtundation and depressed consciousness, ventilatory assistance is almost invariably required, and should be instigated urgently.

Investigations

Arterial blood gases and pulse oximetry

Pulse oximetry should be used early. Arterial blood-gas measurements may not be necessary in mild asthma, but must be undertaken in moderate to severe asthma. Arterial hypoxaemia is attributed to *V*/*Q* mismatching[16] and is almost invariably present in a patient with severe asthma breathing room air.

Ventilation is initially increased in an acute attack, leading to hypocarbia and respiratory alkalosis. As asthma severity and *V*/*Q* mismatch worsen, the minute ventilation required to achieve the same alveolar ventilation and *P*aCO_2 increases, but the capacity to achieve this increased ventilatory requirement diminishes, because of increased work of breathing, hyperinflation and fatigue. Thus a *P*aCO_2 rising towards normal may represent clinical deterioration rather than improvement, leading eventually to hypercarbia. The presence of hypercarbic acidosis is associated with forced expiratory volume in 1 s (FEV_1) < 20% of predicted or <1.2 l,[10] and reliably indicates that asthma is severe. Nevertheless, absence of hypercarbia does not necessarily exclude very severe airflow obstruction.[10]

Serum bicarbonate levels may also be disturbed in acute asthma. Patients with poorly controlled asthma days before presentation may develop a mild non-anion gap metabolic acidosis[17] (serum bicarbonate 22 ± 2 mmol/l), which is presumed to be due to renal compensation for persisting hypocarbia. More severely ill asthmatics may develop lactic acidosis – the most consistent cause appears to be high-dose parenteral *β*-agonists.[18] Lactic acidosis may result in serum bicarbonate concentrations <20 mmol/l, which further increases ventilatory demand.

Ventilatory function tests

The asthmatic patient may be too breathless or distressed to perform even simple bedside ventilatory function tests. However, FEV_1 or peak expiratory flow (PEF) rate are useful indicators of severity and response to treatment if they can be obtained. $FEV_1 < 1.0$ l or PEF < 100 l/min indicates severe asthma. Such tests should be performed as soon as possible after presentation, and used to follow progress. In some patients with highly reactive airways, symptoms may transiently worsen following forced expiration, and may rarely result in respiratory decompensation.[19] Patients should be carefully observed and measurements discontinued if problems occur.

Chest X-ray

A chest X-ray should be performed when asthma is severe or refractory to treatment, when barotrauma or infection is suspected, or when diagnosis is in doubt. It is usually not necessary in milder attacks that respond to treatment. Classical radiological features of severe asthma are a narrow central heart shadow, flattened diaphragms, raised bucket-handle ribs, and generalized hyperinflation. Any associated pulmonary parenchymal infection may be detected.

Electrocardiogram (ECG)

Although the ECG is usually normal, young patients with severe asthma may show transient ECG changes of right heart strain, i.e. right axis deviation, P pulmonale, right bundle branch block, $S_1Q_3T_3$ pattern, and inverted T waves in anterior leads.

Differential diagnosis

The diagnosis of asthma is usually obvious. However, wheeze and dyspnoea may be caused by other illnesses such as left ventricular failure, aspiration, upper airway obstruction, inhaled foreign body and pulmonary embolism. Wheeze and dyspnoea arising in hospitalized patients who were not admitted with asthma are less likely to be due to asthma.

Management

If acute asthma is judged to be severe, urgent treatment is warranted. Information on the dose and type of prior bronchodilator use should be obtained, especially sympathomimetics and theophylline preparations.

Established treatment

Initial pharmacotherapy of acute severe asthma should include the following:

Oxygen

Hypoxaemia contributes to life-threatening events that complicate acute severe asthma.[20] Although high inspired oxygen may increase hypercarbia in patients with severe chronic airflow obstruction, this is highly questionable in acute asthma and adequate oxygen

should not be withheld. A pulse oximeter enables accurate titration of oxygen therapy to achieve $Sao_2 > 96\%$. Oxygen may be titrated to a lower Sao_2 if there is concern about severe chronic airways disease, without risking significant hypoxaemia (see Chapter 22).

Nebulized β-agonists

Nebulized β-agonist remains the first-line bronchodilator therapy. Agents include salbutamol, terbutaline, orciprenaline, fenoterol and isoprenaline. Salbutamol remains the agent of first choice.[21] It acts rapidly and causes fewer side-effects than the non-selective agents, but tremor and tachycardia may be problems. The standard nebulizing dose is 5–10 mg (in 2.5–5.0 ml diluent volume) every 2–4 h, but more frequent (and larger total) doses are required in severe asthma because of impaired airway penetration. Initially, the minimum frequency should be 5–10 mg hourly, but this may be increased to 5 mg in 2.5 ml each 20 min or given continuously up to 20–25 mg in an hour.[22] A minimum reservoir volume of 2–4 ml and an oxygen flow rate of 6–8 l/min are advocated for optimal nebulizer output.[23]

Other β-agonists, terbutaline (1.0% solution), orciprenaline and fenoterol (0.1% solution) are alternative drugs. Fenoterol is less preferred because of a higher incidence of cardiac side effects, hypokalaemia and an association with increased asthma mortality.[20] Longer-acting salmeterol is less desirable because of its slower onset of action.

β-Agonists may also be delivered by metered dose inhaler (MDI). MDI delivery appears to be as effective as nebulization[24] and is cheaper. The inhalation technique is important.[25] After exhalation, one puff of the inhaler is taken (either into the open mouth or with lips closed around the inhaler) just after the start of a slow, deep breath through the mouth. The breath is then held at full inspiration for 2–10 s. Those who cannot coordinate this manoeuvre can try tube spacers and a dry powder inhaler (salbutamol Rotacaps). Less than 10% of the dose is delivered to the airways by these methods, but is enough to be effective. During mechanical ventilation, MDI delivery, even with spacers, may not be as effective as nebulization,[26] which remains the method of choice.

Excessive inhaled β-agonists may cause tremor, tachycardia, hypokalaemia and tachyarrhythmias. Bronchodilators may transiently increase hypoxaemia by increasing $\dot{V}/Q$ mismatch,[27] but this is readily overcome with supplementary oxygen; therapy should not be withheld for this reason. Long-term high-dose β-agonist use has been associated with increased mortality.[20] Whether this is merely a marker of more severe asthma or is due to adverse effects (e.g. cardiotoxicity, arrhythmia genesis, increased hypoxaemia or increased allergen load from bronchodilatation) remains uncertain.

Some studies conclude that β-agonists given IV are less effective than nebulization, and are hence seldom indicated.[28,29] However, nebulized salbutamol followed by IV infusion (5–20 μg/min) has added benefit.[30] The infusion rate is limited by side-effects, e.g. tachycardia, tremor, lactic acidosis (usually with infusions >10 μg/min), hyperglycaemia and hypokalaemia. Salbutamol 100–300 μg may also be given IV to non-intubated patients in extremis, or delivered down an endotracheal tube if emergencies do not permit time to establish IV access.

Anticholinergics

Ipratropium bromide is an anticholinergic bronchodilator with no systemic atropine-like effects and no inhibition of mucociliary clearance. Although its bronchodilator action is variable and not potent, it has good synergy with β-agonists[31] and can be nebulized concurrently (e.g. adding 0.5 mg in 2 ml every 2–6 h to a salbutamol nebule of 5 mg in 2.5 ml). Preservative-induced bonchoconstriction reported in a few patients may be prevented by using preservative-free solutions.[32] Nebulized glycopyrrolate may also be as effective as β-agonists and with fewer side-effects,[33] but has not been extensively studied. Anticholinergics can be recommended for routine use with β-agonists in acute severe asthma.

Steroids

Steroids reduce the inflammatory cell response and increase the sensitivity of β-receptors.[34] Their role in acute severe asthma is now well-established.[35] Failure to administer steroids is cited as contributing to asthma mortality,[5,36] and is now considered questionable practice. Parenteral steroids are given soon after presentation, if asthma is severe or does not rapidly respond to β-agonists. Such early administration does not mandate hospital admission; indeed it contributes to reducing severity and hospital admission.[37] Peak response to IV steroids is 6–12 h, but may be seen as early as 1 h after IV administration:[38] full effects must be assessed over several days.[34]

A suitable regimen is: hydrocortisone 200 mg (or 3–4 mg/kg) IV statim, followed by 800–1000 mg during the next 24 h by continuous infusion (0.5 mg/kg per h) or 6-hourly boluses (3–4 mg/kg). Alternately methylprednisolone may be used. High doses offer no added benefit.[39] Steroids are usually given over several days. Treatment may be withdrawn abruptly if of short duration, but usually IV therapy is replaced by tapering doses of oral steroids (e.g. prednisolone starting at 40–60 mg/day). Steroids may still be used in pregnancy. The risk of fetal anoxia from the asthma is greater than any risk associated with correct use of steroids. Side-effects include hyperglycaemia, hypokalaemia, occasional euphoria or psychosis and myopathy (see below).

Aminophylline

The role of aminophylline in acute asthma is controversial. It is less effective as a single agent than β-agonists.[40] Synergy with β-agonists is debatable[41] and it has potentially serious side-effects. Reported benefits and side-effects of adding aminophylline to β-agonists with or without steroids are conflicting.[42–47] Other potentially beneficial effects include increasing cardiac output and diaphragmatic contractility,[48] and possibly an anti-inflammatory effect.[49] Toxic effects include headache, nausea, vomiting and restlessness, with life-threatening arrhythmias and convulsions at concentrations above 40 mg/l (200 μmol/l).

Aminophylline is not universally recommended for use in acute asthma. However, with careful administration and monitoring, it can be given to patients who have failed to respond to β-agonists and steroids, as it may confer benefit. The IV loading dose is 3 mg/kg (half the traditional recommendation of 5–6 mg/kg)[50] over 20–30 min. It is continued as an infusion of 0.5 mg/kg per h, but reduced in patients with cirrhosis congestive heart failure, chronic obstructive lung disease, acute fevers or receiving cimetidine, erythromycin or antiviral vaccines. The dose may need to be increased in young patients, smokers without chronic airflow obstruction, or regular drinkers without liver disease.

Prior therapy requires measurement of serum theophylline concentration to modify or omit the loading dose. Measurement of serum concentrations should be repeated 1–2 h after loading to titrate to the therapeutic range of 5–20 mg/l (30–110 μmol/l). Subsequent measurements are made 12 and 24 h later, and daily thereafter. Pharmacokinetic predictions of serum concentrations may optimize aminophylline infusions.[51] Effects of aminophylline should be assessed over more than 12–24 h,[52] and evaluation should not be limited to spirometry.[47]

Non-established treatment

Many other therapies in acute severe asthma are not advocated for routine use, not always necessary, or not widely accepted.

Adrenaline

Interest in adrenaline has recently recurred because its α-agonist actions of vasoconstriction and mucosal shrinkage may potentially increase airway diameter beyond the effects of β-agonists.[53] However, no benefit of subcutaneous or nebulized adrenaline has been demonstrated over β-agonists.[54,55] Hence adrenaline should not be routinely used, but may be tried in severe asthma which is refractory to standard therapy. The nebulized dose is 20–40 mg in 2–4 ml (1% solution, 0.05 ml/kg per dose) 1–4-hourly. The subcutaneous dose is 0.2–0.5 mg (0.2–0.5 ml of 1:1000 adrenaline), repeated, if necessary, 2–3 times at 30–min intervals. Adrenaline by infusion may avert mechanical ventilation in very severe cases, but has to be used with extreme caution with ECG monitoring. An initial IV dose of 0.2–1.0 mg (2–10 ml of 1:10 000 adrenaline) is given slowly over 3–5 min. This may be followed by a continuous infusion of 1–20 μg/min[56] which is weaned when the acute attack subsides.

Magnesium sulphate

Magnesium sulphate may bronchodilate through blocking calcium-channel-mediated bronchoconstriction and inhibiting parasympathetic acetylcholine release. Current data do not support routine use in acute asthma,[57,58] but magnesium may be tried in severe asthma refractory to standard therapy. Recommended doses are 5–10 mmol (1.25–2.5 g, 2.5–5 ml of 50% solution) given slowly over 20 min, but doses up to 40–80 mmol (10–20 g) have been given.[59] Side-effects include hypotension, flushing and mild sedation. Serum concentrations should be measured if repeated or high doses are used.

Helium

Inhalation of a helium:oxygen mixture (heliox) reduces gas density and turbulence, with reduced airflow resistance.[60] Work of breathing is decreased,[60] and pulmonary access of inhaled bronchodilators may be improved. The role of heliox in acute asthma is not yet established, but it is safe provided adequate oxygenation is maintained. It may be tried in critical asthma to avert intubation or during difficult mechanical ventilation.

Antibiotics

The majority of acute severe asthma occurs in the absence of bacterial lower respiratory tract infection. Antibiotics are only indicated if there is clear evidence of purulent bronchitis preceding the asthma attack or if pneumonia is present.

Hydration

Patients with more prolonged severe attacks prior to presentation may become dehydrated because of poor fluid intake. The role of fluids in decreasing sputum tenacity is uncertain and care must be taken not to overload patients who were not previously dehydrated. Replacement of electrolytes, especially potassium, is given according to serum biochemical results.

Anaesthetic agents

Ketamine, a dissociative anaesthetic agent, has been used in severe asthma.[61] It decreases airways resistance but the mechanism is not understood. Halothane, isoflurane and enflurane have been successively used in mechanically ventilated patients with severe asthma.[62,63] Halothane can give rise to serious arrhythmias. These inhalational anaesthetic agents must be used with great care and only during mechanical ventilation, or as a prelude to intubation. None of the anaesthetic agents have an established place in standard therapy.

Other drug therapies

Calcium-channel blockers,[64] nitroglycerin,[65] inhaled clonidine,[66] and IV glucagon[67] have all been shown to improve bronchospasm, but none can be currently recommended for use.

Bronchoalveolar lavage

Whole-lung or bronchopulmonary lavage to remove tenacious mucus plugs has been reported to improve airflow.[68,69] It may, however, transiently worsen bronchospasm and hypoxaemia and aggravate dynamic hyperinflation during mechanical ventilation (the fibrescope partially occludes the endotracheal tube). Bronchopulmonary lavage may have a role in ventilated patients without critical hyperinflation, whose recovery is delayed by resistant mucus impaction.

Therapies not recommended

Antihistamines and mucolytic agents are not considered to be effective. No sedative is safe in acute asthma. Patients with severe asthma should never be sedated unless being intubated or mechanically ventilated.

Monitoring progress

Patients with severe asthma must not be left unattended. Instead, their progress should be closely monitored after initiation of treatment. Major contributors to deterioration and mortality are inadequate observation and measurement.

1 *Regular measurement of asthma severity* by a peak flow meter or portable spirometer 2–4-hourly during initial management. Clinical estimation is not always reliable, whereas deterioration in peak expiratory flow or FEV_1 can provide early warning of deterioration.
2 *Regular assessment of oxygenation* using a pulse oximeter $\pm$ arterial blood gases.
3 *Regular assessment of treatment* including assessing serum theophylline concentrations, frequency and dose of nebulized agents, and side-effects (e.g. tachycardia, arrhythmias and tremor).

Non-invasive ventilatory assistance

1 Continuous positive airways pressure (CPAP), by face or nasal mask or endotracheal tube, has been advocated in acute asthma to improve dyspnoea and reduce work of breathing,[70] by overcoming end-expiratory alveoli positive pressure due to gas trapping, i.e. auto-positive end-expiratory pressure (PEEP) or intrinsic PEEP.[71,72] Low levels of CPAP may be used in an attempt to avert mechanical ventilation. The effects on dyspnoea, respiratory rate and blood gases should be carefully assessed before CPAP is continued.

2 *Non-invasive ventilation* by occlusive nasal or facemask in acute asthma remains to be evaluated, but has been reported to be useful (see Chapter 26).

3 *External chest compression* has been advocated to assist expiration in patients with a marginal respiratory status from severe asthma. Data on its use are lacking, but no improvement was found when applied during mechanical ventilation.[73]

Mechanical ventilation

Mechanical ventilation in acute severe asthma may be life-saving, but is associated with significant morbidity and mortality (Table 32.1).[74] Inadvertent pulmonary hyperinflation[74-76] (see below) contributes significantly to morbidity and mortality. Initiation of mechanical ventilation should be considered carefully. Criteria based on blood gases and respiratory variables are unreliable. Avoiding unnecessary mechanical ventilation must be balanced against the risks of delayed intubation. Bedside assessment by an experienced clinician of deteriorating patient status despite aggressive treatment is the most important determinant for intubation. The need for ventilatory support is usually due to extremely severe airflow obstruction and pulmonary hyperinflation (e.g. fulminating hyperacute asthma); respiratory muscle fatigue in severe, prolonged asthma; and cardiorespiratory arrest on presentation.

Pulmonary hyperinflation and intrinsic PEEP

When starting mechanical ventilation in severe asthma, airflow obstruction significantly prolongs expiratory airflow and leads to incomplete exhalation before the next mechanical breath. This progressive hyperinflation continues until the lung reaches an equilibrium after 6–12 mechanical breaths (Fig. 32.1). Equilibrium occurs because increasing lung volume increases airway calibre and lung elastic recoil pressure, both of which improve expiratory airflow and allow each subsequent inspired tidal volume (V_T) to be exhaled in the expiratory time available (T_E). The gas volume retained has been called pulmonary hyperinflation or gas trapping, and may be measured during a period of apnoea long enough to allow complete passive exhalation of trapped gas (30–60 s; Fig. 32.2).[76,77] The pressure exerted on the alveoli by this trapped gas is termed auto-PEEP or intrinsic PEEP ($PEEP_i$),[72,75] measured as the airway pressure during transient airway occlusion at the end of expiration.

Hyperinflation in severe airflow obstruction can lead to hypotension (due to increased intrathoracic pressure and decreased venous return) and barotrauma. The extent of hyperinflation is dependent on V_T, T_E and severity of airflow obstruction. Increasing minute ventilation by increasing V_T or rate (i.e. reducing T_E) or both is the biggest factor which increases pulmonary hyperinflation.[76] End-inspiratory lung volume (V_{EI}) above functional residual capacity (FRC) is a good predictor of total lung

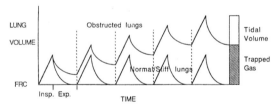

Fig. 32.1 Dynamic hyperinflation. The volume history of normal acutely injured lungs compared with that of obstructed lungs when commenced on controlled mechanical ventilation. This shows initial lung volume to be at the passive relaxation volume of the respiratory system or functional residual capacity (FRC).

Table 32.1 Cause of death in 99 patients requiring mechanical ventilation for acute severe asthma

No.		No.	
Cerebral ischaemia/hypoxia	40	Gastrointestinal complication	3
Hypotension	15	Suspected pulmonary embolus	3
Pneumonia or sepsis with hypotension	10	Arrest postextubation	3
Tension pneumothorax	6	Arrest post-intensive care unit	2
Technical complications with ventilation	6	Treatment withdrawn (end-stage)	2
Arrhythmia	4	Unknown	3
Respiratory complication	3	Total	99

capacity (TLC)[77] (Fig. 32.3), and the best predictor of complications during mechanical ventilation.[74] V_{EI} below 18–20 ml/kg (1.4 l in a.70 kg adult) is safe.[74]

Technique of mechanical ventilation

Initial ventilator settings

The initial stages of ventilatory support are the most critical, as CO_2 production is high and excretion poor. A low level of minute ventilation ($\leqslant 115$ ml/kg per min or < 10 l/min in a 70-kg adult) is started, using

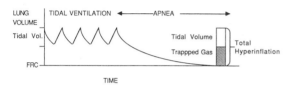

Fig. 32.2 Assessment of pulmonary hyperinflation. The assessment of the degree of pulmonary hyperinflation above functional residual capacity (FRC) during steady-state tidal ventilation. Total exhaled gas volume is measured in a volumetric measuring device during a period of apnoea long enough for observable expiratory gas flow to cease (30–60 s).

a low V_T ($\leqslant 8$ ml/kg) and high inspiratory flow rate (> 80 l/min). The rate is adjusted to achieve the desired minute ventilation ($\leqslant 14$ breaths/min). Inspired oxygen of 50% is usually sufficient. This level of ventilation will usually result in hypercarbic acidosis, and sedation $\pm$ paralysis is needed. Paralysis has the additional benefit of reducing CO_2 production, but should be discontinued after 24 h because of possible associated myopathy (see below). If significant hypotension occurs, minute ventilation is reduced by rate reduction and fluid loading given.

Assessment of ventilation

Once mechanical ventilation has started, the degree of pulmonary hyperinflation should be assessed by measurement of:

1 *Plateau airway pressure* (P_{plat}) during 0.5 s end-inspiratory exhale occlusion. This represents the alveolar pressure at the end of inspiration, which is directly proportional to the degree of hyper-inflation, and should be maintained < 20 cm H_2O.[76]

2 *PEEP$_i$* represents the alveolar pressure at the end of expiration, and is proportional to the trapped gas volume. Unfortunately, $PEEP_i$ can under-estimate the degree of hyperinflation,[78] and does

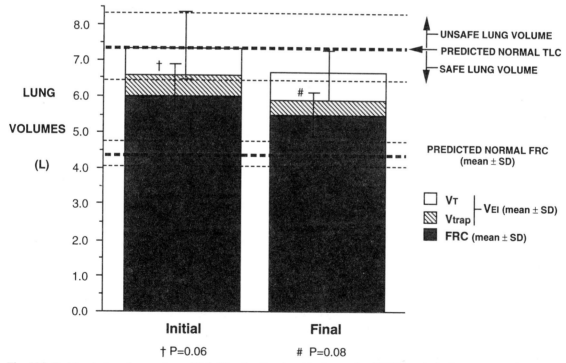

† P=0.06   # P=0.08

Fig. 32.3 End-inspiratory lung volume (V_{EI}). The functional residual capacity (FRC) reached after 60–80 s of apnoea compared with predicted normal values at the beginning of paralysed controlled mechanical ventilation and after asthma had recovered. Trapped gas (V_{trap}) and V_T at the safe level of V_{EI} have been added to this to form the total lung volume at end-inspiration (TLV$_{EI}$) and this has been compared with the predicted normal total lung capacity (TLC).

not account for the size of V_T used, which also determines the risk of barotrauma. $PEEP_i$ is not recommended, but if measured, must be done with a small constant V_T and should be maintained <12 cm H_2O.

3 V_{EI} is assessed in a paralysed patient by measuring the total exhaled volume during a period of apnoea[76] long enough (30–60 s) for exhalation to be completed and the lungs to return to FRC (Fig 32.3). This volume should be maintained <20 ml/kg. Measurement is unfortunately complex and labour-intensive.

4 *Central venous* or *oesophageal balloon pressures* reflect pulmonary hyperinflation. The extent of central venous pressure decrease and blood pressure increase during a period of apnoea will indicate the degree of circulatory tamponade due to hyperinflation.

Adjustment of ventilation

Minute ventilation is adjusted according to the degree of pulmonary hyperinflation, irrespective of $Paco_2$ or pH (except for patients with cerebral oedema). Attempts to correct pH or Pco_2 by increasing minute ventilation will lead to excessive hyperinflation. A low pH is generally well-tolerated and does not depress cardiac function.[79] Sodium bicarbonate may be given if pH is 7.1 or lower, but its usefulness is questioned.[79] PEEP is contraindicated as it increases hyperinflation.[80]

Complications of mechanical ventilation

1 *Hypotension* may be caused by sedation, hyperinflation, pneumothoraces or arrhythmias,[74,76] but rarely by hypovolaemia.

2 *Pneumothoraces* occur up to 10% of mechanically ventilated asthmatic patients, and may be fatal.[74] Once developed, airflow obstruction favours continued gas loss through the ruptured alveoli. A unilateral tension pneumothorax redistributes ventilation to the contralateral lung, increasing its dynamic hyperinflation, thereby increasing the propensity for bilateral pneumothoraces.

3 *Lactic acidosis* has recently been recognized as a complication of parenteral β-agonists,[81] probably through stimulation of muscle glycolytic pathways. It may compound respiratory acidosis and distress and should be avoided. IV salbutamol should be ceased or reduced, if serum lactate concentrations reach 4 mmol/l.

4 *Acute asthma myopathy* is being reported with increasing frequency in acute severe asthma. It is manifested by clinical and electromyographic myopathy, increased serum creatine kinase concentrations and rhabdomyolysis with muscle cell vacuolation on muscle biopsy. Recovery is slow but

weaning from mechanical ventilation and hospital stay are prolonged; incomplete recovery after 12 months has been reported in a few patients.[82] The aetiology is unclear, but steroids appear to be an essential component.[82,83] Neuromuscular blockers appear to play an aggravating role.[82,84,85] Use of lower parenteral steroid doses, early introduction of nebulized steroid (e.g. budesonide 1 mg 12-hourly) and avoidance or early discontinuation of neuromuscular blockers can be recommended.

Mortality and long-term outcome

Mortality of asthma is significantly higher in Australia and New Zealand than in North America, and has been increasing since the 1970s.[3] Most deaths occur before medical help and in older patients, but a significant proportion still occurs after medical intervention and in patients under 35 years. End-stage disease is not a common feature; mortality could probably have been prevented if appropriate therapy had been given 1–2 days prior to death. Life-threatening events can recur in patients previously identified as severe asthmatics. Mortality in patients who have previously required mechanical ventilation is between 7 and 24%.[86–88] Careful follow-up and management of patients who have had a life-threatening event are worthwhile.

References

1 Bauman A, Young L, Peat JK, Hunt J and Larkin P (1992) Asthma under-recognition and under-treatment in an Australian community. *Aust NZ J Med* **22**:36–40.

2 Seale JP (1991) Asthma deaths: where are we now? *Aust NZ J Med* **21**:678–679.

3 O'Donnell TV (1988) Asthma – Australia and New Zealand. *Aust NZ J Med* **18**:303–310.

4 Bellamy D and Collins JV (1979) Acute asthma in adults. *Thorax* **34**:36–39.

5 Benatar SR (1986) Fatal asthma. *N Engl J Med* **314**:423–429.

6 Wasserfallen JB, Schaller MD, Feihl F and Perret CH (1990) Sudden asphyxic asthma: a distinct entity? *Am Rev Respir Dis* **142**:108–111.

7 Burdon JGW, Juniper EF, Hargreave FE and Campbell EJM (1982) The perception of breathlessness in asthma. *Am Rev Respir Dis* **126**:825–828.

8 Ferrer A, Torres A, Roca J, Sunyer J, Anto JM and Rodriguez-Roisin R (1990) Characteristics of patients with soybean dust-induced acute severe asthma requiring mechanical ventilation. *Eur Respir J* **3**:429–433.

9 Kallenbach JM, Frankel AH, Lapinski SE *et al.* (1993) Determinants of near fatality in acute severe asthma. *Am J Med* **95**:265–272.

10 Rebuck AS and Read J (1971) Assessment and management of severe asthma. *Am J Med* **51**:788–798.

11 Shim CS and Williams MH Jr (1993) Relationship of wheezing to the severity of obstruction in asthma. *Arch Intern Med* **143**:890–892.

12 Goss GA, Hayes JA and Burdon JGW (1988) Deoxyhaemoglobin concentrations in the detection of central cyanosis. *Thorax* **43**:212–213.

13 Cooke NJ, Crompton GK and Grant IWB (1979) Observations on the management of acute bronchial asthma. *Br J Dis Chest* **73**:157–162.

14 Shim CS and Williams MH Jr (1980) Evaluation of the severity of asthma: patients versus physicians. *Am J Med* **68**:11–13.

15 Fitzgerald JM and Hargreave FE (1989) The assessment and management of life-threatening asthma. *Chest* **95**:888–894.

16 Roca J, Ramis LI, Rodriguez-Roisin R, Ballester E, Montserrat JM and Wagner PD (1988) Serial relationships between ventilation–perfusion inequality and spirometry in acute severe asthma requiring hospitalization. *Am Rev Respir Dis* **137**:1055–1061.

17 Mountain RD, Heffner JE, Brackett NC and Sahn SA (1990) Acid–base disturbances in acute asthma. *Chest* **98**:651–655.

18 Tuxen DV (1996) Mechanical ventilatory support in acute severe asthma. In: Evans T, Hinds C (eds) *Advances in Critical Care*. Edinburgh: Churchill Livingstone (in press).

19 Lemarchrand P, Labrune S, Herer B and Huchon GJ (1991) Cardiorespiratory arrest following peak expiratory flow measurement during attack of asthma. *Chest* **100**:1168–1169.

20 Beasley R, Pearce N, Crane J, Windom H and Burgess C (1991) Asthma mortality and inhaled beta agonist therapy. *Aust NZ J Med* **21**:753–763.

21 Gern JE and Lemanske RF (1993) Beta-adrenergic agonist therapy. *Immunol Allergy Clin North Am* **13**:839–860.

22 Colacone A, Wolkove N, Stern E, Afilalo M, Rosenthal TM and Kreisman H (1990) Continuous nebulization of albuterol (salbutamol) in acute asthma. *Chest* **97**:693–697.

23 Clay MM, Pavia D, Newman SP, Lennard-Jones T and Clarke S (1983) Assessment of jet nebulizers for lung aerosol therapy. *Lancet* **2**:592–594.

24 Idris AH, McDermott MF, Raucci JC, Morrabel A, McGorray S and Hendeles L (1993) Emergency department treatment of severe asthma: metered-dose inhaler plus holding chamber is equivalent in effectiveness to nebulizer. *Chest* **103**:665–672.

25 Newman SP, Pavia D and Clarke SW (1981) How should a pressurized β-adrenergic bronchodilator be inhaled? *Eur J Respir Dis* **62**:3–21.

26 Manthous CA, Hall JB, Schmidt GA and Wood LDH (1993) Metered-dose inhaler versus nebulized albuterol in mechanical ventilated patients. *Am Rev Respir Dis* **148**:1567–1570.

27 Webb-Johnson DC and Andrews JL Jr (1977) Bronchodilator therapy (first of two parts). *N Engl J Med* **297**:476.

28 Williams SJ, Winner SJ and Clark TJH (1981) Comparison of inhaled and intravenous terbutaline in acute severe asthma. *Thorax* **36**:629–631.

29 Salmeron S. Brochard L, Mal H *et al.* (1994) Nebulized versus intravenous albuterol in hypercapnic acute asthma: a multicenter, double-blind, randomized study. *Am J Respir Crit Care Med* **149**:1466–1470.

30 Cheong B, Reynolds SR, Rajan G and Ward MJ (1988) Intravenous β-agonist in severe acute asthma. *Br Med J* **297**:448–450.

31 Fitzgerald JM (1994) A study of the efficacy and safety of nebulization therapy combining ipratropium bromide 0.5 mg with salbutamol sulphate 3.0 mg alone in acute asthma. *Am J Respir Crit Care Med* **149**:A190.

32 Bryant DH and Rogers P (1992) Effects of ipratropium bromide nebuliser solution with and without preservatives in the treatment of acute and stable asthma. *Chest* **102**:742–747.

33 Gilman MJ, Meyer L, Carter J and Slovis C (1990) Comparison of aerosolized glycopyrrolate and metaproterenol in acute asthma. *Chest* **98**: 1095–1098.

34 Barnes NC (1992) Effects of corticosteroids in acute severe asthma. *Thorax* **47**:582–583.

35 Rowe BH, Keller JL and Oxman AD (1992) Effectiveness of steroid therapy in acute exacerbations of asthma: a meta-analysis. *Am J Emerg Med* **10**:301–310.

36 Cochrane GM and Clark TJH (1975) A survey of asthma mortality in patients between ages 35 and 64 in the Greater London hospitals in 1971. *Thorax* **51**:788–798.

37 Littenberg B and Gluck EH (1986) A controlled trial of methylprednisolone in the emergency treatment of acute asthma. *N Engl J Med* **314**:150–152.

38 Editorial (1975) Corticosteroids in acute severe asthma. *Lancet* **2**:166–167.

39 Raimondi AC, Figueroa-Casas JC and Roncoroni AJ (1986) Comparison between high and moderate doses of hydrocortisone in the treatment of status asthmaticus. *Chest* **89**:832–835.

40 Rossing TH, Fanta CH, Goldstein DH, Snapper JR and McFadden Jr ER (1980) Emergency therapy of asthma: comparison of the acute effects of parenteral and inhaled sympathomimetics and infused aminophylline. *Am Rev Respir Dis* **122**:365–371.

41 Ward MJ, MacFarlane JT and Davies D (1982) Treatment of acute severe asthma with intravenous aminophylline and nebulized ipratropium after salbutamol. *Thorax* **37**:785.

42 Murphy DG, McDermott MF, Rydman RJ, Sloan EP and Zalenski RJ (1993) Aminophylline in the treatment of acute asthma when β_2 adrenergics and steroids are provided. *Arch Intern Med* **153**:1784–1788.

43 Coleridge J, Epstein J, Cameron P and Teichtahl H (1993) Intravenous aminophylline confers no benefit in acute asthma treated with intravenous steroids and inhaled bronchodilators. *Aust NZ J Med* **23**:348–354.

44 Rodrigo C and Rodrigo G (1994) Treatment of acute asthma: lack of therapeutic benefit and increase of the toxicity from aminophylline given in addition to high doses of salbutamol delivered by metered-dose inhaler with a spacer. *Chest* **106**: 1071–1076.

45 Huang D, O Brien RG, Harmen E *et al.* (1993) Does aminophylline benefit adults admitted to the hospital for an acute exacerbation of asthma? *Ann Intern Med* **119**:1155–1160.

46 Lalla S, Saleh A, Faroog J, Lombardo G, Gudi M and Anandarao N (1991) Intravenous aminophylline in acute, severe bronchial asthma. *Chest* **100**:60S.

47 Wrenn K, Slovis CM, Murphy F and Greenberg RS (1991) Aminophylline therapy for acute bronchospastic disease in the emergency room. *Ann Intern Med* **115**:241–247.

48 Aubier M, DeTroyer A, Sampson M, Macklem PT and Roussos C (1981) Aminophylline improves diaphragmatic contractility. *N Engl J Med* **305**:249–252.

49 Pauwels RA (1989) New aspects of the therapeutic potential of theophylline in asthma. *J Allergy Clin Immunol* **83**:548–553.

50 Mitenko PA and Ogilvie RI (1973) Rational intravenous doses of theophylline. *N Engl J Med* **289**:600.

51 Ilett KF, Nation RL, Silbert B and Oh TE (1983) Pharmacokinetic optimisation of aminophylline infusions in critically ill patients. *Anaesth Intens Care* **11**:220–227.

52 Kelly HW and Murphy S (1989) Should we stop using theophylline for the treatment of the hospitalized patient with status asthmaticus? *DICP* **23**:995–998.

53 Appel D, Karpel JP and Sherman M (1989) Epinephrine improves expiratory flow rates in patients with asthma who do not respond to inhaled metaproterenol sulfate. *J Allergy Clin Immunol* **84**:90–98.

54 Uden DL, Goetz DR, Kohen DP and Fifield GC (1985) Comparison of nebulized terbutaline and subcutaneous epinephrine in the treatment of acute asthma. *Ann Emerg Med* **14**:229–232.

55 Spiteri MA, Millar AB, Pavia D and Clarke SW (1988) Subcutaneous adrenaline vs terbutaline in the treatment of acute severe asthma. *Thorax* **43**:19–23.

56 Tirot P, Bouachour G, Varache N *et al.* Use of intravenous adrenaline in severe acute asthma. *Rev Mal Respir* **9**:319–323.

57 Green SM and Rothrock SG (1992) Intravenous magnesium for acute asthma: failure to decrease emergency treatment duration or need for hospitalization. *Ann Emerg Med* **21**:260–265.

58 Tiffany BR, Berk WA, Todd IK and White S (1993) Magnesium bolus or infusion fails to improve expiratory flow in acute asthma exacerbations. *Chest* **104**:831–834.

59 Sydow M, Crozier TA, Zielman S, Radke J and Burchardi H (1993) High-dose intravenous magnesium sulfate in the management of life threatening status asthmaticus. *Intens Care Med* **19**:467–471.

60 Manthous CA, Hall JB, Caputo ME, Walter J, Schmidt GA and Wood LDH (1992) The effect of heliox on pulsus paradoxus and peak flow in non-intubated patients with severe asthma. *Chest* **104**:29S.

61 Fisher MMcD (1977) Ketamine hydrochloride in severe bronchospasm. *Anaesthesia* **32**:771–772.

62 Parnass SM, Feld JM, Chamberlin WH and Segil LJ (1987) Status asthmaticus treated with isoflurane and enflurane. *Anesth Analg* **66**:193–195.

63 Saulnier FF, Durocher AV, Deturck RA, Lefevre MC and Wattell FE (1990) Respiratory and hemodynamic effects of halothane in status asthmaticus. *Intens Care Med* **16**:104–107.

64 Cuss FM and Barnes PJ (1985) The effect of inhaled nifedipine on bronchial reactivity to histamine in man. *J Allergy Clin Immunol* **76**:718–723.

65 Goldstein JA (1981) Nitroglycerin therapy of asthma. *Chest* **3**:449–450.

66 Lindgren ER, Ekstrom T and Andersson RG (1986) The effect of inhaled clonidine in patients with asthma. *Am Rev Respir Dis* **34**:266–269.

67 Wilson JE and Nelson RN (1990) Glucagon as a therapeutic agent in the treatment of asthma. *J Emerg Med* **8**:127–130.

68 Lang DM, Simon RA, Mathison DA and Timms RM (1991) Safety and possible efficacy of fibreoptic bronchoscopy with lavage in the management of refractory asthma with mucous impaction. *Ann Allergy* **67**:324–330.

69 Smith DI and Deshazo RD (1993) Bronchoalveolar lavage in asthma. State of the art. *Am Rev Respir Dis* **148**:523–532.

70 Mathieu M, Tonneau MC, Zarka D and Sartene R (1987) Effects of positive end-expiratory pressure in severe acute asthma. *Crit Care Med* **15**:1164.

71 Martin JG, Shore S and Engel LA (1982) Effect of continuous positive airway pressure on respiratory mechanics and pattern of breathing in induced asthma. *Am Rev Respir Dis* **126**:812–817.

72 Gottfried SB, Rossi A and Milic-Emili J (1986) Dynamic hyperinflation, intrinsic PEEP and the mechanically ventilated patient. *Intensive Crit Care Dig* **5**:30–33.

73 Van der Touw T, Mudaliar M and Nayyer V (1995) Cardiorespiratory effects of expiratory ribcage compression during mechanical ventilation for severe acute asthma. *Anaesth Intens Care* **23**:387.

74 Williams TJ, Tuxen DV, Scheinkestel CD, Czarny D and Bowes G (1992) Risk factors for morbidity in mechanically ventilated patients with acute severe asthma. *Am Rev Respir Dis* **146**:607–615.

75 Pepe PE and Marini JJ (1982) Occult positive end-expiratory pressure in mechanically ventilated patients with airflow obstruction. *Am Rev Respir Dis* **126**:166–170.

76 Tuxen DV and Lane S (1987) The effects of ventilatory pattern on hyperinflation, airway pressures, and circulation in mechanical ventilation of patients with severe airflow obstruction. *Am Rev Respir Dis* **136**:872–879.

77 Tuxen DV, Williams TJ, Scheinkestel CD, Czarny D and Bowes G (1992) Use of a measurement of pulmonary hyperinflation to control the level of mechanical ventilation in patients with severe asthma. *Am Rev Respir Dis* **146**:1136–1142.

78 Leatherman J, Ravenscraft SA, Iber C and Davies S (1993) Does measured auto-PEEP accurately reflect the degree of dynamic hyperinflation during mechanical ventilation of status asthma? *Am Rev Respir Dis* **147**:877A.

79 Cooper DJ, Cailes JB, Scheinkestel CD and Tuxen DV (1993) Acute severe asthma and acidosis – effect of bicarbonate on cardiac and respiratory function. *Anaesth Intens Care* **22**:212–213.

80 Tuxen DV (1989) Detrimental effects of positive end-expiratory pressure during controlled mechanical ventilation of patients with severe airflow obstruction. *Am Rev Respir Dis* **140**:5–9.

81 Totaro RJ and Raper R (1994) Lactic acidosis post cardiopulmonary bypass. Randomised prospective study of adrenaline and noradrenaline as causative factors. *Anaesth Intens Care* **11**:220.

82 Hirano M, Ott BR, Raps EC *et al.* (1992) Acute quadriplegic myopathy: a complication of treatment with steroids, nondepolarizing blocking agents, or both. *Neurology* **42**:2082–2087.

83 Lacomis D, Smith TW and Chad DA (1993) Acute myopathy and neuropathy in status asthmaticus: case report and literature review. *Muscle Nerve* **16**:84–90.

84 Douglass JA, Tuxen DV, Horne M *et al.* Myopathy in severe asthma. *Am Rev Respir Dis* **146**:517–519.

85 Hansen-Flaschen J, Cowen J and Raps EC (1993) Neuromuscular blockade in the intensive care unit. More than we bargained for. *Am Rev Respir Dis* **147**:234–236.

86 Marquette CH, Saulnier F, Leroy O *et al.* (1992) Long-

term prognosis of near-fatal asthma. *Am Rev Respir Dis* **146**:76–81.

87 Richards GN, Kolbe J, Fenwick J and Rea HH (1993) Demographic characteristics of patients with severe life threatening asthma: comparison with asthma deaths. *Thorax* **48**:1105–1109.

88 Seddon PC and Heaf DP (1990) Long term outcome of ventilated asthmatics. *Arch Dis Child* **65**: 1324–1328.

33 | Lung infections

CD Gomersall and TE Oh

Pneumonia

Pneumonia remains a common and major cause of critical illness and death. Increasing use of immuno-suppressive drugs, spread of human immunodeficiency virus (HIV) infection and the emergence of anti-microbial-resistant strains have ensured that management of pneumonia remains a difficult ICU problem.

Community-acquired pneumonia

Aetiology (Tables 33.1 and 33.2)[1-3]

Pneumococcal infection is by far the commonest cause, and is also the most frequent cause of severe pneumonia and of death. Its prevalence is probably underestimated, and most cases in which no organism is identified are probably due to pneumococcal infection.[4] Other causes of community-acquired pneumonia are relatively uncommon.

Haemophilus influenzae can cause pneumonia in fit patients as well as those with chronic lung disease.[5] Pneumonia due to both *Mycoplasma pneumoniae* and influenza virus tends to occur in epidemics.[6,7] *M. pneumoniae* epidemics usually last for three winters, while influenza epidemics tend to occur annually. *Mycoplasma* infections commonly occur in teenagers and young adults, but may affect older patients. Influenza virus infection is commonly associated with secondary bacterial infection, usually *Streptococcus pneumoniae* or, more seriously, *Staphyloccus aureus*. Half of all staphylococcal pneumonias occur in association with influenza infection.[8]

Gram-negative infection is unusual in community acquired pneumonia, except possibly in the elderly (especially in old-age homes). In the USA, 6–37% of infections in the elderly were attributed to Gram-negative bacilli,[9] but no such cases were found in patients aged 65–97 years in the UK.[10]

Clinical presentation

Pneumonia produces both systemic and respiratory manifestations. Common clinical findings include fever, sweats, rigors, cough, sputum production, pleuritic chest pain, dyspnoea, tachypnoea, pleural rub and inspiratory crackles. Classic signs of consolidation occur in less than 25% of cases. Other organ systems may be involved depending on the type and severity of pneumonia. Hypotension from dehydration or septic shock may occur, and result in prerenal renal failure or acute tubular necrosis. In addition, confusion, obtundation, abdominal pain, diarrhoea, paralytic ileus, disturbed liver function and electrolyte abnormalities may be present.

The infective organism cannot be identified from either clinical or radiological features in an individual case.[11,12] Herpes labialis was previously thought to be a particular feature of pneumococcal pneumonia, but is equally commonly associated with other causes of pneumonia.[4] The presence of two of three clinical features associated with severe pneumonia (Table 33.3) suggests a 9–21-fold increase in mortality, but this has poor specificity and the positive predictive value is only 19%.[13]

Diagnosing pneumonia may be more difficult in the elderly. Although the vast majority of elderly patients with pneumonia have respiratory symptoms and signs, over 50% may also have non-respiratory symptoms and over a third may have no systemic signs of infection.[10]

Investigations

Investigations should not delay administration of antibiotics. Important investigations include:

1 chest X-ray: radiological changes may lag behind the clinical course in the acute and recovery phases;
2 arterial blood gases;
3 full blood count: significant leukocytosis (over 15×10^9/l with a high neutrophil count) is seen in

Table 33.1 Aetiology of pneumonia based on host status:[1-3,13,23] **known prevalence is given**

Host status	Usual pathogens	Prevalence (%)
Normal adult	*Streptococcus pneumoniae*	30
	Mycoplasma pneumoniae	
	Haemophilus influenzae	
	Legionella spp.	
	Influenza and other viruses	
	Staphylococcus aureus	
	Chlamydia pneumoniae and *C. psittaci*	
Adults with severe community-acquired pneumonia requiring artificial ventilation	*Streptococcus pneumoniae*	36
	Legionella spp.	28
	Staphylococcus aureus	9
	Haemophilus influenzae	8
	Mycoplasma pneumoniae	6
	Chlamydia spp.	1
	Viral (of these, 60% are due to varicella)	10
	Dual infection, even dual bacterial infection, is common	
Hospital patients and possibly elderly residents of old-age homes	Gram-negative bacilli	59
	Pseudomonas aeruginosa	17
	Enterobacter spp.	10
	Klebsiella pneumoniae	7
	Escherichia coli	6
	Serratia marcescens	5
	Proteus mirabilis	3
	Acinetobacter spp.	3
	Haemophilus influenzae	6
	Gram-positive bacilli	17
	Staphylococcus	14
	Streptococcus pneumoniae	3
	Candida albicans	4
Granulocytopenia	*Aspergillus*	
	Mucor	
Cell-mediated immune defect	Herpes group of viruses	
	Pneumocystis carinii	
	Nocardia	
	Cryptococcus	
	Legionella spp.	
	Mycobacterium spp.	
	Aspergillus	
Hypogammaglobulinaemia or splenectomy	*Streptococcus pneumoniae*	
	Haemophilus influenzae	
Artificial ventilation (not originally for pneumonia)	Gram-negative bacteria	75
	Pseudomonas aeruginosa	30
	Acinetobacter spp.	15
	Proteus spp.	15
	Branhamella catarrhalis	10
	Haemophilus spp.	10
	Escherichia coli	8
	Klebsiella spp.	4
	Gram-positive bacteria	52
	Staphyloccus aureus	33
	Streptococcus pneumoniae	6
	Other streptococci	15
	Corynebacterium spp.	8

Table 33.2 Rare pneumonias associated with unusual exposure

Disease	Organism	Exposure
Psittacosis	*Chlamydia psittaci*	Handling birds and bird excreta
Q fever	*Coxiella burnetii*	Handling cattle or sheep or their hides
Anthrax	*Bacillus anthracis*	Handling infected wool
Pertussis	*Bordatella pertussis*	Pneumonia complicating whooping cough
Brucellosis	*Brucella* spp.	Handling infected cattle, pigs, goats or sheep or their milk
Plague	*Yersinia pestis*	Transmitted by insect bites or scratches from infected rodents or cats to laboratory workers and hunters
Tularaemia	*Francisella tularensis*	Transmitted by insect bite from rodents and wild animals to laboratory workers, farmers and hunters
Histoplasmosis	*Histoplasma capsulatum*	North America: contact with infected bats or birds or their excreta
Blastomycosis	*Blastomyces dermatitidis*	USA: inhalation of spores from soil
Melioidosis	*Pseudomonas pseudomallei*	Asia, Pacific, Caribbean, North Australia: contact with local animals or contaminated skin abrasions
Glanders	*Pseudomonas mallei*	Contact with infected horses (very rare)

Table 33.3 Factors associated with increased mortality in patients with community-acquired pneumonia

Clinical
Age > 60 years
Respiratory rate >30 breaths/min*
Low diastolic blood pressure (<60 mmHg, 8 kPa)*
New atrial fibrillation
Lung contusion
Underlying chronic disease

Investigations
Urea >7 mmol/l*
White cell count <4 or >20 × 10^9/l
Albumin <35 g/l
PaO_2 < 60 mmHg (8 kPa)
Multiple lobes involved on chest X-ray
Bacteraemia
Staphylococcal infection

* Presence of two of these three features indicates a 9–21 fold increased risk of death.

the majority of pneumococcal infections, but in only about 10% of *Mycoplasma* or *Legionella* pneumonia;
4 urea and electrolytes;
5 liver function tests;
6 blood culture;
7 blood for serology (see below);
8 sputum (if immediately available) for urgent Gram stain, culture and pneumococcal antigen. The usefulness of sputum tests remains debatable, because of contamination by upper respiratory tract commensals. However, a single or predominant organism on a Gram stain of a fresh sample, or a heavy growth on culture of purulent sputum is likely to be the organism responsible.
9 pleural fluid (if present) for Gram stain and culture.

Further investigations may be necessary. Pneumococcal antigen detection is particularly useful in patients who have already received antibiotics. It is insensitive when serum is tested, but both sensitive and specific when applied to purulent sputum in patients with clinical features of pneumonia.[13] *Mycoplasma* antibodies (immunoglobulin M (IgM) and IgG) may be positive in acute and recovery samples. Cold agglutinins present in about half of *Mycoplasma* infections. *Legionella* antibodies can be detected by immunofluorescent studies.

Percutaneous fine-needle aspiration is a useful method of obtaining lower airway secretions,[1,14] with a reported sensitivity of 43–83% and a false-positive rate of up to 8%. Major risks are haemorrhage and pneumothorax. The incidence of pneumothorax is about 3% but data in mechanically ventilated patients are very limited.

Transtracheal injection of saline is a useful technique in patients unable to produce a sputum sample. Sterile isotonic solution, 5 ml, is injected through the cricothyroid membrane, with immediate withdrawal of the needle. This results in production of lower respiratory tract secretions in most patients.[15]

Fibreoptic bronchoscopy with use of a protected specimen brush and bronchoalveolar lavage are methods of choice to investigate mechanically ventilated patients with pneumonia. Complications include hypoxaemia, arrhythmias, transient worsening in pulmonary infiltrates, bleeding (particularly following protected specimen brushing) and fever (more common after bronchoalveolar lavage). These techniques need to be combined with quantitative culture to minimize the effect of respiratory tract organisms contaminating the bronchoscope sampling channel. The procedure for obtaining microbiological samples using bronchoscopy and protected specimen brushing and/or bronchoalveolar lavage is as follows.[16]

General precautions

Suction through the endotracheal tube should be performed before bronchoscopy. Suctioning or injection of lignocaine through the working channel of the bronchoscope should be avoided. Protected specimen brushing should be performed before bronchoalveolar lavage.

Ventilated patients

Inspired oxygen is set at 100%(Fio_2 1.0). Respiratory rate is set at 15–20 breaths/min and peak inspiratory flow at or below 60 l/min. The peak airway pressure alarm is set at a level that allows adequate ventilation. Ventilator settings are titrated against exhaled tidal volume. Neuromuscular blockade is given with sedatives to patients at high risk of complications who are undergoing prolonged bronchoscopy.

Protected specimen brushing

Sampling at a subsegmental level is recommended. If purulent secretions are not seen, the brush is advanced until it is no longer visible (but wedging in a peripheral position must be avoided). The brush is moved back and forth and rotated several times.

Bronchoalveolar lavage

The bronchoscope tip is wedged into a subsegment of lung. Sterile isotonic saline (20 ml) is injected and then aspirated. This sample is not to be used for quantitative microbiology or identification of intracellular organisms, but can be used for other analyses. Additional aliquots of 20–60 ml are injected and aspirated for sampling. The total volume of saline injected should be at least 140 ml.

Lung biopsy

This may be indicated when empirical treatment and other investigations are unsuccessful, and histological examination is required. Transtracheal biopsy is performed with bronchscopy and forceps, but has a lower diagnostic yield and higher risk of pneumothorax and haemorrhage than an open lung biopsy.

Management

General supportive measures

Oxygen and intravenous fluids are given. Mechanical ventilatory support is instituted when indicated (see Chapter 26).

Antibiotics

Until the organism is known antibiotics are given on a best-guess basis. A guide is given in Table 33.4[1,17] but requires modifications for local variations in prevalence and antibiotic sensitivity.

Hospital-acquired pneumonia

This is generally defined as pneumonia developing more than 2–3 days after admission to hospital.[18] It occurs in 0.5–5.0% of hospital patients, with a higher incidence in certain groups (e.g. postoperative patients and patients in ICU). Diagnosis may be difficult; clinical features of pneumonia are non-specific and many non-infectious conditions (e.g. atelectasis, pulmonary embolus, aspiration, congestive heart failure and cancer) can cause infiltrates on a chest X-ray. Identification of the organism responsible is even more difficult than community-acquired pneumonia, due to frequent colonization of the oropharynx by Gram-negative bacteria. Approximately 30–40% of non-critically ill and 70–75% of moribund and chronically ill patients become colonized within 48 h. Blood cultures are only positive in about 6 of cases of nosocomial pneumonia.

Pathogenesis

Nosocomial pneumonia is thought to result from aspiration of bacteria colonizing the upper respiratory tract and stomach.[19] It is postulated that antacids and H_2 antagonists (used to prevent stress ulceration) increase the risk, by allowing bacterial overgrowth in the stomach, which subsequently colonize the oropharynx and trachea.[20] However, there are doubts on this theory.[21]

Ventilator-associated pneumonia is a proposed subset of hospital-acquired pneumonia.[22,23] It has a much higher incidence of *Pseudomonas* and *Acinetobacter* pneumonia (Table 33.1). It is defined by a new or persistent pulmonary infiltrate on chest X-ray and purulent tracheal secretions in a ventilated patient plus one other criterion. To make a definitive diagnosis, this criterion may be:

1 radiographic evidence of pulmonary abscess and positive needle aspirate culture from the abscess or
2 histological evidence of pneumonia in lung tissue obtained by open lung biopsy *plus* positive quantitative culture of lung parenchyma (i.e. >10 000 microorganisms/g lung tissue).

Table 33.4 Empirical antibiotics for community-acquired pneumonia[1,17]

Type of patient or situation	Comments	Drugs of choice	Alternatives
Most patients	Must cover *Streptococcus pneumoniae*	Amoxycillin 250–500 t.d.s.	Erythromycin *or* co-trimoxazole
Elderly, and chronic lung disease	*Haemophilus influenzae* possible	Amoxycillin 250–500 t.d.s.	Co-trimoxazole
As above but ampicillin-resistant *Haemophilus influenzae* or *Branhaemella catarrhalis* prevalent locally		Cefuroxime	Co-amoxiclav *or* co-trimoxazole
Young, healthy patient, *Mycoplasma* epidemic, little change with aminopenicillin or epidemiological clues	*Mycoplasma* or other atypical infection possible	Erythromycin 500 mg q.d.s.	Tetracycline *or* ciprofloxacin
During influenza epidemic	*Staphylococcus aureus* possible	Co-amoxiclav ± cloxacillin	Co-trimoxazole
Cavitating lesions		Cefuroxime and metronidazole	
Severe community-acquired pneumonia	Cover *Streptococcus pneumoniae, Haemophilus influenza, Mycoplasma, Staphylococcus* and *Legionella*	Cefuroxime or cefatazdime and erythromycin ± gentamicin	Ampicillin, erythromycin and cloxacillin *or* co-amoxiclav and erythromycin

To diagnose probable ventilator-associated pneumonia, this criterion may be one of the following:

1 positive quantitative culture of a sample of lower respiratory tract secretions obtained by a technique which minimizes contamination with upper respiratory tract flora;
2 positive blood culture unrelated to another source, and obtained within 48 h before and after respiratory sampling. The microorganism recovered should be identical to the organism recovered from a culture of lower respiratory tract secretions;
3 positive pleural fluid culture in the absence of previous pleural instrumentation. The microorganism recovered should be identical to the organism recovered from a culture of lower respiratory tract secretions;
4 histological evidence of pneumonia in lung tissue obtained by open lung biopsy or postmortem examination immediately after death, but *negative* quantitative culture of lung parenchyma (i.e. < 10 000 microorganisms/g lung tissue).

Investigations[24,25]

Accurate microbiological diagnosis is important, as the prognosis of nosocomial pneumonia is probably improved by appropriate antibiotics.[26] Microbiological analysis of expectorated sputum and endotracheal aspirates is of little value, although results from protected brush endotracheal sampling and quantitative culture are more promising. The presence of *Staphylococcus aureus* in the sputum is a more reliable indicator of *S. aureus* pneumonia than the presence of Gram-negative bacteria is of Gram-negative pneumonia.

Techniques for collection of distal airway secretions include aspiration, brushing and bronchoalveolar lavage. These can be performed blindly via an endotracheal tube or under direct bronchoscopic vision. Blind techniques are less invasive, available to patients with small-diameter endotracheal tubes, and have less effect on gas exchange. However, there is an inherent risk of sampling errors. None the less, correlation between blind and bronchoscopic techniques is good. Bronchoscopic techniques are discussed above.

Management

Possible antimicrobial regimens (Table 33.5)[26] must be modified for local variations in prevalence and antibiotic sensitivity. Granulocyte-stimulating factor improves survival in animals with bacterial infections, and human clinical studies are currently in progress.[27]

Prevention

Simple measures such as hand-washing are the most effective means of preventing nosocomial pneumonia. Other proposed measures includes elective decontamination of the digestive tract, use of sucralfate stress ulcer prophylaxis and aspiration of subglottic

Table 33.5 Recommendations for empiric antimicrobial treatment of nosocomial pneumonia[20]

Situation	Likely organisms	Therapeutic options
No specific risk factors, mild–moderate illness	Core organisms: *Staphylococcus aureus* *Klebsiella* spp. *Enterobacter* spp. *Escherichia coli* *Proteus* spp. *Serratia marcescens* *Haemophilus influenzae*	Core antibiotics: Cefazolin plus gentamicin Second-generation cephalosporin (cefuroxime) Non-pseudomonal third-generation cephalosporin (e.g. cefotaxime) β-Lactam/β-lactamase inhibitor (e.g. ampicillin/sulbactam) Fluoroquinoline (e.g. ciprofloxacin)
Mild–moderate illness with specific risk factors		
Gross aspiration or thoracoabdominal surgery	Core organisms plus anaerobes	Core antibiotics plus clindamycin or metronidazole *or* β-lactam/β-lactamase inhibitor alone (e.g. ampicillin/sulbactam or ticarcillin/clavulanic acid)
Diabetes, coma, head injury	Core organisms especially *Staphylococcus aureus*	Core antibiotics plus vancomycin if methicillin-resistant infection likely
High-dose corticosteroids	Core organisms plus *Legionella* spp.	Core antibiotics plus a macrolide (e.g. erythromycin)
Multiple risk factors, including prior antibiotics, prolonged hospital admission, ICU stay	Core organisms plus *Pseudomonas aeruginosa*	Treat as severe pneumonia
Severe pneumonia	Core organisms plus *Pseudomonas aeruginosa* and *Acinetobacter* spp.	Antipseudomonal penicillin (e.g. piperacillin) plus aminoglycoside *or* antipseudomonal third-generation cephalosporin (e.g. ceftazidime) plus aminoglycoside *or* imipenem/cilastin

ICU = Intensive care unit.

secretions. A meta-analysis of selective decontamination reported a reduced incidence of nosocomial pneumonia but with no effect on mortality.[28] Sucralfate is associated with a lower incidence of nosocomial pneumonia than ranitidine or antacids in some, but not all, studies.[29,30] Aspiration of subglottic secretions which pool above the cuff of the endotracheal tube may reduce the incidence of ventilator-associated pneumonia.[31]

Fungal pneumonia[32]

Fungi are rare but important causes of pneumonia. They can be divided into two main groups based on the immune response required to combat infection. *Histoplasma*, blastomycosis, coccidioidomycosis, paracoccidioidomycosis, and *Cryptococcus* require specific cell-mediated immunity for their control. In contrast to infections controlled by phagocytic activity, these organisms can infect otherwise healthy individuals (although more severely in patients with impaired cell-mediated immunity, e.g. organ transplant recipients and HIV patients). With the exception of *Cryptococcus* these organisms are rarely seen outside North America.

Aspergillus and *Mucor* spores are killed by non-immune phagocytes, and rarely result in clinical illness in individuals with normal neutrophils. Candidiasis is effectively a combination of the two types of fungal infection. Impaired cell-mediated immunity predisposes to mucosal overgrowth with *Candida*, but impaired phagocytic function is usually required before deep invasion of tissues occurs. Primary *Candida* pneumonia (i.e. isolated lung infection) is uncommon.[32]

Tuberculosis

Tuberculosis (TB) is undergoing a worldwide resurgence, exacerbated by the appearance of strains

Table 33.6 Risk factors for pulmonary tuberculosis

Living in or originating from a developing country
Age (<5 years, middle-aged and elderly men)
Alcoholism and/or drug addiction
Human immunodeficiency virus infection
Diabetes mellitus
Lodging-house dwellers
Immunosuppression
Close contact with smear-positive patients
Silicosis
Poverty and/or malnutrition
Previous gastrectomy
Smoking

resistant to first-line therapy.[33] The main risk factors are listed in Table 33.6.

Clinical presentation

Vague ill health over weeks, lassitude, anorexia, weight loss, fever and cough (with mucoid, purulent or blood-stained sputum) are typical features. The patient may complain of chest wall pain, night sweats and frequent 'colds'. Signs may include dypsnoea, localized wheeze, apical crackles, pleural effusions, spontaneous pneumothorax, and hoarseness with enlarged cervical nodes or other manifestations of extrapulmonary disease. Clinical disease is seldom found in asymptomatic individuals, even those with strongly positive tuberculin test (Heaf grade III or IV). Older patients, who may have coexistent chronic bronchitis, can be missed unless a chest X-ray is taken. The prognosis of TB patients requiring ICU admission is poor, with a mortality of 67% rising to 81% if accompanied by acute respiratory failure.[34]

Investigations[35]

Isolation of Mycobacteria

Multiple sputum samples should be collected for microscopy for acid-fast bacilli (Ziehl–Neelsen stain) and culture. Bronchial washings taken at bronchoscopy and gastric lavage samples should be obtained if sputum is not available. Bronchoscopy and transbronchial biopsy may be useful in suspected patients with negative sputum results. A pleural biopsy may be helpful. Mediastinoscopy may be needed in patients with mediastinal lymphadenopathy. A part of any biopsy specimen should always be sent for culture.

Chest X-ray

A normal chest film almost excludes TB except in HIV-infected patients, but endobronchial lesions may not be apparent and early apical lesions can be missed. Common appearances include patchy/nodular shadowing in the upper zones (often bilateral),

cavitation, calcification, hilar or mediastinal lymphadenopathy (in the primary complex and may cause segmental or lobar collapse), pleural effusion, dense round or oval shadows (tuberculomas), and diffuse fine nodular infiltrates in miliary TB. Chest X-ray alone cannot infer inactivity of disease. This requires three negative sputum samples and failure of any lesion on chest film to progress. Chest X-ray appearances in HIV-positive patients with TB differ from non-HIV-infected patients.

Management[36]

Drug treatment for 6 months is most important. Long hospitalization is not usually required. Bed rest does not affect outcome. the 6-month drug regimen is:

1 Rifampicin 600 mg (450 mg if <50 kg weight) and
2 isoniazid 300 mg, both taken daily 30 min before breakfast.

For the first 2 months, this combination is supplemented daily with:

1 pyrazinamide 2.0 g (1.5 g if <50 kg weight) and
2 ethambutol 25 mg/kg.

Steroids are also recommended for severely ill patients and to treat severe drug reactions.[36] Liver and renal function should be checked before starting treatment, and visual acuity must be assessed if ethambutol is to be used (i.e. causes dose-related retrobulbar neuritis). Ethambutol is not necessary for patients at low risk of infection with resistant organisms.

Pneumonia in the immunocompromised

Lungs are frequent target organs for infectious complications in the immunocompromised. The incidence of pneumonia is highest amongst patients with haematological malignancies, bone marrow transplant recipients and patients with acquired immunodeficiency syndrome (AIDS).

Possible infective organisms and causes of fever and lung infiltrates in immunocompromised patients are shown in Tables 33.1 and 33.7. The speed of progression of pneumonia may suggest the aetiology (e.g. bacterial pneumonias progress rapidly in 1–2 days, while fungal and protozoal pneumonias take days to weeks). Viral pneumonias are usually not fulminant, but may develop rapidly.

Management

Empirical treatment is based on the chest X-ray findings. The EORTC regimen may be used for the febrile neutropenic patient.[37] Broad-spectrum antibiotics of a third-generation cephalosporin and aminoglycoside (e.g. ceftriaxone 30 mg/kg and amikacin

Table 33.7 Causes of fever and pulmonary infiltrates in immunocompromised patients

Focal infiltrates	Diffuse infiltrates
Gram-negative rods	Bacteria (uncommon)
Staphylococcus aureus	Cytomegalovirus
Tuberculosis	Herpesviruses
Aspergillus	*Aspergillus* (advanced)
Cryptococcus	*Cryptococcus* (uncommon)
Pneumocystis carinii (uncommon)	*Pneumocystis carinii*
Nocardia	Leukoagglutinin reaction
Legionella or legionella-like organisms	Pulmonary infarction
Mucor	Pulmonary haemorrhage
Malignancy	Malignancy
Non-specific interstitial pneumonitis	Non-specific interstitial pneumonitis
Radiation pneumonitis	Radiation pneumonitis (uncommon)
	Drug reaction
	Bleomycin
	Cyclophosphamide
	Busulphan (after very long periods of treatment)
	Bis-chloroethylnitrosurea (BCNU)
	Cyclohexylnitrosurea (CCNU)
	Mitamycin
	Chlorambucil
	Melphalan
	Procarbazine

20 mg/kg IV daily) are given and reevaluated after 72 h:

1 if fever subsides, the antibiotics are continued for up to 1–2 weeks;
2 if fever persists, but the patient is improving, the antibiotics are continued for 7 days and amphotericin B is added if the patient is still febrile;
3 if the patient deteriorates, vancomycin is added, and amphotericin B is added on day 7.

Co-trimoxazole plus erythromycin is added to the initial regimen if the chest infiltrate is diffuse. Vancomycin is indicated if methicillin-resistant *Staphylococcus aureus* is a problem, or if coagulase-negative staphylococcus is probable (e.g. patients with indwelling central venous catheters). Ceftazidime 33 mg/kg 8-hourly is substituted for ceftriaxone if *Pseudomonas* spp. are a concern. Monotherapy ceftazadime has recently been shown to be as effective as, and safer than, a standard piperacillin/tobramycin combination empirical therapy in febrile neutropenic patients.[38] Invasive procedures to obtain microbiological samples (discussed above) may be used in 48–72 h if the patient can tolerate the procedure.

Pneumonia in patients with HIV infection[39–43]

Pneumocystis carinii pneumonia (PCP)

This is the most common opportunistic infection in AIDS patients in Europe and North America, but is unusual in Africa. Onset is insidious in a background of fatigue and weight loss. Dry cough, breathlessness, tachypnoea, and fever are common. Sputum production and chest crackles are rare. Cyanosis is present in severe cases. Recently, the prognosis of these patients admitted to ICU has improved markedly, with survival to hospital discharge being 38–55%. The mean survival time after hospital discharge in most studies is 7–10 months, but a recent study found that 74% are alive at 1 year. The length of ICU stay appears to be unrelated to outcome.

Useful investigations in patients with suspected PCP are:

1 *Chest X-ray*: this may show diffuse bilateral perihilar interstitial shadowing. In early stages this is very subtle and easily missed. Radiological changes are not specific for PCP, and may be seen in other lung diseases associated with AIDS. Chest X-ray may be normal in 10% and atypical in another 10% with focal consolidation of coarse patchy shadowing. Pleural effusions and hilar or mediastinal lymphadenopathy are unusual in PCP, but common in mycobacterial infection, lymphoma or Kaposi's saroma.
2 *Induced sputum*: Neubulized hypertonic 3% saline is inhaled to provoke bronchorrhoea and coughing; coughed material contain cysts and trophozoites. It is time-consuming and requires meticulous care, but may obviate the need for bronchoscopy.
3 *Bronchoscopy and bronchoalveolar lavage* lead to cytological diagnosis in over 90%. Transbronchial biopsy is not necessary in most cases.

Treatment is started as soon as diagnosis is suspected. Response to treatment of the first episode is generally good, with a mortality under 10%. Azidothymidine (AZT) is stopped as AZT and anti-PCP treatment are myelotoxic. First-line agents are *either*

1 trimethoprim plus sulphamethoxazole (co-trimoxazole) – the treatment of choice. Side-effects are common (i.e. nausea, vomiting, skin rash and myelotoxicity). Dose is (20 mg : 100 mg)/kg per day for 3 weeks. if white cell count falls, dose is reduced by 25%
    plus
    glucocorticoids; to begin at the onset of anti-PCP therapy. Prednisolone 40 mg orally b.d. is given for 5 days, followed by 20 mg b.d. for 5 days, and then 20 mg daily until the end of anti-PCP treatment
    or
2 pentamidine 4 mg/kg per day IV for 3 weeks; this has more severe side-effects (i.e. hypoglycaemia, hyperglycaemia, pancreatitis, nephrotoxicity, and hepatotoxicity)
    plus
    glucocorticoids, as the same regimen above.

Second-line drugs are:

1 clindamycin (600 mg q.d.s.–900 mg t.d.s. IV) plus primaquine 15–30 mg base orally daily) *or*
2 trimetrexate (45 mg/m^2 IV plus leucovorin (20 mg/ m^2 IV q.d.s.).

Bacterial pneumonia

This is the most common cause of acute respiratory failure in HIV positive patients. Bacterial pneumonia is more common in HIV-infected patients than in the general population, and tends to be more severe. *Streptococcus pneumoniae, Haemophilus influenzae, Branhamella catarrhalis* and *Staphylococcus aureus* are the commonest organisms. *Nocardia* and Gram-negative organisms should also be considered. Response to appropriate antibiotics is usually good, but may require protracted courses of antibiotics because of a high tendency to relapse.

Tuberculosis

TB may be the initial presentation of AIDS. The pattern of TB in HIV-positive patients is more commonly lymphatic or disseminated. Pulmonary disease is more commonly non-cavitatory and sputum smear-negative. It often presents with unusual features. The chest X-ray often shows atypical features, and the tuberculin test may be negative. Response to treatment is usually rapid.

Cytomegalovirus (CMV) pneumonitis

CMV is often isolated from lung washings, but only occasionally causes pneumonitis (cf. transplant patients).

Empyema[44,45]

Empyema is a collection of pus in the pleural space. It is a complication of chest trauma or infection of structures surrounding the pleural space, including subdiaphragmatic structures. Diagnosis is usually simple. The patient is 'toxic' with a productive cough and chest pain. The chest X-ray has a characteristic appearance with a posterior D-shaped opacity extending to the hemidiaphragm. Confirmation of the diagnosis can be obtained by aspirating pus. The mainstay of treatment is drainage by intercostal drain or by surgery (open or thoracoscopically). The latter is thought to be suitable for acute loculated empyema. Antibiotics have only an adjunctive role. Broad-spectrum antibiotic regimens with anaerobic cover should be used until the results of microbiological identification are available.

Lung abscess

This is a localized cavitating suppuration, often with a fluid level, seen on chest X-ray. The commonest cause is aspiration, but lung abscesses may develop from pneumonias, particularly if caused by *Staphylococcus* or *Klebsiella pneumoniae*. Other abscess may be due to TB or an infected cavitating carcinoma. Clinical features include worsening pneumonia, rigors, foul-smelling sputum and finger clubbing. Invasive techniques may be required for microbiological examinations. Treatment is physiotherapy and antibiotics for aerobic and anaerobic organisms, as there is usually a mixed flora. Prolonged courses may be necessary. Surgery may be indicated.

References

1 Woodhead MA (1992) Management of pneumonia. *Respir Med* **86**:459–469.
2 Woodhead MA, Macfarlane JT, Rodgers FG, Laverick A, Pilkington R and Macrae AD (1985) Aetiology and outcome of severe community acquired pneumonia. *J Infection* **10**:204–210.
3 Horan T, Culver D, Jarvis W *et al.* (1988) Pathogens causing nosocomial infections. *Antimicrob Newslett* **5**:657.
4 Farr BM, Kaiser DL, Harrison BDW and Connolly CK (1989) Prediction of microbial aetiology at admission to hospital for pneumonia from the presenting clinical features. *Thorax* **44**:1031–1035.
5 Woodhead MA and Macfarlane JT (1987) *Haemophilus*

influenzae pneumonia in previously fit adults. *Eur J Respir Dis* **70:**218–220.

6 Foy HM, Cooney MK, Allan I and Kenny GE (1979) Rates of pneumonia during influenza epidemics in Seattle, 1964–1975. *JAMA* **241:**253–258.

7 Report from the PHLS Communicable Disease Surveillance Centre (1987) *Br Med J* **295:**1123–1125.

8 Woodhead MA, Radvan J and Macfarlane JT (1987) Adult community acquired staphylococcal pneumonia in the antibiotic era: a review of 61 cases. *Q J Med* **64:**783–790.

9 Verghese A and Berk SL (1983) Bacterial pneumonia in the elderly. *Medicine (Baltimore)* **62:**271–285.

10 Venkatesan P, Gladman J, Macfarlane JT *et al.* (1990) A hospital study of community acquired pneumonia in the elderly. *Thorax* **45:**25–48.

11 Woodhead MA and Macfarlane JT (1987) Comparative clinical and laboratory features of legionella with pneumococcal and *Mycoplasma* pneumonias. *Br J Dis Chest* **81:**133–139.

12 Fang G-D, Fine M, Orloff J *et al.* (1990) New and emerging etiologies for community acquired pneumonia with implications for therapy. A prospective multicenter study of 359 cases. *Medicine* **69:**307–316.

13 British Thoracic Society (1987) Community-acquired pneumonia in adults in British hospitals in 1982–1983: a survey of aetiology, mortality, prognostic factors and outcome. *Q J Med* **62:**195–220.

14 Torres A, Jimenez P, de la Bellacosa JP, Celis R, Gonzalez J and Gea J (1990) Diagnostic value of non-fluoroscopic percutaneous lung needle aspiration in patients with pneumonia.*Chest* **98:**840–844.

15 Macfarlane JT and Ward MJ (1984) Transtracheal injection of saline in the investigation of pneumonia. *Br Med J* **288:**974–975.

16 Meduri GU and Chastre J (1992) The standardization of bronchoscopic techniques for ventilator-associated pneumonia. *Chest* **102** (suppl):557S–564S.

17 British Thoracic Society (1993) Guidelines for the management of community-acquired pneumonia in adults admitted to hospital. *Br J Hosp Med* **49:**346–350.

18 Scheld WM (1991) Developments in the pathogenesis, diagnosis and treatment of nosocomial pneumonia. *Surg Gynecol Obstet* **172** (suppl):42–53.

19 Dal Nogare AR (1994) Nosocomial pneumonia in the medical and surgical patient. *Med Clin North Am* **78(5):**1081–1090.

20 du Moulin GC, Paterson DG, Hedley-Whyte J *et al.* (1982) Aspiration of gastric bacteria in antacid-treated patients: a frequent cause of postoperative colonization of the airway. *Lancet* **1:**24–25.

21 Bonten MJM, Gaillard CA, van Tiel FH, Smeets HG, van der Geest S and Stobberingh EE (1994) The stomach is not a source for colonization of the upper respiratory tract and pneumonia in ICU patients. *Chest* **105:**878–884.

22 Pingleton SK and Leeper KV (1992) Patient selection for clinical investigation of ventilator-associated pneumonia. Criteria for evaluating diagnostic techniques. *Chest* **102** (suppl 1):553S–556S.

23 Fagon J-Y, Chastre J, Domart Y *et al.* (1989) Nosocomial pneumonia in patients receiving continuous mechanical ventilation. *Am Rev Respir Dis* **139:**877–884.

24 Griffin JJ and Meduri GU (1994) New approaches in the diagnosis of nosocomial pneumonia. *Med Clin N Am* **78:**1091–1122.

25 Scheld WM and Mandell GL (1991) Nosocomial pneumonia: pathogenesis and recent advances in diagnosis and therapy. *Rev Infect Dis* **13** (suppl 9): S743–S751.

26 Niederman MS (1994) An approach to empiric therapy of nosocomial pneumonia. *Med Clin N Am* **78:**1123–1141.

27 Nelson S (1994) Role of granulocyte colony-stimulating factor in the immune response to acute bacterial infection in the nonneutropenic host: an overview. *Clin Infect Dis* **18** (suppl 2):S197–S204.

28 Heyland DK, Cook DJ, Jaeschke R, Griffith L, Lee HN, Guyatt GH (1994) Selective decontamination of the digestive tract. *Chest* **105:**1221–1229.

29 Prodhom G, Leuenberger P, Koerfoer J *et al* (1994) Nosocomial pneumonia in mechanically ventilated patients receiving antacid, ranitidine, or sucralfate as prophylaxis for stress ulcer. *Ann Intern Med* **120:**653–662.

30 Fabian TC, Boucher BA, Cruce MA *et al.* (1993) Pneumonia and stress ulceration in severely injured patients. A prospective evaluation of the effects of stress ulcer prophylaxis. *Arch Surg* **128:**185–191.

31 Mahul P, Auboyer C, Jospe R *et al.* (1992) Prevention of nosocomial pneumonia in intubated patients: respective role of mechanical subglottic secretions drainage and stress ulcer prophylaxis. *Intensive Care Med* **18:**20—25.

32 Haron E, Vartivarian S, Anaissie E, Dekmezian R and Bodey GP (1993) Primary *Candida* pneumonia. Experience at a large cancer center and review of the literature. *Medicine* **72:**137–142.

33 Frieden TR, Sterling T, Pablos-Mendez A, Kilburn JO, Cauthen GM and Dooley SW (1993) The emergence of drug resistant tuberculosis in New York City. *N Engl J Med* **328:**521–526.

34 Frame RN, Johnson M, Eichenhorn MS, Bower GC and Popovich J (1987) Active tuberculosis in the medical intensive care unit: a 15 year retrospective analysis. *Crit Care Med* **15:**1012–1014.

35 Schluger NW and Rom WN (1974) Current approaches to the diagnosis of active pulmonary tuberculosis. *Am J Respir Crit Care Med* **149:**264–267.

36 Ormerod L (1990) Chemotherapy and management of tuberculosis in the United Kingdom: recommendations of the Joint Tuberculosis Committee of the British Thoracic Society. *Thorax* **45:**403–408.

37 The International Antimicrobial Therapy Cooperative Group of the EORTC (1993) Efficacy and toxicity of single daily doses of amikacin and ceftriaxone versus multiple daily doses of amikacin and ceftazidime for infection in patients with cancer and granulocytopenia. *Ann Intern Med* **119:**584–593.

38 De Pauw BE, Deresinski SC, Feld R *et al.* (1994) Ceftazidime compared with piperacillin and tobramycin for the empiric treatment of fever in neutropenic patients with cancer: a multicenter randomized trial. *Ann Intern*

Med **120:** 834–844.

39 Rosen MJ (1994) Pneumonia in patients with HIV infection. *Med Clin N Am* **78:**1067–1079.

40 Wachter RM, Luce JM and Hopewell PC (1992) Critical care of patients with AIDS. *JAMA* **267:**541–547.

41 Lane HC, Laughton BE, Falloon J *et al.* (1994) Recent advances in the management of AIDS-related opportunistic infections. *Ann Intern Med* **120:**945–955.

42 White DA and Zaman MK (1992) Pulmonary disease.

Med Clin N Am **76:**19–44.

43 Bernard EM, Sepkowitz KA, Telzak EE and Armstrong D (1992) Pneumocystosis. *Med Clin N Am* **76:**107–119.

44 Odell JA (1994) Management of empyema thoracis. *J Roy Soc Med* **87:**466–470.

45 Ferguson MK (1993) Thoracoscopy for empyema, bronchopleural fistula, and chylothorax. *Ann Thorac Surg* **56:**644–645.

34 | Aspiration syndromes

DJ Cooper

Aspiration of fluid and/or solids into the lower respiratory tract is a common clinical problem. Aspiration is causative in about 25% of patients with acute respiratory distress syndrome,[1] and usually has a high mortality (40–60%). Outcome depends on the volume and type of aspirate, associated clinical conditions and possibly therapy.[2]

Aetiology

Normal breathing, speaking and swallowing are accompanied by efficient defence mechanisms against aspiration. Aspiration can only occur when these defences are overwhelmed,[1] and when fluids or solids are present in the pharynx.[2] Passive regurgitation may occur whenever there is decreased conscious state or decreased cough and gag reflexes. Table 34.1 lists conditions which increase the risk of aspiration of gastric contents.

Wide-bore nasogastric tubes prevent the closure of both upper and lower oesophageal sphincters, and so impair coughing and clearing of the pharynx. Endotracheal intubation protects against large-volume aspiration, but may predispose to micro-aspiration of small volumes of pharyngeal fluid collecting below the vocal cords and above the endotracheal tube cuff. This fluid may enter the lung; consequently, bacterial colonization of endotracheal aspirates in intubated critically ill patients is almost universal. Microaspiration does not cause major lung injury, but has been suggested as an aetiological factor in nosocomial pneumonia.[3,4]

Pathophysiology

Aspiration of solids

Aspiration of foreign bodies is a common cause of accidental death in children under 1 year of age. Large inhaled particles (e.g. partly masticated meat) may also

Table 34.1 Conditions with aspiration risk

Decreased conscious states
Head trauma
Drug (or alcohol) overdose
Anaesthesia
Sepsis
Metabolic coma
Seizures
Hypoxia, hypercapnia
Cerebrovascular accidents

Impaired cough and gag reflexes
Recent extubation of larynx
Guillain–Barré syndrome, myasthenia, multiple sclerosis, motor neurone disease
Neck or pharyngeal trauma and surgery
Elderly patients

Passive regurgitation
Pregnancy
Emergency surgery with full stomach and for bowel obstruction
Nasogastric tubes
Gastro-oesophageal reflux
Oesophagectomy
Oesophageal obstruction
Achalasia, scleroderma
Raised intra-abdominal pressure (e.g. with succinylcholine)

be immediately life-threatening in adults by causing major airway obstruction. Patients are typically unable to speak or breathe and immediate removal (e.g. Heimlich manoeuvre) is required (see Chapter 25).

Smaller objects may cause partial airway obstruction. Examples include bone, teeth or amalgam fragments (e.g. after facial trauma), peanuts, children's toys, gravel and coins. These smaller inhaled objects may cause atelectasis distal to the obstruction. Some irritative particles (e.g. meat, vegetable products) may cause a localized peritonitis which may progress to bronchiectasis. The inflammatory reaction is initially a neutrophilic response which then progresses to a granulomatous reaction with macrophages and giant cells appearing from 48 to 72 h.[5] By 21 days, there remains a patchy bronchiolitis, some residual granulomas and minimal residual fibrosis. Non-obstructive particulate aspiration (e.g. fine food particles) causes a clinical and radiological picture similar to that of acid aspiration.

Aspiration of liquids

Acid aspiration

Acid aspiration causes extensive lung damage. Lung injury is dependent upon aspirate volume and pH. The most severe injury to the respiratory epithelium occurs with an aspirate pH < 2.5,[6] and 100% mortality is reported in patients with gastric pH < 1.8 at the time of aspiration.[7] Similar but less severe pulmonary injury occurs with aspiration of gastric contents having a pH > 2.5.[8]

Gastric contents in previously healthy patients are acidic and free from microbial colonization. Infection is not important in the early stages of acid aspiration lung injury.[6,9,10] Initial tracheal cultures are usually negative, although later airway colonization often occurs. Severe dyspnoea and shock following major aspiration of gastric contents with pH < 2.5 is termed Mendelson's syndrome.[11] Acid aspiration causes immediate vagally-mediated bronchospasm, followed by damage within minutes[10] to the alveolar epithelium and endothelium, and atelectasis from surfactant dysfunction. Fluid and protein leak into the alveoli and bronchi occurs immediately, becoming severe in about an hour, and is manifest clinically as permeability pulmonary oedema. Alveolar consolidation then progresses with polymorphonuclear infiltration. Hyaline membrane formation occurs by 48 h, and the acute inflammatory reaction usually resolves by 72 h.[9]

Non-acid liquid aspiration

Aspiration of blood, isotonic solutions and salt or fresh water produces limited pulmonary injury which typically resolves over several days. However, large-volume aspirations (e.g. near drowning) may be associated with severe pulmonary dysfunction, due to shunting, surfactant damage and wash-out, and alveolar collapse with oedema formation.[12,13]

Aspiration of infected fluids

Initial damage following infected fluid aspiration is similar to that following acid aspiration, but respiratory tract infection and pneumonia supervene. Later changes depend on the volume of aspirate and the efficacy of antibiotic treatment. Aspiration may be either macroscopic or microscopic. Macroscopic

Table 34.2 Lung colonization patterns following aspiration

Previously well, non-hospitalized	Previously unwell, hospitalized, antacid use
Anaerobes/aerobes = 10/1	Gram-negative and opportunists
Bacteroides melanogenicus	*Escherichia coli, Klebsiella* spp.
Fusobacterium nucleatum	*Pseudomonas* spp., *Proteus* spp.
Peptostreptococcus spp.	Other enteric flora
Bacteroides fragilis and *B. oralis*	*Staphylococcus aureus*
Microaerophilic streptococci	*Candida albicans*
Pneumococcus spp.	Anaerobes

aspiration is less common, but in ill patients, a heavy inoculum of pathogenic bacteria may cause infection, and necrotizing bacterial pneumonia may occur.[14] Infective organisms depend on the clinical background of the host. In non-hospitalized patients, anaerobic oral flora sensitive to penicillin dominate, whereas cultures of hospitalized patients are dominated by gastrointestinal Gram-negative aerobes and anaerobes (Table 34.2).

Microscopic aspiration is more common in critically ill patients. Bacterial colonization of gastric contents is universal within 4 days of commencing antacids or H_2 antagonists for gastric ulcer prevention.[15] Organisms are predominantly Gram-negatives and anaerobes (i.e. overgrowth of bowel flora), but colonization of oral flora also occurs;[15,16] *Candida* sp. has also been reported.[15] Microaspiration of these gastric organisms to the lower respiratory tract can be demonstrated in 50–80% of patients,[4,16] and is encouraged by impaired peristalsis (e.g. by drugs) and sphincter action (by nasogastric tube), supine position and the endotracheal tube (with pooling of secretions above the cuff).

Aspiration of hydrocarbons

Almost 20% of aspiration accidents in children under 5 years involve hydrocarbons (e.g. kerosene, petrol and furniture polish). Pulmonary damage results from dissolution of membrane lipids and surfactant inactivation.[17] Large aspirates are associated with pulmonary oedema and haemoptysis.

Clinical presentation

In acute aspiration syndromes, there is often a history of vomiting or evidence of vomitus, blood or secretions around the mouth. However, their absence does not exclude the diagnosis. Acute aspiration is typically manifested by a sudden onset of cough, dyspnoea, wheeze, tachypnoea, stridor, crepitations, rhonchi, cyanosis, hypotension, tachycardia and fever. Risk factors (Table 34.1) are usually present.

Chronic recurrent aspiration is most commonly seen in patients with subtle abnormalities of bulbar function, and may present with an insidious deterioration of respiratory function in association with intermittent respiratory symptoms and signs. There may be a history of coughing or choking after food or fluid ingestion. Careful neurological examination is required if the risk factor for aspiration is not obvious.

Acute aspiration of obstructive solids leads rapidly to hypoxaemia and death if the obstruction is not relieved. The patient is unable to speak or breathe. Aspiration of smaller, partially obstructive solids presents with dyspnoea, persistent coughing, wheeze and stridor, and various degrees of hypoxaemia. Wheezing may be due both to the inhaled object and to reflex bronchospasm. If inhaled solids are not removed, secondary infection, necrotizing pneumonia, abscess formation and empyema may result. Chronic infection (e.g. bronchiectasis) often then develops. Chest X-ray will commonly show focal consolidation or collapse and radiopaque obstructing particles.

Acid aspiration in large volumes produces Mendelson's syndrome, characterized by severe dyspnoea, wheeze, hypoxaemia and shock.[18] Exudation of protein-rich fluid into the alveoli leads to pulmonary oedema and a fall in dynamic compliance, often accompanied by hypovolaemia and hypotension. Chest X-ray usually shows diffuse bilateral pulmonary infiltrates (more marked at the lung bases) frequently indistinguishable from the acute respiratory distress syndrome (ARDS). Importantly, acid aspiration is also a precipitant of ARDS. The clinical course is characterized by severe pulmonary injury requiring prolonged mechanical ventilation with high inspired oxygen concentrations (Fio_2) and positive end-expiratory pressure (PEEP). Sepsis, multiple organ failure and mortality (25–100%) are all high, depending both on the severity of aspiration and the underlying disease states.

The clinical course of infected, non-acid aspiration depends on the volume of aspirate, efficacy of antibiotics and whether lower respiratory infection becomes established. Although initial hypoxia may be as severe as that of acid aspiration, initial alveolar injury is not as great, and hypotension and a prolonged ARDS-like picture are less common. The lung injury may gradually resolve or pneumonia may develop, giving rise to a more severe, prolonged illness.

With aspiration of other fluids, hydrocarbons cause severe pulmonary damage and ARDS, whereas non-acidic fluids (including blood) usually give rise to a rapidly resolving clinical course (over days) with few complications.

Diagnosis and investigations

In most cases, gastric aspiration is witnessed, and the diagnosis is confirmed by finding gastric contents in the airway or pharynx during endotracheal intubation and tracheal suction. If aspiration is not witnessed in a patient presenting with unexplained deteriorating respiratory function, a history of vomiting and presence of risk factors (Table 34.1) must be sought. Radiological findings of focal changes (in the right upper lob in supine aspiration, and the right middle and lower lobes in sitting or semirecumbent aspiration) suggest aspiration. In most patients, however, radiological appearances are non-specific, i.e. showing diffuse infiltrates, collapse or severe pulmonary oedema. Aspiration is commonly misdiagnosed as acute pulmonary oedema, asthma, sputum retention or ARDS, but the following interventions may assist in making the diagnosis:

1 endotracheal suctioning to detect gastric contents or acidic pH on specific testing. Aspirates should all be Gram-stained and cultured. Testing for glucose in aspirate samples is unreliable, and not useful;[19]
2 fibreoptic bronchoscopy to identify particulate matter;
3 clinical examination to detect laryngeal incompetence;
4 barium swallow in difficult diagnostic situations of recurrent aspiration.

Management

Immediate measures

The Heimlich manoeuvre is indicated in complete airway obstruction (see Chapter 25). With other aspiration, the patient is turned on to the right side and tilted head-downwards. This may localize aspiration to the right lung and prevent further aspiration. Suction and oxygenation can then be applied. If consciousness is reduced, the trachea is intubated and aspirated as quickly as possible. Inhaled fluid quickly disperses, but suction will clear any solid or semisolid material. Bronchoscopy should be performed if clinical and radiological signs of airway obstruction are present. If aspiration is minor, it is reasonable to rely on chest physiotherapy to clear the tracheobronchial tree. However, if significant respiratory distress is present, tracheal intubation and suction is indicated. A nasogastric tube to empty the stomach and reduce the risk of further aspiration is usually indicated. Bronchial lavage is not useful, because pulmonary epithelial damage occurs early and bronchial secretions quickly buffer any aspirated material.[20]

Oxygen therapy

A high Fio_2 should be used initially to ensure a safe Pao_2. Continuous pulse oximetry and arterial blood gases are used to monitor lung function.

Mechanical ventilatory support

There should be a low respiratory distress threshold for intubation and mechanical ventilation because delay may impair outcome.[21] PEEP is usually indicated to maintain alveolar recruitment after surfactant wash-out and inactivation, and to enable reductions in Fio_2. Tidal volumes of 5–7 ml/kg are recommended, as large tidal volumes are associated with pressure- and volume-mediated pulmonary damage in experimental aspiration pneumonia.[22]

Bronchodilator therapy

Bronchospasm may be severe in acid aspiration. Although bronchodilators are not very efficacious in this condition, inhaled β_2-adrenergic agents should be given. Aminophylline is usually not recommended, as additive bronchodilator effects are minimal and side-effects can be significant.

Cardiovascular support

In severe acid aspiration, an acute outpouring of protein-rich fluid into the lungs may reduce preload, impair cardiac output and cause severe hypotension. This is treated by expanding the intravascular volume. Crystalloids, colloids or blood are all suitable solutions, with 5% normal serum albumin, or Haemaccel being the most efficient. Pulmonary artery catheterization is indicated in severe cases. Whether optimal fluid management is achieved by generous fluid administration[2] or fluid restriction[23,24] is controversial. Pulmonary capillary wedge pressure (PCWP) must be individualized for each patient as that associated with an adequate cardiac output, best mixed venous oxygen saturation and adequate tissue perfusion. Fluid balance must be carefully monitored. Inotropic drugs are often necessary. Adrenaline (1–10 μg/min) or dopamine (5–20 μg/kg per min) is usually effective. Diuretics are indicated if an adequate cardiac output is associated with an elevated PCWP.

Bronchoscopy

Therapeutic bronchoscopy is indicated if there is particulate aspiration, focal pulmonary collapse suggesting large airway obstruction, or chest X-ray evidence of foreign bodies. Rigid bronchoscopy allows wide-bore suctioning and access of large grasping instruments, and is usually the procedure of choice to remove semisolid material and most inhaled objects. Flexible fibreoptic bronchoscopy, through an existing endotracheal tube, is usually the procedure for small solid particles (e.g. tooth or amalgam fragments).[25,26] Rigid bronchoscopy requires general anaesthesia and re-intubation, and is limited by its size and rigid nature.

Antibiotics

Prophylactic use of antibiotics without any sign of infection is controversial. Recommendations have been made against[2,27] and for their use, even despite uncertainty about their efficacy.[28,29] Use of antibiotics should be considered under three situations:

Out-of-hospital aspiration

This usually occurs in previously well patients and involves predominantly oral flora (Table 34.2). Penicillin-sensitive aerobes and anaerobes are frequently involved, but there is no evidence for improved outcome with prophylactic antibiotics.[27] Early antibiotic therapy may increase overgrowth of resistant organisms. Indeed, the best reported outcome for aspiration pneumonia used management which excluded early use of antibiotics.[2] Secondary bacterial infection, however, occurs in 20–30% of cases and requires specific antibiotic therapy. Broad-spectrum antibiotics should be started while awaiting culture results of specimens obtained from tracheal suctioning or protected brush catheters. Flucloxacillin and a third-generation cephalosporin (to cover Gram-negative organisms) and either clindamycin or metronidazole (to cover anaerobes) are appropriate combinations. Vancomycin and imipenem will provide better cover against hospital-acquired organisms and if methicillin-resistant *Staphylococcus aureus* is likely (see Chapters 33 and Chapter 64) when culture results are available, specific antibiotics should be instituted.

Infected fluid aspiration

This usually occurs in previously unwell, hospitalized patients. When faecal material is aspirated (e.g. in bowel obstruction) immediate broad-spectrum antibiotics are indicated. A combination of an aminoglycoside and clindamycin has been recommended,[30] but other combinations, particularly an aminoglycoside and imipenem, are equally efficient. Since use of antacids and H_2-antagonists is associated with colonization of gastric contents,[15] aspiration of gastric contents in ICU patients should be assumed to be infected and treated as such.

Secondary infection in obstructing particulate aspiration

Primary therapy remains relief of the obstructed airway and drainage of any infected fluid collections. However, the pathogenetic role of anaerobic bacteria in necrotizing pneumonia and empyema is well-accepted. Penicillin and clindamycin are equally efficacious.[31]

Corticosteroids

Steroids are not of proven benefit in any aspiration syndrome. They may slow pulmonary healing and are not recommended.[5,27]

Experimental approaches

Numerous recent innovative therapies for acute lung injury have been applied to patients with severe aspiration. These include exogenous surfactant, extracorporeal membrane oxygenation, intravascular oxygenator (IVOX), tracheal gas insufflation and systemic antioxidants. None has reached widespread clinical acceptance or application. In contrast, permissive hypercapnia has been widely adopted – both for aspiration pneumonia and for ARDS[32,33] (see Chapter 26).

Prevention

Posture

An unconscious patient should be placed in a head-down, semiprone position, until endotracheal intubation is achieved. Following intubation, nursing in a semirecumbent (45°) rather than supine position has recently been suggested to decrease microaspiration and airway colonization.[34]

Suction

Efficient suction must readily be available whenever unconscious patients are being nursed.

Cricoid pressure

During rapid-sequence induction of anaesthesia for endotracheal intubation in a patient at risk, cricoid pressure should be applied. Staff should be trained to apply this technique effectively and safely.[35] Awake intubation techniques should always be considered when difficulty with intubation is anticipated.

Airway protection

Endotracheal intubation or long-term tracheostomy should be instituted in patients unable to protect their airway or spontaneously clear pharyngeal fluids. Similar to endotracheal intubation, microaspiration commonly occurs with tracheostomies, and is associated with increased patient age.[36] Continuous aspiration of subglottic secretions (using a specially designed endotracheal tube incorporating a second lumen for suctioning) has recently been attempted.[37] The technique decreased the incidence of nosocomial pneumonia but did not influence patient outcome.[37] The laryngeal mask airway is now widely used in anaesthesia, but it does not protect against regurgitation and should not be used in patients at risk.[38]

Nasogastric tube

Although nasogastric tubes increase aspiration risk by impairing the efficiency of upper and lower oesophageal sphincters, they are essential in mechanically ventilated patients to prevent accumulation of gastric secretions. Nasogastric tubes must be aspirated regularly (2–4 h) and left on free drainage. Fine-bore nasogastric feeding tubes which do not allow suctioning must not be used until gastric emptying is assured. In contrast, fine-bore nasojejunal feeding tubes can safely feed patients enterally without creating an aspiration risk.[39] They are usually used in association with a nasogastric tube to drain gastric secretions.

Antacid therapy, H$_2$ receptor antagonists and sucralfate

Until recently, antacids and H$_2$-receptor antagonists were widely used to prevent stress ulceration. However, bacterial colonization of gastric contents and airway colonization due to recurrent microaspirations are now recognized.[40] Hence antacids and H$_2$-antagonists may possibly lead to increased nosocomial pneumonia and mortality in ICU patients.[3,41,42] Because of this concern, many intensivists have adopted selective decontamination of the digestive tract (SDD) with non-absorbable antibiotics, and/or use of sucralfate (a gastric cytoprotective agent which does not alter gastric pH) instead of antacids and H$_2$-antagonists. Sucralfate does not cause major pulmonary damage when aspirated,[43] but it is associated with an acidic gastric pH, and thus does not protect against acid aspiration. Reported SDD studies show decreased incidences of nosocomial pneumonia, but do not convincingly demonstrate decreased patient mortality or length of stay.[44,45] Similarly, improved ICU mortality has not been shown with sucralfate, and reports of its effect on nosocomial pneumonia are conflicting.[42,46] Therefore at present, SDD is not recommended for routine use. Theoretical advantages of sucralfate in nosocomial pneumonia are unproven.

Antacids are used in perioperative patients, particularly in obstetrics, to reduce the risk of acid aspiration. Experimental studies favour non-particulate antacids (e.g. 0.3 molar sodium citrate, 15–30 ml).[47,48] Sodium citrate increases gastric pH during elective and emergency surgery, but varies widely in efficacy and duration of action.[49–51] due partly to differences in gastric emptying.

The risk of acid aspiration is reduced in emergency obstetric anaesthesia by giving 50 mg rantidine IV in addition to sodium citrate, at least 30 min beforehand. Ranitidine, a H$_2$-antagonist, increases gastric pH and decreases the volume of gastric juice by the volume of acid no longer secreted. Ranitidine may be given 8–12-hourly and has a longer duration of action than cimetidine. It is free of the side-effects encountered with IV cimetidine (e.g. hypotension and cardiac arrest).[52] Effective alternatives to ranitidine for emergency obstetric anaesthesia include the proton pump inhibitor omeprazole 40 mg IV,[53] and an oral combination of cimetidine 800 mg and sodium citrate 1.8 g as an effervescent preparation, which is given immediately before surgery. This combination has rapid onset and is more effective than sodium citrate alone.[54] For elective anaesthesia, ranitidine 300 mg or famotidine 40 mg both orally, on the night before and morning of surgery, are equally effective.[55] Omeprazole 40 mg orally is less effective.[55]

Metoclopramide and cisapride

Metoclopramide improves gastric emptying and increases lower oesophageal sphincter tone. However, opioids and atropine counteract these favourable effects.[56] Cisapride is a recently available prokinetic agent, which accelerates gastroduodenal emptying more effectively than metoclopramide.[57] It is also largely devoid of the central depressant and antidopaminergic effects observed with metoclopramide.[58] Cisapride 10 mg 6-hourly via a nasogastric tube improves gastric emptying in critically ill patients receiving enteral feeding,[59] and is suggested to minimize the risk of aspiration pneumonia in long-term enteral feeding patients.[60] Although promising, the role of cisapride against aspiration pneumonia needs to be clarified.

References

1 Hudson L, Milberg J, Anardi D and Maunder R. (1995) Clinical risks for the development of the acute respiratory distress syndrome. *Am J Respir Crit Care Med* **151**: 293–301.

2 Hickling K and Howard R (1988) A retrospective survey of treatment and mortality in aspiration pneumonia. *Intensive Care Med* **14**:617–22.

3 Tryba M (1991) The gastropulmonary route of infection – fact or fiction? *Am J Med* **91**(suppl 2A): 135S–146S.

4 Stoutenbeck C, Van-Saene H, Miranda D and Zandstra D (1983) A new technique of infection prevention in the intensive care unit by selective decontamination of the digestive tract. *Acta Anaesthesiol Belg* **3**:209–221.

5 Wynne J, Reynolds J, Hood C, Auerbach D and Ondrasick J (1979) Steroid therapy for pneumonitis induced in rabbits by aspiration of food stuff. *Anesthesiology* **51**:11–19.

6 Teabeaut J (1952) Aspiration of gastric contents, an experimental study. *Am J Physiol* **28**:51–67.

7 Lewis R, Burgess J and Hampson L. (1971) Cardio-respiratory studies in critical illness. Changes in aspiration pneumonia. *Arch Surg* **103**:335–340.

8 Schwartz D, Wynne J, Gibbs C, Hood C and Kuck E (1980) The pulmonary consequences of aspiration of gastric contents at pH values greater than 2.5. *Am Rev Respir Dis* **121**:119–126.

9 Downs J, Chapman RJ, Modell J and Hood C (1974) An evaluation of steroid therapy in aspiration pneumonitis. *Anesthesiology* **40**:129–135.

10 Wynne J and Modell J (1977) Respiratory aspiration of stomach contents. *Ann Intern Med* **87**:466–474.

11 Mendleson C (1946) The aspiration of stomach contents into the lungs during obstetric anaesthesia. *Am J Obstet Gynecol* **52**:191–205.

12 Modell J, Moya F and Williams H (1968) Changes in blood gases and and $A-aDo_2$ during near drowning. *Anesthesiology* **29**:456–465.

13 Nieman G and Bredenberg C (1985) High surface tension pulmonary edema induced by detergent aerosol. *J Appl Physiol* **58**:129–136.

14 Bartlett J and Gorbach S (1975) The triple threat of aspiration pneumonia. *Chest* **68**:560–566.

15 Garvey B, McCambley J and Tuxen D (1989) Effects of gastric alkalinisation on bacterial colonization in critically ill patients. *Crit Care Med* **17**:211–216.

16 Ledingham I, Eastaway A, McKay I, Alcock S, McDonald J and Ramsay G (1988) Triple regimen of selective decontamination of the digestive tract, systemic cefotaxime, and microbiological surveillance for prevention of acquired infection in intensive care. *Lancet* **i**:785–790.

17 Zucker A, Sznajder J and Becker C (1989) The pathophysiology and treatment of canine kerosene pulmonary injury: effects of plasmapheresis and positive end–expiratory pressure. *J Crit Care* **4**:184–193.

18 Mendelson C (1946) The aspiration of stomach contents into the lungs during obstetric anaesthesia. *Am J Obstet Gynecol* **52**:191–205.

19 Kinsey G, Murray M, Swensen S and Miles J (1994) Glucose content of tracheal aspirates: implications for the detection of tube feeding aspiration. *Crit Care Med* **2**:1557–1562.

20 Taylor G and Pryse–Davies J (1968) Evaluation of endotracheal steroid therapy in acid pulmonary aspiration (Mendelson's syndrome). *Anesthesiology* **29**: 17–21.

21 Cameron J, Sebor J, Anderson R and Zuidema G (1968) Aspiration pneumonia. Results of treatment by positive pressure ventilation in dogs. *J Surg Res* **8**:447–457.

22 Corbridge T, Wood L, Crawford G, Chudoba M, Yanos J and Sznajder J (1990) Adverse effects of large tidal volume and low PEEP in canine acid aspiration. *Am Rev Respir Dis* **142**:311–315.

23 Sznajder J, Zucker A, Wood L and Long G (1986) The effects of plasmapheresis and hemofiltration on canine acid aspiration pulmonary edema. *Am Rev Respir Dis* **34**:222–228.

24 Humphrey H, Hall J, Sznajder J, Silverstein M and Wood L (1990) Improved survival in ARDS patients associated with a reduction in pulmonary capillary wedge pressure. *Chest* **97**:1176–1180.

25 Clark P,Williams T,Teichtahl H,Bowes G and Tuxen D (1989) Removal of proximal and peripheral endotracheal foreign bodies with the flexible fibreoptic bronchscope. *Anaesth Intens Care* **17**:205–208.

26 Cunanan O (1978) The flexible fibreoptic bronchoscope in foreign body removal. Experience in 300 cases. *Chest* **73**:5.

27 Wynne J and Modell J (1977) Clinical review: rspiratory aspiration of stomach contents. *Ann Intern Med* **87**:466–474.

28 Murray H (1979) Antimicrobial therapy in pulmonary aspiration. *Am J Med* **66**:188–190.

29 Arms R, Dines D and Tinstman T (1997) Aspiration pneumonia. *Chest* **65**:136–139.

30 Murray H (1979) Antimicrobial therapy in pulmonary aspiration. *Am J Med* **66**:188–190.

31 Bartlett J and Gorbach S (1975) Treatment of aspiration pneumonia and primary lung abscess. *JAMA* **234:** 935–937.

32 Tuxen D (1994) Permissive hypercapnic ventilation. *Am J Respir Crit Care Med* **150**:870–874.

33 Feihl F and Perret C (1994) Permissive hypercapnia. How permissive should we be? *Am J Respir Crit Med* **150**:1722–1737.

34 Torres A, Serra–Batlles J, Ros E, *et al.* (1992) Pulmonary aspiration of gastric contents in patients receiving mechanical ventilation: the effect of body position. *Ann Intern Med* **116**:540–543.

35 Howells T, Chamney A, Wraight W and Simons R (1983) The application of cricoid pressure. *Anaesthesia* **38:** 457–460.

36 Elpern E, Scott M, Petro L and Ries M (1994) Pulmonary aspiration in mechanically ventilated patients with tracheostomies. *Chest* **105**:563–566.

37 Valles J, Artigas A, Rello J, Bonsoms N, Fontanals D and Blanch L (1995) Continuous aspiration of subglottic secretions in preventing ventilator associated pneumonia. *Ann Intern Med* **122**:179–186.

38 Griffin R and Hatcher I (1990) Aspiration pneumonia and the laryngeal mask airway. *Anaesthesia* **45:** 1039–1040.

39 Montecalvo M, Steger K, Farber H (1992) *et al.* Nutritional outcome and pneumonia in critical care patients randomised to gastric versus jejunal tube feedings. *Crit Care Med* **20**:1377–1387.

40 Atherton S and White D (1978) Stomach as a source of bacteria colonization in the respiratory tract during artifical ventilation. *Lancet* **2**:968–969.

41 Tryba M (1987) Risk of acute stress bleeding and nosocomial pneumonia in ventilated intensive care unit patients: sucralfate versus antacids. *Am J Med* **83**:117–123.

42 Driks M, Craven D and Celli B (1987) Nosocomial pneumonia in intubated patients given sucralfate as compared with antacids or histamine type 2 blockers: the role of gastric colonization. *N Engl J Med* **317:** 1376–1382.

43 Shepherd K, Faulkner C, Thal G and Leiter J (1995) Acute, subacute, and chronic histologic effects of simulated aspiration of a 0.7% sucralfate suspension in rats. *Crit Care Med* **23**:532–536.

44 Heyland D, Cook D, Jaeschke R, Griffith L, Lee H and Guyatt G (1994) Selective decontamination of the digestive tract. An overview. *Chest* **105**:1221–1229.

45 Selective Decontamination of the Digestive Tract Collaborative Group (1993) Meta-analysis of randomised controlled trials of selective decontamination of the digestive tract. *Br Med J* **307**:525–532.

46 Pickworth K, Falcone R, Hoogeboom J, and Santanello S (1993) Occurrence of nosocomial pneumonia in mechanically ventilated trauma patients: a comparison of sucralfate and ranitidine. *Crit Care Med* **21**:1856–1862.

47 Bond V, Stoelting R and Gupta C (1979) Pulmonary aspiration syndrome after inhalation of gastric fluid containing antacids. *Anesthesiology* **51**:452–453.

48 Gibbs C, Schwartz D, Wynne J, Hood C and Kuck E (1979) Antacid pulmonary aspiration in the dog. *Anesthesiology* **51**:380–385.

49 Wrobel J, Koh T and Saunders J. (1982) Sodium citrate: an alternative antacid for prophylaxis against aspiration pneumonitis. *Anaesth Intens Care* **10**:116–119.

50 Dewan D, Floyd H, Thistlewood J, Bogard T and Spielman F (1985) Sodium citrate pretreatment in elective Cesarean section patients. *Anaesth Analg* **64**:34–37.

51 Gibbs C, Spohr L and Schmidt D (1982) The effectiveness of sodium citrate as an antacid. *Anaesthesiology* **57**:44–46.

52 Shaw R, Mashford M and Desmond P (1980) Cardiac arrest after intravenous injection of cimetidine. *Med J Aust* **2**:629–630.

53 Rocke D, Rout C and Gouws E (1994) Intravenous administration of the proton pump inhibitor omeprazole reduces the risk of acid aspiration at emergency cesarian section. *Anaesth Analg* **78**:1093–1098.

54 Ormezzano X, Francois T, Viaud J–Y *et al.* (1990) Aspiration pneumonitis prophylaxis in obstretric anaesthesia: comparison of effervescent cimetidine–sodium citrate mixture and sodium citrate. *Br J Anaesth* **64**:503–506.

55 Boulay K, Blanloeil Y, Bourveau M, Geay G, and Malinovsky J. (1994) The effects of oral ranitidine, famootidine, and omeprazole on gastric volume and pH at induction and recovery from general anaesthesia. *Br J Anaesth* **73**:475–478.

56 Brock-Utne J, Rubin J, Downing J, Dimopolous G, Moshal M and Naiker M (1976) The administration of metoclopramide with atropine. *Anaesthesia* **31**:1186–1190.

57 Orihata M and Sarna S (1994) Contractile mechanisms of gastroprokinetic agents: cisapride, metoclopramide, and domperidone. *Am J Physiol* **266**:G665–G676.

58 Wiseman L and Faulds D (1994) Cisapride. An updated review of its pharmacology and therapeutic efficacy as a prokinetic agent in gastrointestinal motility disorders. *Drugs* **47**:116–152.

59 Spapen H, Duinslaeger L, Diltoer M, Gillet R, Bossuyt A and Huyghens L (1995) Gastric emptying in critically ill patients is accelerated by adding cisapride to a standard enteral feeding protocol: results of a prospective, randomised, controlled trial. *Crit Care Med* **23**:481–485.

60 Sartori S, Trevisani L, Tassinari D *et al.* (1994) Prevention of aspiration pneumonia during long term feeding by percutaneous endoscopic gastrostomy: might cisapride play any role? An open pilot study. *Supp Care Cancer* **2**:188–190.

Part IV

Gastroenterological disorders

35 | Acute gastrointestinal bleeding

JJY Sung

Acute gastrointestinal (GI) bleeding is a common admission to the ICU and a major cause of morbidity and mortality. Peptic ulcer disease accounts for 75% of upper GI bleeding.[1] Bleeding from varices, oesophagitis, duodenitis and Mallory–Weiss syndrome each account for between 5% and 15% of cases. About 20% of GI bleeding arises from the lower GI tract. Common aetiological causes for GI bleeding are listed in Table 35.1. Mortality from upper GI bleeding has remained at approximately 10% for decades,[1] but recent reports suggest that mortality from bleeding ulcers has fallen substantially to about 5%.[2] On the other hand, variceal bleeding has a much higher mortality of about 30%. Risk factors for mortality include old age, associated medical problems, coagulopathy and magnitude of bleeding.[3]

Table 35.1 Common causes of acute gastrointestinal bleeding

Upper gastrointestinal bleeding
Peptic ulcers (DU:GU ≈ 3:1)
Varices (oesophageal varices:gastric varices ≈ 9:1)
Portal hypertensive gastropathy
Mallory–Weiss syndrome
Gastritis, duodenitis and oesophagitis

Lower gastrointestinal bleeding
Diverticular bleeding
Angiodysplasia and arteriovenous malformation
Colonic polyps or tumours
Meckel's diverticulum
Inflammatory bowel diseases

DU = Duodenal ulcer; GU = gastrointestinal ulcer.

Upper gastrointestinal bleeding

Clinical presentation

Haematemesis and melaena are the most common presentations of acute upper GI bleeding. Haematochezia is the passage of bright red or maroon blood from the rectum, in the form of pure blood or admixed with stool. It usually represents a lower intestinal source of bleeding, but can also be a feature of massive upper GI bleeding. Symptoms of hypovolaemia such as tachycardia, pallor, sweating, cyanosis, mental confusion and oliguria may be present in massive GI bleeding. Bleeding ulcers can be painless, especially in elderly patients and users of non-steroidal anti-inflammatory drugs. A history of vomiting and retching preceding haematemesis suggests Mallory–Weiss syndrome.

Investigation

Endoscopy or barium study

As history and physical examination are seldom useful in identifying the source of bleeding, investigations are necessary in most cases of GI bleeding. Endoscopy has replaced barium studies as the investigation of choice. It should be performed as soon as the patient is haemodynamically stabilized, and adequate supportive personnel is available. Endoscopy is preferred to barium X-rays for the following reasons:

1 Endoscopy allows more precise identification of the site and nature of bleeding.
2 Endoscopic appearance often predicts the risk of recurrent bleeding from ulcer and varices (see below).
3 Lesions such as gastritis, portal hypertensive gastropathy and duodenitis are difficult to diagnose by barium X-ray.
4 Barium X-ray is notoriously unreliable in patients with previous gastric surgery.

However, endoscopy can induce serious hypoxia in patients with cardiorespiratory diseases. Continuous monitoring of blood pressure, pulse and oxygen saturation with a pulse oximeter is mandatory. Oxygen should be administered by nasal cannula when necessary.

Angiography

Angiography is seldom used for the diagnosis of upper GI bleeding. Theoretically, when the bleeding is very brisk and obscures the endoscopic view, angiography may help to identify the source of bleeding. In practice, however, most patients with this degree of haemorrhage should be considered for emergency laparotomy.

Management of non-variceal upper GI bleeding

The goals of managing a patient with acute GI bleeding are first to resuscitate, second, to control active bleeding; and third, to prevent recurrence of haemorrhage.

Resuscitation

Blood and plasma expanders should be given through large-bore intravenous cannulae. Vital signs should be closely monitored. In patients with hypovolaemic shock, central venous pressure and hourly urine output should also be observed (see Chapter 14). Following adequate resuscitation, management is directed to identify the high-risk patient and lesion, i.e. those likely to require early endoscopic or surgical treatment.

The high-risk patient

Significant GI bleeding is indicated by syncope, haematemesis, systolic blood pressure below 100 mmHg (13.3 kPa), postural hypotension, and if more than 4 units of blood have to be transfused in 12 h. Patients over 60 years old and with multiple underlying diseases are of even higher risk.[3] Those admitted for other medical problems (e.g. heart or respiratory failure, or cerebrovascular bleed) and who have GI bleeding during hospitalization also have a higher mortality.

The high-risk ulcer

Peptic ulcers which are actively bleeding or have bled recently may show stigmata of haemorrhage on endoscopy. These include localized active bleeding (i.e. pulsatile, arterial spurting or simple oozing), an adherent blood clot, a protuberant vessel or a flat

Table 35.2 Stigmata of haemorrhage and risk of recurrent bleeding in peptic ulcers

Stigmata of haemorrhage	% Recurrent bleeding
Spurter or oozer	85–90
Protuberant vessel	35–55
Adherent clot	30–40
Flat spot	5–10
None	<5

pigmented spot on the ulcer base. Stigmata of haemorrhage are important predictors of recurrent bleeding (Table 35.2).[4–6] The proximal posteroinferior wall of the duodenal bulb and the high lesser curve of the stomach are common sites for severe recurrent bleeding, due probably to their respective large arteries (gastroduodenal and left gastric arteries).

Treatment

Pharmacological control

Acid-suppressing drugs such as H_2-receptor antagonists and proton-pump inhibitors (see below) are very effective drugs to promote ulcer healing. An acidic environment impairs platelet function and haemostasis. Therefore, reducing the secretion of gastric acid should reduce bleeding and encourage ulcer healing. Unfortunately, clinical studies have failed to show that acid suppression can influence the outcome of upper GI bleeding.[7] Similarly, antifibrinolytic agents such as tranexamic acid have not been effective in reducing the operative rate and mortality of acute GI haemorrhage.

Endoscopic therapy

Most patients with acute upper GI haemorrhage stop bleeding spontaneously and have an uneventful recovery. No specific intervention is required in these patients. Endoscopic haemostasis should be used in patients with a high risk of persistent or recurrent bleeding.[8] In the last decade, endoscopic haemostasis, with its high efficacy and low morbidity, has resulted in a dramatic decrease in emergency surgery, and has reduced the mortality of ulcer bleeding. The three most popular methods of haemostasis are:

1 *Adrenaline injection*: Endoscopic injection of adrenaline (1:10 000 dilution) at 0.5–1.0 ml aliquots (up to 10–15 ml) into and around the ulcer bleeding point has achieved successful haemostasis in over 90% of cases.[9] Debate exists as to whether the haemostatic effect is a result of local tamponade by the volume injected, or vasoconstriction by adrenaline. Absorption of adrenaline into the systemic ciculation has been doumented, but without any significant effecton the haemodynamic status of the patient.[10] Adrenaline injection is an effective, cheap, portable and easy-to-learn method of haemostasis, and has acquired a worldwide popularity.

2 *Coaptive coagulation*: This method uses direct pressure and heat energy (heater probe) or electrocoagulation (BICAP probe) to control ulcer bleeding. The depth of tissue injury induced by these devices is minimized, as the bleeding vessel is tamponaded prior to coagulation. The overall efficacy of the adrenaline injection, heater probe and BICAP probe methods is comparable.[11–13] Occasionally, it is not possible to obtain an *en face*

view of the bleeding ulcers, particularly those on the lesser curve or on the posterior wall of the duodenal bulb. In these situations, direct pressure cannot be applied, and the failure rate of coaptive coagulation will be higher.

3 *Laser photocoagulation*: Neodymium:yttrium aluminium garnet (Nd:YAG) laser can been used for the treatment of ulcer bleeding.[14] The interaction between laser energy and tissue results in generation of heat. Laser therapy is a non-contact treatment, and is thus unable to tamponade the vessel during heating. Other disadvantages of laser include cost and the lack of portability. Although Nd:YAG laser can probably achieve a comparable success in haemostasis,[15] enthusiasm has declined due to these limiting factors.

Surgery

Surgery remains the most definitive method of stopping haemorrhage. However, there is little agreement on the exact indications and best timing for surgical intervention. These issues are even less clear now that endoscopic treatment is available. Accordingly, good cooperation among intensivists, gastroenterologists and surgeons is essential. Indications for surgery can be:

1 arterial bleeding that cannot be controlled by endoscopic haemostasis;
2 massive transfusion (i.e. total of 6–8 units of blood);
3 recurrent clinical bleeding after initial success with endoscopic therapy;
4 evidence suggestive of GI perforation.

Surgical procedures include underrunning of the ulcer, underrunning plus vagotomy and drainage, and various types of gastrectomy. The overall mortality of emergency surgery for GI bleeding is about 15–20%. Results of surgery are better if patients are operated on early.

Acute stress ulceration

Acute stress ulceration is associated with sepsis, shock, burns, polytrauma, head injuries, spinal injuries and respiratory, renal and hepatic failure. Respiratory failure and coagulopathy are two strong independent factors in critically ill patients.[17] The incidence in ICU varies from insignificant to 8–45%[17] and has probably decreased in the last decade. Bleeding may be occult or overt from 'coffee grounds' aspirates to frank haemorrhage. Lesions are most commonly seen in the gastric fundus, and range from mild multiple erosions to acute ulcerations.

Prophylaxis and treatment

Significant ulcerations are managed as above. Minor bleeding and *prophylactic* treatment are considered together. Prophylactic treatment aims for gastric alkalinization (gastric pH > 3.5), on the rationale that gastric acidity is the main cause of stress ulceration. However, ulcerations can still occur despite prophylactic treatment,[18] and gastric bacterial overgrowth (with possible nosocomial pneumonia) may be a complication.[19] None the less, the incidence of stress ulcerations appears to be lower with prophylactic gastric alkalinization than with placebos, although an improvement in survival has not been shown.[18,20] On balance, prophylactic treatment should probably be reserved for at-risk patients. Scoring systems to estimate the risk of stress-ulcer bleeding have been proposed, i.e. Zinner[21] and Tryba scores.[19] The mainstay of prophylaxis and treatment for minor bleeding remain supportive–optimize oxygenation and tissue perfusion and reduce infection. Enteral feeding may reduce the risk.[22] Drugs given include the following:

Antacids

Antacids given hourly via a nasogastric tube can maintain gastric alkalinization. Gastric pH monitoring is necessary. Antacids contain magnesium, aluminium, calcium or sodium, and complications may arise from excessive intake of these minerals. Bowel stasis and diarrhoea can also be problems. They are used less commonly now.

H_2-receptor antagonists

These drugs suppress acid secretion by competing for the histamine receptor on the parietal cell. Cimetidine is less potent and has interactions with anticonvulsants, theophyllines and warfarin. Famotidine and nizatidine are newer agents but have no particular advantage over ranitidine. Ranitidine is commonly used, given as 50 mg bolus IV, followed by an infusion of 0.12–0.24 mg/kg per h. The dose is halved in severe renal dysfunction.

Sucralfate

This is a basic aluminium salt of sucrose octasulphate. It is effective in healing ulcers by increasing mucus secretion, mucosal blood flow and local prostaglandin production. These effects promote mucosal resistance against acid and pepsin (i.e. cytoprotective). As it does not alter gastric pH, Gram-negative bacterial colonization of gastric juice is less likely. The incidence of nosocomial pneumonia may be less with sucralfate than with antacids or H_2-receptor antagonists,[19] but this is debatable.[23] There is no proven advantage over the latter. Sucralfate is given via the nasogastric tube as 1.0 g/4–6 h. Constipation is a side-effect, and aluminium toxicity may arise from renal dysfunction.

Other drugs

Other ulcer-healing drugs have been used as prophylactic treatment in stress-related ulcers. Their efficacy and role in this setting are unclear. *Omeprazole* is a proton-pump inhibitor, i.e. it inhibits hydrogen–potassium adenosine biphosphatase, the enzyme responsible for acid secretion. An oral dose of 40 mg can sustain achlorhydria for 24 h. It is used for resistant peptic ulcers. *Pirenzepine* is a muscarinic M_1 antagonist used occasionally to treat peptic ulcers. A dose of 100 mg/day still has minimal anticholinergic side-effects. *Misoprostol* is a prostaglandin PGE_1 analogue with antacid secretory and cytoprotective actions, given as 200 μg 6-hourly. *Dopamine* improves splanchnic circulation. *Vasodilators* ketanserin and clonidine experimentally inhibit gastric lesions.[18] *Corticosteroids* may have a cytoprotective effect through various mechanisms.[17,18] Antibiotic selective decontamination of the gut (see Chapter 62) may be helpful, postulated through an antiendotoxin effect.[17]

Management – variceal bleeding

Acute variceal bleeding is a serious complication of portal hypertension, with a high mortality. About 50% of patients with bleeding varices have had an earlier bleed during hospitalization. The degree of liver failure, i.e. Child–Pugh's classification (see Chapter 37) is the most important prognostic factor for early rebleeding and survival.

Resuscitation

Immediate resuscitation with whole blood and fluids is mandatory. Overtransfusion may cause a rebound increase in portal pressure (with a consequent increased risk of rebleeding) and must be avoided. Fresh frozen plasma may be indicated. A nasogastric cannula is often inserted for the removal of blood (and also drug administration). Forceful aspiration through the nasogastric tube should be avoided as bleeding may be induced. Lactulose (15–30 ml every 4–6 h) should be given to prevent or correct hepatic encephalopathy. A colonic wash-out can be used, but a magnesium-containing enema should be avoided in the presence of renal failure. Close attention must be given to haemodynamic monitoring.

When the patient is haemodynamically stable, upper endoscopy should be performed to identify the source of bleeding. Patients with portal hypertension could bleed from oesophageal or gastric varices, peptic ulcers and portal hypertensive gastropathy.

Pharmacological control

Vasopressin (0.2–0.4 u/min) has been the most widely used agent to reduce portal blood pressure and control variceal bleeding. Cardiac ischaemia (in about 10% of patients) and worsening coagulopathy (by release of plasminogen activator) are important adverse effects. These side-effects can be reduced by adding glyceryl trinitrate to vasopressin.[24] Terlipressin, a triglycyl synthetic analogue of vasopressin, has a

longer half-life and fewer cardiac side-effects, and may be also effective.[25] Somatostatin infusion (250 μg/h) reduces portal blood pressure and azygous blood flow, and is safe and effective in acute variceal bleeding.[26,27] Octreotide, the longer acting synthetic analogue of somatostatin (given as a 50 μg bolus IV followed by an infusion of 50 μg/h), is as effective as emergency sclerotherapy.[28] These drugs are valuable stop-gap therapies to control acute variceal bleeding before endoscopic treatment is available, and probably reduce early recurrence of haemorrhage.

Endoscopic therapy

Endoscopic sclerotherapy

Endoscopic injection sclerotherapy is the mainstay treatment. At endoscopy, a sclerosant can be injected directly into the variceal columns (intravariceal injection) or into the mucosa adjacent to the varices (paravariceal injection) to cause venous thrombosis, inflammation, and tissue fibrosis Commonly used sclerosants are ethanolamine oleate, sodium tetradecyl sulphate (1–3% STD), polidocanol and alcohol. None has appreciable advantages over the others.[29] Endoscopic sclerotherapy controls 80–90% of acute variceal bleeding. Complications such as ulcer formation, fever, chest pain and mediastinitis are common. Bleeding from gastric varices is more difficult to control by injection sclerotherapy because of difficult access. Butylcyanoacrylate (Histoacryl) has been used recently for gastric variceal injections, with a claimed superior haemostatic effect.[30] It is generally mixed with lipiodol to delay the rate of polymerization and allow radiological monitoring of the injection.

Endoscopic variceal ligation

Endoscopic variceal ligation is a recently introduced technique for the treatment of variceal bleeding.[31] Rubber bands mounted on the banding device at the tip of the endoscope are released to strangulate the bleeding varices. The technique is as effective as injection sclerotherapy in acute bleeding.[32,33] Procedure-related complications are significantly fewer as there is no tissue chemical irritation. An overtube to facilitate banding avoids aspiration during the procedure, but may result in serious oesophageal injury if used improperly.[33] The tunnel vision produced by the banding device restricts visibility, and thus makes the procedure technically difficult when bleeding is heavy.

Balloon tamponade

Variceal bleeding can be controlled by exerting pressure directly on the bleeding point using a balloon. The Sengstaken–Blackmore tube has been replaced by the four-lumen Minnesota tube which allows aspiration of gastric and oesophageal contents. Inflation of the gastric balloon (by 250–350 ml of water) is often sufficient to stop the bleeding by occluding the feeding veins to the oesophageal varices. If bleeding continues, the oesophageal balloon can be inflated by air and kept at a pressure of 50–60 mmHg (6.7–8.0 kPa). Use of balloon tamponade should be limited to under 24 h to avoid tissue pressure necrosis.

Transjugular intrahepatic portosystemic shunt (TIPS)

Using a transjugular approach, a catheter is inserted into the hepatic vein, and advanced under fluoroscopic guidance into a branch of the portal vein. By means of a guide wire and dilators, a stent is introduced to create an intrahepatic portosystemic shunt[34] (Fig. 35.1). In good hands, success can be achieved in over 90% of cases[35]. This procedure significantly reduces portal blood pressure and thus bleeding from varices.

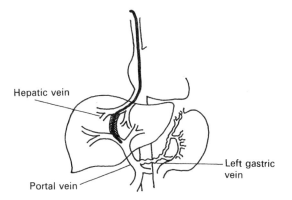

Left gastric vein

Hepatic vein

Portal vein

Fig. 35.1 Transjugular intrahepatic portosystemic shunt (TIPS)

Major complications include intra-abdominal haemorrhage and stent occlusion. Hepatic encephalopathy in 25% of patients has been reported.[35] Nevertheless, this is an effective salvage treatment for uncontrolled variceal bleeding. Unlike shunt surgery, TIPS will not reduce the chance of a future liver transplantation.

Surgery

The role of surgery has diminished since the advent of endoscopic treatment and TIPS.[36] Surgery is now used as a second-line treatment, when bleeding continues or recurs after two sessions of injection sclerotherapy or banding ligation. Both staple transection of the oesophagus and portocaval shunt surgery are highly effective emergency measures. Despite successful control of bleeding, long-term survival is not significantly improved. Hepatic encephalopathy is one of the major complications of shunting operations. Expectations that the Warren distal splenorenal shunt will preserve antegrade portal flow and avoid accelerated deterioration of liver function have not been realized.[37,38] The Warren shunt is technically more difficult, especially if performed as an emergency. Choice of surgery should be carefully made in those who are potential transplant candidates, as it may complicate subsequent surgery. A protocol to manage variceal bleeding is shown in Figure 35.2.

Lower gastrointestinal bleeding

Lower GI bleeding arises from a source distal to the ligament of Treitz. It accounts for 10–20% of acute GI bleeding. Common causes of colonic bleeding

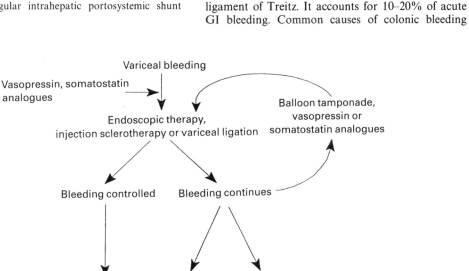

Fig. 35.2 Management of variceal bleeding. TIPS = Transjugular intrahepatic portosystemic shunt.

include diverticular haemorrhage and angiodysplasia (both occur on the right-sided colon), colonic polyps and carcinoma, and inflammatory bowel diseases.[39,40]

Clinical presentation

Haematochezia is the most common presentation of lower GI bleeding. However, bleeding from small intestine and right colon may also present as melaena. Abdominal pain preceding a massive bleeding episode suggests either ischaemia or inflammatory bowel disease. Painless massive bleeding is common in diverticulosis, angiodysplasia or from a Meckel's diverticulum. In a patient with portal hypertension, haemorrhoids may present with massive haematochezia.

Investigations

Haemorrhoids and rectal tumour can easily be identified by proctosigmoidoscopy, which should always be performed. Since upper GI bleeding is about five times as common as lower GI bleeding, the former should be excluded. When both proctosigmoidoscopy and gastroscopy are negative, the lower GI tract should be examined by colonoscopy, angiography or radionuclide scan. Barium enema plays no role in the management of acute rectal bleeding.

Colonoscopy

Patients with mild to moderate haematochezia can be safely examined by colonoscopy. Colonoscopy is difficult in an actively bleeding patient, and may carry an increased risk of perforation. Visualization is often unsatisfactory due to the dark discoloration of blood.[41] Colonoscopy yields much better results with adequate bowel preparation once bleeding has stopped.

Angiography or radionuclide scan

The diagnostic efficacy of radionuclide scan and angiography varies in different studies. ^{99m}Tc sulphur colloid is quickly removed from the blood stream after injection. Its diagnostic yield is low because of its short circulatory half-life. ^{99m}Tc labelling of red cells prolongs the duration of radioactivity in the body. Red cell scan has been reported to detect the source of active bleeding in over 80% of cases.[42]

Diagnostic angiography is helpful in two situations:

1 when the view of endoscopy is completely obscured by active haemorrhage;
2 angiography is more sensitive in defining abnormal vasculatures, even if extravasation of contrast material is not seen. These lesions include angiodysplasia, arteriovenous malformation and various inherited vascular anomalies (e.g. Rendu–

Osler–Weber syndrome, pseudoxanthoma elasticum and Ehlers–Danlos syndrome). Angiography may localize the site of bleeding in 80–85% of patients when the bleeding rate is more than 0.5 ml/min.[43] Both superior and inferior mesenteric angiograms are often needed.

Management
Endoscopy

Bleeding from vascular anomalies can be treated by electrocoagulation, heater probe and laser photocoagulation, unless they are too large or too diffuse.[44] Bleeding colonic polyps can be removed by polypectomy or coagulated by hot biopsy forceps.

Angiography

Angiographic intra-arterial infusion of vasopressin or occlusion of the bleeding artery with embolic agents such as an absorbable gelatin sponge (Gelfoam) may be used in lower GI bleeding pathologies.[45] Both diverticular bleeding and bleeding from angiodysplasia can be stopped by vasopressin infusion during angiography, but recurrence of bleeding occurs frequently with diverticular disease.

Surgery

Diverticular bleeding usually arises from a relatively large vessel, and is thus not controllable with endoscopic or angiographic therapy. Partial resection of the colon is warranted after localization of the bleeding site. Surgery is also indicated in vascular anomalies when endoscopic treatment fails. When an obvious and refractory massive lower GI bleed is not identified by endoscopic or angiographic examina-

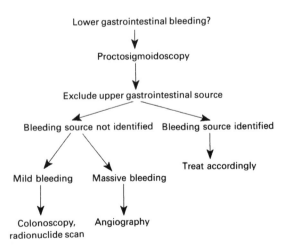

Fig. 35.3 Management of lower gastrointestinal bleeding.

tions, immediate laparotomy with possible subtotal colectomy should be offered. A protocol to manage lower GI bleeding is shown in Figure 35.3.

References

1 Silverstein FE, Gilbert DA, Tedesco FJ *et al.* (1981) The National ASGE survey on upper gastrointestinal bleeding. I. Study design and baseline data. *Gastrointest Endosc* **27**:73–79.

2 Holman RAE, Davis M, Gough KR *et al.* (1990) Value of a centralized approach in the management of haemetemesis and melaena: experience in a district general hospital. *Gut* **31**:504–508.

3 Silverstein FE, Gilbert DA, Tedesco FJ *et al.* (1981) The national ASGE survey on upper gastrointestinal bleeding. II. Clinical prognostic factors. *Gastrointest Endosc* **27**:80–93.

4 Swain CP, Storey DW, Bown SG *et al.* (1986) Nature of bleeding vessel in recurrently bleeding gastric ulcers. *Gastroenterology* **90**:595–608.

5 Foster DN, Miloszewski K, Losowsky MS *et al.* (1978) Stigmata of recent haemorrhage in diagnosis and prognosis of upper gastrointestinal bleeding. *Br Med J* **1**:1173–1177.

6 Griffiths WJ, Neumann DA, and Welsh JD (1979) The visible vessel as an indicator of uncontrolled or recurrent gastrointestinal haemorrhage. *N Engl J Med* **300**:1411–1413.

7 Daneshmend TK, Hawkey CJ, Langman MJS *et al.* (1992) Omeprazole versus placebo for acute upper gastrointestinal bleeding: randomized double blind controlled trial. *Br Med J* **304**:143–147.

8 NIH Consensus Conference (1989). Therapeutic endoscopy and bleeding ulcers. *JAMA* **262**:1369–1372.

9 Chung SCS, Leung JWC, Steele RJ *et al.* (1988) Endoscopic injection of adrenaline for actively bleeding ulcers: a randomized trial. *Br Med J* **296**:1631–1633.

10 Sung JY, Chung SCS, Low JM *et al.* (1993) Systemic absorption of epinephrine after endoscopic submucosal injection in patients with bleeding peptic ulcers. *Gastrointest Endosc* **39**:20–22.

11 Chung SCS, Leung JWC, Sung JY *et al.* (1991) Injection or heat probe for bleeding ulcer. *Gastroenterology* **100**:33–37.

12 Jensen DM, Machicado GA, Kovacs TG *et al.* (1988) Controlled, randomized study of heater probes and BICAP for haemostasis of severe ulcer bleeding. *Gastroenterology* **94**:A208.

13 Laine (1987) L. Multipolar electrocoagulation in the treatment of active upper gastrointestinal haemorrhage: a prospective controlled trial. *N Engl J Med* **316**:1613–1617.

14 Laurence BH, Valloon AG, Cotton PB *et al.* (1980) Endoscopic laser photocoagulation for bleeding peptic ulcers. *Lancet* **1**:124–125.

15 Hui WM, Ng MMT, Lok ASF *et al.* (1991) A randomized comparative study of laser photocoagulation, heater probe, and bipolar electrocoagulation in the treatment of actively bleeding ulcers. *Gastrointest Endosc* **37**:299–304.

16 Cook DJ, Fuller HO, Guyatt GH *et al.* (1994) Risk factors for gastrointestinal bleeding in critically ill patients. *N Engl J Med* **330**:377–381.

17 Zandstra DF and Stoutenbeek CP (1994) The virtual absence of stress-ulceration related bleeding in ICU patients receiving prolonged mechanical ventilation without any prophylaxis – a prospective cohort study. *Intensive Care Med* **20**:335–340.

18 Tryba M (1994) Stress ulcer prophylaxis – quo vadis? *Intensive Care Med* **20**:311–313.

19 Tryba M (1987) Risk of acute stress bleeding and nosocomial pneumonia in ventilated intensive care patients: sucralfate versus antacids. *Am J Med* **83**(suppl 3B):117–124.

20 Cook DJ, Witt LJ, and Guyatt GH (1991) Stress ulcer prophylaxis in the critically ill: a meta-analysis. *Am J Med* **91**:519–527.

21 Zinner MJ, Zuidema GD, Smith PL, Mignosa M. (1981) The prevention of upper gastrointestinal tract bleeding in patients in an intensive care unit. *Surg Gynecol Obstet* **153**:214–220.

22 Pingleton SK. (1986) Gastric bleeding and/or enteral feeding. *Chest* **90**:2–3.

23 McCarthy DM (1991) Sucralfate. *N Engl J Med* **325**:1018–1025.

24 Bosch J, Groszmann RJ, Garcia–Pagan JC *et al.* (1989) Association of transdermal nitroglycerin to vasopressin infusion in the treatment of variceal haemorrhage: a placebo-controlled clinical trial. *Hepatology* **10**:962–968.

25 Soderlund C, Magnusson I, Tongren S *et al.* (1990) Terlipressin (triglycyl-lysine vasopressin) controls acute bleeding oesophageal varies: a double-blind randomized placebo-controlled trial. *Scand J Gastroenterol* **25**:622–630.

26 Burroughs AK, McCormick PA, Hughes MD *et al.* (1990) Randomized, double-blind, placebo-controlled trial of somatostatin for variceal bleeding: emergency control and prevention of early variceal bleeding. *Gastroenterology* **99**:1388–1395.

27 Shields R, Jenkins SA, Baxter JN *et al.* (1992) A prospective randomized controlled trial comparing the efficacy of somatostatin with injection sclerotherapy in the control of bleeding oesophageal varices. *J Hepatol* **16**:128–137.

28 Sung JY, Chung SCS, Lai CW *et al.* (1993) Octreotide infusion or emergency sclerotherapy for variceal haemorrhage. *Lancet* **342**:637–641.

29 Sarin SK and Kumar A (1990) Sclerosant for variceal sclerotherapy: a critical appraisal. *Am J Gastroenterol* **85**:641–649.

30 Soehendra N, Grimm H, Nam VC *et al.* (1987) N-butyl-2-cyanoacrylate: a supplement to endoscopic sclerotherapy. *Endoscopy* **19**:221–224.

31 Van Stiegmann GV and Goff JS (1988) Endoscopic oesophageal varix ligation: preliminary clinical experience. *Gastrointest Endosc* **34**:113–117.

32 Van Stiegmann GV, Goff JS, Michaletz-Onody PA *et al.* (1992) Endoscopic sclerotherapy as compared with endoscopic ligation for bleeding oesophageal varices. *N Engl J Med* **326**:1527–1532.

33 Laine L, El-Newihi HM, Migikovsky B *et al.* (1993) Endoscopic ligation compared with sclerotherapy for the treatment of bleeding oesophageal varices. *Ann Intern Med* **119**:1–7.

34 Conn HO (1993) Transjugular intrahepatic portalsystemic shunts: the state of the art. *Hepatology* **17**:148–158.

35 Rossle M, Haag K, Ochs A *et al.* (1994) The transjugular

intrahepatic portosystemic stent-shunt procedure for variceal bleeding. *N Engl J Med* **330:**165–171.

36 Bornman PC, Krige JEJ and Terblanche J. (1994) Management of oesophageal varices. *Lancet* **343:** 1079–1084.

37 Millikan WJ, Warren WD, Henderson JM *et al.* (1985) The Emory prospective randomized trial: selective versus nonselective shunt to control variceal bleeding. *Ann Surg* **201:**712–722.

38 Langer B, Taylor BR, MacKenzie DR *et al.* (1985) Further report of a prospective randomized trial comparing distal splenorenal shunt with end-to-side portacaval shunt: an analysis of encephalopathy, survival, and quality of life. *Gastroenterology* **88:**424–429.

39 Boley SJ, Brandt LJ and Frank MS (1981). Severe lower intestinal bleeding: diagnosis and treatment. *Clin. Gastroenterol* **10:**65–91.

40 Leitman IM, Paull DE Shires GT (1989) Evaluation and management of massive lower gastrointestinal haemorrhage. *Ann Surg* **209:**175–180.

41 Jensen DM and Machicado GA Diagnosis and treatment of severe haematochezia: the role of urgent colonoscopy after purge. *Gastroenterology* **95:**1569–1574.

42 Bunker SR and Lull RJ. (1984) Scintigraphy of gastrointestinal bleeding: superiority of ^{99m}Tc red blood cells over ^{99m}Tc sulfur colloid. *Am J Radiol* **143:**543–548.

43 Wright HK (1980) Massive colonic haemorrhage. *Surg Clin North Am* **60:**1297–1304.

44 Rutgeerts P, Van Gompel F, Geboes K *et al.* (1985) Long term results of treatment of vascular malformations of the gastrointestinal tract by neodymium YAG laser photocoagulation. *Gut* **26:**586–593.

45 Sherman LM, Shenoy SS and Cerra FB (1979) Selective intra-arterial vasopressin: clinical efficacy and complications. *Ann Surg* **189:**298–302.

36 | Acute pancreatitis

JD Santamaria

Acute pancreatitis remains a relatively common disorder with significant morbidity and mortality.[1-3] It may affect patients of all ages and often becomes a multisystem disorder requiring facilities within ICUs for optimal management.

Aetiology[4,5]

There are many causes of acute pancreatitis (Table 36.1) but in most studies these can be divided into four common categories:

1 biliary tract disease;
2 excessive alcohol ingestion over many years;
3 idiopathic;
4 miscellaneous;

Biliary disease and alcohol account for 70% of cases. Although incidences vary from one location to another, biliary disease is more commonly reported in British papers while alcohol predominates in American studies. Cases with no discernible cause (idiopathic) may account for up to 30% of some series. Several drugs are known to cause pancreatitis and many others are implicated, but without conclusive evidence. Pancreatitis has been described following endoscopic retrograde cholangiopancreatography (ERCP), abdominal and thoracic surgery and cardiopulmonary bypass.

Pathophysiology

As with many body systems, the pancreas reacts in a limited number of ways to an acute insult. The pancreas is rich in enzymes which have the potential to cause extensive tissue damage. Under normal circumstances, several mechanisms protect the pancreas from damage. These include containment within storage granules, potent enzyme inhibitors, and the production of enzymes in an inactive precursor form

Table 36.1 Aetiology of acute pancreatitis

Excess alcohol ingestion
Biliary tract disease
Idiopathic
Metabolic
   Hyperlipidaemia
   Hyperparathyroidism
   Diabetic ketoacidosis
   End-stage renal failure
   Pregnancy
   Post renal transplant
Mechanical disorders
   Post-traumatic
   Postoperative
   Post-ERCP
   Penetrating duodenal ulcer
   Duodenal obstruction
Infections
   Mumps, Epstein–Barr virus, HIV, *Mycoplasma*, hepatitis, *Campylobacter*, *Legionella*, ascariasis
Vascular
   Necrotizing vasculitis – SLE, TTP
   Atheroma
   Shock
Drugs
   Definite: azathioprine, thiazides, frusemide, tetracyclines, oestrogens, sulphonamides, valproic acid, metronidazole, pentamidine, nitrofurantoin, erythromycin, methyldopa, cimetidine, ranitidine, salicylates, paracetamol
   Possible: chlorthalidone, ethacrynic acid, procainamide, L-asparaginase, anticoagulants, propranolol, diazoxide
Toxins
   Scorpion venom, methyl alcohol, organophosphates
Associations
   Hypothermia, histocompatibility antigens, α_1-antitrypsin deficiency
   Hereditary

ERCP = Endoscopic retrograde cholangiopancreatography; HIV = human immunodeficiency virus; SLE = systemic lupus erythematosus; TTP = thrombotic thrombocytopenic purpura.

(zymogens). Inappropriate activation of these enzymes within the pancreas will lead to extensive damage by autodigestion (Fig. 36.1).

Although the proteolytic enzymes such as trypsin,

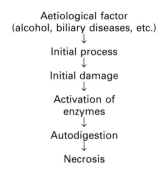

Aetiological factor
(alcohol, biliary diseases, etc.)
↓
Initial process
↓
Initial damage
↓
Activation of
enzymes
↓
Autodigestion
↓
Necrosis

Fig. 36.1 Pathogenesis of acute pancreatitis.

chymotrypsin and elastase were initially considered to be the main destructive agents, there is increasing evidence that the lipolytic enzyme, phospholipase A_2, may be important. Furthermore, this enzyme has been implicated in extrapancreatic complications.[6,7]

Several mechanisms have been proposed to explain the initial processes by which autodigestion begins. These include the reflux of duodenal contents (although evidence in humans is inconclusive), reflux of bile into the pancreatic duct when the common bile duct is obstructed, activation of the complement system and overstimulation of pancreatic secretions (e.g. from scorpion stings and hyperparathyroidism).

The coincidental release of vasoactive substances such as bradykinin from the pancreas into the circulation may explain the increased vascular permeability, hypotension and organ dysfunction, which accompany some episodes of acute pancreatitis.

Acute *oedematous pancreatitis* results in a congested and swollen pancreas, as seen in patients with mild to moderate pancreatitis. On the other hand, *necrotizing pancreatitis* causes severe inflammation with necrosis and haemorrhage. Fat necrosis may be seen in adjacent tissues, and there is a tendency to suppuration. The superficial third of the gland is usually involved and mortality is increased. However, upon recovery, survivors tend to have normal function. Pancreatic ischaemia from hypovolaemia and disturbances of the microcirculation have been suggested to cause this transition from oedema to necrosis.[8] Necrotic tissue provides a suitable environment for growth of microorganisms; clinical infections develop in 40–60% of patients with necrosis observed at operation[9] or on computed tomography (CT) guided aspirations.[10]

Many attempts have been made to classify pancreatitis so that treatments can be better evaluated.[11] At a recent consensus conference,[12] 40 international authorities provided definitions of acute pancreatitis, severe acute pancreatitis, mild acute pancreatitis, acute fluid collection, pancreatic necrosis, acute pseudocysts and pancreatic abscess. These definitions are based on clinical manifestations and pathological findings.

Clinical presentation

Symptoms[13]

The patient may be any age. Alcoholic pancreatitis usually occurs in patients less than 40 years, and males predominate. There may be a history of heavy alcohol intake over several years. On the other hand, pancreatitis associated with biliary tract disorders occurs in middle to later life, and a female to male ratio of 3:1 is usually described. It is important to take a detailed drug history.

Pain comes on relatively quickly and is classically central in position, radiating to the back and eased by sitting forward. Variations do occur, with pain initially confined to the right upper quadrant or felt diffusely over the abdomen; isolated left upper quadrant pain is uncommon. Nausea and vomiting occur in 90% of cases.

Signs

On examination, the patient is usually agitated and restless. Generalized abdominal tenderness and guarding are often noted; marked rigidity can occur and may simulate a ruptured viscus. Fever is common but usually less than 39°C; hypothermia has been described.[14] Abnormal respiratory findings of basal wheezes or pleural effusions are seen in 10–20%. In the severe attack, the patient may be shocked with tachycardia and hypotension or in acute respiratory failure. Erythematous nodules from fat necrosis have been described. Retroperitoneal haemorrhage is evidenced by a brown discoloration in the flanks (Grey Turner sign) or in the umbilicus (Cullen's sign). The abdomen is usually distended due to an associated ileus or the presence of complications.

Acute pancreatitis may simulate other acute abdominal conditions and up to 20% of cases were first diagnosed at laparotomy. However, the greater availability of CT scanning has reduced this percentage dramatically. Differential diagnoses include perforated viscus, cholecystitis, bowel obstruction, vascular occlusions, renal colic, myocardial infarction, pneumonia and diabetic ketoacidosis.

Complications
Local

Local changes contribute to the mortality from pancreatitis. A phlegmon or swelling of the pancreas may be seen on ultrasound or CT in 30–50% of cases, and is palpable in 15–20%. Pancreatic abscesses usually develop after the second week, and may lead to septicaemia. Pseudocysts likewise occur after 2–3 weeks, and are more commonly seen on scans (ultrasound, CT) than found on palpation; they may cause compression of adjacent structures. Spontaneous resolution of pseudocysts may occur. The surrounding inflammation can lead to fistula formation, haemorrhage and infection – all more common with severe necrotizing disease. Pancreatic ascites has been described, as has involvement of contiguous organs with massive intraperitoneal bleeding, vascular thrombosis and infarction of bowel.

Systemic

As noted above, respiratory complications are frequent and include effusions, atelectasis, pneumonitis, and the acute respiratory distress syndrome (ARDS). Cardiac abnormalities include hypotension, sudden death, ST–T-wave changes and pericardial effusions. Renal function may be impaired with acute tubular necrosis progressing to acute renal failure requiring dialysis. Disseminated intravascular coagulation may be noted on coagulation studies. Gastrointestinal haemorrhage may be due to acute peptic ulceration.

Investigations[15–17]

Serum amylase and lipase

A two- or three-fold elevation of serum amylase is usually diagnostic of acute pancreatitis, but absolute levels do not correlate with severity or mortality. Concentrations rise within 2–3 h and return to normal in 3–10 days. Quicker changes are seen in mild oedematous forms and severe necrotizing pancreatitis, where enzyme concentrations diminish because of extensive damage to the gland. Unless concentrations are estimated early and frequently, rises in amylase may be missed. Serum concentrations may also rise in patients with perforated or infarcted bowel, and in conditions affecting other organs which secrete amylase (e.g. salivary glands, ovaries, etc.). Although it is possible to separate the isoenzymes of amylase into pancreatic (P-type) and others (S-type), these tests are not routinely available. Steinberg *et al.* suggest that the best sensitivity (92–95%) and specificity (98–100%) of serum amylase occurs when a cut-off of 1.5–2.0 times the upper limit of normal is used.[18]

Serum lipase concentrations parallel those of serum amylase, but may remain higher for longer, and are not increased by extrapancreatic disorders. The cut-off which results in the best sensitivity (86.5%) and specificity (99%) for serum lipase occurs at the upper limit of the normal range.[18] Lipase concentrations are now available in many laboratories, and may help to diagnose pancreatitis in difficult clinical situations.

CT scanning

CT scanning has become extremely useful in the diagnosis and management of patients with pancreatitis.[19,20] Sequential contrast-enhanced scans now permit more accurate diagnosis, and have reduced the number of cases of pancreatitis found at exploratory laparotomy. The detection of necrosis within the pancreas indicates greater severity. The course of the disease can be followed with subsequent scans which also allow the detection of complications such as abscesses and pseudocysts. Some collections can be aspirated at the time of imaging.

Ultrasound

In general terms, definition of the gland with ultrasonography is more difficult, and it is not visualized in up to 40% of patients.[21] However, an abdominal ultrasound is particularly useful in demonstrating gallstones as the cause of acute pancreatitis. Collections such as cysts and pseudocysts are not reliably found.

Other enzymes and fluids

Amylase concentrations within pleural or ascitic fluid may be elevated in acute pancreatitis. Urinary excretion of amylase and the ratio of urinary amylase clearance to creatinine clearance (C_{am}/C_{cr}) are rarely measured. Plasma trypsin-like immunoreactivity and phospholipase A_2 increase but are not routinely estimated.

Haematology

The white cell count is typically raised to $15–20 \times 10^3/mm^3$ with neutrophilia and left shift. Haemoglobin levels may increase if sufficient haemoconcentration occurs or the levels may decrease if there is bleeding from the gland.

Chemical pathology

Liver function tests

Transient elevations in serum bilirubin are seen in 10% of patients. Concentrations return to normal within 4 days. Increases in alkaline phosphatase and transaminases are also observed.

Glucose

Hyperglycaemia is observed, with incidences varying from 25 to 75%. These rises have been attributed to decreased concentrations of circulating insulin and increased concentrations of glucagon, catecholamines and steroids.

Calcium and magnesium

Serum calcium falls in 25% of patients. The change is usually due to concomitant hypoproteinaemia, although ionized concentrations of calcium may decrease, possibly due to intraperitoneal saponification. Hypocalcaemia may occasionally require treatment. Hypomagnesaemia may also occur and is more common in alcohol-induced pancreatitis.

Electrocardiography

Widespread ST–T-wave changes may simulate acute myocardial ischaemia. Arrhythmias have been observed in pericarditis associated with pancreatitis.

Imaging

Abdominal X-rays

Many changes have been described but are not specific for pancreatitis. These include localized jejunal ileus, generalized small bowel ileus, colon cut-off sign (from isolated peripancreatic dilatation) and duodenal distension. A swollen pancreas or associated cyst/pseudocyst may displace the stomach anteriorly or widen the duodenal loop. These changes can be seen when a dye such as Gastrografin is administered prior to plain erect and lateral abdominal radiographs.

Chest X-rays

May be abnormal in up to 40% of cases. An elevated left hemidiaphragm with pleural effusion, basal atelectasis or alveolar infiltrates, consistent with a diagnosis of ARDS, may be noted.

Assessment of severity

In the majority of cases, acute oedematous pancreatitis is a self-limiting disease of 3–7 days' duration and with a low mortality. Necrotizing pancreatitis occurs in 20–30% with an estimated mortality of 50%. Abscesses are seen in 5–10% of patients, but have a mortality approaching 100% without surgery. Chronic pancreatitis is a rare complication of an isolated episode of acute pancreatitis.

Table 36.2 Early prognostic signs of morbidity and mortality

At admission
Age >55 years
White cell count >16000/mm^3
Blood glucose >11 mmol/l
Serum LDH >twice normal
Serum AST >6 times normal

During initial 48 h
Haematocrit decrease by >10%
Increase in blood urea >2.0 mmol/l
Serum calcium <2.0 mmol/l
Pao_2 <60 mmHg (8 kPa)
Base deficit >4 mmol/l
Estimated fluid sequestration >6 l

Adapted from Ranson *et al.*[22]
LDH = Lactate dehydrogenase; AST = aspartate transaminase.

Several attempts have been made to define high-risk patients upon admission and during hospital stay. In 1974, Ranson *et al.* published a severity score based upon factors present or absent on admission or during the initial 48 h (Table 36.2).[22] The prognostic factors were used in a subsequent study of 200 patients with pancreatitis. Of 162 patients with fewer than three factors present, one had severe disease; 24 of 38 patients with more than three factors had severe disease and 100% mortality.[23] Imrie *et al.* proposed a simplified score based on the presence of nine clinical and laboratory factors within the first 48 h.[24] This scoring system, with a minor modification, predicted severity in 76.6% of 145 episodes of pancreatitis.[25] Both criteria take 48 h before classification can be made.

CT scans have also been used to assess severity and outcome.[19] The presence and degree of pancreatic necrosis (<30%, 50%, >50%) correlated with increased mortality, complications, hospital length of stay, and Ranson's original criteria. APACHE II scores have also been evaluated with complication rates, mortality and clinical outcome associated with high initial and rising values.[26,27]

Management

In general terms, acute management consists of medical therapies, with surgical intervention reserved for complications. Patients with necrotizing pancreatitis should be admitted to an ICU where major complications can be detected and treated with minimal delay.

Medical therapies

Fluid replacement

The inflammatory exudate around the pancreas resembles that of an internal burn, and huge volumes of fluid may be sequestered into the retroperitoneal and peritoneal spaces. Rapid fluid loss may occur with deficits of many litres recorded. Blood, plasma expanders and crystalloid should be administered to restore these deficits. The choice of solution is determined by the clinical signs, haemoglobin and packed cell volume results and serum albumin. Volumes and rates of infusion must be adjusted according to central venous pressures, urine output and blood pressure. As with other multisystem disorders, pulmonary artery catheters can be very useful in patients with myocardial or respiratory disorders, especially if ARDS develops.

Pain relief

Adequate analgesia can be achieved by parenteral narcotics in most patients. Pethidine has often been prescribed in preference to morphine on the basis that the latter constricts the sphincter of Oddi. However, this preference is more theoretical than practical, as both drugs affect the sphincter, and pancreatic secretions are minimal. Epidural anaesthesia by intermittent or continuous infusion may be very helpful, especially in patients with impaired respiratory function from pain and basal atelectasis.

Metabolic and electrolyte balance

Hyperglycaemia usually requires insulin therapy. Under most conditions, insulin infusions provide rapid and better control, but a dextrose infusion should be administered concurrently to prevent inadvertent hypoglycaemia. Calcium gluconate is occasionally required to treat symptomatic hypocalcaemia. Plasma magnesium and phosphate concentrations should be checked, and major deficits corrected.

Antibiotics

The role of antibiotics in the treatment of pancreatitis is complex. Patients with abscesses or other sepsis require drainage and therapeutic administration of drugs based on results of cultures. Routine administration of antibiotics is generally not recommended. Early studies with ampicillin[28,29] found no benefit. However, for those with necrotizing pancreatitis, recent trials demonstrated a decrease in infective complications with prophylactic imipenem,[30] and in mortality with prophylactic cefuroxime.[31]

ERCP

Patients with acute pancreatitis due to gallstones may benefit from ERCP and sphincterotomy. In a randomized trial of 121 patients with gallstone pancreatitis, morbidity was significantly reduced in patients who underwent ERCP with sphincterotomy and removal of stones within 72 h of presentation.[32]

Nutrition

Total parenteral nutrition (TPN) is often seen as an adjunct to other therapies. Its safety in pancreatitis has been established.[33,34] Whether or not TPN can alter outcome remains unclear. In a randomized study on 73 patients with severe pancreatitis, TPN improved nutritional indices in 81%; greater mortality was seen in patients who failed to achieve a positive nitrogen balance (21.4 versus 2.5%).[35] None of these studies has been randomized or controlled. Despite the association between hyperlipidaemia and pancreatitis, lipid infusions (Intralipid) appear safe.[36]

Jejunal feeding may be an alternative and would avoid the septic risks of TPN. It is well-known that oral or intraduodenal food will increase pancreatic secretions while nutrients placed in the jejunum do not have the same effect.

Suppression of pancreatic secretion

All patients should be fasted. A nasogastric tube is required if there is gastric distension, vomiting, paralytic ileus or when the patient requires endotracheal intubation. Somatostatin and the somatostatin analogue octreotide have been extensively studied in recent years with conflicting results.[37–42] A recent meta-analysis of six individual studies suggests reduced mortality in patients receiving somatostatin, as well as a reduction in pain and analgesic requirements.[43] Additional studies involving larger numbers of patients are required before this therapy can be routinely recommended.

Enzyme inhibitors

Although initially used enthusiastically, aprotinin (Trasylol) is no longer recommended, as results of trials have been disappointing. Newer antiproteases such as gabexate mesilate have been used in randomized clinical trials, but have not reduced mortality, need for surgery or length of stay.[44]

Surgery
Early intervention

There are very few indications for early surgery in the course of acute pancreatitis. Early cholecystectomy (within 48 h) for gallstone pancreatitis is associated with greater morbidity for mild and severe disease when compared to conservative management, with cholecystectomy performed between 4 and 10 days after presentation.[45]

Peritoneal lavage

Early peritoneal lavage using ordinary peritoneal dialysis catheters has been recommended for patients with moderate and severe pancreatitis,[14,23,46] but its use has declined in the past 10 years. Two randomized trials of peritoneal lavage in severe pancreatitis did not show any benefit on morbidity or mortality.[47,48] However, a recent trial in patients with severe pancreatitis suggested a reduction in frequency and mortality of sepsis in those randomized to long-term (7 days) versus short-term (2 days) lavage.[49] Although it does not treat the underlying pathology nor alter the eventual mortality, it may result in better haemodynamic stability.[2]

Management of complications

Surgery is often necessary for complications which may develop days to weeks after the acute event. Extensive necrosis may require debridement and the placement of large drain tubes within the pancreatic bed.[2] Patients with a pancreatic abscess (sometimes difficult to separate from necrotic tissue) must undergo surgery as mortality is 100% with antibiotics alone and 20–40% with surgery. Attempts to drain these collections by percutaneous catheters placed under CT control have only been moderately successful.[10] Complications such as bleeding, vascular obstruction and fistulae require correction. Pseudocysts may also require drainage which can be undertaken many days after the acute changes have subsided, unless the cyst has become infected.

References

1 Marshall JB (1993) Acute pancreatitis. A review with an emphasis on new developments. *Arch Intern Med* **153**:1185–1198.
2 Fernandez-del Castillo C, Rattner DW and Warshaw AL (1993) Acute pancreatitis. *Lancet* **342**:474–479.
3 Steinberg W and Tenner S (1994) Acute pancreatitis. *N Engl J Med* **330**:1198–1210.
4 Battersby C and Chapius P (1977) Acute pancreatitis: the Queensland scene. *Aust NZ J Surg* **47**:205–209.
5 Bockus H. (1985) Gastroenterology. In: Berk J (ed.) *Gastroenterology*. Philadelphia: W.B. Saunders.
6 Lankish P, Rahif G and Koop H (1983) Pulmonary complications in fatal acute hemorrhagic pancreatitis. *Dig Dis Sci* **28**:111–116.
7 Schroder T, Kivilaakso E, Kinnunen PK *et al.* (1980) Serum phospholipase A₂ in human acute pancreatitis. *Scand J Gastroenterol* **15**:633–636.
8 Klar E, Messmer K, Warshaw AL *et al.* (1990) Pancreatic ischaemia in experimental acute pancreatitis: mechanism, signficance and therapy. *Br J Surg* **77**:1205–1210.
9 Beger HG, Bittner R, Block S *et al.* (1986) Bacterial contamination of pancreatic necrosis. A prospective clinical study. *Gastroenterology* **91**:433–438.
10 Gerzof SG, Banks PA, Robbins AH *et al.* (1987) Early diagnosis of pancreatic infection by computed tomography-guided aspiration. *Gastroenterology* **93**:1315–1320.
11 Singer MV, Gyr K and Sarles H (1985) Revised classification of pancreatitis. Report of the Second International Symposium on the Classification of Pancreatitis in Marseille, France, March 28–30, 1984. *Gastroenterology* **89**:683–685.
12 Bradley E. (1993) A clinically based classification system for acute pancreatitis. Summary of the International Symposium on Acute Pancreatitis, Atlanta, Ga, September 11–13, 1992. *Arch Surg* **128**:586–590.
13 Amman R and Warshaw A (1985) Acute pancreatitis: clinical aspects and medical management. In: Berk J (ed.) *Bockus Gastroenterology*. Philadelphia: WB Saunders, pp. 3993–4009.
14 Paroulakis M, Fischer S, Vellar ID *et al.* (1981) Problems in the diagnosis and management of acute pancreatitis. *Aust NZ J Surg* **51**:257–263.
15 Bell J and Go V. Laboratory diagnosis of pancreatic disease. In: Berk J (ed.) *Bockus Gastroenterology*. Philadelphia: WB Saunders, pp. 3877–3892.
16 Klein G and Stein G (1985) Conventional radiography of the pancreas. In: Berk J (ed.) *Bockus Gastroenterology*. Philadelphia: WB Saunders, pp. 3893–3906.
17 Scheible W and Leopold G (1985) Pancreatic ultrasound In: Berk J (ed.) *Bockus Gastroenterology*. Philadelphia: WB Saunders, pp. 3907–3912.
18 Steinberg WM, Goldstein SS, Davis ND *et al.* (1985) Diagnostic assays in acute pancreatitis. A study of sensitivity and specificity. *Ann Intern Med* **102**:576–580.
19 Balthazar EJ, Robinson DL, Megibow AJ *et al.* (1990) Acute pancreatitis: value of CT in establishing prognosis. *Radiology* **174**:331–336.
20 Hill MC and Huntington DK. (1990) Computed tomography and acute pancreatitis. *Gastroenterol Clin North Am* **19**:811–842.
21 Silverstein W, Isikoff MB, Hill MC *et al.* (1981) Diagnostic imaging of acute pancreatitis: prospective study using CT and sonography. *Am J Roentgenol* **137**:497–502.
22 Ranson JH, Rifkind KM, Roses DF *et al.* (1974) Prognostic signs and the role of operative management in acute pancreatitis. *Surg Gynecol Obstet* **139**:69–81.
23 Ranson JH, Rifkind KM and Turner JW. (1976) Prognostic signs and operative peritoneal lavage in acute pancreatitis. *Surg Gynecol Obstet* **143**:209–219.
24 Imrie CW, Benjamin IS, Ferguson JC *et al.* (1978) A single-centre double-blind trial of Trasylol therapy in primary acute pancreatitis. *Br J Surg* **65**:337–341.
25 Blamey SL, Imrie CW, O'Neill J *et al.* (1984) Prognostic factors in acute pancreatitis. *Gut* **25**:1340–1346.
26 Larvin M and McMahon MJ. (1989) APACHE-II score for assessment and monitoring of acute pancreatitis. *Lancet* **2**:201–205.
27 Wilson C, Heath DI and Imrie CW (1990) Prediction of outcome in acute pancreatitis: a comparative study of APACHE II, clinical assessment and multiple factor scoring systems. *Br J Surg* **77**:1260–1264.
28 Finch WT, Sawyers JL and Schenker S (1976) A prospective study to determine the efficacy of antibiotics in acute pancreatitis. *Ann Surg* **183**:667–671.
29 Howes R, Zuidema GD and Cameron JL. (1975) Evaluation of prophylactic antibiotics in acute pancreatitis. *J Surg Res* **18**:197–200.
30 Pederzoli P, Bassi C, Vesentini S *et al.* (1993) A randomized multicenter clinical trial of antibiotic prophylaxis of septic complications in acute necrotizing pancreatitis with imipenem. *Surg Gynecol Obstet* **176**:480–483.
31 Saino V, Kemppainen E, Puolakkainen P *et al.* (1995) Early antibiotic treatment in acute necrotising pancreatitis. *Lancet* **346**:664–667.
32 Neoptolemos JP, Carr-Locke DL, London NJ *et al.* (1988) Controlled trial of urgent endoscopic retrograde cholangiopancreatography and endoscopic sphincterotomy versus conservative treatment for acute pancreatitis due to gallstones. *Lancet* **2**:979–983.
33 Kalfarentzos FE, Karavias DD, Karatzas TM *et al.* (1991) Total parenteral nutrition in severe acute pancreatitis. *J Am Coll Nutr* **10**:156–162.
34 Robin AP, Campbell R, Palani CK *et al.* (1990) Total parenteral nutrition during acute pancreatitis: clinical experience with 156 patients. *World J Surg* **14**:572–579.
35 Sitzmann JV, Steinborn PA, Zinner MJ *et al.* (1989) Total parenteral nutrition and alternate energy substrates in treatment of severe acute pancreatitis. *Surg Gynecol Obstet* **168**:311–317.
36 Van Gossum A, Lemoyne M, Greig PD *et al.* (1988) Lipid–associated total parenteral nutrition in patients with severe acute pancreatitis. *J Parenter Enteral Nutr* **12**:250–255.
37 Beechey-Newman N. (1993) Controlled trial of high-

dose octreotide in treatment of acute pancreatitis. Evidence of improvement in disease severity. *Dig Dis Sci* **38**:644–647.

38 Binder M, Uhl W, Friess H *et al.* (1994) Octreotide in the treatment of acute pancreatitis: results of a unicenter prospective trial with three different octreotide dosages. *Digestion* **55** (Suppl): 20–23.

39 Binmoeller KF, Harris AG, Dumas R *et al.* (1992) Does the somatostatin analogue octreotide protect against ERCP induced pancreatitis? *Gut* **33**:1129–1133.

40 Gjorup I, Roikjaer O, Andersen B *et al.* (1992) A double-blinded multicenter trial of somatostatin in the treatment of acute pancreatitis. *Surg Gynecol Obstet* **175**:397–400.

41 Luengo L, Vicente V, Gris F *et al.* (1994) Influence of somatostatin in the evolution of acute pancreatitis. A prospective randomized study. *Int J Pancreatol* **15**:139–144.

42 Sternlieb JM, Aronchick CA, Retig JN *et al.* (1992) A multicenter, randomized, controlled trial to evaluate the effect of prophylactic octreotide on ERCP-induced pancreatitis. *Am J Gastroenterol* **87**:1561–1566.

43 Buchler MW, Binder M and Friess H. (1994) Role of somatostatin and its analogues in the treatment of acute and chronic pancreatitis. *Gut* **35**:S15–S19.

44 Buchler M, Malfertheiner P, Uhl W *et al.* (1993) Gabexate mesilate in human acute pancreatitis. German Pancreatitis Study Group. *Gastroenterology* **104**:1165–1170.

45 Kelly TR and Wagner DS (1988) Gallstone pancreatitis: a prospective randomized trial of the timing of surgery. *Surgery* **104**:600–605.

46 Warshaw A. (1980) Surgical pros and cons: peritoneal lavage in acute pancreatitis. *Surg Gynecol Obstet* **151**:547–548.

47 Ihse I, Evander A, Gustafson I *et al.* (1986) Influence of peritoneal lavage on objective prognostic signs in acute pancreatitis. *Ann Surg* **204**:122–127.

48 Mayer A, McMahon M and Corfield A. (1985) Controlled clinical trial of peritoneal lavage for the treatment of severe acute pancreatitis. *N Engl J Med* **312**:399–404.

49 Ranson JH and Berman RS (1990). Long peritoneal lavage decreases pancreatic sepsis in acute pancreatitis. *Ann Surg* **211**:708–716; discussion 716–718.

37 | Hepatic failure

FH Hawker

Acute liver failure

In acute liver failure (ALF), massive necrosis of hepatocytes leads to severely impaired liver function and hepatic encephalopathy.[1-4] Several subgroups are recognized, although the nomenclature remains non-standardized.[5] The term *fulminant hepatic failure* (FHF) should be reserved for patients who develop hepatic encephalopathy within 8 weeks of first symptoms, whereas *late-onset hepatic failure* (LOHF) is used when encephalopathy appears between 8 and 26 weeks. Patients with LOHF have a lower incidence of cerebral oedema, develop renal failure more frequently and have a worse prognosis without liver transplantation.[6]

Aetiology (Table 37.1)

Viral hepatitis

Acute viral hepatitis accounts for 40–70% of ALF. Clinical characteristics of the hepatitis viruses are shown in Table 37.2.

Acute hepatitis A (HAV)
HAV infection is common but rarely leads to ALF (0.35%).[7] It is diagnosed by the presence of the immunoglobulin M (IgM) antibody to HAV. Patients with ALF caused by HAV infection have a relatively good prognosis; survival is approximately 60% without liver transplantation.[8]

Acute hepatitis B (HBV)
HBV is the cause of approximately 70% of ALF from viral hepatitis. Liver injury is immunologically mediated. Mortality is around 60–70% with medical treatment.[8] It is diagnosed by the presence of the IgM antibody (HBcAb) to hepatitis B core antigen, with or without hepatitis B surface antigen (HbsAg). Co-infection with hepatitis D virus (HDV) increases the risk and severity of ALF.

Table 37.1 Causes of acute liver failure

		Incidence (% of cases)
Viral hepatitis		40–70
Hepatitis A	5–30	
Hepatitis B	25–75	% of all
Hepatitic C	<1	viral cases
Hepatitis E	0–20	
Drug-induced hepatitis		15
Poisoning (including paracetamol)		5*
Miscellaneous		10
Unknown		20–30

*Incidence of paracetamol-induced acute liver failure is much higher in the UK.

Hepatitis C (HCV)
HCV infection is commonly associated with chronic liver disease. It is detected by the presence of antibodies to HCV in serum. ALF very rarely results.[9]

Hepatitis E (HEV)
HEV is a recently described virus responsible for outbreaks of enterically transmitted hepatitis, particularly in the Indian subcontinent, Asia and Africa. Mortality is high among pregnant women.[10] It can be diagnosed by detection of antibodies to HEV in serum. HEV infection may account for as many as 20% of instances of non-A, non-B hepatitis (NANB) in the western world, particularly if there has been recent travel to endemic areas.[11]

New hepatitis viruses
New hepatitis viruses will doubtless be described. A major proportion of sporadic cases of ALF remain of uncertain cause (formerly called NANB). Even with sophisticated molecular biological techniques, known hepatitis viruses cannot be incriminated in many cases.[9]

Table 37.2 Clinical characteristics of the hepatitis viruses

	Hepatitis A	Hepatitis B	Hepatitis C	Hepatitis D	Hepatitis E
Spread	Faecal–oral	Parenteral Sexual Perinatal	Parenteral ?Sexual Perinatal	Parenteral ?Sexual	Faecal–oral
Incubation period					
Mean	28 days	70–80 days	6–12 weeks	?	42 days
Range	14–49 days	28–160 days	2–26 weeks	28–140 days	14–63 days
Acute mortality	0.2%	0.2–1%	0.2%	2–20%	0.2%
Mortality from ALF	30–40%	50–60%	85%	(See HBV)	20% (pregnant women)
Chronicity	None	2–10%	>20%	2–70%	None
Antigens	HAVAg	HBsAg HBcAg HBeAg	HCVAg	HDVAg	HEVAg
Antibodies	Anti-HAV	Anti-HBs Anti-HBc Anti-HBe	Anti-HCV	Anti-HDV	Anti-HEV

ALF = Acute liver failure.

Other viruses

Other viruses such as herpes simplex 1 and 2, varicella-zoster virus, cytomegalovirus (CMV), Epstein–Barr virus and measles virus are all rare causes of ALF, particularly in the immuno-compromised patient. Infections such as Rift Valley fever, dengue, yellow fever, Lassa fever and the haemorrhagic fevers should be considered in those returning from endemic areas.

Acute drug-induced hepatic necrosis

Drug-induced hepatitis is responsible for approximately 15–25% of ALF. In some patients, there appears to be true hypersensitivity. Symptoms develop after a sensitization period of 1–5 weeks, recur promptly with readministration of the drug, and may be accompanied by fever, rash and eosinophilia. In other patients, toxic drug metabolites are believed to be responsible. Many drugs have been implicated. However isoniazid, phenytoin, salazopyrine, non-steroidal anti-inflammatory agents, antidepressants and allopurinol are reported frequently. Only approximately 12% of patients with drug-induced ALF survive without liver transplantation.[8]

Halothane hepatitis is the rare fulminant liver injury associated with administration of the volatile anaesthetic agent halothane.[12] It is believed to be caused by an allergic reaction to a reactive intermediate of oxidative halothane metabolism.

Hepatic necrosis from poisoning (see Chapter 77)

Paracetamol poisoning

Paracetamol poisoning is a more common cause of ALF in the UK than anywhere else. Early nausea and vomiting are usual, followed by signs of liver failure 48–72 h after ingestion. Hepatotoxic effects are caused by a reactive metabolite that is normally efficiently detoxified by glutathione. Treatment is with N-acetylcysteine to increase hepatic stores of glutathione. The recommended dosage schedule is 150 mg/kg in 5% dextrose over 15 min, followed by 50 mg/kg in 5% dextrose over 4 h, followed by 100 mg/kg in 5% dextrose over 16 h. Even late administration (up to 36 h after ingestion) may improve outcome.[13]

Mushroom poisoning

Signs of hepatic necrosis can develop 2–3 days after ingestion of some mushrooms, of which *Amanita phalloides* is the most toxic.[14] There are severe gastrointestinal symptoms, resulting in dehydration and electrolyte imbalance. Liver injury is caused by amatoxins. The most useful treatment is forced diuresis, as large amounts of toxin are excreted in urine. Thioctic acid, silibinin and penicillin have been advocated, but have not been subjected to controlled trials.

Other poisonings

Acute yellow phosphorus, carbon tetrachloride, chloroform, trichloroethylene, xylene (in glue sniffers) and some herbal remedies are very rare causes of ALF.

Miscellaneous

Miscellaneous causes account for a small proportion of ALF. These include fulminant Wilson's disease, microvesicular steatosis (Reye's syndrome and acute fatty liver of pregnancy), hyperthermia, ischaemic liver necrosis, hepatic venous obstruction (Budd–Chiari syndrome), reactivation of chronic HBV infection, and complications of liver transplantation and hepatic resection surgery.

Clinical features

There may be a history suggestive of a cause. In many cases no such history is available. The disease typically evolves over several days, but deep coma can occur in hours or may develop over months in LOHF.[2] Most patients become deeply jaundiced. The liver is usually small and impalpable. Signs of chronic liver disease (e.g. palmar erythema, spider naevi, spleno-megaly and hypoalbuminaemia) are absent, but ascites may develop in patients with LOHF.

Encephalopathy

Encephalopathy is a characteristic feature of ALF. It is classified by severity into four grades (Table 37.3).

Table 37.3 Clinical features of grade of encephalopathy

Grade	Features
I	Mild or episodic drowsiness, impaired intellect, concentration and pychomotor function, but rousable and coherent
II	Increased drowsiness with confusion and disorientation; rousable and conversant
III	Very drowsy, disorientated, responds to simple verbal commands, often agitated and aggressive
IV	Responds to painful stimuli at best, but may be unresponsive. May be complicated by evidence of cerebral oedema

Cerebral oedema is present in over 80% of grade IV encephalopathy, and is the major cause of death. Although documentation of the grade of encephalopathy is important, the clinical course can be followed more accurately by repeated clinical examination (Fig. 37.1). An early sign of progression of encephalopathy is a generalized increase in muscle tone, which may progress to full decerebrate posturing. There is a parallel increase in briskness of the deep tendon reflexes, and an extensor plantar response; sustained clonus may be present as encephalopathy progresses. Lateralizing signs are virtually never present, and suggest an alternative or additional diagnosis, such as intracerebral haemorrhage. Spontaneous hyper-ventilation is also common, and can result in significant respiratory alkalosis. The pupils may become dilated in advanced encephalopathy, particu-larly in response to noxious stimuli, and may subsequently become sluggishly reactive. Despite the cerebral oedema, papilloedema is unusual. If the pupils become dilated and unreactive, brainstem coning is likely. In such situations, metabolic derangements preclude diagnosis of death by clinical brainstem tests, and death should be confirmed by absence of cerebral blood flow as demonstrated by radiological or nuclear medicine techniques.

The precise cause of encephalopathy in ALF is unknown. It is generally attributed to accumulation of circulating toxic substances which can cause both coma and cerebral oedema. Substances arising from

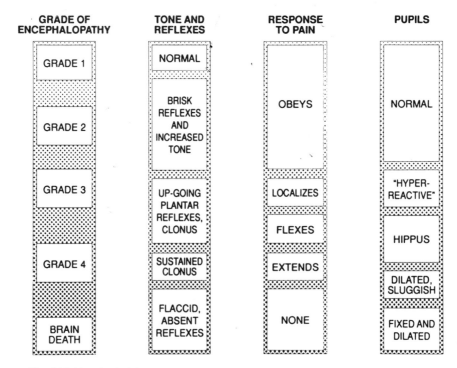

Fig. 37.1 Neurological features of acute liver failures.

the gut (e.g. ammonia, mercaptans, fatty acids, phenols and γ-aminobutyric acid (GABA)), endogenous benzodiazepines, glutamine and other neurotransmitters (e.g. octopamine) have been implicated. No useful specific treatment for encephalopathy or cerebral oedema has resulted from antagonizing effects of these substances.

Bleeding diathesis

The liver plays a central role in haemostasis, and ALF results in a complex coagulopathy. All coagulation factors except factor VIII are synthesized in hepatocytes, and in ALF circulating concentrations of fibrinogen, prothrombin and factors V, VII, IX and X are reduced. The international normalized ratio (INR) for prothrombin or prothrombin time (PT) is prolonged, primarily because of reduced synthesis of factors of the extrinsic coagulation pathway (see Chapter 89). Prolongation of the INR is a useful prognostic indicator. There is low-grade disseminated vascular coagulation (DIC) in most patients,[15] but a fulminant disorder is unusual. Principal causes are endotoxaemia and sepsis, although impaired synthesis of the naturally occurring inhibitors of coagulation (e.g. antithrombin III and protein C) may contribute. Quantitative and qualitative defects of platelet function occur.[16] About two-thirds of patients have platelet counts under $100\,000 \times 10^6$ cells/l. Platelet aggregation is impaired but there is increased platelet adhesiveness.

Older studies report severe bleeding in 30% of ALF patients,[16] but this complication appears to be less common in recent years. Deficiency of coagulation factors does not correlate with risk of bleeding. Haemorrhage is most likely with thrombocytopenia, and with frank DIC. The most common site of haemorrhage is the gastrointestinal tract. Other sites include the nasopharynx, respiratory tract, skin puncture sites or the retroperitoneal space. Spontaneous intracerebral haemorrhage is unusual.

Cardiovascular disturbances

Patients with ALF characteristically have a high cardiac index (>5 l/min per m^2) and low systemic vascular resistance.[17] A flow murmur is commonly present. Hypotension from peripheral vasodilatation is usually responsive to volume loading. Pathogenetic mediators of this high-output state are not known with certainty; nitric oxide may be involved. Hypertension may occur in patients with advanced encephalopathy, and is probably an attempt to maintain cerebral perfusion pressure (CPP) in response to an increased intracranial pressure.

Respiratory failure

The decreased level of consciousness may compromise the airway. Hyperventilation (leading to respiratory alkalosis) is a characteristic feature of hepatic encephalopathy. The indication for mechanical ventilation is cerebral oedema in most patients, and hypoxaemia in approximately one-third.[18] Complications of coma, such as bronchopneumonia, aspiration or atelectasis are the usual causes of hypoxaemia.

Renal failure

Renal failure occurs in approximately 75% of patients with grade IV encephalopathy following paracetamol poisoning (largely due to drug nephrotoxic effects). The incidence is lower with other aetiologies ($<30\%$),[8] when renal failure may present as the hepatorenal syndrome. This condition of unknown pathogenesis is believed to be functional in nature. It is characterized by a progressive oliguria, increased plasma creatinine concentration, low urine sodium concentration (<10 mmol/l) and histologically normal kidneys (see Chapter 38). Acute tubular necrosis (ATN) may also occur as a result of hypotension, hypovolaemia or severe sepsis. Differentiation between the two disorders may be difficult.

In the past, associated renal failure requiring renal replacement therapy had a dismal prognosis. However, more recently, survival rates of 50% for renal failure associated with paracetamol-induced ALF, and 30% with viral hepatitis-induced ALF have been reported.[8]

Infective complications

Severe infections may complicate ALF. Early infections are usually caused by Gram-positive and Gram-negative aerobes. The respiratory and urinary tracts are the most common sites. Spontaneous bacterial peritonitis is rare, since ascites is uncommon. Infections occurring after the first week of ICU treatment are often fungal.[20] Sepsis worsens liver function[19,20] and may directly cause death. Death from sepsis typically occurs after the first week, and is most common in patients with LOHF. Fever and increased white blood cell counts are not good indices of infection in ALF. They are absent in 30% of patients with documented bacterial infection.

Metabolic disturbances

Hypoglycaemia is usual, and results from impaired gluconeogenesis, reduced glycogen stores and increased circulating insulin concentrations. It should be considered whenever the mental state deteriorates, but clinical signs may be masked in established encephalopathy.

Both hypernatraemia and hyponatraemia may be present. The former results from treatment of cerebral oedema with dehydration and the large salt load in blood products. Hyponatraemia appears to be dilutional. Hypokalaemia is present in about half the patients. It may be both the cause and the result of metabolic alkalosis. Decreased plasma concentrations of magnesium, phosphate and zinc occur frequently.[21]

Primary respiratory alkalosis is usual in spontaneously breathing patients. It is a consequence of hepatic encephalopathy but the mechanism is unknown. Metabolic alkalosis occurs in 25–50% of patients, and predisposing factors are hypokalaemia and inability of the liver to synthesize urea. Gastric aspiration and vomiting do not seem to be important causes. Metabolic acidosis is common in paracetamol poisoning, and is the most reliable indicator of poor prognosis in these patients. In other patients, it is almost always associated with severe circulatory compromise.

Impaired drug metabolism

Patients with ALF are particularly sensitive to the depressant effects of sedative and analgesic drugs. This is chiefly the result of impaired drug breakdown, but increased cerebral sensitivity and changes in plasma protein binding contribute.

Rare complications

Rare complications of viral hepatitis include myocarditis, atypical pneumonia, aplastic anaemia, transverse myelitis and peripheral neuropathy.

Investigations

Laboratory investigations

These should include serological investigations for hepatitis (hepatitis A, B, C and E, CMV, Epstein–Barr virus and herpes simplex) and a drug screen, specifically for paracetamol. Plasma caeruloplasmin concentration and 24-h urinary copper excretion exclude Wilson's disease.

Coagulation studies

The INR is a sensitive index of liver function and an important determinant of prognosis and the need for liver transplantation. It should be measured every 6 h.

Liver function tests

These should be performed at least daily. A plasma bilirubin concentration of $>300 \, \mu mol/l$ is a poor prognostic sign and is a criterion for transplantation. Peak plasma aminotransferase concentrations (alanine aminotransferase, ALT, and aspartate aminotransferase, AST) are always high, but these enzymes may be only mildly elevated at ICU admission if massive loss of hepatocytes had already occurred. Plasma alkaline phosphatase (ALP), γ-glutamyl transpeptidase (GGT), albumin and globulin concentrations are usually normal on presentation.

Other investigations

Blood glucose levels should be measured at least 4-hourly. Plasma electrolytes, urea and creatinine concentrations, arterial blood gases and full blood count should be measured at least twice daily. Regular cultures are undertaken of sputum and urine, and of blood if indicated. A chest X-ray and 12-lead electrocardiogram (ECG) should be performed daily. Computed tomography (CT) scan to estimate intracranial pressure (ICP) is of limited value, as signs of cerebral oedema on CT correlate poorly with the ICP until very late in the clinical course.[22] It is useful, however, to confirm intracerebral haemorrhage. Liver biopsy may occasionally be necessary. If indicated, the transjugular route is preferred, because of a decreased risk of haemorrhagic complications.

Management

The mainstay of treatment in ALF is supportive care and appropriate selection of transplant candidates. Early transfer of suitable candidates to a liver transplant unit should be considered. When the need for transplantation is being considered, drugs that may obscure the true neurological state and clotting factors that would affect coagulation tests should be avoided. These agents can be given once the decision is made to proceed with transplantation. The indications for liver transplantation are discussed in Chapter 93.

Monitoring

Oxygenation indices, ECG, haemodynamic variables, and temperature should be monitored continuously, and urine output measured hourly. Pulmonary artery catheterization may be indicated. ICP monitoring is now well-established in the management of ALF and advanced encephalopathy. It allows early recognition and treatment of intracranial hypertension (also during liver transplantation). However, risk of intracranial bleeding is considerable in these coagulopathic patients; the incidence is as high as 5%.[23] Fresh frozen plasma should be given prior to placement of the device, during which the patient should be anaesthetized, to avoid increases in ICP caused by pain and stimulation. ICP over 25–30 mmHg (3.3–4.0 kPa) requires urgent treatment (see below). The risk–benefit ratio should be considered for each patient, as excellent results have been obtained without ICP monitoring.[24]

Supportive care

Mechanical ventilation at normocarbia is usually necessary in grade III encephalopathy. An infusion of 10% dextrose will help avert hypoglycaemia. Lactulose (30 ml t.d.s. via the nasogastric tube) is widely used, although there is no evidence that it will improve encephalopathy in ALF. Bowel distension associated with its use may complicate liver transplantation. Use of neomycin is not recommended because of its nephrotoxicity and ototoxicity.

In general, normovolaemia should be maintained. Fluid overload may precipitate or worsen cerebral oedema, and hypovolaemia may result in hypotension with disastrous effects on the liver, other organs and CPP. If hypotension on presentation is not controlled by fluid replacement, inotrope infusions are indicated. The first aim of inotropic support is to maintain the CPP; the second is to improve tissue perfusion. N-acetylcysteine improves tissue perfusion, oxygen extraction ratio and mean arterial pressure (MAP) in ALF, but its effect on outcome has yet to be evaluated.

Infusions of clotting factors are indicated before invasive procedures or if there is overt bleeding. Fresh frozen plasma is not given routinely unless transplantation has been decided. Vitamin K should be administered daily. Blood losses are replaced by blood transfusion. Platelet transfusions are indicated if the platelet count falls below $50\,000 \times 10^6$ cells/l. H_2-antagonists or omeprazole are given because of the high risk of gastrointestinal bleeding.

Oliguria is managed initially with volume loading, but balanced against the risk of worsening cerebral oedema. Renal failure has a worse prognosis, but this is obviously better than brainstem coning. Low-dose dopamine is commonly used to increase urine output and promote diuresis, but true benefits are unproven. If oliguric renal failure develops, early dialysis is indicated. Continuous dialytic techniques are preferred because of greater haemodynamic stability and beneficial effects on the ICP.[25]

Infective complications should be anticipated. Appropriate antibiotic therapy is instituted early. If empirical antibiotics are necessary, these should be effective against both Gram-positive and Gram-negative bacteria. Antifungal agents should be considered after a week of ICU care. Aminoglycosides should be avoided because of the increased risk of nephrotoxicity in patients with liver disease. Application of topical antifungal agents to the mouth and skin creases is useful to reduce colonization (particularly important before liver transplantation). Some centres use selective decontamination of the digestive tract[26] (see Chapter 61).

Nutritional therapy is indicated, preferably by the enteral route. There is no evidence that protein restriction improves outcome in ALF. Branched chain amino acid solutions have not been demonstrated to improve encephalopathy or overall mortality.

Management of cerebral oedema

Patients should be nursed with the head elevated to $20°$[27] and venous return from the head must be unimpeded. Mannitol is the most effective treatment of cerebral oedema in ALF.[28] A dose of 0.5 g/kg should be infused using a burette, but maximum reductions in ICP may not occur for 20–60 min. The dose can be repeated for further episodes of intracranial hypertension, provided that serum osmolality remains < 320 mosmol/kg. In patients with renal failure, mannitol should only be used in conjunction with haemodialysis or haemofiltration, since fluid overload may exacerbate cerebral oedema. Frusemide may be useful adjunctive therapy to maintain the initial osmotic gradient established by mannitol.

Hyperventilation may be effective during an acute increase in ICP, but does not reduce the incidence or severity of cerebral oedema in the longer term.[29] Barbiturates (specifically thiopentone by infusion) have been used to control ICP in ALF,[30] but controlled trials are unavailable. Although ICP is reduced, the concomitant decrease in MAP from barbiturate cardiovascular depression can result in no change, or a decrease in CPP. Barbiturates may have a place in treating cerebral oedema refractory to mannitol therapy when liver transplantation is imminent, but only when ICP (and therefore CPP) is monitored. Corticosteroids do not influence the incidence and severity of cerebral oedema.[28] The usefulness of benzodiazepine antagonists has not been established.

Measures to improve liver function

There are no drugs which reverse the effects of hepatic failure. Drugs with cytoprotective properties (e.g. corticosteroids[31] and prostaglandin E_1) do not have beneficial effects. Interest has been recently shown on experimental treatments to stimulate hepatic regeneration. Insulin and glucagon therapy appears to have no benefit, but specific growth factors, such as hepatocyte growth factor, may have therapeutic potential.[32]

Artificial liver support

Exchange transfusion, plasma exchange, human cross-circulation, porcine liver cross-perfusion, haemofiltration through large-pore membranes and haemoperfusion have not improved survival. However, bioartificial means of hepatic support are now being investigated.[33] These devices involve perfusion through columns or plates of living hepatocytes,[34] and may become available for clinical use in the future.

Liver transplantation

Liver transplantation for ALF is discussed in Chapter 93. It should be considered early in the course of ALF.

Prognosis

Overall survival from ALF is approximately 20–25% with medical therapy alone, and 70% with liver transplantation. The aetiology of ALF is particularly important. In general, the prognosis for spontaneous recovery is relatively good for HAV infection, paracetamol poisoning and acute fatty liver of pregnancy; intermediate for HBV infection; and poor for idiosyncratic drug reactions, fulminant Wilson's disease and when the aetiology is unknown (previously termed NANB).[8]

Precautions against hepatitis

All ICU staff should be vaccinated against HBV. More than 90% of healthy adults achieve protective antibody levels.[35] Routine post-vaccination testing is recommended so that additional doses of vaccine can be given to those without an adequate response. Booster doses are usually necessary after 4 years. Vaccination against HAV is also recommended.[36] There is no vaccine against HCV or HEV.

All patients with ALF should be initially regarded as infectious. They should be barrier-nursed unless an alternative non-infectious diagnosis is proven. Blood, urine, faeces and other biological samples should be handled carefully and labelled prominently. All precautions should be taken to avoid puncture by contaminated needles or other sharp instruments.

The procedure for needlestick or permucosal exposure to blood or high-risk body fluids from a patient infected with HBV depends on whether the exposed individual has antibodies (HBsAb) to HBsAg. These may be acquired by vaccination or by previous subclinical infection. If HBsAb is present, no further action is necessary. If HBsAb status is unknown, hepatitis B immune globulin (HBIG; 0.06 ml/kg) should be administered as early as possible within 7 days, and the person tested for HBsAb. If HBsAb is negative, vaccination should also be started immediately, and the first dose of HBV vaccine (20 μg IM at a different site) should be given within 7 days of exposure and repeated 1 and 6 months later. Passively acquired HBsAb does not interfere with the immune response to the vaccine.

For HAV, immune globulin markedly reduces attack rate both pre- and postexposure in non-vaccinated individuals. A single IM dose of 0.02 ml/kg is advised within 2 weeks of exposure. Immune globulin does not offer protection against HCV or HEV infection.

Chronic liver failure

Chronic liver failure is most often the result of chronic infection with the HBV and HBC, autoimmune diseases (i.e. primary biliary cirrhosis, chronic active hepatitis and primary sclerosing cholangitis), alcoholic liver disease or, occasionally, cryptogenic cirrhosis.

Clinical signs include jaundice, ascites and encephalopathy, which may be present in isolation or in combination. Spider angiomata and palmar erythema

Table 37.4 Complications of portal hypertension

Bleeding
Oesophageal varices
Portal hypertensive gastropathy

Ascites
Spontaneous bacterial peritonitis

Hypersplenism
Thrombocytopenia
Neutropenia

Portal–systemic shunting
Prolonged half-life of drugs metabolized by the liver
Systemic spread of gut-derived microorganisms and endotoxin
Hypergammaglobulinaemia
Probable role in hepatic encephalopathy by allowing systemic spread of ammonia and gut-derived amines
?Role in circulatory manifestation of chronic liver disease
?Role in hepatorenal syndrome
?Role in hepatopulmonary syndrome

are usually present. There is usually a high cardiac output and low-resistance haemodynamic state.[37] Hypoxaemia caused by intrapulmonary shunting (the hepatopulmonary syndrome)[38] occurs in some patients. The hepatorenal syndrome (see above) also occurs in patients with chronic liver disease and is often a terminal complication.[39,40] Many of these clinical manifestations are the result of portal hypertension (Table 37.4). Plasma albumin concentration is usually low and the INR or PT may be prolonged, reflecting a reduced capacity of the liver to synthesize proteins. Other liver function tests are often unremarkable.

Acute episodes of decompensation may be caused by insults such as gastrointestinal bleeding, sepsis or dehydration. It is therefore important to recognize and treat these precipitants. Unlike ALF, patients with chronic liver disease have minimal potential for hepatic regeneration, and ICU management has little to offer unless there is an acute reversible complication or if liver transplantation is feasible. Complications are as described below.

Oesophageal varices

Variceal haemorrhage is a major cause of acute decompensation in chronic liver disease, and a common reason for admission to the ICU. This is discussed in Chapter 35.

Ascites[41,42]

Ascites is almost invariably present in patients with advanced chronic liver disease. Portal hypertension, hypoalbuminaemia, excessive hepatic lymph formation and abnormalities of sodium and water balance all contribute to its pathogenesis. Ascites increases intra-abdominal pressure and may decrease cardiac output, compromise pulmonary function and contribute to renal impairment. Although treatment of ascites traditionally includes salt and water restriction and diuretic therapy, these measures are usually unsuccessful or impractical in the critically ill. Paracentesis is the safest and most effective treatment in this setting. The total volume of ascites can be removed at a single paracentesis,[43] although blood pressure, urine output and central venous pressure should be closely monitored. Paracentesis has been shown to have beneficial effects on cardiac output,[44] pulmonary function[45] and portal venous pressure.[44] As ascites rapidly reaccumulates after paracentesis, colloid administration is usually required to prevent the consequent decrease in intravascular volume.

Sepsis

Sepsis is a common cause of decompensation in patients with chronic liver disease. The site of infection may be known, but spontaneous bacterial peritonitis is common in patients with ascites, and should be suspected if there are signs of sepsis, worsening encephalopathy, or an unexplained general deterioration. The diagnosis is made by ascitic tap, which should be performed in all patients with ascites requiring ICU admission. If the white cell count is $>250 \times 10^6$ cell/l, antibiotics should be commenced. The ascitic fluid should also be cultured. The infecting microorganism is usually a Gram-negative aerobe, often *Escherichia coli*.

Encephalopathy

Hepatic encephalopathy (termed portal–systemic encephalopathy in patients with chronic liver disease) often develops or worsens after an episode of gastrointestinal bleeding, and may also be precipitated by sepsis, dehydration, protein loading and portal–systemic shunting procedures. It is treated with lactulose (30 ml 3–4 times daily) instilled down the nasogastric tube, the gastric lumen of the balloon tamponade tube, or rectally, and concurrently with treatment of the underlying cause. General management includes airway and ventilatory support, and avoidance, where possible, of sedative drugs. Hepatic encephalopathy is very rarely associated with cerebral oedema in patients with chronic liver failure, and measures to control ICP are not necessary. It usually resolves with time if the precipitating cause can be controlled.

Liver dysfunction in the ICU

Critically ill patients admitted to the ICU with primarily non-hepatic diseases frequently develop liver dysfunction.[46] There may be:

1 direct hepatocellular damage (hepatitis-like pattern) with a marked rise in plasma AST and ALT concentrations, a prolonged INR, and variable but usually minor elevation of the plasma bilirubin concentration; or
2 intrahepatic cholestasis, where there is elevation of the plasma bilirubin concentration, with relatively normal plasma concentrations of AST, ALT, ALP and GGT.

Multiple aetiological factors may be present, and hepatocellular damage and intrahepatic cholestasis may coexist. In patients with unexplained jaundice, ultrasonography of the liver should be performed to exclude extrahepatic bile duct obstruction. Possible causes of liver dysfunction in ICU include the following,

Ischaemic hepatitis

This is the most common cause of direct hepatocellular damage (AST > 1000 IU/l) in the ICU and in the hospital.[47] It results from a critical reduction in liver blood flow in some patients with shock (particularly cardiogenic shock).[48,49] It is characterized biochemically by a marked increase in the plasma concentrations of the aminotransferase enzymes and prolongation of the INR. Other manifestations of shock (e.g. renal failure and metabolic acidosis) are often present. Mortality is approximately 67%, but whether the poor prognosis depends on the liver injury itself or the severity of the underlying disease is unclear. The treatment is aggressive improvement of the low cardiac output state.

'ICU jaundice'

This syndrome is associated with severe trauma and sepsis, and develops approximately 1 week after the onset of critical illness. It is the classic liver failure of the multiple organ failure syndrome, although conventional signs of liver failure are not present. Jaundice is the major clinical and biochemical finding, and other clinical signs reflect the underlying disease. The principal histological finding is intrahepatic cholestasis. The pathogenesis is thought to involve uncontrolled production of inflammatory cytokines by Kupffer cells primed by ischaemia and stimulated by endotoxin, perhaps derived from the gut. These cytokines act on adjacent hepatocytes to produce the classical metabolic changes of sepsis as well as the hyperbilirubinaemia. They may also be responsible for multiple organ dysfunction commonly seen in this setting. Treatment is that of the underlying disease.

Drugs

Jaundice and liver dysfunction have been associated with many drugs. Drugs may impair metabolism of bilirubin or may be hepatotoxic (directly or due to metabolites). Hypersensitivity reactions may also cause hepatocellular dysfunction and, occasionally, massive liver cell necrosis. In such cases there may be other allergic manifestations such as fever, arthralgia, urticaria and eosinophilia. Drugs may cause hepatocellular necrosis or intrahepatic cholestasis. Drug reactions should be considered in any patient with abnormal liver function tests.

Total parenteral nutrition

Increased plasma AST, ALP and bilirubin concentrations may occur with total parenteral nutrition, particularly if excessive calorie intake is prolonged. Histologically, there is fatty infiltration of the liver associated with cholestasis and periportal inflammation. In general, the abnormalities reverse when enteral nutrition is established, although some infants have developed cirrhosis.

Hepatitis

Exposure to viral hepatitis may very occasionally be the cause of abnormal liver function tests in the ICU patient. The clinical picture and management are as discussed above.

References

1 Lee WM (1993) Acute liver fialure. *N Engl J Med* **329**:1862–1863.
2 Hawker F (1993) *The Liver: Critical Care Management*. London: WB Saunders.
3 Munoz SJ (1993) Difficult management problems in fulminant hepatic failure. *Sem Liver Dis* **13**:395–413.
4 Caraceni P and Van Thiel DH (1995) Acute liver failure. *Lancet* **345**:163–169.
5 O'Grady J, Schalm SW and Williams R (1993) Acute liver failure: redefining the syndromes. *Lancet* **342**:273–275.
6 Gimson AES, O'Grady J, Ede RJ, Portmann B and Williams R (1986) Late-onset hepatic failure: clinical serological and histological features. *Hepatology* **6**:288–294.
7 Fagan EA and Williams R (1990) Fulminant viral hepatitis. *Br Med Bull* **46**:462–480.
8 O'Grady JG, Gimson AES, O'Brien CJ, Pucknell A, Hughes RD and Williams R (1988) Controlled trials of charcoal hemoperfusion and prognostic factors in fulminant hepatic failure. *Gastroenterology* **94**:1186–1192.
9 Fagan EA (1994) Acute liver failure of unknown pathogenesis: the hidden agenda. *Hepatology* **19**:1307–1312.
10 Krawczynski K (1993) Hepatitis E. *Hepatology* **17**:932–941.
11 Sallie R, Silva A E, Purdy M *et al.* (1994) Hepatitis C and E in non-A non-B fulminant hepatic failure: a polymerase chain reaction and serological study. *J Hepatol* **20**:580–588.

12 Ray DC and Drummond GB (1991) Halothane hepatitis. *Br J Anaesth* **67**:84–99.
13 Harrison PM, Keays R, Bray GP, Alexander GJM and Williams R (1990) Improved outcome of paracetamol-induced fulminant hepatic failure by late administration of acetylcysteine. *Lancet* **335**:1572–1573.
14 Pinson WC, Daya MR, Benner KG *et al.* (1990) Liver transplantation for severe *Amanita phalloides* mushroom poisoning. *Am J Surg* **159**:493–499.
15 Langley PG, Forbes A, Hughes RD and Williams R (1990) Thrombin–antithrombin 111 complex in fulminant hepatic failure: evidence for disseminated intravascular coagulation and relationship to outcome. *Eur J Clin Invest* **20**:627–631.
16 O'Grady JG, Langley PG, Isola LM, Aledort LM and Williams R (1986) Coagulopathy of fulminant hepatic failure. *Semin Liver Dis* **6**:159–163.
17 Harrison PM, Wendon JA, Gimson AES, Alexander GJM and Williams R (1991) Improvement by acetylcysteine of haemodynamics and oxygen transport in fulminant hepatic failure. *N Engl J Med* **324**:1852–1857.
18 Bihari DJ, Gimson AES and Williams R (1986) Disturbances in cardiovascular and pulmonary function in fulminant hepatic failure. In: Williams R (ed.) *Liver Failure*. Edinburgh: Churchill Livingstone, pp. 47–71.
19 Rolando N, Harvey F, Brahm J *et al.* (1990) Prospective study of bacterial infection in acute liver failure: an analysis of 50 patients. *Hepatology* **11**:49–53.
20 Rolando N, Harvey F, Brahm J *et al.* (1991) Fungal infection: a common, unrecognised complication of acute liver failure. *J Hepatol* **12**:1–9.
21 Nandi SS, Chawla YK, Nath R and Dilawari JB (1989) Serum and urinary zinc in fulminant hepatic failure. *J Gastro Hepatol* **4**:209–213.
22 Munoz SJ, Robinson M, Northrup B *et al.* (1991) Elevated intracranial pressure and computed tomography of the brain in fulminant hepatocellular failure. *Hepatology* **13**:209–212.
23 Blei AT, Olafsson S, Webster S and Levy R (1993) Complications of intracranial pressure monitoring in fulminant hepatic failure. *Lancet* **341**:157–158.
24 Sheil AGR, McCaughan GW, Isai H, Hawker F, Thompson JF and Dorney SFA (1991) Acute and subacute fulminant hepatic failure: the role of liver transplantation. *Med J Aust* **154**:724–728.
25 Davenport A, Will EJ, Davison AM *et al.* (1989) Changes in intracranial pressure during haemofiltration in oliguric patients with grade IV encephalopathy. *Nephron* **53**:142–146.
26 Rolando N, Gimson A, Wade J, Philpott-Howard J, Casewell M and Williams R (1993) Prospective controlled trial of selective parenteral and enteral antimicrobial regimen in fulminant liver fialure. *Hepatology* **17**:196–201.
27 Davenport A, Will EJ and Davison AM (1990) Effect of posture on intracranial pressure and cerebral perfusion pressure in patients with fulminant hepatic failure and renal failure after acetaminophen self–poisoning. *Crit Care Med* **18**:286–289.
28 Canalese J, Gimson AES, Davis C, Mellon PJ, Davis M and Williams R (1982) Controlled trial of dexamethasone and mannitol for the cerebral oedema of fulminant hepatic failure. *Gut* **23**:625–629.
29 Ede RJ, Gimson AES, Bihari D and Williams R (1986) Controlled hyperventilation in the prevention of cerebral

oedema in fulminant hepatic failure. *J Hepatol* **2**:43–51.

30 Forbes A, Alexander GJM, O'Grady JG *et al.* (1989) Thiopental infusion in the treatment of intracranial hypertension complicating fulminant hepatic failure. *Hepatology* **10**:306–310.

31 European Association for the Study of the Liver (1979) Randomised trial of steroid therapy in acute liver failure. *Gut* **20**:620–623.

32 Boros P and Miller CM (1993) Hepatocyte growth factor: a multifunctional cytokine. *Lancet* **345**:293–295.

33 Davies E and Hodgson HJF (1995) Artificial livers – what's keeping them? *Gut* **36**:168–170.

34 Gerlach JC, Encke J, Hole O, Muller C, Ryan CJ and Neuhaus P (1994) Bioreactor for a larger scale hepatocyte *in vitro* perfusion. *Transplantation* **58**:984–988.

35 Roome AJ, Walsh SJ, Cartter ML and Hadler JL (1993) Hepatitis B vaccine responsiveness in Connecticut public safety personnel. *J Am Med Assoc* **270**:2931–2934.

36 Editorial (1992) Hepatitis A: a vaccine at last. *Lancet* **339**:1198–1199.

37 Groszmann RJ (1994) Hyperdynamic circulation of liver disease 40 years later: pathophysiology and clinical consequences. *Hepatology* **20**:1359–1363.

38 Krowka MJ and Cortese DA (1994) Hepatopulmonary syndrome: current concepts in diagnostic and therapeutic considerations. *Chest* **105**:1528–1537.

39 Badalamenti S, Graziani G, Salerno F and Ponticelli C (1993) Hepatorenal syndrome: new perspectives in pathogenesis and treatment. *Arch Intern Med* **153**:1957–1967.

40 Gines A, Escorsell A, Gines P *et al.* (1993) Incidence,

predictive factors, and prognosis of the hepatorenal syndrome in cirrhosis with ascites. *Gastroenterology* **105**:229–236.

41 Runyon BA (1994) Care of patients with ascites. *N Engl J Med* **330**:337–342.

42 Aiza I, Perez GO and Schiff ER (1994) Management of ascites in patients with chronic liver disease. *Am J Gastroenterol* **89**:1949–1956.

43 Tito L, Gines P, Arroyo V *et al.* (1990) Total paracentesis associated with intravenous albumin management of patients with cirrhosis and ascites. *Gastroenterology* **98**:146–151.

44 Luca A, Feu F, Garcia-Pagan JC *et al.* (1994) Favorable effects of total paracentesis on splanchnic hemodynamics in cirrhotic patients with tense ascites. *Hepatology* **20**:30–33.

45 Angueira CE and Kadakia SC (1994) Effects of large-volume paracentesis on pulmonary function in patients with tense cirrhotic ascites. *Hepatology* **20**:825–828.

46 Hawker F (1991) Liver dysfunction in critical illness. *Anaesth Intens Care* **19**:165–181.

47 Hickman PE and Potter JM (1990) Mortality associated with ischaemic hepatitis. *Aust NZ J Med* **20**:32–34.

48 Mohacsi P and Meier B (1994) Hypoxic hepatitis in patients with cardiac failure. *J Hepatology* **21**:693–695.

49 Henrion J, Descamps O, Luwaert R, Schapira M, Parfonry A and Heller F (1994) Hypoxic hepatitis in patients with cardiac failure; incidence in a coronary care unit and measurement of hepatic blood flow. *J Hepatol* **21**:696–703.

Part V

Renal failure

38 | Acute renal failure

R Bellomo

Acute renal failure is a syndrome characterized by a rapid increase in the metabolic waste products that are normally excreted by the kidney. This acute failure of the normal excretory function of the kidney is typically associated with a marked decrease in urinary output (oliguria or anuria) but can sometimes be accompanied by normal or slightly increased urinary output (so called polyuric acute renal failure). Acute renal failure is relatively frequent in the ICU[1,2] but occurs as a continuum of functional injury, from mild or moderate rise in plasma urea and serum creatinine, to anuric renal replacement-dependent acute renal failure. The former should probably be called acute renal dysfunction, the term acute renal failure being more correctly applied to the latter condition.

The mortality associated with the syndrome of acute renal failure depends on its severity and clinical associations. In patients who are not critically ill and who have isolated acute renal failure, mortality remains below 10%.[3] Those with acute renal failure in the setting of multiorgan failure have a 60–100% mortality.[4-7]

Classification

It is clinically useful to classify acute renal failure or dysfunction on the basis of its probable aetiology. Three broad categories exist: prerenal, postrenal and intrarenal (intrinsic).

Prerenal kidney dysfunction

This form is most commonly seen in the ICU. It refers to a clinical syndrome in which kidney dysfunction is thought to be largely due to diminished perfusion, but established tissue injury has not yet occurred. Several clinical situations can result in diminished kidney perfusion. They include any cause of a significantly reduced cardiac output (e.g. myocardial ischaemia, tamponade and valvular disease) and any cause of severe hypotension or intravascular volume depletion (e.g. haemorrhagic or septic shock, pancreatitis and peritonitis). These conditions typically result in oliguric renal dysfunction. Regardless of the aetiology, prerenal oliguria is often associated with laboratory findings (Table 38.1) which may help differentiate diminished kidney perfusion from established renal failure, even before such difference is realized by the course of the illness.

In the ICU, however, many of the laboratory markers of prerenal oliguria have limited practical implications. The aetiology is usually readily apparent, and optimal haemodynamic-guided resuscitation is typically initiated without delay. Thus, measurement of the laboratory markers in Table 38.1 is infrequently performed.

Postrenal kidney dysfunction

This is the most common cause of functional renal impairment in the community[8] but is rarely seen in the ICU. It is due to obstruction to renal outflow. Common causes include bladder neck obstruction from prostatic hyperplasia or malignancy, and ureteric obstruction by pelvic tumours, calculi, papillary necrosis or retroperitoneal fibrosis. The clinical presentation may be acute or acute on chronic, with urinary output being variable. Obstructive renal failure can occur in the absence of anuria. Although an uncommon cause of kidney failure in the ICU, the presence of obstruction must always be excluded in a patient with acute renal failure, because it can usually be relieved. It is sometimes difficult to evaluate the clinical significance of an obstruction when other causes of renal dysfunction are associated. Management is then best achieved in consultation with a urologist and nephrologist.

Intrinsic renal failure

This term implies that renal parenchymal damage is responsible for inadequate renal function. *Acute tubular necrosis* is often loosely used to describe

Table 38.1 Biochemical features of prerenal and intrinsic acute renal failure

Index	*Prerenal*	*Intrinsic*
Sediment	Normal	Tubular cells, casts, granular casts
Specific gravity	High 1.020	Fixed 1.010–1.020
Urine [Na]	Low <20 mmol/l	High >40 mmol/l
U:P urea ratio	High 20	Low 10
U:P creatinine ratio	High 40	Low 10
U:P osmolality ratio	High 2.1	Low 1.2
U osmolality	High >(serum + 100) mosmol/l	Low <(serum + 100) mosmol/l
P urea creatinine ratio	>Normal (depends on units used)	Normal

U = urine; P = plasma.

Table 38.2 Intrinsic acute renal failure

Acute tubular necrosis (so-called)

Other causes
Bilateral cortical necrosis
Acute glomerulonephritis
Acute interstitial nephritis
Malignant hypertension
Severe pyelonephritis
Acute activation of chronic renal disease
Severe, unrelieved prerenal failure
Raised intra-abdominal pressure

Tables 38.3 Nephrotoxic drugs

Radiocontrast agents
Aminoglycosides
β-Lactam antibiotics
Acyclovir
Amphotericin
Pentamidine
Heavy metals
Sulphonamides
Cisplatin
Methotrexate
Non-steroidal anti-inflammatory drugs

established renal replacement-dependent renal failure which has resulted from severe, inadequately treated prerenal injury (Table 38.2). As parenchymal damage is postulated, this condition is considered a form of intrinsic renal failure. However, evidence that extensive tubular necrosis underlies established severe acute renal failure following decreased renal perfusion is lacking in humans, as no pathological studies of the kidneys of such patients have been performed.[9] The term acute tubular necrosis is borrowed from experimental animal studies of severe renal ischaemia, and renal biopsies of Korean war victims performed days after haemorrhagic-shock injury. It probably inaccurately describes the histology of the clinical condition now seen in the ICU, which current data suggest to be one of patchy focal tubular damage.[10]

Apart from acute tubular necrosis, other disorders can induce intrinsic renal damage either by principally involving the glomerulus, renal vasculature or interstitium (Table 38.2). Amongst these, iatrogenic renal failure is particularly important for two reasons: it is the most common cause of hospital-acquired acute renal failure,[11] and it can often be prevented or successfully treated by removal of the offending agent. Thus, it is very important to take an accurate drug history in all patients presenting to the ICU with acute renal failure. A list of drugs frequently responsible for renal dysfunction is given in Table 38.3.

Hepatorenal syndrome

The hepatorenal syndrome is a form of acute renal failure occurring in patients with severe liver disease for which a specific cause cannot be found. Progressive oliguria and an extremely low urinary sodium concentration (<10 mmol/l) characterize this entity, which is believed to be functional in nature. The pathogenesis is unknown, but several points should be noted. Most patients with severe liver disease are hypotensive because of hypoalbuminaemia, decreased intravascular volume, vasodilatation and shunting. Intravascular filling is further decreased by frequent doses of diuretics to treat oedema, and by lactose-induced diarrhoea. Ascites and increased intra-abdominal pressure are also often present. Thus, baseline renal perfusion is low in these patients. Acute renal failure in this setting may well fit into the hepatorenal syndrome, but it also has many features of prerenal failure. As more attention is paid to physiological abnormalities, the diagnosis of hepatorenal failure is likely to decrease in future.

Pathogenesis of acute renal failure

The mechanisms responsible for the development of acute renal failure vary according to its aetiology, from immune-mediated glomerular damage to drug-induced interstitial inflammation. In the case of so-called acute tubular necrosis, several mechanisms may be involved. They include:

1 *medullary ischaemia* (particularly of the thick ascending loop of Henle),[12] with activation of the tubuloglomerular feedback,[13] and subsequent decrease in glomerular filtration rate and urinary output;
2 *tubular obstruction* due to casts of damaged tubular cells, with associated build-up in intratubular pressure and inhibition of glomerular filtration;[14]
3 *interstitial oedema* secondary to back-diffusion of ultrafiltrate from the tubular lumen through damaged tubular cells;[14]
4 *severe, humorally mediated vasoconstriction* due to the systemic release of vasoactive substances in the context of sepsis and organ injury.[15,16]

Clinical presentation

Acute renal failure secondary to inadequate renal perfusion is by far the commonest form of kidney failure seen in the ICU. The patient has usually received a serious insult (eg haemorrhage, burn, bacteraemia and trauma) which has resulted in a shock-like state. Despite successful resuscitation, severe oliguria or anuria and a rapid rise in serum creatinine and plasma urea levels have resulted. In other cases, the patient remains unstable following the initial insult, and has ongoing hypotension, sepsis and inadequate tissue perfusion, which progressively lead to multiple organ dysfunction, including kidney failure.

Once renal failure becomes established and supportive care is initiated, the duration of oliguria and inadequate excretory function is variable, and depends on the resolution of the initial injury, its severity, and the premorbid condition of the kidneys. Generally, a period of 2 weeks is required before sufficient renal function returns. However, recovery can take a few days to many weeks.

Recovery occurs gradually. Initially, urinary output returns but excretory function remains limited. Slowly, urea clearance improves and (provided no further insults occur and fluid and haemodynamic management is optimal) near normal renal function returns over a period of days to weeks. At times, urinary output increases to above normal levels, e.g. 3–5 l/day, for a period of time (i.e. polyuric phase). During this phase, great care should be taken to avoid volume depletion, as this will cause further renal injury and delay recovery.

Current evidence also indicates that the type of renal replacement therapy offered during the period of established renal failure may influence the rate of renal recovery. In particular, continuous forms of renal replacement (i.e. haemofiltration or haemodiafiltration) or haemodialysis using biocompatible mem-branes appear superior to conventional intermittent haemodialysis.[17]

Prevention of acute renal failure

Careful implementation of several resuscitation measures below, simultaneously with treatment of the initial insult, may prevent loss of renal function.

Intravascular volume

The first and foremost step in preventing the development of acute renal failure is to rapidly restore and maintain intravascular volume at optimal levels. In critically ill patients, this should always be done under haemodynamic monitoring (i.e. arterial pressure, central venous pressure and pulmonary capillary wedge pressure and often, cardiac output). Once intravascular volume has been restored, some patients may remain hypotensive, i.e. mean arterial pressure (MAP) below 65–70 mmHg or 8.7–9.3 kPa. In these patients, restoration of MAP to levels that optimally preserve renal perfusion pressure (i.e. above 75–80 mmHg or 10.0–10.6 kPa) is likely to increase renal blood flow and prevent further ischaemia. Such elevations in MAP often require the addition of vasopressor drugs (e.g. noradrenaline or adrenaline).[18]

Drugs

Once fluid replacement and haemodynamic targets have been achieved and are being maintained, it is unclear whether additional measures are of further benefit to the kidneys. A number of drugs, however, have been proposed as having a protective effect on the kidneys.

Dopamine

Of these, dopamine is the one most commonly used in the ICU. It is usually administered at a low infusion rate (i.e. low-dose dopamine 2 µg/kg per min), in the belief that, as in normal individuals, renal blood flow will be significantly augmented. Evidence of this in critically ill patients is lacking.[19,20] None the less, because of the lack of major risks and the significance of any potential benefit, administration of this drug remains widespread. In addition to being a potential cause of increased renal blood flow, low-dose dopamine is a natriuretic and diuretic agent. An increase in urine output can therefore be expected in most patients after several hours of drug infusion. However, such an increase does not necessarily indicate improved renal perfusion, and can be similarly obtained with the infusion of another diuretic agent.

Diuretics

Diuretics, including mannitol and frusemide, have been used to diminish renal injury in this context. No controlled trials, however, exist to support their use, although there are good arguments for their use in this situation. These include the potential usefulness of maintaining urine output, decreasing renal medulla workload and decreasing tubular cell oedema. These drugs may be particularly helpful in situations where a renal insult is unavoidable and can be predicted. Examples are the need for radiocontrast agent infusion in a diabetic patient with chronic renal impairment, major surgery involving the abdominal aorta and hepatobiliary surgery in a patient with obstructive jaundice. In these situations, their infusion in association with the administration of intravenous fluids may offer further protection to the kidneys.

Many clinicians use drugs such as mannitol, frusemide or even low-dose dopamine, in the unproven hope of preventing established renal failure and of converting oliguric to polyuric renal failure in some patients. (Polyuric renal failure was reported in the 1970s as being associated with a better prognosis.) Data supporting this clinical approach are uncontrolled, do not take into account overall illness severity, and apply to a time when only conventional dialytic techniques were in use.[21] Their clinical relevance in critically ill patients treated with continuous haemofiltration techniques in a modern ICU is doubtful.

Other agents

Finally, several agents have been shown to be protective in animal models of experimental ischaemic renal injury. They include calcium antagonists, low-dose theophylline, leukotriene antagonists, the hormone urodilatin, endothelin antagonists and atrial natriuretic factors. They still remain beyond the realm of clinical practice.

Assessment of renal function

It is difficult to measure excretory renal function in critically ill patients accurately, because of the dynamic nature of renal blood flow and because of the variable nature of renal injury.

Serum creatinine

Serum creatinine, however, is a clinically useful gauge of glomerular filtration rate, because great precision is rarely needed in clinical practice. However, serum creatinine concentrations do not simply depend on the glomerular filtration rate, but also on the volume of distribution, rate of production, intestinal degradation and tubular secretion of creatinine, and on the patient's muscle mass. Thus, the steady-state relationship of serum creatinine to creatinine clearance (see below) is not easily predicted in intensive care patients. Early in the course of renal injury, serum creatinine concentrations are insensitive predictors of changes in glomerular filtration rate; a 30% decrease in filtration rate often results in no abnormality. When injury is established, the serum creatinine concentration will continue to rise to a new steady state, even though no further renal injury is taking place. These facts need to be taken into account when interpreting the significance of serum creatinine concentrations.

Creatinine clearance

A more accurate way of gauging renal function is to measure a patient's creatinine clearance. This is not commonly done in the ICU, as it is somewhat laborious and findings rarely offer major clinical advantages. At times, however, short urine collection periods (e.g. 4 h) can be used to gauge response to therapy more closely. Such short collection periods are similar in accuracy to the standard 24-h urine collection.

Serum urea

Serum urea concentrations are also widely used clinically to assess excretory renal function. They are less accurate markers of glomerular filtration rate than serum creatinine, and are modified by many variables (e.g. diet, catabolic state, steroid use and presence of gastrointestinal blood). None the less, serum urea concentrations continue to be used, despite lack of controlled data, as clinically useful markers of uraemic intoxication, and as a guide to determine the need for dialysis. Serum urea, with serum creatinine concentrations, remain part of the routine laboratory assessment of renal function in the ICU.

Other tests of renal function

Other more expensive and sophisticated tests of excretory renal function are rarely performed. They include the measurement of renal blood flow with paraaminohippurate, and of glomerular filtration rate with ^{99m}Tc diethylenetriaminepentaacetic acid (DTPA). Both are used in the ICU for research purposes only.

Serum electrolytes and acid–base balance

Several derangements of serum electrolytes and acid–base balance develop during acute renal failure. They include hyperkalaemia, hyperphosphataemia and metabolic acidosis. Such abnormalities are insensitive and non-specific markers of renal failure and are typically monitored with the aim of preventing complications.

Diagnostic investigations

The diagnosis of acute renal failure secondary to decreased renal perfusion is usually based on the typical clinical picture of rapidly deteriorating renal function in the setting of hypotension, volume depletion, and/or severely impaired cardiac output. When renal damage becomes established (so-called acute tubular necrosis), several laboratory features confirm the diagnosis: urine osmolality similar to that of serum due to inability to concentrate urine; urine sodium concentration above 40 mmol/l; epithelial cell casts; degenerative cell casts; coarse granular casts; and free tubular epithelial cells in the urinary sediment.

Irrespective of the likely clinical diagnosis, laboratory and microscopic examination and culture of the urine are important in all patients with acute renal failure. Urinary sepsis must always be excluded. The urine must be assessed for proteinuria or haematuria, the latter being inconsistent with simple acute tubular necrosis. The sediment must be examined microscopically for white cells, white and red cell casts, and fragmented red cells. Their presence suggests glomerular disease and inflammation, and other investigations for glomerulonephritis should be undertaken. The presence of urine eosinophilia suggests the diagnosis of interstitial nephropathy. In cases of severe rhabdomyolysis, urine testing may yield a misleading finding of haematuria. Measurement of free myoglobin and serum muscle enzyme activity is diagnostically useful in this situation.

If a pulmonary–renal syndrome or a form of acute glomerulonephritis is suspected, a chest X-ray, tests for specific autoantibodies (e.g. antiglomerular basement membrane antibodies, antineutrophil cytoplasmic antibodies, and collagen disease-related antibodies) and serological tests for inflammatory markers (e.g. sedimentation rate, C-reactive protein, complement and immune complexes) become necessary. If the haemolytic–uraemic syndrome or thrombotic thrombocytopenic purpura are suspected, blood films must be examined microscopically for evidence of red cell fragmentation, and laboratory tests for haemolysis performed (e.g. lactic dehydrogenase activity, haptoglobin concentration, free haemoglobin concentration and serum bilirubin concentrations). In some patients, intrinsic inflammatory renal disease is suspected, but the cause and nature remain unclear. A kidney biopsy then becomes necessary, and can be performed in ventilated patients with ultrasonographic guidance.

Renal imaging in the ICU

The clinical and laboratory assessment of the patient described above should frequently be complemented by imaging techniques. Renal imaging often provides important information on the aetiology of renal failure and the degree of any previous renal damage, if premorbid renal function is unknown. A plain X-ray of the abdomen, for example, permits assessment of renal size, and detects parenchymal calcification. Small kidneys, with or without calcifications, strongly suggest chronic renal disease.

An ultrasound of the kidneys is mandatory in all cases of acute renal failure, because renal outflow obstruction cannot reliably be diagnosed clinically. The technique has no morbidity and can easily be performed at the bedside. Kidney size can be assessed with great accuracy; the parenchyma can clearly be imaged, and any pelvicaliceal obstruction detected. Rarely, renal ultrasonography may miss a clinically significant obstruction. In this situation, further investigations, e.g. retrograde pyelography and cystoscopy, and (rarely) intravenous pyelography, must be performed if obstruction is strongly suspected. Contrast-dependent imaging techniques are now rarely indicated to investigate acute renal failure in ICU patients, because of the risks associated with infusion of contrast, and the availability of other imaging modalities. Ultrasonography and CT scanning (without contrast) are usually sufficient. Also, ^{99m}Tc-DTPA isotope scanning can demonstrate the adequacy of renal perfusion and excretion without the risks of infusing contrast. Renal angiography may be necessary but is rarely indicated, e.g. suspected acute renal artery or renal vein thrombosis.

Complications of acute renal failure

Typical complications of acute renal failure are related to the loss of excretory function, the first being the development of the uraemic state. This condition is characterized by the retention of metabolic toxins, bleeding diathesis, pericardial inflammation and progressive encephalopathy. Biochemical derangements frequently develop, and involve all major electrolytes. Hyperkalaemia can be potentially life-threatening. Untreated patients typically develop hyperphosphataemia, hypocalcaemia, hypermagnesaemia and hyponatraemia. Sodium and water retention lead to peripheral oedema (and pulmonary oedema if severe). Inadequate acid excretion and buffering result in progressive metabolic acidosis. The bleeding tendency and the common association with sepsis and multiorgan failure result in an increased risk of gastrointestinal haemorrhage.

Management of acute renal failure

The most important aspect of management is prevention. Several strategies have been discussed above, e.g. fluid resuscitation, drugs and maintaining adequate renal perfusion pressure. However, their prompt application and the individualization of resuscitation targets must be emphasized. For example, the target MAP in an elderly, previously hypertensive patient with intra-abdominal bleeding and increased intra-abdominal pressure is likely to be 15–20 mmHg (2.0–2.7 kPa) higher than that needed in a previously healthy young man with pneumonia and septic shock. Equally, fluid resuscitation in acute respiratory distress syndrome needs to take into account the adverse consequences of increased lung water. Once appropriate resuscitation goals have been achieved, other aspects of management require attention.

Nutrition

Adequate nutritional support in acute renal failure is vital to organ recovery, maintenance of near-neutral nitrogen balance, and avoidance of the serious muscular and immunological sequelae of malnutrition. Administration of a low-protein diet to delay inevitable dialytic therapy or to lengthen the interval between dialytic sessions is physiologically unsound. It leads to severe protein depletion[22] and should be avoided. Critically ill patients with acute renal failure should receive aggressive, protein-rich (e.g. >1.5 g/kg per day) nutritional support, either enterally or parenterally. Their caloric requirements are essentially no different to those of other ICU patients without renal failure.[23]

Electrolyte control

Hyperkalaemia is the most serious electrolyte derangement seen in acute renal failure and can be life-threatening. High concentrations of potassium (e.g. >6 mmol/l) should immediately be treated with a rapid IV infusion of insulin (10 units) with dextrose (50 ml of 50% solution), an infusion of bicarbonate if acidosis is present (usually 150 mmol), and/or a nebulized inhalation of salbutamol (20 mg in saline). If the serum potassium concentration exceeds 7 mmol/l, or if there are electrocardiogram signs of cardiac potassium toxicity, calcium gluconate (10 ml of 10% solution IV) should also immediately be administered to counter the cardiotoxic effects. The safest approach, however, is prevention of such problems by early institution of renal replacement therapy.

Metabolic acidosis

Metabolic acidosis is invariably present in patients with established acute renal failure. In most cases, no correction is required. Occasionally, its severity is such that the patient's minute ventilation is markedly increased by the resultant cerebrospinal fluid acidosis. In these cases, renal replacement therapy is clearly indicated, and there is no compelling evidence to support the use of bicarbonate. It is physiologically unsound and clinically unwise to wait for significant metabolic acidosis (e.g. pH<7.2) to develop before initiating renal replacement therapy.

Anaemia

Many critically ill patients develop a normochromic normocytic anaemia, particularly if complicated by acute renal failure. Blood transfusion is necessary in most patients to maintain a haematocrit above 0.3.

Infection

The uraemic state is associated with disordered immune function. Double-lumen haemodialysis catheters or surgical arteriovenous shunts further expose the patient to infection. If peritoneal dialysis is used, the dialysis catheter is an important route of infection, and peritonitis is a relatively frequent complication. The urinary catheter should be removed if oliguria or anuria is present, and periodic catheterization every 24 or 48 h performed instead. There is no place for prophylactic antibiotics.

Drug administration

The majority of drugs used in the ICU are excreted via the kidneys. Thus doses must be modified in patients with acute renal failure. This is particularly true for toxic drugs such as aminoglycosides and vancomycin. Drug dose can be decreased or the interval between doses increased. Since peak concentrations correlate with bactericidal activity and trough concentrations with toxicity, aminoglycosides are best administered over extended intervals (e.g. once daily).[24,25]

Stress ulcer prophylaxis

Patients with acute renals failure and multiorgan failure are at high risk of developing stress ulcers. Oral or nasogastric administration of sucralfate or IV infusion of H_2-receptor antagonists should be given (see Chapter 35). Antacids are best avoided in these patients because of the risks of inducing serum calcium or magnesium derangements.

Renal replacement therapy

Traditional indications for initiating renal replacement therapy (i.e. continuous haemofiltration, continuous haemodiafiltration, intermittent haemodialysis and peritoneal dialysis) are inappropriate in critically ill patients with acute renal failure. It is pointless to wait for complications such as hyperkalaemia, acidosis, pulmonary oedema and uraemia to develop, before implementing artificial renal support. The current trend is towards early and aggressive renal replacement therapy. In most ICUs in Europe and Australia, this is now achieved by continuous haemofiltration-based techniques. Peritoneal dialysis is uncommonly used because of its shortcomings with fluid removal and solute clearances, as well as its increased risk of intra-abdominal infection. Conventional intermittent haemodialysis using cuprophane membranes has serious short-comings in critically ill patients, and its clinical use is diminishing[26,27] (see Chapter 39).

Prognosis

Critically ill patients with acute renal failure continue to have a high mortality because acute renal failure is, in fact, a marker of extreme illness severity. Most patients die *with* renal failure rather than *of* it. Until therapies are developed to deal with the pathogenesis of multiple organ dysfunction and systemic sepsis, the grim prognosis of acute renal failure is unlikely to change. Despite these considerations, there are several patients in whom careful management and safe renal support contribute significantly to survival. In particular, the use of biocompatible membranes and continuous forms of renal replacement appears to offer some hope.[17,26,27]

References

1 Chew SL, Lins RL, Daelemans R and De Broe ME (1993) Outcome in acute renal failure. *Nephrol Dial Transplant* **8**:101–107.
2 Groeneveld ABJ, Tran DD, van der Meulen J, Nauta JJP and Thjis LG (1991) Acute renal failure in the medical intensive care unit: predisposing, complicating factors and outcome. *Nephron* **59**:602–610.
3 Corwin HL and Bonventre JV (1989) Factors influencing survival in acute renal failure. *Semin Dial* **2**:220–225.
4 Lohr JW, McFarlane MJ and Grantham JJ (1988) A clinical index to predict survival in acute renal failure patients requiring dialysis. *Am J Kidney Dis* **11**:254–259.
5 Liano F, Garcia-Martin F, Gallego A *et al.* (1989) Easy and early prognosis in acute tubular necrosis: a forward analysis of 228 cases. *Nephron* **51**:307–313.
6 Lien J and Chan V. (1985) Risk factors influencing survival in acute renal failure treated by hemo-dialysis. *Arch Intern Med* **145**:2067–2069.
7 Spiegel DM, Ullian ME, Zerbe GO and Berl T (1991) Determinants of survival and recovery in acute renal failure patients dialysed in intensive care units. *Am J Nephrol* **11**:44–47.
8 Feest TG, Round A and Hamad S (1993) Incidence of severe acute renal failure in adults: results of a community-based study. *Br Med J* **306**:481–483.
9 Solez K (1992) Acute renal failure. In: Heptinstall RH (ed) *Pathology of the Kidney,* 4th edn. Boston: Little, Brown.
10 Racusen CR, Trpkov K and Solez K (1995) The

pathology of acute renal failure. In: Bellomo R and Ronco C (eds) *Acute Renal Failure in the Critically Ill.* Heidelberg: Springer-Verlag.
11 Rasmussen HH and Ibels LS (1992) Acute renal failure: multivariate analysis of causes and risk factors. *Am J Med* **73**:211–218.
12 Brezis M, Rosen SN, Silva P and Epstein FH (1984) Selective vulnerability of the medullary thick ascending limb to anoxia in the isolated perfused rat kidney. *J Clin Invest* **73**:182–190.
13 Osswald H, Muhlbauer B and Schenk F (1991) Adenosine mediates tubuloglomerular feedback response: an element of metabolic control of kidney function. *Kidney Int* **39**:S12831.
14 Burke TJ, Cronin RE, Duchin KL, Peterson LN and Schrier RW (1980) Ischemia and tubule obstruction during acute renal failure in dogs: mannitol in protection. *Am J Physiol* **238**: F305–314.
15 Sugiura M, Inagami T and Kon V (1989) Endotoxin stimulates endothelin-release *in vivo* and *in vitro* as determined by radioimmunoassay. *Biochem Biophys Res Commun* **161**:1220–1227.
16 Tomita K, Ujiie K, Nakanishi T *et al.* (1989) Plasma endothelin levels in patients in acute renal failure. *N Engl J Med* **321**:1127–1131.
17 Bellomo R, Mansfield D, Rumble S, Shapiro J, Parkin G and Boyce N (1992) Acute renal failure in critical illness. Conventional dialysis versus acute continuous hemodiafiltration. *ASAIO J* **38**:M654–M657.
18 Redl-Wenzl EM, Armbruster C, Edelman G *et al.* (1993) The effects of norepinephrine on hemodynamics and renal function in severe septic shock. *Intensive Care Med* **19**:151–154.
19 Myles PS, Buckland MR, Schenk NJ *et al.* (1993) Effect of renal-dose dopamine on renal function following cardiac surgery. *Anaesth Int Care* **21**:56–61.
20 Polson RJ, Park GR, Lindop MJ *et al.* (1987) The prevention of renal impairment in patients undergoing orthotopic liver grafting by infusion of low-dose dopamine. *Anaesthesia* **42**:15–19.
21 Anderson RJ, Linas SL, Berns A *et al.* (1977) Non oliguric renal failure. *N Engl J Med* **296**:1134–1138.
22 Bouffard Y, Viale JP, Annat G, Delafosse B, Guillame G and Motin J (1987) Energy expenditure in the acute renal failure patient mechanically ventilated. *Intensive Care Med* **13**:401–404.
23 Bellomo R, Martin H, Parkin G, Love J and Boyce N (1991) Continuous arteriovenous hemodiafiltration in the critically ill. Influence on major nutrient balances. *Intensive Care Med* **17**:399–402.
24 Prins JM, Bueller H, Kuijper E, Tange R and Speelman P (1993) Once versus thrice a day gentamicin in patients with serious infections. *Lancet* **341**:335–339.
25 Gilbert DN (1991) Once-daily aminoglycoside therapy. *Antimicrob Agents Chemother* **35**:399–405.
26 Hakim RM (1993) Clinical implications of hemodialysis membrane biocompatibility. *Kidney Int* **44**:484–494.
27 Schiffl H, Lang SM, Koenig A, Strasser T, Haider MC and Held E (1994) Biocompatible membranes in acute renal failure prospective case-controlled study. *Lancet* **344**:570–572.

Dialytic therapies

R Bellomo

In patients with severe acute renal failure, renal excretory function is lost. Resolution can often take several weeks, catabolism is marked and the need for nutritional support is immediate and important. Also, multiple drugs and fluids have to be infused. Thus in these patients, a procedure which replaces renal excretory function is necessary to avoid inevitable complications of water and salt overload, electrolyte and acid–base derangements and accumulation of toxic waste products. Various techniques developed to do this include peritoneal dialysis (continuous or intermittent), intermittent haemodialysis and continuous haemofiltration/haemodiafiltration. They all rely on the principle of allowing solute and water clearance through a semipermeable membrane, which is either natural (peritoneum) or artificial (haemodialysis or haemofiltration), and then discarding the waste products thus obtained.

Principles[1–5]

Water removal

Water is removed during dialytic procedures by a mechanism called ultrafiltration. This process is essentially that performed in the kidney by the glomerulus. It requires a driving force (e.g. hydrostatic pressure) to move fluid across a semipermeable membrane. Such fluid would normally be retained within the circulation by the patient's oncotic pressure. In the artificial kidney, the equivalent of such hydrostatic pressure is achieved by:

1 applying a negative pressure to the non-blood (dialysate) side of the membrane, as in haemo-dialysis;
2 using a hyperosmolar solution, as in peritoneal dialysis, or;
3 using the patient's blood pressure (or a pump-dependent pressure) and a highly permeable

membrane, as in haemofiltration/haemodiafiltration.

Solute removal

If poorly permeable membranes made of cellulose are used (e.g. standard haemodialysis), convection of solutes associated with the process of ultrafiltration will only result in small amounts of electrolytes and other molecules being removed. Consequently, effective solute removal can only be achieved if an electrochemical gradient is generated by the rapid countercurrent flow of a dialysis fluid (dialysate). This fluid must have the appropriate concentration of electrolytes and none of the waste solutes that require extraction. This principle of solute removal is called diffusion. The rate of diffusion for small molecules during haemodialysis depends on the blood flow rate, the dialysate flow rate, duration of the dialytic procedure, concentration gradient across the membrane and the size of the membrane. For larger molecules (> 500 Da molecular weight), such diffusion is poor. Their extraction can only effectively occur in the presence of highly porous membranes. Even with such membranes, however, because of their thickness, removal by diffusion is relatively poor and convection is required. When a technique like haemofiltration is applied (in which solute removal depends on net ultrafiltrate production), such solute removal is said to occur by convection. Convective solute extraction through the highly porous membranes used for continuous haemofiltration occurs for all molecules up to the size of the membrane pores (approximately 30 kDa in molecular weight).

In peritoneal dialysis, even larger molecules (such as albumin) are removed, because of the extraordinary permeability of the peritoneum. However, due to the limited blood flow-to-dialysate contact and the rapidly decreasing waste product gradient across this natural membrane, solute removal is much less efficient. This is why peritoneal dialysis is often performed continuously.

Indications for dialytic and blood purification therapies in the ICU

These techniques are typically used in the ICU to manage acute renal failure. They may also be indicated for other conditions (Table 39.1).

Renal failure

Patients may require dialytic therapy because of acute renal failure, or if they have dialysis-dependent end-stage renal failure and have developed an acute illness requiring ICU admission. Traditionally, several principles of management have been followed in these patients:

1 The cause of acute renal failure should clearly be established, and renal outflow obstruction excluded.
2 Renal perfusion should be optimized and maintained at physiologically safe levels.
3 Any sepsis should be aggressively treated.
4 Drug doses should be altered according to the degree of renal dysfunction and the type of renal replacement therapy in use.

Other concepts embraced in the past include restriction of water, sodium and protein intake. Such concepts are outmoded in the ICU where continuous

Table 39.1 Indications for and modes of dialytic therapy

Renal failure
Continuous haemofiltration
Continuous haemodiafiltration
Intermittent haemodialysis
Peritoneal dialysis

Diuretic-resistant pulmonary oedema
Continuous haemofiltration
Machine ultrafiltration
Peritoneal dialysis

Detoxification
Haemoperfusion
Intermittent haemodialysis
Haemofiltration

Severe hepatic failure
Continuous haemofiltration
Haemoperfusion
Haemodiabsorption

Sepsis (?)
Continuous haemofiltration
Haemoperfusion
Haemadsorption with polymyxin B

haemofiltration is used as the dialytic technique of choice.

Initiation and frequency of dialysis

Dialysis should be initiated early in the course of the patient's illness. It is physiologically unsound and clinically perilous to wait for complications of uraemia to develop before dialytic therapy is undertaken. Wariness of early dialysis stems from the adverse effects of standard intermittent haemodialysis with cuprophane membranes. Such effects unfavourably influence haemodynamics, lung function, the immune system and the kidney itself.[6-9] Such concerns, however, are probably irrelevant if biocompatible membranes and continuous haemofiltration are used.

There are no scientifically established criteria to initiate dialysis. Time-honoured criteria are simply complications of renal failure (i.e. pulmonary oedema, severe hyperkalaemia, refractory metabolic acidosis, and a plasma urea concentration above 35 mmol/l). In the ICU, maintenance of homeostasis is a major therapeutic goal, and such criteria are thus inappropriate. Modern criteria to initiate dialytic therapy in the ICU are presented in Table 39.2.

Once dialysis is initiated, there is no scientifically established biochemical measure of dialytic adequacy. None the less, most clinicians seek to maintain plasma urea concentration below 30 mmol/l. To achieve this, intermittent haemodialysis may have to be applied daily; the duration and frequency are partly dependent on the severity of catabolism and the nutritional intake of nitrogen. If aggressive nutritional support with amino acids is undertaken, continuous peritoneal dialysis is usually insufficient to maintain control of urea levels.[10] Continuous haemofiltration or haemodiafiltration, on the other hand, can control uraemia in all patients, if adequate amounts of ultrafiltrate are produced (>20 ml/min) or if sufficient amounts of dialysate are delivered (>20 ml/min) in combination with ultrafiltration.[11-14]

Table 39.2 Modern criteria for the initiation of dialytic therapy in the ICU*

Oliguria (urinary output <5 ml/kg per day)
Anuria (no urinary output for 12 h)
Plasma urea concentration >35 mmol/l
Serum creatinine concentration >600 μmol/l
Hyperkalaemia (serum potassium concentration >6.5 mmol/l)
Pulmonary oedema not responsive to diuretics
Metabolic acidosis (pH <7.2)
Uraemic encephalopathy
Uraemic pericarditis
Uraemic neuropathy

*The presence of one criterion is sufficient to justify the initiation of dialytic therapy. The presence of two criteria strongly indicates the need for dialytic therapy

Mode of dialysis

The choice between peritoneal dialysis, intermittent haemodialysis and continuous haemofiltration/haemodiafiltration depends on local resources and expertise. No randomized trials have so far been performed comparing these three techniques in acute renal failure, and such trials are unlikely.[15] In the absence of direct comparisons, arguments favouring continuous haemofiltration/haemodiafiltration include the following:

1 greater haemodynamic stability;[16]
2 ability to remove fluids at will;
3 use of biocompatible membranes;
4 avoidance of acid–base disorders;
5 prevention of brain oedema and increases in intracranial pressure;[17–18]
6 ease of administration of nitrogen-rich nutritional support,[19]
7 the additional blood purification effect in sepsis.[20–22]

The expertise to run continuous haemofiltration-based therapies is relatively easily acquired, and these techniques are now commonly used in ICUs.

Other indications for dialytic therapies

Occasional patients with severe cardiac failure and renal dysfunction are unable to respond to large doses of diuretics. Under these circumstances, fluid removal can easily be achieved by continuous haemofiltration. The technique is haemodynamically well-tolerated, and by reducing left ventricular dilatation may improve haemodynamics. In all cases, removal of salt and water is achieved to the desired physiological targets without any adverse consequences.

Dialytic therapies have been used in the management of drug overdose and for the removal of poisons,[23] but without documented increased survival. However, their immediate effect on drug or poison concentrations in blood, as well as their demonstrable ability to remove these substances, make them the only viable therapeutic option in addition to the usual supportive measures. For standard haemodialysis to remove drugs and poisons, the substances must not be significantly protein-bound, they must have a molecular weight under 500 Da, and must be water-soluble. Similar principles apply if continuous haemofiltration/haemodiafiltration therapies are used, except that even larger water-soluble molecules can be removed. Haemoperfusion, however, can remove lipid-soluble and protein-bound compounds, and is more effective than haemodialysis with compounds such as barbiturates, tricyclic antidepressants, theophylline and some poisons (e.g. organophosphates, parathion, benzene and paraquat). Haemodialysis remains indicated for life-threatening poisoning with alcohols, ethylene glycol and salicylates.

Other factors affect the removal of drugs or poisons from the body. Drugs with large volumes of distribution will require prolonged blood purification therapy, as the plasma volume is the only compartment available for purification at any given time, and equilibration from tissue to plasma proceeds at a constant, relatively slow pace. With such compounds (e.g. lithium), continuous therapies may be superior.[24] Protein-binding and half-life will also determine the rate of drug removal; protein-binding impedes removal by dialytic techniques, and liver and kidney dysfunction profoundly influence disposal of several drugs.

Dialytic and blood purification techniques have also been applied in acute severe hepatic failure.[25,26] Results have been mixed, and there is presently no clear-cut indication for the use of haemoperfusion under these circumstances. Continuous haemofiltration, however, appears to be the technique of choice in these patients as, unlike other dialytic techniques, it does not induce increases in intracranial pressure.[27,28]

Other forms of biological and non-biological artificial livers are now under development. Biological artificial livers rely on a combination of membrane technology and immobilization of hepatocytes on to different types of matrices, including dialysis hollow fibre membranes.[29] Non-biological artificial livers may now combine the features of both haemodiafiltration and charcoal haemoperfusion in a technique known as haemodiabsorption[30].

Continuous haemofiltration (Fig. 39.1)

This is now the commonest form of renal replacement therapy in Australian and European ICUs. It has undergone technical improvements since it was first described in the late 1970s. All technical modifications rely on the principle of using a highly permeable membrane to act as an artificial glomerulus, by allowing spontaneous hydrostatic pressure-driven ultrafiltration. Such ultrafiltration results in the loss of large amounts of water and solutes (including urea and other waste products). Replacement of the losses with solutions containing necessary amounts of water and electrolytes results in a sufficient degree of blood purification. This mechanism of solute renal clearance is called convective clearance.

Continuous arteriovenous haemofiltration (CAVH)

CAVH is the simplest form of continuous haemofiltration. In CAVH, blood is driven through the filter by the patient's own blood pressure, either via the arterial limb of an arteriovenous Scribner shunt, or via a large-bore femoral artery cannula. The blood traverses the biocompatible and highly permeable filter (polysulphone or polyacrylonitrile membrane),

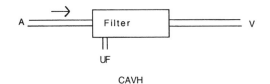

(a)

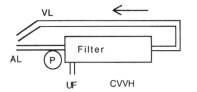

(b)

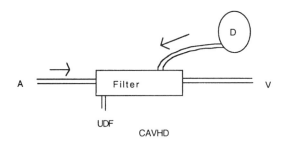

(c)

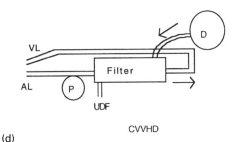

(d)

Fig. 39.1 Four principal techniques of continuous renal replacement therapy. (a) In continuous arteriovenous haemofiltration (CAVH), blood flows from an artery (A) through the filter into a vein (V), producing ultrafiltrate (UF). (b) In continuous venovenous haemofiltration (CVVH), blood flows from the arterial limb (AL) of a double-lumen central venous catheter to the venous limb (VL). Flow through the filter is driven by a roller pump (P) and ultrafiltrate (UF) is produced in the same way as in CAVH. (c) In continuous arteriovenous haemodiafiltration (CAVHD), the circuit is the same as in CAVH, but dialysate (D) is delivered countercurrent to blood into the non-blood compartment of the filter. The combination of diffusive and convective clearance results in the production of ultradiafiltrate (UDF). (d) In continuous venovenous haemofiltration (CVVHD), the circuit is the same as in CVVH, but modified to deliver dialysate (D) as in CAVHD.

undergoes ultrafiltration and returns to the circulation via the venous limb of the shunt or a femoral vein cannula (Fig. 39.1a). Although simple, CAVH requires a surgical shunt or insertion of two femoral cannulas, and vascular complications are relatively common.[31] Furthermore, solute clearance is inadequate in up to 20% of patients, and supplemental haemodialysis has to be applied. None the less, CAVH is associated with excellent haemodynamic stability and ample fluid removal.

Continuous arteriovenous haemodiafiltration (CAVHD)

To improve solute clearance, the CAVH circuit has been modified in a number of ways. If suction is applied to the ultrafiltrate port of the filter, greater ultrafiltration is achieved with an associated increase in solute removal. If the replacement fluids are administered proximal to the filter (i.e. predilution), oncotic pressure is diminished and ultrafiltration and solute extraction increased. The most effective way of increasing solute clearance is to add countercurrent dialysate flow to the haemofiltration circuit. This countercurrent flow permits solute removal by diffusion, with the process being driven by an electrochemical gradient. Such modification, at a dialysate flow rate of 1 l/h, results in a near doubling of small solute clearance. The technique is now called continuous arteriovenous haemodiafiltration (CAVHD; Fig. 39.1c). However, CAVHD still requires insertion of cannulas in the arterial and venous circulation.

Continuous venovenous haemofiltration (CVVH) and haemodiafiltration (CVVHD)

In order to decrease the morbidity associated with arterial cannulation, pump techniques of continuous haemofiltration have now been developed and applied. Access to the circulation is obtained via a double-lumen catheter which is inserted in a central vein (femoral, subclavian or jugular). Blood is then pumped by a peristaltic roller pump at a set rate (100–200 ml/min) into the filter and returns to the circulation via the venous limb of the double-lumen catheter. The pump typically incorporates some mandatory safety features, e.g. an air trap, pressure monitors and alarms. This technique is now called continuous venovenous haemofiltration (CVVH; Fig. 39.1b). If countercurrent dialysate flow is added as in CAVHD, to increase clearances further, the technique is then called continuous venovenous haemodiafiltration (CVVHD; Fig. 39.1d).

Slow continuous ultrafiltration with dialysis (SCUF-D)

With CVVH and CVVHD, minimal invasiveness is achieved with full control of uraemia.

The large amounts of fluids removed, however, require extreme attention to fluid balance and intravascular pressures. Continuous uncontrolled ultrafiltrate production also requires at least hourly measurements of net fluid losses. This is often cumbersome and always time-consuming. For this reason, volumetric pumps are now frequently used to control ultrafiltrate production at a set rate of 1.0, 1.5 or 2.0 l/h. Fluid replacement also proceeds at a similar rate, and allowances are made for other fluids (e.g. nutrition, drugs, blood and blood products). With such degrees of control available, several further technical variations have been used. One of these is based on higher dialysate flows (e.g. 2.0 l/h), minimal controlled ultrafiltration (100–200 ml/h), and no requirements for fluid replacement. This technique is more correctly termed slow continuous ultrafiltration with dialysis (SCUF-D). It provides excellent small-molecular-weight solute removal, but, being based on diffusion rather than convection, significantly fails to remove larger (> 500 Da) molecules. In this regard, and since convective middle molecular clearance is both desirable and achievable in septic acute renal failure,[32,33] convective clearance techniques such as CVVH may be more suitable for septic patients.

Circuit anticoagulation

Blood flow through the extracorporeal circuit for 24 h results in activation of the coagulation cascade. Filter clotting eventually results (but can also occur due to mechanical problems with the circuit). Circuit anticoagulation can be achieved by different means and at varying degrees (Table 39.3). However, circuit anticoagulation is not always necessary in patients with severe endogenous coagulopathies. In many of these patients, an adequate filter life can be achieved

Table 39.3 Approaches to extracorporeal anticoagulation during continuous haemofiltration[48]

Low-dose (≤500 IU/h) pre-filter heparin

Mid-range pre-filter heparin (500–1000 IU/h)

Full systemic heparinization

Regional anticoagulation (pre-filter heparin at full anti-coagulation dose and post-filter protamine to prevent systemic anticoagulation; usual heparin-to-protamine ratio is 100:1)

Regional citrate anticoagulation (pre-filter citrate and post-filter calcium to prevent systemic anticoagulation)

Low-molecular-weight heparin

Prostacyclin and prostacyclin analogues

Serine proteinase inhibitors (nafamostat mesylate)

No anticoagulation in patients with endogenous coagulopathy

with pumped and non-pumped techniques without any anticoagulants.[34]

Clinical effects

The clinical consequences of continuous haemofiltration are well-established.[13] Access-related complications are minimal, if double-lumen venous catheters are used. Outstanding haemodynamic stability can be achieved in inotrope-dependent multiorgan failure patients, even when fluid removal is being implemented. Uraemia can be controlled in all patients by changing the intensity of ultrafiltration or the rate of dialysate flow. Such control is steady, and can take place even during aggressive nutritional protein supplementation (i.e. > 2 g/kg per day).[19] Hormonal and trace element losses are minimal and clinically insignificant. Folate and vitamin C are the only vitamins that are likely to require supplementation during long-term therapy. Continuous haemofiltration may also have a blood purification effect in sepsis, and thus may be seen as an adjunctive therapy in septic patients[35,36] (see below).

Haemodialysis

Intermittent haemodialysis remains the traditional dialytic technique for acute renal failure, and is the dominant form of renal replacement therapy outside the ICU.

Vascular access is currently almost invariably a double-lumen central venous catheter, as in venovenous haemofiltration. Increasingly sophisticated haemodialysis machines able to vary dialysate electrolyte concentrations and to monitor patient haematocrit are now available.

Dialysate

Dialysate is produced by mixing a concentrated solution and purified water to achieve the desired electrolyte concentrations. Dialysate is then delivered to the dialyser at rates varying between 300 and 500 ml/min depending on the technique, while blood flow is typically maintained at 200–300 ml/min. Traditionally, dialysate sodium concentrations are 130–140 mmol/l, but higher concentrations of 140–145 mmol/l should be used in haemodynamically unstable patients, or those at risk of the disequilibrium syndrome. Acetate is the most commonly used dialysate buffer. It may induce vasodilatation and hypoventilation, and is best replaced with bicarbonate in patients at risk of hypotension.[37]

Water and solute removal

Fluid removal in intermittent haemodialysis has to occur over a short period of time. If it is too rapid or too great, hypotension will be induced. A longer duration of dialysis at a lesser ultrafiltration rate is then more appropriate. In all patients, particularly the critically ill, the effectiveness of compartmental blood purification is variable. Vascular beds with poor blood flows are slow to equilibrate with the central circulation, so that toxin extraction from certain organs (especially the splanchnic area) is suboptimal. Consequently, the plasma urea concentration obtained just after dialysis is often 20–30% less than that measured 30–45 min later (due to post-dialysis tissue to plasma equilibration). These swings in the concentrations of circulating toxins have unknown effects on metabolism and immune function, but are probably physiologically undesirable. Thus, intermittent procedures will always replace renal function less adequately than continuous therapies.

Anticoagulation

Anticoagulation of the circuit is typically needed during haemodialysis, but may not be necessary in patients with endogenous coagulopathies. In patients at risk of bleeding, regional anticoagulation using heparin and protamine, or citrate and calcium infusion, may be safer.

Complications

Several well-recognized complications of standard intermittent haemodialysis include those associated with central venous catheters, bleeding from heparin, hypotension, arrhythmias, hypoventilation and hypoxaemia, inability to deliver sufficient nutritional support and the disequilibrium syndrome. Other more subtle but important problems associated with the most commonly used dialyser membrane, i.e. cellulose-based cuprophane, have only recently become widely appreciated. This type of membrane can cause immunological derangement and activation of multiple inflammatory pathways,[38] contributing to the systemic inflammatory response syndrome, delayed renal recovery and increased mortality.[39-41] Hence, it seems strongly advisable exclusively to use biocompatible membranes (e.g. polysulphone and polyacrylonitrile) in critically ill patients.

Despite all available information, it is still unknown whether continuous haemofiltration or intermittent haemodialysis should preferentially be used in the ICU. Retrospective studies suggest that continuous haemofiltration may increase survival in critically ill acute renal failure patients,[36] but no prospective randomized studies have yet been performed. At present, clinicians continue to individualize therapy on the basis of available resources and current information.

Peritoneal dialysis

This simple technique has been used frequently in the past to manage acute renal failure, but is now uncommonly used in the critically ill. Typically, dialytic access is achieved by the surgical insertion of an intraperitoneal Tenckhoff catheter. Blind insertion is inadvisable, as the chance of inducing injury to intra-abdominal organs and vessels is significant. Dialysate is inserted into the peritoneal cavity for 'dwell times' which are initially short, but are then prolonged to 3–4 h if continuous peritoneal dialysis is required. Dialysate volumes are progressively increased to 2 l per exchange. Machine peritoneal dialysis allows intermittent dialysate infusion at shorter dwell times and in larger amounts.

If increased dialysis is desired, more exchanges are performed. Any manipulation will increase the risk of peritonitis. If increased fluid removal is desired, tonicity of the dialysate is increased by increasing its glucose concentration. This draws more fluid from the peritoneal membrane, and the fluid is then removed with the bag exchange. The physiological price of increasing the dialysate glucose concentration is the frequent development of hyperglycaemia.

A number of shortcomings and complications make this technique relatively unsuited to critically ill patients:

1 Small solute clearances are often inadequate, and supplemental haemodialysis has to be applied[10] to control uraemia.
2 Electrolyte removal is often unsatisfactory and uncontrolled hyperkalaemia may require haemodialysis.
3 The incidence of peritonitis remains high (20%).
4 Other clinically significant problems include hyperglycaemia, abdominal fluid leaks, hydrothorax, respiratory embarrassment from abdominal distension, mechanical complications from the catheter and significant protein loss from the peritoneal membrane.

Haemoperfusion

This blood purification technique is based on the absorptive capacity of activated charcoal granules or ion exchange resins. Blood passes through an extracorporeal circuit, which contains a cartridge of activated coated charcoal or an ion exchange resin. Many free molecules and even lipid or protein-bound molecules are adsorbed to this large active surface during blood transit. A number of systems use charcoal encapsulated with cellulose nitrate, cellulose acetate, acrylic hydrogel, or as fixed beads. An amberlite ion exchange resin cartridge is also available. Charcoal microcapsules effectively remove molecules of 300–500 Da molecular weight, and are thus able to extract some renal and hepatic toxins. Urea removal, however, does not take place, and the cartridges have no significant effect on acid–base balance and electrolytes.

Vascular access uses a double-lumen central venous catheter. A haemodialysis extracorporeal circuit is used, except that a carbon cartridge is substituted for the dialyser. Heparinization is necessary to prevent clotting within the cartridge. Attention must be paid to the patient's intravascular volume at the start, because of the large priming volume of the cartridge (up to 260 ml). The technique tends to induce hypoglycaemia, and monitoring of serum glucose is mandatory. Thrombocytopenia is also common and may be reduced by the use of prostacyclin.

The role of haemoperfusion in the treatment of critically ill patients is not formally established. In cases of life-threatening poisoning with drugs that can be removed by this technique, it seems unreasonable to withhold its application because of the lack of controlled data. The role of haemoperfusion remains unclear in fulminant hepatic failure. A randomized study[26] showed no difference in outcome between a control group and those treated for 5 and 10 h/day.[26] However, benefits may be possible if larger, more biocompatible surfaces are used on a 24-h basis, alone or in conjunction with other blood purification techniques. Advances in membrane and charcoal or resin technology will require further investigations in this area.

Blood purification in sepsis

The recently popular humoral theory of sepsis supports the effect of several 'soluble mediators of injury' on a variety of target organs.[42] Such mediators are a heterogeneous group of molecules which include cytokines, platelet activating factor, leukotrienes, prostanoids, histamine, bradykinin, thromboxane, etc. (see Chapters 61 and 85). Most are small to mid molecules, and their removal from the circulation by haemofiltration techniques has now been demonstrated.[33] Experimental evidence indicates that continuous haemofiltration may be protective in animal models of sepsis.[43] Consequently, there is growing interest in using blood purification techniques in sepsis. Apart from haemofiltration, such techniques would include extracorporeal endotoxin elimination by means of polymyxin B-bound polystyrene fibres, polymyxin adsorbent acrylic particles or haemoperfusion.[44-46] No controlled studies have yet been performed, and all reports are confined to small series, but this area will attract much research and development in the near future. At present, blood purification techniques cannot be recommended for routine application in the ICU.

Drug prescription during dialytic therapy

Acute renal failure and dialytic therapy profoundly affect drug disposition. Appropriate adjustments must be made in the prescription of most of the drugs administered to critically ill patients. Many factors affect the removal of drugs by dialytic therapy. They include drug properties (i.e. volume of distribution,

Table 39.4 ICU drug therapy during various dialytic therapies

Drug	Haemofiltration	Haemodialysis	Peritoneal dialysis
Amikacin	80–100% normal D q. 32 h	50% normal D q. 48 h Two-thirds redose post-dialysis	15–20 mg/l per day
Gentamicin	80–100% normal D q. 32 h	50–70% normal D q. 48 h Two-thirds redose post-dialysis	3–4 mg/l per day
Tobramycin	80–100% normal D q. 32 h	50–70% normal D q. 48 h Two-thirds redose post-dialysis	3–4 mg/l per day
Cefotaxime	1 g q. 8–12 h	1 g q. 12–24 h and after dialysis	1 g/day
Ceftazidime	1 g q. 8–12 h	1 g q. 12–24 h and after dialysis	1 g/day
Ceftriaxone	1–2 g q. 24 h	1 g q. 24 h and after dialysis	750 mg q. 12 h
Clavulanic acid	100 mg q. 4–6 h	75 mg q. 6 h and after dialysis	50 mg q. 6 h
Imipenem	250–500 mg q. 6 h	200 mg q. 6 h and after dialysis	150 mg q. 6 h
Metronidazole	500 mg q. 6 h	250 mg q. 6 h and after dialysis	250 mg q. 6 h
Co-trimoxazole	Normal D q. 18 h	Normal D q. 24 h and after dialysis	Normal D q. 24 h
Amoxycillin	500 mg q. 8 h	500 mg q. 24 h and after dialysis	250 mg q. 12 h
Vancomycin	0.5–1.0 g q. 24 h	1 g q. 96–120 h	1 g q. 96–120 h
Piperacillin	3–4 g q. 6 h	3–4 g q. 8 h and after dialysis	3–4 g q. 8 h
Ticarcillin	1–2 g q. 8 h	1–2 g q. 12 h and after dialysis	1–2 g q. 12 h
Ciprofloxacin	200 mg q. 12 h	250 mg q. 12 h	250 mg q. 12 h
Fluconazole	200 mg q. 24 h	200 mg q. 48 h and after dialysis	200 mg q. 48–72 h
Acyclovir	3.5 mg/kg q. 24 h	2.5 mg/kg per day and after dialysis	2.5 mg/kg per day
Ganciclovir	5 mg/kg per q. 24–48 h	5 mg/kg per 48–96 h and after dialysis	5 mg/kg per 96 h
Ranitidine	100–150 mg/day	75 mg/day and after dialysis	75 mg/day

N.B. The above values represent dosing guidelines. Potentially toxic drugs require monitoring of their blood concentrations as clinically indicated. For many other drugs, little or no information is available. In many cases, titration of infusion is to desired physiologic target. D = Dose; q. = indicates frequency.

protein binding, electrical charge, molecular weight and water-solubility), the dialytic therapy being applied, duration of application and the type of artificial membrane used. Despite the multiplicity of variables, working approximations can be made to allow safe and effective drug prescribing.

If peritoneal dialysis is used, the clearance of a free drug can be approximately predicted by multiplying urea clearance (20 ml/min for a 1.0 h dwell, 8 ml/min for a 4.0 h dwell) by the ratio of the square root of the molecular weight of urea (60 Da) over the square root of the drug's molecular weight.[47]

If haemofiltration is used, drug extraction depends on its sieving coefficient (i.e. drug concentration in the ultrafiltrate divided by the mean of its concentrations in the pre- and post-filter blood). Clearance of the drug is the product of its sieving coefficient and the ultrafiltration rate. For most drugs, the sieving coefficient for the unbound drug is close to 1.0. If countercurrent dialysate flow is used (i.e. CAVHD or CVVHD), small solute clearance is the simple sum of diffusive and convective clearance. The clearance of larger molecules, on the other hand, is unlikely to be substantially affected by the addition of diffusive clearance.

During intemittent haemodialysis with cuprophane membranes, molecules larger than 500 Da in molecular weight are not removed from the circulation. For smaller molecules, overall extraction depends on the urea clearance achieved during the procedure and the duration of the procedure. For a number of drugs used in the ICU, post-dialysis redosing is necessary. The effect of different dialytic techniques on drugs commonly used in the ICU is summarized in Table 39.4.

References

1. Sargent J and Gotch F (1989) Principles and biophysics of dialysis. In: Maher J (ed.) *Replacement of Renal Function by Dialysis*. Dordrecht: Kluwer Academic Publishers, p.87.

2. Henderson L (1989) Biophysics of ultrafiltration and hemofiltration. In: Maher J (ed.) *Replacement of Renal Function by Dialysis*. Dordrecht: Kluwer Academic Publishers, p.300.

3. Nolph KD (1986) Peritoneal dialysis. In: Brenner BM and Rector FC (eds) *The Kidney*, 3rd edn. Philadelphia: WB Saunders, pp. 1791–1845.

4. Henderson LW (1976) Hemodialysis: rationale and physical principles. In: Brenner BM and Rector FC (eds) *The Kidney* 1st edn. Philadelphia: WB Saunders, pp. 1643–1671.

5. Colton CK, Smith KA and Merrill W (1971) Diffusion of urea in flowing blood. *Am Inst Chem Eng J* **17**:800–808.

6. Korchik WP, Brown DC and De Master EG (1978) Hemodialysis induced hypotension. *Int J Artif Intern Organs* **1**:151–156.

7. Aurigemma NM, Feldman NT, Gottlieb M, Ingram RH, Lazarus JM and Lowrie EG (1977) Arterial oxygenation during hemodialysis. *N Engl J Med* **279**:871–875.

8. Goldblum SE and Reed WP (1980) Host defenses and immunologic alterations associated with chronic haemodialysis. *Ann Intern Med* **93**:597–613.

9. Schulman G, Fogo A, Gung A, Badr K and Hakim R (1991) Complement activation retards resolution of ischemic renal failure in the rat. *Kidney Int.* **40**:1069–1074.

10. Howdieshell TR, Blalock WE, Bowen PA, Hawkins ML and Hess C (1992) Management of post-traumatic acute renal failure with peritoneal dialysis. *Am Surg* **6**:378–382.

11. Canaud B, Garred LJ, Christol JP, Anbas S, Beraud JJ and Mion C (1988) Pump-assisted continuous venovenous hemofiltration for treating acute uremia. *Kidney Int* **33**:S154–S156.

12. Bellomo R, Parkin G, Love J and Boyce N (1992) Management of acute renal failure in the critically ill with continuous veno-venous hemodiafiltration. *Renal Fail* **14**:183–186.

13. Barton IK, Hilton PJ, Taub NA *et al.* (1993) Acute renal failure treated by hemofiltration: factors affecting outcome. *Q J Med* **86**:81–90.

14. Bellomo R and Boyce N (1993) Acute continuous hemodiafiltration: a prospective study of 110 patients and a review of the literature. *Am J Kidney Dis* **21**:508–518.

15. Bellomo R and Boyce N (1993) Does continuous hemodiafiltration improve survival in acute renal failure? *Semin Dial* **6**:16–19.

16. Paganini E (1993) Continuous renal replacement is the preferred treatment for all acute renal failure patients receiving intensive care. *Semin Dial* **6**:176–179.

17. Arieff AI (1994) Dialysis disequilibrium syndrome: current concepts on pathogenesis and prevention. *Kidney Int* **45**:629–635.

18. Davenport A, Will EJ and Davidson AM (1993) Improved cardiovascular stability during continuous modes of renal replacement therapy in critically ill patients with acute hepatic and renal failure. *Crit Care Med* **21**:328–338.

19. Bellomo R, Martin H, Parkin G, Love J, Kearley Y and Boyce N (1991) Continuous arteriovenous haemodiafiltration in the critically ill: influence on major nutrient balances. *Intensive Care Med* **17**:399-402.

20. Gomez A, Wang R, Unruh H *et al.* (1990) Hemofiltration reverses left ventricular function during sepsis in dogs. *Anesthesiology* **73**:671–685.

21. Grootendorst AF, van Bommel EFH, van der Hoven B, van Leengoed LAMG and van Osta ALM (1992) High volume hemofiltration improves right ventricular function in endotoxin-induced shock in the pig. *Intensive Care Med* **18**:235–240.

22. Ossenkoppele GJ, van der Meulen J, Bronsveld W and Thijs LG (1985) Continuous arteriovenous hemofiltration as an adjunctive therapy for septic shock. *Crit Care Med* **13**:102–104.

23. Garella S (1988) Extracorporeal techniques in the treatment of exogenous intoxications. *Kidney Int* **33**:735-754.

24. Bellomo R and Boyce N (1992) Current approaches to the treatment of severe lithium intoxication. *Lithium* **3**:245–248.

25. Silk DBA, Trewby PN, Chase RA *et al.* (1977) Treatment of fulminant hepatic failure by polyacrylonitrile-membrane haemodialysis. *Lancet* **ii**:1–3.

26. O'Grady JG, Gimson AES, O Brien CJ, Pucknell A, Hughes RD and Williams R (1988) Controlled trials of charcoal hemoperfusion and prognostic factors in

fulminant hepatic failure. *Gastroenterology* **94:**1186–1192.

27 Davenport A, Will E and Davison AM (1993) Effect of renal replacement therapy on patients with combined acute renal failure and fulminant hepatic failure. *Kidney Int.* **43:**S245–S251.

28 Davenport A, Will E and Davison AM (1993) Improved cardiovascular stability during continuous modes of renal replacement therapy in critically ill patients with acute hepatic and renal failure. *Crit Care Med* **21:**328–338.

29 Shin-ichi Kasai, Masyuki Sawa and Michio Mito. Is the biological artificial liver clinically applicable? A historic review of biological artificial liver support systems. *Artificial Organs* **18:**348–354.

30 Ash SR (1994) Hemodiabsorption in treatment of acute hepatic failure and chronic cirrhosis with ascites. *Artif Organs* **18:**355–362.

31 Bellomo R, Ernest D, Love J *et al.* (1990) Continuous arteriovenous haemodiafiltration: optimal therapy for acute renal failure in an intensive care setting? *Aust NZ J Med* **20:**237–242.

32 Grootendorst AF, van Bommel EFH, van der Hoven B *et al.* (1992) High volume haemofiltration improves right ventricular function in endotoxin-induced shock in the pig. *Intensive Care Med* **18:**235–240.

33 Bellomo R, Tipping P and Boyce N (1993) Continuous veno-venous hemofiltration with dialysis removes cytokines from the circulation in septic patients. *Crit Care Med* **21:**508–513.

34 Bellomo R, Teede H and Boyce N 1993 Anticoagulant regimens in acute continuous hemodiafiltration: a comparative study. *Intensive Care Med* **19:**329–332.

35 Barzilay E, Kessler D, Berlot G *et al.* (1989) Use of extracorporeal supportive techniques as additional treatment for septic-induced multiple organ failure patients. *Crit Care Med* **17:**634–637.

36 Bellomo R, Mansfield D, Rumble S *et al.* (1992) Acute renal failure in critical illness: conventional dialysis vs. acute continuous hemodiafiltration. *ASAIO J* **38:**M654–M657.

37 Wolff J, Pendersen T, Rossen M and Cleeman-Rasmussen K (1986) Effects of acetate and bicarbonate dialysis on cardiac performance, transmural myocardial perfusion and acid–base balance. *Int J Artif Organs* **9:**105–110.

38 Hakim RM (1993) Clinical implications of hemodialysis membrane biocompatibility. *Kidney Int* **44:**484–494.

39 Hakim R. Wingard RL, Lawrence P, Parker A and Schulamn G (1992) Use of biocompatible membranes improves outcome and recovery from acute renal failure. *J Am Soc Nephrol* **3:**367 (abstract).

40 Schiffl H, Lang SM, Koenig A, Strasser T, Haider MC and Held E (1994) Biocompatible membranes in acute renal failure: prospective case-controlled study. *Lancet* **344:**570–572.

41 Hakim RM, Wingard R and Parker RA (1994) Effect of dialysis membrane in the treatment of patients with acute renal failure. *N Engl J Med* **331:**1338–1342.

42 The ACCP/SCCM Consensus Conference Committee (1992) Definitions for sepsis and organ failure and guidelines for the use of innovative therapies in sepsis. *Chest* **101:**1644–1655.

43 Lee P, Matson JR, Pryor RW and Hinshaw LBH (1993) Continuous arteriovenous hemofiltration therapy for *Staphylococcus aureus*-induced septicemia in immature swine. *Crit Care Med* **21:**914–924.

44 Kodama M, Tani T, Aoki H, Hanasawa K and Yoshioka T (1991) Treatment of sepsis with extracorporeal elimination of endotoxin. *Circ Shock* **34:**115.

45 Staubach KH, Kooistra A, Otto V, Konstantin P and Bruch HP (1991) Extracorporeal adsorption of endotoxin in blood – a feasible method in sepsis. *Circ Shock* **34:**115.

46 Bende S and Bertok L (1991) Extracorporeal hemoperfusion in endotoxin shock. *Circ Shock* **34:**116.

47 Maher JF (1984) Pharmacokinetics in patients with renal failure. *Clin Nephrol* **21:**39–46.

48 Mehta R, Dobos GJ and Ward DM (1992) Anticoagulation procedures in continuous renal replacement. *Semin Dial* **5:**61–68.

Part VI

Neurological disorders

40 | Disorders of consciousness

JA Myburgh and TE Oh

Consciousness depends on the interaction of the cerebral hemispheres and the reticular activating system of the upper brain. Any process that disrupts this interaction may lead to an altered level of consciousness, with impaired physiological arousal. Various levels of consciousness are defined in Table 40.1.[1] In the critically ill patient, impaired consciousness is usually a neurological expression of a wide range of medical and surgical illnesses.

Aetiology

Although the aetiology is invariably multifactorial, disorders of consciousness may be due to a structural disturbance of the activating system or to a more diffuse disturbance of neuronal metabolism (Table 40.2).

Initial assessment

Initial assessment of a patient with impaired conscious level takes place at the same time as resuscitative measures.

History

A detailed history from the patient, relatives, ambulance staff, passers-by, medic-alert bracelets and usual medical attendants will yield the cause of impaired consciousness in the vast majority of patients. Important factors in the medical history are outlined in Table 40.3.

Examination

Examination of patients with impaired consciousness must be directed at neurological assessment to quantify the degree of impaired consciousness and to elicit signs of the possible cause.[2-4] The principles of neurological assessment are outlined in Table 40.4,

Table 40.1 Definitions of impaired consciousness

Condition	Definition
Consciousness	Awareness of self and environment
Confusion	Reduced awareness, disorientation
Delirium	Disorientation, fear, irritability, misperception, hallucination
Obtundation	Reduced alertness, psychomotor retardation, drowsiness
Stupor	Unresponsiveness with arousal only by vigorous and repeated stimuli
Coma	Unarousable unresponsiveness
Vegetative state	Prolonged coma (> 1 month), some preservation of brainstem and motor reflexes
Akinetic mutism	Prolonged coma with apparent alertness and flaccid motor tone
Locked-in state	Total paralysis below third cranial nerve nuclei; normal or impaired mental function

and the examination may be divided into cranial and general (extracranial) components.

Cranial examination

Level of consciousness
This is assessed by the patient's response to command and to physical stimuli. The Glasgow coma scale (GCS; Table 40.4) was developed to grade the severity and outcome of traumatic head injury,[5] and its use has been extended for all causes of impaired consciousness and coma. This was not the intended purpose of the GCS, and it should only be used as an assessment of the depth of unconsciousness. It is important to define the responses in descriptive terms rather than emphasizing the numerical score attached to each response. This is particularly important when transferring details between health providers, as inter-observer variation in scoring may be misleading.

Table 40.2 Differential diagnosis of disorders of consciousness

STRUCTURAL DISORDERS	METABOLIC CAUSES
Vascular	*Alteration of neuronal metabolism*
Haemorrhage	Ischaemia (any cause)
Extradural	Hypoxia
Subdural	Hypotension
Subarachnoid	Hypoglycaemia
Intracerebral	Hypothermia
Infarction	Hyperthermia
Thrombosis	Coenzyme deficiency
Embolism	Thiamine
Vasospasm	Nicotinic acid
	Endocrinopathies
Infection	Hypothyroidism
Meningitis	Adrenal insufficiency
Encephalitis	Hypopituitarism
Abscess	
	Alteration of neuronal membrane activity
Herniation syndrome (*mass effect*)	Hypo–osmolar states
Tumour	Hyperosmolar states
Vascular causes (q.v.)	Acid-base disturbance
Cerebral oedema	Seizure disorders
Neurotrauma	Neurotrauma (concussion)
Hypoxia	
Reye's syndrome	MULTIFACTORIAL CAUSES
Metabolic causes (q.v.)	*Organ failure*
	Severe sepsis
TOXIC/DRUG CAUSES	Hepatic encephalopathy
	Uraemic encephalopathy
Sedatives	Multiple organ failure
Narcotics	
Alcohol	*Behavioural*
Poisons (q.v.)	Sleep deprivation
Psychotropic drugs	Psychiatric disorders
Carbon monoxide	Conversion reactions
	Catatonia

Table 40.3 Important factors in the medical history in patients with impaired consciousness

Known systemic disease
Cardiac disease
Respiratory disease
Renal failure
Liver disease
Endocrine disease
  Diabetes mellitus
  Hypothyroidism
Psychiatric disorders
Medications

Previous neurology
Epilepsy
Cerebrovascular disease
Subarachnoid haemorrhage

Risk factors
Depression
Alcohol abuse
Drug abuse

Circumstances of onset
Sudden/subacute preceding headache
Visual disturbances
Trauma
Environmental factors
  Drugs in vicinity
  Gas
  Poisons
  Temperature

If possible, the GCS should be determined prior to intubation or administration of sedative drugs, and always be defined with regard to the patient's vital signs, namely blood pressure, pulse rate and temperature. Concomitant or previous drug therapy must be noted, as the pharmacokinetics of commonly used drugs in the ICU (especially sedatives and analgesics) may be markedly altered in patients with underlying liver or renal disease. This may be manifest as reduced level of consciousness or as cerebral agitation due to drug withdrawal. The presence of alcohol should always be stated.

Pupillary responses

The response of the pupils to light, both directly and consensually, must be assessed. Changes in responses must be assessed in conjunction with the GCS. Factors that affect pupillary responses must be considered. These include traumatic mydriasis, drugs causing pupillary dilatation (e.g. tricyclics, sympathomimetics and topical mydriatics) or constriction (e.g. narcotics, organophosphates and topical β-blockers. Horner's syndrome and prosthetic eyes.

The unilateral, unresponsive pupil suggests ipsilateral third nerve compression, and is usually due to uncal herniation. Bilateral unresponsive dilated pupils suggest posterior midbrian compression or excessive sympathetic stimulation. Bilateral pupillary constriction is a marker of bilateral hemispheric dysfunction or pontine damage.

Eyes

Corneal reflexes are preserved until coma is very deep. The loss of corneal responses when drug-induced or local anaesthetic causes are excluded is a poor prognostic sign of brainstem function. Upward rolling of the eyes after corneal stimulation (Bell's phenomenon) implies intact midbrain and pontine function. The resting position of the eyes and presence and nature of spontaneous eye movements must be noted. Conjugate deviation of the eyes implies ipsilateral hemispheric or contralateral brainstem lesions. The responses of the eyes to oculovestibular stimuli (e.g. injection of cold water in the ear) and oculocephalic stimuli (e.g. rapid changes in head position) assess brainstem function. Intermittent downward-jerking eye movements (ocular bobbing) are seen in destructive pontine and cerebellar lesions and in hydrocephalus.[1,2] Spontaneous roving horizontal eye movements exclude brain stem pathology as a cause of coma.

Table 40.4 Neurological assessment of impaired consciousness

GLASGOW COMA SCALE

Eye opening	*Points*
Spontaneous	4
To speech	3
To pain	2
Nil	1

Best verbal response	
Oriented	5
Confused	4
Inappropriate	3
Incomprehensible	2
Nil	1
Intubated	T

Best motor response	
Obeys commands	6
Localizes to pain	5
Withdraws to pain	4
Abnormal flexion	3
Extensor response	2
Nil	1

Brainstem function	*Motor function*
Pupillary reactions	Muscle tone
Corneal reflexes	Decorticate or
Spontaneous eye movements	decerebrate rigidity
Oculocephalic response	Tendon reflexes
Oculovestibular response	Seizures
Respiratory pattern	

The fundi should be examined for subhyaloid haemorrhages (subarachnoid haemorrhage) and for evidence of hypertensive and diabetic retinopathy. Papilloedema is indicative of intracranial hypertension, but is frequently absent when the lesion is acute. Periorbital haematomas are common following trauma and may indicate an anterior cranial basal skull fracture, particularly if there is associated cerebrospinal fluid rhinorrhoea.

Head, ears and neck

The tympanic membrane should be examined for evidence of perforation or otitis interna. Signs of meningeal irritation include neck rigidity, Kernig's (inability to fully extend the legs) and Brudzinski's (hip and knee flexion in response to neck flexion) signs. Patients in deep coma may exhibit no neck rigidity despite meningeal irritation.

The head should be inspected for trauma, and lacerations carefully explored for an underlying skull fracture. Drainage of cerebrospinal fluid from the ear and a retroauricular haematoma (Battle's sign) indicate a posterior basal skull fracture. The breath may smell of alcohol or poisons (e.g. organophosphates). Patients with severe uncontrolled diabetes mellitus may exhibit a sweet smell of ketones when examined, but this may not be a reliable sign. Hepatic and uraemic foetor are rare.

General examination

Respiratory rate and pattern

Abnormalities in respiratory rate and pattern are common, and must be determined as a marker of respiratory distress for the level of cerebral dysfunction. At lighter levels of impaired consciousness, tachypnoea may predominate. This may be seen in patients with head injury (neurogenic hyperventilation), delirium from drug withdrawal, poisoning from salicylates or tricyclic antidepressants, or in other acidotic states such as diabetic ketoacidosis and sepsis. As a general rule, respiratory depression increases with depth of coma. Abnormal breathing patterns such as Cheyne–Stokes respiration indicate bilateral hemispheric dysfunction; apneustic breathing is a feature of pontine dysfunction, and ataxic or Biot respiration represents medullary dysfunction. Drug-induced coma (e.g. opioids) usually causes a dose-dependent bradypnoea.

Lungs

Patients with impaired consciousness are at risk of pulmonary aspiration. Any cause of respiratory failure may result in impaired consciousness, although this is usually due to hypercapnia. Processes such as pneumonia, asthma and chronic airways disease should be excluded. Neurogenic pulmonary oedema is a sympathetic nervous system-mediated phenomenon that occurs in severe brain injury.[6] Coincidental chest problems in the multiple-traumatized patient should always be considered.

Cardiovascular

Any cause of hypotension below a critical cerebral perfusion pressure will result in impaired consciousness and must be identified. Hypertensive patients may require a higher than normal mean arterial pressure to maintain adequate cerebral perfusion. Patients with cardiac pacemakers should be assessed for pacemaker malfunction or Stokes–Adams attacks. The traditional Cushing response of hypertension and bradycardia in intracranial hypertension is variable, and any heart rhythm may be present.

Abdomen and skin

Signs of liver disease may indicate an hepatic cause, and other organomegaly or evidence of intra-abdominal malignancy should be established. The presence of polycystic kidneys raises the possibility of subarachnoid haemorrhage. Needle puncture marks may indicate substance abuse. Skin changes may be seen in porphyria, diabetes, hypoadrenalism, hypothyroidism and panhypopituitarism. Skin rashes may indicate infectious causes of meningoencephalitis.

Investigations

The order of investigations depends on the clinical circumstance. In the majority of cases, history and examination will provide enough information. Investigations should be directed at the likely cause and may be grouped into the following:

Routine investigations

Conventional routine investigations include measurements of plasma glucose, serum electrolytes, arterial blood gases, blood count and examination of blood film, and urinary electrolytes and glucose. Hypoglycaemia commonly produces coma. Attention should be paid to electrolyte disturbances that may result in impaired consciousness (e.g. hypo- and hyperosmolal states, hyperkalaemia and hypocalcaemia).

Neuroimaging (see Chapter 99)

Relevant imaging investigations include computed tomography (CT), magnetic resonance imaging (MRI), single-photon emission with computed tomography (SPECT), positron emission tomography (PET) and cerebral angiography. These investigations are performed in areas where patient access is limited, and should not precede adequate resuscitation or careful neurological examination. Cerebrally agitated or comatose patients generally require endotracheal intubation and sedation before proceeding to imaging.

Advances in neuroimaging such as CT and MRI have greatly improved diagnostic ability. These scans accurately diagnose space-occupying lesions, stroke and cerebral oedema. Angiography will often identify cerebral aneurysms or arteriovenous malformations in patients presenting with subarachnoid haemorrhage. Newer nuclear medicine techniques such as SPECT and PET help to assess cerebral blood flow and oxygen utilization, and, possibly, to prognosticate neurotrauma, but have no role in the management of acute disorders of consciousness.[7]

Other investigations

1 *Lumbar puncture* gives information on the presence of meningeal inflammation, haemorrhage, infection and cerebrospinal fluid cytology. If clinical or CT scan evidence of raised intracranial pressure is present, a neurosurgical opinion should be sought prior to lumbar puncture. In general, lumbar puncture should not be performed under this circumstance.
2 *Electroencephalography:* This is rarely used in the ICU due to difficulties in interpretation and electrical interference. It may have a limited role in identifying patients who are in subclinical status epilepticus.[8]
3 *Evoked potentials:* Visual, brainstem and somatosensory evoked potential test the integrity within the brain and spinal cord. They may be used in the diagnosis of blindness in comatose patients, and in the assessment of locked-in patients. There is little

conclusive evidence that these tests improve prognostication in patients with coma.[9]
4 *Toxicology:* When drug overdose is suspected, samples of blood, gastric contents and urine should be analysed. Carboxyhaemoglobin may be measured by co-oximetry or direct assay.

Resuscitation

Hypoxia and hypotension, both as primary causes of impaired consciousness and as secondary insults, are associated with adverse outcome and must be assiduously avoided.[10]

Airway

The airway must be assessed for overt or potential obstruction. This is best done by assessing the patient's response to command and physical stimulation, and whether a gag reflex is present. Securing the airway will depend on the level of consciousness. This may entail simple manoeuvres such as jaw thrust and chin lift, use of oropharyngeal airways, or in the comatose patient mandate endotracheal intubation. All of these patients are at risk of pulmonary aspiration, and there must be a low threshold for establishing a definitive airway (endotracheal intubation).

As a general rule, patients presenting with medical causes of coma may be nursed on their side (coma position) if the airway is adequate. However, all traumatized patients should be assumed to have a potential cervical spine injury, and must be nursed with the cervical spine in the neutral position and/or with a rigid collar, until an injury is excluded by definitive radiological views[11] (see Chapter 69). All patients with disordered consciousness must receive supplemental oxygen.

Ventilation

Once the airway is secure, ventilation must be assessed so that gaseous exchange is optimal for that particular patient. Generally, a $Pa_{O_2}>80$ mmHg (10.6 kPa) and $Pa_{CO_2}<40$ mmHg (5.3 kPa) is desirable. In mild disorders of consciousness, spontaneous ventilation may be adequate or even increased, but with increasing depth of coma, artificial support either by hand or mechanical ventilation may be necessary.

Circulation

Adequacy of circulation by pulse rate, blood pressure and perfusion must be assessed, and efforts directed at prompt restoration of appropriate mean arterial blood pressure. Dehydration and hypovolaemia must be corrected with appropriate fluids and inotropes used where appropriate. Attention to life-threatening causes of shock (e.g. haemorrhage or sepsis) must take precedence over the diagnosis of coma.

Treatment

Following initial assessment and resuscitation, treatment is directed at the underlying cause. Principles of treatment may be considered as emergency treatment, specific treatment and preventive care.

Emergency treatment

Hypoglycaemia and thiamine deficiency are the greatest concern, since most other metabolic causes of coma are reversible if vital functions are supported. If there is any suspicion of hypoglycaemia, 50 ml of 50% dextrose should be injected IV immediately after the blood for glucose estimation is drawn. Care should be exercised when administering carbohydrate-rich fluids to a patient with incipient or overt thiamine deficiency (Wernicke–Korsakoff syndrome or beriberi). Empirical parenteral thiamine (100 mg IV) is safe in any patient with a history of alcoholism who presents in impaired consciousness.[12]

The use of drug antagonists in drug overdose, such as naloxone for opioids, flumazenil for benzodiazepine, and benztropine for anticholinergics, is to be cautioned, and limited to diagnostic evaluation only due to their short half-lives. In most cases, supportive measures suffice and are safer (see Chapter 77).

Specific treatment

This refers to the specific treatment of the underlying cause and is discussed in the relevant chapters. Principles to consider here are the maintenance of an appropriate cerebral perfusion pressure and oxygenation, so that secondary hypoxic or ischaemic insults are avoided.

Preventive care

Assessment and evaluation

A modified neurological examination, with emphasis on the GCS criteria, is important in the ongoing assessment. Alterations in coma score warrant immediate patient reassessment. Sedatives and analgesics should be used when appropriate, but withdrawn as soon as possible to facilitate this assessment.

Nursing care

Meticulous eye and mouth care, regular changes in patient position, limb physiotherapy, bronchial toilet and psychological support are mandatory. Nosocomial infections and iatrogenic complications are associated with an increased mortality and morbidity in these patients, and must be promptly diagnosed and treated. The rational use of invasive procedures such as intravascular and urinary catheters and prescription of antibiotics is essential.

Nutrition

Early establishment of enteral feeding via a duodenal tube is preferable. Exclusion of a basal skull fracture is recommended before insertion of a nasoenteric tube. Patients at risk of gastric bleeding should receive stress ulcer prophylaxis if enteral feeding has not been established.

Prognosis

Patients with a potential for recovery should be managed in ICUs or specialist wards. However, patients in whom prognosis is hopeless should not be exposed to prolonged or inappropriate intensive care. Acute confusional states and delirium from drug-induced or metabolic causes will generally respond to correction of the underlying disorder, provided that secondary hypoxic insults do not supervene.[2] Patients who develop deeper levels of stupor and coma may remain unconscious for a variable time, and prognosis will depend on the degree of permanent brain damage. Clinical markers and scoring systems at various time intervals following the onset of coma have been used to predict outcome. These include cause (medical or traumatic), depth of coma, and the presence or absence of neurological signs.[13–15]

Studies analysing outcome from medical causes have concentrated on outcome following cardiac arrest,[13,14] but coma due to metabolic causes, infection and multiple organ failure generally have a better prognosis.[2] The best predictor of poor outcome following cardiac arrest (i.e. progression to a persistent vegetative state or death) is the absence of motor responses to painful stimuli after 3 days.[16] Absence of pupillary responses and other brainstem reflexes are further predictors of poor outcome.[2,9]

Following traumatic causes of coma, correlation between CT appearance and initial GCS with outcome has been described. The best prognostic factors are age, motor score and pupillary response.[15] If patients in deep coma progress to a persistent vegetative state, the chances of recovery from traumatic coma are more favourable than from medical causes. However, for such patients, the outlook is bleak, with a mean life expectancy of 2–5 years.[17,18]

References

1 Plum F and Posner J (1980) *The Diagnosis of Stupor and Coma*, 3rd edn. Philadelphia: FA Davis.
2 Bates D (1993) The management of medical coma. *J Neurol Neurosurg Psych* **56**:589–598.
3 Hawkes CH (1991) How to perform a rapid neurological examination. *Hosp Update* **2**:125–130.

4 Peterson PL (1993) Disorders of consciousness. In: Carlson RW and Geheb MA (eds) *Principles and Practice of Intensive Care Medicine*. Philadelphia: WB Saunders, pp. 631–639.

5 Teasdale G and Jennett B (1974) Assessment of coma and impaired consciousness: a practical scale. *Lancet* **2**:81–83.

6 Demling R and Riessen R (1990) Pulmonary dysfunction after cerebral injury. *Crit Care Med* **18**:768–774.

7 Lewis SB, Reilly PL and Myburgh JA (1994) Developments in intracranial pressure monitoring and investigation of head injured patients. In: Dobb GJ, Bion J, Burchardi H and Dellinger RP (eds). *Current Topics in Intensive Care*. London: WB Saunders, pp 1–19.

8 Engel J, Ludwig BI and Fetell M (1978) Prolonged partial complex status epilepticus: EEG and behavioural observations. *Neurology* **28**:863–869.

9 Diringer MN (1992) Early prediction of outcome from coma. *Curr Opin Neurol Neurosurg* **5**:826–830.

10 Chesnut RM, Marshall LF, Klauber MR *et al.* (1993) The role of the secondary brain injury in determining outcome from severe head injury. *J Trauma* **34**:216–222.

11 Trauma Committee, Royal Australasian College of Surgeons (1992) *Early Management of Severe Trauma* Melbourne: EMST.

12 Harris JO and Berger JR (1991) Clinical approach to stupor and coma. In: Bradley WG, Daroff RB, Fenichel GM and Marsden CD (eds) *Neurology in Clinical Practice*. London: Butterworths pp. 47–54.

13 Sacco RL, Vangool R, Mohr JP *et al.* (1990) Non-traumatic coma: Glasgow Coma Score and coma etiology as predictors of 2 week outcome. *Arch Neurol* **47**:1181–1184.

14 Niskanen M, Kari A, Nikki P *et al.* (1991) Acute physiology and chronic health evaluation (APACHE II) and Glasgow Coma Scores as predictors of outcome from intensive care after cardiac arrest. *Crit Care Med* **19**:1465–1473.

15 Born JD, Albert AA, Hans P *et al.* (1985) Relative prognostic value of best motor response and brain stem reflexes in patients with severe head injury. *Neurosurgery* **16**:595–601.

16 Edgren E, Hedstrand U, Kelsey S *et al.* (1994) Assessment of neurological progress in comatose survivors of cardiac arrest. *Lancet* **343**:1055–1059.

17 Multi-Society Task Force on PVS (1994) Medical aspects of the persistent vegetative state (first part). *N Engl J Med* **330**:1499–1508.

18 Multi-Society Task Force on PVS (1994) Medical aspects of the persistent vegetative state (second part). *N Engl J Med* **330**:1572–1579.

41 | Status epilepticus

CD Gomersall and TE Oh

Status epilepticus or epilepsy is a medical emergency requiring prompt intervention to prevent the development of irreversible brain damage. It is generally defined as 'recurrent epileptic seizures without full recovery of consciousness before the next seizure begins' or 'continuous clinical and/or electrical seizure activity lasting for more than 30 minutes whether or not consciousness is impaired'.[1]

Various types of status epilepticus can be classified:[2]

1 Repeated generalized tonic and/or clonic convulsive seizures where the patient does not fully recover neurological function between attacks.
2 Non-convulsive status epilepticus which can be seen as a prolonged twilight state. This may be absence seizures and complex partial seizures (see below). These conditions commonly have an element of tonic–clonic or myoclonic activity, either at presentation or at a subsequent examination.
3 Continuous focal epileptic activity without alteration of consciousness.

Pathophysiology

The pathophysiological effects of seizures on the brain are thought to result from both direct excitotoxic neuronal injury and secondary injury due to systemic complications such as hypotension and hypoxia. It is postulated that seizures result in excessive pre-synaptic release of glutamate. This activates post-synaptic glutamate receptors, resulting in calcium influx into cells via receptor-gated calcium channels and release of intracellular calcium stores. The increase in intracellular calcium ions activates calcium-dependent enzymes that are responsible for irreversible neuronal injury.

Aetiology

Status epilepticus may occur *de novo* or, less commonly, in a previously diagnosed epileptic. The most common causes of generalized convulsive status in a previously diagnosed epileptic are as listed:[3]

1 poor compliance with medication;
2 change in antiepileptic drug or dosage;
3 withdrawal of the effects of alcohol;
4 pseudostatus.

In patients without any history of epilepsy, conditions which should be considered as possible causative factors are shown in Table 41.1[1,4,5]

Generalized convulsive status epilepticus

The most common and dangerous form of status epilepticus is generalized convulsions. It includes

Table 41.1 Status epilepticus causes with no previous history of epilepsy[1,4,5]

Cerebral tumour, primary or secondary
Stroke of all varieties
Intracranial infection, i.e. meningitis, meningoencephalitis or cerebral abscess
Hypoxic encephalopathy (e.g. post cardiac arrest)
Drug abuse and overdose, e.g. tricyclic antidepressants, theophylline, cocaine or other stimulants
Electrolyte disturbances, including:
  Hyponatraemia
  Hypocalcaemia
  Hypomagnesaemia
Hypoglycaemia
Human immunodeficiency virus infection
First presentation of primary epilepsy (by exclusion)

Table 41.2 Systemic complications of generalized convulsive status epilepticus[6,9,20]

Hypoxia
Lactic acidosis
Hypercarbia
Rhabdomyolysis, hyperkalaemia, and acute renal failure
Hyperpyrexia
Hypoglycaemia
Hypertension (early)
Hypotension (late)
Cardiac arrhythmias
Neurogenic pulmonary oedema
Aspiration pneumonitis
High-output cardiac failure
Intracranial hypertension

Table 41.3 Clinical features of pseudostatus

More common in females
History of psychosocial disturbance
Consciousness may be retained in the presence of bilateral jerking
Resistance to examination
Vocalization
Pelvic thrusting
Gaze aversion
Normal pupillary response during convulsion
Normal tendon reflexes and plantar responses immediately after convulsion

a wide range of presentations, from repeated overt generalized seizures to very subtle focal twitches of a localized part of the body (e.g. rhythmic nystagmoid eye jerks and twitching of an eyelid). The latter may superficially appear to be a form of focal epilepsy, but can clearly be distinguished from focal epilepsy, by the fact that the patient has profound impairment of conscious level and bilateral electroencephalogram (EEG) changes. It should be noted that if a patient with generalized tonic–clonic convulsions is inadequately treated, the generalized convulsions may stop despite continued ictal EEG discharges.[1] The morbidity and mortality associated with generalized convulsive status epilepticus relates in part to the neuronal injury (which may result from inadequate treatment), in part to the systemic complications (Table 41.2), and in part to the aetiology.[6,7]

The most important differential diagnosis of generalized convulsive epilepsy is pseudoseizures.[8] Clinical features suggestive of pseudoseizures are listed in Table 41.3.[6,9,10] Distinction between the two may be extremely difficult, and can only be made with complete certainty using EEG monitoring.[11,12] Serum prolactin concentrations are often increased following a single true fit, and can be used to distinguish a single fit from a pseudoseizure, but concentrations are not usually raised in status epilepticus.[13]

Non-convulsive status epilepticus[14]

This accounts for at least 25% of status epilepticus cases. Its incidence is probably underestimated, because of failure to recognize and diagnose the condition. Non-convulsive status epilepticus is divided into absence status epilepticus and complex partial status epilepticus.

Absence status epilepticus

This condition is characterized by a prolonged confusional state associated with generalized 3 Hz spike and slow-wave EEG activity. Coma is almost never caused by this condition. It is not a life-threatening condition, unlike generalized convulsive status epilepticus. Although it is a relatively common form of status epilepticus, patients rarely require admission to ICU. However, it is important to differentiate between absence status epilepticus and the unresponsive state associated with prolonged, generalized convulsive status epilepticus.

Complex partial status epilepticus

Diagnosis of this condition may be difficult, due to its variable presentation and the need for EEG confirmation. Ictal activity may be continuous or cyclical, with failure to regain consciousness between seizures. The characteristic manifestation of ictal activity is altered mentation, with variable responsiveness and amnesia. Patients may demonstrate automatism and complex motor activity, bizarre behaviour and lateralizing or localizing neurological deficits (e.g. aphasia or paresis). The duration of complex partial status epilepticus is usually several minutes to hours. Prompt diagnosis is significant, as early treatment appears to be important in preventing neurological morbidity.

Investigations

Not all of the investigations (Table 41.4) need be performed in every patient. Selection of tests depends on both the patient's history and presentation. Most patients with status epilepticus should have a computed tomography (CT) scan performed at some stage, but patients with established epilepsy who have already had a CT scan do not usually require another scan.

Central nervous system (CNS) infection must be seriously considered in all patients, especially young children with a fever. Lumbar puncture is indicated in patients with fits not controlled with a benzodiazepine and phenytoin, evidence of craniofacial infection (e.g. otitis or mastoiditis), or nuchal rigidity.[11] It is contraindicated in those in whom an intracranial space-occupying lesion is suspected. Although CT

Table 41.4 Investigations in status epilepticus

Initial investigations
Blood glucose and serum urea, creatinine, sodium, potassium, calcium
Antiepileptic drug concentrations
Complete blood count
Oximetry Sao_2 or arterial blood gases
Urinalysis

Further investigations after stabilization
Liver function tests
Serum magnesium
Toxicology screen
Computed tomography scan
Lumbar puncture
Electroencephalogram

Table 41.5 Protocol to treat generalized convulsions

Make the diagnosis
Assess airway, breathing and circulation
Place in left lateral position
Give oxygen by facemask
Consider tracheal intubation, especially if patient is cyanosed
Insert IV cannula and draw blood for investigations
If hypoglycaemic, or if blood glucose estimation is not available, give glucose
  In adults, give 100 mg thiamine first, then 50 ml 50% IV bolus glucose
  In children, give glucose 25% 2 ml/kg
Give diazepam 0.2 mg/kg IV at 5 mg/min *or* lorazepam 0.1 mg/kg at 2 mg/min
  If diazepam is given to stop status epilepticus, phenytoin should be given next to prevent recurrence
If status persists, give phenytoin
  In adults, 15–20 mg/kg IV at a rate ≤ 50 mg/min, and
  In children, 1 mg/kg per min
  Monitor ECG and blood pressure during infusion. If hypotension or arrhythmias develop, slow the rate of phenytoin infusion
If status persists after 20 mg/kg phenytoin, give extra doses of 5 mg/kg, to a maximum of 30 mg/kg
If status still continues, give phenobarbitone 20 mg/kg IV at 100 mg/min
Be prepared for tracheal intubation and ventilatory support as the risk of apnoea is high
If status is still not controlled, give anaesthetic doses of thiopentone (3–5 mg/kg), and intubate and ventilate the patient

IV = Intravenous; ECG = Electrocardiogram.

scanning prior to lumbar puncture may not be considered mandatory,[15] one should remember that, in adults, CNS tumours are more common causes of epilepsy than infections.[1,5] Lumbar puncture is never a life-saving procedure. Even in suspected meningitis, lumbar puncture should be delayed for 30 min after a fit, because of the accompanying transient cerebral oedema.[16] Patients with cerebrospinal fluid (CSF) leukocytosis should be treated for suspected meningitis until the diagnosis is excluded by microbiological culture or antibody assays, even though CSF leukocytosis occurs in 20% of status epilepticus cases.[17]

Management

Generalized convulsive status epilepticus

An accurate history, with particular emphasis on eye-witness accounts of the onset and nature of the seizures, should be obtained, and a full physical examination performed. However, neither must delay initial emergency management. There is evidence that the longer status epilepticus goes untreated, the harder it is to control with drugs. In animals, the risk of brain damage is directly related to the duration of status epilepticus.[18,19]

Management of continuing generalized convulsions involves control of the seizures to prevent neuronal damage and other secondary complications (Table 41.3), and treatment of complications and the underlying pathology. The latter is beyond the scope of this chapter. A treatment protocol to control the seizures is outlined in Table 41.5.[15]

Absence status epilepticus

These patients do not usually require admission to ICU and thus management will depend to some extent on the availability of staff and equipment. If resuscitation equipment is at hand, IV diazepam or lorazepam are suitable first-line drugs. Acetazolamide (IV 500 mg in adults or 250 mg in children and adults under 35 kg) is safer but less effective. Once absence status epilepticus has been terminated, a long-acting oral anticonvulsant should be started (e.g. valproate, ethosuximide or clonazepam).

Complex partial status epilepticus

Treatment should be instituted urgently, as soon as the diagnosis has been confirmed with an EEG. Management is essentially the same as for generalized convulsive status epilepticus.

Drugs for status epilepticus

Benzodiazepines

The most commonly used first-line drugs in the control of status epilepticus are benzodiazepines. They achieve high brain levels rapidly when given IV, and will usually terminate an attack of seizures within minutes (33% at 3 min and 80% within 5 min). The most commonly used benzodiazepine for this purpose is diazepam. It terminates status more rapidly (1–3 min) than lorazepam, but fits often recur if used alone, because brain concentrations fall rapidly due to rapid redistribution. Lorazepam has a slower onset of action but longer duration of action. There is some evidence in children that midazolam may terminate status in cases where adequate doses of diazepam and phenytoin have failed, without causing severe respiratory depression.[20]

Diazepam and lorazepam can also be given rectally when IV administration is not possible. If a rectal preparation is not available, a Foley catheter can be inserted into the rectum and the balloon inflated. Either drug can then be simply diluted with an equal amount of saline and flushed into the rectum. The catheter balloon prevents the drug leaking out of the rectum. Doses of 0.2–0.7 mg/kg of diazepam given rectally control status epilepticus in most patients within 1–10 min.[21] Absorption after intramuscular injection is erratic and this route should not be used.

Phenytoin

Phenytoin can cause hypotension and cardiac arrhythmias, especially in patients with pre-existing heart disease. Both blood pressure and ECG should be monitored during infusion of phenytoin. The rate of infusion must be slowed if the patient develops hypotension, prolonged QT interval or cardiac arrhythmias. If status epilepticus stops before the complete dose is given, the infusion rate should be slowed to decrease the risk of adverse effects. When the patient's plasma phenytoin concentration is known, the additional dose of phenytoin required to achieve a therapeutic plasma concentration can be calculated using the following formula:[22]

Loading dose (mg) $= 0.65$ weight ((kg) $\times (C_{desired} - C_{current})$

where C is the phenytoin concentration in mg/l (divide by 4 if in μmol/l).

Phenytoin is not stable in dextrose solutions, and is only stable in saline for 30 min. Its absorption is unpredictable when given intramuscularly, and therefore this route should not be used in emergencies. Intramuscular injection has the additional disadvantage that it may cause sterile abscesses.

Fosphenytoin is a water-soluble disodium phosphate ester of phenytoin, which can be given intramuscularly. Its use in the treatment of status epilepticus is currently under investigation.

Sodium valproate

Valproate is now available in an intravenous form, but there are as yet no controlled data on its efficacy in the treatment of status epilepticus. There are, however, case reports of valproate being used to treat status epilepticus successfully.[23]

Paraldehyde

Paraldehyde, given intramuscularly, followed by massaging the injection site, may be of use in situations where intravenous access is limited or difficult (e.g. children). The dose is 5 ml every 30 min as necessary. Time to peak plasma level is 0.5–1.0 h. Reported adverse effects include right heart failure, pulmonary oedema, pulmonary haemorrhage and hypotension. Damage to adjacent nerves and sterile muscle abscesses may occur following intramuscular injection.[11]

Barbiturates

Thiopentone sodium (Pentothal) is a rapidly effective anticonvulsant. It should be used in cases of refractory status epilepticus (Table 41.5). Endotracheal intubation must be performed, and ventilatory facilities must be available. An initial IV dose of 3–5 mg/kg is given for intubation, with aliquots of 50–100 mg after a few minutes if the seizures remain uncontrolled. Following bolus IV administration, the drug is rapidly taken up in the brain, but high concentrations are not sustained due to its rapid redistribution into peripheral fat stores. For this reason, an IV infusion should follow – a dose of about 50 mg/h. When fat stores are saturated, disposition of the drug may take days, consistent with its long half-life. Thiopentone should be regarded as a general anaesthetic, capable of predictable respiratory and cardiac depression. Hypotension is usually managed with intravenous fluids, but inotropes may be needed due to the combined effects of the numerous drugs used to control the seizures.

Phenobarbitone (IV or IM) has a slower speed of action and a longer duration. Intubation, ventilatory and resuscitative facilities must also be available with its use (Table 41.5).

Neuromuscular blocking agents

Paralysis is indicated if uncontrolled fitting causes respiratory embarrassment or severe lactic acidosis. Neuromuscular blockade should only be used if continuous EEG monitoring is also used, as the clinical expression of seizure activity is abolished.[11] Blind use of muscle relaxants without control of seizures will result in cerebral damage.

Intensive care monitoring

In status epilepticus refractory to treatment with phenytoin and phenobarbitone, the monitoring procedures listed in Table 41.6 may be necessary.[16] In prolonged status epilepticus or in patients paralysed with muscle relaxants, motor activity may not be present. In these cases, continuous EEG monitoring is necessary. This can be performed using EEG leads or a form of cerebral function monitor. Continuous intracranial pressure monitoring is indicated in the presence of persisting, severe or progressive elevated intracranial pressure.

Table 41.6 Monitoring in status epilepticus

Intra-arterial blood pressure
Capnography
Pulse oximetry
Central venous pressure
Pulmonary artery wedge pressure
Electroencephalogram
Intracranial pressure

Table 41.7 Commonest causes of status epilepsy in children

Fever or infection
Medication change
Idiopathic
Metabolic
Congenital
Anoxia
Central nervous system infection
Cerebrovascular disease
Drug-related
Tumour

Outcome[7,15]

The prognosis of patients with status epilepticus is related to the aetiology, age, duration of status, occurrence of systemic complications (especially anoxia) and the type of treatment given. Estimated mortality ranges from 3 to 35%.

Status epilepticus in children

The majority of cases of status epilepticus occur in young children,[24] with 21% occurring in the first year of life and 64% in the first 5 years. More than 90% of cases are convulsive and the majority are generalized.[25] The commonest causes of status epilepticus in children under 16 years old are listed in order of frequency in Table 41.7. The overall mortality in recent paediatric series is 3–10%. Neurological sequelae in children with idiopathic or febrile status epilepticus are rare. This favourable outcome may be due to advances in therapy and to the relative resistance of the immature brain to damage from seizures. The risk of subsequent seizures in a child who presents with idiopathic status epilepticus is no greater than a child who presents with a brief fit, and the risk of another status episode is very low.[24]

References

1 Treiman DM (1993) Generalized convulsive status epilepticus in the adult. *Epilepsia* **34**(suppl. 1):S2–S11.

2 Gastaut H (1983) Classification of status epilepticus. *Adv Neurol* **34**:15–35.

3 Brodie MJ (1990) Status epilepticus in adults. *Lancet* **336**:551-552.

4 Aminoff MJ and Simon RP (1980) Status epilepticus: Causes, clinical features and consequences in 98 patients. *Am J Med* **69**:657–666.

5 DeLorenzo RJ, Towne AR, Pellock JM and Ko D (1992) Status epilepticus in children, adults, and the elderly. *Epilepsia* **33**(suppl 4): S15–S25.

6 Wasterlain CG, Fujikawa DG, Penix L and Sankar R (1993) Pathophysiological mechanisms of brain damage from status epilepticus. *Epilepsia* **34**(suppl 1):S37–S53.

7 Towne AR, Pellock JM, Ko D and DeLorenzo RJ (1994) Determinants of mortality in status epilepticus. *Epilepsia* **35**:27–34.

8 Wills AJ and Stevens DL (1994) Epilepsy in the accident and emergency department. *Br J Hosp Med* **52**:42–45.

9 Walton NY (1993) Systemic effects of generalized convulsive status epilepticus. *Epilepsia* **34**(suppl 1): S54–S58.

10 Shorvon S (1993) Tonic clonic status epilepticus. *J Neurol Neurosurg Psychiatry* **56**:15–140.

11 Ramsay RE (1993) Treatment of status epilepticus. *Epilepsia* **34**(suppl 1): S71–S81.

12 Betts T (1990) Pseudoseizures: seizures that are not epilepsy. *Lancet* **336**:163–164.

13 Tomson T, Lindborn U, Nilsson BY, Svanborg E and Anderson DHE (1989) Serum prolactin during status epilepticus. *J Neurol Neurosurg Psychiatry* **52**:1433–1437.

14 Cascino GD (1993) Nonconvulsive status epilepticus in adults and children. *Epilepsia* **34**(suppl 1): S21–S28.

15 Working Group on Status Epilepticus (1993) Treatment of convulsive status epilepticus. Recommendations of America's Working Group on Status Epilepticus. *JAMA* **270**:854–859.

16 Mellor DH (1992) The place of computed tomography and lumbar puncture in suspected bacterial meningitis. *Arch Dis Child* **67**:1417–1419.

17 Simon RP (1985) Physiological consequences of status epilepticus. *Epilepsia* **26**(suppl 1):S58–S66.

18 Walton NY and Treiman DM. (1988) Response of status epilepticus induced by lithium and pilocarpine to treatment with diazepam. *Exp Neurol* **101**:267–275.

19 Treiman DM and Mayers PD (1991) The DVA Status Epilepticus Cooperative Study Group. Utility of the EEG pattern as a predictor of success in the treatment of generalized convulsive status epilepticus. *Epilepsia* **32**(suppl 3):93-98.

20 Rivera R, Segnini M, Baltodano A and Perez V (1993) Midazolam in the treatment of status epilepticus in children. *Crit Care Med* **21**:991–994.

21 Albano A, Reisdorff EJ and Wiegenstein JG (1989) Rectal diazepam in pediatric status epilepticus. *Am J Emerg Med* **70**:168–172.

22 Winter ME and Tozer TN (1986) Phenytoin. In: Evans WE, Schentag JJ and Jusko WJ (eds). *Applied Pharmacokinetics*. Spokane: *Applied Therapeutics*, pp. 493–539.

23 Snead OC and Miles MV. (1985) Treatment of status epilepticus in children with rectal sodium valproate. *J Pediatr* **106**:323–325.

24 Maytal J, Shinnar S, Moshe SL and Alvarez LA (1989) Low morbidity and mortality of status epilepticus in children. *Pediatrics* **83**:323–331.

25 Gross–Tsur V and Shinnar S (1993) Convulsive status epilepticus in children. *Epilepsia* **34**(suppl. 1): S12–S20.

42 | Acute cerebrovascular complications

WR Thompson

Cerebrovascular disease is common, and its acute complications – thrombosis, embolism, intracerebral haemorrhage and subarachnoid haemorrhage (SAH) – produce transient ischaemic attacks (TIA) and stroke syndromes. The worldwide incidence of stroke is about 150-200/100 000 population.[1] Strokes are the third most common cause of death (10% of all deaths) in the USA, with an annual incidence of 140/100 000 population.[2] The National Survey of Stroke reported survival rates of 69.7% for 30 days and only 52.4% for 12 months.[3] Some recent studies have demonstrated a decline in the incidence[4] of and mortality[4,5] from strokes. However, with the ageing of the population, the prevalence may be increasing. Age and hypertension remain important aetiological and prognostic factors.[4] Thromboembolism accounts for some 85% of all strokes; up to 23% of those are due to cardiac emboli.[6] Spontaneous intracranial haemorrhage accounts for some 15% of strokes (Table 42.1).

Advances in basic neurosciences and neuro-pharmacology offer hope that more active early management may improve outcome.[7] In some circumstances, particularly following SAH and TIA, intensive care management may improve functional outcome.

Cerebral infarction

Cerebral infarction refers to occlusion of a cerebral blood vessel in association with an inadequate collateral circulation. The occlusion may be due to cerebral thrombosis or cerebral embolism (Table 42.1).

Aetiology

Cerebral thrombosis

The most common arterial causes are atherosclerosis and hypertension. Rarer causes include arteritis, arterial dissection, aortic arch syndromes, syphilis, angiography, infection, trauma to the head and neck and haematological disorders. Venous thrombosis is

Table 42.1 Stroke manifestations

Strokes
Cerebral infarction
Thrombosis
Embolism
Spontaneous intracranial haemorrhage
Intracranial haemorrhage
Subarachnoid haemorrhage

not common, but may occur with raised intracranial pressure (ICP), malignancy, dehydration, septicaemia and hyperviscosity syndromes.

Cerebral embolism

This is generally from a left atrial thrombus associated with mitral stenosis or atrial fibrillation, a mural thrombosis following myocardial infarction or bacterial endocarditis.

In addition, the risk factors for cerebral infarction include advanced age, hypertension, hypotension, heart disease, diabetes mellitus, obesity, hyperlipidaemia, cigarette smoking and the use of some oral contraceptives.

Pathology

Cerebral thrombosis

Atherosclerosis leads to plaque formation and progressive narrowing at the origins and bifurcations of arteries. Hypertension can aggravate this process, and may also produce lipohyaloid changes in the arteries. In addition, the plaques may ulcerate due to ischaemic necrosis. Thrombus formation occurs in the areas of reduced blood flow around the atheroma or on the ulcerated plaques. The thrombus may then occlude the vessel, become incorporated into the plaque or embolize.

Cerebral embolism

Cardiac disorders which produce thrombi, valvular disease or tumours may lead to cerebral embolism. The emboli may be platelet aggregates, fibrin, debris from atheromatous plaques, calcified valve fragments, bacterial vegetations or tumour tissue. Emboli may become impacted and produce thrombosis, or may fragment and travel further. TIA may be due to atheroma, variable blood flow across a stenotic area or to emboli.

Clinical presentation

Cerebral thrombosis

The initial stroke is commonly preceded by TIA. There is generally no headache and no loss of consciousness. The neurological deficit may come on suddenly. However, more commonly, it gradually progresses to its full extent over a matter of hours. The symptoms and signs are dependent on the size of the lesion and the artery that is affected.

Cerebral embolism

Cerebral embolism is characterized by sudden onset and rapid development of the complete neurological deficit. Occasionally, fragmentation of the embolus may lead to resolution of the neurological deficit. Neurological deficit is dependent on the artery involved.

Investigations

The investigations required will be determined by the history, examination and differential diagnosis. The following are useful:

1 urinalysis;
2 urea, electrolytes and blood sugar;
3 full blood picture and erythrocyte sedimentation rate;
4 coagulation profile;
5 serum cholesterol and triglycerides;
6 syphilis serology;
7 electrocardiogram (ECG): to detect arrhythmias or myocardial infarction;
8 skull X-rays and cervical spine X-ray: if trauma or cervical abnormalities are suspected or if the patient is comatose.
9 computed tomography (CT) scan: cerebral infarction may not be seen on the scan in the first 2 days. However, the scan may indicate intracerebral haemorrhage, SAH, hydrocephalus, chronic subdural haematoma or a malignancy. Haemorrhage must be excluded if anticoagulants are planned to be administered. Magnetic resonance imaging (MRI) scanning, if feasible, may allow earlier detection of the changes associated with cerebral infarction.[7]

10 cerebrospinal fluid (CSF) examination is indicated if haemorrhage needs to be excluded and a CT scanner is not available. It is also required if there is a possibility of infection, multiple sclerosis or neurosyphilis;
11 angiography; particularly following TIA or when the CT scan has not provided a diagnosis;
12 echocardiography may assist in diagnosing unusual cardiac conditions;
13 transcranial Doppler.

Management

1 *General care*: Most of these patients may not be comatose, but they may have major neurological deficits. Their general care may therefore need to be similar to that of the unconscious patient.
2 *Blood pressure control*: The patient's clinical condition and neurological function are the appropriate determinants of treatment, rather than the measured blood pressure. Severe hypertension ($>180/120$ mmHg or $>23.9/16$ kPa) should be treated, but blood pressure must be reduced slowly to prevent further cerebral ischaemia due to hypotension. More aggressive treatment is required in hypertensive encephalopathy.
3 *Oxygen therapy*: Supplemental oxygen is important to prevent hypoxaemia. A positive role for hyperbaric oxygen has not been confirmed.
4 *Cardiac disorders*: It is important to maintain adequate cardiac output. Treatment may be required for myocardial infarction, cardiac failure, ventricular arrhythmias, atrial fibrillation and bacterial endocarditis.
5 *Haemorrheology:* Animal experiments have suggested that early haemodilution may reduce infarct size. While haemodilution increases cerebral blood flow, to date clinical studies[8,9] have failed to demonstrate a clinical advantage. To ensure optimal cerebral oxygen delivery and cerebral blood flow, it is important to correct any existing volume depletion, polycythaemia or anaemia. The optimum haematocrit is probably in the range of 0.30–0.35.[10] However, the relative values and efficacy of hypervolaemia versus isovolaemic haemodilution have yet to be determined.[10] In order to reduce the risk of cerebral oedema and intracranial hypertension, colloid solutions may be preferable to crystalloid solutions for isovolaemic haemodilution.[11] Cardiac and cerebral functions are carefully monitored during fluid loading. Pentoxifylline increases red-cell deformability and reduces whole-blood viscosity, but its role in the treatment of strokes has yet to be established.
6 *Anticoagulation*: This remains a controversial and unproven treatment in acute stroke.[7,10,12] Intracranial haemorrhage and non-ischaemic causes of

stroke must be excluded before anticoagulation is commenced. Anticoagulation may be indicated for:

(a) TIAs,[10,12] particularly recent or crescendo TIAs and/or tight stenoses of the carotid or vertebrobasilar systems;
(b) progressing strokes;
(c) embolic strokes, with the exception of bacterial endocarditis. Anticoagulation has been recommended for patients with small or moderate embolic strokes, who are not hypertensive and who have no evidence of haemorrhage on CT scan at 24–48 h after the stroke.[13–15]

While it has been suggested that patients seen within 6 h with a progressing stroke should be anti-coagulated,[16] a large randomized study of all forms of acute ischaemic stroke only demonstrated minimal benefit.[17]

7 *Antiplatelet therapy:* Inhibition of platelet aggregation using acetylsalicylic acid (aspirin) has been shown to reduce the incidence[10,18] and severity[19] of strokes in patients with TIAs. The optimum dose of aspirin has not been determined[10] and no effect on mortality from TIAs has been demonstrated to date.[20] There may be an increased risk of moderate/severe haemorrhagic strokes associated with the use of aspirin.[21] The efficacy of dipyridamole or sulphinpyrazone to prevent further strokes is as yet unproven.

8 *Thrombolytic therapy:* There are anecdotal reports of good results with thrombolytic therapy and further trials are in progress, particularly using tissue plasminogen activator (tPA). A pilot study of tPA initiated within 90 min of symptoms showed neurological improvement in 30% of patients.[22] In another study,[23] angiographic recanalization occurred in 26–30% of proximal and middle cerebral artery occlusion, when tPA was commenced within 8 h of symptoms of focal ischaemia. Haemorrhagic transformation tended to occur with higher doses of tPA and in patients treated later.

9 *Cerebral protection:* There is probably no indication for the use of steroids in cerebral ischaemia.[24] The benefit of hyperventilation in acute stroke remains unproven. No positive effects of barbiturates have been demonstrated in stroke patients.

Calcium channel-blocking agents may have a role in the management of acute cerebral ischaemia. In a randomized double-blind trial nimodipine did not improve mortality or overall neurological outcome.[25] However, in that study, the patients treated within 18 h of symptoms, particularly those with no abnormality on CT scan, had a better outcome.

The roles of hypothermia, naloxone, *N*-methyl-D-aspartate (NMDA) receptor blockers, laza-

roids, free radical scavengers and gangliosides have yet to be determined (see Chapter 44).

10 *Surgery:* TIAs and symptomatic carotid artery disease are indications for carotid endarterectomy (CEA).[7,10] The NASCET[26] and ECST[27] studies demonstrated the benefits of CEA in symptomatic patients with high-grade (>70%) stenoses. In addition, the ACAS group[28] recently showed that, provided perioperative morbidity/mortality is less than 3%, CEA will reduce the 5-year risk of ipsilateral stroke in good-risk patients with asymptomatic carotid artery stenoses of 60% or greater. Further comparisons of early and delayed surgery are required, but emergency CEA may be indicated in:[7]

(a) crescendo TIAs;
(b) the first few hours of an abrupt severe neurological deficit;
(c) the first 48 h of a complete carotid occlusion;
(d) patients with recent-onset mild-to-moderate neurological deficits with normal conscious level and normal CT scan.

The Extracranial–Intracranial (EC–IC) bypass study group failed to demonstrate a reduction in the risk of ischaemic stroke, when EC–IC bypasses were compared to standard therapy for stroke prevention in patients with carotid occlusion or surgically inaccessible stenoses.[29] However, much debate has centred on the eligibility criteria of the trial and the large number of EC–IC bypasses performed outside the trial.

11 *Physiotherapy and rehabilitation.*

Complications of strokes

Local complications are cerebral oedema and cerebral haemorrhage. General complications include bronchopneumonia, deep venous thrombosis, pulmonary embolism, urinary tract infection, pressure sores, contractures and depression.

Spontaneous intracranial haemorrhage

Spontaneous intracranial haemorrhage may be either intracerebral haemorrhage or SAH (Table 42.1).

Intracerebral haemorrhage

This incidence of intracerebral haemorrhage is about 9/100 000 population.[2] It generally affects adults 40–70 years old. Sex distribution is approximately equal, although some studies have reported a female predominance.

Aetiology

Spontaneous intracerebral haemorrhage is generally the result of systemic hypertension. Other causes include:

1 intracranial tumours, both primary and metastatic;
2 supratentorial space-occupying lesions and transtentorial herniation;
3 inflammatory arterial disease;
4 mycotic aneurysms associated with bacterial endocarditis;
5 haemorrhagic disorders and complications of anticoagulation;
6 vasopressor drugs;
7 amyloidosis and sarcoidosis.

Pathology

Common sites of intracerebral haemorrhage are putamen (55%), thalamus (10%), cerebral cortex (15%), pons (10%) and cerebellum (10%).[30] The rupture of microaneurysms occurs at the bifurcation of small perforating arteries, but they are not always the source of the bleeding. Hypertension and lipohyalinosis are considered to be important pathogenetic factors.[31] Lipohyalinosis can produce vascular occlusion or vascular rupture. The haemorrhage is generally due to the rupture of a single vessel.

The size of the haemorrhage depends on the volume that can be tolerated in relation to the anatomical site. Cortical haemorrhages tend to be larger and less devastating than those in the pons. The haemorrhage may extend into adjacent structures. Large supratentorial haemorrhages may be complicated by pontine haemorrhages.

Clinical presentation

Usually there are no prodromal symptoms. There is a sudden onset of coma or stupor and neurological deficit, with the rate of evolution of the deficit depending on the rate of bleeding. Headache and nuchal rigidity are generally only associated with cortical haemorrhages or bleeding into the ventricles. The clinical syndromes referable to the site of haemorrhage have been described.[30,32]

Investigations

These include:

1 CT scan – investigation of choice;
2 coagulation profile;
3 lumbar puncture, if CT scan is unavailable and there is no clinical evidence of raised ICP or transtentorial herniation. It is important to exclude a traumatic spinal tap;
4 angiography, where it is considered likely that an aneurysm, an arteriovenous malformation or a

tumour are the cause of the haemorrhage, and if surgery for such a lesion is contemplated.

Management

Principles of management include:

1 bed rest and general supportive care as for an unconscious patient, including mechanical ventilatory support;
2 physiotherapy;
3 relief of headache;
4 treatment of respiratory disorders, especially pneumonia;
5 treatment of cardiovascular disorders;
6 control of blood pressure;
7 correcting coagulation disorders;
8 maintaining fluid and electrolyte balance;
9 control of ICP. Raised ICP may be due to mass effect of the haematoma, oedema of adjacent brain or obstructive hydrocephalus. Steroids are generally ineffective. Hyperventilation is probably of no benefit in primary intracerebral haemorrhage without cerebral oedema. Mannitol will reduce the oedema. Operative treatment is required for hydrocephalus and intracerebellar mass lesions, where it is often life-saving. Early (within 6 h) removal of putaminal haemorrhage has been shown to improve outcome,[33] and there are hopes that stereotactic or endoscopic evacuation of the clot may improve outcome;[7]
10 antifibrinolytics have no proven benefit in treating intracerebral haemorrhage.

Subarachnoid haemorrhage

SAH refers to bleeding which occurs principally within the subarachnoid space, rather than into the brain parenchyma. In approximately 75% of cases, the cause is the rupture of an intracranial aneurysm. About 5% of cases are due to bleeding from an arteriovenous malformation (AVM) and in up to 20% of cases no cause is found, even with adequate angiography.

Ruptured intracranial aneurysm

The incidence of aneurysmal rupture is 11/100 000 of population in North America,[34] and this occurs most commonly in the 40–60-year age group. The ratio of males to females is approximately 2:3 due to a female preponderance after the age of 40.

Aetiology and pathogenesis

The vast majority of intracranial aneurysms are saccular (berry) aneurysms. The other, less common types include atherosclerotic, mycotic and traumatic aneurysms. Saccular aneurysms occur in the bifurcations of the arteries which form the circle of Willis, and in the bifurcations of the major arteries which arise from the circle of Willis. Most (90–95%) occur in the anterior part of the circle of Willis and 5–10% in the vertebrobasilar system. Saccular aneurysms were initially thought to be congenital and due to a defect in the tunica media. It now appears likely that they are acquired, due to degeneration of the internal elastic membrane at the apex of the bifurcation as a result of haemodynamic stress.[35] This produces the initial aneurysmal sac. Hypertension and turbulent flow within the sac produce further degeneration of the aneurysm wall, and this leads to enlargement of the sac.[35] This in turn increases the risk of rupture of the aneurysm, which usually occurs when the aneurysm is 5–15 mm in diameter. Rupture commonly occurs in association with activities that increase the blood pressure.

Clinical presentation

1 Prodromal symptoms may be absent. However, many patients may experience headache, dizziness, orbital pain or transient neurological symptoms. Unfortunately, complaints are often vague and they are misdiagnosed. Gillingham[36] and Drake[37] have emphasized the importance of headache and the 'warning leak'.
2 Sudden onset of severe headache.
3 Loss of consciousness which often follows the onset of the headache. The depth and duration of coma are dependent on the site and extent of the haemorrhage.
4 Meningism – neck stiffness, photophobia, vomiting and Kernig's sign.
5 Transient neurological deficits, related to the site of the aneurysm and size of the haemorrhage. Early gross deficits are often due to cerebral ischaemia or intracerebral haematoma.

Patients are graded on the basis of their conscious state and neurological deficit. The grade score increases from I to V as the level of responsiveness falls and the neurological deficits become more severe (Table 42.2). In general, coma and major deficits indicate a poor prognosis. A universal SAH grading scale, based on the Glasgow coma scale (GCS) and major focal deficits has been proposed by the World Federation of Neurological Surgeons (Table 42.3).[38]

Complications

Cerebral

Rebleeding

The chance of rebleeding is dependent on the site of the aneurysm, presence of clot, degree of vasospasm, age and sex of the patient.[39] Kassell and Torner[40] reported a 19% cumulative rebleeding rate in the first 2 weeks after the initial SAH – 4.1% occurred within

Table 42.2 Clinical neurological classification of subarachnoid haemorrhage

Grade	Signs
I	Conscious patient with or without meningism
II	Drowsy patient with no significant neurological deficit
III	Drowsy patient with neurological deficit – probably intracerebral clot
IV	Deteriorating patient with major neurological deficit (because of large intracerebral clot)
V	Moribund patient with extensor rigidity and failing vital centres

Table 42.3 Proposed WFNS SAH scale[38]

WFNS grade	GCS score	Motor deficit
I	15	Absent
II	14–13	Absent
III	14–13	Present
IV	12–7	Present or absent
V	3–6	Present or absent

WFNS = World Federation of Neurological Surgeons; SAH = subarachnoid haemorrhage; GCS = Glasgow coma scale score.

the first 24 h, then approximately 1.5% per day for the next 13 days. Other authors[41–43] have reported rebleeding rates of 16–25% in the first 2 weeks with a peak incidence around days 4–9. The rebleed rates can be reduced by 30–50% in patients who receive antifibrinolytic therapy.[42,44] However, overall mortality has remained unchanged because of the problems of cerebral ischaemia, hydrocephalus and thrombosis associated with antifibrinolytic therapy.[39,45] There is a 40% mortality from the second haemorrhage.[46] Late (after 6 months) rebleeding occurs at an average of 3% per year and is fatal in 67% of cases.[39]

Cerebral vasospasm[47]

Angiographic evidence of vasospasm can be demonstrated in 40–70% of patients between days 4 and 12 following SAH. Clinical vasospasm is the most important cause of morbidity and mortality following SAH, and occurs in some 40% of patients between 4 and 12 days after SAH, with a peak incidence at 6–7 days. Diagnosis is based on the time of onset (days 4–9), rate of development (over hours) of neurological deficits (impaired orientation and decreased level of consciousness preceding focal deficits) plus exclusion of other causes (e.g. rebleeding, hydrocephalus, hypoxia, hyponatraemia, cerebral oedema and intracranial haemorrhage). There is an association between the amount of blood in the subarachnoid space and the development of vasospasm.[48] Numerous other aetiological factors have been proposed, but none has been proven, and it is now recognized that structural changes within the arterial wall are responsible for the arterial narrowing after SAH.[49]

Hydrocephalus[46,50]

Seizures

General complications

Non-neurological complications include ECG changes (e.g. T-wave inversion, ST segment changes, U waves and Q-T prolongation), arrhythmias, sympathetic hyperactivity, hyponatraemia and reductions in total blood volume and red cell mass.

Investigations

General investigations are as above for cerebral ischaemia. More specific investigations include the following:

1 *CT scan* may indicate the site of bleeding, blood in CSF, mass lesions, hydrocephalus or cerebral oedema.
2 *Lumbar puncture* is required if blood is not seen on CT scan, and ICP is not raised, and there is a strong suspicion of SAH. Xanthochromia is usually present within 6 h of SAH. Lumbar puncture may be required to rule out bacterial meningitis.
3 *Skull X-rays:* displacement of a calcified pineal gland will indicate intracranial shifts if a CT scan is not available.
4 *Angiography* will confirm the diagnosis of the lesion and its position prior to surgery. It may also indicate areas of vasospasm.
5 *Cerebral blood flow studies* may assist in the timing of surgery.
6 *ICP monitoring* is useful in comatose patients, and in patients with cerebral oedema or hydrocephalus.
7 *Transcranial Doppler*[51,52] allows non-invasive detection of increases in mean arterial velocities and these can be correlated with vasospasm.
8 *Somatosensory evoked potentials*[52] may be indicative of clinical grades and neurological deficits, particularly intraoperatively.

Management

Management will be influenced by the SAH grading of the patient, pre-existing medical problems and the relationship to surgery. Preoperative management includes:

1 *Bed rest* with oxygen, sedation and analgesia as required.

2 *General care* of the poorer-grade SAH patients as per care of the unconscious patient.
3 *Blood pressure control:* Except for patients with cerebral vasospasm, hypertension should be controlled with sedation, analgesics and antihypertensives. Drugs that produce cerebral vasodilatation should be used cautiously as they may increase the ICP. β-adrenergic blockers, methyldopa and hydralazine have been used. Calcium-channel blockers may have potential advantages with reference to vasospasm. Circulating volume should be maintained and hypotension avoided.
4 *Antifibrinolytics:* ε-Aminocaproic acid (EACA) and tranexamic acid, which inhibit clot lysis, have been shown to reduce the rate of recurrent haemorrhage. but because of their disadvantages (see above) their usefulness has been questioned.[53] These considerations, together with the trend to earlier surgery for grade I and II SAH patients, have largely led to the abandonment of antifibrinolytics.
5 *Treatment of vasospasm:* Angiographic evidence of vasospasm occurs in 60–70% of patients following SAH, but only 30% develop symptomatic delayed cerebral ischaemic deficits. Numerous approaches to the prevention and treatment of vasospasm have been advocated.[54] Both oral and IV nimodipine[55,56] have been shown to reduce the mortality and morbidity of aneurysmal SAH by reducing the incidence and severity of cerebral ischaemia.

   Another effective treatment adjuvant is hypervolaemia and/or induced hypertension.[49,57] For hypervolaemia to be undertaken safely, the aneurysm should be isolated from the circulation – early surgery is required. If that is not feasible, then moderate hypervolaemia (e.g. pulmonary capillary wedge pressure (PCWP) 12–14 mmHg or 1.6–1.9 kPa) and normotension with meticulous monitoring of neurological and cardiovascular status are required. Complications include pulmonary oedema, myocardial infarction, haemorrhagic cerebral infarction and cerebral oedema.
6 *Treatment of seizures.*
7 *Treatment of cerebral oedema:* Steroids are often used prophylactically.
8 *Prevention of gastric erosions.*
9 *Maintenance of fluid and electrolyte balance.*
10 *Treatment of hydrocephalus.*
11 *Surgery:* Clipping of the aneurysm is the preferred definitive approach. Other methods include reinforcement of the sac, trapping, proximal ligation, bypass graft and intravascular occlusion. Surgical mortality for good-risk patients should be less than 5%.

   Timing of surgery remains a matter of debate.[10] Many centres favour late surgery (i.e. at 7–10 days) because the aneurysm is less fragile, less retraction is required, and late surgery is associated with less vasospasm and a lower mortality.[37] Early surgery (within 3 days) was initially the method employed, and is once again being advocated for good-risk patients, as it may reduce postoperative mortality.[59,60] However, there may increased postoperative ischaemic complications after early surgery,[61] particularly in grades III–IV patients. Hence, the measured benefits of early surgery may not be as great as was predicted. Nevertheless, it is now an option for grades I and II patients. Delayed surgery is still recommended for the poorer-grade SAH patients.

Postoperative management includes:

1 *analgesia and general supportive care*;
2 *ICP measurement* and raised ICP therapy in patients with operative complications, cerebral oedema or vasospasm.
3 *medical complications*, e.g. seizures, inappropriate antidiuretic hormone secretion, hyponatraemia, cardiac arrhythmias, myocardial infarction, cardiac failure, pneumonia, pulmonary emboli and urinary tract infections require individual treatment.
4 *surgical complications*, e.g. rebleeding, subdural and extradural haematomas, hydrocephalus and intracranial hypertension must be diagnosed and treated appropriately;
5 *vasospasm:* postoperative vasospasm is treated with nimodipine and/or hypervolaemia. Preferred fluids are blood and colloids,[11] which are infused to a central venous pressure of 8–12 mmHg (1.1–1.6 kPa) or a PCWP of 10–12 mmHg (1.3–1.6 kPa). Normal serum electrolytes and a haematocrit of 0.30–0.35 are maintained. Should the patient's condition not improve, PCWP should be cautiously increased to 16–20 mmHg (2.1–2.7 kPa); patients with heart disease may require inotropic support and/or digitalis. If there is no neurological improvement, further inotrope support and induced hypertension (e.g. systolic pressure of 140–180 mmHg or 18.6–23.9 kPa) should be attempted. Bradycardic patients may respond to vagolytic agents. Hypervolaemia may produce a marked diuresis, and antidiuretics and/or mineralocorticoids may then be useful. Patients with cerebral oedema and vasospasm may require mannitol, judicious volume loading and mechanical ventilation.

Arterial blood pressure, PCWP, ICP and cerebral perfusion pressure, arterial blood gases, urine output, haemaglobin, haematocrit and serum electrolytes are monitored. CT scans will indicate areas of oedema or infarction. Hypervolaemia is reported to produce transient improvement in 80–90% of cases and permanent improvement in 60%. Complications include pulmonary oedema, cerebral oedema, cerebral haemorrhagic infarction, electrolyte imbalance and those related to the insertion of monitoring devices.

Arteriovenous malformation

AVMs are congenital and enlarge during life. They may present with epilepsy, haemorrhage or headache (often migrainous), and sometimes as cranial bruits in children. Investigations will depend on the mode of presentation, but should include CT scan, electroencephalogram, skull X-rays and angiography. Surgery is the treatment of choice if resection is feasible, but the risk of serious neurological deficits must be kept in mind. Proximal ligations of feeding vessels or intra-arterial embolization are other methods which can be used. Rebleeding is less likely to occur than with ruptured aneurysms and therefore antifibrinolytics are not required.

Prognosis in cerebrovascular disease

The survival rate from stroke is related to the patient's age, cardiovascular status and the type of stroke. In general, 30% of patients with stroke die within 30 days, and 43% are dead within 6 months.[3] Prognosis is worse for haemorrhagic strokes than for ischaemic strokes.[3] Stroke units may improve the functional outcome and reduce the need for long-term hospital care,[62-64] but selection criteria have yet to be verified.

The benefits of carotid endarterectomy in symptomatic patients with high-grade stenoses have been confirmed.

There have been improvements in the surgical management and the treatment of rebleeding and vasospasm. Unfortunately, only one-third of patients with a ruptured aneurysm ever receive surgery.[46,54] Among SAH patients who survive to reach hospital, a favourable outcome has been reported in 43% of surgical cases.[54] Approximately 60% of grade I and II SAH patients will have a favourable outcome.[64] Among aneurysm patients without major preoperative neurological deficits a surgical mortality of less than 5% is possible.[46,64] Intensive care management is of benefit to SAH patients and patients following carotid endarterectomy.

References

1 Viriyavejakul A (1990) Stroke in Asia. An epidemiological consideration. *Clin Neuropharmacol* 1990; **13**:526–533.
2 Robins M and Baum HM (1981) Incidence. In: Weinfeild FD (ed.) The National Survey of Stroke. *Stroke* **12**:145–157.
3 Baum HM and Robins M (1981) Survival and prevalence. In: Weinfeild FD (ed.) The National Survey of Stroke. *Stroke* **12**:159–168.
4 Whisnant JP (1984) The decline of stroke. *Stroke* **15**:160–168.
5 Doyon B, Serrano G and Marc–Vergnes JP (1988) Trends in mortality from cerebrovascular disease in France from 1968 to 1978. With reference to

cardiovascular and all causes of death. *Stroke* **19**: 330–334.

6 Cerebral Embolism Task Force (1989) Cardiogenic brain embolism. *Arch Neurol* **46**:727–743.

7 Camratta PJ, Heros RC and Latchaw RE (1994) 'Brain attack': The rationale for treating stroke as a medical emergency. *Neurosurgery* **34**:144–158.

8 Italian Acute Stroke Study Group (1988) The Italian haemodilution trial on acute stroke. *Stroke* **19**:145.

9 Scandinavian Stroke Study Group (1987) Multicentre trial of haemodilution in acute ischaemic stroke. Results in the total population. *Stroke* **18**:691–699.

10 Grotta JC (1987) Current medical and surgical therapy for cerebrovascular disease. *N Engl J Med* **317**:1505–1516.

11 Tommasino C, Moore S and Todd MM (1988) Cerebral effects of isovolemic hemodilution with crystalloid or colloid solutions. *Crit Care Med* **16**:862–868.

12 Miller VT and Hart RG (1988) Heparin anti-coagulation in acute brain ischemia. *Stroke* **19**:403–406.

13 Cerebral Embolism Task Force (1988) Cardiogenic brain embolism. *Arch Neurol* **43**:71–84.

14 Cerebral Embolism Study Group (1983) Immediate anticoagulation of embolic stroke: a randomised trial. *Stroke* **14**:668–676.

15 Yatsu FM, Hart RG, Mohr JP and Grotta JC (1988) Anticoagulation of embolic strokes of cardiac origin: an update. *Neurology* **38**:314–316.

16 Sherman DG, Dyken MJ, Fisher M, Harrison MJ and Hart RG (1992) Antithrombotic therapy for cerebrovascular disorders. *Chest* **102**:529S–537S.

17 Duke RJ, Bloch RF, Turpie AG, Trebilcock R and Bayer N (1986) Intravenous heparin for the prevention of stroke progression in acute partial stable stroke. *Ann Intern Med* **105**:825–828.

18 The Canadian Co-operative Study Group (1978) A randomised trial of aspirin and sulfinpyrazone in threatened stroke. *N Engl J Med* **299**:53–59.

19 Grotta JC, Lemak NA, Gary H, Fields WS and Vital D (1985) Does platelet antiaggregant therapy lessen the severity of stroke? *Neurology* **35**:632–636.

20 Ramirez–Lassepas M and Cipolle RJ (1988) Medical treatment of transient ischemic attacks: does it influence mortality? *Stroke* **19**:397–400.

21 The Steering Committee of the Physicians Health Study Research Group (1988) Special report. Preliminary report: findings from the aspirin component of the ongoing physician health study. *N Engl J Med* **318**:262–264.

22 Brott TG, Haley EC, Levy D *et al.* (1992) Urgent therapy for stroke. Part 1. Pilot study of tissue plasminogen activator administered within 90 minutes. *Stroke* **23**:632–640.

23 Del Zoppo GJ, Poeck K, Pessin MS *et al.* (1992) Recombinant tissue plasminogen activator in acute thrombotic and embolic stroke. *Ann Neurol* **32**:78–86.

24 Mulley G and Wilcox RG (1978). Dexamethasone in acute stroke. *Br J Med* **2**:994–996.

25 American Nimodipine Study Group (1992) Clinical trial of nimodipine in acute ischaemic stroke. *Stroke* **23**:3–8.

26 NASCET Collaborators (1991) Beneficial effect of carotid endarterectomy in symptomatic patients with high-grade carotid stenosis. *N Engl J Med* **325**:445–453.

27 European Carotid Surgery Trial (ECST) Collaborative Group (1991) MRC European carotid surgery interim results for symptomatic patients with severe (70–90%) or mild (0–29%) carotid stenosis. *Lancet* **337**:1235–1243.

28 Executive Committee for the Asymptomatic Carotid Atherosclerosis Study (1995) Endarterectomy for asymptomatic carotid artery stenosis. *JAMA* **273**:1421–1428.

29 The EC/IC Bypass Study Group (1985) Failure of extracranial–intracranial arterial bypass to reduce the risk of ischemic stroke: results of an international randomised trial. *N Engl J Med* **313**:1191–1200.

30 Fisher CM (1975) Clinical syndromes in cerebral thrombosis, hypertensive haemorrhage and ruptured saccular aneurysm. *Clin Neurosurg* **22**:117–147.

31 Feigin I and Prose P (1959) Hypertensive fibrinoid arteritis of the brain and gross cerebral haemorrhage. A form of 'hyalinosis'. *Arch Neurol* **1**:98–110.

32 Mohr JP, Miller Fisher C and Adams RD (1980) Cerebrovascular disease. In: Adams RD, Braunwald E, Petersdorf RG and Wilson JD (eds) *Harrison's Principles of Internal Medicine*, 9th edn. New York: McGraw-Hill, pp. 1933–1934.

33 Kanno T, Sano H, Shinomiya Y *et al.* (1984) Role of surgery in hypertensive intracerebral haematoma: a comparative study of 305 non surgical and 154 surgical cases. *J Neurosurg* **61**:1091–1099.

34 Phillips LH, Whisnant JP, O'Fallon WM and Sundt TM (1980) The unchanging pattern of subarachnoid haemorrhage in a community. *Neurology* **30**:1034–1040.

35 Ferguson GG (1982) The pathogenesis of intracranial saccular aneurysms. In: Varkey GP (ed.) *Anaesthetic Considerations in the Surgical Repair of Intracranial Aneurysm. International Anesthesiology Clinics*, vol. 20. Boston: Little, Brown, pp. 19–24.

36 Gillingham FJ (1967) The management of ruptured intracranial aneurysm. *Scot Med J* **12**:377–383.

37 Drake CG (1981). Management of cerebral aneurysm. *Stroke* **12**:273–283.

38 Drake CG, Hunt WE, Kassell N *et al.* (1988) Report of the World Federation of Neurological Surgeons Committee on a universal subarachnoid hemorrhage grading scale. *J Neurosurg* **68**:985–986.

39 Winn HR, Richardson AE and Jane JA (1980) The assessment of the natural history of single cerebral aneurysms that have ruptured. In: Hopkins LN and Long DM (eds). *Clinical Management of Intracranial Aneurysms*. New York: Raven Press, pp. 1–10.

40 Kassell NF and Torner JC (1993) Aneurysmal rebleeding:a preliminary report from the Cooperative Aneurysm Study. *Neurosurgery* **13**:479–481.

41 Rosenorn J, Eskesen V, Schmidt K and, Ronde F. (1987) The risk of rebleeding from ruptured intracranial aneurysm. *J Neurosurg* **67**:329–332.

42 Nibbelink DW, Torner JC and Henderson ISG (1975) Intracranial aneurysms and subarachnoid haemorrhage: a cooperative study. Antifibrinolytic therapy in recent onset subarachnoid haemorrhage. *Stroke* **6**:622–629.

43 Muller S, Hanlon K and Brown F (1978) Management of 136 consecutive supratentorial berry aneurysms. *J Neurosurg* **49**:794–804.

44 Adams HP, Nibbelink DW, Torner JC and Sahs AL (1981) Antifibrinolytic therapy in patients with aneurysmal subarachnoid haemorrhage. *Arch Neurol* **38**: 25–29.

45 Vermeulen M, Lindsay KW, Murrary GD et al. (1984) Antifibrinolytic treatment in subarachnoid haemorrhage. *N Engl J Med* **311**:432–437.

46 Hitchcock ER (1983) Ruptured aneurysms. *Br Med J* **286**:1299–1301.

47 Kassell NF, Sasaki T, Colohan ART and Nazar G (1985) Cerebral vasospasm following aneurysmal subarachnoid hemorrhage. *Stroke* **16**:562–572.

48 Fisher CM, Kistler JP and Davis JM (1980) Relation of cerebral vasospasm to subarachnoid haemorrhage visualized by computerised tomographic screening. *Neurosurgery* **6**:1–9.

49 Ausman JI, Diaz FG, Malik GM, Fielding AS and Son CS (1985) Current management of cerebral aneurysms: is it based on facts or myths? *Surg Neurol* **24**:625–635.

50 Black P McL (1986) Hydrocephalus and vasospasm after subarachnoid haemorrhage from ruptured intracranial aneurysms. *Neurosurgery* **18**:12–16.

51 De Witt LD and Wecusler LR (1988) Transcranial Doppler. *Stroke* **19**:915–921.

52 Symon L (1987) Current management of aneurysmal subarachnoid haemorrhage. In: Jewkes DA (ed.) *Baillière's Clinical Anesthesiology – Anaesthesia for Neurosurgery,* London: Baillière Tindall, pp. 295–315.

53 Ramirez-Lassepas M (1981) Antifibrinolytic therapy in subarachnoid haemorrhage caused by ruptured intracranial aneurysm. *Neurology* **31**:316–322.

54 Wilkins RH (1986) Attempts at prevention or treatment of intracranial arterial spasm: an update. *Neurosurgery* **18**:808–825.

55 Allen, GS, Ahn HS, Preziosi TJ et al. (1983) Cerebral arterial spasm – a controlled trial of nimodipine in patients with subarachnoid haemorrhage. *N Engl J Med* **308**:619–624.

56 Pickard JD, Murray GD, Illingworth R et al. (1989) Effect of oral nimodipine on cerebral infarction and outcome after subarachnoid haemorrhage: British Aneurysm Nimodipine Trial (BRANT). *Br J Med* **298**: 636–642.

57 Kassell NJ, Peerless SJ, Durward QJ, Beck DW, Drake CG and Adams HP (1982) Treatment of ischemic deficits from vasospasm with intravascular volume expansion and induced arterial hypertension. *Neurosurgery* **11**:337–341.

58 Finn SS, Stephensen SA, Miller CA, Drobnich L and Hunt WE (1986) Observations on the perioperative management of aneurysmal subarachnoid haemorrhage. *J Neurosurg* **65**:48–62.

59 Vapalahti M, Ljunggren B, Saveland H et al. (1984) Early aneurysm operation and outcome in two remote Scandinavian populations. *J Neurosurg* **60**:1160–1162.

60 Disney L, Weir B and Petruk K (1987) Effect on management mortality of a deliberate policy of early operation on supratentorial aneurysms. *Neurosurgery* **20**:695–701.

61 Chyatte D, Fode NC and Sundt TM (1988) Early versus late intracranial aneurysm surgery in subarachnoid haemorrhage. *J Neurosurg* **69**:326–331.

62 Strand T, Asplund K, Eriksson S, Hagg E, Lithner F and Wester PO (1986) Stroke unit care – who benefits? *Stroke* **17**:377–381.

63 Dombovy ML, Sandok BA and Basford JR (1986) Rehabilitation for stroke: a review. *Stroke* **17**:363–369.

64 Saveland H, Sonesson B, Ljunggren B et al. (1986) Outcome evaluation following subarachnoid haemorrhage. *J Neurosurg* **64**:191–196.

43 | Intracranial hypertension

D Hanley

Intracranial pressure (ICP) is an important parameter to monitor in the ICU. Guillaume and Janny were the first to describe continuous ICP monitoring in a patient using an intraventricular catheter in 1951.[1] Nine years later, Lundberg published the first systematic observations of ICP and its response to medical and physiological interventions.[2] In the following three decades, raised ICP (intracranial hypertension) has been widely recognized as an important contributor to injury and death in head trauma, cerebral haemorrhage, large ischaemic infarctions, tumours and hydrocephalus.

ICP measurement devices

ICP monitoring techniques are divided between fluid-coupled systems with external transducers, such as intraventricular catheters (IVC) and subarachnoid (SA) bolts, and solid-state systems that utilize a self-contained pressure transducer embedded in a catheter placed in the cranial vault. The actual practice of monitoring ICP via an IVC or SA bolt has changed little in 40 years.

Fluid-coupled catheters

For an IVC, the most common skull insertion site is over the posterior frontal lobe, preferably in the non-dominant hemisphere. The catheter is passed to a depth of 6 cm. Once cerebrospinal fluid (CSF) is encountered, this fluid catheter is connected to a three-way stopcock that leads to a transducer through one port and to an external drainage collection system through the other. Therefore, the IVC can be used both for ICP monitoring and for CSF drainage.

Fluid-coupled surface devices

The SA bolt technique for ICP monitoring was developed out of concern for the infection rate associated with IVCs, and because small ventricular size after head trauma often made catheter insertion difficult.[3] Thus, the SA bolt is indicated for ICP monitoring when CSF drainage is neither feasible nor desired. The skull insertion site is similar to the IVC, except that there is more freedom to place the SA bolt at different sites because the brain parenchyma is not punctured and eloquent cortex not at risk for injury during placement. The hollow self-tapping bolt is inserted into a burr hole in the skull, and the dura at the base of the bolt is perforated to allow SA CSF to fill the bolt. Saline-filled pressure tubing is then connected to the bolt to establish communication to a transducer.

Solid-state devices

These devices use miniature transducers that are coupled by wire or fibreoptic cables to an external instrument. The miniature transducers most commonly consist of a solid wire or fibreoptic cable configuration for ICP monitoring alone, but they can also be incorporated into an IVC for simultaneous ICP monitoring and CSF drainage. Solid-state devices can be inserted in the lateral ventricle, the brain parenchyma, the subarachnoid space or the epidural space. One of the better-known fibreoptic systems (Camino Laboratories, San Diego, CA) operates by projecting light through an optic fibre to a miniature, displaceable mirror in the catheter tip.[4] The amount of light reflected to a collecting optic fibre depends on the mechanical displacement of the mirror which, in turn, is a function of ICP. Recently introduced solid-state ICP devices include a fibreoptic system that relates change in ICP to shift in the interference pattern of a Fabry-Perot interferometer[5] (Inner Space Medical, Irvine, CA), and a miniature semiconductor strain-gauge transducer[6] (Codman & Shurtleff, Randolph, MA).

Use of ICP measurement devices in the ICU

Fluid-coupled catheters

The IVC is generally considered to be the most precise and accurate method of measuring ICP. Additionally, it is a therapeutic device providing the ability to drain CSF when intracranial hypertension is present. The IVC system provides accurate ICP measurements as long as it is free of air, blood or debris, the ventricles are not collapsed about the catheter fenestrations and the three-way stopcock in the drainage system is set so that no drainage occurs.

The stopcock can be set so that CSF is drained while the pressure waveform is displayed simultaneously for monitoring purposes; however, the ICP displayed will be erroneously low because the drainage system is open to the atmosphere.[7] With this configuration, accurate trending of ICP measurements during CSF drainage can be attained only by temporarily closing the stopcock to the atmosphere for fixed periods at frequent intervals, and recording the ICP on a flow sheet. All externally transduced ICP systems require an atmospheric pressure reference that should be zero-balanced to account for variations in patient head position. A commonly used anatomical reference point for adjusting the vertical position of the transducer is the external auditory meatus (EAM), although Lundberg originally suggested a point 1.5 cm below the uppermost part of the head regardless of position[2]. For active or confused patients, variation in patient position with respect to the external reference accounts for the shift of ICP baseline pressure of 0.7–2.0 kPa (5–15 mmHg) often seen in detailed clinical recordings. Where an unanticipated change in ICP is noted, a reassessment of the relation between skull reference and external transducer is recommended.

Fluid-coupled surface devices

The SA bolt is only a monitoring instrument; CSF cannot be withdrawn from it reliably. It usually provides a reliable ICP wave form and pressure reading, but is susceptible to error if the dural perforations become plugged with blood or debris, or if brain swelling obliterates communication with the CSF space.[8] This type of error is identified when the wave form becomes damped. Flushing debris from the open bolt surface with 0.2 ml of preservative-free (non-bacteriostatic) saline solution may restore accurate ICP readings, and does not cause dangerous ICP elevation in most circumstances.[8]

SA bolts are susceptible to referencing error in the same manner as IVCs. They tend to underestimate ICP, particularly when ICP is elevated.[8,9] Because the SA bolt measures the local ICP at the surface of the hemisphere, it can be inaccurate if there is a pressure gradient between the left and right supratentorial compartments.[8] The importance of compartmental pressure differences has been debated, but such gradients occur between the left and right hemispheres or the supratentorial and infratentorial compartments, and sometimes are only transient.[8-11] This is an important phenomenon to consider, and if there is a discrepancy between the apparent ICP and the patient's clinical condition, emergency computed tomographic (CT) scanning or treatment of elevated ICP may be warranted.

Solid-state devices

The greatest advantage of solid-state devices is that they do not require fluid coupling for pressure transduction, which avoids the problems of wave-form damping and artifacts from poor coupling. Additionally, they are air-referenced and thus do not require repositioning of the external transducer element. A major disadvantage is that the transducer cannot be calibrated to zero once it has been inserted. The performance of the Camino system has been evaluated more extensively than the newer systems. The Camino system accuracy, as compared to the IVC, has been demonstrated in the subdural space, the brain parenchyma and the ventricles. Parenchymal fibre-optic pressures may consistently exceed IVC pressures by nearly 1.3 kPa (10 mmHg).[12-15] The Camino fibreoptic device has substantial baseline drift after 5 days use (± 0.8 kPa or 6 mmHg). This is enough to cause significant inaccuracy and may necessitate replacement.[14] None of the solid-state ICP monitoring devices is directly compatible with common ICU bedside monitoring and patient data management systems. A separate module requiring an additional interface with the ICU monitoring system for recording and trending is necessary. This additional equipment increases the cost of ICP monitoring.

Physiology

Cranial vault

Water makes up the majority of the intracranial vault volume. Tissue water approaches 80% of tissue weight and is the major component of blood and CSF. A four-compartment model is the simplest and most practical way of conceptualizing the intracranial vault and its mechanics during health and disease. These compartments are brain cells, interstitial fluid, blood and CSF. The entire intracranial contents account for about 1400 – 1600 ml, with brain cellular space 65–70%, interstitial space 10–15%, blood 5% and CSF 5%. Since the intracranial volume remains constant, the volume relationships between these spaces are reciprocal. An increase in volume of one space must lead to decreases in the others. Blood and CSF are displaceable to a certain extent and provide a buffer. When this ability to buffer is overwhelmed, small additions of volume create large increases in ICP. Increases of cellular or interstitial water are the most common increases. Addition of a mass, either tumour or haematoma, is another major type of volume expansion. Early on in this process the CSF space decreases in size, leaving ICP stable. As volume is added rapidly to the closed cranial vault, the ability to decompress this change becomes limited and ICP rises rapidly as compliance fails. For masses that occur near the ventricular system, obstruction to outflow of CSF occurs, and this rise in ICP occurs even more rapidly. As ICP approaches mean arterial pressure (MAP), ischaemia occurs and results in cerebral vasodilatation. This homeostatic mechanism produces a rapid increase of cerebral blood volume and consequent ICP elevation. The attendant failure of cerebral perfusion pressure (CPP) leads to significant secondary brain injury.

Vascular mechanisms

The amount of blood in the cerebral vasculature accounts for approximately 5% of the intracranial contents. The absolute cerebral blood volume (CBV) at a given time is dependent on cerebral blood flow (CBF) and changes in this volume may have important effects on ICP and dynamics. The pial arterioles are the main resistance vessels in the cerebral vasculature and determine the CBV and CBF. When arteriolar tone is low, CBV and CBF increase, producing an increase in ICP. Conversely, when arteriolar tone is high, CBV and CBF are low and ICP decreases.

Several factors affect the arteriolar tone and, in turn, the CBV. The most important factor governing CBV and CBF is cerebral oxygen delivery. Cerebrovascular resistance changes in normal brain occur to maximize oxygen delivery. In instances where relative cerebral ischaemia or hypoxia occurs, CBF and CBV increase causing a concomitant increase in ICP. Ensuring adequate oxygenation, then, is an important step in controlling ICP.

Another factor influencing arteriolar tone is MAP. CBF is maintained constant over a wide range of MAP (6.7–20 kPa or 50–150 mmHg) by changes in cerebrovascular resistance (autoregulation). Above a MAP of 20 kPa (150 mmHg), however, autoregulation fails and arterioles become maximally dilated. The CBF then becomes a direct function of MAP. Increases in MAP cause increases in CBF and ICP. In areas of injured brain, autoregulation may be lost, although MAP remains in the range of 6.7–20 kPa (50–150 mmHg). In these cases, CBV may become directly related to MAP even though arterial pressure remains in the normal autoregulatory range.

Pa_{CO_2} has a direct effect on arteriolar calibre, and this effect has been used clinically for years to treat acute intracranial hypertension. Decreased Pa_{CO_2} results in vasoconstriction and a decrease in ICP. Hypercarbia causes vasodilatation and an increase in ICP. It is thus important to avoid hypercarbia in patients with increased ICP.

Cellular mechanisms

The central nervous system is a protected environment where oxidative energy-derived cellular ionic concentration gradients are modulated to produce neuronal work. A stable ionic milieu allows afferent, integrative and efferent signal processing to occur without interference. Ischaemia leads rapidly to energy failure and increased intracellular water. Thus, with ischaemia, cranial vault pressure regulation is further compromised by excess water accumulation as the ischaemic process progresses.

The cellular mechanisms for volume/water control are particularly important because both ionic transport systems and membrane integrity are at risk with excessive cellular swelling. Two distinct types of cellular volume buffering mechanisms are well-described:

Osmolar buffering mechanisms

These function by cells regulating the cytoplasmic concentration of low-molecular-weight amino acids such as taurine and sarcosine. For example, if excessive cellular shrinking has occurred because of systemic hyperosmolarity, the cell will increase its concentration of these substances to bring the cellular osmolarity into equilibrium with the systemic osmolarity. In this way, extracellular water passively returns to the cell and its prior volume state is restored. This system is active in mammalian brain, and it is important in preventing excessive shrinkage of central nervous system cells during systemic dehydration. As baseline levels of these amino acids or 'idiogenic osmoles' are low, it is thought that this system does not have a major influence on the ability of the cell to decrease its volume. Data regarding the function of this system with brain oedema states do not exist.

Ionic transporter buffering mechanisms

These exist in a wide variety of cells from red cells to brain cells. The best studied are the haematopoietic red and white cell lines. The principles of red cell volume regulation appear to apply to brain tissues; however, more work is required to define completely the exact mechanisms for neurones, glia and brain vasculature. Shrunken cells activate at least two ionic transporter systems – the Na^+/H^- antiporter system and the Na^+-K^+/Cl^- symporter system. Both of these ion pumps are energy-dependent, of neutral charge and produce a net flux of ions into the cell, to increase intracellular water. In many cell systems, they are activated by a protein kinase and deactivated by a protein phosphatase. The specific molecular site of the sensors for this activation is not known. Overall, these regulatory actions are thought of as a regulatory volume increase system.

Cellular swelling activates K^+/Cl^- transport from the cell or a regulatory volume decrease system. This system appears to complement the regulatory volume increase system, in that it is activated by phosphatases and inactivated by kinases. Recent studies suggest that chloride ion transport may be the key element of this process. Because KCl represents the largest concentration of intracellular ions, this system has potential as a major regulator of oedematous cells. Its role in the physiological and pathological regulation has not been evaluated in brain tissue.

Treatment of ICP

The precise importance of elevated ICP probably varies among disease processes. Until further research defines these differences, this section will address ICP as an adverse influence, and use head injury as a treatment scenario. Clinical data suggest that the threshold for mechanical brain injury is an ICP of 2.7–4.0 kPa (20–30 mmHg).[16,17] Treatment requires rapid onset of pressure control, long-term (3–10 days) stabilization, and in certain situations, definitive surgical revision of cranial vault anatomy. The selection and removal of these treatments are best guided by direct measurement of the ICP.

Rapid onset treatments

Hyperventilation

Hyperventilation presents the most rapid time action profile of the ICP treatments. Two steps are necessary: intubation and increased minute ventilation. The effect of increased minute ventilation on cerebral blood volume and ICP has been known for decades.[18,19] This has been successfully used to produce lowered ICP and intracranial relaxation as a routine measure in ICUs and operating rooms for the last 40 years. The effect of lowered arterial Pa_{CO_2} occurs immediately and is maximal within minutes. In the subsequent 6–24 h, this effect is diminished by buffering of the respiratory alkalosis that produces cerebral vascular vasoconstriction.[20] This occurs via the loss of intracerebral bicarbonate and a decrease in brain alkalosis. During this time frame, the cerebral vessels relax and CBV returns to normal. This tachyphylaxis to hyperventilation is a universal physiological event. Thus, hyperventilation is an excellent acute treatment, but the effect on ICP is not well-sustained.[21] Conversely, discontinuation of hyperventilation is accompanied by a greater than anticipated increase in brain pH, because the intracerebral pool of bicarbonate is decreased after prolonged hyperventilation; the same increase in Pa_{CO_2} produces a larger increase in ICP than if it occurred in a patient who had not received prolonged hyperventilation.

Ideally, hyperventilation should be to a Pa_{CO_2} of about 3.3 kPa (25 mmHg). This produces a near maximal immediate response, but is usually accompanied by a systemic alkalosis and potentially increased cerebral ischaemia.[20,21] After ICP has been controlled, a stabilizing treatment and a long-term definitive treatment plan should be developed. Usually the first-order stabilizing treatment is an osmotic treatment; with effective initiation of this osmotic treatment hyperventilation can be withdrawn. Withdrawal is best accomplished over 24 h in approximately 0.7 kPa (5 mmHg) Pa_{CO_2} increments between 5.3 and 6.0 kPa (25–40 mmHg). This time period should be longer if tachyphylaxis has developed. Additional reasons to avoid prolonged hyperventilation are haemodynamic instability, arrhythmia and barotrauma with increased ventilation. The former have been demonstrated to relate to long-term complications in the ICU.[21]

Bolus osmotic treatments

This can be initiated with mannitol, glycerol, urea, hypertonic saline or THAM buffer. Each of these agents may have specific sites of action that alter their potency profile. However, the main mode of cation action is the production of an osmotic gradient across an intact blood–brain barrier. This action depends on the existence of an intact barrier that impedes the diffusion of osmotic equivalents across the systemic and the brain compartments. Thus a bolus infusion of mannitol that presents to the blood–brain barrier a hypertonic environment, will lead to the efflux of water from the normal tissue inside the blood–brain barrier to the vascular compartment outside the barrier. Mannitol is usually administered as an initial bolus of 0.25–1.0 g/kg. This produces a decrease in the amount of water in normal brain tissue.[22] Usually the brain is 76–78% water. After hypertonic treatments, this decreases by 1–3% to the 74–76% range. Within 30–60 min of administration, an osmotic agent produces a diuresis and initial decline in ICP. This is usually maximal at 2–4 h. The effect on both urine output and ICP is extended if the osmotic agent is administered with a loop diuretic. Prolonged use of this regimen leads to decreased cardiac preload and an increased likelihood of hypotension.[23]

Stabilizing treatments
Osmotherapy

Prolonged use of osmotic therapy has been reported to effectively assist the treatment of cerebral masses and raised ICP.[22,24] Mannitol is often chosen if intravenous agents are required, although hypertonic saline and THAM buffer have also been used. When mannitol is used, it is usually given as intermittent boluses of 0.25 g/kg every 4–6 h.[25] Glycerol has the advantage of being well-absorbed orally; it is usually administered every 4 h if a continuous effect is desired. Case-controlled studies have suggested that hyperosmolar treatments that raise the osmolality to greater than 320 mosmol/kg are not increasingly effective, and are associated with frequent patient death.[23] Whether this is a measure of effect of ICP or is a clinical marker for severe brain injury is not clear from current data.

As hyperosmolarity is maintained over a prolonged period, the benefit may decrease with time. After initial dehydration, upregulation of cell volume is also known to occur. Although this process is substantially longer in onset than hyperventilation tachyphylaxis, this type of tachyphylaxis to increased osmolality does occur over a 3–5-day period. When brain tissue is exposed to an elevated serum osmolality, neurones and glia accumulate an increased amount of osmotic equivalents or taurine idiogenic osmoles. With this accumulation, the passage of water back into the brain occurs. Additionally, the osmotic equivalents that have been added as a treatment accumulate in the brain areas that do not have an intact blood–brain barrier. Thus, as systemic osmolality drops with tapering or discontinuation of treatments, water reaccumulates in the brain, increasing the overall volume of brain tissue and potentially increasing the ICP. Hence, if ICP is stabilized with continuous hyperosmolar therapy, this treatment is best withdrawn slowly and with ICP monitoring and/or close neurological observation.

Other stabilizing treatments

Several other treatments have been used in the stabilization of patients with elevated ICP. Corticosteroids are perhaps the most important drug to have beneficial effect. Where brain oedema from a tumour such as a glioma or meningioma is associated with elevated ICP, a significant reduction in brain water content and a decrease in ICP can be produced over 24–72 h with the initiation of treatment.[26] Dexamethasone in doses of 4–10 mg every 4–6 h is the initial treatment. The regimen is then tapered or increased depending on patient response.[27] Ischaemic and traumatic causes of oedema are not likely to benefit from corticosteroids. Barbiturate coma has been used to control elevated ICP when hyperventilation and osmotic agents have not been effective. Pentobarbitone, thiopentone and, occasionally, phenobarbitone have been used. When a flat electroencephalogram (EEG) is produced, most evidence suggests that these anaesthetics are equipotent agents that produce their effect by decreasing the cerebral metabolic rate and CBV. Hypothermia and hypotension are additional physiological properties of general anesthetics that may produce a decrease in ICP. A recent study suggested that moderate hypotension leads to a more effective control of tissue oedema and ICP.[28] Similarly, head-injured patients

may have improved ICP control and decreased mortality with early hypothermia.[29]

Surgical treatments

Cerebral masses

A major cause of raised ICP is the presence of a mass within the cranial vault. Both intra-axial and extra-axial masses are associated with intracranial hypertension. The former includes haemorrhages, glial and non-glial tumours and metastases. The latter includes meningeal tumours, subdural haematomas and epidural haematomas. Excision of a mass lesion is a simple and straightforward method of improving ICP, and producing a normalization of cranial vault mechanics. The timing and selection of candidates for craniotomy and excision are surgical decisions that require trained judgement, and frequently are preceded by supportive medical treatments directed at minimizing the impact of surgery on a compromised cranial vault with intracranial hypertension. Conversely, the decision to treat an intracranial mass surgically may primarily be to diagnose the aetiology, rather than to treat ICP, which may be elevated but well-compensated and represent no acute threat. In general, the longer a mass has existed, the greater the remodelling of normal brain structures and the lower the ICP. In contrast, with acute masses such as spontaneous haematomas and rapidly expanding tumours, the ICP is higher and less well-compensated with incremental additions of intracranial volume.

As a general guideline, the removal of brain that allows for the closure of dura without tension on the suture line is an effective decompression of mass effect. Delayed swelling after surgery, particularly with gliomas, and when significant intracurrent brain contusion has occurred, may require a larger than anticipated removal of tissue. Generally, removal of 30–50 ml of brain tissue effects a significant reduction in ICP and dynamics. Larger volumes of decompression are common when brain tumours and haematomas produce significant shift and secondary tissue damage.

Removal of CSF

Acute obstructive hydrocephalus is the main indication for inserting a lateral ventricular catheter. This syndrome occurs when there is a mass lesion involving the aqueduct at the third or the fourth ventricle level. Most commonly, tumours or haemorrhages produce this syndrome, which is accompanied by rapid loss of consciousness, impaired volitional motor control and focal cranial nerve deficits. Compression of the tegmental structures of the brainstem produces impaired consciousness, independent of the precise location of the mass lesion. Thus the insertion of a catheter will produce a rapid return to normal consciousness.

The insertion of a ventricular catheter may be accomplished at the bedside or in the operating room. Considerations include the need for a sterile environment, presence of an appropriately trained assistant and the availability of advanced imaging or image-localizing devices (for use in situations of ventricular distortion). With a skilled operator, an assistant and an ICU-type sterile environment, a lateral ventricular catheter may be inserted in less than 15 min under emergency situations.

Removal of CSF accompanies the successful localization of the lateral ventricle. The rate of removal of subsequent fluid is a function of the clinical situation. Where an unruptured aneurysm is the probable cause of obstruction, the need for control of intracranial hypertension is tempered by the clinical goal of slowly reducing the transmural pressure gradient across the aneurysm wall. In this situation, a reservoir pressure of 3.3–4.0 kPa (25–30 mmHg) is initially used. Sedation is undertaken to avoid transient ICP increases due to cough or Valsalva manoeuvres. For all clinical indications, the ventricular catheter should have its reservoir height designated, hourly CSF drainage recorded and ICP measured with the drainage turned off for 5 min every hour.[7] These assessments are central to achieving the goal of normal ICP. Under most conditions, CSF production is 0.35 ml/min or 20 ml/h and 500 ml/day. Drainage is continued until normal CSF resorptive pathways reconstitute themselves or permanent shunt pathways are established. Persistent low ICP and volumes of CSF less than 100 ml/day are consistent with normal CSF flow, and merit a trial of no drainage. This may be accomplished by either removing the catheter or discontinuing drainage and monitoring the pressure.

Bony decompression

A final type of decompression is the alteration of the cranial vault itself. This has not been a widely advocated treatment. However, when used successfully[30] there is wide removal of skull bone and the expansion of the dura mater that usually constrains the brain. With both mechanical barriers removed, expansion of the brain into the spaces normally occupied by these rigid structures occurs. Widespread acceptance of this technique awaits a controlled trial. Complications of this treatment include cranial deformity and low-pressure herniation syndromes.

Complications of ICP monitoring

Infection

The most significant risk of IVC usage is infection, with rates varying from 0 to 27%.[8,31–35] The risk of IVC-associated meningitis or ventriculitis appears to be related to the duration of catheter insertion,

increasing significantly after 5 days.[33,34] Some studies, however, have reported no association of infection with catheter duration.[31,33] Additional risk factors for infection are irrigation of the catheter or drainage system, and intraventricular blood.[33–35] Clearly, operator skill and technique are important to successful antiseptic use of the IVC. However, detailed study of the importance of technical factors is limited. Inserting the IVC in the operating room does not reduce the risk of infection compared to insertion in the ICU, but tunnelling the catheter subcutaneously to a distant skin exit site appears to reduce the infection risk.[33,34,36] The role of prophylactic antibiotics during external CSF drainage is still unclear.[34,35,37] One practice is to give prophylactic antibiotics as long as an IVC is in place; to remove or replace an IVC within 5 days whenever possible; never to flush or irrigate an IVC (except in emergencies such as occlusion during signs of brain herniation), and to sample CSF infrequently (every other day).

The infection risk for SA bolts is extremely low (consistently below 5%), and infections are nearly always superficial and rarely involve the brain or meninges.[34,38] Risk of SA bolt infection is increased when it is opened and flushed to improved the wave form.[34] SA bolts should be flushed only when their accuracy is seriously in doubt and ICP monitoring is essential to direct therapy. Prophylactic antibiotics for SA bolts are not recommended.

There are few reports on complications associated with solid-state devices. With epidural monitoring, one report found no infections in 140 patients monitored for an average of 9.2 days.[39] The risk of infection with these devices at other insertion sites has not been reported, but should be similar to the risk for IVCs or SA bolts depending on the site.

Placement injuries

Injury to brain parenchyma is another important consideration in ICP monitoring. Complications attending direct brain puncture can occur with IVC usage. Parenchymal or subdural haemorrhage occur, but fortunately are uncommon. Bleeding probably occurs, because during placement it is possible to tear unseen pial vessels. Rarely, injury of vital structures such as the thalamus, hypothalamus or midbrain occurs if the IVC is passed too deeply. SA bolts are rarely associated with brain injury, but cortical laceration or puncture can occur if the needle used to puncture the dura is passed too deeply. Epidural or subdural haemorrhage can also occur at the SA bolt site, but this usually happens when coagulation is disordered. With solid-state devices, the risk of cerebral injury probably depends on the insertion site, but no studies have compared injury rates. The risk should be higher with intraventricular or parenchymal insertion, and lower with subarachnoid or epidural insertion – an important consideration when monitoring patients with bleeding disorders and high ICP (e.g. fulminant hepatic failure).[40]

References

1 Guillaume J and Janny P (1951) Manométrie intra-cranienne continue. Intérét de la méthode et premiers résultats. *Rev Neurol (Paris)* **84:**131–142.

2 Lundberg N (1960) Continuous recording and control of ventricular fluid pressure in neurosurgical practice. *Acta Pyschiatr Neurol Scand* **36** (suppl 149):1–193.

3 Vries JK, Becker DP and Young HF (1973) A sub-arachnoid screw for monitoring intracranial pressure. *J Neurosurg* **39:**416–419.

4 Barnett GH and Chapman PH (1988) Insertion and care of intracranial pressure monitoring devices. In: Ropper AH and Kennedy SK (eds) *Neurological and Neuro-surgical Intensive Care*, 2nd edn. Rockville, MD, Aspen, p. 43.

5 Yablon JS, Lantnes HJ, McCormack TM, Nairs S, Barker F and Black P (1993) Clinical experience with a fiber optic intracranial pressure monitor. *J Clin Monit* **9:**171–175.

6 Piek J and Bock WJ (1990) Continuous monitoring of cerebral tissue pressure in neurosurgical patients: preliminary results. *Acta Neurochir* **87:**144–149.

7 Wilkinson HA, Yarzebski J, Wilkinson EC and Anderson FA (1989) Erroneous measurement of intracranial pressure caused by simultaneous ventricular drainage: a hydrodynamic model study. *Neurosurgery* **24:**348–354.

8 Mendelow AD, Rowan JO, Murray L *et al.* (1983) A clinical comparison of subdural screw pressure measure-ments with ventricular pressure. *J Neurosurg* **58:**45–50.

9 Yano M, Ikeda Y, Kobayashi S *et al.* (1987) Intracranial pressure in head-injured patients with various intra-cranial lesions is identical throughout the supratentorial intracranial compartment. *Neurosurgery* **21:**688–692.

10 Gambardella G, d'Avella D and Tomasello F (1992) Monitoring of brain tissue pressure with a fiberoptic device. *Neurosurgery***31:**918–922.

11 Johnston IH and Rowan JO (1974) Raised intracranial pressure and cerebral blood flow. *J Neurol Neurosurg Psychiatry* **37:**585.

12 Crutchfield JS, Narayan RK, Robertson CS and Michael LH (1990) Evaluation of a fiberoptic intracranial pressure monitor. *J Neurosurg* **72:**482–487.

13 Chambers IR, Mendelow AD, Sinar EJ and Modha P. (1990) A clinical evaluation of the Camino subdural screw and ventricular monitoring kits. *Neurosurgery* **26:** 421–423.

14 Ostrup RC, Luerssen TG, Marshall LF and Zornow MH (1987) Continuous monitoring of intracranial pressure with a miniaturized fiberoptic device. *J Neurosurg* **67:**206–209.

15 Schickner DJ and Young RF (1992) Intracranial pressure monitoring: fiberoptic monitor compared with the ventricular catheter. *Surg Neurol* **27:**251–254.

16 Eisenberg H, Frankowski R, Contant C *et al.* (1988) High-dose barbiturate control of elevated intracranial pressure in patients with severe head injury. *J Neurosurg* **69:**15–23.

17 Marmarou A, Anderson RL, Ward JD *et al.* (1991) Impact of ICP instability and hypotension on outcome in patients with severe head trauma. *J Neurosurg* **75:**S159–S166.

18 Obrist WD, Langfitt TW, Jagg JL, Cruz J and Generarelli TA (1984) Cerebral blood flow and metabolism in comatose patients with acute head injury. *J Neurosurg* **61:**241–252.

19 Raichle ME and Plum F (1972) Hyperventilation and cerebral blood flow. *Stroke* **3:**566–75.

20 Robertson CS, Contant CF, Gokaslan ZL *et al.* (1992) Cerebral blood flow, arteriovenous oxygen difference and outcome in head injured patients. *J Neurol Neurosurg Psychiatry* **55:**594–603.

21 Muizelaar JP, Marmarou A, Ward JD *et al.* (1991) Adverse effects of prolonged hyperventilation in patients with severe head injury: a randomized clinical trial. *J Neurosurgery* **75:**731–739.

22 Nath F and Galbraith S (1966) The effect of mannitol on cerebral white matter content. *J Neurosurg* **65:**41–43.

23 Becker DP and Vries JK (1972) The alleviation of increased intracranial pressure in the chronic administra-tion of osmotic agents. In: Brock M and Deitz H (eds) *Intracranial Pressure*. Berlin: Springer-Verlag, pp. 309–315.

24 Schwartz MI, Tator CH and Rowed DW (1989) The University of Toronto head injury treatment study: a prospective randomized comparison of pentobarbital and mannitol. *Can J Neurol Sci* **11:**434–440.

25 Smith HP, Kelley DL, McWhorter JM *et al.* (1986) Comparison of mannitol regimens in patients with severe head injury undergoing intracranial monitoring. *J Neurosurg* **65:**820–824.

26 French LA and Galicich JH (1964) The use of steroids for control of cerebral edema. *Clin Neurosurg* **10:** 212–223.

27 Renaudin J, Fewer D, Wilson CB *et al.* (1973) Dose dependency of decadron in patients with partially excised brain tumors. *J Neurosurgery* **39:**302–305.

28 Asgeirsson B, Grände PO and Nordström CH (1994) A new therapy of post-trauma brain edema based on haemodynamic principles for brain volume regulation. *Intensive Care Med* **20:**260–267.

29 Marion DW, Obrist WD, Carlier PM, Penrod LE and Darby JM (1993) The use of moderate therapeutic hypothermia for patients with severe head injuries: a preliminary report. *J Neurosurg* **79:**354–362.

30 Rieke K, Schwab S, Krieger D *et al.* (1995) Decompressive surgery in space-occupying hemispheric infarction: results of an open, prospective trial. *Crit Care Med* **23:**1576–1587.

31 Öhrström JK, Skou JK, Ejlertsen T *et al.* (1989) Infected ventriculostomy: bacteriology and treatment. *Acta Neurochir (Wien)* **100:**67.

32 Smith RW and Alksne JF (1976) Infections complicating the use of external ventriculostomy. *J Neurosurg* **44:**567–570.

33 Mayhall CG, Archer NH, Lamb A *et al.* (1988) Ventriculostomy-related infections. *N Engl J Med* **310:**553–559.

34 Aucoin PJ, Kotilainen HR, Gantz NM, Davidson R, Kellogg P and Stone B (1986) Intracranial pressure monitors. Epidemiologic study of risk factors and infections. *Am J Med* **80:**369–76.

35 Wyler AR and Kelly WA (1972) Use of antibiotics with external ventriculostomies. *J Neurosurg* **37:**185–187.

36 Friedman WA and Vries JK (1980) Percutaneous tunnel ventriculostomy. Summary of 100 procedures. *J Neurosurg* **53:**662–665.

37 Rosner MJ and Becker DP (1976) ICP monitoring: complications and associated factors. *Clin Neurosurgery* **23:**494–519.

38 Winn HR, Dacey RG and Jane JA (1977) Intracranial subarachnoid pressure recording: experience with 650 patients. *Surg Neurol* **8:**41–47.

39 Levin AB (1977) The use of a fiberoptic intracranial pressure monitor in clinical practice. *Neurosurgery* **1:**266–271.

40 Blei AT, Olafsson S, Webster S and Levy R (1993) Complications of intracranial pressure monitoring in fulminant hepatic failure. *Lancet* **341:**157–158.

44 | Cerebral protection

J Ulatowski

The concept of cerebral or neural protection has taken on many forms, from prophylaxis in stroke prevention to resuscitation in the treatment of ongoing ischaemia or recent infarction. A complete review is beyond the scope of this chapter, but current understanding of cerebral protection is beneficial to intensivists in treating cerebral insults.

Normal physiology

The brain is an energetic tissue utilizing approximately 3–5 ml O_2/min per 100 g tissue (45–75 ml O_2/min per 1500 g brain) and 5 mg glucose/min per 100 g tissue (75 mg glucose/min per 1500 g brain). It has little ability to store precursors of metabolism, and thus depends on a constant supply of nutrients from the blood. At a cerebral blood flow (CBF) of 50 ml/min per 100 g tissue (750 ml/min per 1500 g brain) and a normal oxygen content of 20 ml O_2/100 ml blood, the brain receives approximately 150 ml O_2/min per 1500 g brain, or 2–3 times the amount needed for normal brain activity. On pass, the brain extracts 35–50% of the oxygen delivered to fuel metabolism. Similarly, assuming the same CBF of 50 ml/min per 100 g tissue and a blood glucose concentration of 5.5 mmol/l (100 mg/100 ml blood), then there is 50 mg/min per 100 g tissue (750 mg/min per 1500 g brain) delivery of glucose. Glucose extraction by the brain, as 5 mg/min per 100 g brain tissue, is minimal by comparison to that of oxygen.

Cerebral injury has many aetiologies but the mechanisms of injury are thought to be few. The most common by far is caused by the lack of essential nutrients, oxygen and glucose. This can occur separately with preserved blood flow (i.e. hypoxia or hypoglycaemia), or more often together, because of reduced/absent perfusion (i.e. ischaemia or infarction). Reduced supply of these energy precursors is a major contributor in the mechanism of brain injury, regardless of the aetiology.

Natural protective mechanisms

The importance of the brain to the whole being is highlighted by the mechanisms in place to protect cerebral elements from ischaemia.

Collateral blood supply

There is an elaborate vascular architecture designed to ensure adequate cerebral blood flow. Circulation to the head is divided into anterior (carotid arteries) and posterior (vertebral arteries) systems, each providing bilateral supply. Carotid arteries divide before entering the skull to form the external carotid branches (feeding the face and scalp) and the internal branches supplying the anterior cerebrum (frontal, parietal and temporal lobes) and anterior diencephalon (basal ganglia and hypothalamus). Vertebral arteries join once inside the cranium to form the basilar artery, which runs the length of the posterior fossa, supplying the brainstem, cerebellum and posterior portion of the cerebrum (occipital lobes) and diencephalon (thalamus). Adequacy of arterial blood supply is ensured by connections between these two cirulations called collaterals. The circle of Willis, which joins the large branches of the anterior and posterior circulations at the base of the brain, is the major component of this collateral network in humans. Between these arterial distributions are watershed zones fed by leptomeningeal connections. In addition, persistent fetal arteries can infrequently provide collateral routes between the anterior and posterior arterial systems in the brain.

Cerebral blood flow

Cerebral perfusion pressure

The amount of blood delivered to the brain is highly regulated, and is determined by several factors. CBF is determined in part by the perfusion pressure across the brain, called cerebral perfusion pressure (CPP).

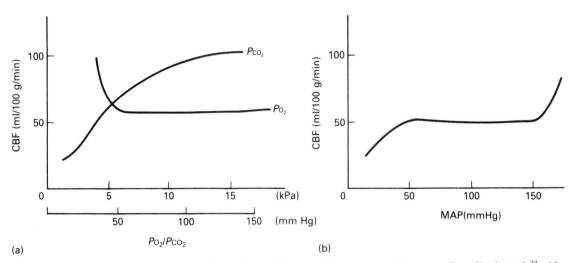

Fig. 44.1 Cerebral blood flow relationship with (a) Pao_2 and $Paco_2$ and (b) mean arterial pressure. From Yentis *et al.*,[74] with permission. MAP = Mean arterial pressure.

CPP, in fact, is the difference between the arterial pressure in the feeding arteries as they enter the subarachnoid space, and the pressure in the draining veins before they enter the major dural sinuses. Because these pressures are difficult to measure, CPP is derived from the difference between the systemic mean arterial pressure (MAP) and the intracranial pressure (ICP), which is an estimate of tissue pressure.

The cerebral vessels change diameter inversely with changing perfusion pressure; as CPP rises, the vessels constrict and as CPP falls the vessels dilate, such that blood flow is kept constant over a wide range of CPP (Fig. 44.1). This pressure autoregulation is thought to be controlled by local myogenic responses of the vessel wall to changes in intra-arterial pressure. At pressures above and below this range of 6.7–20 kPa (50–150 mmHg), cerebral perfusion becomes pressure-passive and increases or decreases in direct proportion to changes in CPP. The autoregulatory range varies with age, being shifted to the left in newborns and to the right with chronic hypertension. The latter is important to remember, to avoid overtreating systolic blood pressure in such patients, and thus incur the risk of cerebral ischaemia at the lower limits of autoregulation. Alternatively, cerebral perfusion above normal can be caused by acute hypertension overcoming the upper limits of autoregulation. This may lead to cerebral oedema secondary to increased hydrostatic pressures (hypertensive encephalopathy) and potentially lead to seizures or cerebral haemorrhage.

Pao₂ and *Paco₂* effects

A second group of factors control CBF through an influence on the local metabolic milieu. Prominent in this mechanism are oxygen and carbon dioxide. Arterial content or partial pressure of oxygen in the normal or hyperoxic range causes very little change in CBF. Perhaps this represents a demand for another nutrient (i.e. glucose) or a need to remove waste products (i.e. carbon dioxide or metabolic acid). With the onset of hypoxaemia ($Pao_2 < 8$ kPa or 60 mmHg), there is a prompt increase in CBF proportional to the decrease in blood oxygen content, in order to maintain oxygen delivery constant (Fig. 44.1).

There is also a direct relationship between CBF and $Paco_2$ such that cerebral perfusion increases with increasing $Paco_2$ (Fig. 44.1). This probably represents the need of the brain to maintain homeostatic pH by removing metabolic breakdown products more efficiently by increased blood flow. Unlike the response to oxygen, the CBF response to changes in $Paco_2$ is dramatic in the physiological range, such that for every 0.13 kPa (1.0 mmHg) change in $Paco_2$ there is a 1–2 ml/min per 100 g tissue change in CBF. Therefore, an increase in $Paco_2$ to 10.6 kPa (80 mmHg) will increase CBF to approximately 100 ml/min per 100 g, and a decrease in $Paco_2$ to 2.7 kPa (20 mmHg) will decrease CBF to 25 ml/min per 100 g. Briefly, a doubling of $Paco_2$ doubles CBF, and halving $Paco_2$ halves CBF within this range. Understanding this basic physiology will make treatment logical (see below), as increases in CBF often lead to increases in cerebral blood volume, which in turn can increase ICP – a common cause of cerebral ischaemia.

Pathophysiology

There are many aetiologies of injury to the nervous system, including vascular insufficiency or disruption, trauma, tumour, infection/inflammation and metabolic and nutritional derangement. However, there are few mechanisms of injury, the most common of which is hypoxic and/or ischaemic injury. The protective mechanism afforded by the ability to increase CBF manyfold in response to hypoxaemia allows for sufficient blood flow with maintenance of oxygen delivery and supply of other nutrients in many cases. This assumes an ability to increase CBF, which may be precluded in those with cerebrovascular disease as a baseline. Ultimately, severe or prolonged hypoxaemia will eventually disturb systemic circulatory homeostasis, leading to hypotension and eventual ischaemia. Intracranial masses, oedema and increased ICP all exert excess force on surrounding tissue, causing hypoxic/ischaemic injury. Thus, this chapter will consider hypoxic and ischaemic injury as being synonymous, although there are differences between them. Perhaps a more important distinction is to be made between global and focal hypoxic/ischaemic insults.

Global hypoxic/ischaemic insults

Global insults and hypoxic and low/no-flow states are caused by hypoxaemia and cardiovascular insufficiency or arrest respectively. These are usually sudden, short and severe. If there is to be recovery, prompt return of oxygen delivery and spontaneous circulation are necessary. The recovery may be variable depending on the severity and duration of the insult, and the selective vulnerability of certain cell types. After 5–6 min of complete global ischaemia, there are signs of permanent histological damage in selective neuronal populations, and the beginnings of neurological deficits in survivors. Outcome worsens significantly after 15 min of global ischaemia.[1]

Focal hypoxic/ischaemic insults

Although just as sudden, focal hypoxic/ischaemic insults are usually of more prolonged duration, but are less severe because the surrounding brain is preserved by collateral blood supply. Even if perfusion does not return to the area in jeopardy, patient survival initially is not a concern, because a subtotal area of the brain is affected. However, the centre of the focal ischaemic area supplied by end arteries will result in cell death unless reperfusion is established rapidly. The periphery of an infarcted area is the ischaemic penumbra. Here, CBF is greater than the infarcted core, but less than the normal tissue around it. The time course for infarction and irreversible damage to brain from a focal hypoxic/ischaemic event is around 30–60 min based on animal studies. The penumbral area after a focal infarction receives the most attention for therapeutic intervention. If blood flow can be normalized in this region, or pharmacological agents can be delivered despite reduced flow,

there is a potential for recovery. Conversely, failure to maintain this area will result in a coalescing of the penumbra into the infarcted area as the ischaemic stimulus continues. Despite these differences, it is possible that the transiently ischaemic whole brain (during early cardiac arrest, low flow cardiopulmonary resuscitation (CPR) or elevated ICP states) and the ongoing ischaemic penumbral area of a focal insult undergo similar pathophysiological processes. As these events are sudden and without forewarning, prevention and treatment of the secondary insults often become the focus in neuroprotection and tissue salvage paradigms.

Brain ischaemic and infarction processes

As blood flow is reduced below 50 ml/min per 100 g, changes begin to occur in the normal physiology (Table 44.1). Neurological function is impaired and there is slowing of the electroencephalogram (EEG). CBF in the range 15–25 ml/min per 100 g results in loss of electrical activity. At approximately 10 ml/min per 100 g there is membrane failure due to a critical loss of adenosine triphosphate (ATP), which causes ionic imbalance between the cell and the extracellular milieu. If prolonged or worsened, blood flow at this level will lead to permanent neurological impairment due to cell death. However, blood flow between 10 and 15 ml/min per 100 g is sufficeint to maintain ATP to support ionic pump function for a time, despite the lack of electrical activity and normal neurological function.

With ischaemia, there is reduced available oxygen and glucose to support aerobic production of ATP. Based on animal studies, ATP is depleted within 2–3 min of complete ischaemia. Since there is little brain storage of either glucose or oxygen, ATP production during ischaemia relies on anaerobic glycolysis for as long as these stores last. Unfortunately, this results in suboptimal production of ATP and accumulation of lactic acid. This in turn leads to an acidotic environment with worsening brain function and less chance of recovery if oxidative metabolism is not restored. Loss of ATP causes failure of membrane ionic pump function, leading to an efflux of potassium

Table 44.1 Brain ischaemic thresholds

Cerebral blood flow (ml/min per 100 g brain)	Changes
50	Normal
25–30	Abnormal EEG
15–25	Isoelectric EEG
10–15	Absent evoked potentials
<10	Membrane failure
<10 prolonged (min)	Cell death

EEG = Electroencephalogram.

and an influx of sodium, calcium and chloride ions. This begins a cascade of events resulting in eventual cell death.

The potassium leakage probably causes cell depolarization, with voltage-sensitive ion channel opening and release of excitatory amino acid (EAA) neurotransmitters. EAA neurotransmitters will begin a wave of further depolarization that affects neighbouring cells and parts of the brain removed from the initial injury. These depolarizations (agonist-operated) will allow influx of sodium and chloride through activation of kainate (K) and quisqualate (Q) receptors, and influx of calcium by activation of the N-methyl-D-aspartate (NMDA) receptors. Influx of sodium (and chloride) is followed by water, leading to intracellular oedema. Calcium influx or release from intracellular stores can lead to further release of excitatory transmitters, conversion of phosphorylases with uncoupling of oxidative phosphorylation in the mitochondria, activation of proteases with degradation of cytosolic protein and stimulation of lipases with liberation of arachidonic acid and other free fatty acids which cause tissue damage via production of oxygen radicals and prostaglandins.

Other effects occur at the nuclear level, interfering with the machinery to replicate DNA and produce RNA necessary for further protein production. This may explain why cellular and clinical recovery is partial, even with restoration of ionic equilibrium and near normal ATP levels after successful reperfusion.

In addition, there may be injury from outside the cell. The immune system, predominantly the leucocytes, are thought to be major contributors to reperfusion injury. Leukocytes may plug up small capillaries under conditions of low blood flow and prevent reflow in certain areas, thus hindering restoration of perfusion. Furthermore, leukocytes appear to enhance production of oxygen radicals and begin a cascade of inflammatory mediators, which may potentiate cell destruction in injured tissue. Most injury to tissue involves some form of tissue oedema. This can affect the core lesion by narrowing blood vessels and worsening chances of reperfusion, and can alter function in neighbouring tissue by mechanical compression of tissue or its blood supply. This is of extreme importance in the adult brain because the cranial vault is non-distensible, preventing accommodation to an expanding lesion.

Although there have been many advancements in the understanding of the above systemic and cellular events, the application of this knowledge is still awaited. Progress is hampered by the likelihood that no one treatment will suffice to prevent cellular dysfunction or restore function. The lesions caused by hypoxic/ischaemic insults are only partially remediable, because there is little forewarning and the process is usually well-established when clinicians intervene.

Management

The first approach to neurological injury is to establish adequate vital function. Airway management and protection become a priority. Early attention to the airway also facilitates the use of hyperventilation to reduce cerebral blood volume and ICP. Management includes the following:

Revascularization

For global ischaemia from cardiac arrest, this entails re-establishing systemic blood pressure and consideration of the no-reflow phenomenon in certain areas of the brain. Current research is addressing variations in CPR to include high-dose adrenaline and simultaneous ventilation–chest compression in an attempt to increase blood pressure during CPR and to open up capillaries that may be collapsed during the arrest period. No clinical trials have indicated benefit (see Chapter 7).

Treatment for focal ischaemia has been limited to prevention of recurrences with the use of aspirin and systemic anticoagulants. Recently, there have been attempts to reperfuse tissue undergoing focal ischaemia from vascular insufficiency or occlusion, using cerebral angioplasty[2-4] or endovascular thrombolysis.[5-7]

Haemodilution and hypervolaemia

Decreasing haematocrit and viscosity by haemodilution has the potential of facilitating blood and oxygen delivery to areas that have narrowed arterial supply. This benefit has been shown in animal models of ischaemia but in clinical trials of stroke, results are not impressive. Three major studies have shown no benefit of normovolaemic[8,9] and hypervolaemic[10] haemodilution, mainly because of complications of volume therapy in patients with an associated risk of heart disease. Whether the experimental benefits can ever be reproduced in humans will require further studies.

Hypervolaemic haemodilution and deliberate hypertension with augmentation of cardiac output using vasopressors and inotropic agents are currently being used in many centres for the treatment of delayed ischaemic deficits after subarachnoid haemorrhage related to vasospasm. This therapy can be administered safely with intensive monitoring, but benefits are anecdotal as it has not been tested with concurrent controls.[11,12] (see Chapter 42). If nothing else, this therapeutic approach has changed the long-held belief that dehydration is best for patients with central nervous system disease.

Intracranial pressure management

Global ischaemia from raised ICP requires adequate systemic blood pressure management and simultaneous treatment of the ICP to ensure adequate CPP. MAP should be raised to a level at or above the usual pressure for that patient, within the zone of pressure autoregulation. If a majority of the vasculature is autoregulating, raising the blood pressure may decrease vascular diameter and reduce blood volume within the cranium. When the inciting event cannot be treated (e.g. blood clot or brain tumour), often the only alternative is to prevent secondary injury around the lesion. Since an increased ICP can cause further ischaemia, reducing ICP should facilitate adequate perfusion to areas in jeopardy. Treating ICP requires knowledge of the three compartments within the intracranial vault (brain, blood and cerebrospinal fluid (CSF)). Whenever possible, the offending compartment should be treated primarily (e.g. tumour extraction, blood evacuation and drainage of hydrocephalus). If this is not advisable, reducing the relative volumes of other compartments may improve compliance overall and reduce ICP.

Brain compartment

Reduction in the parenchymal compartment relies on removal of free water across an intact blood–brain barrier, using osmotic agents – mannitol (20% solution 0.25–1.0 g/kg) and glycerol (10% solution 250–500 ml/4 h). Hypertonic saline has been attempted with early success.[13–15] The ease and apparent lack of side-effects make this an interesting alternative therapy; however, outcome studies are necessary to determine safety and efficacy. Mannitol may have a beneficial rheological effect on blood to facilitate flow.[16] Removal of tumour or blood clot, drainage of abscess, extirpation of infarcted brain or, in the final form, removal of viable brain are all potential therapies aimed at improving compliance. Temporary craniectomy to relieve the focal pressure of a life-threatening stroke (e.g. middle cerebral artery infarction) has gained renewed interest.[17–19]

Blood compartment

Although a small component of intracranial volume, the blood compartment is the most compliant. Reduction in blood volume is useful in the treatment of raised ICP, especially in the acute setting. As explained above, hypoxia and hypercarbia can lead to hyperaemia and an increase in cerebral blood volume, potentially worsening ICP. Alternatively, there are very rapid changes in blood flow and blood volume to induced hypocarbia. Initial levels of Pa_{CO_2} 3.3–3.7 kPa (25–28 mmHg) are desirable. Since post ischaemic cerebral blood vessels have less vasoconstriction from hypocarbia, the ischaemic area is likely spared the risk of further ischaemia, and may benefit from shunting of blood flow from areas of normal brain that vasoconstrict during hyperventilation. Prolonged hyperventilation may be detrimental in treating

patients with head trauma, and it is recommended that a secondary treatment for ICP be instituted as soon as possible to allow slow withdrawal of hyperventilation.[20] If adaptation to hypocapnia has not occurred, hyperventilation can be reinstituted with the same effect. Finally, CBF and volume are reduced by lowering the need for blood supply and nutrients to the brain, through prevention and treatment of seizures and hyperthermia and by deliberate hypothermia.

CSF compartment

The CSF compartment is quickly reduced by drainage whenever possible. Care is taken regarding the route and rate of CSF drainage to avoid herniation of a mass lesion, either towards the other side of the brain or through the tentorium. Slower means of reducing ICP by changing the production/removal quotient for CSF can be achieved by the use of acetazolamide, but this is only effective in subacute and chronic ailments (e.g. pseudotumour cerebri).

Metabolic therapy
Hypothermia

Injury to the central nervous system is temperature-dependent. Fever can make an existing neurological dysfunction more apparent and may worsen an ongoing insult. Cooling the body, and in turn the brain, has been known for years to offer protection. Drowning victims who were cold have survived long periods of ischaemia. Therefore, treatment of fever should be aggressive, using cooling blankets, cool water or alcohol baths, cool intravenous fluids, fans and antipyretic medications. Induced hypothermia (28–30°C) is commonplace for coronary bypass surgery, and deep hypothermia (<20°C) has allowed prolonged circulatory arrest times necessary to complete repair of high thoracic and giant cerebral aneurysms. In addition, it has been shown that histological injury can be lessened by mild (<6° change from normal) passive and induced hypothermia in animals before or after ischaemia. This has led to ongoing studies of mild hypothermia (32–33°C) after severe brain injury in humans.[21] It has been assumed that the benefits of hypothermia rest in its ability to suppress baseline energy requirements and prevent the build-up of toxic metabolites. However, the benefits of hypothermia in the post ischaemic period raise the possibility that efficacy may also be due to reduction in the no-reflow state, improved cell membrane and ion channel integrity, amelioration of the effects of oxygen radicals, prostanoids and phospholipase induction or reduction in EAA.

Anaesthetic agents

Pharmacological reduction in cerebral metabolism with general anaesthetics has received much interest over the years. Suppression of EEG activity and an associated 50% reduction in the cerebral metabolic rate has been used in many animal models of global and focal ischaemia. Studies using barbiturates in many animal species have showed some convincing benefit, especially for focal ischaemia. However, only one clinical study has shown reduction in focal deficits using the induction of barbiturate coma during coronary bypass surgery.[22] Opponents have criticized the few patient numbers in this study, and this use of barbiturates has not become common practice. There have been no proven benefits of barbiturates for global ischaemia in near-drowning[23] or during CPR.[24] Prophylactic barbiturate coma for cerebral aneurysm,[25] carotid end-arterectomy[26] and extracranial vertebral[27] or extra–intracranial[28] vascular surgery has been postulated to be safe and an important component of the anaesthetic technique, but comparison has been made only to historical controls.

Etomidate which has fewer associated cardiovascular side-effects than barbiturates, and propofol which has a shorter effective half-life than the other agents, have both been proposed as alternatives for induction of electrical silence and neuroprotection during aneurysm surgery. However, neither of these agents has been tested against routine anaesthetic management.[29,30]

Barbiturates rapidly decrease ICP[31] and are used in patients with central nervous system injury to control the rise in ICP associated with intubation. Barbiturate coma has been advocated for the treatment of ICP elevations refractory to primary therapy. Although there seems to be efficacy in lowering ICP, the outcome of patients treated with barbiturates has not been reproducibly improved.[32–34]

Calcium antagonists

The influx of calcium from the extracellular space and from intracellular organelles, which is normally in minute quantities unbound within the cytosol, has been implicated as the common mediator of cell death from a variety of causes. The data on use of calcium-channel blockers for treatment of global ischaemia after cardiac arrest are mixed, and their use has not become routine.[35–37] Use in focal ischaemia is somewhat better. Nimodipine appears to provide a slight improvement in outcome from focal ischaemia.[38,39] Furthermore, nimodipine has become standard therapy in the prophylactic treatment of cerebral vasospasm after subarachnoid haemorrhage.[40–42] Benefits appear to be due to an effect on smaller penetrating vessels not seen by angiography, or a neuroprotective effect at the cell level,[41] rather than cerebral vasodilatation as determined by angi-

ography. The potential for hypotension and worsening of CPP is a disadvantage of calcium-channel blockers.

Steroids and anti-inflammatory therapy

Glucocorticoids are thought to decrease cerebral oedema associated with breakdown of the blood–brain barrier (i.e. vasogenic oedema). In this regard, improvement in central nervous system function has been seen with brain tumours and abscesses.[43,44] High-dose methylprednisolone for 24 h has been shown to offer some benefit in the treatment of acute spinal cord injury, if treatment begins within 8 h of injury.[45,46] Unfortunately, this has translated into steroid therapy for many other kinds of injury to the spine without controlled studies to justify such use. However, treatment for only 1 day means that prolonged use of steroids for these other injuries has lessened and may be an overall saving (see Chapter 69). Glucocorticoids are not effective for cytotoxic oedema, which is seen with ischaemic disease, whether focal[47] or global[48] in aetiology. Patients with head trauma also do not benefit from the use of steroids[49,50], which may be detrimental by suppressing the immune system.[51]

Tirilazad, a 21-aminosteroid without glucocorticoid activity, is a potent inhibitor of lipid peroxidation and a scavenger of oxygen radicals. It is currently under investigation in the treatment of a variety of neurological injuries including stroke, head trauma and spinal cord injury. However, to date the only reported benefit seems to be in the prophylactic treatment of vasospasm from subarachnoid haemorrhage.[52] Other anti-inflammatory agents, such as indomethacin, while inhibiting cyclooxygenase and subsequent prostanoid production, have not been beneficial in clinical studies. Specific prostaglandin therapy designed to inhibit vasoconstriction and platelet aggregation with prostacyclin has not proven beneficial in acute stroke.[53]

Experimental therapy

Oxygen radical production after neural injury probably results in secondary injury. Several drugs may inhibit this injury, but none has been studied in humans. Allopurinol blocks the production of superoxide anion by inhibiting xanthine oxidase, and appears to decrease focal ischaemic injury and result in improved outcome after global ischaemia.[54] Iron catalyses the conversion of hydrogen peroxide to hydroxyl radical. Deferoxamine inhibits this reaction, and has been shown to improve survival after global ischaemia in dog and rat, but neurological outcome is not changed.[55,56] Dimethyl sulfoxide (DMSO) and mannitol are hydroxyl radical scavengers, and they reduce ICP. DMSO improves neurological outcome in the brain after short periods of focal cerebral ischaemia[57,58] and during reperfusion after spinal cord ischaemia.[59] Mannitol lessens the histological damage after focal ischaemia[60] and improves the milieu in the ischaemic penumbra.[61] Superoxide dismutase (SOD) converts superoxide to hydrogen peroxide, which is eventually detoxified to water by catalase. SOD reduces the tissue damage associated with acute hypertension[62] and head trauma,[63] and reduces infarct volume prior to focal cerebral ischaemia[64,65] and injury during reperfusion after spinal cord ischaemia.[66] Human studies are anticipated for many of the above.

Inhibition of EAA in an attempt to interrupt the cascade of secondary injury already provides useful information. NMDA receptor antagonists have been shown to reduce damage when given before focal cerebral ischaemia[67,68] and after head[69] and spine injury.[70] NMDA[71] and quisqualate[72] receptor antagonists have even been demonstrated to offer a degree of neuroprotection when administered shortly after the onset of ischaemia. Although studies in global ischaemia are not as promising, this may be due to a matter of dosage.[73] Side-effects may eventually limit the usefulness of these compounds in humans.

References

1 Bedell S, Delbanco T, Cook E and Epstein P (1983) Survival after cardiopulmonary resuscitation in the hospital. *N Engl J Med* **309**:569–576.

2 Zubkov YN, Nifkiforov BM and Shustin VA (1984) Balloon catheter technique for dilatation of constricted cerebral arteries after aneurysm SAH. *Acta Neurochir* **70**:65–79.

3 Higashida RT, Halbach VV, Cahan LD et al. (1989) Transluminal angioplasty for treatment of intracranial arterial vasospasm. *J Neurosurg* **71**:648–653.

4 Newell DW, Eskridge JM, Mayberg MR et al. (1989) Angioplasty for the treatment of symptomatic vasospasm following subarachnoid hemorrhage. *J Neurosurg* **71**: 654–660.

5 Zeumer H, Freitag H-J, Zanella F et al. (1993) Local intra-arterial fibrinolytic therapy in patients with stroke: urokinase versus recombinant tissue plasminogen activator (r-TPA). *Neuroradiology* **35**:159–162.

6 Brott T, Broderick J and Kothari R (1994) Thrombolytic therapy for stroke. *Curr Opin Neurol* **7**:25–35.

7 Sipos EP, Kirsch JR, Nauta HJ et al. (1992) Intra-arterial urokinase for treatment of retrograde thrombosis following resection of an arteriovenous malformation. Case report. *J Neurosurg* **76**:1004–1007.

8 Scandinavian Stroke Study Group (1987) Multicenter trial of hemodilution in acute ischemic stroke. Results in the total patient population. *Stroke* **18**:691–699.

9 Italian Acute Stroke Study Group (1988) Hameodilution in acute stroke: results of the Italian haemodilution trial. *Lancet* **1**:318–321.

10 The Hemodilution in Stroke Study Group (1989) Hypervolemic hemodilution treatment of acute stroke.

Results of a randomised multicenter trial using pentastarch. *Stroke* **20**:317–323.

11 Solomon R, Fink M and Lennihan L (1988) Early aneurysm surgery and prophylactic hypervolemic hypertensive therapy for the treatment of aneurysmal subarachnoid hemorrhage. *Neurosurgery* **23**:699–704.

12 Medlock M, Dulebohn S and Elwood P (1992) Prophylactic hypervolemia without calcium channel blockers in early aneurysm surgery. *Neurosurgery* **30**:12–16.

13 Worthley LI, Cooper DJ and Jones N (1988) Treatment of resistant intracranial hypertension with hypertonic saline. Report of two cases. *J Neurosurg* **68**:478–481.

14 Henschen S, Busse MW, Zisowsky S et al (1991) Short term volume effects of a hypertonic saline bolus during neurosurgery. *Neurochir* **34**:163–165.

15 Fisher B, Thomas D and Peterson B (1992) Hypertonic saline lowers raised intracranial pressure in children after head trauma. *J Neurosurg Anesthesiol* **1**:4–10.

16 Muizelaar JP, Wei EP, Kontos HA and Becker DP (1983) Mannitol causes compensatory cerebral vasoconstriction and vasodilation in response to blood viscosity changes. *J Neurosurg* **59**:822–828.

17 Chen HJ, Lee TC and Wei CP (1992) Treatment of cerebellar infarction by decompressive suboccipital craniectomy. *Stroke* **23**:957–961.

18 Hornig CR, Rust DS, Busse O et al. (1994) Space-occupying cerebellar infarction. Clinical course and prognosis. *Stroke* **25**:372–374.

19 Forsting M, Reith W, Shabitz WR et al. (1995) Decompressive craniectomy for cerebellar infarction. An experimental study in rats. *Stroke* **6**:259–264.

20 Muizelaar JP, Marmarou A, Ward JD et al. (1991) Adverse effects of prolonged hyperventilation in patients with severe head injury: a randomized clinical trial. *J Neurosurg* **75**:731–739.

21 Clifton GL (1995) Systemic hypothermia in treatment of severe brain injury. *J Neurosurg Anesthesiol* **7**:152–156.

22 Nussmeier NA, Arlund C and Slogoff S (1986) Neuropsychiatric complications after cardiopulmonary bypass: cerebral protection by a barbiturate. *Anesthesiology* **64**:165–170.

23 Rockoff MA, Marshall LF and Shapiro HM (1979) High-dose barbiturate therapy in humans: a clinical review of 60 patients. *Ann Neurol* **6**:194–199.

24 Brain Resuscitation Clinical Trial I Study Group (1986) Randomized clinical study of thiopental loading in comatose survivors of cardiac arrest. *N Engl J Med* **314**:397–403.

25 Spetzler RF, Hadley MN, Rigamonti D et al. Aneurysms of the basilar artery treated with circulatory arrest, hypothermia, and barbiturate cerebral protection. *J Neurosurg* **68**:868–879.

26 Spetzler RF, Martin N, Hadley MN et al. (1986) Microsurgical endarterectomy under barbiturate protection: a prospective study. *J Neurosurg* **65**:63–73.

27 Spetzler RF, Hadley MN, Martin NA et al. (1987) Vertebrobasilar insufficiency. Part I: Microsurgical treatment of extracranial vertebrobasilar disease. *J Neurosurg* **66**:648–661.

28 Hadley M and Spetzler R (1987) Contemporary application of the extracranial–intracranial bypass for cerebral revascularization. *Contemp Neurosurg* **9**:1–6.

29 Batjer HH, Frankfurt AI, Purdy PD *et al.* (1988) Use of etomidate, temporary arterial occlusion, and intraoperative angiography in surgical treatment of large and giant cerebral aneurysms. *J Neurosurg* **68**:234–240.

30 Ravussin P and De Tribolet N (1993) Total intravenous anesthesia with propofol for burst suppression in cerebral aneurysm surgery. Prelminary report of 42 patients. *Neurosurgery* **32**:236–240.

31 Shapiro HM (1985) Barbiturates in brain ischaemia. *Br J Anaesth* **57**:82–95.

32 Schwartz ML, Tator CH, Rowed DW *et al.* (1984) The University of Toronto head injury treatment study: a prospective, randomized comparison of pentobarbital and mannitol. *Can J Neurol Sci* **11**:434–440.

33 Ward JD, Becker DP, Miller JD *et al.* (1985) Failure of prophylactic barbiturate coma in the treatment of severe head injury. *J Neurosurg* **62**:383–388.

34 Eisenberg HM, Frankowski RF, Contant CF *et al.* (1988) High-dose barbiturate control of elevated intracranial pressure in patients with severe head injury. *J Neurosurg* **69**:15–23.

35 Schwartz A (1985) Neurological recovery after cardiac arrest: clinical feasibility trial of calcium blockers. *Am J Emerg Med* **3**:1–10.

36 Roine RO, Kaste M, Kinnunen A *et al.* (1990) Nimodipine after resuscitation from out-of-hospital ventricular fibrillation. A placebo-controlled, double-blind, randomized trial. *J Am Med Assoc* **264**:3171–3177.

37 Forsman M, Aarseth H, Nordby H *et al.* (1989) Cerebral blood flow, intracranial pressure and neurologic outcome after cardiac arrest: effects of nimodipine. *Anesth Analg* **68**:436–443.

38 Gelmers HJ, Gorter K, de Weerdt CJ and Wiezer HJ (1988) A controlled trial of nimodipine in acute ischemic stroke. *N Engl J Med* **318**:203–207.

39 The American Nimodipine Study Group (1992) Clinical trial of nimodipine in acute ischemic stroke. *Stroke* **23**:3–8.

40 Allen GS, Ahn HS, Preziosi TJ *et al.* (1983) Cerebral arterial spasm – a controlled trial of nimodipine in patients with subarachnoid hemorrhage. *N Engl J Med* **308**:619–624.

41 Petruk KC, West M, Mohr G *et al.* (1988) Nimodipine treatment in poor-grade aneurysm patients. Results of a multicenter double-blind placebo-controlled trial. *J Neurosurg* **68**:505–517.

42 Pickard JD, Murray GD, Illingworth R *et al.* (1989) Effect of oral nimodipine on cerebral infarction and outcome after subarachnoid haemorrhage: British aneurysm nimodipine trial. *Br Med J* **298**:636–642.

43 Reulen H (1976) Vasogenic brain oedema. New aspects in its formation, resolution and therapy. *Br J Anaesth* **48**:741–752.

44 French LA and Galicich JH (1964) The use of steroids for control of cerebral edema. *Clin Neurosurg* **10**:212–223.

45 Bracken M, Shepard M, Collins W *et al.* (1992) Methylprednisolone or naloxone treatment after acute spinal cord injury: one-year follow-up data. *J Neurosurg* **76**:23–31.

46 Bracken MB, Shepard MJ, Collins WP *et al.* (1990) A randomized, controlled trial of methylprednisolone or naloxone in the treatment of acute spinal-cord injury. Results of the second national acute spinal cord injury study. *N Engl J Med* **322**:1405–1411.

47 Patten BM, Mendell J, Bruun B *et al.* (1972) Double-blind study of the effects of dexamethasone on acute stroke. *Neurology (Minneapolis)* **22**:377–383.

48 Jastremski M, Sutton Tyrrell K, Vaagenes P *et al.* (1989) Glucocorticoid treatment does not improve neurological recovery following cardiac arrest. Brain Resuscitation Clinical Trial I Study Group. *J Am Med Assoc* **262**:3427–3430.

49 Braakman R, Schouten JHA, Blaauw-Van Dischoeck M and Minderhoud JM (1983) Megadose steroid in severe head injury. *J Neurosurg* **58**:326–330.

50 Cooper PR, Moody S, Clark WK *et al.* (1979) Dexamethasone and severe head injury. A prospective double-blind study. *J Neurosurg* **51**:307–316.

51 DeMaria EJ, Reichman W, Kenney PR *et al.* (1985) Septic complications of corticosteroid administration after central nervous system trauma. *Ann Surg* **202**:248–252.

52 Haley E, Kassell N, Alves W *et al.* (1995) Phase II trial of tirilazad in aneurysmal subarachnoid hemorrhage. *J Neurosurg* **82**:786–790.

53 Hsu C, Fraught R, Furlan A *et al.* (1987) Intravenous prostacyclin in acute nonhemorrhagic stroke: a placebo-controlled double-blind trial. *Stroke* **18**:352–358.

54 Itoh T, Kawakami M, Yamauchi Y *et al.* (1986) Effect of allopurinol on ischemia and reperfusion-induced cerebral injury in spontaneously hypertensive rats. *Stroke* **17**:1284–1287.

55 Fleischer JE, Lanier WL, Milde JH and Michenfelder JD (1987) Failure of deferoxamine, an iron chelator, to improve neurologic outcome following complete cerebral ischemia in dogs. *Stroke* **18**:124–127.

56 Kompala SD, Babbs CF and Blaho KE (1986) Effect of deferoxamine on late deaths following CPR in rats. *Ann Emerg Med* **15**:405–407.

57 Albin MS, Bunegin L and Helsel P (1983) Dimethyl sulfoxide and other therapies in experimental pressure-induced cerebral focal ischemia. *Ann NY Acad Sci* **411**:261–268.

58 de la Torre JC and Surgeon JW (1976) Dexamethasone and DMSO in experimental transorbital cerebral infarction. *Stroke* **7**:577–583.

59 Coles JC, Ahmed SN, Mehta HU and Kaufmann JC (1986) Role of free radical scavenger in protection of spinal cord during ischemia. *Ann Thorac Surg* **41**:551–556.

60 Little JR (1976) Treatment of acute focal cerebral ischemia with intermittent, low dose mannitol. *Neurosurgery* **5**:687–691.

61 Meyer FB, Sundt TM, Yanagihara T and Anderson RE (1987) Focal cerebral ischemia: pathophysiologic mechanisms and rationale for future avenues of treatment. *Mayo Clin Proc* **62**:35–55.

62 Zhang XM and Ellis EF (1990) Superoxide dismutase reduces permeability and edema induced by hypertension in rats. *Am J Physiol* **259**:H497–H503.

63 Chan PH, Longar S and Fishman RA (1987) Protective effects of liposome-entrapped superoxide dismutase on posttraumatic brain edema. *Ann Neurol* 1987 **21**:540–547.

64 Imaizumi S, Woolworth V, Fishman RA and Chan PH (1990) Liposome-entapped superoxide dismutase reduces cerebral infarction in cerebral ischemia in rats. *Stroke* **21**:1312–1317.

65 Matsumiya N, Koehler RC, Kirsch JR and Traystman RJ (1991) Conjugated superoxide dismutase reduces extent of caudate injury after transient focal ischemia in cats. *Stroke* **22**:1193–1200.

66 Lim KH, Connolly M, Rose D *et al.* (1986) Prevention of reperfusion injury of the ischemic spinal cord: use of recombinant superoxide dismutase. *Ann Thorac Surg* **42**:282–286.

67 Park CK, Nehls DG, Graham DI *et al.* The glutamate antagonist MK-801 reduces focal ischemic brain damage in the rat. *Ann Neurol* **24**:543–551.

68 Ozyurt E, Graham DI, Woodruff GN and McCulloch J (1988) Protective effect of the glutamate antagonist, MK-801 in focal cerebral ischemia in the cat. *J Cereb Blood Flow Metab* **8**:138–143.

69 McIntosh TK, Vink R, Soares H *et al.* (1990) Effect of noncompetitive blockade of *N*-methyl-D-aspartate receptors on the neurochemical sequelae of experimental brain injury. *J Neurochem* **55**:1170–1179.

70 Faden AI, Lemke M, Simon RP and Noble LJ (1988) *N*-methyl-D-aspartate antagonist MK-801 improves outcome following traumatic spinal cord injury in rats: behavioral, anatomic, and neurochemical studies. *J Neurotrauma* **5**:33-45.

71 Park CK, Nehls DG and Graham DI *et al.* (1988) Focal cerebral ischaemia in the cat: treatment with the glutamate antagonist HK-801 after induction of ischemia. *J Cereb Blood Flow Metab* **8**:757–762.

72 Sheardown MJ, Nielsen EO, Hansen AJ *et al.* (1990) 2,3-Dihydroxy-6-nitro-7-sulfamoyl-benzo(F)quinoxaline: a neuroprotectant for cerebral ischemia. *Science* **247**: 571–574.

73 Stevens MK and Yaksh TL (1990) Systematic studies on the effects of the NMDA receptor antagonist MK-801 on cerebral blood flow and responsivity, EEG, and blood–brain barrier following complete reversible cerebral ischemia. *J Cereb Blood Flow Metab* **10**:77–88.

74 Yentis SM, Hirsch NP and Smith GB (1993) *Anaesthesia A to Z.* Oxford: Butterworth-Heinemann, p. 91.

45 | Brain death

TE Oh

Today, ICUs can maintain cardiopulmonary function by artificial means, and death cannot always be equated with cessation of spontaneous heart beat. It has become necessary to reappraise death based on the integrity of the central nervous system.[1] The ability to certify death when there is irrecoverable cessation of brain function enables intensivists to withdraw treatment on ethical, humanitarian and utilitarian grounds. Relatives are relieved of unnecessary prolonged anxiety and false hopes, and the burden on expensive medical resources is reduced. A potential benefit for the community is a greater availability of physiologically sound organs for transplantation. The role of intensivists is vital in diagnosing brain death and supporting organ donation.

Brain death and persistent vegetative state

Comatose patients may recover (albeit with various degrees of disability) or remain in persistent coma (Fig. 45.1). Those who remain in a persistent vegetative state (PVS) have lost cortical (higher brain) activity, but are able to breathe spontaneously. If properly cared for, PVS patients can live a considerable time. Patients with permanent structural brain damage with 'irreversible loss of consciousness and of the capacity to breathe' are brain dead. Brain death is associated with death of the brainstem and needs to be diagnosed with absolute certainty. Causes of brain death usually involve catastrophic intracerebral events such as trauma and haemorrhage. Infections (e.g. encephalitis) are less common causes. Hypoxia may be the sole cause (e.g. cardiac arrest or drowning) or a complicating factor. Cerebral oedema may be a contributory or principal cause (e.g. secondary to hypoglycaemia).

Establishment of brain death criteria

The concept of accepting a clinical state of brain death as death was proposed by Harvard Medical School (the Harvard criteria) in 1968.[2] Two neurosurgeons in 1971 introduced the diagnostic importance of irreversible brainstem damage and emphasized that an electroencephalogram (EEG) was not necessary (the Minnesota criteria).[3] The memoranda on brain death by the UK Medical Royal Colleges and their Faculties in 1976 and 1979, [4,5] stated that 'death of brain stem is a necessary and sufficient component of brain death' and 'brain death equates with death'.[6] In the USA, the President's Commission in 1981[7] established death as 'irreversible cessation of circulatory and respiratory functions' or 'irreversible cessation of all functions of the entire brain, including the brain stem'. Current practices in Australasia,[8] the UK, and many countries are based on the UK and US guidelines.

Role of the brainstem

The brainstem maintains consciousness and the sleep–waking cycle. Pathways through the brainstem are required for cranial nerve reflexes and voluntary and coordinated trunk and limb movement. The pathways serving eye movements pass through both the midbrain and pons. Spontaneous ventilation is dependent on medullary nuclei. Brainstem death has always been followed by cardiac asystole within days (0.5–9 days).[9,10] Apart from heralding asystole,

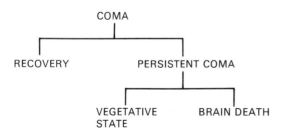

Fig. 45.1 The outcome of coma.

brainstem death nearly always precedes isoelectric EEG recordings.[10] Why asystole occurs is unclear; it may be related to the increased sympathetic activity secondary to gross intracranial damage.[11]

Clinical procedure to diagnose brain death

Preconditions[12]

Certain preconditions and exclusions must be fulfilled before considering a diagnosis of brain death.

1 *The patient is deeply comatose.*

(a) The effects of depressant drugs must be excluded. The drug history should be obtained or reviewed; if suspicion so indicates, a toxicology screen is obtained. If depressant drugs are present, then adequate time must be allowed for their effects to be excluded. This is especially important when pharmacological toxic effects were the cause of the coma and resultant hypoxic brain damage. The observation period depends on the drug pharmacokinetics, dose used, half-life and the patient's renal and hepatic status. Most commonly used drugs would be adequately cleared within 8–12 h. Assays of the drug in blood or urine may be necessary.

(b) Hypothermia as a cause of coma must be excluded. Body temperature may be low because of depression of temperature regulation by drugs or brainstem damage. Core temperature should be at least 35°C before diagnostic tests are performed. A low-reading thermometer should be used.

(c) Metabolic or endocrine disturbances that may cause or contribute to coma must be excluded. Possible factors should be carefully assessed. There must be no profound abnormality of serum urea and electrolytes, acid–base or blood glucose concentrations.

2 *The patient is apnoeic.* The patient must be on a ventilator with no spontaneous breathing efforts. Effects of muscle relaxants (if used) must be excluded, e.g. by eliciting spinal reflexes (flexion or stretch), or by demonstrating adequate neuromuscular conductance with a nerve stimulator. Persistent effects of opioids and central depressants on respiration must also be excluded.

3 *The patient's condition is due to irreversible structural brain damage.* The diagnosis of a disorder which can lead to brain death must be established. This is fairly straightforward in head injuries and cerebrovascular bleeds, but confirmation of the diagnosis may take longer in coma of hypoxic or other causes.

Diagnostic tests to confirm brain death[12]

These tests are intended to demonstrate the absence of brainstem reflexes in brain death. They should not

be performed in the presence of seizures. Facial trauma or obstruction to both external ear canals may preclude assessment of all reflexes.

1 Both pupils are fixed in diameter and unresponsive to bright light (direct and consensual responses). Pupil size is irrelevant, although most will be dilated. (Tests oculomotor III cranial nerve.)

2 Corneal reflexes are absent in response to a firm pressure on the cornea using a cotton-wool swab. (Tests trigeminal V cranial nerve.)

3 Vestibulo-ocular reflexes (caloric response) are absent. No eye movement occurs during or after a slow injection of 20 ml of ice-cold water into one, or preferably each ear canal. Clear access to the tympanic membrane must be confirmed by direct inspection with an auroscope. (Tests vestibulo-cochlear VIII cranial nerve.)

4 Motor responses within the cranial nerve distribution (e.g. grimacing) are absent when painful stimuli are applied to any somatic area. (Tests trigeminal V sensory supply to upper face and facial VII cranial nerves). Tendon stretch reflexes and plantar reflexes are of spinal cord origin, and may persist in the presence of brainstem death[3].

5 The gag and cough reflexes are absent in response to pharyngeal, laryngeal or tracheal stimulation. (Tests glossopharyngeal IX and vagus X cranial nerves.)

6 Spontaneous ventilation is absent. Testing for apnoea involves disconnecting from the ventilator when $Paco_2$ is near normal, ensuring that $Paco_2$ reaches the threshold required to stimulate the medullary centre, and observing for respiratory movements. Normally, a $Paco_2$ of 50 mmHg (6.7 kPa) would be sufficient to stimulate the medullary centre, but a threshold of 60 mmHg (8 kPa) is recommended.[7,13-15] Arterial blood-gas analysis must be used to assess $Paco_2$. A decrease in arterial pH to 7.30 will also confirm that respiratory stimulus is adequate.

Ventilation with 5% carbon dioxide in oxygen can be used to increase $Paco_2$ and achieve some denitrogenation before ventilator disconnection. Alternatively, $Paco_2$ is allowed to rise with apnoea, after first ventilating with 100% oxygen. Hypoxia is avoided during apnoea by diffusion oxygenation via a catheter delivering 4–6 l/min of oxygen into the trachea. These patients are often mildly hypothermic and flaccid with a depressed metabolic rate, so that the usual rate of rise of $Paco_2$ during apnoea may be reduced to about 2 mmHg/min (0.27 kPa/min). The threshold $Paco_2$ in patients with chronic obstructive airways disease needs to be increased accordingly.

Other considerations

1 *Two full and separate examinations must be performed.* The first should be undertaken following

Table 45.1 Indications for objective tests to demonstrate absence of cerebral blood flow to diagnose brain death

No clear cause for coma exists
Possible drug or metabolic effect on coma
Cranial nerves cannot be adequately tested
Cervical vertebra or cord injury is present
Cardiovascular instability which precludes testing for apnoea

at least 4 h of observed coma and absent cough, gag and muscle activity. However, the observation period before the first examination should be at least 12 h for victims of primary hypoxic brain damage. The second formal test is carried out after an interval of at least 2 h.[8,12] *Time of death for certification purposes will be the time after the second confirmatory examination.*

2 *Testing for brain death should be performed by two doctors* who have the expertise and are designated by the hospital. Each must actually perform one examination, although both may be present at both examinations. Neither doctor should be principally involved in organ removal or transplant.

3 *Objective demonstration of absent cerebral blood flow is required* if the preconditions cannot be satisfied or doubt about the diagnosis exists (Table 45.1), but this is unusual. A preceding 6-h observation period is necessary. Angiography is used, either three-vessel (i.e. one basilar and both carotid arteries) or four-vessel (i.e. arch aortography of both vertebral and carotid arteries). Digital subtraction,[16] radionuclide[17,18] and xenon-enhanced computed tomography techniques[19] can also be used.

4 *The oculocephalic reflex and EEG are not necessary tests* to diagnose brain death. (Absence of the oculocephalic reflex is denoted by the eyes remaining fixed when the head is briskly turned side to side.) An EEG is believed to be 'of great confirmatory value' in the USA,[2] but EEG activity may be present in brain death or absent in some comatose patients who eventually recover.[20,21]

5 *A hospital policy and protocol* for diagnosing brain death are recommended. This should include educational information, a list of designated doctors, a standard form (to be signed by both examining doctors) and organ donation procedures.

6 *Relatives must be supported* (see Chapter 1). It is a medical decision to withdraw life support and the relatives must be helped to accept this situation. Organ donation will occasionally influence the timing of stopping mechanical ventilation. The legal statutory definition and diagnosis of brain death will obviously apply in each institution.

Brain death diagnosis in young children and infants

Caution is recommended in applying the above brain death testing criteria in children under 5 years old,

on the assumption that the young brain has a greater capacity for recovery after acute damage.[7] The following modifications have been recommended.[22]

1 *Newborns*: A waiting period of 7 days after the acute injury must elapse before testing.
2 *Under 2 months*: Two examinations and an EEG, separated by 48 h, need to be performed.
3 *2 months to 1 year*: Two examinations and an EEG. separated by 24 h, need to be performed. The second examination and EEG can be omitted if absent cerebral blood flow is demonstrated by radionuclide angiography.
4 *Over 1 year*: Criteria are the same as those for older children and adults.

References

1 Pallis C (1982) ABC of brain stem death. Reappraising death. *Br Med J* **285**:1409–1412.
2 Ad Hoc Committee of the Harvard Medical School. A definition of irreversible coma. *J Am Med Assoc* **205**:85–88.
3 Mohandas A and Chou SN (1971) Brain death – a clinical and pathological study. *J Neurosurg* **35**:211–218.
4 Conference of Medical Royal Colleges and their Faculties in the UK (1976) Diagnosis of brain death. *Br Med J* **2**:1187–1188.
5 Conference of Medical Royal Colleges and their Faculties in the UK (1979) Diagnosis of brain death. *Br Med J* **i**:3320.
6 Pallis C (1982) From brain death to brain stem death. *Br Med J* **285**:1487–1490.
7 Report of the medical consultants on the diagnosis of death to the President's commission for the study of ethical problems in medicine and biomedical and behavioural research (1981) Guidelines for the determination of death. *J Am Med Assoc* **246**:2184–2186.
8 Report of the ANZICS working party on brain death and organ donation (1993) *Statement and Guidelines on Brain Death and Organ Donation – 1993*. Melbourne: Australian and New Zealand Intensive Care Society.
9 Jennet B, Gleave J and Wilson P (1981) Brain death in three neurosurgical units. *Br Med J* **282**:533–539.
10 Pallis C (1983) Prognostic significance of a dead brain stem. *Br Med J* **286**:123–124.
11 McLeod AA, Neil-Dwyer G, Meyer CHA *et al.* (1982) Cardiac sequelae of acute head injury. *Br Heart J* **47**:221–226.
12 Pallis C (1982) Diagnosis of brain stem death I and II. *Br Med J* **285**:1558–1560, 1641–1644.
13 Belsh JM, Blatt R and Schiffman PL (1986) Apnea testing in brain death. *Arch Intern Med* **146**:2385–2388.
14 Benzel EC, Gross CD, Hadden TA, Kesterson L and Lendreneau MD (1989) The apnea test for the determination of brain death. *J Neurosurg* **71**:191–194.
15 Schafer JA and Coronna JJ (1978) Duration of apnoea needed to confirm brain death. *Neurology* **28**:661–666.

16 Vatne K, Nakstad P and Lundar T. Digital subtraction angiography (DSA) in the evaluation of brain death. *Neuroradiology* **27**:155–157.

17 Galake RG, Schober O and Heyer K (1988) ^{99m}Tc-HM-PAO and 123-I-amphetamine cerebral scintigraphy: a new non invasive method in determination of brain death in children. *Eur J Nucl Med* **14**:446–452.

18 Reid RH Gulenchyn KY and Ballinger JR (1989) Clinical use of technetium-99m HM-PAO for determination of brain death. *J Nucl Med* **249**:246–247.

19 Ashwal S, Schneider S and Thompson J (1989) Xenon computed tomography measuring cerebral blood flow in the determination of brain death in children. *Ann Neurol* **25**:539–546.

20 Pallis C (1983) The arguments about EEG. *Br Med J* **286**:286–287.

21 Pallis C Prognostic value of brain stem lesions. *Lancet* **i**:379.

22 Task force for the determination of brain death in children (1987). Guidelines for the determination of brain death in children. *Neurology* **37**:1077–1078.

J Lipman

Infections of the cranial contents can be divided into those affecting the meninges and those affecting the brain parenchyma. Chronic, insidious or rare infections are beyond the scope of this chapter, which will concentrate on acute bacterial and viral infections. Definitions that can be applied to these different entities are:[1-4]

1 *Meningitis* – an acute inflammatory response of the meninges (pia-arachnoid mata) and/or the surrounding fluid, usually initiated by bacteria, viruses, fungi or protozoa. Meningeal inflammation may, occasionally, be caused by vaccines (e.g. measles) or be a manifestation of other multiorgan diseases such as collagen vascular diseases (e.g. systemic lupus erythematosus), sarcoid or lymphomas.[1-6]
2 *Subdural empyema* is a suppurative process in the space between the pia and dura mata.[2,7]
3 *Brain abscess* is a collection of pus within the brain tissue.[2,7]
4 *Aseptic meningitis*[3,4] loosely describes any meningeal irritation where bacteria are not isolated. It incorporates partially treated meningitis of bacterial, tuberculous or fungal origin, as well as viral meningitis and central nervous system (CNS) manifestations of other diseases (e.g. some collagen vascular diseases, sarcoidosis and certain drug reactions).

General points

1 The inflammatory response to all infecting organisms is not only limited to the brain and meninges. It usually has a systemic component,[1-8] which often requires specific treatment (e.g. severe sepsis, shock, acute respiratory distress syndrome (ARDS), and bleeding disorders such as disseminated intravascular coagulation (DIC)).
2 A variety of different pathogens are able to cause parenchymal and/or meningitic inflammation, resulting in a very similar clinical presentation.

However, bacterial infections must be treated urgently and appropriately, to limit ongoing CNS damage.[1,2,7-9] It is also important to treat complications of these diseases, such as seizures and raised intracranial pressure (ICP).
3 Urgent investigation includes lumbar puncture, which is dangerous if ICP is raised (see below). An urgent computed tomography (CT) scan is required to exclude a mass lesion in such patients, as cerebral herniation is a life-threatening complication of lumbar puncture.[1,7,9-13]

Bacterial meningitis[1,2]

Aetiology[5,8,10,12,14,15]

General infections

Virtually any species of bacteria can cause meningitis, although three organisms are consistently reported – *Haemophilus influenzae*, *Streptococcus pneumoniae* and *Neisseria meningitidis*. Their incidence varies, especially in different age groups. *N. meningitidis* and *H. influenzae* are common pathogens in childhood meningitis, with *S. pneumoniae* being most common in adult community-acquired meningitis. *N. meningitidis* and *H. influenzae* account for most of the other bacterial adult meningitis. However, vaccines against *H. influenzae* became available in 1992, and its incidence has fallen.[1,5] There is a higher incidence of group B streptococcus and *Listeria monocytogenes* meningitis in the very young, and of the latter organism in the elderly.

Nosocomial infections

Common systemic nosocomial pathogens such as *Escherichia coli*, *Pseudomonas* spp., *Klebsiella* and *Acinetobacter* spp. account for a high percentage of nosocomial infections of the meninges.

Immunocompromised hosts

Similar to systemic infections, fungi and viruses (e.g. human immunodeficiency virus, HIV) are common CNS pathogens in the immunocompromised patient with meningitis.

Neurosurgery and trauma

Infections following skull trauma are frequently caused by *Staphylococcus aureus*, and in those following neurosurgery, by *S. epidermidis*. These patients may also have nosocomial infection from other organisms listed above.

Pathogenesis and pathophysiology[11,12,16–18]

Most bacteria obtain entry into the CNS via the haematogenous route. Factors that result in meningeal localization of the bacteria are largely unknown. Bacteria seem to settle on the walls of the venous sinuses and vessels with slow blood flow. Subsequently, the bacteria penetrate the dura to enter the subarachnoid space. It seems that release of cytokines (particularly interleukin-1, and tumour necrosis factor-α) and other endogenous mediators then cause an inflammatory response in the CNS, with vasculitis, infarctions, vasogenic oedema, permeability of the blood–brain barrier, raised ICP and decreased cerebral blood flow (Fig. 46.1).[1,11,16–18]

Any infection can haematologically 'seed' the meninges, but typical associated infections are those of the upper respiratory tract, pneumonia and otitis media. Other important infections documented to precede meningitis are endocarditis and osteomyelitis. Contiguous spread from compound cranial fractures and surgery is another common path of entry of organisms into the CNS.

Clinical presentation[5,6,8,11,15]

An accurate history may reveal recent trauma or contact with cases of meningitis, upper respiratory tract infection or ear infection. The disease entities may take hours to days from prodrome to full-blown presentation (and from presentation to death).

Although suspicion of meningitis is usually obvious, clinical presentation may resemble subarachnoid haemorrhage and severe migraine. Malaise, photophobia, rigors, nausea, vomiting, fever and headache are common complaints. Most patients will present with the triad of fever, headache and neck stiffness.[1,2,5,6] Altered mental status (from irritability and delirium to drowsiness and coma) is probably the next most common sign. A variety of neurological signs can present with meningitis, but signs of meningeal irritation include neck rigidity, positive Brudzinski's sign (neck flexion produces flexion of lower limbs), thoracolumbar rigidity and positive Kernig's sign (pain and hamstring spasm result from

attempts to straighten, e.g. with the hip flexed). Focal neurological signs may be present with isolated cranial nerve lesions. Seizures can be the presenting feature, especially in children.

Systemic signs are common. Classically, meningococcal disease presents with a haemorrhagic, petechial or purpuric rash, but petechiae may also be seen with infection by other organisms. Severe sepsis, septic shock, ARDS and DIC may be present or ensue as complications.[8,15]

Investigations[1,2,5,8,10,13]

1 *CT scan*: A CT scan is advocated before a lumbar puncture to assess ICP and exclude a cerebral abscess.[8]
2 *Lumbar puncture*: A lumbar puncture will confirm the diagnosis and help in the choice of antibiotics. Cerebrospinal fluid (CSF) in bacterial meningitis is often turbid with a raised pressure, and shows polymorphonuclear leukocytes and a low glucose and high protein content (Table 46.1). An urgent Gram stain and microbiological culture of the CSF specimen must be ordered. Latex particle agglutination of CSF is specific for bacterial meningitis, although C-reactive protein levels have also been reported to be sensitive.[19]

Lumbar puncture incurs a risk of cerebral herniation. About 5% of children with meningitis are reported to have cerebral herniation, although not all could be attributed to lumbar puncture.[20] Therefore, apart from premature infants and patients with raised ICP, a lumbar puncture should be performed to enable an accurate and early diagnosis.[5,9–12]
3 *Blood cultures*: The spread of organisms in meningitis is haematogenous. Thus, blood cultures of infected patients should be undertaken.
4 *Other investigations*: Other tests should be undertaken according to clinical need (e.g. full blood count, chest and any other relevant X-rays, and cultures of infected specimens and tissues).

Management

1 *Antibiotics*[5,7,9,10,12,14,15,21] should be started as early as possible. Empirical choice is complicated by the development of resistance by the three common causative organisms. Unless local resistance patterns are a problem, standard regimens of penicillin (or ampicillin) and chloramphenicol can be used. In the young and elderly, ampicillin covers prevalent *Listeria monocytogenes*. *Haemophilus* meningitis and infection of uncertain aetiology (or resistant pneumococci in some areas) often require broad-spectrum third-generation cephalosporins. Suggested regimens and doses of antibiotics are given in Table 46.2.

Nosocomial meningitis or infection in the

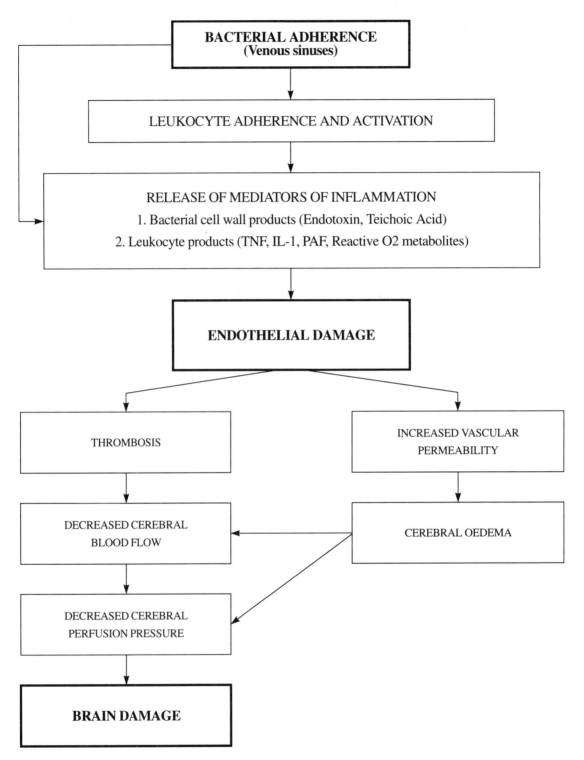

Fig. 46.1 Pathogenesis of inflammatory response in bacterial meningitis.

Table 46.1 Cerebrospinal fluid changes in meningitis

	Normal	*Bacterial*	*Viral*
Appearance	Clear	Turbid/purulent	Clear/turbid
White cell count	<5/mm³ mononuclear	200–10 000/mm³ predominantly polymorphonuclear	<500/mm³ mainly lymphocytes
Protein	0.2–0.4 g/l	0.5–2.0 g/l	0.4–0.8 g/l
Glucose	$>\frac{1}{2}$ Blood glucose	$<\frac{1}{3}$ Blood glucose	$>\frac{1}{2}$ Blood glucose

Table 46.2 Empirical antibiotic regimens for bacterial meningitis

Patient categories	*First choice*	*Alternative*
Neonate	Ampicillin plus cefotaxime or ceftriaxone	Ampicillin plus chloramphenicol (or gentamicin)
Child	Cefotaxime or ceftriaxone	Ampicillin plus chloramphenicol (or gentamicin)
Adolescent and adult	Penicillin	Cefotaxime or ceftriaxone
Penicillin-sensitive individual	Cefotaxime or ceftriaxone	Vancomycin plus gentamicin, depending on age group
Penicillin-resistant organism	Vancomycin	Ampicillin plus cefotaxime or ceftriaxone

Drug doses	*Paediatrics*	*Adults*
Penicillin 2- or 4-hourly IV	80 000 U/kg per day	24 M U/day
Ampicillin 6-hourly IV	50–200 mg/kg per day	12 g/day
Cefotaxime 6–8-hourly IV	200 mg/kg per day	6–8 g/day
Ceftriaxone 12–24-hourly IV	100 mg/kg per day	2–4 g/day
Vancomycin 12-hourly IV	40 mg/kg per day	2 g/day
Chloramphenicol 6-hourly IV	50–100 mg/kg per day	4 g/day
Gentamicin daily IV	4–5 mg/kg per day	5 mg/kg per day

IV = Intravenous.

immunocompromised patient[12,14] presents a greater difficulty for choosing the correct antibiotic. It is often only after the organism is identified and sensitivity results are obtained that the optimal antibiotic choice can be made.

Antibiotics should be reviewed and appropriately changed, once antibiotic sensitivities are known or if the patient is not improving. Antibiotics are traditionally given for 10–14 days, although a shorter course is adequate for meningococcal meningitis.[5] The use of intrathecal antibiotics is controversial. It can be considered in certain cases[22] but should not be routinely used.

2 *Steroids*:[9,10,16,21,22] Experimentally, steroids can block some of the inflammatory response of bacterial meningitis. A few large clinical trials have shown some benefit of early steroid administration in paediatric meningitis.[9,10,16,21,23] the recommendations are for dexamethasone 0.15 mg/kg IV 6-hourly for 4 days, to begin with or just before the first dose of antibiotic. However, steroids are *not recommended* for adult meningitis.[16]

3 *Anticonvulsants*:[5,8,10,13,24] Focal or generalized fitting should be treated with benzodiazepines (e.g. diazepam 10 mg IV repeated every 5 min until seizure is controlled) or phenytoin (15 mg/kg IV). Although there is no direct evidence to show benefits, it may be prudent to give prophylactic anticonvulsants to the high-risk patient.

4 *Treatment of raised ICP*:[8,13,16,19] Intracranial hypertension is a common feature or complication of meningitis, and can potentiate other complications to cause permanent neurological impairment. Raised ICP is treated by standard measures (hyperventilation, mannitol or glycerol therapy, and drainage of CSF). To maintain adequate cerebral perfusion pressure, systemic blood pressure must be maintained and hypotension avoided[25] (see Chapter 43).

5 *Fluid therapy*:[8,16,25] Inappropriate antidiuretic hormone secretion has been documented in meningitis. Although this may be treated by fluid restriction, it is more beneficial to provide adequate amounts of fluid to maintain blood pressure, thereby maintaining adequate cerebral perfusion pressures.

Table 46.3 Neurological sequelae from meningitis

Sequela	Occurrence
Deafness	30%
Cerebral palsy	30%
Hydrocephalus	10–15%
Cerebrovascular complications	10–15%
Focal neurological defects	10–15%
Mental retardation	10%
Behavioural disorders	10%
Paraesthesias	10%
Visual disorders	10%
Brain abscess	1%

6 *Supportive therapy*[5,8,13,15] Airway patency and toilet must be maintained in the comatosed or confused patient. Appropriate fluid, inotropic and ventilatory supportive therapy must be given to patients with severe sepsis, shock or ARDS. Nutritional support is given. Necessary precautions are taken against nosocomial infections.

7 *Therapy for contacts:*[1,2,5,10] Close contacts of patients with meningococcal and *Haemophilus* meningitis, both of which can be droplet spread (i.e. to family and staff involved in airway management) should be advised to take rifampicin. Contacts of meningococcus require 10 mg/kg 12-hourly for 2 days, and those of *Haemophilus* require 20 mg/kg daily for 4 days (with maximal doses of 600 mg/day).[5]

Outcome[1,2,8,15,21]

Untreated bacterial meningitis is usually fatal. Appropriate therapy significantly reduces mortality, but less so in those with unusual presentations, late antibacterial therapy and resistant organisms. The very old and young have the worst prognosis – up to 40% mortality. In adult patients, pneumococcal meningitis still has the poorest outcome.[8] Long-term neurological complications of bacterial meningitis are shown in Table 46.3.

Viral encephalomyelitis (also known as meningoencephalitis)[3,4]

Acute viral CNS infections often involve the meninges (i.e. viral meningitis), the brain tissue (i.e. encephalitis) and the spinal cord (i.e. myelitis). This anatomical grouping is often impossible to differentiate clinically, as more than one site is usually affected. Hence the terms meningoencephalitis or encephalomyelitis are commonly used.

Aetiology

The most common causes of viral encephalomyelitis worldwide are probably the arboviruses.[3] Other common viruses causing CNS infections include the echoviruses, mumps, Coxsackie and even polio.

Clinical presentation

Viral encephalomyelitis is a relatively common disease. In some patients, meningeal irritation may predominate, whilst in others, encephalitic involvement may be more striking. Regardless of the aetiology, the onset of the encephalomyelitis usually consists of abrupt fever, headache, neck stiffness, retrobulbar pain, photophobia, vertigo and nausea and vomiting. When encephalitis is prominent, confusion, seizures, coma, respiratory depression, cranial nerve palsies and even paralysis can occur. Cerebral infection may be the only manifestation of viral disease, but often other peripheral manifestations are present, such as parotitis, herpangina, pleurodynia, myopericarditis, lymphadenopathy and hepatosplenomegaly.

Investigations

Although a peripheral blood smear may show a lymphopenia or a lymphocytosis, CSF changes are often typical, with fewer than 500 leukocytes/mm^3, most being mononuclear. CSF proteins and glucose are normal (Table 46.1). To aid identification of causative organisms, swabs should be obtained from other suspected infected sites, e.g. mucous membranes, throat, skin and rectum.

Management

Therapy is largely supportive. Hyperimmune globulins may have potential value, but there are no definitive reports of their benefit.

Outcome

In most cases of viral meningitis, complete recovery within days is the rule. With encephalitis, however, recovery varies from complete to severe neurological impairment.

Subdural empyema[2,7]

This entity may be mistaken for meningitis. The subdural space is infected either from nasal sinuses or from neurosurgical drainage. Signs of raised ICP are common. The diagnosis is made on CT scan, which shows a collection of fluid around the dura. Treatment is urgent surgical drainage and antibiotics against the causative organisms (usually polymicrobial, e.g. streptococci, staphylococci and Gram-negative organisms). Penicillin and chloramphenicol (plus possibly gentamicin) or a third-generation cephalosporin should be used. Doses similar to those for meningitis are appropriate, but should be continued for 3–6 weeks. Good supportive therapy is important. Neurological sequelae are common and mortality is 10–20%.

Brain abscess[2,7,26,27]

Brain abscesses are primarily bacterial, originating via haematogenous spread or from direct entry across bone or dura mata. Conditions predisposing to cerebral abscesses are chronic ear or sinus disease, suppurative lung disease, congenital heart disease and cranial trauma. The organism varies with aetiology of the sepsis. *Staphylococcus* spp. would be common in trauma, and *Streptococcus*, *Bacteroides* and Gramnegative bacteria are common with lung disease.

Common clinical features are severe headache, vomiting, obtundation, seizures and focal neurological signs. Neck stiffness is often absent. The diagnosis depends on first, an obvious primary source of infection; second, evidence of raised ICP; and third, focal cerebral or cerebellar signs. Lumbar puncture is dangerous. A CT scan is the most valuable procedure, although magnetic resonance imaging is becoming more widely used.[7]

There is no consensus on when surgical intervention should be undertaken, but indications for surgery include large single lesions, relief of raised ICP and the need for tissue diagnosis. Antibiotics are the mainstay of therapy. Penicillin plus chloramphenicol (as for meningitis) and metronidazole 500 mg IV 8-hourly or 1 g rectally 12-hourly should be empirical therapy until culture and sensitivity results are obtained. Better intracranial drug penetration may be obtained from cefotaxime 1–2 g IV 6–8-hourly and metronidazole 500 mg IV 8-hourly.[27] If recent cranial trauma or neurosurgery is the primary factor, cloxacillin or vancomycin should be used in doses as for meningitis. Antibiotics should be continued for 3–6 weeks. Supportive therapy limits morbidity. Morbidity is high, and mortality from cerebral abscesses is 10–20% in most studies.

References

1 Harter DH and Petersdorf RG (1991) Bacterial meningitis and brain abscess. In: Wilson JD, Braunwald E, Isselbacher KJ *Harrison's Principles of Internal Medicine*, 12th edn. New York: McGraw-Hill, pp. 2023–2031.

2 Overturf GD (1994) Bacterial meningitis. In Hoeprich PD, Jordan MC and Ronald AR (eds) *Infectious Diseases. A Treatise of Infectious Processes*, 5th edn. Philadelphia: JB Lippincott, pp. 1107–1123.

3 Harter DH and Petersdorf RG (1991) Viral diseases of the central nervous system: aseptic meningitis and encephalitis. In: Wilson JD, Braunwald E, Isselbacher KJ *Harrison's Principles of Internal Medicine*, 12th edn. New York: McGraw-Hill, pp. 2031–2038.

4 Doherty RL and Jordan MC (1994) Viral meningoencephalitis. In: Hoeprich PD, Jordan MC and Ronald AR (eds) *Infectious Diseases. A Treatise of Infectious Processes*, 5th edn. Philadelphia: JB Lippincott, pp. 1092–1100.

5 Lambert HP (1994) Meningitis. *J Neurol Neurosurg Psychiatry* **57**:405–415.

6 Isenberg H (1992) Bacterial meningitis: signs and symptoms. *Antibiot Chemother* **45**:79–95.

7 Anderson M (1993) Management of cerebral infection. *J Neurol Neurosurg Psychiatry* **56**:1243–1258.

8 Pfister H-W, Feiden W and Einhaupl K-M (1993) Spectrum of complications during bacterial meningitis in adults: results of a prospective clinical study. *Arch Neurol* **50**:575–581.

9 Baraff L, Oslund S and Prather M (1993) Effect of antibiotic therapy and etiologic microorganism on the risk of bacterial meningitis in children with occult bacteremia. *Pediatrics* **92**:140–143.

10 Booy R and Kroll S (1994) Bacterial meningitis in children. *Curr Opin Pediatr* **6**:29–35.

11 Lipton JD and Schafermeyer RW (1993) Evolving concepts in pediatric bacterial meningitis – Part I: pathophysiology and diagnosis. *Ann Emerg Med* **22**:1602–1615.

12 Neu HC (1992) Microbiology of bacterial meningitis pathogens. *Antibiot Chemother* **45**:52–67.

13 Lipton JD and Schafermeyer RW (1993) Evolving concepts in pediatric bacterial meningitis – Part II: current management and therapeutic research. *Ann Emerg Med* **22**:1616–1629.

14 Sepkowitz K and Armstrong D (1992) Bacterial meningitis in the immunocompromised host. *Antibiot Chemother* **45**:262–269.

15 Durand ML, Calderwood SB, Weber DJ *et al.* (1993) Acute bacterial meningitis in adults. A review of 493 episodes. *N Engl J Med* **328**:21–28.

16 Pfister H-W, Fontana A, Tauber MG, Tomasz A and Scheld WM (1994) Mechanisms of brain injury in bacterial meningitis: workshop summary. *Clin Infect Dis* **19**:463–479.

17 Goh D and Minns RA (1993) Cerebral blood flow velocity monitoring in pyogenic meningitis. *Arch Dis Child* **68**:111–119.

18 Ashwal S, Stringer W, Tomasi L, Schneider S, Thompson J and Perkin R (1990) Cerebral blood flow and CO_2 reactivity in children with bacterial meningitis. *J Pediatr* **117**:523–530.

19 Roine I, Foncea LM, Cofre J, Ledermann W and Peltola H (1992) Serum C-reactive protein vs tumor necrosis factor alpha and interleukin 1 beta of the cerebrospinal fluid in the diagnosis of bacterial meningitis with low cerebrospinal fluid cell count. *Pediatr Infect Dis J* **11**:1057–1058.

20 Rennick G, Shann F and de Campo J (1993) Cerebral herniation during bacterial meningitis in children. *Br Med J* **306:**953–955.

21 Baraff LJ, Lee SI and Schriger DL (1993) Outcomes of bacterial meningitis in children: a meta-analysis. *Pediatr Infect Dis J* **12:**389–394.

22 Luer MS and Hatton J (1993) Vancomycin administration into the cerebrospinal fluid: a review. *Ann Pharmacother* **27:**912–921.

23 Waagner D, Kennedy W and Hoyt M (1990) Lack of adverse effects of dexamethasone therapy in aseptic meningitis. *Pediatr Infect Dis J* **9:**922–923.

24 Handrick W and Wasser S. Seizures during bacterial meningitis. *Antibiot Chemother* **45:**239–253.

25 Powell KR, Sugarman LI, Eskenazi AE *et al.* (1990) Normalisation of arginine vasopressin concentration when children with meningitis are given maintenance plus replacement fluid therapy. *J Pediatr* **117:**515–522.

26 Domingo Z and Peter JC (1994) Brain abscess in childhood. A 25-year experience. *S Afr Med J* **84:**13–15.

27 Sjolin J, Lilja A, Eriksson N, Arneborn P, and Cars O (1993) Treatment of brain abscess with cefotaxime and metronidazole: prospective study on 15 consecutive patients. *Clin Infect Dis* **17:**857–863.

47 | Tetanus

J Lipman and TE Oh

Tetanus is a preventable, often Third-World disease, frequently requiring expensive First-World technology to treat. It is an acute, often fatal disease caused by exotoxins produced by *Clostridium tetani,* and is characterized by generalized muscle rigidity, autonomic instability and sometimes convulsions.

Epidemiology

Recently, tetanus has become a disease of the elderly and debilitated in developed countries, as younger people are likely to have been immunized.[1] In the USA, its incidence decreased from 0.23 per 100 000 in 1955 to 0.04 per 100 000 in 1975, and remained stable thereafter.[2] The annual world mortality from tetanus is estimated to be 400 000–2 000 000.[3] Tetanus claimed the lives of over 433 000 infants in 1991, and accounts for 5 deaths for every 1000 live births in Africa.[4] It is geographically prevalent in rural areas with poor hygiene and medical services. Thus, tetanus remains a significant public health problem in the developing world, primarily because of poor access to immunization programmes.[5] In addition, modern management requires ICU facilities, which are rarely available in the most severely afflicted populations.[6] Therefore, tetanus will continue to afflict developing populations in the foreseeable future.

Pathogenesis

C. tetani is an obligate anaerobic, spore-bearing, Gram-positive bacillus. Spores exist ubiquitously in soil and in animal and human faeces. After gaining access to devitalized tissue, spores proliferate in the vegetative form, producing toxins, tetanospasmin and tetanolysin. Tetanospasmin is extremely potent; an estimated 240 g could kill the entire world population,[6] with 0.1 mg being lethal for an average man. Tetanolysin is of little clinical importance.

C. tetani is non-invasive. Hence, tetanus occurs only when the spores gain access into tissues to produce vegetative forms. The usual mode of entry is through a puncture wound or laceration, although tetanus may follow surgery, burns, gangrene, chronic ulcers, dog bites, injections such as with drug users, dental infection, abortion and childbirth. Tetanus neonatorum usually follows infection of the umbilical stump. The injury itself may be trivial, and in 20% of cases there is no history or evidence of a wound.[1] Germination of spores occurs in oxygen-poor media (e.g. in necrotic tissue), with foreign bodies, and with infections. *C. tetani* infection remains localized, but the exotoxin tetanospasmin is distributed widely via the blood stream, taken up into motor nerve endings, and transported into the nervous system. Here, it affects motor neurone end-plates in skeletal muscle (to decrease release of acetylcholine), the spinal cord (with dysfunction of polysynaptic reflexes) and the brain (with seizures, inhibition of cortical activity and autonomic dysfunction). Tetanus is not communicable from person to person.

The symptoms of tetanus appear only after tetanospasmin has diffused from the cell body through the extracellular space, and gained access to the presynaptic terminals of adjacent neurons.[1] Tetanospasmin spreads to all local neurons, but is preferentially bound by inhibitory interneurons, i.e. glycinergic terminals in the spinal cord, and γ-aminobutyric acid (GABA) terminals in the brain.[6] Its principal effect is to block these inhibitory pathways. Hence stimuli to and from the central nervous system (CNS) are not 'damped down'.

Active immunoprophylaxis[1,2,7]

Natural immunity to tetanus does not occur. Tetanus may both relapse and recur. Victims of tetanus must be *actively immunized.* Tetanus toxoid is a cheap and effective vaccine, which is thermally stable.[8] It is a non-toxic derivative of the toxin which, nevertheless, elicits and reacts with antitoxic antibody. By consensus, an antibody titre of 0.01 u/ml serum is protective.[9] None the less, tetanus has been reported in a few victims with much higher serum antibody titres.[2]

In adults, a full immunization course consists of three toxoid doses, given at an optimal interval of 6–12 weeks between the first and second doses, and 6–12 months between the second and third doses. A single dose will offer no immediate protection in the unimmunized, but a full course should never be repeated. Neonates have immunity from maternal antibodies. Children over 3 months should be actively immunized, and need four doses in total. Two or more doses to child-bearing females over 14 years will protect any child produced within the next 5 years. Pregnant females who are not immunized should thus be given two spaced-out doses 2 weeks to 2 months before delivery. Booster doses should be given routinely every 10 years.

Side-effects of tetanus toxoid are uncommon and not life-threatening. They are associated with excessive levels of antibody due to indiscriminate use.[10] Common reactions include urticaria, angio-oedema and diffuse, indurated swelling at the site of injection.

Clinical presentation[1,2,9,11,12]

The incubation period (i.e. time from injury to onset of symptoms) varies from 2 to 60 days. The period of onset (i.e. from first symptom to first spasm) similarly varies. Nearly all cases (90%), however, present within 15 days of infection.[11,12] The incubation period and the period of onset are of prognostic importance, with shorter times signifying more severe disease.

Presenting symptoms are pain and stiffness. Stiffness gives way to rigidity, and there is difficulty in mouth opening – trismus or lockjaw. Most (75%) on non-neonatal generalized tetanus present with trismus.[11,12] Rigidity becomes generalized, and facial muscles produce a characteristic clenched-teeth expression called risus sardonicus. The disease progresses in a descending fashion. Typical spasms, with flexion and adduction of the arms, extension of the legs and opisthotonos, are very painful, and may be so intense that fractures and tendon separations occur.[1] Spasms are caused by external stimuli, e.g. noise and pressure. As the disease worsens, even minimal stimuli produce more intense and longer-lasting spasms. Spasms are life-threatening when they involve the larynx and/or diaphragm.

Neonatal tetanus presents most often on day 7 of life,[9] with a short (1-day) history of failure of the infant to feed. The neonate displays typical spasms that can be easily misdiagnosed as convulsions of another aetiology. In addition, because these infants vomit (as a result of the increased intra-abdominal pressure) and are dehydrated (because of their inability to swallow), meningitis and sepsis are often considered first.

Autonomic dysfunction occurs in severe cases,[11–15] and begins a few days after the muscle spasms. (The toxin has further to diffuse to reach the lateral horns of the spinal cord.) There is increased basal sympathetic tone, manifesting as tachycardia and bladder and bowel dysfunction. Also, episodes of marked sympathetic overactivity involving both α- and β-receptors occur. Vascular resistance, central venous pressure and, usually, cardiac output are increased, manifesting clinically as labile hypertension, pyrexia, sweating, and pallor and cyanosis of the digits.[13] These episodes are usually of short duration and may occur without any provocation. They are caused by reduced inhibition of postsynaptic sympathetic fibres in the intermediolateral cell column, as evidenced by very high circulating noradrenaline concentrations.[1,15] Other postulated causes of this variable sympathetic overactivity include loss of inhibition of the adrenal medulla with increased adrenaline secretion, direct inhibition by tetanospasmin of the release of endogenous opiates, and increased release of thyroid hormone.[1,6]

The role of the parasympathetic nervous system is debatable. Episodes of bradycardia, low peripheral vascular resistance, low central venous pressure and profound hypotension are seen, and are frequently preterminal.[13] Sudden and repeated cardiac arrests occur, particularly in intravenous drug abusers.[15] These events have been attributed to total withdrawal of sympathetic tone, since it is unresponsive to atropine.[16] However they may be caused by catecholamine-induced myocardial damage[15,17] or direct brainstem damage.[15] Whatever the mechanism, patients afflicted with the autonomic dysfunction of tetanus are at risk of sudden death.

Local tetanus is an uncommon mild form of tetanus with a mortality of 1%. The signs and symptoms are confined to a limb or muscle, and may be the result of immunization. *Cephalic tetanus* is also rare. It results from head and neck injuries, eye infections and otitis media. The cranial nerves, especially the seventh, are frequently involved, and the prognosis is poor. This form may progress to a more generalized form. Tetanus in heroin addicts seems to be severe, with a high mortality, but numbers are small.[15,18,19]

Diagnosis

The diagnosis is clinical and often straightforward. There are no laboratory tests specific to tetanus. *C. tetani* is cultured from the wound only in a third of cases. The most common differential diagnosis is dystonic reaction to tricyclics. Other differential diagnoses include strychnine poisoning, local temporomandibular disease, local oral disease, convulsions, tetany, intracranial infections or haemorrhage and psychiatric disorders.

Management

Initial objectives of treatment are to neutralize circulating toxin (i.e. passive immunization) and prevent it from entering peripheral nerves (i.e. wound care), as well as eradicating the source of the toxin (i.e. extensive surgery, hygiene, wound care and antibiotics). Treatment then aims to minimize the effect of toxin already bound in the nervous system, and to provide general supportive care.

Passive immunization[1,2,20]

Human antitetanus toxin has now largely replaced antitetanus serum (ATS) of horse origin, as it is less antigenic. Antitetanus toxin will at best neutralize only circulating toxin, but does not affect toxins already fixed in the CNS, i.e. it does not ameliorate symptoms already present. Although never prospectively tested, present recommendations for human antitetanus toxin in tetanus are IV 3000–6000 units. It has been suggested that unimmunized patients or those whose immunization status is unknown should be given human rich antiserum on presentation with contaminated wounds . No controlled study has shown this to be more effective than wound toilet and penicillin administration.

Intrathecal administration of antitetanus toxin is still controversial.[21] A large meta-analysis reported it to be ineffective.[22] Moreover, suitable intrathecal preparations are not widely available. Side-effects of human antitetanus toxin include fever, shivering and chest or back pains. Cardiovascular parameters need to be monitored, and the infusion may need to be stopped temporarily if significant tachycardia and hypotension present.[1,2,10,20] If human antiserum is not available, equine ATS can be used after testing and desensitization.[2]

Eradication of the organism
Wound care

Once human antitetanus toxin has been given, the infected site should be thoroughly cleaned and all necrotic tissue extensively debrided.

Antibiotics

Tetanus spores are destroyed by antibiotics. The vegetative form (bacillus) is sensitive to antibiotics *in vitro*. However, *in vivo* efficacy depends on the antibiotic concentration at the wound site, and large doses may be required. Recommended antibiotic regimens include:

1 Metronidazole 500 mg IV 8-hourly for 10 days: The drug has a spectrum of activity against anaerobes, is able to penetrate necrotic tissue, and has been shown to be more effective than penicillin in this situation.[23]
2 Penicillin G 1–3 Mu IV 6-hourly intervals for 10 days: penicillin is a GABA antagonist in the CNS,[24] and may aggravate the spasms. Nevertheless, it is still often used in this situation.
3 Erythromycin has been used, but should not be routinely used.

Suppression of effects of tetanospasmin
Controlling muscle spasms

In the early stages of tetanus, the patient is most at risk from laryngeal and other respiratory muscle spasm. Therefore, if muscle spasms are present, airway should be urgently secured by endotracheal intubation or tracheostomy. If respiratory muscles are affected, mechanical ventilation is instituted. In severe tetanus, spasms usually preclude effective ventilation, and muscle relaxants may be required. Pancuronium bromide may cause tachycardia and hypertension[25] by stimulating noradrenaline release from sympathetic nerve endings,[26] but has been used safely in tetanus.[27] Heavy sedation alone may prevent muscle spasms and improve autonomic dysfunction (see below).

Management of autonomic dysfunction

Autonomic dysfunction manifests in increased basal sympathetic activity[28,29] and episodic massive outpourings of catecholamines.[28–31] During these episodes, noradrenaline and adrenaline may be up to 10 times basal levels.[28,30] The clinical picture is variable.[31] Hypertension, tachycardia and sweating do not always occur concurrently.

Traditionally, a combination of α- and β-adrenergic blockers has been used to treat sympathetic overactivity. Phenoxybenzamine, phentolamine, bethanidine and chlorpromazine have been used as α-receptor blockers. Ganglion blockers and nitroprusside have occasionally been used. Propranolol and labetalol have had limited success.[32–34] However, unopposed β-adrenergic blockade cannot be advised. Deaths from acute congestive cardiac failure have resulted.[32,33] Removal of β-mediated vasodilatation in limb muscle causes a rise in systemic vascular resistance, and β-blocked myocardium may not be able to maintain adequate cardiac output. Also, with β-blockade, hypotension follows when sympathetic overactivity abates. Esmolol, a very short-acting β-adrenergic blocker given IV, has been reported to be useful.[35] However, although sympathetic crises can be controlled by esmolol, catecholamine levels remain raised.[31]. This raises concern, because excessive catecholamine secretion is associated with myocardial damage.[17]

From above, it appears more logical to decrease catecholamine output. This can be done with sedatives. Benzodiazepines and morphine are success-fully used.[30] Morphine and diazepam act centrally to minimize the effects of tetanospasmin. Morphine probably acts by replacing deficient endogenous opioids.[1] Benzodiazepines increase the affinity and efficacy of GABA.[1] Very large doses of these agents, e.g. diazepam 3400 mg/day[30] and morphine 235 mg/day,[36] may be required, and are well-tolerated.

Magnesium has been used as an adjunct to sedation[30,37]. Magnesium sulphate infusions to keep serum concentrations between 2.5 and 4.0 mmol/l have decreased systemic vascular resistance and pulse rate, with a small decrease in cardiac output.[30,37] In animal studies, magnesium inhibits release of adrenaline and noradrenaline, and reduces the sensitivity of receptors to these neurotransmitters.[38] Magnesium also has a marked neuromuscular blocking effect, and may reduce the intensity of muscle spasms. However, magnesium sulphate must be used with sedatives,[30] and calcium supplements may be needed when it is infused. Anecdotally, clonidine, a central α^2 stimulant, has successfully produced sedation with control of autonomic dysfunction.[39] Intrathecal baclofen has produced the same result in 15 cases, but significant respiratory depression occurred in a third.[40]

Supportive treatment

Steps should be taken to prevent contractures, nosocomial pneumonias and deep vein thrombosis. The patient (including the mother if a neonate is afflicted) must be actively immunized. Where possible, supportive psychotherapy should be offered to both patient and family.

Complications[1,2,9,11,12,17,41]

Muscle spasms disappear after 1–3 weeks, but residual stiffness may persist. Although most survivors recover completely by 6 weeks, cardiovascular complications, including cardiac failure, arrhythmias, pulmonary oedema and hypertensive crises can be fatal. No obvious cause of death can be found at autopsy in up to 20% of deaths. Other complications include those associated with factors shown in Table 47.1.

Outcome

Recovery from tetanus is thought to be complete. However, in 25 non-neonatal patients followed for up to 11 years,[42] 15 were reported to have one or more abnormal neurological features, such as intellectual or emotional changes, fits and myoclonic jerks, sleep disturbance, and decreased libido. Of the 10 apparently normal survivors, 6 had electroencephal-ogram changes. Some of these symptoms resolved within 2 years.

Mortality figures depend on the availability of

Table 47.1 Factors contributing to death in tetanus

Hypoxia

Complications of mechanical ventilation

Myoglobinuria and its attendant problems

Sepsis, particularly pneumonia

Fluid and electrolyte problems
(including inappropriate antidiuretic hormone secretion)

Deep vein thrombosis and embolic phenomena

Bed sores

Bony fractures

intensive care. In neonates, the mortality from African countries with no ICU facilities is 79% of cases,[43] but falls to 11% when artificial ventilation is used.[44] In the USA, mortality in non-neonates relates directly to age, with rates from 0% in patients under 30 years to 52% in those 60 years or older.[45] An average of 10% mortality would seem to be reasonable for most ICUs.[46] However, as this disease is easily and completely preventable, loss of life is unacceptable.

References

1 Bleck TP (1987) Tetanus: dealing with the continuing clinical challenge. *J Crit Illness* **2**:41–52.
2 Bleck TP (1991) Tetanus: pathophysiology, management and prophylaxis. *Dis Mon* **37**:556–603.
3 Warrell DA (1978) Tetanus and rabies. *Med J Aust* **5**:289–302.
4 Whitman C, Belgharbi L, Gasse F, Torel C, Mattei V, Zoffman H (1992) Progress towards the global elimina-tion of neonatal tetanus. *World Health Stat Quart* **45**:248–256.
5 Babaniyi OA, Parakoyi BD, Muhammad D (1991) Prospects of eliminating neonatal tetanus in Nigeria by the year 1995 (letter). *J Trop Pediat* **37**:264–266.
6 Ackerman AD (1987) Immunology and infections in the pediatric intensive care unit. Part B: Infectious diseases of particular importance to the pediatric intensivist. In: Rogers MC (ed.) *Textbook of Pediatric Intensive Care*, Baltimore: Williams and Wilkins, pp. 866–875.
7 Editorial (1983) Prevention of neonatal tetanus. *Lancet* **1**:1253–1254.
8 Da Silveira CM and De Quadros CA (1991) Neonatal tetanus: Countdown to 1995. *World Health Forum* **12**:289–296.
9 Stoll BJ (1979) Tetanus. *Pediatr Clin North Am* **26**:415–431.
10 Editorial (1974) Reactions to tetanus toxoid. *Br Med J* **1**:48.
11 Alfery DD and Rauscher LA (1979) Tetanus: a review. *Crit Care Med* **7**: 176–181.
12 Trujillo MJ, Catillo A, Espana JV, Guevarra P and Eganez H (1980) Tetanus in the adult: intensive care and

management experience with 233 cases. *Crit Care Med* 1980; **8**:419–423.

13 Kerr JH, Corbett JL, Prys-Roberts C, Crampton Smith A and Spalding JMK (1968) Involvement of the sympathetic nervous system in tetanus. *Lancet* **2**:236–241.

14 Wright DK, Lalloo UG, Nayiager S and Govender P (1989) Autonomic nervous system dysfunction in severe tetanus. Current perspectives. *Crit Care Med* **17**:371–375.

15 Tsueda K, Oliver PB and Richter RW (1974) Cardiovascular manifestations of tetanus. *Anesthesiology* **40**:588–592.

16 Kerr J (1979) Current topics in tetanus. *Intensive Care Med* **5**:105–110.

17 Rose AG (1974) Catecholamine-induced myocardial damage associated with phaeochromocytomas and tetanus. *S Afr Med J* **48**:1285–1289.

18 Weinstein L (1973) Tetanus. *N Engl J Med* **289**: 1293–1297.

19 Sun KO, Chan YW, Cheung RT, So PC, Yu YL and Li PC (1994) Management of tetanus: a review of 18 cases. *J R Soc Med* **87**:135–137.

20 Annotation (1976) Antitoxin in treatment of tetanus. *Lancet* **1**:944.

21 Benson CA and Harris AA (1986) Acute neurologic infections. *Med Clin North Am* **70**:1001–1002.

22 Abrutyn E and Berlin JA (1991) Intrathecal therapy in tetanus: a meta-analysis. *J Am Med Assoc* **266**:2262–2267.

23 Ahmadsyah I and Salim A (1985) Treatment of tetanus: an open study to compare the efficacy of procaine, penicillin and metronidazole. *Br Med J* **291**:648–650.

24 Clarke G and Hill RG (1972) Effects of a focal penicillin lesion on responses of rabbit cortical neurones to putative neurotransmitters. *Br J Pharmacol* **44**:435–441.

25 Buchanan N, Cane RD, Wolfson G and De Andrade M (1979) Autonomic dysfunction in tetanus: the effects of a variety of therapeutic agents, with special reference to morphine. *Intensive Care Med* **5**:65–68.

26 Barnes PK, Brindle Smith G, White WD and Tennant R (1982) Comparison of the effects of Org NC 45 and pancuronium bromide on heart rate and arterial pressure in anaesthetized man. *Br J Anaesth* **54**:435–439.

27 Spelman D and Newton-John H (1980) Continuous pancuronium infusion in severe tetanus. *Med J Aust* **1**:676.

28 Domenighetti GM, Savary G and Stricker H (1984) Hyperadrenergic syndrome in severe tetanus: extreme rise in catecholamines responsive to labetalol. *Br Med J* **288**:1483–1484.

29 Corbett JL, Kerr JH, Prys-Roberts C, Crampton Smith A and Spalding JMK (1969) Cardiovascular disturbances in severe tetanus due to overactivity of the sympathetic nervous system. *Anaesthesia* **4**:198–212.

30 Lipman J, James MFM, Erskine J, Plit ML and Eidelman J (1987) Autonomic dysfunction in severe tetanus: magnesium sulphate as an adjunct to deep sedation. *Crit Care Med* **15**:987–988.

31 Beards SC, Lipman J, Bothma P and Joynt GM (1994) Esmolol in a case of severe tetanus: adequate haemodynamic control despite markedly elevated catecholamine levels. *S Afr J Surg* **32**:33–35.

32 Buchanan N, Smit L, Cane RD and De Andrade M (1978) Sympathetic overactivity in tetanus: fatality associated with propranolol. *Br Med J* **2**:254–255.

33 Wesley AG, Hariparsad D, Pather M and Rocke DA (1983). Labetalol in tetanus. *Anaesthesia* **38**:243–249.

34 Edmondson RS and Flowers MW (1979) Intensive care in tetanus: management, complications and mortality in 100 cases. *Br Med J* **1**:1401–1404.

35 King WW and Cave DR (1991) Use of esmolol to control autonomic instability of tetanus. *Am J Med* **91**:425–428.

36 Rocke DA, Wesley AG, Pather M, Calver AD and Hariparsad D (1986) Morphine in tetanus – the management of sympathetic nervous system overactivity. *S Afr Med J* **70**:666–668.

37 James MFM and Manson EDM (1985) The use of magnesium sulphate infusions in the management of very severe tetanus. *Intensive Care Med* **11**:5–12.

38 Von Euler VS and Lishajko F (1973) Effects of Mg^{++} and Ca^{++} on noradrenaline release and uptake in adrenergic nerve granules in different media. *Acta Physiol Scand* **89**:415–422.

39 Sutton DN, Tremlett MR, Woodcock TE and Nielsen MS (1990) Management of autonomic dysfunction in severe tetanus: the use of magnesium sulphate and clonidine. *Intensive Care Med* **16**:75–80.

40 Saissy JM, Demaziere J, Vitris M *et al.* (1992) Treatment of severe tetanus by intrathecal injections of baclofen without artificial ventilation. *Intensive Care Med* **18**:241–244.

41 Potgieter PD (1983) Inappropriate ADH secretion in tetanus. *Crit Care Med* **11**:417–418.

42 Illis LS and Taylor FM (1971) Neurological and electroencephalographic sequelae of tetanus. *Lancet* **1**:826–830.

43 Einterz EM and Bates ME (1991) Caring for neonatal tetanus patients in a rural primary care setting in Nigeria: a review of 237 cases. *J Trop Pediatr* **37**:179–181.

44 Khoo BH, Lee EL and Lam KL (1978) Neonatal tetanus treated with high dosage diazepam. *Arch Dis Child* **53**:737–739.

45 MMWR CDC (1985) 34:43 Tetanus–United States 1982–1984. *J Am Med Assoc* **254**:2873–2878.

46 Fisher MM (1990) The luck paradox. *Crit Care Med* **18**:783–784.

48 Disorders of peripheral and motor neurones

GA Skowronski

Generalized disorders of the peripheral nervous system may require admission to the ICU. Some of these primarily affect the cell bodies of lower motor neurones in the anterior horns, such as motor neurone disease and poliomyelitis, while others reflect disturbances of peripheral nerve conduction, such as Guillain–Barré syndrome (GBS) and various similar polyneuropathies.

Guillain–Barré syndrome and related disorders

In 1834 James Wardrop reported a case of ascending sensory loss and weakness in a 35-year-old man, leading to almost complete quadriparesis over 10 days, and complete recovery over several months.[1] In 1859, Landry described an acute ascending paralysis occurring in 10 patients, 2 of whom died. Guillain, Barré and Strohl in 1916[2] reported 2 cases of motor weakness, paraesthesiae and muscle tenderness in association with increased protein in the cerebrospinal fluid (CSF; lumbar puncture for CSF examination was first described only in the 1890s).

Many variants of this syndrome have since been reported, and this is largely responsible for the confusion in nomenclature. The lack of specific diagnostic criteria has also been a problem. However, criteria proposed by the National Institute of Neurological and Communicative Disorders and Stroke (NINCDS) in 1978 are now widely accepted (Table 48.1).[3] The NINCDS systematic name for the disorder is acute inflammatory demyelinating polyradiculopathy (AIDP). Nevertheless, GBS remains an acceptable and more widely recognized alternative.

Incidence

Since the incidence of poliomyelitis has markedly declined due to mass immunization programmes, GBS has become the major cause of rapid-onset flaccid paralysis in previously healthy people, with

Table 48.1 Criteria to diagnose Guillain–Barré syndrome defined by the National Institute of Neurological and Communicative Diseases and Stroke (NINCDS)[48]

Features required for diagnosis
Progressive motor weakness of more than one limb
Areflexia or marked hyporeflexia
Cerebrospinal fluid cell counts of no more than 50 monocytes or 2 polymorphonuclear leukocytes

Features strongly supportive of the diagnosis
Progression over days to a few weeks
Relative symmetry
Mild sensory signs or symptoms
Cranial nerve involvement
Onset of recovery 2–4 weeks after halt of progression
Autonomic dysfunction
Initial absence of fever
Elevated cerebrospinal fluid protein after 1 week of symptoms
Abnormal electrodiagnostics with slowed conduction or prolonged F waves

Features required to rule out other diagnoses
No history of hexacarbon abuse
No evidence of porphyria
No history or culture evidence of diphtheria
No history or evidence of lead intoxication
Symptoms not purely sensory
No evidence for polio, botulism, toxic neuropathy, organophosphates or tick paralysis

an incidence of approximately 1.7 per 100 000.[4] Epidemics have occurred in large populations exposed to viral illness or immunization.[5] Immunosuppression and concurrent autoimmune disease may also be predisposing factors.[6,7] The disorder is twice as common in females, and commoner in the elderly. No consistent seasonal or racial predilection has been demonstrated.[8]

Aetiology

Most recent evidence supports the proposition that GBS is caused by immunologically mediated nerve injury.[9] Cell-mediated immunity, in particular, probably plays a significant role, and inflammatory cell infiltrates are often seen in association with the demyelination, which is generally regarded as the primary pathologic process.[10] Antibodies to a number of nervous system components have been demonstrated in GBS patients, but none is of clear diagnostic or pathogenic importance.[9]

Although the precise mechanism of sensitization is not known, clinical associations suggest that antecedent viral infections or immunizations are commonly involved. Infective agents implicated include influenza A, parainfluenza, varicella-zoster, Epstein–Barr, chickenpox, mumps, human immunodeficiency virus (HIV),[11] and measles virus, cytomegalovirus and *Mycoplasma. Campylobacter jejuni* gastroenteritis commonly precedes GBS and may be associated with a more severe clinical course.[12] Immunization against viral infections, tuberculosis, tetanus,[13] and typhoid have all preceded the development of GBS. Most of these associations are anecdotal and of doubtful aetiological significance, but 65% of patients present within a few weeks of a minor respiratory (43%) or gastrointestinal (21%) illness.

Pathogenesis[10]

The peripheral nerves of patients who have died of GBS show infiltration of the endoneurium by mononuclear cells, which tend to be distributed in a perivenular distribution. This inflammatory process may be distributed throughout the length of the nerves, but with more marked focal changes in the nerve roots, spinal nerves and major plexuses. Electron micrographs show macrophages actively stripping myelin from the bodies of Schwann cells and axons. In some cases, Wallerian degeneration of axons is also seen, and failure of regeneration in these cases may correspond with a poor clinical outcome. However, axonal degeneration is generally regarded as a 'bystander' effect of the primary demyelinating process.

The underlying immune response is complex and poorly understood, but serum from GBS patients produces myelin damage *in vitro* when complement is present.[14] Although antibodies to various glycolipids have been demonstrated in GBS, these are generally in low titre and can occasionally be seen in controls. Nevertheless, the basis of the effectiveness of plasma exchange and immunoglobulin therapy is likely to be blocking of demyelinating antibodies by several mechanisms.[15]

Clinical presentation

The majority of patients describe a minor illness in the 8 weeks prior to presentation, with a peak incidence 2 weeks beforehand. Approximately half the patients initially experience paraesthesiae, typically beginning in the hands and feet. One-quarter complain of motor weakness, and the remainder have both.[16] Motor weakness proceeds to flaccid paralysis, which becomes the predominant complaint. Objective loss of power and reduction or loss of tendon reflexes usually commence distally and ascend, but a more haphazard spread may occur. Cranial nerves are involved in 45% of cases, most commonly the facial nerve, followed by the glossopharyngeal and vagus nerves. In the Miller–Fisher syndrome, which may or may not be a variant of GBS,[17,18] cranial nerve abnormalities predominate, with ataxia, areflexia and ophthalmoplegia as the predominant features.

Sensory loss is generally mild, with paraesthesiae or loss of vibration and proprioception, but occasionally sensory loss, pain or hyperaesthesia can be prominent features. Autonomic dysfunction is common, and a major contributor to morbidity and mortality in ventilator-dependent cases.[19,20] Orthostatic or persistent hypotension, paroxysmal hypertension, and bradycardia are all described, as are fatal ventricular tachyarrhythmias. Adynamic ileus, urinary retention and abnormalities of sweating are also commonly seen. Central nervous system involvement, producing pyramidal or cerebellar signs, may occur rarely.

Differential diagnosis

Most of the important alternative diagnoses are listed as exclusion criteria in Table 48.1. A major differential diagnostic concern is that of a rapidly progressing spinal space-occupying lesion (e.g. epidural abscess). Of particular relevance to intensive care is the variant called critical illness polyneuropathy.[21,22] This disorder usually presents in the recovery phase of a severe systemic illness with persistent weakness, hyporeflexia and difficulty in weaning from respiratory support. There appear to be specific associations with severe sepsis, shock states and the acute respiratory distress syndrome (ARDS). There is also a possible link with the long-term use of steroidal muscle relaxants (pancuronium or vecuronium).[23] Electrophysiological and pathological features are those of purely axonal degeneration (features of a myopathy may also be seen when relaxants are implicated), in contrast with the demyelination seen in classical GBS, and the CSF protein level is normal. In addition, the prognosis appears worse than for classical GBS. It is not yet clear whether there is any effective treatment.

In patients with prolonged illness, the possibility of chronic inflammatory demyelinating polyradiculopathy (CIDP) should be considered.[24] In this condition, which is usually distinguished from GBS (AIDP), preceding viral infection is uncommon, the onset is more insidious and the course is one of slow worsening or stepwise relapses. Corticosteroids and plasma exchange are possibly effective in this disorder, but adequate studies of immunosuppressive drugs have not been carried out.

An intermediate subacute polyradiculopathy (SIDP) as well as a recurrent form of GBS are also described, and all of these variants may be part of the spectrum of a single condition.[24] However, a recently described purely motor axonal neuropathy (acute axonal motor neuropathy, AAMN), which causes seasonal childhood epidemics mimicking classical GBS in China and elsewhere,[25] appears to be a distinct entity.

Investigations

In over 90% of patients, CSF protein is increased (greater than 0.4 g/l), within a week of onset of symptoms.[26] The level does not correlate with the clinical findings. A pleocytosis with lymphocytes and monocytes in the CSF may be seen in a small proportion of patients, especially later in the disease. Nerve conduction studies may demonstrate reduced conduction velocity and prolonged distal latencies.[27] Again, there is no correlation between the severity of electrophysiological changes and the clinical findings.

Management

The management of the patient with severe and protracted GBS provides a major challenge, as the prognosis is generally excellent if complications can be treated early or avoided. These complications may be life-threatening, affect any of the major organ systems or result in permanent disability, and can be prevented only by meticulous attention to detail.

Specific therapy

Plasma exchange (plasmapheresis) is of value in GBS. Two large controlled trials showed a reduction in patients requiring mechanical ventilation, reduced duration of mechanical ventilation for those who required it, and reduced time to motor recovery and time to walking without assistance.[28,29] Mortality, however, was not altered. Plasma exchange was most effective when carried out within 7 days of onset of symptoms. The plasma exchange schedules consisted of three to five exchanges of 1–2 plasma volumes each, over 1–2 weeks. Adverse events are common, and some relate to the disease itself.[30] Fresh frozen plasma is reported to have more side effects than albumin as the replacement fluid.[30] Immunoglobulin therapy was as effective as plasmapheresis in a randomized study,[31] but deterioration and more relapses have recently been reported.[32,33] Insufficient data currently exist to justify its routine use. Available studies suggest that low- or high-dose corticosteroids are of no value.[34,35] However, large multicentre controlled trials have not been carried out.

Supportive care

Respiratory

In the spontaneously breathing patient, chest physiotherapy and careful monitoring of respiratory function are of paramount importance. Regular measurement of vital capacity is probably the best way to predict respiratory failure, and is more reliable than arterial blood gases[36] (which should also be performed regularly). Any patient with a vital capacity less than 15 ml/kg or 30% of the predicted level, or a rising arterial P_{CO_2} is likely to require mechanical ventilation.

Bulbar involvement should be carefully sought, as there is a significant risk of aspiration of upper airway secretions, gastric contents or ingested food. The cough reflex may be inadequate, and airway protection by tracheal intubation or tracheostomy is then required. Oral feeding should be stopped in any patient in whom bulbar involvement is suspected.

Mechanical ventilation is mandatory if coughing is inadequate, pulmonary collapse or consolidation are present, arterial blood gases are significantly abnormal, vital capacity is less than predicted tidal volume (approximately 10 ml/kg), or the patient is dyspnoeic, tachypnoeic or appears exhausted. Mechanical ventilation, if necessary, will probably be required for several weeks (although there is wide variation), and early tracheostomy should be considered.

Cardiovascular

Cardiac rhythm and blood pressure should be monitored. Induction of anaesthesia appears particularly likely to induce serious arrhythmias. Use of suxamethonium may contribute significantly to this,[37] and, as with many other neuromuscular disorders, should be avoided. Cardiovascular instability may also be exacerbated by a number of other drugs (Table 48.2). These should be avoided or used with great care.

Table 48.2 Drugs associated with cardiovascular instability in Guillain–Barré syndrome

Exaggerated hypotensive response
Phentolamine
Nitroglycerin
Hexamethonium
Edrophonium
Thiopentone
Morphine
Frusemide

Exaggerated hypertensive response
Phenylephrine
Ephedrine
Dopamine
Isoprenaline

Arrhythmias
Suxamethonium

Cardiac arrest
General anaesthesia

Modified from Dalos *et al.*,[19] with permission.

Mild hypotension and bradycardia may require no treatment, particularly if renal and cerebral function are maintained. However, blood volume expansion or inotropic drugs may be required in some cases, and occasionally pulmonary artery catheterization may be helpful.[36] Hypertension is often transient, but may occasionally require appropriate drug therapy. Hypoxia and hypercarbia should be excluded as causes.

Fluids, electrolytes and nutrition

Paralytic ileus is not uncommon, especially immediately following the institution of mechanical ventilation, and a period of parenteral nutrition may be required. However, wherever possible, nasoenteric feeding should be instituted because of its significantly greater safety. Energy and fluid requirements are considerably reduced in these patients.

Sedation and analgesia

In non-ventilated patients, sedation should be avoided because of the potential for worsening respiratory and upper airway function. In ventilated patients, sedation becomes less necessary as the patient becomes accustomed to the ventilator, but night sedation may help to preserve diurnal rhythms. Limb pain, particularly with passive movement, is very common and may be quite severe. Quinine, minor and non-steroidal analgesics and antidepressant drugs may all be tried, but opioids are often required. Methadone given twice daily by nasogastric tube is usually effective.

General and nursing care

A comprehensive programme of physiotherapy should be implemented by nurses and physiotherapists, with careful attention to pressure area care, and the maintenance of joint mobility and pulmonary function. Opportunistic infection should be actively sought with culture of urine and respiratory secretions at least twice weekly. Sites of vascular access should be inspected frequently, and changed whenever necessary. It may be possible to manage stable long-term patients without venous access. Care should be taken to prevent corneal ulceration and faecal impaction.

Prophylaxis against venous thromboembolism should be given, and enterally administered low-dose warfarin may be preferable to twice-daily heparin injections in long-stay patients. Psychological problems, especially depression, are common, and some patients are helped by antidepressant drugs. Good rapport between the patient and staff, the provision of television, radio and reading aids, and where possible, occasional trips outdoors, are all of great value.

Prognosis

Death in up to 25% of GBS patients has been reported in those requiring intensive care.[38] Many of these deaths were due to potentially avoidable problems such as respiratory arrest, ventilator malfunction and intercurrent sepsis, and considerably better results have been achieved.[28,39] Approximately 16% of patients suffer permanent disability. Those requiring mechanical ventilation (except for children),[40] those who show improvement after more than 3 weeks from maximum deficit, and those who have not improved within 1 month of onset have a greater risk of a poor outcome.[41] However, even in patients ventilated for more than 2 months, gradual improvement may continue for 18 months to 2 years.[42]

Motor neurone disease

This term refers to a large group of related disorders (Table 48.3), some of which are clearly genetically determined, while others arise sporadically, are of completely unknown aetiology, and are generally untreatable. The most common variant is the sporadic form known as amyotrophic lateral sclerosis, a relentlessly progressive degenerative disease which most commonly affects males over 50 years of age.[43]

Pathogenesis

The disease affects both upper and lower motor neurones. The involvement of either can predominate early on, giving rise to several clinically recognizable subgroups (Table 48.3). The cerebral cortex as well as the anterior horns of the spinal cord are involved, with shrinkage, degenerative pigmentation and, eventually, disappearance of the affected cells. As muscles are denervated, there is progressive atrophy of muscle fibres (amyotrophy), but, remarkably, sensory neurones as well as those concerned with autonomic function, coordination and higher cerebral function are all spared. The precise cause remains unknown. Postulated pathogenetic causes include oxygen free radicals, excess excitatory neurotrans-

Table 48.3 Degenerative motor neurone diseases

Amyotrophic lateral sclerosis
Spinal muscular atrophy
Bulbar palsy
Primary lateral sclerosis
Pseudobulbar palsy

Heritable motor neurone diseases
Autosomal recessive spinal muscular atrophy
Familial amyotrophic lateral sclerosis
Other

Associated with other degenerative disorders

Modified from Beal *et al.*,[48] with permission.

mitters and growth factor and immunological abnormalities.[44]

Clinical presentation

The earliest symptoms are those of insidiously developing limb weakness, often asymmetrical, accompanied by obvious muscle wasting. This classically affects the small muscles of the hand and may be accompanied by fasciculation. As time passes, the disease becomes more generalized and more symmetrical, with a mixture of upper and lower motor neurone signs (i.e. spasticity and hyperreflexia in addition to gross wasting). Bulbar and respiratory muscles are affected, but awareness and intellect are completely preserved. Death occurs in 50% of cases within 3–5 years, usually due to respiratory infection, aspiration or ventilatory failure from profound weakness. However, there is wide variability, and a few patients may survive for many years.

Diagnosis

There are no specific investigations, and the diagnosis must be made on clinical grounds together with electromyogram (EMG) evidence of denervation. The differential diagnosis includes high cervical cord or brainstem compression and chronic heavy metal poisoning. Poliomyelitis can also result in a syndrome of progressive weakness, wasting and fasciculation, beginning many years after the initial illness (the post-polio syndrome), and leading occasionally to respiratory failure and death.[45,46]

Management

Treatment is essentially symptomatic and supportive. No benefit has been shown with antioxidants, neurotransmitter inhibitors, growth factors and immunosuppressants.[44] Admission to ICU is sometimes requested when these patients present with an acute deterioration. The intensivist may be asked to assist with ambulatory or home respiratory support for gradually worsening chronic respiratory failure. Such cases present major ethical as well as clinical problems, but the provision of continuous positive airways pressure, pressure support or other modes of assisted ventilation can result in an improved quality of life, and possibly prolonged survival for carefully selected individuals.[47] Respiratory support may be given by facemask, nasal mask or, rarely, by tracheostomy using simple, compact ventilators. Some patients require only intermittent support, particularly at night or during periods of acute deterioration due to intercurrent illness. Long-term respiratory support outside the ICU is a major undertaking, requiring specific equipment and extensive liaison with the patient, the family and numerous specialized support services.

References

1 Wardrop J (1834) Clinical observations on various diseases. *Lancet* **1**:380.
2 Guillain G, Barré JA and Strohl A (1916) Sur un syndrome de radiculo-nevrites avec hyperalbuminose du liquide cephalorachidren sans reaction cellulaire. Remarques sur les caracteres cliniques et graphiques des reflexes tendineaux. *Bull Soc Med Hop Paris* **40**:1462.
3 Asbury AK, Aranson BG, Karp HR and MacFarlin DE (1978) Criteria for diagnosis of Guillain–Barré syndrome. *Ann Neurol* **3**:565–567.
4 Kennedy RH, Danielson MA, Mulder DW and Kurland LT (1978) Guillain–Barré syndrome: a 42 year epidemiological and clinical study. *Mayo Clin Proc* **53**:93–99.
5 Sliman NA (1978) Outbreak of Guillain–Barré syndrome associated with water pollution. *Br Med J* **1**:751–752.
6 Lisak RP, Mitchell M, Zweiman B, Orrechio E and Asbury AK (1977) Guillain–Barré syndrome and Hodgkin's disease. Three cases with immunological studies. *Ann Neurol* **1**:72–78.
7 Korn-Lubetzki I and Abramsky O (1986) Acute and chronic demyelinating inflammatory polyradiculoneuropathy: association with auto-immune diseases and lymphocyte response to human neuritogenic protein. *Arch Neurol* **43**:604–608.
8 Alter M (1990) The epidemiology of Guillain–Barré syndrome. *Ann Neurol* **27**(suppl):S7–S12.
9 Kornberg AJ and Pestronk A (1993) Immune-mediated neuropathies. *Curr Opin Neurol* **6**:681–687.
10 Honavar M, Tharakan JK, Hughes RA, Leibowitz S and Winer JB (1991) A clinicopathological study of the Guillain–Barré syndrome. Nine cases and literature review. *Brain* **114**:1245–1269.
11 Simpson DM and Olney RK (1992) Peripheral neuropathies associated with human immunodeficiency virus infection. *Neurol Clin* **10**:685–711.
12 Lees JH, Gregson NA, Griffiths PL and Hughes RA (1993) *Campylobacter jejuni* and Guillain–Barré syndrome. *Q J Med* **86**:623–634.
13 Newton N and Janoti A (1987) Guillain–Barré syndrome after vaccination with parified tetanus toxoid. *South Med J* **80**:1053–1054.
14 Sawant S, Clark MB and Koski CL (1991) *in vitro* demyelination by serum antibody from patients with Guillain–Barré syndrome requires terminal complement complexes. *Ann Neurol* **29**:397–404.
15 Steck AJ (1992) Inflammatory neuropathy pathogenesis and clinical features. *Curr Opin Neurol* **5**:633–637.
16 Loffel NB, Rossi LN, Mumethaler M, Lashig J and Ludin HP (1977) Landry–Guillain–Barré syndrome: complications, prognosis and natural history in 123 cases. *J Neurol Sci* **33**:71–79.
17 Fisher CM (1956) Unusual variant of acute idiopathic polyneuritis (syndrome of ophthalmoplegia, ataxia and areflexia). *N Engl J Med* **255**:57–65.
18 Najim al-Din AS, Anderson M, Eeg-Olofsson O and Trontelj JV (1994) Neuroophthalmic manifestations of the syndrome of ophthalmoplegia ataxia and areflexia.

Observations on 20 patients. *Acta Neurol Scand* **89:**87–94.

19 Dalos NO, Borel C and Hanley DF (1988) Cardiovascular autonomic dysfunction in Guillain–Barré syndrome. Therapeutic implications of Swan Ganz monitoring. *Arch Neurol* **45:**115–117.

20 Truax BT (1984) Autonomic disturbances in the Guillain–Barré syndrome. Semin Neurol **4:**462–468.

21 Leijten FS and de Weerd AW (1994) Critical illness polyneuropathy. A review of the literature, definition and pathophysiology. *Clin Neurol Neurosurg* **96:**10–19.

22 Bolton Ch F (1993) Neuromuscular abnormalities in critically ill patients. *Intensive Care Med* **19:**309–310.

23 Margolis B, Kachikian D, Friedman Y *et al.* (1991) Prolonged reversible quadriparesis in mechanically ventilated patients who received long-term infusions of vecuronium. *Chest* **100:**877–878.

24 Hughes RA (1994) The spectrum of acquired demyelinating polyradiculopathy. *Acta Neurol Belg* **94:**128–132.

25 McKhann GM, Cornblath DR, Griffin JW *et al.* (1993) Acute motor axonal neuropathy: a frequent cause of acute flaccid paralysis in China. *Ann Neurol* **33:**333–342.

26 Moore P and James O. (1981) Guillain–Barré syndrome: incidence, management and outcome of major complications. *Crit Care Med* **9:**549–555.

27 Olney RK and Aminoff MJ (1990) Electrodiagnostic features of the Guillain–Barré syndrome: the relative sensitivities of different techniques. *Neurology* **40:**471–475.

28 French cooperative group on plasma exchange in Guillain–Barré syndrome (1987) EEfficiency of plasma exchange in Guillain–Barré syndrome: role of replacement fluids. *Ann Neurol* **22:**753–761.

29 The Guillain–Barré study group (1985) Plasmapheresis and acute Guillain–Barré syndrome. *Neurology* **35:**1096–1104.

30 Bouget J, Chevret S, Chastang C *et al.* Plasma exchange morbidity in Guillain–Barré syndrome: results from the French prospective, double-blind, randomized, multicenter study. *Crit Care Med* **21:**651–658.

31 Van der Mech FGA and Schmitz PIM (1992) The Dutch Guillain–Barré study group. A randomised trial comparing intravenous immune globulin and plasma exchange in Guillain–Barré syndrome. *N Engl J Med* **326:**1123–1129.

32 Irani DN, Cornblath DR, Chaudry V and Borel C (1993) Hanley DF Relapse in Guillain–Barré syndrome after treatment with human immune globulin. *Neurology* **45:**872–875.

33 Castro LH and Ropper AH (1993) Human immune globulin infusion in Guillain–Barré syndrome: worsening during and after treatment. *Neurology* **43:**875–878.

34 Hughes RAC, Newsom-Davis JM and Perkins GD (1978) Controlled trial of prednisolone in acute polyneuropathy. *Lancet* **ii:**750–753.

35 Guillain–Barré syndrome steroid trial group (1993) Double-blind trial of intravenous methylprednisolone in Guillain–Barré syndrome. *Lancet* **341:**586–590.

36 Hund EF, Borel CO, Cornblath DR, Hanley DF and McKhann GM (1993) Intensive management and treatment of severe Guillain–Barré syndrome. *Crit Care Med* **21:**433–466.

37 Fergusson RJ, Wright DJ, Willey RJ, Crompton GK and Grant WB (1981) Suxamethonium is dangerous in polyneuropathy. *Br Med J* **282:**298–299.

38 Scott IA, Seeley G, Wright M, Boyle RS and Ravenscroft PJ (1988) Guillain–Barré syndrome: a retrospective review. *Aust NX J Med* **18:**149–155.

39 Ropper AH and Kehne SM (1985) Guillain–Barré syndrome: management of respiratory failure. *Neurology* **35:**1662–1665.

40 Cole GF and Matthew DJ (1987) Prognosis in severe Guillain–Barré syndrome. *Arch Dis Child* **62:**288–291.

41 Winer JB, Greenwood RJ, Hughes RAC, Perkin GD and Healy MJR (1985) Prognosis in Guillain–Barré syndrome. *Lancet* **1:**1202–1203.

42 Ropper AH (1986) Severe acute Guillain–Barré syndrome. *Neurology* **36:**429–432.

43 Williams DB and Windebank AJ (1991) Motor neuron disease (amyotrophic lateral sclerosis). *Mayo Clin Proc* **66:**54–82.

44 Orrell RW, Lane RJM and Guiloff (1994) Recent developments in the drug treatment of motor neurone disease. *Br Med J* **309:**140–141.

45 Fischer DA (1985) Poliomyelitis: late respiratory complications and management. *Orthopedics* **8:**891–894.

46 Halstead LS and Rossi CD (1985) New problems in old polio patients: results of a survey of 539 polio survivors. *Orthopedics* **8:**845–850.

47 Edwards PR and Howard P (1993) Methods and prognosis of non-invasive ventilation in neuromuscular disease. *Monaldi Arch Chest Dis* **48:**176–182.

48 Beal MF, Richardson EP and Martin JB (1991) Degenerative diseases of the nervous system. In: Wilson JD, Braundwald E, Isselbacher KJ *et al.* (eds) *Harrison's Principles of Internalk Medicine.* New York: McGraw-Hill, pp. 2060–2075.

GA Skowronski

Myasthenia gravis (MG), botulism and periodic paralysis are a group of disorders of muscles and the neuromuscular junction which may require ICU care.

Myasthenia gravis

MG is an autoimmune disorder caused by antibodies directed against acetylcholine (ACh) receptors in skeletal muscle. Despite its relative rarity, it is the most studied and best understood clinical disorder of neuroreceptor function, and arguably the best understood organ-specific autoimmune disease. It is characterized clinically by weakness or exaggerated fatigability on sustained effort. Intensive care is most commonly required because of severe involvement of the bulbar or respiratory muscles, which may be the result of a spontaneous exacerbation of the disease, complication of drug therapy, intercurrent illness or surgery, or following surgical thymectomy – the treatment of choice for most patients.

Incidence

The incidence of MG is approximately 1 in 20 000 in the USA. There is no racial or geographic predilection. Although MG can occur at any age, it is very rare in the first 2 years of life, and the peak incidence is in young adult females. Overall, females are affected about twice as often as males. This sexual preference decreases with increasing age, and there is a smaller, second incidence peak in elderly males.[1]

Aetiology and pathophysiology

In 75% of cases, there is histological evidence of thymic abnormality. Thymic hyperplasia is present in the majority of patients, but approximately 10% have a thymoma. The latter appears more common in the older age group. The precise role of the thymus is uncertain, but ACh receptors are present in myoid cells in the normal thymus, and there is evidence that anti-ACh receptor antibody production is mediated by both B and T lymphocytes of thymic origin. Other organ-specific autoimmune disorders, most commonly thyroid disease,[2] but also rheumatoid arthritis, lupus erythematosus and pernicious anaemia, are significantly associated with MG, and autoantibodies to other organs may be seen in MG patients without evidence of disease.

Children born to mothers with MG demonstrate transient weakness ('neonatal MG') in about 15% of cases. A number of congenital myasthenic syndromes exist, in which symptoms develop in infancy, without evidence of autoantibody production.[3] A familial tendency is more common in this group, and structural changes at the neuromuscular junction have been demonstrated.

The stimulus to autoantibody production is not known, but these can be detected in about 90% of patients with generalized myasthenia. They may interfere with neuromuscular transmission by competitively blocking receptor sites, by initiating immune-mediated destruction of receptors, or by binding to portions of the receptor molecule which are not part of the ACh receptor site, but which, nevertheless, are important in allowing ACh to bind.

Clinical presentation

Ptosis and diplopia are the most common initial symptoms, and in 20% of cases, the disorder remains confined to the eye muscles (ocular MG).[4] Bulbar muscle weakness is common and may result in nasal regurgitation, dysarthria and dysphagia. Limb and trunk weakness can occur with varying distribution, and is usually asymmetrical. Some patients complain of fatigue rather than weakness, and may be misdiagnosed as having psychogenic symptoms. However, weakness can be elicited by sustained effort of an involved muscle group, e.g. sustained upward gaze is often worse at the end of the day and improves with rest.

Investigations

Impairment of neuromuscular transmission may be confirmed by a positive edrophonium (Tensilon) test. Atropine 0.6 mg is given IV to prevent muscarinic side-effects, and this is followed by 1 mg edrophonium. If there is no obvious improvement within 1–2 min, a further 5 mg may be given. Some authors recommend the use of a saline placebo injection, and the presence of a second doctor as a 'blinded' observer. Resuscitation facilities should be available, as profound weakness may ensue, especially in patients already receiving anticholinesterase drugs. Intramuscular neostigmine, 1–2 mg, may produce a positive response in 5–10% of patients who do not respond to edrophonium.[5]

The presence of autoantibodies against ACh receptors is quite specific, but false positives occur in patients with penicillamine-treated rheumatoid disease, other autoimmune diseases and in some first-degree relatives of myasthenic patients.[6] Electromyography shows characteristic changes in 90% of patients with generalized MG, and also in many patients with ocular symptoms only.

A syndrome of myasthenic weakness occurs in association with malignancy and other autoimmune diseases (Eaton–Lambert syndrome). Although fatigability is present, the pelvic and thigh muscles are predominantly affected, whereas ocular and bulbar involvement are rare. Tendon reflexes are reduced or absent, and there are specific electromyographic changes.

Management

1 *Symptomatic treatment* is provided by anticholinesterase drugs which potentiate the action of ACh at receptor sites. Pyridostigmine (Mestinon) is the most commonly used, and is usually commenced at a dose of 60 mg orally four times daily. Considerable adjustment of dosage may be required.

2 *Thymectomy* produces the best results, and early thymectomy is now advocated as the treatment of choice in virtually all patients, regardless of the severity of disease or the presence of a thymoma. Compared with medical therapy, thymectomy results in an earlier onset of remission, lower mortality and greater delay in the appearance of extrathymic recurrences.[7]

Preoperative optimization of neuromuscular function is essential, using anticholinesterase drugs, supplemented by plasma exchange if necessary. Though anticholinesterase requirements are usually reduced in the immediate postoperative period to about three-quarters of the preoperative dose, sustained improvement following thymectomy may not be seen for many months. A transcervical approach has been advocated, but doubts remain about the completeness of excision by this route.

The traditional sternotomy approach continues to be much more widely used.[8]

3 *Corticosteroids* are effective in approximately 70% of patients, and give best results when high doses (e.g. prednisolone 100 mg/day) are used initially, and then gradually reduced. However, transient exacerbation upon commencement of steroids is very common,[9] and severely affected patients are often hospitalized for the initiation of therapy. Older patients are more likely to respond, but an average of 4 months' treatment is required to achieve clinical stability, and the majority will require continuing treatment indefinitely.[10]

4 *Azathioprine and cyclophosphamide* are both effective adjuncts to corticosteroid therapy, especially in patients with thymoma. Overall, 80% of patients are helped, but improvement may be seen only after some months. A few patients may achieve complete remission.[11] Cyclosporin is also effective, and patients may show benefit more quickly than with azathioprine.[12]

5 *Plasma exchange* is effective in producing short-term clinical improvement.[13] It is mainly used in myasthenic crisis or to improve severely affected patients before thymectomy. Its use should be considered, particularly in patients with severe respiratory failure refractory to conventional therapy (see below).[14] Typically, five exchanges of 3–4 l each are performed over a 2-week period, and this results in improvement within days. However, the benefits are short-lived, lasting only weeks.[15]

6 *IV γ-globulin* has similar effects to those of plasma exchange. A dose of 400 mg/kg per day is usually given for 5 successive days, and occasional patients derive long-term benefit.[16] Interestingly, γ-globulin has no consistent effect on ACh receptor antibody concentrations, and its mechanism of action is unknown.

Myasthenic and cholinergic crisis

Patients with known MG may undergo life-threatening episodes of acute deterioration. These may follow intercurrent infection, pregnancy or the administration of various drugs (Table 49.1). Such episodes, known as myasthenic crises, usually resolve over several weeks, but occasionally last months. The incidence of myasthenic crisis increases markedly with age.[17]

These patients should be admitted directly to the ICU, as there is a significant risk of pulmonary aspiration due to bulbar involvement, bacterial pneumonia due to stasis, and acute respiratory failure or cardiorespiratory arrest. After stabilization and resuscitation, if necessary, an edrophonium (Tensilon) test should be performed. This will indicate whether the patient can be expected to respond to increased dosage of anticholinergic drugs.

If the condition is worsened by edrophonium, the

Table 49.1 Drugs which may exacerbate myasthenia gravis

Antibiotics
Streptomycin
Kanamycin
Tobramycin
Gentamicin
Polymyxin group
Tetracycline

Antiarrhythmics
Quinidine
Quinine
Procainamide

Local anaesthetics
Procaine
Lignocaine

General anaesthetics
Ether

Muscle relaxants
Curare
Suxamethonium

Analgesics
Morphine
Pethidine

patient is likely to be suffering from overadministration of anticholinesterase drugs (i.e. cholinergic crisis). Abdominal cramps, diarrhoea, excessive pulmonary secretions, sweating, salivation and bradycardia may be present; the patient may improve if anticholinesterase drugs are reduced in dosage or withdrawn temporarily and restarted after 1–2 days. Frequent estimations of vital capacity and maximum inspiratory force should be made and recorded. Tracheal intubation and mechanical ventilation should be considered in patients with significant bulbar involvement or clinical evidence of worsening respiratory failure. As with other neuromuscular disorders, deterioration of blood gases may occur late, and is an unreliable sign of progressive respiratory failure.[18] Aggressive chest physiotherapy, urinary drainage and nasogastric feeding may be required. Hypokalaemia, hypocalcaemia and hypermagnesaemia should be avoided, as all may exacerbate muscle weakness.

If the patient's clinical status cannot be rapidly improved by the adjustment of anticholinesterase dosage and aggressive treatment of intercurrent illness, high-dose corticosteroids and plasma exchange should be commenced simultaneously, and may produce some benefit within as little as 24 h.

Perioperative management

MG patients often require intensive care in relation to surgery for intercurrent illness or, more often, thymectomy. Unstable patients should be admitted to hospital some days in advance for stabilization. In severely affected patients, preoperative high-dose corticosteroids and/or plasma exchange may be used to improve the patient's fitness for surgery. It may be prudent to omit premedication, and an anaesthetic technique which avoids the use of non-depolarizing muscle relaxants is usually advocated, though vecuronium and atracurium are probably acceptable in reduced dosage.[19,20] Suxamethonium can be used safely in normal dosage.[21]

Up to one-third of patients require continuing mechanical ventilation postoperatively following thymectomy. Predictive factors include a long preoperative duration of myasthenia, coexistent chronic respiratory disease, high anticholinesterase requirements (e.g. pyridostigmine > 750 mg/day), and a preoperative vital capacity of less than 2.9 l.[22] In those cases requiring mechanical ventilation, some authors advocate temporary cessation of anticholinesterase drugs to reduce respiratory secretions[23] but in all other cases they should be continued, though dosage requirements must be reassessed carefully and repeatedly.

Botulism

Botulism is a widespread but very uncommon potentially lethal disease caused by preformed exotoxins produced by *Clostridium botulinum* – an anaerobic, spore-forming Gram-positive bacillus. Food-borne, wound and infantile forms of botulism are described.

Aetiology

Strains of *C. botulinum* produce seven antigenically distinct exotoxins, types A to G,[24] but human botulism is caused mostly by types A, B and E. *C. botulinum* spores are widely distributed in soil, especially aquatic soil. The spores are moderately resistant to heat (e.g. they withstand boiling for several hours).

The vast majority of botulism is food-borne and outbreaks are largely due to home-preserved vegetables (type A toxin), meat (type B) or fish (type E), but high-risk foods also include low-acid fruit and condiments. Wound botulism[25] arises rarely, when wounds (typically open fractures) are contaminated by soil containing type A or B organisms. Chronic intravenous drug abusers are also at risk.[26] Signs and symptoms are caused by toxin production *in vivo*.

Pathophysiology[24]

Food-borne botulism is caused by ingestion of preformed botulinum exotoxin. The exotoxin is absorbed (primarily in the upper small intestine), and carried by the blood stream to cholinergic nerves at the neuromuscular junction, postganglionic parasympathetic nerve endings and autonomic ganglia, to which it irreversibly binds. The toxin enters the nerve endings to interfere with ACh release. No predisposing factors leading to infection have been identified.

Clinical presentation[27]

With food-borne botulism, most patients become ill about 3 days after ingestion of toxin, but symptoms may appear from 12 h to 16 days. The commonest presenting features include gastrointestinal (nausea, vomiting, abdominal pain, diarrhoea or constipation) and ocular symptoms (blurred vision, mydriasis, diplopia or ptosis), dryness of the eyes and mouth, dysphagia and generalized weakness. The severity of illness is related to early onset. Patients are alert and afebrile in the absence of complications. Cranial nerve dysfunction is manifested by ptosis and extraocular muscle palsies, impaired gag reflex, facial muscle and tongue weakness. Muscle weakness progresses in a symmetrical descending fashion. In severe cases, respiratory insufficiency and flaccid weakness of upper and lower limbs are present. Deep tendon reflexes are normal or decreased.

Wound botulism is similar to food-borne botulism, except that gastrointestinal tract (GIT) manifestations do not occur.

Diagnosis and investigations

The differential diagnosis of botulism includes food poisoning from other causes, MG and the Guillain–Barré syndrome. Botulism is diagnosed on clinical grounds, and confirmed by the presence of toxin (either in the patient or in contaminated food) in about two-thirds of cases. This may be detected by a mouse bioassay or enzyme-linked immunosorbent assay.

The following investigations may be helpful in eliminating alternative diagnoses:

1 *Cerebrospinal fluid examination* will be normal, in contrast to typical cases of Guillain–Barré syndrome (although the protein level may be mildly elevated in a few cases, and conversely, may be normal in the early course of the Guillain–Barré syndrome).
2 An *edrophonium (Tensilon) test* may help exclude MG although transient, less impressive responses may be seen with botulism patients.
3 A *12-lead electrocardiogram (ECG)* may show minor conduction disturbances and non-specific T wave and S-T changes.
4 *Nerve conduction studies* will be normal.
5 *Electromyography* of affected muscles demonstrates evidence of a presynaptic block in only about one-third of cases.[27]
6 *Isolation of C botulinium* from stool is considered confirmatory, as it is rarely found in stools of normal individuals.

Management

Treatment for botulism is mainly supportive.

1 *Respiratory care*: Close monitoring and support of respiratory function are of paramount importance. Monitoring techniques and the indications for intervention are as for other neurological and neuromuscular diseases. Endotracheal intubation and mechanical ventilation should be initiated if bulbar palsy is significant, or when respiratory failure is present (e.g. where vital capacity is less than 10–15 ml/kg with hypoxaemia and hypercarbia). The risk for respiratory failure is greatest within the first 2 days of hospitalization.[28]
2 *Metabolic support*: Close attention must be paid to fluid balance, electrolyte homeostasis (especially if diarrhoea is severe) and the provision of nutrition. Parenteral or enteral nutrition is frequently necessary.
3 *Prevention and treatment of complications*: These principles are similar to those for other neurological and neuromuscular diseases.
4 *GIT toxin removal*: In the absence of profound ileus, removal of unabsorbed toxin from the GIT may be attempted by water, saline or cathartic enemas. Magnesium-containing cathartics should probably not be used, as increased magnesium levels may theoretically enhance the toxin.
5 *Antitoxin*: If the toxin type is known, and symptoms are severe, monovalent antitoxin should be used if available. Otherwise equine trivalent (ABE) botulinus antitoxin can be given, although its efficacy in humans has not been proven by prospective data. Significant efficacy has only been reported for type E toxin illness; hypersensitivity reactions occur in 9% of recipients.[29] As a result, there is little justification for the use of antitoxin in milder cases.[27] If used, it must be given early, since only circulating toxin is neutralized. A history of asthma, hay fever or previous administration of equine serum are relative contraindications. Adrenaline and full resuscitation facilities must be available, and the precautions and technique of administration are similar to those used with other equine antivenoms. Doses of antitoxin may be repeated 4-hourly if signs and symptoms continue to worsen.
6 *Guanidine/antibiotics*: Guanidine hydrochloride, which enhances the release of ACh from nerve terminals, has been reported to improve muscle strength, especially in ocular muscles, and may be more appropriate than antitoxin for milder cases.[30] It appears to have less efficacy for respiratory than for ocular muscles. Antibiotics should be reserved for specific infectious complications. Aminoglycosides may worsen muscle weakness.
7 *Treatment of wound botulism*: Apart from supportive measures, wound debridement should be performed. Penicillin is generally given, although its efficacy is not proven.

Prognosis

Most patients begin to improve within a week or so, and only a small minority require ventilatory support. Prognosis is influenced adversely by a short incubation period, early involvement of cranial nerves and respiratory muscles, and possibly by age and race (it is more severe in Asian people). Evidence regarding the influence of toxin serotype is conflicting. Overall mortality figures vary from extremely low up to as high as 50%, but with modern intensive care very few (if any) botulism patients should die, as the outlook for complete recovery is excellent once the patient survives the paralytic illness. However, general weakness, constipation and mild cranial nerve abnormalities may persist for some months.

Infant botulism[31-34]

Botulism infections have been reported in infants aged from 1 week to 9 months, with 95% of victims aged under 6 months. Type A and B strains are associated, and honey ingestion is considered a risk factor. In contrast to adult food-borne botulism, infant botulism results from ingestion of spores which germinate and produce toxins in the infant's GIT.

The clinical picture may vary from mild constipation to sudden death, which is indistinguishable from the sudden infant (cot) death syndrome. Usually, neurological signs (e.g. weak cry, impaired sucking, drooling and floppy head) follow 1–3 weeks after constipation. The differential diagnosis includes other diseases which produce hypotonia in infants (e.g. sepsis, infectious mononucleosis, virus infections or diphtheria). The diagnosis is confirmed by isolation of toxin or organism from stools. Unlike adult disease, infants rarely have toxin detected in serum. Treatment is supportive, and the mortality rate is about 2%.

Periodic paralysis

This term describes a group of rare primary disorders, mostly inherited as autosomal dominant traits, producing episodic weakness. They must be distinguished from other causes of intermittent weakness, including electrolyte abnormalities, MG and transient ischaemic attacks. In the inherited disorders, symptoms begin early in life (before age 25), and follow rest or sleep rather than exertion. Alertness during attacks is completely preserved, and muscle strength between attacks is normal. Treatment is usually successful in preventing both the attacks and the chronic weakness, which can develop after many years in untreated patients.

Hypokalaemic periodic paralysis[35]

This disorder is predominantly inherited, but one-third of cases are sporadic. Hypokalaemic periodic paralysis can also occur in young men,

particularly those of Latin American or oriental origin, in association with thyrotoxicosis. The underlying cause appears to be a disturbance in the adenosine triphosphate-sensitive potassium channel in skeletal muscle.[36] The degree of hypokalaemia during attacks is not profound, and total body potassium is normal, but there seems to be excessive potassium transport into muscle, especially in response to insulin.

Symptoms usually commence in adolescence, with attacks of with widely varying frequency and duration. These may be precipitated by meals high in carbohydrate or sodium, and paralysis may rarely involve bulbar or respiratory muscles, with an attendant risk of death. Cardiac arrhythmias may also occur during attacks. Examination between attacks is normal, as is the serum potassium concentration, and suspicion is usually aroused on the basis of history alone. Provocative testing with glucose and insulin can be done if necessary, but may be hazardous.

Acute attacks respond to potassium administration, which can be given orally if the patient can swallow, or IV, with careful monitoring of the serum potassium concentration. Paradoxically, potassium administration is not effective in prophylaxis, for which the best agent appears to be acetazolamide. This may block the flux of potassium into muscle, and its effectiveness may be related to the metabolic acidosis it produces.

Potassium-sensitive (hyperkalaemic or normokalaemic) periodic paralysis

In these disorders, attacks are briefer, more frequent, and much less severe (never fatal). Clear evidence of autosomal dominant transmission is more common, and many patients demonstrate myotonia. Attacks are usually precipitated by fasting, or by rest following exercise, and provocative testing with potassium administration is positive. Serum potassium may be modestly elevated during attacks, but is often normal. Bulbar and respiratory involvement is less likely than in the hypokalaemic form. The underlying mechanism appears to be a point mutation in the gene encoding the α-subunit of the sodium channel of skeletal muscle, located on chromosome 17.[37]

Acute attacks can be managed with oral glucose or carbohydrate, while prophylaxis with either acetazolamide or thiazide diuretics is effective.

References

1 Kurtze JF and Kurland LT (1992) The epidemiology of neurologic disease. In: Joynt RJ (ed.) *Clinical Neurology*, vol. 4. Philadelphia: JB Lippincott, pp. 80–88.

2 Osserman KE, Tsairis P and Weiner LB (1967) Myasthenia gravis and thyroid disease. Clinical and immunological correlation. *Mt Sinai J Med* **34**:469–483.

3 Penn AS, Richman DP, Ruff RL and Lennon VA (eds) (1993) Myasthenia gravis and related disorders: experi-

mental and clinical aspects. *Ann NY Acad Sci* **681**:425–514.

4 Grobb D, Arsura EL, Brunner NG and Namba T. (1987) The course of myasthenia gravis and therapies affecting outcome. *Ann NY Acad Sci* **505**:472–499.

5 Osserman KE and Genkins G (1966) Critical reappraisal of the use of edrophonium (Tensilon) chloride tests in myasthenia gravis and significance of clinical observation. *Ann NY Acad Sci* **135**:312–326.

6 Vincent A and Newsom-Davis J (1985) Acetylcholine receptor antibody as a diagnostic test for myasthenia gravis: results in 153 validated cases and 2967 diagnostic assays. *J Neurol Neurosurg Psychiatry* **48**:1246–1252.

7 Papatestas AE, Genkins G, Kornfeld P *et al.* (1987) Effects of thymectomy in myasthenia gravis. *Ann Surg* **206**:79–88.

8 Younger DS, Jaretzky A III, Penn AS *et al.* (1987) Maximum thymectomy for myasthenia gravis. *Ann NY Acad Sci* **505**:832–835.

9 Johns TR (1987) Long-term corticosteroid treatment of myasthenia gravis. *Ann NY Acad Sci* **505**:568–583.

10 Sghirlanzoni A, Peluchetti D, Mantegazza R, Fiacchino F and Cornelio F (1984) Myasthenia gravis: prolonged treatment with steroids. *Neurology* **34**:170–174.

11 Niakan E, Harati Y and Rolak LA. Immunosuppressive drug therapy in myasthenia gravis. *Arch Neurol* **43**:155–156.

12 Schalke BCG, Kappos L, Rohrbach E *et al.* (1988) Ciclosporin A vs azathioprine in the treatment of myasthenia gravis: final results of a randomised, controlled double-blind clinical trial. *Neurology* **38** (suppl 1):135 (abstract)

13 Dau PC, Lindstrom JM, Cassel CK, Denys Eh, Shev EE and Spitler LE (1977) Plasmapheresis and immunosuppressive drug therapy in myasthenia gravis. *N Engl J Med* **297**:1134–1140.

14 Gracey DR, Howard FM and Divertie MB (1984) Plasmapheresis in the treatment of ventilator-dependent myasthenia gravis patients. Report of four cases. *Chest* **85**:739-743.

15 Drachman DB (1994) Myasthenia gravis. *N Engl J Med* **330**:1797–1810.

16 Arsura E (1989) Experience with intravenous immunoglobulin in myasthenia gravis. *Clin Immunol Immunopathol* **53**:(suppl)S170–S179.

17 Sellman MS and Mayer RF (1985) Treatment of myasthenic crisis in late life. *South Med J* **78**:1208–1210.

18 Harrison BDW, Collins JV, Brown KGE and Clark THJ (1971) Respiratory failure in neuromuscular diseases. *Thorax* **26**:579–584.

19 Bell CF, Florence AM, Hunter JM, Jones RS and Utting JE (1984) Atracurium in the myasthenic patient. *Anaesthesia* **39**:691–698.

20 Eisenkraft JB, Sawkney RK and Papatestas AE (1986) Vecuronium in the myasthenic patient. *Anaesthesia* **41**:666–667.

21 Wainwright AP and Broderick PM (1987) Suxamethonium in myasthenia gravis. *Anaesthesia* **42**:950–957.

22 Eisenkraft JB, Papatestas AE, Kahn CH, Mora CT, Fagerstrom R and Genkins G (1986) Predicting the need for postoperative mechanical ventilation in myasthenia gravis. *Anesthesiology* **65**:79–82.

23 Gracey DR, Divertie MB, Howard FM, Payne WS (1984) Postoperative respiratory care after transternal thymectomy in myasthenia gravis. *Chest* **1**:67–71.

24 Simpson LL (1982) The origin, structure, and pharmacological activity of botulinum toxin. *Pharmacol Rev* **33**:155–188.

25 Fullerton P, Gogna N and Stoddart R (1980) Wound botulism. *Med J Aust* **1**:662–663.

26 MacDonald KL, Rutherford GW, Friedman SM *et al.* (1984) Botulism and botulism-like illness in chronic drug abusers. *Ann Intern Med* **102**:616–618.

27 Roblot P, Roblot F, Fauchere JL *et al.* (1994) Retrospective study of 108 cases of botulism in Poitiers, France. *J Med Microbiol* **40**:379–384.

28 Schmidt-Nowara WW, Samet JM and Rosario PA (1983) Early and late pulmonary complications of botulism. *Arch Intern Med* **143**:451–456.

29 Black RE and Gunn RA (1980) Hypersensitivity reactions associated with botulinal antitoxin. *Am J Med* **65**:567–570.

30 Puggiari M and Cherington M (1978) Botulism and guanidine. Ten years later. *J Am Med Assoc* **240**:2276–2277.

31 Arnon SS (1980) Infant botulism. *Ann Rev Med* **31**:541–560.

32 Arnon SS, Damus K and Chin J (1981) Infant botulism: epidemiology and relation to sudden infant death syndrome. *Epidemiol Rev* **3**:45–60.

33 Brown LW (1981) Infant botulism. *Adv Pediatr* **28**:141–157.

34 Morris JG, Snyder JD, Wilson R and Feldman RA (1983) Infant botulism in the United States: an epidemiological study of cases occurring outside of California. *Am J Public Health* **73**:1385–1388.

35 Links TP, Smit AJ, Molenaar WM, Zwarts MJ and Oosterhuis HJ (1994) Familial hypokalemic periodic paralysis. Clinical, diagnostic and therapeutic aspects. *J Neurol Sci* **122**:33–43.

36 Links TP, Smit AJ Oosterhuis HJ and Reitsma WD (1993) Potassium channels in hyperkalemic periodic paralysis: a key to the pathogenesis? *Clin Sci (Colch)* **85**:319–325.

37 Rudel R, Ricker K and Lehmann-Horn F (1993) Genotype–phenotype correlations in human skeletal muscle sodium channel disease. *Arch Neurol* **50**:1241-1248.

Part VII

Endocrine disorders

50 | Diabetic emergencies

KK Young and TE Oh

Diabetes mellitus produces an array of pathologies involving many organ systems. Morbidity and mortality result from end-organ damage, or directly from severe metabolic derangements of insulin deficiency, e.g. diabetic ketoacidosis and hyperosmolar non-ketotic coma. Severe hypoglycaemia may complicate therapy, especially with insulin. All three conditions may present as altered states of consciousness or coma, and constitute acute diabetic emergencies.

Definitions of diabetes[1]

The most widely accepted classification of diabetes is that of the World Health Organization, which describes three clinical classes:[1] diabetes mellitus; impaired glucose tolerance; and gestational diabetes mellitus. Diabetes mellitus consists of four subgroups:

1 insulin-dependent;
2 non-insulin-dependent;
3 malnutrition-related;
4 diabetes associated with other conditions.

The first two subgroups comprise the great majority of cases.

Insulin-dependent diabetes mellitus (IDDM)

This is also called *juvenile-onset* or *type I* diabetes. Insulin deficiency leads to hyperglycaemia and poorly controlled lipolysis, producing elevated concentrations of ketone bodies. This manifests as classical symptoms of thirst, polyuria, wasting and/or ketoacidosis. Insulin is required to control the hyperglycaemia and spontaneous occurrence of acidosis. Fasting plasma glucose concentration is over 7.8 mmol; glucose and ketones are present in urine. In the asymptomatic patient, or when fasting glucose concentration is not diagnostic, an oral glucose tolerance test should be performed.

Non-insulin-dependent diabetes mellitus (NIDDM)

This may present with classical symptoms, but is more commonly asymptomatic. Diagnosis may be incidental from a blood or urine sugar screen. It may present as a diabetic emergency or through complications such as ischaemic heart disease, nephropathy, neuropathy or retinopathy. NIDDM patients may require insulin to provide better blood sugar control. Ketoacidosis does not develop spontaneously, but may occur in the presence of concomitant disease.

Aetiology

In most cases of IDDM, there is autoimmune destruction of the pancreatic β cells, resulting in absolute insulin deficiency. There is an association with certain human leukocyte antibody (HLA) types.[2] Familial clustering occurs, and environmental events are postulated to trigger an autoimmune response in susceptible patients.[3]

NIDDM is aetiologically diverse. There is insulin resistance with elevated insulin concentrations early in the disease. Hyperglycaemia and overt NIDDM develop when a decline in insulin production occurs.[4,5] There is also familial clustering, but no single gene locus has been identified.[1] Truncal obesity is a risk factor.

Epidemiology[6]

IDDM has a peak incidence in the young, rising from 9 months to 14 years, then declining. It is rare before the age of 6 months. Incidence varies across race and countries, being highest in northern Europe and lowest in Asia and Australasia.[7] Ketoacidosis remains a common initial presentation (around 25%), especially under the age of 5.[8]

NIDDM is prevalent in the elderly, but may occur at any age. A form called *maturity-onset diabetes of the young* (MODY) shows an autosomal dominant inheritance, and affects young adults. Risk varies across racial groups. Caucasians fall in a low-risk group (about 7%) and Asians are intermediate.[9] Only about half of NIDDM cases are diagnosed. There is a high prevalence of risk factors for vascular disease (e.g. hypertension, hypertriglyceridaemia and obesity). NIDDM often remains undiagnosed for years.[10]

Pathogenesis

Diabetic ketoacidosis

Patients with IDDM have minimal secretory response to glucose and non-glucose stimuli.[11] This can be demonstrated by an intravenous glucose tolerance test.[12] Lack of insulin, especially concomitant with increases in counterregulatory hormones (i.e. glucagon, catecholamines, cortisol and growth hormone) promotes lipolysis, free fatty acid (FFA) mobilization and ketogenesis, resulting in ketoacidosis.

Hyperglycaemia results mainly from accelerated hepatic glucose production (i.e. gluconeogenesis and glycolysis), and also from decreased peripheral uptake and utilization by tissues.[13] The renal threshold for glucose (10 mmol/l) is exceeded, and there is loss of glucose, up to 200 g/day. Glycosuria imposes a large osmolar solute load on the kidneys (up to 2000 mosmol/day), causing impaired renal tubular resorption of water and electrolytes, and volume contraction.[14]

Increased circulating FFAs are taken up by the liver as substrate to form acetyl coenzyme A (CoA) by β-oxidation in the mitochondria. The FFA oxidation exceeds the capacity of Krebs' cycle to oxidize acetyl CoA, which is then used to synthesize ketone bodies (β-hydroxybutyrate, acetoacetate and acetone). Normal ketone blood concentration is 0.1–0.2 mmol/l, which may increase 10-fold in diabetic ketoacidosis.[15] Kidneys have a low threshold for ketones, and ketonuria accounts for up to half the osmotic diuresis.[14]

Ketoacids β-hydroxybutyrate and acetoacetate result in metabolic acidosis,[14] (see Chapter 80). Typically, there is an anion gap in the range 25–35 mmol/l (normal = 10–17 mmol/l). The anion gap reflects unmeasured acid anions. If lactic acid is present (e.g. in conditions with ischaemia, hypoxia or sepsis) the mixed keto/lactic acidosis will give a large anion gap (e.g. over 40 mmol/l). The increase in anion gap will be matched by a decrease in bicarbonate, unless a metabolic alkalosis is superimposed (e.g. caused by vomiting). In this case, the decrease in bicarbonate will be less than the increase in the anion gap.

Hyperosmolar non-ketotic coma

This condition, in which severe hyperglycaemia develops without significant ketosis, is a metabolic emergency characteristic of uncontrolled NIDDM, and is thus more prevalent in the elderly. Nevertheless, non-ketotic coma and ketoacidosis represent two ends of a spectrum rather than two distinct diseases. There are three interrelated factors in the development of non-ketotic coma: insulin deficiency, dehydration and renal impairment. Absence of significant ketosis is not completely understood[13,16] Insulin deficiency is less severe and reasonably sufficient to restrain hepatic ketogenesis, but glucose production is uninhibited. However, ketosis is present in most patients, but minor relative to the severity of diabetic ketoacidosis.[17,18]

Clinical presentation

Diabetic ketoacidosis

Diabetic ketoacidosis is the clinical triad of hyperglycaemia, ketosis and metabolic acidosis. There is no universal definition, but these criteria are widely accepted:

pH <7.30, HCO_3^- <15 mmol/l, blood glucose >14 mmol/l

A history of infection, intercurrent illness and inadequate or omitted insulin therapy is common.[19] Patients using continuous subcutaneous insulin infusion devices are known to be at risk.[20] Classical symptoms are polyuria, polydipsia, weight loss, vomiting and abdominal pain. Clinical findings include Kussmaul respirations, dehydration, hypotension, tachycardia, muscular weakness and acetone odour on the breath. Blood glucose concentration varies, depending on hydration, nutritional status, concentrations of counterregulatory hormones and insulin administration, and is not a good determinant of severity.[21] Although the most common cause is infection, many patients are normothermic or hypothermic. Coma indicates severe metabolic derangement or may reflect the precipitating event, such as stroke.[21]

Hyperosmolar non-ketotic coma[21]

The incidence is 10:1000000 population – six times less than ketoacidosis. About 30% are previously undiagnosed diabetics. The typical patient is elderly and socially isolated or a nursing-home patient. Infection, intercurrent cardiovascular disease, corticosteroids, diuretics, and intake of glucose-rich fluids are precipitant causes.[13] Onset is more insidious. The patient may present with non-specific symptoms of anorexia, malaise or weakness, or with symptoms

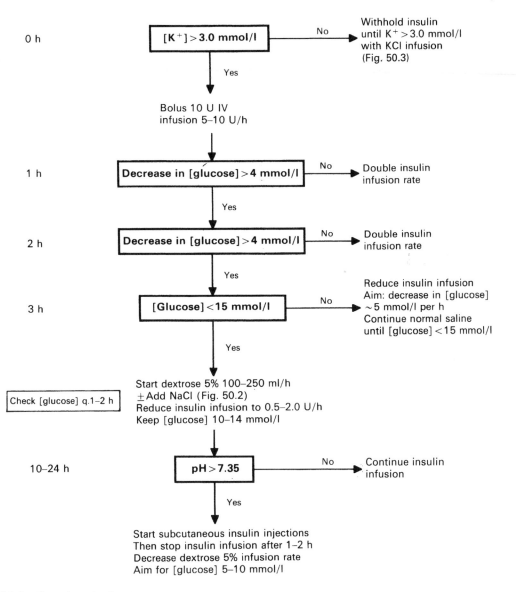

Fig. 50.1 Insulin regimen in diabetic ketoacidosis

attributable to the precipitating event (e.g. neurological deficit). Coma may be present, and impairment of consciousness is proportional to the severity of hyperosmolality. The degree of hyperglycaemia exceeds that typically found in ketoacidosis – often exceeding 50 mmol/l.[22] Dehydration is severe. An increased anion gap indicates the possibility of ketoacidosis, lactic acidosis, uraemic acidosis or drug ingestion. Clinical differences between diabetic ketoacidosis and hyperosmolar non-ketotic coma are shown in Table 50.1.

Investigations are discussed under Monitoring below.

Table 50.1 Differences between diabetic ketoacidosis and hyperosmolar non-ketotic coma

	Diabetic ketoacidosis	*Hyperosmolar non-ketotic coma*
Prodromal illness	Days	Weeks
Coma	+ +	+ + +
Blood glucose	+ +	+ + +
Ketones	+ + +	0, +
Acidaemia	+ + +	0, +
Anion gap	+ +	0, +
Osmolality	+ +	+ + +

Management[13,14,21]

ICU admission is required for diabetic ketoacidosis and non-ketotic coma. Therapy involves supplementing deficient insulin, replacing fluid and electrolyte losses, restoring acid–base imbalance and supplying energy requirements.

Insulin therapy

Short-acting insulins (bovine, porcine or human) are given as an infusion (Fig. 50.1). They have small pharmacodynamic differences and identical biological potency.[23] Standard therapy uses low-dose insulin infusion (5–10 U/h) to achieve blood insulin concentrations in the high physiological to low pharmacological range. High dose therapy (25–50 U/h) is associated with a higher incidence of hypokalaemia, and has no advantage. Severe insulin resistance in 10% of cases will necessitate the use of higher doses. Insulin infusion is also applicable in hyperosmolar non-ketotic coma, but the dose is reduced to about half. It is important to titrate therapy to each individual.

Fluid and electrolyte replacement

Average deficits in diabetic ketoacidosis are 5–7 l water and 300–450 mmol sodium. Resuscitation is started with normal (0.9%) saline. If severe hypernatraemia exists (i.e. over 155 mmol/l), half normal (0.45%) saline is indicated initially. Severe hypotension may be treated with colloids, but use of colloid in severe uncontrolled diabetes is not well-studied.[24] Dextrose 5% is started when blood glucose falls below 15 mmol/l. Hyperglycaemia is more rapidly corrected (in 4–8 h) than ketoacidosis (in 10–20 h). Hence, a glucose infusion is necessary while insulin infusion continues. Figure 50.2 shows an algorithm for fluid and sodium therapy. A central venous pressure line is indicated to aid volume replacement, and a pulmonary artery catheter is useful in complicated circumstances. Potassium replacement is shown in Figure 50.3. Magnesium and phosphate are given when appropriate (see below).

Correction of acidosis

Use of sodium bicarbonate to treat the metabolic acidosis of diabetic ketoacidosis is controversial.

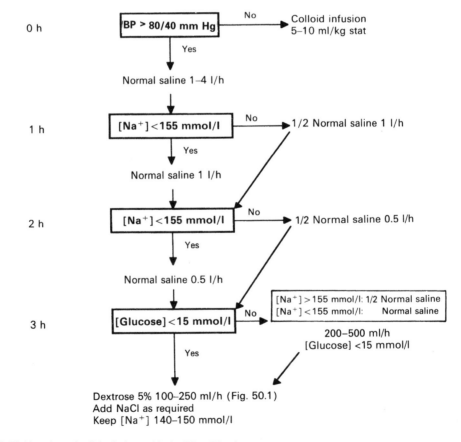

Fig. 50.2 Fluid regimen in diabetic ketoacidosis. BP = Blood pressure.

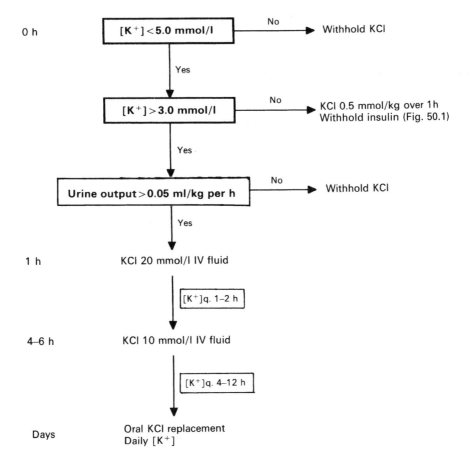

Fig. 50.3 Potassium replacement regimen in diabetic ketoacidosis.

Sodium bicarbonate is associated with numerous side-effects which may overshadow any benefits. These include increased CO_2 production, cerebrospinal fluid acidosis, hypokalaemia, rebound alkalosis, volume overload and altered tissue oxygenation. Despite these reservations, most authorities would give sodium bicarbonate for severe ketoacidosis. The recommended threshold for treatment varies: pH less than 6.9,[13] 7.1,[21] and 7.10–7.15,[14] with an aim to increase the pH up to the threshold, rather than normal level. Life-threatening hyperkalaemia is, of course, a clear indication for using bicarbonate.[25]

Monitoring[14]

The following monitoring parameters are also undertaken as investigations on presentations.

1 Blood glucose concentration: initially every hour, then less frequently.
2 Blood urea and creatinine concentrations: on admission and at least daily. Acetoacetate interferes with the alkaline picrate assay of serum creatinine, giving a false elevation.[13]

3 Serum electrolytes:
  (a) *Serum sodium*: on admission and at least daily. Serum sodium reflects relative water and electrolyte losses, and may be normal (50% of cases), raised or decreased. It cannot be used to infer the state of hydration. Each 1.0 mmol/l rise in blood glucose will decrease the serum sodium concentration by approximately 0.3 mmol/l, so hypernatraemia will represent a profound loss of water.
  (b) *Serum potassium*: initially every hour, then less frequently (2–4-hourly). Diabetic ketoacidosis patients have a potassium deficit of 3–5 mmol/kg. However, serum concentrations are usually normal or raised, because of the shift of intracellular potassium into the extracellular space, due to acidaemia, insulin deficiency and hypertonicity. Hypokalaemia on admission is a sign of severe total body depletion, exceeding 600–800 mmol. This represents an emergency, and necessitates potassium administration before starting insulin therapy.
  (c) *Serum chloride*: as indicated.
  (d) *Serum phosphate*: on admission and every 1–2

days. About 75–150 mmol phosphate is lost in the urine, but serum concentrations will usually be normal or only slightly decreased. Insulin treatment will induce shift of phosphate into cells, and hypophosphataemia is inevitable. Phosphate replacement was previously given routinely, because of reports of decreased erythrocyte 2,3-diphosphoglycerate.[13] Severe hypophosphataemia (i.e. concentration under 0.4 mmol/l) may manifest as muscle weakness, ventilatory failure, rhabdomyolysis, acute renal failure and altered consciousness. However, recent studies fail to demonstrate any benefit of routine phosphate supplementation, and the risk of hypocalcaemia is documented.[26,27]

(e) *Serum magnesium*: on admission and every 1–2 days. In IDDM and NIDDM disease, chronic hypomagnesaemia may be present,[28] and may contribute to insulin resistance, carbohydrate intolerance and hypertension. However the benefits of replacement therapy have not been demonstrated.[29] In severe uncontrolled diabetes, magnesium depletion also occurs, but routine replacement is not recommended, and there is a risk of acute hypermagnesaemia with renal impairment.[13,16] It may be indicated if arrhythmias are present.

4 Serum ketones (if available): on admission. The ketostix test relies on the nitroprusside reaction, and reacts strongly with acetoacetate but not with β-hydroxybutyrate. A 2+ reaction corresponds with a total serum ketone concentration of about 3 mmol/l; a 3+ reaction with about 5 mmol/l.[30] In severe diabetic ketoacidosis with lactic acidosis, β-hydroxybutyrate predominates and the test is unreliable.

5 Urinary glucose and ketones: 4-hourly. Ketonuria may persist up to 2 days after correction of acidosis due to the presence of acetone, which is not an acid anion, and is highly fat-soluble.

6 Arterial blood gases: frequently as indicated.

7 Serum osmolality and anion gap: initially and as indicated.

Serum osmolality can be measured with an osmometer or calculated from the equation:

Osmolality (normal = 285-300 mosmol/l) = $2(Na^+ + K^+)$ + glucose + urea (all values in mmol/l).

Anion gap is calculated by the equation:

Anion gap (normal = 10–17 mmol/l = Na^+ + K^+) − (Cl^- + HCO^{3-}) (all values in mmol/l).

8 Serum lactate: if acidosis is severe and anion gap is large.

9 Full blood count and coagulation studies: daily and as indicated. Leukocytosis with left shift may occur in the absence of sepsis.[21]

10 Chest X-ray.

11 Blood cultures, urine and sputum microscopy and culture, and culture of relevant specimens as indicated.

12 Pulse oximetry continuously.

13 Electrocartdiogram – 12-lead recording and continuous monitoring.

14 Invasive haemodynamic monitoring as indicated.

15 Neurological status and observations: including Glasgow coma scale and computed tomography scans as indicated for persistent coma or worsening neurological state.

16 Other investigations as indicated (e.g. liver function tests, serum amylase, cardiac enzymes and creatinine clearance).

Complications

Complications of therapy

1 Hypoglycaemia.

2 Hypokalaemia.

3 Hypophosphataemia.

4 Hyperchloraemic acidosis, usually mild, may develop during therapy.[31,32] Metabolic acidosis persists, although the anion gap has returned to normal, and serum chloride is raised.

5 Cerebral oedema is attributed to rapid correction of hyperosmolality, causing a shift of water into neurones.[21] Diminished conscious level improves and then deteriorates, when hyperglycaemia and acidosis are improving. It is rare in adults and best described in children and adolescents.[33] Prevention is by avoiding precipitous falls in serum osmolality (i.e. by avoiding hyponatraemia and maintaining blood glucose above 10 mmol/l for the first 8–10 h). Treatment aims to increase osmolality with mannitol (1 g/kg).[14]

Complications of associated medical conditions

1 Deep venous thrombosis and pulmonary embolism: diabetes is associated with a higher risk of thromboembolic events.[34] Thromboembolism is a significant cause of mortality in hyperosmolar non-ketotic coma.[35] Prophylaxis with subcutaneous heparin (5000 units 6–8-hourly) is advisable.[13]

2 Aspiration pneumonitis.

3 Erosive gastritis.

Hypoglycaemia

Hypoglycaemia is the commonest cause of diabetic coma. It may be precipitated in known diabetics (up to 10% of IDDM patients each year) by missed meals, exercise and overdose of insulin or oral hypoglycaemic agents.[20] Changing therapy or insulin preparations are susceptible periods. There is an increased risk with long-acting sulphonylurea agents. Alcohol inhibits gluconeogenesis, and binges may precipitate hypoglycaemia. Alcoholic ketoacidosis is a syndrome of hypoglycaemia, ketoacidosis and dehydration associated with starvation, vomiting, upper abdominal pain and neurological changes including seizures and coma.[36] Hypoglycaemia may complicate other disease states (e.g. liver and renal failure or adrenocortical insufficiency).[16] Severe hypoglycaemia (e.g. blood glucose less than 1 mmol/l) is a medical emergency. Brain metabolism uses half the glucose produced by the liver. Neuronal store of glycogen is depleted in 2 min, after which the brain is susceptible to damage.[37] Clinically, there is confusion, agitation, coma and fitting. Tremor, tachycardia and sweating may be blunted by diabetic autonomic neuropathy. Treatment is with intravenous glucose (50 ml of 20%) without delay. Hypoglycaemia due to long-acting oral hypoglycaemic agents or insulins will require an ongoing glucose infusion.

Lactic acidosis[38] (see Chapter 80)

Lactate is formed as the end-product of the anaerobic metabolism of glucose. Lactic acidosis complicates fewer than 10% of cases of diabetic ketoacidosis, and usually reflects tissue hypoperfusion and anaerobic metabolism (type A).[14] However, lactic acidosis can also exist in diabetes without obvious clinical hypoperfusion, such as that associated with sepsis, biguanide therapy and alcohol ingestion (type B).

Prognosis

IDDM is associated with a high risk of mortality – eight times more that the general population. There are significant differences in mortality rates across countries.[39] Mortality from diabetic ketoacidosis is 1–10%, and 40–70% in hyperosmolar non-ketotic coma.[14,39] Most deaths are due to medical conditions which precipitate the episode, especially sepsis.

References

1 National Diabetes Data Group (1979) Classification and diagnosis of diabetes mellitus and other categories of glucose intolerance. *Diabetes* **28**:1039–1057.
2 Bennett PH (1994) Definition, diagnosis, and classification of diabetes mellitus and impaired glucose tolerance. In: Kahn CR and Weir GC (eds) *Joslin's Diabetes Mellitus*. Philadelphia: Lea & Febiger, pp. 193–200.
3 Leslie. RDG and Elliott RB (1994). Early environmental events as a cause of IDDM. *Diabetes* **43**:843–849.
4 DeFronzo RA (1992) Pathogenesis of type 2 (non-insulin dependent) diabetes mellitus: a balanced overview. *Diabetologica* **35**:389–397.
5 Taylor SI, Accili D and Imai Y (1994) Insulin resistance or insulin deficiency: which is the primary cause of NIDDM? *Diabetes* **43**:735–740.
6 Warram JH, Rich SS and Krolewski AS (1994) Epidemiology and genetics of diabetes mellitus. In: Kahn CR and Weir GC (eds) *Joslin's Diabetes Mellitus*. Philadelphia: Lea & Febiger, pp. 201–215.
7 Karvonen M, Tuomilehto J, Libman I and LaPorte R (1993) A review of the recent epidemiological data on worldwide incidence of type 1 (insulin-dependent) diabetes mellitus. *Diabetologica* **36**:883–892.
8 Pinkney JH, Bingley PJ, Sawtell PA, Dunger DB and Gale EAM (1994) Presentation and progress of childhood diabetes mellitus: a prospective population-based study. *Diabetologica* **37**:70–74.
9 Zimmet PZ (1992) Kelly West lecture 1991: challenges in diabetes epidemiology – from west to the rest. *Diabetes Care* **15**:232–252.
10 Harris MI (1993) Undiagnosed NIDDM: clinical and public health issues. *Diabetes Care* **16**:642–652.
11 O'Meara NM and Polonsky KS (1994) Insulin secretion in vivo. In: Kahn CR and Weir GC (ed) *Joslin's Diabetes Mellitus*. Philadelphia: Lea & Febiger, pp. 81–96.
12 Ziegler AG, Herskowitz RD, Jackson RA *et al.* (1990) Predicting type 1 diabetes. *Diabetes Care* **13**:762–775.
13 Marshall SM, Walker M and Alberti KGMM (1992) Diabetic ketoacidosis and hyperglycaemic non-ketotic coma. In: Alberti KGMM, DeFronzo RA, Keen H and Zimmet P (eds) *International Textbook of Diabetes Mellitus*. Chichester: John Wiley, pp. 1151–1171.
14 DeFronzo RA, Matsuda M and Barrett EJ (1994) Diabetic ketoacidosis. *Diabetes Rev* **2**:209–238.
15 Hood VL and Tannen RL (1994) Maintenance of acid–base homeostasis during ketoacidosis and lactic acidosis. *Diabetes Rev* **2**:177–194.
16 Rossini AA and Mordes JP (1991) The diabetic comas. In: Rippe JM, Irwin RS, Alpert JS and Fink MP (eds) *Intensive Care Medicine*. Boston: Little, Brown, pp. 963–975.
17 Papadakis M and Grunfeld C (1986) Ketonuria in hospitalised patients with non-insulin-dependent diabetes. *Diabetes Care* **9**:596–600.
18 Nosadini R, Avogaro A and Scognamiglio R (1994) Regulation of ketone body metabolism in IDDM and NIDDM. *Diabetes Rev* **2**:156-167.
19 Kitabchi AE, Fisher JN, Matteri R and Murphy MB (1983) The use of continuous insulin delivery systems in the treatment of diabetes mellitus. *Adv Int Med* **28**:449–490.
20 Frier BM (1991) Hypoglycaemia and diabetes mellitus. In: Pickup JC and Williams G (eds) *Textbook of Diabetes*. London: Blackwell Scientific Publications, pp. 495–506.
21 Kitabchi AE, Fisher JN, Murphy MB and Rumbak MJ (1994) Diabetic ketoacidosis and the hyperglucemic, hyperosmolar, nonketotic state. In: Kahn CR and Weir GC (eds) *Joslin's Diabetes Mellitus*. Philadelphia: Lea & Febiger, pp. 738–770.

22 Krentz AJ and Nattras M (1991) Diabetic comas. In: Pickup JC and Williams G (eds) *Textbook of Diabetes*. London: Blackwell Scientific Publications, pp. 479–494.

23 Heinemann L and Richter B (1993) Clinical pharmacology of human insulin. *Diabetes Care* **16**:90–100.

24 Fein IA, Rackow EC, Sprung CL and Goodman R (1982) Relation of colloid osmotic pressure to arterial hypoxemia and cerebral edema during crystalloid volume loading of patients with diabetic ketoacidosis. *Ann Intern Med* **96**:570–575.

25 Emergency Cardiac Care Committee and Subcommittees, American Heart Association (1992) Guidelines for cardiopulmonary resuscitation and emergency cardiac care, III. Adult advanced cardiac life support. *J Am Med Assoc* **268**:2199–2241.
care, III. Adult advanced cardiac life support. *JAMA* **268**: 2199–2241.

26 Clerbaux T, Reynaert M, Willems E and Frans A (1989) Effect of phosphate on oxygen–hemoglobin affinity, diphosphoglycerate and blood gases during recovery from diabetic ketoacidosis. *Intensive Care Med* **15**: 995–998.

27 Fisher JN and Kitabchi AE (1983) A randomized study of phosphate therapy in the treatment of diabetic ketoacidosis. *J Clin Endocrinol Metab* **57**:177–180.

28 Schnack C, Bauer I, Pregant P, Hopmeier P and Schernthaner G (1992) Hypomagnesaemia in type 2 (non-insulin-dependent) diabetes mellitus is not corrected by improvement of long-term metabolic control. *Diabetologia* **35**:77–79.

29 Clinical practice recommendations: American Diabetes Association (1993) Consensus statement: magnesium supplementation in the treatment of diabetes. *Diabetes Care* **16**:79–81.

30 Alberti KG and Hockaday TD (1972) Rapid blood ketone estimation in the diagnosis of diabetic ketoacidosis. *Br Med J* **2**:565–568.

31 Androgu HJ, Wilson H, Boyd AE *et al.* (1982) Plasma acid–base patterns in diabetic ketoacidosis. *N Engl J Med* **307**:1603–1610.

32 Kitabchi AE, Murphy MB, Matteri R and Spencer J (1991) Contributing factors in the development of hyperchloremic metabolic acidosis during treatment of diabetic ketoacidosis. *Diabetes* **40**:42A.

33 Rosenblood AL (1990) Intracerebral crises during treatment of diabetic ketoacidosis. *Diabetes Care* **13**:22–33.

34 Ceriello A (1993) Coagulation activation in diabetes mellitus: the role of hyperglycaemia and therapeutic prospects. *Diabetologia* **36**:1119–1125.

35 Whelton MJ, Walde D and Harvard CWH (1971) Hyperosmolar nonketotic coma: with particular reference to vascular complications. *Br Med J* **1**:85–86.

36 Cusi K and Consoli A (1994) Alcoholic ketoacidosis and lactic acidosis. *Diabetes Rev* **2**:195–208.

37 Guyton AC (1991) *Textbook of Medical Physiology*, 8th edn. Philadelphia: Saunders.

38 Arieff AI (1994) Pathogenesis of lactic acidosis: current concepts. *Diabetes Rev* **2**:168–176.

39 Songer TJ, DeBerry K, LaPorte RE and Tuomilheto J (1992) International comparisons of IDDM mortality. *Diabetes Care* **15**:15–21.

51 | Diabetes insipidus

AE Vedig

Diabetes insipidus (DI) is a syndrome characterized by polyuria, excessive thirst and polydipsia. *Central* or *neurogenic* DI results from a lack of antidiuretic hormone (ADH) being released into the circulation in response to an osmotic stimulus. Persistent severe central DI occurs rarely, as does the syndrome of DI which is precipitated by excessive intake of water caused by abnormalities of thirst mechanisms or psychological function (*dipsogenic* or *psychogenic* DI). Transient, usually incomplete, central DI is noticed frequently by intensivists in patients with severe head injuries. *Nephrogenic* DI, caused by deficient action of ADH, occurs very uncommonly in its classical form, but may be recognized frequently, often as an acquired, less severe form, in patients on lithium therapy. A vasopressin-resistant, transient pregnancy-related disorder of water metabolism is recognized where the polyuria is responsive to vasopressin analogues.

Basic physiology[1–6]

Water balance and body fluid tonicity are maintained by the double-negative system of feedback involving thirst, ADH secretion and action on the kidney. The basic mechanisms of stimulating and decreasing thirst are not as well-understood, but involve neuroendocrine reflexes, mediation by ADH, angiotensin II, osmotic mechanisms and pharyngeal distension. Thirst is stimulated by plasma osmolalities in excess of 290 mosmol/kg. Cold fluids held in the oropharynx inhibit ADH release. Ageing and drugs affect these processes.

Normally, plasma osmolality is maintained in a very narrow range, $\pm 1\%$ for an individual, with a population range of 275–295 mosmol/kg. As plasma osmolality increases from 280 mosmol/kg, there is a steady increase in ADH secretion. Small changes (1% increase or decrease) in plasma osmolality influence ADH secretion. Stress, disease states, many drugs and the ageing process can influence the hypothalamic osmostat and the ADH-secretory response to an osmotic change (Table 51.1). Hormonal release is also mediated by peripheral stretch receptors (in atria, great veins, arterial vasoreceptors and lungs). Hypotension or depletion of effective blood volume will stimulate the release of very large amounts of ADH, overriding any osmotic stimulus.

ADH (8-arginine vasopressin), a nonapeptide, is synthesized in neurones of the hypothalamus, predominantly in the paired supraoptic and paraventricular nuclei. It has structural and some functional similarities to oxytocin. ADH is transported intra-axonally to the pituitary gland (neurohypophysis). Here, the hormone is stored in granules bound to the

Table 51.1 Factors influencing antidiuretic hormone (ADH) secretion or action

ADH secretion is *increased* by:
  Hyperosmolality, hypotension
  Stress, emotional stimuli
  Trauma, surgery, pain
  Exercise, increased temperature
  Positive-pressure ventilation
  Cholinergic and β-adrenergic drugs
  Nicotine, angiotensin II, barbiturates
  Chlorpropamide

ADH action is *potentiated* by:
  Chlorpropamide, carbamazepine
  Clofibrate, thiazide diuretics
  Prostaglandin synthetase inhibitors

ADH secretion is *inhibited* by:
  Causes of central diabetes insipidus (Table 51.2)
  Diphenylhydantoin
  Opioid antagonists
ADH action is *antagonized* by:
  Hypokalaemia
  Hypercalcaemia
  Prostaglandin E_2
  Drugs: e.g. demeclocycline, lithium carbonate, amphotericin B
  Excess vasopressinase

carrier protein neurophysin. Some neurones containing ADH terminate in the median eminence, where adrenocorticotrophic hormone release may be stimulated. The half-life in blood is 10–15 min, with metabolism undertaken by hepatic and renal peptidases. Seven to 10% of active hormone is excreted in the urine. Plasma concentrations range from 1–5 pg/ml (antidiuretic action) to greater than 40 pg/ml with 20% blood volume depletion. Nausea is also a potent stimulus for ADH secretion.

Actions of ADH

Antidiuresis

Antidiuresis results from ADH action on V_2 receptors in the distal renal tubule, mainly in the collecting duct. The V_2 agonist action stimulates adenylcyclase generation of 3,5 cyclic adenosine monophosphate (AMP) within the tubular cytoplasm, which allows a protein kinase to open microtubular passages for water ingress from the renal filtrate. Up to 12% of glomerular filtrate may be reabsorbed. This regulation of free water excretion maintains osmotic and volume homeostasis. Severe DI may result in the excretion of very large amounts of dilute urine (e.g. 20 l/day). Stimulation of V_2 receptors also results in tachycardia, facial flushing, decreased blood pressure and increased plasma renin concentration.

ADH stimulates renal prostaglandin E_2 synthesis, which in turn modulates the antidiuresis by inhibiting ADH-induced cyclic AMP generation. Prostaglandin E_1, hypokalaemia, hypercalcaemia and drugs such as demeclocycline and lithium antagonize the ADH effect on adenyl cyclase.

Vasoconstriction

Vasoconstriction results from V_{1a} receptor stimulation, which occurs when higher concentrations of ADH exist. This is clinically significant in hypotensive states, where high concentrations of ADH contribute to the maintenance of blood pressure. The skin, mesenteric and coronary vessels are particularly sensitive to this vasoconstriction. This action is not antagonized by α-adrenergic blocking agents or by vascular denervation. Intravenous infusions of ADH have been used to diminish bleeding from oesophageal varices. Other V_{1a} effects include glycogenolysis, stimulation of renal prostaglandin synthesis and inhibition of renal renin secretion.

Coagulation

Coagulation effects are extrarenal V_2 receptor-mediated. Prostacyclin generation is stimulated; tissue-type plasminogen activator activity, factor VIII-related antigen activity, factor VIII coagulant activity and von Willebrand factor multimers all increase. ADH and its analogues, in pharmacological doses, induce coagulant activity in healthy individuals as well as disease states (e.g. haemophilia, renal and hepatic disease[7,8] and after cardiac surgery.[9,10]

Other actions

ADH via V_{1a} receptors affects learning, memory and water permeability of the brain. V_{1b} receptors are found in the pituitary. Activation results in secretion of corticotrophin.

Central diabetes insipidus[2–5,11–14]

Aetiology

Causes of persistent central DI invariably involve destruction of the hypothalamus or pituitary gland, and sometimes produce defects in thirst mechanisms. Permanent, complete or incomplete central DI may follow severe head injury,[15] and, rarely, quite minor trauma.[16] Transient complete or incomplete central DI occurs quite commonly with severe head injuries and particularly brain death.[17,18] Fatal central diabetes mellitus and insipidus resulting from untreated hyponatraemia has recently been described.[19]

Pituitary apoplexy continues to be described after hypovolaemic[20,21] and septic shock.[22] The enlarged pituitary that occurs with pregnancy may be more vulnerable to vasospasm. Obvious polyuria is unusual; the first sign may be inability to lactate. Transient central DI has been described as a sequela to infectious meningitis,[23,24] chemical meningitis,[25] electric burns[26] and associated with amiodarone therapy.[27] Transient DI has also been described with penetrating thoracic trauma[28] and coronary artery bypass surgery.[29] Some causes (e.g. lithium and sarcoidosis) may have variable components of central and nephrogenic DI and thirst disorders.

The nature and level of interruption of the neurohypophyseal tract will influence the time course and severity of central DI. Almost complete lesions, at or above the median eminence, or lesser lesions of the neural stalk, will probably result in a permanent state of DI. However, localized cerebral oedema and lower lesions are more likely associated with milder or temporary deficiency in ADH secretion.

Pathophysiology[2–5,11–14,30]

The syndrome of DI results from a failure of appropriate ADH secretion or action, in response to the physiological stimulus of water deficiency which is characterized by relative plasma hyperosmolality. If the ADH deficiency is complete, over 20 l/day of very dilute urine may be passed. Frequently, the ADH deficiency is relative, with a reduction in the slope and sensitivity of the ADH response to a change in plasma tonicity, resulting in lesser amounts of hypotonic urine output (3–6 l/day). Nocturia may be the major symptom. Even if the ADH limb of the regulatory feedback is completely lost, the excess thirst mechanism ensures that plasma osmolality stabilizes at a level only slightly above normal, no matter how severe the polyuria. Hyperosmolaemia and hypernatraemia are associated with a defect in thirst or water intake. If the thirst mechanism or water intake is very impaired in severe ADH deficiency, plasma will become hyperosmotic and grossly depleted in volume. Extra fluid losses such as vomiting and diarrhoea will complicate management. Death may result from the hypernatraemia and cardiovascular collapse.

Conceptually, four types of permanent central DI may be considered.

1 Type 1 – where there is complete lack of ADH, i.e. no rise in urine osmolality with increasing plasma osmolality secondary to dehydration or infusion of hypertonic saline.
2 Type 2 – where there is very little or no ADH, i.e. no increase in urine osmolality until moderate or severe hyperosmolaemia occurs. This occurs during a persistent dehydration test which produces hypovolaemia.
3 Type 3 – shows increasing plasma ADH concentrations and urine osmolality, but the responses are markedly inadequate.
4 Type 4 – where there is an ADH and urine response to a normal increase in plasma osmolality, but the magnitude of this response is abnormally low as the osmotic stimulus increases.

Types 2–4 may respond with antidiuresis to a number of physiological or pathological events or drug therapy (Table 51.1).

Central DI is less severe in the presence of simultaneous failure of the anterior pituitary. A deficiency of adrenocorticotrophic hormone and cortisol results in a lower metabolic rate, renal solute load and glomerular filtration rate, and inhibition of free water excretion. Corticosteroid replacement therapy may exacerbate DI. The converse situation, of relative ADH excess, is the syndrome of inappropriate antidiuretic hormone (SIADH; see Chapter 81).

Clinical presentation and diagnosis[2-5,11-14,30,31]

The usual clinical manifestations of DI are sudden onset of polyuria (sometimes the major complaint is nocturia), resultant thirst and excessive intake of (usually) cold drinks. Lack of thirst, inability to drink, inadequate water replacement or excessive saline administration may result in signs of hypovolaemia and hypernatraemia (e.g. lethargy, confusion, delirium and coma; convulsions are uncommon).

Urine volumes over 4–6 l/day or 3 ml/kg for 2 consecutive hours in neurosurgical patients point towards DI. In severe forms, urine is very hypotonic (SG 1.001–1.005, urine osmolality 50–200 mosmol/kg), but in incomplete forms, particularly if hypovolaemia is present, urine osmolality may rise well above plasma osmolality (up to 700 mosmol/kg). The essential feature is that urine osmolality is inappropriately low compared to the plasma osmolality.

Following neurosurgery on the hypothalamus and pituitary, four patterns of urine output have been observed:[32]

1 temporary polyuria, which may last several days;
2 the classic triphasic pattern, which consists of transient polyuria, an interphase of essentially normal urine output which may last a week, and then permanent polyuria;
3 an immediate and permanent polyuria, without an interphase;
4 a variation of the triphasic pattern. There is a diminution of urine output during the interphase, but it does not return to normal and is followed by worsening polyuria which becomes permanent.

Evidence suggests that the early polyuria is not due to decreased concentrations of circulating ADH, but may be related to the release of the biologically inactive precursor neurophysin I.[33] It is hypothesized that this may lead to renal refractoriness to effects of ADH.

Additional signs relating to an underlying disease state (e.g. neoplasia, sarcoid and intracranial haemorrhage) may be evident, as may signs of anterior hypopituitarism (particularly after hypophyseal radiotherapy or transsphenoidal operative procedures). Central DI must be distinguished from other causes of polyuria (Table 51.2). Solute diuresis can be recognized and quantified by specific measurements (e.g. glucose in plasma and urine) or measurement of total daily urine osmolality (eg salts and urea) or measurement and calculation of plasma or urine osmolar gaps (e.g. mannitol and IV contrast agents).

Other causes of polyuria, such as primary defects in thirst or psychogenic polydipsia, will present very rarely to the intensivist, but endogenous or exogenous fluid overload may occur much more frequently. Plasma osmolality generally remains low in fluid overload[34] after water deprivation, as opposed to becoming hyperosmolar with incomplete central DI. Recovery from fluid overload in association with SIADH has a similar pattern of plasma and urine osmolality changes. However, unrecognized excess exogenous solute administration may complicate the diagnosis.

A predictor of the development of the triphasic pattern of ADH deficit and osmoreceptor impairment is the absence or impairment of thirst in hypernatraemic patients (especially after hypothalamic surgery).[35]

Table 51.2 Major polyuric syndromes

EXCESS WATER LOAD
Exogenous:
Iatrogenic
Thirst disorders
    Hypothalamic disease
    Drugs: thioridazine, chlorpromazine, anticholinergics
Psychogenic polydipsia
Endogenous
Recovery from unrecognized overload

SOLUTE (OSMOTIC) DIURESIS
Exogenous or endogenous solute load
Glucose, urea
Mannitol, IV contrast media
Sodium chloride
Abnormal solute handling
Chronic renal disease
Diuretics

RENAL TUBULAR UNRESPONSIVENESS TO ADH
Nephrogenic DI
Congenital and familial
Acquired nephrogenic DI
Drug-induced:
    Lithium, demeclocycline, methoxyflurane, foscarnet, gen-
    tamicin, rifampicin, frusemide
Chronic electrolyte disturbances
    Hypercalcaemia (hyperparathyroidism)
    Hypokalaemia (primary hyperaldosteronism)
Renal disease
    Postobstructive, pyelonephritis
    Post acute tubular necrosis
    Post renal transplant
Systemic disorders
    Amyloid, multiple myeloma, Sjögren's syndrome
    Polycystic disease, sickle-cell disease
Pregnancy
    Excess vasopressinase
    Acquired nephrogenic

CENTRAL DI
*Neoplastic, infective or infiltrative lesions of hypothalamus or
pituitary*
Primary and secondary neoplasms
Granulomatous diseases
Tuberculosis, mycoses, toxoplasmosis, encephalitis, basal
meningitis
Pituitary or hypothalamic surgery or ablative radiotherapy
Head injuries
Vascular lesions
Postpartum necrosis
Aneurysm, haemorrhage
Hyperviscosity syndrome
Idiopathic
Familial (usually autosomal dominant)

IV = Intravenous; ADH = antidiuretic hormone; DI = diabetes insipidus.

Nephrogenic DI is recognized by a failure to concentrate urine even after ADH administration. Where acquired partial nephrogenic DI exists, together with incomplete central DI in patients with an altered conscious state, the precise diagnosis is irrelevant to the central aim of maintaining plasma volume and osmolality within appropriate limits.

Investigations[2–5,11–14,30]

Random plasma and urine osmolality (with liberal water intake)

Subjects with DI have higher plasma osmolalities, but there is considerable overlap with the normal range, and this determination is not diagnostic in individual patients. Urine osmolality is low – often 50–100 mosmol/kg – but the degree varies inversely with the severity of the polyuria. Solute diuresis may be suspected if urine SG > 1.010 or urine osmolality is measured between 250 and 320 mosmol/kg, and particularly if an abnormal plasma or urine osmolar gap exists. Plasma osmolality may be calculated from determinations of serum sodium, potassium glucose and urea:

mosmol/kg = $1.86 (Na^+ + K^+)$ + glucose + urea (where all values are in mmol/l).

A diagnosis of DI may usually be made when there is an elevated plasma osmolality due to increased sodium, and an inappropriately low urine osmolality (see below). Often, there is no need for a dehydration test, and desmopressin (DDAVP) may be given to examine the renal response.

Blood chemistry

Blood glucose, 24-h urinary osmolality and electrolytes, blood and urine electrolytes, urea and creatinine are useful for determining solute load and renal function.

Plasma and urine osmolality relationships, and water deprivation

If required, comparison of simultaneously determined plasma and urine osmolality during dehydration may be conducted at any time. Fluid replacement regimens are simply ceased (or restricted if laboratory reports take too long). The rate of change of plasma osmolality is proportional to the degree of continuing polyuria. In normal subjects, there is a relationship between increasing plasma osmolality and increasing urine osmolality. Provided solute diuresis has been excluded and assuming blood urea and glucose are normal, failure to concentrate urine adequately suggests either central or nephrogenic DI.

The normal plasma/urine osmolality relationship is shown in Table 51.3

Where there is an elevated urea (e.g. renal failure), a corrected osmolality may be calculated substituting a urea measurement of 5 mmol/l. Allowances can be made with hyperglycaemia, but corrections are less helpful. The hypothalamic–pituitary axis responds to tonicity changes rather than strictly osmolality.

Table 51.3 Normal plasma/urine osmolality relationship

Plasma osmolality (mosmol/kg)	Urine osmolality (mosmol/kg)
>288	>125
>290	>200
>292	>400
>294	600

During pregnancy, there is a resetting of the osmostat, resulting in generally lower plasma sodium concentrations and plasma osmolality for a corresponding urine osmolality.

The degree of failure to concentrate urine and an examination of the relationship may indicate the type of DI and its severity. Excess water load states usually manifest a hypotonic urine (e.g. osmolality <150 mosmol/kg) with persistently low plasma osmolality (e.g. <288 mosmol/kg). Following demonstration of failure to concentrate urine adequately in response to water deprivation, renal response to exogenous ADH should be examined.

ADH test

If dehydration exists, as indicated by elevated plasma osmolality, and there is inadequate urine concentration, then ADH (as 10 μg DDAVP nasally, or 1 μg SC or IV) should be given. A rise in urine osmolality of 50% following ADH is almost always sufficient to differentiate central from nephrogenic diabetes insipidus if type 1 DI is present, i.e. severe DI. Unfortunately, if urine is able to be concentrated greater than 300 mosmol/kg with dehydration, then ADH administration in supraphysiological amounts does not reliably differentiate between chronic severe excess water loads, chronic incomplete central DI or partial nephrogenic DI.

ADH assay[36]

Reliable, simple and highly sensitive radioimmunoassays are commercially available.[37] Plasma ADH can be measured before and during dehydration tests, and results analysed together with plasma and urine osmolality changes. Basal plasma ADH is normal or high in the presence of polyuria associated with nephrogenic DI. Basal concentrations are low and remain clearly subnormal with central DI. ADH concentrations rise appropriately in response to hyperosmolaemia with thirst disorders and psychogenic polydipsia.

Plasma ADH may be related to plasma and urine osmolality (sampling having been taken during dehydration). Nomograms are available to compare these relationships. Careful studies using reliable and sensitive ADH assays have cast doubt on the diagnostic veracity of the classical dehydration and ADH administration test. It has been found that the maximum concentrating capacity of the kidney in all types of DI is decreased equally in proportion to the polyuria. Furthermore, for partial nephrogenic DI, incomplete central DI and primary polydipsia, the relationships between urine osmolality and plasma ADH differ only at submaximal concentrations of plasma ADH. It is possible that these relationships may not be precise with acute DI because of the release of inactive precursors.

ADH trial

If the diagnosis is unclear after clinical assessment and the above investigations, then a carefully conducted clinical trial is indicated for both diagnostic and therapeutic purposes. DDAVP (1–2 μg SC 12-hourly) is administered for several days. If thirst and polydipsia are abolished without excessive fluid retention, then the patient probably has incomplete central DI. Administration of larger amounts of ADH may decrease polyuria in partial nephrogenic DI.

Hypertonic saline

Infusions of hypertonic saline, according to a specific protocol, may be used to evaluate the 'set-point' of the osmoreceptor mechanism.

Specific investigations

Special investigations, including magnetic resonance imaging (MRI) and assessment of anterior pituitary function, may be required for suspected lesions of the hypothalamus and pituitary gland. MRI studies demonstrate the anatomy and provide insights into the underlying pathology. T_1-weighted imaging may differentiate primary polydipsia from central DI. The presence of a hyperintense signal is consistent with a diagnosis of primary polydipsia, whereas it is absent with central DI.[38]

Management[3–5,11–14,39]

Management problems in ICU are usually polyuria and hypovolaemia, associated with varying states of plasma osmolality. Priorities in diagnosis and treatment have to be balanced carefully. Water restriction and administration of ADH may be required. Rapid return to normal' plasma osmolality is not always the major objective, particularly where an increase in cerebral volume is undesirable.

Provided there is cardiovascular stability, mild polyuria (e.g. 3 ml/kg per h) is often best observed with frequent determinations of plasma and urine osmolality, unless hyperosmolaemia occurs. Even if a provisional diagnosis of incomplete central DI is made, at this level of urine output it is often advantageous simply to replace output with an appropriate solution or allow the patient to drink rather than initiate specific drug therapy. If the polyuria is persistent (>24 h) or severe (>7 ml/kg per h for 4–6 h), drug therapy should be considered as specific replacement therapy or as part of a diagnostic and therapeutic trial. Resuscitation may be necessary in dehydrated patients in shock. The priority is almost always restoration of circulatory stability rather than reversal of hyperosmolaemia. If parasellar pathology is suspected, then one should assume anterior pituitary deficiency and routinely use stress-dose steroids.

Routine management will require accurate fluid balance with daily patient weighing, and at least daily plasma and urine osmolality and electrolytes in the acute phase. Water is lost far in excess of electrolytes, so IV replacement fluid as 5% dextrose is generally satisfactory. Large volumes of 5% dextrose may cause hyperglycaemia and further exacerbate polyuria, particularly if corticosteroids are being administered. Large sodium inputs are unnecessary and may confuse the diagnosis. Dextrose 4% with 0.18% saline is often a convenient way of supplying daily sodium requirements. Potassium requirements are generally small. Disturbances of thirst, whether due to primary polydipsia or habit, can complicate management. Hormone therapy other than ADH will be required in panhypopituitarism.

ADH therapy

ADH replacement is the most effective means of reducing the polyuria, nocturia and polydipsia of central DI. Significant regeneration of ADH secretion may occur even months postoperatively, allowing a decrease in ADH supplementation. The volume of IV replacement must be decreased with the onset of ADH action or water overload will result.

Short-acting agents

Aqueous vasopressin (arginine)
The dose is 5–10 IU either IM or SC. Duration of action is 4–6 h. It has been given IV by continuous infusion[40] and in ultra-low doses (e.g. 1–2 IU/24 h).[41] Although vasopressin is a V_1 and V_2 agonist, small IV doses are not associated with undesirable V_1 effects (e.g. coronary vasoconstriction, abdominal and uterine cramps). There is a role for aqueous vasopressin parenterally in low doses because of its short duration of action.

Lysine vasopressin:
Lysine vasopressin and vasopressin tannate in oil also act on V_1 and V_2 receptors. These preparations are longer-acting and have been superseded by desmopressin.

Long-acting agents

DDAVP,[42] 1-deamino-8-D-arginine-vasopressin (desmopressin), is an analogue of arginine vasopressin with specific V_2 agonist effects. It has generally been given intranasally in doses of 0.1–0.4 ml (10–40 μg) in adults, but may be administered parenterally (1–4 μg) and as a continuous infusion.[43] Dosing is less flexible with metered-dose inhalers (minimum dose 10 μg), but is preferred by many patients. The duration of action of 12–24 h, when given intranasally, is due to slow absorption, resistance to enzymatic breakdown and an enhanced effect on the kidney. In individuals, the duration of effect is relatively constant, although there is inconsistency between patients. Larger doses are sometimes required in the very early phase of central DI, possibly due to receptor blockade by biologically active precursors of ADH released by the acutely damaged hypothalamic–pituitary tract.[33]

Although DDAVP is a polypeptide, it has been successfully administered sublingually (0.4 μg/kg)[44] and orally,[45–47] when about 10–20 times the intranasal dose is required (100–400 μg t.d.s. in adults). In young children below the age of 6 months, an initial dose of 5–10 μg orally 2–3 times a day is recommended.

There are problems with nasal absorption, storage and compliance, particularly in children. Doubts have been raised concerning the safety of its use during pregnancy.[48] Antibodies to vasopressin have occasionally occurred in patients treated with arginine and lysine vasopressin, causing secondary resistance. in these patients the antidiuretic response to DDAVP is normal.[49]

Non-hormonal therapy (not for emergency management)

These agents either increase renal sensitivity to ADH or potentiate ADH release, and are only considered in partial central DI. Usually, these patients do not require antidiuretic therapy or may be managed with small doses of DDAVP.

Thiazide diuretics

These have a paradoxical action in decreasing diuresis. Treatment, including salt restriction, causes contraction of circulatory volume, decreased glomerular filtration rate, and enhanced proximal tubular sodium chloride reabsorption such that less chloride is available for reabsorption in the diluting segment.

Chlorpropamide

This oral hypoglycaemic agent enhances the release and potentiates the renal action of residual ADH in incomplete DI. It may also restore thirst perception. Dosage is 200–500 mg daily. Hypoglycaemia still occurs despite frequent meals. Its latency of action is 3 days.

Clofibrate (Atromid-S)

This hypolipaemic agent is also thought to enhance ADH release. Dosage is 500 mg q.i.d. Combined treatment with chlorpropamide is sometimes successful. The complications of myositis, cholelithiasis and malignancy have limited its use.

Carbamazepine (Tegretol)

This anticonvulsant is thought to stimulate ADH release, but is not used in the long term because of toxicity at the dose required (400–600 mg daily).

Nephrogenic diabetes insipidus[5,50]

Congenital nephrogenic DI

The congenital form is X-linked, affecting males from birth. This form is rare and unlikely to present undiagnosed to an intensivist. These patients are V_2 receptor-deficient in the kidneys and often lack V_2 receptors extrarenally.[51,52] Hypercalcaemia, hypokalaemia and drugs (e.g. lithium, methoxyflurane and amphotericin) are likely to exacerbate the disorder and should be avoided. ADH and its analogues are ineffective in this disorder. However, thiazide diuretics and salt restriction decrease the diuresis. Additional benefit is obtained with prostaglandin synthetase inhibitors[53] (e.g. indomethacin and tolmetin sodium), especially in children where severe salt restriction is difficult.

Acquired nephrogenic DI

Acquired nephrogenic DI occurs commonly. Nephrogenic DI to some degree occurs in 20–70% of patients receiving long-term lithium therapy,[54] even when plasma lithium concentrations are kept within the normal range. Lithium causes relative unresponsiveness to exogenous ADH. Larger doses of ADH will increase renal concentrating ability. Lithium decreases renal cyclic AMP production, which may, in turn, be increased by non-steroidal anti-inflammatory drugs. Unfortunately, amelioration of lithium-induced nephrogenic DI by indomethacin[55] may produce its own complications of increasing plasma lithium concentrations and potentiating toxicity.[56] Amiloride, rather than thiazides, has been advocated for lithium-induced DI.[57] Lithium-induced nephrogenic DI may be persistent and occasionally permanent. Chronic renal failure may predispose to persistence of the DI.[58]

Nephrogenic DI has long been recognized as a side-effect of amphotericin B. Resolution of the DI has been described shortly after commencing therapy with its liposomal counterpart.[59]

Demeclocycline, which inhibits cyclicAMP accumulation and action, may be used deliberately in doses 600–1200 mg/day in the management of SIADH.

Transient diabetes insipidus of pregnancy

A vasopressin-resistant DI of pregnancy has been recognized.[60–63] This is a transient condition caused by excessive placental-generated vasopressinase,[63] an aminopeptide that metabolizes ADH. There is a brisk response with DDAVP which is not metabolized by vasopressinase.[64] Associated acute fatty liver[65,66] and liver failure have been described. Transient nephrogenic DI of pregnancy unresponsive to DDAVP has also been recognized.[67] The normal pregnancy-induced elevation in vasopressinase may unmask partial central or nephrogenic DI.[68,69] Vasopressinase concentrations decrease rapidly after delivery.

References

1 Robertson GL (1984) Abnormalities of thirst regulation. *Kidney Int* **25**:460–469.

2 Robertson GL and Berl T (1991) Pathophysiology of water metabolism. In: Brenner BM and Rector FC Jr (eds). *The Kidney* vol. 1. Philadelphia: WB Saunders, pp. 699–703.

3 Robertson GL (1987) Posterior pituitary. In: Felig P, Baxter JD, Broadus AE and Frohman LA (eds) *Endocrinology and Metabolism*, 2nd edn. New York: McGraw-Hill, pp.338–385.

4 Czernichow P and Robinson AG (1989) Neurohypophysis. In: Collu R, Ducharme JR and Guyda HJ (eds) *Paediatric Endocrinology* 2nd edn. New York: Raven Press, pp. 581–614.

5 Moses AM and Streeten DHP (1994) Disorders of the neurohypophysis. In: Isselbacher KJ, Braunwald E, Wilson JD, Martin JB, Fauci AS and Kasper DL (eds) *Harrison's Principles of Internal Medicine*, 13th edn. New York: McGraw-Hill, pp. 1921–1928.

6 Lightman SL (1993) Molecular insights into diabetes insipidus. *N Engl J Med* **328**:1562–1563.

7 Mannucci PM, Canciani MT, Rota L and Donovan BS (1981) Response of factor VIII/von Willebrand factor to dDAVP in healthy subjects and patients with haemophilia A and von Willebrand's disease. *Br J Haematol* **47**:283–293.

8 Mannuci PM, Remuzzi G, Pusineri F *et al.* (1983) Deamino-8-D-arginine vasopressin shortens the bleeding time in uremia. *N Engl J Med* **308**:8–12.

9 Salzman EW, Weinstein MJ, Weintraub RM *et al.* (1986) Treatment with desmopressin acetate to reduce blood loss after cardiac surgery. *N Engl J Med* **314**:1402–1406.

10 Czer LSC, Bateman TM and Gray RJ (1987) Treatment of severe platelet dysfunction and hemorrhage after cardiopulmonary bypass: reduction in blood product usage with desmopressin. *J Am Coll Cardiol* **9**:1139–1147.

11 Ober KP (1991) Endocrine crises. Diabetes insipidus. *Crit Care Clin* **7**:109–125.

12 Buonocore CM and Robinson AG (1993) The diagnosis and management of diabetes insipidus during medical emergencies. *Endocrinol Metab Clin North Am* **22**:411–423.

13 Blevins LS and Wand GS (1992) Diabetes insipidus. *Crit Care Med* **20**:69–79.

14 Greger NG, Kirkland RT, Clayton GW and Kirkland JL (1986) Central diabetes insipidus. 22 years' experience. *Am J Dis Child* **140**:551–554.

15 Notman DD, Mortek MA and Moses AM (1980) Permanent diabetes insipidus following head trauma: observations on 10 patients and an approach to diagnosis. *J Trauma* **20**:599–602.

16 Kern KB and Meislin HW (1984) Diabetes insipidus: occurrence after minor head trauma. *J Trauma* **24**:69–72.

17 Outwater KM and Rockoff MA (1984) Diabetes insipidus accompanying brain death in children. *Neurology* **34**:1243–1246.

18 Fiser DH, Jimenez JF, Wrape V and Woody R (1987) Diabetes insipidus in children. *Crit Care Med* **15**:551–553.

19 Fraser CL and Arieff AI (1990) Fatal central diabetes mellitus and insipidus resulting from untreated hyponatraemia: a new syndrome. *Ann Intern Med* **112**:113–119.

20 Tulandi T, Yusuf N and Posner BI (1987) Diabetes insipidus; a postpartum complication. *Obstet Gynecol* **70**:492–495.

21 Wickramasinghe LS, Chazan BI, Mandal AR, Baylis PH and Russell I (1988) Cranial diabetes insipidus after upper gastrointestinal haemorrhage. *Br Med (Clin Res)* **296**:969.

22 Jenkins HR, Hughes IA and Gray OP (1988) Cranial diabetes insipidus in early infancy. *Arch Dis Child* **63**:434–435.

23 Christensen C and Bank A (1988) Meningococcal meningitis and diabetes insipidus. *Scand J Infect Dis* **20**:341–343.

24 MacGilvray SS and Billow M (1990) Diabetes insipidus as a complication of neonatal group B streptococcal meningitis. *Pediatr Infect Dis J* **9**:742–743.

25 Garfield JM, Andriole GL, Vetto JT and Richie JP (1986) Prolonged diabetes insipidus subsequent to an episode of chemical meningitis. *Anesthesiology* **64**:253–254.

26 Urquart CK, Craft PD and Nehlawi MM (1994) Transient diabetes insipidus following electrical burns in two patients. *South Med J* **87**:412–413.

27 Palakurthy PR, Iyer V and Klein J (1987) Amiodarone-induced encephalopathy and diabetes insipidus. *J Ky Med Assoc* **85**:373–374.

28 Salky B and Kim US (1978) Aufses AH Jr. (1978) Transient diabetes insipidus following penetrating thoracic trauma. *Mt Sinai J Med (NY)* **45**:545–550.

29 Kuan P, Messenger JC and Ellestad MH (1983) Transient central diabetes insipidus after aortocoronayr bypass operations. *Am J Cardiol* **52**: 1181–1183.

30 Robertson GL (1988) Differential diagnosis of polyuria. *Annu Rev Med* **39**:425–442.

31 Hans P, Stevenaert A and Albert A (1986) Study of hypotonic polyuria after transphenoidal pituitary adenomectomy. *Intensive Care Med* **12**:95–99.

32 Randall RV, Clark EC, Dodge HW and Love JG (1960) Polyuria after operation for tumours in the region of the hypophysis and hypothalamus. *J Clin Endocrinol Metab* **20**:1614–1621.

33 Seckl JR, Dunger DB, Bevan JS *et al.* (1990) insipidus. *Lancet* **335**:1353–1356.

34 Chuecos JM, Gaite FB and Pardos FI (1988) Vasopressin antagonist in early post-operative diabetes Partial ADH deficiency vs endogenous fluid overload in hypotonic polyuria (letter). *Intensive Care Med* **14**: 252–253.

35 Arem R, Rushford FE, Segal J, Robinson A, Grossman RG and Field JB (1986) Selective osmoreceptor dysfunction presenting as intermittent hypernatraemia following surgery for a pituitary chromophobe adenoma. *Am J Med* **80**:1217–1224.

36 Robertson GL (1994) The use of vasopressin assays in physiology and pathophysiology. *Semin Nephrol* **14**:368–383.

37 Sakurai H, Kanai A, Nomura K, Demura H and Shizume K (1986) A simple and highly sensitive radio-immunoassay for 8-arginine vasopressin in human plasma using a reversed-phase C18 silica column. *J Tokyo Wom Med Coll* **56**:394–403.

38 Moses AM, Clayton B and Hochhauser L (1992) The use of T1-weighted magnetic resonance imaging to differentiate between primary polydipsia and central diabetes insipidus. *Am J Neuroradiol* **13**: 1273–1277.

39 Seckl JR and Drager DB (1992) Diabetes insipidus. Current treatment recommendations. *Drugs* **44**: 216–224.

40 Levitt MA, Fleischer AS and Meislin HW (1984) Acute post-traumatic diabetes insipidus: treatment with continuous intravenous vasopressin. *J Trauma* **24**:532–535.

41 Chanson P, Jedynak CP, Dabrowski G *et al.* (1987) Ultra low doses of vasopressin in the management of diabetes insipidus. *Crit Care Med* **15**:44–46.

42 Richardson DW, Robinson AG (1985) Desmopressin. *Ann Intern Med* **103**:228–239.

43 Chanson P, Jedynak CP and Czernichow P (1988) Management of early postoperative diabetes insipidus with parenteral desmopressin. *Acta Endocrinol* **117**: 513–516.

44 Kappy MS and Sonderer E (1987) Sublingual administration of desmopressin. Effectiveness in an infant with holoprosencephaly and central diabetes insipidus. *Am J Dis Child* **141**:84–85.

45 Stick SM and Betts PR (1987) Oral desmopressin in neonatal diabetes insipidus. *Arch Dis Child* **62**: 1177–1178.

46 Fjellestad-Paulsen A, Paulsen O, d-Agay-Abensour L, Lundin S and Czernichow P (1993) Central diabetes insipidus: oral treatment with dDAVP. *Regulatory Peptides* **45**:303–307.

47 Hammer M and Vilhardt H (1985) Peroral treatment of diabetes insipidus with a polypeptide hormone analog, desmopressin. *J. Pharmacol Exp Ther* **234**:754–760.

48 Linder N, Matoth I, Ohel G, Yourish D and Tamir I (1986) L-deamino-8-arginine vasopressin treatment in pregnancy and neonatal outcome. A report of three cases. *Am J Perinatol* **3**:165–167.

49 Vokes TJ, Gaskill MB and Robertson GL (1988) Antibodies to vasopressin in patients with diabetes insipidus. Implications for diagnosis and therapy. *Ann Intern Med* **108**:190–195.

50 Knoers N and Monnens LAH (1992) Nephrogenic diabetes insipidus: clinical symptoms, pathogenesis, genetics and treatment. *Paediatr Nephrol* **6**:476–482.

51 Brenner B, Seligsohn U and Hochberg Z (1988) Normal response of factor VIII and von Willebrand factor to L-deamine-8-D-arginine vasopressin in nephrogenic diabetes insipidus. *J Clin Endocrinol Metab* **67**:191–193.

52 Moses AM, Miller JL and Levine MA (1988) Two distinct pathophysiological mechanisms in congenital nephrogenic diabetes insipidus. *J Clin Endocrinol Metab* **66**:1259–1264.

53 Libber S, Harrison H and Spector D (1986) Treatment of nephrogenic diabetes insipidus with prostaglandin synthesis inhibitors. *J Pediatr* **108**: 305–311.

54 Waller DG (1985) Thyroid function and urine-concentrating ability during lithium treatment. *J Psychiatr Res* **19**:569–571.

55 Allen HM, Jackson RL, Winchester MD, Deck LV and Allon M (1989) Indomethacin in the treatment of lithium-induced nephrogenic diabetes insipidus. *Arch Intern Med* **149**:1123–1126.

56 Grindlinger GA and Boylan MJ (1987) Amelioration by indomethacin of lithium-induced polyuria. *Crit Care Med* **15**:538–539.

57 Batlle DC, von Riotte AB, Graviria M, Grupp M. (1985) Amelioration of polyuria by amiloride in patients receiving long-term lithium therapy. *N Engl J Med* **312**:408–14.

58 Neitherent WD, Spooner RJ, Hendry A, Dagg JH (1990) Persistent nephrogenic diabetes insipidus, tubular proteinuria, aminoaciduria, and parathyroid hormone resistance following long-term lithium administration. *Postgrad Med J* **66**:479–482.

59 Smith OP, Gale R, Hamon M, McWhinney P and Prentice HG (1994) Amphotericin B-induced nephrogenic diabetes insipidus: resolution with its liposomal counterpart. *Bone Marrow Transplant* **13**:107–108.

60 Barron WM, Cohen LH, Ulland LA *et al.* (1984) Transient vasopressin-resistant diabetes insipidus of pregnancy. *N Engl J Med* **310**:442–444.

61 Durr JA (1987) Diabetes insipidus in pregnancy. *Am J Kidney Dis* **9**:276–283.

62 Robinson AG and Amico JA (1991) 'Non-sweet' diabetes of pregnancy. *N Engl J Med* **324**:556–558.

63 Durr JA, Hoggard JG, Hunt JM and Schrier RW (1987) Diabetes insipidus in pregnancy associated with abnormally high circulating vasopressinase activity. *N Engl J Med* **316**:1070–1074.

64 Shah SV and Thakur V (1988) Vasopressinase and diabetes insipidus of pregnancy (letter). *Ann Intern Med* **109**:435–436.

65 Cammu H, Velkeniers B, Charels K, Vincken W and Amy JJ (1987) Idiopathic acute fatty liver of pregnancy associated with transient diabetes insipidus. Case report. *Br J Obstet Gynaecol* **94**:173–178.

66 Kennedy S, Hall P, Seymour AE and Hague WM (1994) Transient diabetes insipidus and acute fatty liver of pregnancy. *Br J Obstet Gynaecol* **101**:387–391.

67 Ford SM Jr. (1986) Transient vasopressin-resistant diabetes insipidus of pregnancy. *Obstet Gynecol* **68**: 288–289.

68 Williams DJ, Metcalf KA, Skingle L, Stock AI, Beedham T and Monson JP (1993) Pathophysiology of transient cranial diabetes insipidus during pregnancy. *Clin Endocrinol* **38**:595–600.

69 Iwasaki Y, Oiso Y, Kondo K *et al.* (1991) Aggravation of subclinical diabetes insipidus during pregnancy. *N Engl J Med* **324**:522–526.

52 | Thyroid emergencies

AE Vedig

Thyroid disease is common in western countries (it occurs in 1–3% of the population). Myxoedema coma and thyroid crisis are rare, but have a high mortality without specific treatment. Abnormal thyroid hormone concentrations commonly occur in critically ill patients.

Basic physiology and pathophysiology[1–4]

The thyroid gland actively uptakes and concentrates iodide, which is oxidized and organified to produce tetraiodothyronine (T_4) and triiodothyronine (T_3). When iodine deficiency exists, the gland increases the efficiency of uptake, whereas excess iodine inhibits synthesis and release of the thyroid hormones. Both T_4 and T_3 are extensively bound to plasma proteins with small amounts (T_4 0.03%, T_3 0.3%) circulating free. The total concentrations of T_4 and T_3 are affected by protein binding. T_4 is produced only by the thyroid gland. T_3 is secreted by the thyroid, but most arises from β-deiodination of T_4 in peripheral tissues (particularly liver and kidney), which also yields an inactive metabolite, reverse T_3 (rT_3), by α-deiodination. Peripheral deiodination of T_4 is decreased in pathological states and by some pharmaceutical agents (Table 52.1). The half-life of T_4 in the circulation is 7 days; the half-life of T_3 is approximately 24 h. Free hormone (FT_3) enters cells and attaches to specific intracellular receptors (TR). The brain, heart, liver and kidney have high concentrations of TR. T_3 has a much greater effect than T_4 on metabolic state, which correlates more closely to concentrations of free hormones rather than total hormones in plasma. The rate of synthesis of a variety of proteins is affected through messenger RNA. Thyroid hormones increase sodium–potassium ATPase activity, stimulate β-adrenergic receptors, increase cycling of fatty acids, and generally increase cell respiration and energy expenditure.

Syndromes with distinctive clinical features of generalized thyroid hormone resistance are recognized.[5] Abnormal function of thyroid receptors results in a euthyroid or hypothyroid state with elevated circulating FT_3 and FT_4.

There are two distinct mechanisms of regulation of thyroid function. First, thyroid hormones regulate in a classic negative feedback manner the secretion of thyroid-stimulating hormone (TSH) from the anterior pituitary. The level of circulating FT_4 and FT_3 and intrapituitary-generated T_3 from T_4 influences TSH secretion, as does thyrotrophin-releasing hormone (TRH), which sets the threshold of feedback. TRH is, in turn, also influenced by circulating thyroid hormones and higher centres in the brain. Dopamine and somatostatin are physiological inhibitors of TRH secretion, as are glucocorticoids. Interleukin and tumour necrosis factor also inhibit TSH secretion.

Autoregulation is the second mechanism of regulating thyroid hormones by maintaining the pool of organic iodine within the thyroid gland. A negative feedback exists between the size of the organic pool of iodine, the sensitivity of the thyroid gland to TSH, and the activity of the iodide transport mechanism in the gland. When autoregulation is unable to sustain normal secretion of thyroid hormone, increased activation of the hypothalamus–pituitary axis occurs. Large amounts of iodine inhibit thyroid hormone synthesis (Wolff–Chaikoff effect), but normal autoregulation permits 'escape'. Failure of escape leads to

Table 52.1 States associated with decreased deiodination of T_4 to T_3 tetraiodothyronine to triiodothyronine

Systemic illness
Fasting
Malnutrition
Postoperative state
Trauma
Drugs – propylthiouracil, glucocorticoids, propranolol, amiodarone
Radiographic contrast agents (ipodate, ipanoate)

continued inhibition of hormone synthesis with consequent TSH-induced goitre and enhanced iodide transport, which further inhibits hormone synthesis, often resulting in hypothyroidism. Neonatal and damaged glands (e.g. Hashimoto's disease, radio-iodine-treated Graves' disease, and patients treated with lithium and phenazone) are susceptible to failure of escape. If there is a basic failure in autoregulation, then iodide excess, rather than inhibiting synthesis of thyroid hormones, will lead to sustained hyper-secretion (Jod–Basedow disease).

Laboratory tests usually available include FT_4, FT_3 concentrations in blood, and sensitive and ultra-sensitive TSH measurements.

Thyroid function with non-thyroidal illness

The sick euthyroid syndrome[6-8] is used to describe clinically euthyroid patients with severe non-thyroidal illness (NTI) who have low T_3, normal or low T_4, elevated rT_3, and a TSH that is normal or low, but occasionally increased in the recovery phase of an illness (Table 52.2). A normal TSH suggests a euthyroid state, but the TSH level is probably inappropriately low for circulating thyroid hormone concentrations, although synthesis of T_3 tissue receptors is increased.[9] Starvation, stress, effects of cytokines and drugs (dopamine, steroids and opioids) reduce thyrotropin secretion and effect.

Conditions such as hepatic cirrhosis and chronic renal failure may elevate TSH. As the underlying illness improves, a TSH concentration that has been low or normal may rise and be transiently elevated. Specific variants of thyroid function abnormality have been described with severe NTI. Low T_4 and/or T_3 and TSH correlate with the severity of illness and mortality in many non-thyroidal disorders.[7,10]

Rarely, euthyroid hyperthyroxinaemia[11] occurs in sick patients. The diagnosis may be difficult in an elderly patient with severe NTI where apathetic hyperthyroidism is a consideration. TSH concentrations are normal, reduced or increased. The mechanism of causation is sometimes uncertain, but is sometimes associated with drugs that inhibit peripheral T_4 conversion to T_3 (e.g. amiodarone, propranolol and contrast agents), hyperemesis, acute psychiatric illness and hyponatraemia. Failure to

recognize these clinical entities may result in inappropriate therapy.

In general, patients who have low thyroid hormone concentrations in blood in the setting of NTI do not benefit from treatment with thyroid hormones.[8,12]

Thyroid crisis (thyroid storm)[1,13–17]

Thyroid crisis is the life-threatening clinical extreme of hyperthyroidism. It is more common in women than in men, and has a mortality rate of 10–20% with treatment. The onset is usually abrupt, and precipitating factors may be identified in about 50% of cases.

FT_3 or FT_4, although usually high in crisis, does not correlate well with the severity of the condi-tion.[18,19] The essential feature of crisis is that it is a condition of decompensation, where target organs lose their ability to modulate their response to excess T_3 or T_4. Pathogenesis is obscure and, curiously, many of the precipitating conditions are normally associated with inhibition of T_4 to T_3 conversion. TSH is undetectable.

Precipitating factors

The majority of patients presenting in crisis have unrecognized or poorly-controlled Graves' disease. Intercurrent illness, particularly infection, trauma, operative procedures, uncontrolled diabetes mellitus, labour and eclampsia, are the most commonly described provoking factors. Crisis is now uncommon as a complication of thyroid surgery, but has been reported following excessive palpation of the thyroid gland, incomplete preparation,[20,21] and inadequate dosage of β-adrenergic antagonists perioperatively. Uncommon factors include the use of radioiodine in unprepared patients, and drugs such as iodides in patients with impaired autoregulation (Jod–Basedow phenomenon), haloperidol, or massive overdose of thyroid hormone preparations. Overdoses of less than 10 mg usually cause few problems, but massive doses may precipitate a thyrotoxic crisis within days.[22,23]

Clinical presentation[13–17]

Exaggerated manifestations of hyperthyroidism (Table 52.3) are usually present. Hyperpyrexia, tachycardia with atrial fibrillation (AF), delirium, agitation or coma, vomiting, diarrhoea and muscle weakness are the main features. Rarely, apathetic hyperthyroidism (occurring usually in the elderly) may present in crisis with the features of profound exhaustion, tachycardia, hyporeflexia, severe myopathy, marked weight loss and hypotension. The usual differential diagnosis is sepsis, but the presentation may be confused with malignant hyperthermia. Clinical presentation may be complicated by the precipitating factors and coexistent disease.

Table 52.2 Changes in thyroid hormone concentrations

	FT_4	T_3	TSH
Euthyroid	N	N	N
Hyperthyroid	↑	↑	↓
Hypothyroid	↓	↓ N	↑
Non-thyroid illness	↑ N ↓	↓	N ↓

FT_4 = Free tetraiodothyronine; T_3 = triiodothyronine; TSH = thyroid-stimulat-ing hormone; N = normal; ↑ = increased; ↓ = decreased.

Table 52.3 Clinical manifestations of hyperthyroidism

Nervousness, insomnia, tremor, hyperkinesis, muscle weakness, hyperactive reflexes

Heat intolerance, hot and moist skin, increased sweating, acropachy, onycholysis

Bowel hyperactivity, increased appetite, weight loss

Eye symptoms, stare, lid retraction, lid lag, ophthalmopathy (if Graves disease)

Dyspnoea, fatigue, tachycardia, atrial fibrillation, congestive cardiac failure, mitral valve prolapse

Goitre, dysphagia, thyroid bruit (if Graves disease)

Fever

Fever may be extreme (>41°C) and is generally regarded as essential to the diagnosis. Pyrexia is not usually present in uncomplicated thyrotoxicosis. The skin is usually moist and warm.

Cardiovascular features

Cardiovascular features are very common, even in patients with the apathetic presentation. Sinus tachycardia (often >160 beats/min), heart failure, AF and ventricular arrhythmias are common. Mitral valve prolapse occurs frequently in patients with treated or active hyperthyroidism. Cardiomegaly and electrocardiogram (ECG) changes of left ventricular hypertrophy may be seen. Decreasing pulse rate and systemic blood pressure with the development of shock are poor prognostic features.

Neurological and muscular disturbances

These are very common. A clinical picture of tremor and increasing restlessness progressing to delirium, coma and death is characteristic of untreated cases. Profound muscular weakness may occur, particularly with apathetic thyrotoxic crisis. Other syndromes of muscle weakness have been described, including descriptions of an upper motor neurone abnormality with asymmetrical reflexes, and sudden-onset episodic thyrotoxic periodic paralysis.[24] Rhabdomyolysis[25] has also occurred.

Gastrointestinal disturbances

Gastrointestinal disturbances of vomiting, nausea and diarrhoea may be present and complicate management, because of the poor bioavailability of orally administered drugs. Severe abdominal pain[26,27] may suggest an underlying abdominal emergency. Jaundice is sometimes present and is a poor prognostic sign.

Hypercalcaemia

Hypercalcaemia is relatively common (15%) in severe thyrotoxicosis, but rarely an independent emergency. Hypokalaemia and leukocytosis occur frequently, and hypomagnesaemia may be severe, particularly with apathetic thyrotoxicosis.

Management[13–17]

Management includes diagnosis of the precipitating event, supportive measures, reducing the synthesis, release, peripheral conversion, and peripheral effects of thyroid hormones, and searching for the cause of hyperthyroidism. The diagnosis of thyroid crisis is clinical and management must be aggressive. A protocol that includes rapid access to required drugs must be formulated in advance. Blood should be collected for thyroid hormone and TSH assays before commencing therapy. Responses to treatment can be monitored by observation of clinical signs (e.g. pulse, temperature and agitation) and serum T_3.

β-Adrenergic blockade

β-Adrenergic blockade antagonizes the effect of thyroid hormones and the hypersensitivity to the action of catecholamines. Propranolol is the drug of choice, as it inhibits the peripheral conversion of T_4 to T_3.[28] Tachycardia, fever, hyperkinesis and tremor respond promptly. Other beneficial effects include improvement in proximal myopathy, periodic thyrotoxic paralysis, bulbar palsy and thyrotoxic hypercalcaemia. Blockade is achieved with IV increments of 0.5 mg, with continuous cardiovascular monitoring, usually to a total of 10 mg. Further amounts are given 4–6-hourly. The usual oral doses are 20–120 mg 6-hourly, but because of the markedly increased clearance, very large doses (>720 mg) may be required to achieve β-blockade.

β_1-Selective antagonists do not inhibit T_4 to T_3 conversion as effectively as propranolol,[29] but may be favoured in the presence of complicating factors, e.g. reactive airways and heart failure. Use of β-blockers should be combined with other therapy, since the basic metabolic abnormalities are not inhibited.

Esmolol[30–32] 250–500 μg/kg IV loading dose followed by an infusion of 50–100 μg/kg per min may be titrated to a desired effect. Because of its ultrashort action, undesirable side-effects will be short-lived.

Reserpine and guanethidine, although largely superseded by the β-adrenergic blockers, may be life-saving, and should be considered in propranolol-resistant hyperthyroidism[33] and if propranolol is contraindicated. Onset of action is slow, and adverse effects include central nervous system depression and diarrhoea. The parenteral formulation of reserpine is no longer manufactured.

Diltiazem reduces pulse rate as effectively as propranolol[34] and could be considered as an alternative to β-blockers in thyroid crisis.

Corticosteroids

Corticosteroids are usually administered during a crisis, because a relative deficiency may be present, and glucocorticoids inhibit the peripheral conversion of T_4 to T_3. Hydrocortisone 100 mg IV 6-hourly or dexamethasone 5 mg IV 12-hourly is suggested. Dexamethasone, together with iodides, can produce a rapid reduction in the degree of thyroxtoxicosis.

Thioamides

Propylthiouracil

Propylthiouracil is given orally or administered as a slurry via a nasogastric tube. Unfortunately, gastro-intestinal absorption is impaired or unreliable in thyroid crisis, but no parenteral preparation of this thioamide is available. It has a rapid onset of action, and exerts its effects by blocking the iodination of tyrosine and partial inhibition of the peripheral conversion of T_4 to T_3. A loading dose of 1 g may be given, followed by 200–300 mg 4–6 hourly.

Methimazole

Methimazole may be less rapidly absorbed, but is longer acting. It does not inhibit peripheral conversion of T_4. Equipotent doses are one-tenth of propyl-thiouracil. A dose of 100 mg may be given orally, followed by 20 mg 8-hourly.

Carbimazole

Carbimazole is metabolized to methimazole (relative potency 0.62 : 1.0).

Transient leukopenia is common (20%) with antithyroid drugs, but agranulocytosis is rare.

Iodine

When given in large doses, iodine inhibits the synthesis and release of thyroid hormones. Its administration is generally delayed for at least an hour after thioamides. Oral iodine/iodide preparations include Lugol's iodine (130 mg total iodine/ml), potassium iodide or sodium iodide. Intravenous preparations are not always available, but can be easily prepared. Sodium iodide, 1 g IV, can be given 12-hourly as either a continuous infusion or a bolus over a few minutes. Equivalent doses of other available preparations are given orally or via a nasogastric tube. There is evidence that the iodine-containing contrast media (Ipodate 1 g orally twice daily for the first day and then 1 g daily for a maximum of 2 weeks) may specifically ameliorate the cardiac effects of thyroxine.[35] In addition they are the most potent blockers of T_4 to T_3 conversion. It has been suggested that these agents are now the drugs of choice rather than simple iodides.[17]

Lithium carbonate

Lithium carbonate is an alternative in patients who are allergic to iodine. It has a similar action in blocking thyroid hormone release. Doses of 500–1500 mg daily have been used. Frequent drug level monitoring is required to maintain lithium concentrations of 0.7–1.4 mmol/l.

Digoxin

Digoxin is indicated following the correction of hypokalaemia when AF is present. Larger doses than usual will be required because of pharmacokinetic and pharmacodynamic changes associated with the hyperthyroid state. Adequate slowing of ventricular responses is not usually achieved with digoxin alone. β-Adrenergic blockers, verapamil, or even reserpine may be considered. Thyrotoxic patients are very sensitive to warfarin, if oral anticoagulants are considered because of AF.

Amiodarone[36-39]

Amiodarone may be useful when given parenterally to control acute arrhythmias, and has been shown to inhibit peripheral deiodination of T_4 to T_3. It has been used by itself and in combination with thioamides to treat thyrotoxicosis. Acute antithyroid hormone effects on the heart are also described.

Supportive measures

Supportive measures include identification and treatment of the precipitating cause. This is complicated by the non-specific symptoms and signs of severe hyperthyroidism. These patients are grossly hypermetabolic and may require large amounts of fluids, electrolytes and glucose. Careful monitoring is required. Vitamins, particularly thiamine, are usually given. Usual measures are used for the treatment of hyperpyrexia, except that salicylates are avoided. They displace thyroid hormones from their binding proteins.[40] Frusemide is also a competitor for binding proteins and causes abrupt increases in FT_3 and FT_4 concentrations,[41] and should be similarly avoided. Ethacrynic acid is a suggested alternative.[42] The markedly increased metabolism and clearance of drugs may complicate management. Specimens should be taken for microbiological purposes and consideration should be given to empiric antibiotics.

Plasma exchange[43-45] and charcoal haemoperfusion have been successfully used in refractory cases following 24–48 h of aggressive conventional therapy. However, lack of efficacy has also been reported.[46]

Dantrolene[47,48] has been used with symptomatic improvement, when thyrotoxic crisis mimicked malignant hyperthermia, and for the treatment of a recognized thyrotoxic crisis.

Myxoedema coma[1,14,15,17,49-52]

Overt hypothyroidism is present in 0.5–0.8% of the population. While hypothyroidism may occur in either sex or at any age, myxoedema coma occurs typically during winter in elderly females. Myxoedema coma represents the terminal stage of decompensated hypothyroidism, and has a high mortality even if recognized. Most patients present in an earlier stage with neither coma nor obvious myxoedema. Patients presenting with decompensated hypothyroidism or coma usually have long-standing unrecognized thyroid hypofunction, most commonly caused by autoimmune thyroiditis, radioiodine therapy or thyroidectomy.

Drugs (e.g. phenytoin, frusemide, non-steroidal anti-inflammatory drugs, glucocorticoids and dopamine) can affect thyroid hormone concentrations, such that hypothyroidism is falsely suggested. Diagnosis of hypothyroidism in patients with critical illness should be made with caution. Thyroid hormone replacement in hypothyroxinaemic sick patients simply to achieve normal levels of circulatory hormone is not recommended.[9] True hypothyroidism may be produced by antithyroid drugs, iodine lithium and amiodarone.[53,54]

Thyroid hormone concentrations will indicate whether the hypothyroidism is probably due to intrinsic thyroid disease (primary and most common), a failure of secretion of TSH (secondary) or hypothalamic dysfunction (tertiary).

Precipitating factors

Coma is often precipitated by hypothermia, sometimes consequent to central nervous system depressant drugs (that inhibit thermogenesis or interfere with neurovascular adaptation to reduced thermogenesis, infections, trauma, cardiac failure or cerebrovascular accident), or drugs with antithyroid actions, including amiodarone.[55] There is usually a long history of pre-existing hypothyroidism.

Clinical presentation

The diagnosis of myxoedema coma is dependent on recognizing the triad of altered mental state, hypothermia, and clinical features of hypothyroidism (Table 52.4). When the typical features of hypothyroidism are present, diagnosis is straightforward. Difficulties arise when the features are atypical, the onset is relatively rapid, or when complicated by

Table 52.4 Clinical manifestations of hypothyroidism

Cold intolerance, decreased energy, muscular weakness, bradykinesia, dementia, delayed tendon reflexes

Dry, yellowish skin, hoarse voice, coarse facial features, lateral eyebrow thinning, periorbital oedema, brittle hair

Constipation, weight gain, pleural and pericardial effusions, ischaemic heart disease, anaemia

precipitating factors. Myxoedemic coma and coma in association with the sick euthyroid syndrome may be difficult to differentiate.

1 *Coma* is due to the combination of hypothermia, hypercarbia, hypoxia, cerebral oedema and other metabolic derangements. Its onset may be quite abrupt. Tendon reflexes are usually symmetrical, but show a slow relaxation phase. Major seizures precede coma in about 25% of patients. Myopathy may be present. Creatine phosphokinase is frequently elevated.

2 *Hypothermia* may be profound, particularly when ambient temperatures are low. A low reading thermometer is required.

3 *Hypoventilation* occurs very frequently. Quantitation and monitoring of hypoxaemia and hypercarbia require blood-gas analysis. Multifactorial contributions to the respiratory failure include decreased ventilatory responsiveness to hypoxia and carbon dioxide, respiratory muscle fatigue, obesity, myxoedematous thickening of the vocal cords and sensitivity to the depressant effects of drugs.[56]

4 *Hypotension* is common and usually accompanied by an inappropriate sinus bradycardia. Baroreceptor dysfunction and reduction in plasma volume contribute. Tissue hypoxia is compounded by shock and anaemia. Myocardial myxoedematous infiltrates occur, but while pericardial effusions are frequently present, cardiac tamponade is uncommon. A small heart suggests adrenal insufficiency secondary to either pituitary hypothyroidism or coincidental primary adrenal failure. Lactic acidosis is frequent and may be severe. Increased creatine kinase MB[57,58] may be due to hypothermia rather than myocardial infarction. The ECG may show a slow-rate, low-voltage trace, with prolongation of Q–T interval and T-wave flattening or inversion.

5 *Hypoglycaemia* is often present and requires rapid recognition and treatment.

6 *Hyponatraemia* with low serum osmolality and increased total body water and sodium associated with oedema will be evident if hypothyroidism is long-standing and severe. Increased antidiuretic hormone concentrations and altered renal clearance of free water contribute to fluid accumulation. Despite excess total body sodium and water, plasma volume is usually depleted by 10–20% of predicted. Azotaemia and hypophosphataemia are common.

7 *Hypofunction of gut and bladder* with paralytic ileus, megacolon[59] and urinary retention are frequent accompaniments.

Management[1,14,15,17,49]

Management of myxoedema coma includes careful assessment, treating precipitating factors and complications, and appropriate administration of thyroid hormone. Treatment should begin once the clinical diagnosis is made without awaiting laboratory confirmation. Rapid availability of appropriate formulations of thyroid hormone is very important. Blood should be collected for thyroid function tests and plasma cortisol determination before thyroid hormone is administered.

Thyroid hormones[60-62]

The emphasis in severe and long-standing hypothyroidism is on initial low doses, with gradual escalation of hormone replacement. This may take months and never reach normal requirements, if complicated by ischaemic heart disease. More rapid replacement has been associated with sudden death due to arrhythmias or myocardial infarction, because of the imbalance in myocardial oxygen supply and demand. Oral T_4 (of variable, but approximately 50% bioavailability) is usually commenced at 50–100 μg/day with 25 μg increments, although 12.5–25.0 μg/day is an appropriate initial dose if ischaemic heart disease is present. There may be advantages in the use of T_3 orally (10 μg/day with 5 μg increments). It has good oral bioavailability and there is rapid cessation of hormone action if arrhythmias occur or angina worsens.

The optimum regimen for thyroid hormone replacement in myxoedema coma is unknown. Intestinal absorption of thyroid hormones, particularly T_4, is very variable with severe hypothyroidism, and the peripheral conversion of T_4 to T_3 is decreased. Larger-dose proponents suggest that loading doses are necessary in myxoedema coma to saturate binding protein, and restore hormone levels to a low-normal euthyroid state. If T_4 is to be used, it must initially be given IV. A bolus of 400–500 μg (300 μg/m^2) followed by 50 μg IV daily is recommended. Changeover to orally administered T_4 may occur when gastrointestinal function resumes. Although a safer, smoother response is claimed for the use of T_4 (because of a gradual increase in the T_4 to T_3 conversion), this response is slow. Improvements in body temperature, heart rate and mental state barely begin within 24 h. Doses of T_4 (300 μg/m^2) have been given to sick euthyroid patients without detectable adverse effects.[12] T_3 may be given IV or via a nasogastric tube as 25–50 μg bolus, followed by 10–20 μg 8-hourly. The clinical response with T_3 is more rapid.

Alternatively, it is argued that large doses are not essential for recovery and may be harmful. A dose of 200–300 μg of thyroxine IV may be quite adequate. Intravenous infusions of T_3, either continuously (20 μg/day) or very slow boluses repeated 8-hourly, may be preferred. The solubility and stability of T_3 in solution can be maintained if albumin 2% is added to the normal saline diluent, and polypropylene syringes and minimum-volume polyvinyl chloride extension tubes are used.[63] The advantage of more rapid onset and cessation of action may be achieved with infusions of T_3, or even repeated smaller doses (5 μg) via nasogastric tube, without getting dangerously high plasma concentrations.

The degree of hypothyroidism (as indicated by thyroid hormone concentrations) is not directly related to the severity of illness (e.g. degree of hypothermia or metabolic acidosis). Hence, initial doses of thyroid hormones should not necessarily relate to illness severity.

Corticosteroids

Corticosteroids are usually administered, as patients with myxoedema coma may have impaired glucocorticoid response to stress, or even frank coexistent adrenal insufficiency (Schmidt's syndrome). Hydrocortisone, at least 200–300 mg/day, should be administered until normal adrenocortical function is demonstrated.

Supportive measures

These patients have reduced ventilatory response to hypoxia and hypercarbia, and are very sensitive to central nervous system depressants. Endotracheal intubation and ventilation will often be required for airway protection and symptomatic management of hypercarbia. An additional benefit of intubation is the provision of warm humidification to treat hypothermia. Delayed gastric emptying and the anatomical abnormalities of the upper airway require specific care with intubation.

Shock is managed in accordance with usual principles, except that thyroid hormone and corticosteroids must be given. Intravascular fluid depletion is common despite oedema. There is resistance to inotropic agents, due to a reduction in β-adrenergic receptor expression.[64] α-Adrenergic activity appears to remain intact. Hyponatraemia usually responds to water restriction. Rarely, rapid onset, severe hyponatraemia (less than 110 mmol/l) in association with coma and convulsions will require hypertonic saline. Sodium bicarbonate (8.4%) should be considered if severe metabolic acidosis coexists.

Intravenous glucose, 25 g statum, is given for hypoglycaemia. Hypertonic (20–50%) glucose may be infused via a central vein commensurate with glucose, and water restriction requirements.

Mild hypothermia (e.g. 34–36°C) requires little more than prevention of further heat loss, treating hypoglycaemia, and warming of inspired gases. Moderate to severe hypothermia ($<$32°C) requires specific active management to bring core temperatures to $>$34°C. Provided there is adequate monitoring of body temperature gradients, appropriate responses to haemodynamic and metabolic changes to prevent rewarming shock and acidosis, there is little to support the often repeated traditional warning against active warming.[65,66]

Precipitating events and complications, e.g. septicaemia and pneumonia, will require specific therapy. Impaired bioavailability and clearance of drugs[67] complicate therapy (e.g. sensitivity to digoxin, but resistance to anticoagulants).

References

1 Wartofsky L (1994) Diseases of the thyroid. In: Isselbacher KJ, Braunwald E, Wilson JD, Martin JD, Fauci AS and Kasper DL (eds) *Harrison's Principles of Internal Medicine,* 13th edn. New York: McGraw-Hill, pp. 1930–1953.

2 Woeber KA (1991) Iodine and thyroid disease. *Med Clin North Am* **75:**169–178.

3 Kaye TB (1993) Thyroid function tests: application of newer methods. *Postgrad Med* **94:**81–90.

4 Kaptein EM (1993) Clinical application of free thyroxine determinations. *Clin Lab Med* **13:**653–672.

5 McDermott MT and Ridgway EC (1993) Thyroid hormone resistance syndromes. *Am J Med* **94:**424–432.

6 Chopra IJ, Hershman JM, Pardridge WM and Nicoloff JT (1983) Thyroid function in nonthyroidal illness. *Ann Intern Med* **98:**946–957.

7 Zologa GP, Chernow B, Smallridge RC *et al.* (1985) A longitudinal evaluation of thyroid function in critically ill surgical patients. *Ann Surg* **201:**456–464.

8 Tibaldi JM and Surks MI (1985) Effects of nonthyroidal illness on thyroid function. *Med Clin North Am* **69:**899–911.

9 Williams GR, Franklyn JA, Neuberger JM and Sheppard MC (1989) Thyroid hormone receptor expression in the 'sick euthyroid' syndrome. *Lancet* **ii:**1477–1481.

10 Slag MR, Morley JE, Elson MK, Crowson TW, Nuttall FQ and Shaffer RB (1981) Hypothyroxinaemia in critically ill patients as a predictor of high mortality. *J Am Med Assoc* **245:**43–45.

11 Jackson JA, Verdonk CA and Spiekerman AM (1987) Euthyroid hyperthyroxinaemia and inappropriate secretion of thyrotropin. Recognition and diagnosis. *Arch Intern Med* **147:**1311–1313.

12 Brent GA and Hershman JM (1986) Thyroxine therapy in patients with severe nonthyroidal illnesses and low serum thyroxine concentrations. *J Clin Endocrinol Metab* **63:**1–8.

13 Franklyn JA (1994) The management of hyperthyroidism. *N Engl J Med* **330:**1731–1738.

14 Stockigt JR (1993) Thyroid disease. *Med J Aust* **158:**770–774.

15 Smallridge RC (1992) Metabolic and anatomical thyroid emergencies. A review. *Crit Care Med* **20:**276–91.

16 Burch HB and Wartofsky L (1993) Life–threatening thyrotoxicosis. Thyroid storm. *Endocrinol Metab Clin North Am* **22:**263–277.

17 Burger AG and Philippe J (1992) Thyroid emergencies. *Bailliere's Clin Endocrinol Metab* **6:** 77–93.

18 Topliss DJ and Stockigt JR (1979) Free thyroxine concentrations in thyroid storm. *N Engl J Med* **300:**92–93.

19 Brooks MH and Waldenstein SS (1980) Free thyroxine concentrations in thyroid storm. *Ann Intern Med* **93:**694–697.

20 Strube PJ (1984) Thyroid storm during beta blockade. *Anaesthesia* **39:**343–346.

21 Reed J and Bradley EL (1985) Postoperative thyroid storm after lithium preparation. *Surgery* **98:**983–986.

22 Nystrom E, Lindstedt G and Lundberg PA (1980) Minor signs and symptoms of toxicity in a young woman in spite of a massive thyroxine ingestion. *Acta Med Scand* 207:135–136.

23 Ratnaike S, Campbell DG and Melick RA (1986) Thyroxine overdose. *Aust NZ J Med* **16:**514.

24 Robson NJ (1985) Emergency surgery complicated by throtoxicosis and thyrotoxic periodic paralysis. *Anaesthesia* 40:27–31.

25 Bennett NR and Huston DP (1989) Rhabdomyolysis in thyroid storm. *Am J Med* **77:**733–735.

26 Coe NP, Page DW, Friedmann P and Haag BL (1982) Apathetic thyrotoxicosis presenting as an abdominal emergency: a diagnostic pitfall. *South Med J* **75:**175–178.

27 Harwood–Nuss AL and Martel TJ (1991) An unusual case of abdominal pain in a young woman. *Ann Emerg Med* **20:**574–582.

28 Wiersinga WM and Touber JL (1977) The influence of beta-adrenoreceptor blocking agents on plasma thyroxine and triiodothyronine. *J Clin Endocrinol Metab* **45:**293–298.

29 Perrild H, Hansen JM, Skovsted L and Christensen LK (1983) Different effects of propranolol, alprenolol, sotalol, atenolol and metoprolol on serum T3 and serum rT3 in hyperthyroidism. *Clin Endocrinol* **18:** 139–142.

30 Brunette DD and Rothong C (1991) Emergency department management of thyrotoxic crisis with esmolol. *Am J Emerg Med* **9:**232–234.

31 Isley WL, Dahl S and Gibbs H (1990) Use of esmolol in managing a thyrotoxic patient needing emergency surgery. *Am J Med* **89:**122–123.

32 Thorne AC and Bedford RF (1989) Esmolol for perioperative management of thyrotoxic goitre. *Anesthesiology* **71:**291–294.

33 Anaisse E and Tohme JF (1985) Reserpine in propranolol-resistant thyroid storm. *Arch Intern Med* **145:**2248–2249.

34 Roti E, Montermini M and Roti S (1988) The effect of diltiazem, a calcium channel-blocking drug, on cardiac rate and rhythm in hyperthyroid patients. *Arch Int Med* **148:**1919–1921.

35 Chopra IJ, Huang TS, Hurd RE and Solomon DH (1984) A study of cardiac effects of thyroid hormones: evidence for amelioration of the effects of thyroxine by sodium ipodate. *Endocrinology* **114:**2039–2045.

36 Sheldon J (1983) Effects of amiodarone in thyrotoxicosis. *Br Med J* **286:**267–268.

37 Unger J, Lambert ML, Jonckheer MH and Denayer PH (1993) Amiodarone and the thyroid: pharmacological, toxic and therapeutic effects. *J Intern Med* **233:**435–443.

38 Gammage MD and Franklyn JA (1987) Amiodarone and the thyroid. *Q J Med* **62**:83–86.

39 Rajatanavin R, Chailurkit L, Kongsuksai A, Teeravaninthorn U and Himathongkam T (1990) The effect of amiodarone on the control of hyperthyroidism by propylthiouracil. *Clin Endocrinol* **33**:193–203.

40 Brooks MH, Waldenstein SS, Bronsky D and Sterling K (1975) Serum triiodothyronine concentrations in thyroid storm. *J Clin Endocrinol Metab* **40**:339–341.

41 Stockigt JR, Lim CF, Barlow JW, Stevens V, Topliss DJ and Wynne KN (1984) High concentrations of furosemide inhibit serum binding of thyroxine. *J Clin Endocrinol Metab* **59**:62–66.

42 Lim CF, Curtis AJ and Barlow JW (1989) Assessment of loop diuretics as inhibitors of thyroid hormone binding in serum. *Proc Endocrinol Soc Aust* **32**:143.

43 Ashkar FS, Katims RB, Smoak WM and Gilson AJ (1970) Thyroid storm treatment with blood exchange and plasmapheresis. *J Am Med Assoc* **214**:1275–1279.

44 Tajiri J, Katsuya H, Kiyokawa T, Urata K, Okamoto K and Shimada T (1984) Successful treatment of thyrotoxic crisis with plasma exchange. *Crit Care Med* **12**:536–537.

45 Derksen RHWM, Van de Wiel A, Poortman J, der Kinderen PJ and Kater L (1984) Plasma-exchange in the treatment of severe thyrotoxicosis in pregnancy. *Eur J Obstet Gynecol Reprod Biol* **18**:139–148.

46 Henderson A, Hickman P, Ward G and Pond SM (1994) Lack of efficacy of plasmapheresis in a patient overdosed with thyroxine. *Anaesth Intens Care* **22**:463–464.

47 Stevens JJ (1983) A case of thyrotoxic crisis that mimicked malignant hyperthermia (letter). *Anesthesiology* **59**:263.

48 Christensen PA and Nissen LR (1987) Treatment of thyroid storm in a child with dantrolene (letter). *Br J Anaesth* **59**:523.

49 Nicoloff JT and LoPresti JS (1993) Myxedema coma a form of decompensated hypothyroidism. *Endocrinol Metab Clin N Am* **22**:279–290.

50 Stockigt JR and Topliss DJ (1986) Diagnosis and management of hypothyroidism. *Med J Aust* **145**:206–210.

51 Mazzaferri EL (1986) Adult hypothyroidism. 1: Manifestations and clinical presentation. *Postgrad Med* **79**:64–72.

52 Mazzaferri EL (1986) Adult hypothyroidism. 2: Causes, laboratory diagnosis and treatment. *Postgrad Med* **79**:75–86.

53 Mechlis S, Lubin E, Laor J, Margaliot M and Strasberg B (1987) Amiodarone-induced thyroid gland dysfunction. *Am J Cardiol* **59**:833–835.

54 Editorial (1987) Amiodarone and the thyroid: the Janus response. *Lancet* **2**:24–25.

55 Mazonson PD, Williams ML, Cantley LK, Dalldorf FG, Utiger RD and Foster JR (1984) Myxedema coma during long-term amiodarone therapy. *Am J Med* **77**:751–754.

56 Murkin JM (1982) Anaesthesia and hypothyroidism: a review of thyroxine. Physiology, pharmacology, and anaesthetic implications. *Anesth Analg* **61**:371–383.

57 Hickman PE, Silvester W, Musk AA, McLellan GH and Harris A (1987) Cardiac enzyme changes in myxedema coma. *Clin Chem* **33**:622–624.

58 Nee PA, Scane AC, Lavelle PH, Fellows IW and Hill PG (1987) Hypothermic myxedema coma erroneously diagnosed as myocardial infarction because of increased creatine kinase MB. *Clin Chem* **33**:1083–1084.

59 Solano FX Jnr, Starling RC and Levey GS (1985) Myxedema megacolon (editorial). *Arch Intern Med* **145**:231.

60 Ladenson PW, Goldenheim PD and Ridgway EC (1983) Rapid pituitary and peripheral tissue responses to intravenous L–triiodothyronine in hypothyroidism. *J Clin Endocrinol Metab* **56**:1252–1259.

61 Chernow B, Burman KD, Johnson DL (1983) T_3 may be a better agent that T_4 in the critically ill hypothyroid patient: evaluation of transport across the blood–brain barrier in a primate model. *Crit Care Med* **11**:99–104.

62 McCullock W, Pricie P, Hinds CJ and Wass JAH (1985) Effects of low dose oral triiodothyronine in myxoedema coma. *Intens Care Med* **11**:259–262.

63 Odgers CL, Phillips PJ and Shanks G (1984) Intravenous liothyronine sodium (T_3) for myxoedema coma – pharmaceutical considerations. *Aust J Hosp Pharm* **14**:181–188.

64 Ros M, Northup JK and Malbon CC (1988) Steady state levels of G-proteins and beta-adrenergic receptors in rat fat cells. Permissive effects of thyroid hormones. *J Biol Chem* **263**:4362–4368.

65 Frank DH and Robson MC (1980) Accidental hypothermia treated without mortality. *Surg Gynecol Obstet* **151**:379–381.

66 Fitzgerald FT and Jessop C (1982) Accidental hypothermia: a report of 23 cases and review of literature. *Adv Intern Med* **27**:127–150.

67 O'Connor P and Freely J (1987) Clinical pharmacokinetics and endocrine disorders. Therapeutic implications. *Clin Pharmacokin* **13**:345–364.

53 | Adrenocortical insufficiency

AE Vedig

Adrenocortical insufficiency may present as an insidious, occult disorder, unmasked by conditions of stress, or as a catastrophic syndrome that may result in death. Empirical treatment may be required before the diagnosis is confirmed by investigations.

Physiology and pathophysiology[1-7]

The adrenal cortex synthesizes and secretes three major types of hormones: first, glucocorticoid (cortisol); second, mineralocorticoids (aldosterone and 11-deoxycorticosterone); and third, adrenal androgens. The major pathogenic effects of disease result from cortisol and aldosterone deficiency.

Anatomically, the adrenal gland is unique in that the arteries and veins do not run in parallel. There is a very rich autonomic innovation and vascular supply. Venous drainage is limited to one or two veins which have an eccentric muscular arrangement, making the gland sensitive to stress states and coagulopathy. Histologically, the adrenal cortex is divided into three major zones: zona fasciculata, zona glomerulosa and zona reticularis.

Zona fasciculata

This is the thickest, intermediate layer which secretes cortisol. The hormone affects intermediary metabolism via a type II glucocorticoid receptor. It regulates protein, carbohydrate, lipid and nucleic acid metabolism, resulting in increased gluconeogenesis and enhanced catabolism and lipolysis. Anti-inflammatory activity is related to the inhibition of neutrophil and macrophage migration, resulting in a microvascular stabilizing effect. Free water clearance is facilitated, and there is a permissive effect on peripheral vascular responses to endogenous vasoconstrictors.

Cortisol secretion is directly controlled by adrenocorticotropic hormone (ACTH) which is, in turn, regulated by corticotrophin-releasing hormone (CRH).

Release of these hypothalamic–pituitary hormones is influenced by circulating levels of cortisol or cortisol-like steroids, stress antidiuretic hormone (ADH), sleep–wake cycles and circulating levels of interleukin-1. ACTH is derived from a precursor molecule pro-opiomelanocortin (POMC). β-Lipotropin and several other POMC derivatives have melanocyte-stimulating activity.

Zona glomerulosa

This is the thin outermost layer which secretes aldosterone. The hormone increases sodium conservation and potassium loss by the kidney, sweat glands and gastrointestinal tract. These actions are mediated by the type 1 glucocorticoid receptor. It is a major regulator of extracellular fluid volume. Fluid and electrolyte abnormalities of primary adrenal gland insufficiency are mostly due to aldosterone deficiency. Most glucocorticoids have some mineralocorticoid-like activity. Prolonged administration of glucocorticoids results in adrenal atrophy and hyposecretion of endogenous glucocorticoid and androgens, although aldosterone responsiveness to sodium depletion is maintained. Aldosterone secretion is controlled by the renin–angiotensin system, serum potassium concentration and ACTH (which plays a minor role).

Zona reticularis

This is the inner layer which secretes androgens. Deficiency produces a decrease in body hair in female patients, while male patients notice little or no change because of gonadal testosterone production. Androgen deficiency in females may contribute to anaemia and osteoporosis.

Primary adrenocortical insufficiency (Addison's disease)[1,2,4,8]

This is a rare disorder that occurs equally in males or females at any age. Most of the adrenal gland (90%)

is destroyed if symptoms are present. More than 80% of cases are idiopathic, of whom 50% have antiadrenal antibodies present. Other immune disorders are commonly associated with adrenocortical insufficiency. Specific polyglandular autoimmune syndromes and other associated neurological disorders are rare. Tuberculosis accounts for a lesser proportion than previously, but is more likely (50%) if adrenal calcification is present.[9] Cryptococcosis, other fungi and cytomegalovirus (CMV) infections occur rarely, except in patients with acquired immunodeficiency syndrome (AIDS).[10,11] CMV adrenalitis is a common abnormality present in autopsy specimens of patients with AIDS,[12] although clinically less than 5% have overt adrenal insufficiency. Individual patients with known CMV infection have a higher rate of adrenal infarction.[13]

Destruction of the gland may occur with metastic neoplasms,[14,15] and rarely with granulomatous or amyloid infiltration, irradiation or haemochromatosis. Other causes include haemorrhage, congenital adrenal hyperplasia and drugs such as ketoconazole,[16,17] fluconazole,[18] and those used to treat hyperadrenalism (e.g. metyrapone). More recently, thrombosis and infarction of the adrenal glands have been recognized in patients with the antiphospholipid (anticardiolipin) syndrome,[19–21] who may present in ICU with thromboembolic disease. Physical destruction of the adrenal glands will result in varying degrees of glucocorticoid, mineralocorticoid and androgen deficiency. Specific diseases and drugs may result in a preponderance of glucocorticoid or mineralocorticoid insufficiency.

Secondary adrenocortical insufficiency[1,2,4,8]

This condition may be due to ACTH deficiency from pituitary and hypothalamic disease, or to hypothalamic–pituitary–adrenal (H–P–A) gland suppression by exogenously administered corticosteroid. Adrenocortical insufficiency associated with corticosteroid therapy occurs frequently. The type of steroid, dose, route and duration influence the likelihood of H–P–A suppression. Prednisolone (or other equivalent) in excess of 7.5 mg/day for longer than 2–3 weeks may suppress the H–P–A, and, with continued use, result in adrenal atrophy. Suppression may continue for months after the cessation of therapy, during which time acute deficiency may occur if the patient is stressed. Suppression may occur with topically applied,[22] inhaled,[23] and depot-type preparations.[24] Neither the dose and duration of corticosteroid therapy, nor basal cortisol levels can reliably predict the functional reserve.[25]

Pituitary dysfunction as a cause of secondary adrenocortical insufficiency occurs rarely, and may be due to neoplasms, infections, haemorrhage, infarction, radiation and granulomatous infiltration. Aldosterone secretion continues normally (as it is not controlled predominantly by ACTH), but severe fluid losses may reveal a subnormal aldosterone secretory capacity. Isolated mineralocorticoid deficiency due to reduced renin activity is uncommon. If panhypopituitarism exists, hypogonadism, growth retardation and hypothyroidism may be present. Secondary hormonal deficiencies (e.g. hypothyroidism) may further complicate glucocorticoid metabolism.

Clinical presentation of deficiency states

There may be few symptoms. The only physical sign apparent in Addison's disease may be hyperpigmentation of skin which is exposed to light, friction or pressure. Gingival, scar, nipple, freckle, tongue and genital pigmentation may also be present, secondary to the combined effects of β-lipotropin and melanocyte-stimulating hormone. Clinical features common to primary and secondary adrenocortical deficiency include asthenia, muscle weakness, malaise, fever,[26] anorexia, abdominal pain (which may be severe), vomiting, alternating diarrhoea and constipation and weight loss. Postural and supine hypotension also occur, as do salt craving, myalgias, arthralgias, vitiligo, flexural contractures, alteration in personality, mental confusion and psychosis. There is increased sensitivity to central nervous system depressant drugs, including opioids.

Signs of reactive or fasting hypoglycaemia may be present (more common in pituitary insufficiency). In advanced disease, there may be hyponatraemia and/or hyperkalaemia, which may lead to a form of life-threatening ascending neuromyopathy. Hypercalcaemia is rarely present. A small heart may be demonstrated radiographically. Haemodynamic measurements may reveal increased cardiac output and low systemic vascular resistance.[27,28] Eosinophilia, relative lymphocytosis and normocytic anaemia also occur. Although cortisol has a permissive role in haemosynthesis, androgen deficiency is responsible for the anaemia. Since the features of adrenocortical deficiency are non-specific and common in other severe debilitating disease, it is important to maintain a high index of suspicion.

Secondary insufficiency is more difficult to diagnose than primary insufficiency. Hyperpigmentation is absent. Major findings, in order of prevalence, are hypoglycaemia, weight loss, hypotension, anaemia, weakness and fatigue, hair loss, nausea, vomiting and hyponatraemia.[29] Stiffman syndrome and delirium[30] and fever[31] are also described.

Acute adrenocortical insufficiency (Addisonian crisis)[1,2,4,8]

Aetiology

Acute adrenal insufficiency may present as an intensification of chronic hypoadrenalism, where there is insufficient hormonal resource to meet the stress requirements of trauma, infection and surgery.[32,33] Sudden cessation or too rapid reduction of chronic exogenous steroids may precipitate an acute crisis. Unrecognized, inappropriately low-level therapy with corticosteroid drugs may result from drug interactions which increase steroid metabolism (e.g. with rifampicin, barbiturates and phenytoin).[34–36] Also, drugs such as ketoconazole that inhibit steroid synthesis when given in the setting of stress (it also binds to the glucocorticoid receptor) may precipitate a crisis in patients with congenital adrenal hyperplasia or decreased adrenocortical reserve.

Sudden destruction of glands due to haemorrhage,[37] although unusual, may occur with severe sepsis, anticoagulant therapy (particularly heparin-induced thrombocytopenia),[38–40] burns, surgery, or trauma. The classical Waterhouse–Friederichsen syndrome was associated with meningococcaemia, but may occur with either Gram-positive or Gram-negative septicaemia. Chest,[41] abdominal or investigation trauma has caused an Addisonian crisis secondary to haemorrhage. Surgical removal of a single gland,[42] postpartum pituitary infarction (Sheehan's syndrome) and pituitary apoplexy may cause acute adrenal insufficiency.

Infusions of the anaesthetic agents etomidate[43] and alfathesin (althesin) probably contributed to the adrenocortical insufficiency ascribed to critically ill patients without other recognized precipitating factors. In critically ill patients, there is correlation between cortisol concentrations and the degree of illness and mortality.[44]

Clinical presentation

Patients present usually in a shocked state with a history of worsening prodromal symptoms of hypoadrenalism. Malaise, weakness, tiredness, anorexia, nausea, vomiting, mental disturbance, fever and severe abdominal pain are common presenting complaints. Precipitating events such as surgery or septicaemia may be elicited. Sudden flank or epigastric pain suggest adrenal haemorrhage. Anticoagulant-induced haemorrhage is more common in the middle-aged to elderly and thrombocytopenic patients. Although hypovolaemia is not so obvious with secondary insufficiency, severe dehydration, hypotension and peripheral circulatory failure are evident terminally, and are refractory to treatment without steroid administration. The diagnosis of Addisonian crisis should be suspected in all shocked patients if they remain refractory to usual treatment, and when the cause of their condition is not apparent.

Investigations[1,2,4,8]

Those which assist diagnosis and management include the following.

Plasma pituitary and adrenal hormones

Baseline plasma cortisol levels < 500 nmol/l with marked stress are suggestive of insufficiency. Plasma ACTH (high in primary, but low or normal with secondary adrenocortical insufficiency), plasma aldosterone, plasma renin and other pituitary hormone measurements may be indicated. The short ACTH test will confirm adrenocortical insufficiency.

Biochemical and haematological

Hyponatraemia and hyperkalaemia ($Na^+:K^+$ ratio of < 25:1) are very suggestive of Addison's disease. Hypoglycaemia is common. Serum calcium may be elevated, although the ionized calcium is usually normal (but may rarely be increased). Metabolic acidosis and respiratory failure may be present. Evidence of hypovolaemia is common. High urinary sodium excretion may occur despite hypovolaemia. Moderate neutropenia with relative eosinophilia and lymphocytosis may be seen. Antibodies to adrenal gland and other organs may be detected.

Electrocardiogram

Low voltage and slow conduction are present in severe hypoadrenalism.

Radiology

Chest X-rays may show evidence of old tuberculosis. The heart is small in chronic insufficiency. Abdominal computed tomography scan will indicate adrenal gland size and reveal calcification, haemorrhage, and some infiltrates.

Management[1,2,4,8]

Treatment must be immediate, and should be initiated prior to confirmation of the diagnosis. Precipitating factors, if not apparent, should be sought and treated appropriately (e.g. sepsis and thrombocytopenia).

Corticosteroids

Acute management

If adrenal crisis is suspected, corticosteroids must be given without delay; results of plasma cortisol assays will not readily be available. The short ACTH test may be undertaken together with treatment, provided that there is no undue delay in corticosteroid administration. Blood is taken for baseline cortisol concentrations, and other hormone and electrolyte estimates. Dexamethasone 10 mg IV is given, together with tetracosactrin 250 mg (Synacthen, Cortrosyn). Dexamethasone begins replacement therapy rapidly without interfering with the cortisol assay.

Cortisol concentrations are taken at 0, 30 and 60

min. If there is any delay in blood sampling, basal cortisol concentrations may be suppressed by dexamethasone. Cortisol levels of >700 nmol/l disprove glucocorticoid insufficiency. Basal plasma ACTH concentrations of >200 ng/l establish the diagnosis. The 30-min response to ACTH is the most reliable parameter for assessing adrenal response.[45] Measurement of plasma aldosterone at 0, 30 and 60 min after ACTH may also be helpful. Plasma aldosterone levels less than 14 000 pmol/l indicate insufficiency.[46] Corticosteroid treatment is continued as hydrocortisone 100 mg IV 6-hourly. The initial bolus may be 250 mg IV if the short ACTH test is omitted. On day 2, 100 mg hydrocortisone is given 8-hourly IM, then 12-hourly, and changed to an oral maintenance regimen. Hydrocortisone has sufficient mineralocorticoid activity in higher doses (>120 mg/day) to allow omission of mineralocorticoid replacement.

Maintenance[47,48]

When the crisis has been successfully treated, appropriate investigations help formulate a corticosteroid maintenance regimen, which will involve giving cortisol or its equivalent twice daily (on waking and at 18:00 h) to mimic circadian rhythm. Oral fludrocortisone 50–100 mg daily or every other day provides mineralocorticoid support if required. Concomitant phenytoin may cause adverse effects.[49] The choice of corticosteroid and dosage will depend on the degrees of insufficiency of the two essential hormones. Although adrenal insufficiency is usually permanent when the glands have been destroyed by haemorrhage and infarction, recovery is possible.[50,51]

Prevention

If stress is predictable or occurring (e.g. acute illness, temperature >38°C, and elective operations), the glucocorticosteroid maintenance regimen must be increased. The oral dose may be doubled if this route is appropriate and the stress is mild. Vomiting or diarrhoea are indications for parenteral therapy. Hydrocortisone succinate 50 mg IM every 6 h should be given if the patient is not acutely ill. If stressed (e.g. pneumonia and major operation) 100 mg hydrocortisone is given IM of IV 6-hourly until the recovery phase, or at least for 72 h. For minor operations, 100 mg parentally 6-hourly for 24 h, and for minimal procedures (e.g. cystoscopy), a single dose of 100 mg IM prior to the procedure is given. The doses suggested may have to be doubled if the patient is taking concomitant enzyme-inducing drugs.

Monitoring and general supportive measures

These include oxygen therapy, and assessment and management of metabolic and respiratory acidosis. Opioid and sedative drugs should be avoided. Frequent electrolyte (in particular, potassium) and glucose determinations will be required. Continuous electrocardiogram (ECG) and frequent arterial and central venous pressure measurements and attention to fluid balance are essential. Repeated urinary electrolytes may be helpful. More invasive haemodynamic monitoring and inotropic drugs may be required in managing the precipitating event, or if shock remains unresponsive to appropriate fluid replacement.

Intravenous fluids

Normal saline is infused rapidly, without awaiting monitoring catheter placement. The infusion rate could be 1 l or more in the first 30 min. Subsequent infusion may be in the order of 1 l/h, but is determined by the response to initial infusion and monitoring of clinical signs. The volume deficit in acute adrenal crisis is seldom greater than 10% of total body water. Dextrose should be given at the same time as the saline infusion, as 5% dextrose in normal saline, or separately. Hypertonic dextrose can be given via a central line to treat hypoglycaemia. About 50 g of dextrose may be required in the first 1–2 h.

Corticosteroid therapy[3,52,53]

Apart from substitution therapy in adrenocortical deficiency, the use of corticosteroids is largely empirical and palliative by virtue of the anti-inflammatory effects. A single dose (even a large one) or a few days of therapy is unlikely to produce harm, unless specific contraindications exist. In the long term, the likelihood of disabling and potential lethal effects increases in proportion to the extent that the dose exceeds substitution therapy. Sudden cessation may precipitate an Addisonian crisis, or unmask an underlying disease. This may occur even with topically or rectally applied, inhaled and locally injected glucocorticoids. Alternate-day dosing with the shorter-acting steroids minimizes H–P–A suppression, but in acute situations, at least daily dosing must be used. Selection and dosing regimens are based on anti-inflammatory potency, mineralocorticoid activity and duration of action (Table 53.1). The pharmacodynamic effects of the corticosteroid drugs are more relevant than plasma half-lives when considering dosing schedules.

Hypoaldosteronism[1,4,7]

Inherited hypoaldosteronism

Inherited hypoaldosteronism (congenital adrenal hyperplasia) is most commonly due to 21-hydroxylase deficiency. This autosomal recessive disorder occurs in 1 in 10 000–15 000 births. Infants present with hyponatraemia and hyperkalaemia, which can

Table 53.1 Corticosteroid and synthetic analogues

Drug	Equivalent dose	Sodium-retaining activity	Plasma $T_{1/2}$ (h)	Biological $T_{1/2}$ (h)
Cortisone	25	+ +	1.5	8–12
Hydrocortisone (cortisol)	20	+ +	1.5	8–12
Prednisone, prednisolone	5	+	>3	>18
Methylprednisolone	4	0	>3	>18
Dexamethasone	0.75	0	>3	>36
Betamethasone		0.60	>3	>36

$T_{1/2}$ (h) = half-life in hours

progress to shock and death. Girls usually have masculinized genitalia. Mineralocorticoids and glucocorticoids control the salt wasting. Aldosterone synthase deficiency occurs less commonly, as does pseudohypoaldosteronism.

Acquired hypoaldosteronism

In the presence of normal glucocorticoid synthesis, acquired hypoaldosteronism may occur during prolonged heparin or heparinoid therapy, and following operative removal of aldosterone-secreting adenomas, and is common with critical illness. Patients are unable to increase aldosterone secretion appropriately in response to sodium restriction or hypovolaemia. Unexplained hyperkalaemia is the commonest presenting feature. Once transcellular shifts of potassium have been excluded, hypoaldosteronism must be considered in patients with hyperkalaemia.

Hyporeninaemic hypoaldosteronism[54]

This is most frequently seen in adults with diabetes mellitus and mild renal failure, where the hyperkalaemia and metabolic acidosis are disproportionate to the degree of kidney impairment. Renin production is low, as is the aldosterone level in relationship to the degree of hyperkalaemia. Other associated diseases are gout, pyelonephritis, nephrosclerosis and amyloid.

Hyperreninaemic hypoaldosteronism

Hyperreninaemic hypoaldosteronism is common with prolonged, severe illness.[55,56] Plasma renin activity and angiotensin II levels are elevated.[57] The pathogenesis is unknown, but may result from prolonged stimulation of the adrenal cortex by ACTH, resulting in a shift from mineralocorticoid to glucocorticoid production. The aldosterone precursor 18-hydroxycorticosterone is frequently elevated, hypotension is common, and an increased mortality is associated. Although mild hyponatraemia is often seen, normokalaemia is usual. In the stressed critically ill patient, the high cortical concentrations may inhibit the development of hyperkalaemia. Disorders associated with hyperreninaemic hypoaldosteronism include heparin therapy,[58–60] diabetes mellitus,[61] AIDS,[62] and secondary carcinoma of the adrenal gland.[63] Hyperkalaemia is well-recognized in association with prolonged heparin therapy, and seems more common in less severely ill patients.

Both hyporeninaemic and hyperreninaemic hypoaldosteronism respond to mineralocorticoids. Hydrocortisone administration results in marked improvement in cardiovascular status, with dramatic reduction in inotropic requirement in hypotensive critically ill patients. Basal and ACTH-stimulated plasma cortisol levels are frequently very high. The patients with renal insufficiency often respond to a reduction in sodium intake and to administration of frusemide, which improves the hyperkalaemia and metabolic acidosis.

Plasma cortisols/occult hypoadrenalism in the critically ill

Plasma cortisol concentrations[64] and response to the short ACTH stimulation test have been reported in critically ill patients.[44,65,66] Prognosis in patients with low concentrations has generally been poor.[44,64] Basal cortisol concentrations appear to be related to the degree of stress. Patients with gastrointestinal bleeding have lower concentrations (600 nmol/l) compared with those who have respiratory failure or sepsis (1200 nmol/l).[44,67] Where basal cortisol concentrations are high, no correlation between outcome and cortisol concentrations has been demonstrated.[67]

More recently, a poor response (<250 nmol/l rise in cortisol concentrations) to parenteral ACTH has been linked to very poor outcomes, although basal cortisol concentrations were similar in survivors and non-survivors.[65] A degree of secondary adrenal insufficiency is postulated,[66,68] but where high unstimulated cortisols exist, interpretation is difficult.[69] Certainly, impressive pressor responses to administration of corticosteroids are a frequent clinical observation, and are well-described in both adults[65–67,69] and neonates.[70,71] The precise mechanisms of these physiological responses and how they fit with the pressor responses observed in patients with isolated hypoaldosteronism is presently unclear.

References

1 Williams GH and Dluhy RG (1994) Diseases of the adrenal cortex. In: Isselbacher KJ, Braunwald E, Wilson JD, Martin JD, Fauci AS and Kasper DL (eds) *Harrison's Principles of Internal Medicine*, 13th edn. New York: McGraw-Hill, pp. 1953–1976.

2 Passmore JM. (1985) Adrenal cortex. In: Geelhoed GW and Chernow B (eds) *Clinics in Critical Care Medicine – Endocrine Aspects of Acute Illness*. New York: Churchill Livingstone, pp. 97–134.

3 Haynes Jnr RC (1990) Adrenocorticotropic hormone; adrenocortical steroids and their synthetic analogs; inhibitors of the synthesis and action of adrenocortical hormones. In: Gilman AG, Rall TW, Nies AS and Taylor P (eds) *The Pharmacological Basis of Therapeutics*, 8th edn. New York: Macmillan, pp. 1431–1462.

4 Werbel SS and Ober KP (1993) Acute adrenal insufficiency. *Endocrinol Metab Clin North Am* 22: 303–328.

5 Tsigos C and Chrousos GP (1994) Physiology of the hypothalamic–pituitary–adrenal axis in health and dysregulation in psychiatric and autoimmune disorders. *Endocrinol Metab Clin North Am* 23:451–466.

6 Bertagna X (1994) Proopiomelanocortin–derived peptides. *Endocrinol Metab Clin North Am* 23: 467–485.

7 White PC (1994) Disorders of aldosterone biosynthesis and action. *N Engl J Med* 331:250–258.

8 Burke CW (1985) Adrenocortical insufficiency. *Clin Endocrinol Metab* 14:947–976.

9 Vita JA, Silverberg SJ, Goland RS, Austin JH and Knowlton AI (1985) Clinical clues to the cause of Addison's disease. *Am J Med* 78:461–466.

10 Guenthner EE, Rabinowe SL, Van Niel A, Naftilan A and Dluhy RG (1984) Primary Addison's disease in a patient with the acquired immunodeficiency syndrome. *Ann Intern Med* 100:847–848.

11 Glasgow BJ, Steinsapir KD, Anderes K and Layfield LJ (1985) Adrenal pathology in the acquired immune deficiency syndrome. *Am J Clin Pathol* 84:594–597.

12 Donovan DS and Dluhy RG (1991) AIDS and its effect on the adrenal gland. *Endocrinologist* 1:227–232.

13 Pulakhandam U and Dincsoy HP (1990) Cytomegaloviral adrenalitis and adrenal insufficiency in AIDS. *Am J Clin Pathol* 93:651–656.

14 Redman BG, Pazdur R, Zingas AP and Loredo R (1987) Prospective evaluation of adrenal insufficiency in patients with adrenal metastasis. *Cancer* 60: 103–107.

15 Kung AWC, Pun KK, Lam K, Wang C and Leung CY (1990) Addisonian crisis: a presenting feature in malignancies. *Cancer* 65:177–179.

16 Pont A, Williams PC, Loose DS *et al.* (1982) Ketoconazole blocks adrenal steroid synthesis. *Ann Intern Med* 97:370–372.

17 Best TR, Jenkins JK, Murphy FY, Nicks SA, Bussel KL and Vesely DL (1987) Persistent adrenal insufficiency secondary to low–dose ketoconazole therapy. *Am J Med* 82:676–680.

18 Gradon JD and Sepkowitz DV (1991) Fluconazole-associated acute adrenal insufficiency. *Postgrad Med* 67:1084–1085.

19 Dorling A and Knowles GK (1991) Antiphospholipid syndrome and acute adrenal insufficiency. *R Soc Med* 84:560.

20 Yap AS (1989) Lupus anticoagulant. *Ann Intern Med* 111:262–263.

21 Asherson RA and Hughes GRV (1989) Recurrent deep vein thrombosis and Addison's disease in 'primary' antiphospholipid syndrome. *J Rheumatol* 16:378–380.

22 Flynn MD, Beasley P and Tooke JE (1992) Adrenal suppression with intranasal betamethasone drops. *J Laryngol Otol* 106:827–828.

23 Zwaan CM, Odink RJH, Delemarre-Van De Waal HA and Dankert-Reolse JE (1992) Acute adrenal insufficiency after discontinuation of inhaled corticosteroid therapy. *Lancet* 340:1289–1290.

24 Chernow B, Bigersky R, O'Brian JT and Georges LP (1982) Secondary adrenal insufficiency after intrathecal steroid administration. *J Neurosurg* 56: 567–570.

25 Schlaghecke R, Kornely E, Santen RT and Ridderskamp P (1992) The effect of long-term glucocorticoid therapy on pituitary–adrenal responses to exogenous corticotropin-releasing hormone. *N Engl J Med* 326:226–230.

26 Page RCL and Alford F (1993) Adrenocorticosteroid deficiency: an unusual cause of fever of unknown origin. *Postgrad Med* 69:395–396.

27 Dorin RI and Kearns PJ (1988) High output circulatory failure in acute adrenal insufficiency. *Crit Care Med* 16:296–297.

28 Bonachour G, Tirot P, Varache JP, Harry P and Alquier Ph (1994) Hemodynamic changes in acute adrenal insufficiency. *Intensive Care Med* 20:138–141.

29 Stacpoole PW, Interlandi JW, Nicholson WE and Rabin D (1982) Isolated ACTH deficiency; a heterogeneous disorder. *Medicine* 61:13–24.

30 Fang VS and Jaspan JB (1989) Delirium and neuromuscular symptoms in an elderly man with isolated corticotroph-deficiency syndrome completely reversed with glucocorticoid replacement. *J Clin Endocrinol Metab* 69:1073–1077.

31 Soto-Hernandez JL, Verghese A, Hall BD, Cole CP and Cupp HB Jr (1989) Secondary adrenal insufficiency manifested as an acute febrile illness. *South Med J* 82:384–385.

32 Hertzberg LB and Shulman MS (1985) Acute adrenal insufficiency in a patient with appendicitis during anesthesia. *Anesthesiology* 62:517–519.

33 Jacobson SA, Blute RD Jr, Green DF, McPhedran P, Weiss RM and Lytton B (1986) Acute adrenal insufficiency as a complication of urological surgery. *J Urol* 82:676–680.

34 Kyriazopoulou V, Parparousi O and Vagenakis AG (1984) Rifampicin-induced adrenal crisis in Addisonian patients receiving corticosteroid replacement therapy. *J Clin Endocrinol Metab* 59:1204–1206.

35 Kannan CR (1988) Diseases of the adrenal cortex. *Disease Month* 34:627–638.

36 Wilkins EGI and Cope A (1989) Addisonian crisis induced by treatment with rifampicin. *Tubercle* 70:69–73.

37 Wolverson MK and Kannegiesser H (1984) CT of bilateral adrenal hemorrhage with acute adrenal insufficiency in the adult. *Am J Radiol* **142**:311–314.

38 Souied F, Pourriat J, Le Roux G, Hoang P, Kemeny JL and Cupa M (1991) Adrenal hemorrhagic necrosis related to heparin-induced thrombocytopaenia. *Crit Care Med* **19**:1297–301.

39 Dahlberg PJ, Goellner MH and Pehling GB (1990) Adrenal insufficiency secondary to adrenal hemorrhage. *Arch Intern Med* **150**:905–909.

40 Bleasel JF, Rasko JEJ, Rickard KA and Richards G (1992) Acute adrenal insufficiency secondary to heparin-induced thrombocytopaenia–thrombosis syndrome. *Med J Aust* **157**:192–193.

41 Hardy K, Mead B and Gill G. (1992) Adrenal apoplexy after coronary artery bypass surgery leading to Addisonian crisis. *R Soc Med* **85**:577–578.

42 McLeod MK, Thompson NW, Gross MD, Bondeson AG and Bondeson L (1990) Sub-clinical Cushing's syndrome in patients with adrenal gland incidentalomas: pitfalls in diagnosis and management. *Am Surg* **56**:398–403.

43 Fellows IW, Bastow MD, Byrne AJ and Allison SP (1983) Adrenocortical suppression in multiply injured patients: a complication of etomidate treatment. *Br Med J* **287**:1835–1837.

44 Jurney TH, Cockrell JL Jr, Lindberg JS, Lamiell JM and Wade CE (1987) Spectrum of serum cortisol response to ACTH in ICU patients. Correlation with degree of illness and mortality. *Chest* **92**:292–295.

45 Dickstein G, Shechner C, Nicholson WE *et al.* (1991) Adrenocorticotropin stimulation test. Effects of basal cortisol level, time of day, and suggested new sensitive low dose test. *J Clin Endocrinol Metab* **72**:773–778.

46 Dluhy RG, Himathong Kam T and Greenfield M (1974) Rapid ACTH test with plasma aldosterone levels improve diagnostic discrimination. *Ann Intern Med* **80**:693–696.

47 Khalid BA, Burke CW, Hurley DM, Funder JW and Stockigt JR (1982) Steroid replacement in Addison's disease and in subjects adrenalectomized for Cushing's disease: comparison of various glucocorticoids. *J Clin Endocrinol Metab* **55**:551–559.

48 Mortimer RH (1985) Adrenal corticosteroid replacement therapy. *Med J Aust* **143**:350–354.

49 Keilholz U and Guthrie GP Jr (1986) Adverse effect of phenytoin on mineralocorticoid replacement with fludrocortisone in adrenal insufficiency. *Am J Med Sci* **291**:280–283.

50 Feurstein B and Strecten DHP (1991) Recovery of adrenal functions after failure resulting from traumatic bilateral adrenal hemorrhages. *Ann Intern Med* **115**:785–786.

51 Vengrove MA and Amoroso A (1993) Reversible adrenal insufficiency after adrenal hemorrhage. *Ann Intern Med* **119**:439.

52 Begg EJ, Atkinson HC and Gianarakis N (1987) The pharmacokinetics of corticosteroid agents. *Med J Aust* **146**:37–41.

53 Reynolds JEF, Parfitt K, Parsons AV and Sweetman SC (1996) *Martindale, The Extra Pharmacopoeia*, 31st edn. London: Royal Pharmaceutical Society, pp. 1017–1058.

54 Schambelan M, Stockigt JR and Biglieri EG (1972) Isolated hypoaldosteronism in adults: a renin-deficiency syndrome. *N Engl J Med* **287**:573–578.

55 Zipser RD, Davenport MW, Martin KL *et al.* (1981) Hyperreninemic hypoaldosteronism in the critically ill: a new entity. *J Clin Endocrinol Metab* **53**:867–73.

56 Davenport MW and Zipser RD (1983) Association of hypotension with hyperreninemic hypoaldosteronism in the critically ill patient. *Arch Intern Med* **143**:735–737.

57 Findling JW, Waters VO and Raff H (1987) The dissociation of renin and aldosterone during critical illness. *J Clin Endocrinol Metab* **64**:592–595.

58 O'Kelly R, Magee F and McKenna TJ (1983) Routine heparin therapy inhibits adrenal aldosterone production. *J Clin Endocrinol Metab* **56**:108–112.

59 Levesque H, Verdier S, Cailleux N *et al.* (1990) Low molecular weight heparins and hypoaldosteronism. *Br Med J* **300**:1437–1438.

60 Aull L, Chao H and Coy K (1990) Heparin-induced hyperkalemia. *Drug Intell Clin Pharm* **24**:244–246.

61 Morimoto S, Kyung SK, Yamamoto I, Uchida K, Takeda R and Kornel L (1979) Selective hypoaldosteronism with hyperreninemia in a diabetic patient. *J Clin Endocrinol Metab* **49**:742–747.

62 Guy RJC, Turberg Y, Davidson RN, Finnerty G, MacGregor GA and Wise PH (1989) Mineralocorticoid deficiency in HIV infection. *Br Med J* **298**:496–497.

63 Taylor HC, Shah B, Pillay I and Mayes DM (1988) Isolated hyperreninemic hypoaldosteronism due to carcinoma metastatic to the adrenal gland. *Am J Med* **85**:441–444.

64 Sibbald WJ, Short A, Cohen MP and Wilson RF (1977) Variations in adrenocortical responsiveness during severe bacterial infections. Unrecognized adrenocortical insufficiency in severe bacterial infections. *Ann Surg* **186**:29.

65 Rothwell PM, Udwadia ZF and Lawler PG (1991) Cortisol response to corticotropin and survival in septic shock. *Lancet* **337**:582–583.

66 Baldwin WA and Allo M (1993) Occult hypoadrenalism in critically ill patients. *Arch Surg* **128**:673–676.

67 Schein RMH, Sprung CL, Marcial E, Napolitano L and Chernow B (1990) Plasma cortisol levels in patients with septic shock. *Crit Care Med* **18**:259–263.

68 Kidess AI, Caplan RH, Reynertson RH, Wickus GG and Goodnough DE (1993) Transient corticotropin deficiency in critical illness. *Mayo Clin Proc* **68**:435–441.

69 Martinez E and Marcos A (1991) Cortisol response to corticotropin and survival in septic shock. *Lancet* **337**:1230–1231.

70 Colasurdo MA, Hanna CE, Gilhooly JT and Reynolds JW (1989) Hydrocortisone replacement in extremely premature infants with cortisol insufficiency. *Clin Res* **37**:180A.

71 Helbock HJ, Insoft RM and Coate FA (1993) Glucocorticoid-responsive hypotension in extremely low birth weight newborns. *Pediatrics* **92**:715–717.

54 | Acute calcium disorders

CD Scheinkestel and TE Oh

Calcium is the most abundant cation in the body and principal mineral of the skeleton. It is essential for the integrity and function of cell membranes, cardiac action potentials and pacemaker activity, secretion of neurotransmitters, transmission of nerve impulses, and excitation–contraction coupling in cardiac, skeletal and smooth muscle. Calcium is an essential cofactor in many enzymatic reactions, and is required for extracellular motility (e.g. cilia and flagella), intracellular motility (e.g. filaments and microtubules), mitosis and white blood cell chemotaxis. Calcium is also required for actions of catecholamines at α- and β-adrenergic receptors.

Paradoxically, calcium also plays a pivotal role in a number of harmful processes (e.g. activation of proteases and lipases and production of free oxygen radicals). The entry of calcium into injured cells is considered one of the final steps in the pathogenesis of cell death in reperfusion injury. However, there is no evidence to support the suggestion that calcium-containing solutions (e.g. Hartmann's and polygeline or Haemaccel) in resuscitation may worsen subsequent reperfusion injury.

Calcium distribution

Total body calcium is 1000–1400 g (20–25 g/kg of fat-free tissue), with 99% being in bone and only 1% in the extracellular and intracellular spaces. Bone consists of water (30%), predominantly collagen, organic matrix (30%) and mineral (40%). The skeleton constantly undergoes resorption and formation. Bone resorption depends on the number and activity of osteoclasts, whilst bone formation is dependent on osteoblast activity.

Most intracellular calcium is in complex and sequestered form within the cell membrane. The free intracellular ionized calcium concentration is dependent on energy-requiring processes, which either extrude calcium from the cell or sequester it in

intracellular organelles (e.g. endoplasmic reticulum and mitochondria).

Only 0.03% of total body calcium is present in plasma as three forms[1] (Fig. 54.1). Laboratory determination of calcium concentration is usually the *total serum* fractions: protein-bound (40%), ion-bound complexes (13%), and the unbound, ionized moiety (47%). The unbound, ionized moiety is the biologically active component of calcium, and is normally maintained within a narrow range of values by several regulating mechanisms.[2,3] Complexed calcium, bound to phosphate, citrate and sulphate, is usually of little clinical importance, but is increased

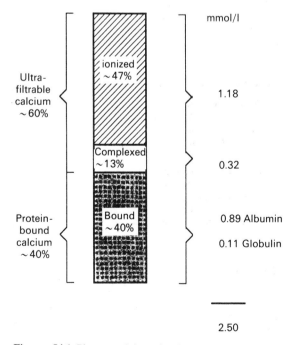

Figure 54.1 Plasma calcium fractions. Modified from Slatopolsky *et al.*[1]

in conditions where these substances are elevated, such as renal failure.

Total calcium estimations may be misleading with hypoalbuminaemia (i.e. total calcium is low, but ionized calcium is normal) and alkalosis (i.e. total calcium is normal but with increased protein binding, and ionized calcium is low). Serum phosphate concentration also influences the calcium concentration (high phosphate causes serum calcium to decrease). Ionized calcium concentration should be requested if available.[4] Otherwise, a correction is made for hypoalbuminaemia by adding to the measured serum calcium concentration 0.02 mmol/l for every 1 g difference in albumin concentration from 40 g/l (a set normal value). However, mathematical corrections of calcium measurements for altered serum proteins and pH correlate poorly with directly measured ionized calcium, and are unreliable in critically ill patients.[5–9]

Heparin forms complexes with the calcium, and hence decreases ionized calcium. Special syringes are recommended for measuring ionized calcium from arterial blood samples. Changes in pH alter the concentration of ionized calcium, and samples must be handled anaerobically. Lactate also chelates calcium; lactic acidosis is associated with hypocalcaemia. The conversion factor to express mg/dl as mmol/l is 0.25.

Calcium homeostasis

There is a complex interrelationship between hormonal and non-hormonal factors regulating calcium homeostasis. The main factors involved in calcium homeostasis are as follows

Parathyroid hormone (PTH)

PTH plays a central role. Minor changes in ionized calcium alter the secretion of PTH, resulting in restoration of ionized calcium to normal concentrations. PTH stimulates osteoclastic bone resorption (requiring vitamin D to do so), thereby increasing serum calcium. It increases renal reabsorption of calcium, and stimulates the renal production of vitamin D (thereby indirectly increasing gut absorption of calcium). High doses of vitamin D are therefore used to treat hypoparathyroidism.

Calcitriol

Calcitriol is the active metabolite of vitamin D. Hypocalcaemia stimulates and hypercalcaemia inhibits the synthesis of vitamin D. Calcitriol increases calcium absorption in the gut, causes minor increases in renal calcium reabsorption, and promotes mineralization of the organic bone matrix.

Calcitonin

Calcitonin is a polypeptide released from the thyroid gland which opposes the actions of PTH. It decreases osteoclast activity and blocks osteoclastic bone resorption, and increases renal excretion of calcium.

Phosphate

In the extracellular fluid, phosphate takes part in the following reaction: $HPO_4^{2-} + Ca^{2+} = CaHPO_4$.

Addition of phosphate shifts the reaction to the right, and causes serum calcium to fall (stimulating increased PTH secretion), whilst $CaHPO_4$ is deposited in bone and tissues. A decrease in phosphate moves the reaction to the left, resulting in a slight increase in calcium concentration and a decrease in PTH.

pH

An increase in pH (alkalosis) causes increased protein binding of calcium and a decrease in the ionized fraction.

Magnesium

Hypomagnesaemia decreases PTH secretion, impairs PTH responsiveness and deranges calcium–magnesium exchange in bone. Low magnesium levels are a cause of hypocalcaemia.

Calcium balance

A normal concentration of ionized calcium is maintained by balancing the input of calcium into the blood from gut and bone, and excretion of calcium into the urine and gut (Table 54.1).

Gastrointestinal tract (GIT) absorption

Occurs predominantly in the duodenum and proximal jejunum. Some absorption is passive, down an electrochemical gradient. Active absorption (some via a carrier protein) is principally influenced by vitamin

Table 54.1 Calcium metabolism

Gastrointestinal tract	
Diet	600–1200 mg/day
Absorbed	200–400 mg/day
Secreted	150–180 mg/day
Renal	
Filtered	~11 000 mg/day
Reabsorbed	~10 800 mg/day
Urinary calcium	~200 mg/day
Bone	
Turnover	600–800 mg/day

D metabolites. GIT absorption is also influenced by non-hormonal factors such as pH, bile salts, fibre, oxalate, lactose and ethanol. Gut adaptation occurs – absorption becomes more efficient with low-calcium diets.

Renal excretion

The glomerulus filters only diffusible calcium, 97–99% of which is reabsorbed (mainly in the proximal convoluted tubule). Reabsorption is predominantly passive. Active reabsorption is energy-dependent (Ca-Mg-ATPase) via calcium channels or carrier proteins. Ionized calcium is more readily reabsorbed; hence 80% of the calcium excreted in urine is complexed. PTH is the major regulator of renal calcium reabsorption.

Bone calcium turnover

Bone resorption and consequent release of calcium into the circulation are predominantly mediated by PTH and vitamin D, and inhibited by calcitonin. Other hormones implicated in bone resorption include prostaglandins, interleukins, tumour necrosis factor and epidermal and transforming growth factors.

Calcium homeostatic control is lost when production of calcium-regulating hormones is deficient, excessive, unresponsive or independent of serum ionized calcium concentration. Even when homeostatic control is intact, hypercalcaemia or hypocalcaemia may develop if regulatory mechanisms are overwhelmed by an abnormal passage of calcium into or from the circulation.

Hypercalcaemia

Clinical presentation

Clinical manifestations of hypercalcaemia (Table 54.2) are encountered when total serum calcium exceeds 3.0 mmol/l.[10] Immobilization and volume depletion worsen mild degrees of hypercalcaemia. The severity of symptoms depends on the degree of hypercalcaemia and the rate at which it develops; the faster the change, the lower the serum concentration at which symptoms develop. Symptoms and signs of the underlying disease process (e.g. bronchogenic carcinoma) may dominate the clinical picture. Coma is a terminal occurrence. Chronic hypercalcaemia stimulates the G cells of the stomach to secrete gastrin, with an increased incidence of peptic ulceration.

Pathophysiology[2,11–18]

The frequency and aetiology of hypercalcaemia vary according to the patient sample. In 90% of hospitalized patients with hypercalcaemia, hyper-parathyroidism or malignant disease is the cause,[16]

Table 54.2 Clinical manifestations of hypercalcaemia

Neuropsychiatric	*General*
Headache	Apathy, lethargy
Impaired concentration	
Loss of memory	*Cardiovascular*
Confusion	Hypertension
Drowsiness	Arrhythmias
Anxiety	Heart block
Mania	Calcification
Psychosis	Enhanced digoxin toxicity
Neuromuscular	*Gastrointestinal*
Weakness	Peptic ulcer
Atrophy	Pancreatitis
Hyporeflexia	Anorexia
Coma	Nausea
	Vomiting
Urological	Constipation
Nephrolithiasis	Abdominal pain
Nephrocalcinosis	
Tubular dysfunction	*Ectopic calcification*
Polyuria	Band keratopathy
Impaired concentration	Conjunctival irritation
Acidosis	Periarticular calcification
Polydipsia	Pruritus
Renal impairment	Pseudogout

Modified from Prielipp *et al.*[10]

with the latter being more common in those over 60 years. Half of those with malignancies are due to direct bone involvement. Causes of hypercalcaemia are listed in Table 54.3. Important ones are described below.

Malignancy

There are three broad clinical categories of malignancy causing hypercalcaemia.

Tumours with bone involvement
Metastatic carcinomas in bone, from breast, bronchus (squamous cell), stomach, kidney and uterus most commonly cause hypercalcaemia in this group. Strangely, carcinoma of the prostate and small-cell carcinoma of the bronchus frequently metastasize to bone, but are rarely associated with hypercalcaemia. Presumably, hypercalcaemia is secondary to bone destruction accompanying the bone metastases. Very often, the metastatic deposits are associated with severe bone pain.

Humoral hypercalcaemia of malignancy (HHM)
This accounts for about 40% of malignancy-associated hypercalcaemia. Cancers may give rise to humoral substances, other than PTH or vitamin D, which inhibit bone formation and stimulate bone resorption. Bronchogenic carcinoma and hyper-nephroma are common examples. Ectopic PTH, polypeptides with PTH-like activity, vitamin D-like sterols, prostaglandins (PGE), growth factors (epidermal and transforming) or osteoclast-activating factors are thought to be released from the tumours.

Table 54.3 Causes of hypercalcaemia

Increased intestinal absorption
Increased vitamin D production/activity
   Vitamin D intoxication
   Granulomatous diseases (production of vitamin D by
   macrophages)
      Sarcoidosis (occurs in ~10%)
      Tuberculosis
      Berylliosis
      Histoplasmosis
      Coccidiomycosis
   Acromegaly (growth hormone stimulation of vitamin D
   production in kidneys)
   Lymphomas (via ectopic production of vitamin D)
Increased absorption of calcium
   Calcium ingestion
   Milk-alkali syndrome (ingestion of calcium and alkali)

Diminished excretion of calcium
Hypovolaemia
Familial hypocalciuric hypercalcaemia
Thiazide diuretics (decrease urinary calcium excretion
by direct action on distal tubule)
Addison's disease (volume depletion, lack of glucocorticoids)

Increased bone reabsorption
Malignancy
   Solid tumours with bone metastases
   Solid tumours without bone metastases (humoral)
   Haematological malignancies (myeloma, lymphoma)
Hyperparathyroidism
   Primary (adenoma, hyperplasia, carcinoma, multiple
   endocrine adenomatosis)
   Secondary
   Tertiary
Other endocrine
   Hyperthyroidism (occurs in ~10%)
   Acromegaly
   Phaeochromocytoma (catecholamine has a direct effect on
   bone resorption and increases PTH release)
   Adrenal insufficiency
Miscellaneous increased bone reabsorption
   Paget's disease
   Prolonged immobilization
   Hypophosphataemia
   Lithium (increases the threshold at which serum calcium
   suppresses PTH)
   Vitamin A intoxication (via increased PTH secretion)
   Aluminium bone disease

Miscellaneous
Recovery from acute renal failure following rhabdomyolysis[17]
Recovery from acute pancreatitis
Parenteral nutrition
Tamoxifen

Modified from Kobrin and Goldfarb.[18]
PTH = Parathyroid hormone.

Haematological malignancies

Hypercalcaemia may be seen in lymphoma and myeloma. As the bony involvement is via osteoclasts and not osteoblasts, serum alkaline phosphatase concentrations are not increased.

Hyperparathyroidism

In primary hyperparathyroidism, excessive PTH is secreted by a parathyroid adenoma, carcinoma or hyperplasia. Adenomas may be part of multiple endocrine adenomatosis. Secondary hyperparathyroidism occurs in renal failure and is complicated by osteodystrophy. It is due to hyperplastic changes within the parathyroid glands as a result of phosphate retention and mild hypocalcaemia, which stimulate PTH release. The hyperplastic glands may, in time, become autonomous and result in tertiary hyperparathyroidism. Secondary hyperparathyroidism is treated medically, whereas primary and tertiary hyperparathyroidism are treated surgically.

In patients with chronic renal failure and bone disease, use of vitamin D analogues may contribute to hypercalcaemia and cause further deterioration of renal function. Hypercalcaemia may also occur following renal transplantation, when the hyperplastic parathyroid glands are slow to involute following restoration of renal function. This usually resolves within a few months.

Immobilization

Immobilization, with lack of postural mechanical stimuli to the skeleton, alters the balance between bone formation and resorption, resulting in excesive loss of bone minerals, hypercalcaemia, hypercalciuria, osteoporosis and increased risk of calculi and renal failure. Usually, the increased calcium released from bone is excreted in urine and hypercalcaemia does not occur. However, if bone turnover is rapid (e.g. in children or adults with hyperparathyroidism or Paget's disease) or renal impairment is present, immobilization may result in severe hypercalcaemia. This has also been described in patients with acute spinal injuries, multiple fractures and Guillain–Barré syndrome.

Hypovolaemia

Hypovolaemia reduces renal calcium excretion by decreasing the glomerular filtration rate and increasing tubular reabsorption. The most consistent renal defect in hypercalcaemia is tubular dysfunction, resulting in a concentrating defect which leads to polyuria, and which aggravates the hypovolaemia. Hypovolaemia may be further aggravated by other sequelae of hypercalcaemia, e.g. poor oral intake secondary to nausea, vomiting and decreased conscious state.

Extrarenal production of vitamin D

This is commonly seen in a number of granulomatous conditions. Corticosteroids are effective in turning off this increased vitamin D production.

Investigations

The following investigations are used to confirm the diagnosis, determine the aetiology and assess complications.

1 *Serum calcium concentration*: Measurement of the ionized calcium fraction is recommended. An increased fasting total serum calcium concentration may be misleading if hyperalbuminaemia or hyperglobulinaemia are present.
2 *Serum phosphate concentration* is low in hyperparathyroidism and in patients with tumours producing ectopic PTH-like substances (unless renal impairment is present).
3 *PTH assay* is of definitive diagnostic value for hyperparathyroidism. Non-PTH-caused hypercalcaemia should result in suppression of PTH concentrations.
4 *Radiology and organ imaging:* Chest X-rays may provide evidence of neoplasms (primary or secondary) or granulomas, whereas bone X-rays may show changes of osteitis fibrosa cystica, myeloma or metastatic deposits. Differentiation between osteolytic and osteoblastic deposits may provide clues on the source of the primary neoplasm. A bone scan may be useful to determine the extent and sites of secondary deposits. Ultrasound and radionucleotide scans may be helpful in finding the parathyroid glands.
5 *Angiotensin-converting enzyme (ACE)*: Raised concentrations are suggestive of granulomatous disease.
6 *Other biochemical investigations* which may be useful include serum alkaline phosphatase and indices of renal function.
7 *Electrocardiogram (ECG)*: Classical Q–T shortening is an uncommon marker of hypercalcaemia.[19]

Management[2,11–14,20,21]

Hyperparathyroidism and malignancy are usually responsible for clinically severe hypercalcaemia. Prompt treatment is necessary to avert a fatal outcome. Hypercalcaemia associated with malignancy may be refractory to treatment. Treatment of hypercalcaemia consists of measures to enhance renal excretion of calcium, decrease calcium efflux from bone, and decrease calcium absorption from GIT, and decrease serum calcium concentration. Treatment may be considered according to the onset of action.[18]

Immediate treatment

Edetate disodium (EDTA)
EDTA 15–50 mg/kg IV rapidly lowers serum ionized calcium. It is a metal chelating agent, with the greatest affinity for calcium to form a stable, soluble complex that is readily excreted by the kidneys. Although total serum calcium concentration will not decrease until the chelated calcium has been excreted by the kidneys, there is an immediate reduction of the ionized fraction which protects against immediate toxic effects of hypercalcaemia. Serum calcium concentration can be reduced so quickly that hypocalcaemic tetany, seizures, severe cardiac arrhythmias and respiratory arrest may occur. Large doses of EDTA have also been associated with renal failure (but EDTA is cleared by dialysis). For these reasons, EDTA is reserved for life-threatening hypercalcaemia only.

Haemo- or peritoneal dialysis
This is effective, particularly if oliguric renal failure is present. Calcium-free dialysate needs to be used.

Treatment within hours

Volume repletion
Volume repletion is achieved with IV saline with central venous pressure (CVP) monitoring. Expansion of the intravascular compartment has a diluting effect on serum calcium. Saline also inhibits proximal tubular reabsorption of calcium where sodium and calcium transport are linked.

Calciuresis
Calciuresis is induced once volume expansion is achieved. Normal saline is given IV with frusemide 20–40 mg 2–4 hourly or by infusion. Calcium loss results from increased glomerular filtration and decreased tubular resorption. A minimum urine volume of about 6 l/day is required for adequate calciuria. Care must be taken so that the diuretic is neither insufficient nor excessive, particularly in elderly patients and those with renal impairment and heart failure. Fluid balance, CVP and serum potassium and magnesium concentrations must be closely monitored. Potassium replacement is usually required. The serum calcium concentration usually falls within 8–12 h of therapy.

Mithramycin
Mithramycin is indicated when volume repletion and diuresis fail to lower the serum calcium concentration. This is an antibiotic cytotoxic agent which inhibits bone resorption. When 25 μg/kg IV is given as a bolus or an infusion, it is effective within 6–12 h and is effective for 4–6 days.[22] A single dose has been shown to reduce hypercalcaemia to normal concentrations in the majority (70%) of patients.[11] Thrombocytopenia and hepatic and renal toxicity are reported complications, but the risks are low when it is used sparingly (1–2 doses). Monitoring of platelet count and hepatic and renal function should be undertaken. Subsequent doses should only be given after careful consideration.

Calcitonin
Calcitonin has proven effective in cases of refractory hypercalcaemia associated with cancer.[3] It inhibits bone resorption and may enhance calcium clearance.

It is given IV 3–4 U/kg initially, followed by 4 U/kg SC at 12-hourly intervals. The maximum recommended dose is 8 U/kg every 6 h. Duration of action is brief and tachyphylaxis usually develops. About 20% of patients do not respond to calcitonin; most who do become resistant after several days of therapy. Concurrent use of corticosteroids may increase calcitonin's effectiveness and duration of action. It is particularly useful in Paget's disease and hypercalcaemia secondary to immobilization from traumatic injuries.

Diphosphonates

Diphosphonates are pyrophosphate analogues which are resistant to phosphatases, and are powerful inhibitors of bone resorption. Aminohydroxypropylidene diphosphonate (APD) given as a single infusion of 60 mg over 8 h is reported to be effective.[23] Other diphosphonates now available include etidronate, clodronate and pamidronate.

Treatment within days

Corticosteroids

Glucocorticoids (e.g. hydrocortisone IV 200–400 mg/day or prednisolone 10–25 mg/day) may be beneficial in hypercalcaemia associated with malignancy, vitamin D overdose and sarcoidosis. Their effect, by inhibiting GIT absorption and bone resorption, and facilitating renal excretion of calcium, may take several days to manifest. Therefore, corticosteroids are of limited value in severe life-threatening hypercalcaemia, and should be used in conjunction with other modes of therapy.

Non-steroidal anti-inflammatory drugs (NSAIDs)

NSAIDs such as indomethacin inhibit synthesis of prostaglandins and may be helpful in patients with neoplasms that secrete (prostaglandin-like) nonparathyroid humoral substances to cause bone resorption and hypercalcaemia. Certainly, they are often of major benefit in controlling bone pain.

Parathyroidectomy

Parathyroidectomy is the treatment of choice for primary and tertiary hyperparathyroidism.[23] The operation is performed following volume repletion and correction of other reversible disturbances. Other cause-oriented therapy includes tumour removal, chemotherapy, deep X-ray therapy to large secondary tumour deposits and mobilization.

Monitoring of cardiac and respiratory function and biochemical status is mandatory during the management of severe hypercalcaemia. Oral or IV phosphates are not recommended as they may increase ectopic calcification. This is likely to occur when the calcium–phosphate solubility product is exceeded (> 5 mmol/l). Thiazide diuretics, vitamin D and absorbable antacids should be avoided. Hypercalcaemia poten-

tiates digitalis effect and dosage should be adjusted accordingly. Endocrinologists should be consulted for further management.

Hypocalcaemia

Pathophysiology[2,13,18,24]

The causes of hypocalcaemia are listed in Table 54.4. It is essential first to confirm the diagnosis; hypoalbuminaemia is common in the critically ill, and the consequent decreased total serum calcium may

Table 54.4 Causes of hypocalcaemia

Decreased parathyroid hormone
Hypoparathyroidism
  Idiopathic
  Post surgical
  Infiltration (malignancy, amyloidosis)
Magnesium deficiency (decreased secretion of PTH)
Sepsis (suppression of parathyroid glands – ? part of multiple organ dysfunction syndrome)
End-organ resistance to PTH
  Pseudohypoparathyroidism
  Magnesium deficiency

Decreased vitamin D
Decreased ingestion
Decreased gastrointestinal absorption
  Gastrectomy
  Bypass surgery
  Sprue
  Pancreatic insufficiency
Decreased conversion
  Lack of exposure to sunlight
  Liver disease (decreased hepatic conversion to $25(OH)D_3$)
  Renal failure (decreased renal conversion to $1,25(OH)_2D_3$)
Increased metabolism (anticonvulsants, barbiturates, alcohol)
Hypoparathyroidism
Pseudohypoparathyroidism
Magnesium deficiency
Vitamin D-resistant rickets (autosomal recessive defect in renal synthesis)

Calcium losses
Excessive skeletal uptake of calcium (hungry bones)
Soft-tissue calcification
  Pancreatitis
  Rhabdomyolysis, renal failure
  Hyperphosphataemia
Citrate
EDTA
Ethylene glycol poisoning (generates oxalate which then chelates with calcium)
Radiographic contrast agents (chelate calcium)

Calcium shifts
Alkalosis (decreases ionized calcium)
Free fatty acids (high levels increase calcium binding to albumin)
Lactate (chelates calcium)

Modified from Kobrin and Goldfarb.[18]
PTH = parathyroid hormone. EDTA = ethylenediaminetetraacetic acid.

suggest hypocalcaemia. In these circumstances, it is important to measure the ionized fraction. Hypocalcaemia may be associated with the following conditions.

Hypoparathyroidism

Cervical surgery resulting in parathyroid gland removal is the most common cause of hypoparathyroidism. In addition, handling of the thyroid gland may release calcitonin. Up to 90% of post thyroid surgery patients develop hypocalcaemia.[25] Unless all parathyroid tissue is removed, hypocalcaemia is usually transient. Permanent hypoparathyroidism occurs with total thyroidectomy or parathyroidectomy, infiltrative disease of the parathyroids, and irradiation of the neck. Idiopathic hypoparathyroidism of autoimmune origin usually appears in childhood and may be associated with candidiasis, Addison's disease and pernicious anaemia. Hypoparathyroidism may also result from end-organ resistance to PTH. This pseudohypoparathyroidism is characterized by hypocalcaemia with high PTH concentrations, and is due to a genetic defect, whereby the kidneys cannot respond to PTH. There are associated skeletal abnormalities.

Hypomagnesaemia impairs PTH responsiveness, decreases PTH secretion and causes defective calcium–magnesium exchange in bone. Correction of hypomagnesaemia restores normal PTH responsiveness. Drugs (e.g. cimetidine) may impair PTH release.

Abnormal vitamin D metabolism

Deficiency of vitamin D results from inadequate intake or GIT malabsorption. Disturbances of vitamin D metabolism may also occur. Production of 1,25 $(OH)_2D$, the active metabolite of vitamin D, is impaired in severe renal disease and in vitamin D-dependent rickets. 25 (OH)D, an intermediate in the conversion of vitamin D to 1,25 $(OH)_2D$, is dependent on intact hepatic function. Its production may be diminished in liver failure or its breakdown accelerated by concurrent use of enzyme-inducing agents such as phenobarbitone, alcohol and phenytoin.

Excessive calcium 'loss'

An acute excess of phosphate in the circulation from massive ingestion, cell lysis or rhabdomyolysis results in calcium–phosphate deposition in tissues, and a fall in serum ionized calcium. Severe acute pancreatitis may also produce hypocalcaemia as a result of intra-abdominal saponification of fat, and possibly from destruction of PTH by proteolytic enzymes released from the pancreas.[26] Transient hypocalcaemia occurs with massive blood transfusion due to chelation of calcium with citrate.[27] The effect is increased by hypothermia and hepatic insufficiency (see Chapter 86).

Hypocalcaemia may occur with osteoblastic metastases, presumably secondary to the osteoblastic activity and increased bone formation. It is a frequent occurrence following parathyroidectomy in patients with severe bone disease; presumably the calcium is 'soaked-up' by the demineralized bones (i.e. the hungry bone syndrome).

Calcium shifts

Hyperventilation with acute respiratory alkalosis may reduce serum ionized calcium and induce symptoms of hypocalcaemia. Respiratory acidosis has no effect on ionized calcium. Metabolic acidosis increases, whereas metabolic alkalosis decreases urinary calcium excretion. Free fatty acids (FFAs) increase calcium binding to albumin.[28] Critically ill patients, as a result of the stress response, lipid infusions and the presence of heparin, may develop high levels of FFAs.

Hypocalcaemia is commonly associated with renal failure, sepsis,[9,29] burns[30] and shock states.[6] Hypoparathyroidism may be a manifestation of endocrine failure, which may be part of multiple organ dysfunction. Hypocalcaemia in acutely ill patients has been associated with a poorer outcome.[9,31] The incidence is more common in critically ill patients than is usually considered, being present in up to 70% of patients.[31,32]

Clinical presentation[2,10,11,13,24,33]

Clinical manifestations of hypocalcaemia vary greatly (Table 54.5). Patients who develop acute hypocalcaemia (e.g. post surgery) may develop severe symptoms with only a modest decline in ionized calcium concentration. Patients with renal failure may develop marked ionized hypocalcaemia, but do so gradually over some time, and do not commonly develop symptoms. The concomitant metabolic acidosis in renal failure may have a protective role.

Reduced serum calcium concentration causes increased neuromuscular irritability. Neurological symptoms and signs generally appear when the serum calcium concentration is < 2 mmol/l. Circumoral and peripheral paraesthesia, carpopedal spasm and muscle cramps may occur. The neuromuscular irritability is evidenced by positive Chvostek's and Trousseau's signs. Chvostek's sign (facial twitch following tapping of the facial nerve) is positive in 10% of the normal population, and is not as specific for latent hypocalcaemia as Trousseau's sign (paraesthesia and carpopedal spasm in the arm following inflation of the blood pressure cuff over systolic pressure for 3 min). Hypocalcaemic tetany may resemble, or be exacerbated by, coexisting hypokalaemia and/or hypomagnesaemia.

Neuromuscular weakness is usually associated with vitamin D deficiency.[33] It may result in laryngeal

Table 54.5 Clinical manifestations of hypocalcaemia

General	*Cardiovascular*
Dry coarse skin	Digitalis resistance
Dermatitis	Impaired β-adrenergic action
Hair loss	ECG
Brittle nails	OT prolongation
Fatigue	ST prolongation
Cataracts	T-wave inversion
Bone pain	Heart failure
Bone deformities	Hypotension
Fractures	Heart block
	Ventricular fibrillation
Respiratory	
Apnoea	*Neuromuscular*
Laryngeal spasm	Neuronal irritability
Bronchospasm	Tetany
	Muscle spasm/cramps
Psychiatric	Papilloedema
Anxiety	Seizures
Dementia	Grand mal
Depression	Petit mal
Psychosis	Focal
Impaired mental function	Weakness
Confusion	Tingling
Hallucinations	Circumoral
Lethargy	Acral
	Movement disorders
	Hyperreflexia

Modified from Prielipp *et al.*[10]
ECG = Electrocardiogram.

spasm, bronchospasm, respiratory muscle weakness and apnoea. Cardiovascular manifestations include arrhythmias, hypotension, heart failure and decreased sensitivity to digitalis. Inotropic agents act by increasing calcium concentrations within cardiac cells, and are therefore dependent on normal circulating calcium concentrations. Hence, hypocalcaemia may render patients unresponsive to these drugs. Electrocardiogram (ECG) abnormalities of long QT and ST intervals and T-wave inversion occur, but do not correlate well with the degree of hypocalcaemia. Mental changes of excitement, irritability and anxiety may occur in the acute stage. Grand mal epileptic fits may be an early feature.[34] Personality changes occur with chronic hypocalcaemia, including anxiety, dementia, depression, irritability and psychosis. Choreoathetosis, cataracts and papilloedema may also be present.

Investigations

1 *Ionized calcium measurement* should be performed if total serum calcium is low.
2 *Phosphate and PTH measurements* are useful. When calcium loss is the problem (i.e. calcium is sequestered by chelation or deposited in soft tissues or bone), the PTH response is normal (increases) and phosphate concentrations decrease (unless hyperphosphataemia is the cause). In PTH deficiency, PTH concentrations are low in gland failure or high in end-organ resistance, and

phosphate concentrations are usually high. Phosphate concentrations are usually low with vitamin D deficiency.
3 *Serum magnesium concentrations* should also be estimated. Hypomagnesaemia may contribute to hypocalcaemia by impairment of the release and action of PTH.
4 *Renal function tests* should also be performed.

Management[2,13,25,30,35]

Acute hypocalcaemia complicated by tetany, seizures or cardiovascular problems requires immediate treatment. Asymptomatic hypocalcaemia should also be treated, but not with the same urgency, because of the potential to produce severe symptoms. Treatment includes:

1 *Airway support* and provision of supplementary oxygen.
2 *Continuous ECG monitoring* to assist detection of arrhythmias during severe hypocalcaemic crisis or during IV calcium administration. Refractory ventricular fibrillation has been reported with profound hypocalcaemia.
3 *Calcium supplements* given slowly IV. Rapid infusion may cause flushing, headache and arrhythmias. Following initial treatment, calcium may be continued by infusion and the rate adjusted according to frequent serum calcium estimations. Calcium ampoules are available as 10% calcium gluconate (1 g or 2.2 mmol in 10 ml) or 10% calcium chloride (0.5 g or 3.4 mmol in 5 ml). The latter is more likely to cause thrombophlebitis and irritation with extravasation.
4 *Magnesium (MgSO$_4$)* given as 1–5 mmol IV over 15 min if magnesium deficiency coexists. Failure of symptoms to resolve following calcium administration may indicate concurrent magnesium deficiency.[36]
5 *Calcitrol* $(1,25(OH)_2D_3)$ as 0.25 μg tablets, is given orally if vitamin D deficiency is present.
6 *Hyperphosphataemia* is controlled if present.

Chronic hypocalcaemia

This is usually managed with oral calcium supplements plus calcitriol. Thiazide diuretics, by reducing urinary calcium excretion and vitamin D requirements, may be useful in these patients.

Effective hypocalcaemia

This occurs as a result of overdose (accidental or deliberate) of calcium-channel blockers. These drugs are highly protein-bound and extensively distributed throughout the body, thus removal by extracorporeal means is limited. Their major side-effects are negative inotropy, bradycardia and vasodilatation and hypotension. Other side-effects include seizures and coma, hyperglycaemia (due to direct inhibition of insulin release), lactic acidosis secondary to hypoperfusion, hypokalaemia and hypomagnesaemia.

Treatment consists of supportive care and high-dose calcium infusion, which has been shown to reverse both the negative inotropy and conduction disturbances. Calcium concentrations of 3mmol/l are often achieved. Glucagon, by increasing cyclic adenosine monophosphate, increases intracellular calcium concentration. Some reports indicate that it reverses the effects of calcium-channel blockers. Transvenous pacing is sometimes required.

References

1 Slatopolsky E, Hruska K and Klahr S (1993) Disorders of phosphorous, calcium, and magnesium metabolism. In: Gottschalk CW and Schrier RW (eds) *Diseases of the Kidney*. Boston: Little, Brown, pp. 2865–2920.

2 Agus ZS and Goldfarb S (1981) Clinical disorders of calcium and phosphate. *Med Clin North Am* **65**:385–399.

3 Austin LA and Heath H (1981) Calcitonin: physiology and pathophysiology. *N Engl J Med* **304**:269–278.

4 Ladenson JH, Lewis JW, Mcdonald JM, Slatopolsky E and Boyd JC (1979) Relationship of free and total calcium in hypercalcemic conditions. *J Clin Endocrinol Metab* **48**:393–397.

5 Zaloga GP, Chernow B and Cook D (1985) Assessment of calcium homeostasis in the critically ill surgical patient. The diagnostic pitfalls of the Mclean-Hastings nomogram. *Ann Surg* **202**:587–594.

6 Drop LJ and Laver MB (1975) Low plasma ionized calcium and response to calcium therapy in critically ill man. *Anesthesiology* **43**:300–306.

7 Baldwin TE and Chernow B (1987) Hypocalcaemia in the ICU: coping with the causes and consequences. *J Crit Illness* **2**:9.

8 Ladenson JH, Lewis J and Boyd JC (1987) Failure of total calcium corrected for protein, albumin, and pH to correctly assess free calcium status. *J Clin Endocrinol Metab* **46**:986–993.

9 Chernow B, Zaloga G, Mcfadden E *et al.* (1982) Hypocalcemia in critically ill patients. *Crit Care Med* **10**:848–851.

10 Prielipp RC, Heyneker TJ and Prough DS (1993) Fluid and divalent cation therapy in the critically ill patient. *Internat Anesthesiol Clinics* **31**:21–47.

11 Bagdade JD (1986) Endocrine emergencies. *Med Clin North Am* **70**:1112–1115.

12 Watson L. (1972) Diagnosis and treatment of hypercalcaemia. *Br Med J* **2**:150–152.

13 Peacock M (1979) The endocrine control of calcium and phosphorus metabolism and its diseases. *Med Aust* **1**:533–548.

14 Chopra D and Clerkin EP (1975) Hypercalcemia and malignant disease. *Med Clin North Am* **59**:441–447.

15 Sherwood LM (1980) The multiple causes of hypercalcemia in malignant disease. *N Engl J Med* **303**:1412–1413.

16 Goodwin FJ (1982) Symptomless abnormalities: hypercalcaemia. *Br J Hosp Med* **28**:50–58.

17 Knochel JP (1981) Serum calcium derangements in rhabdomyolysis. *N Engl J Med* **305**:161–163.

18 Kobrin SM and Goldfarb S (1991) Hypocalcemia and hypercalcaemia. In: Adrogue HJ (ed.) *Acid-Base and Electrolyte Disorders*. New York: Churchill Livingstone, pp. 69–97.

19 Ellman H, Dembin H and Seriff N (1982) The rarity of shortening of the Q-T interval in patients with hypercalcemia. *Crit Care Med* **10**:320–323.

20 Editorial (1978) Management of hypercalcaemic crisis. *Lancet* **2**:617–618.

21 Simpson D (1984) Treatment of hypercalcaemia associated with malignancy. *Br Med J* **288**:812–814.

22 Kiang DT, Loken MK and Kennedy BJ (1979) Mechanism of the hypocalcaemic effect of mithramycin. *J Clin Endocrinol Metab* **48**:341–344.

23 Morton AR, Cantrill JA, Craig AE *et al.* (1988) Single dose versus daily intravenous aminohydroxyporpylidene biphosphonate (Apd) for the hypercalcaemia of malignancy. *Br Med J* **296**:811–814.

24 Thomas DW (1977) Calcium, phosphorus and magnesium turnover. *Anaesth Intens Care* **5**:361–367.

25 Burnett HF, Mabry CD and Westbrook KC (1977) Hypocalcemia after thyroidectomy: mechanisms and management. *South Med J* **70**:1045–1048.

26 Condon JR, Ives D, Knight MJ and Day J (1975) The aetiology of hypocalcaemia in acute pancreatitis. *Br J Surg* **62**:115–118.

27 Denlinger JK, Nahrwold ML, Gibbs PS and Lecky JH (1976) Hypocalcaemia during rapid blood transfusion in anaesthetized man. *Br J Anaesth* **48**:995–999.

28 Zaloga GP and Chernow B (1985) Free fatty acids increase calcium binding to albumin in serum of critically ill patients. *Clin Res* **33**:296a.

29 Aderka D, Schwartz D and Dan M (1987) Bacteremic hypocalcaemia. *Arch Intern Med* **147**:232–236.

30 Szyfelbein SK, Drop LJ and Martyn JAJ (1981) Persistent ionized hypocalcemia in patients during resuscitation and recovery phases of body burns. *Crit Care Med* **9**:454–458.

31 Desai TK, Carlson RW and Geheb MA (1988) Prevalence and clinical implications of hypocalcaemia in acutely ill patients in a medical intensive care setting. *Am J Med* **84**:209–214.

32 Zaloga GP (1992) Hypocalcemia in critically ill patients. *Crit Care Med* **20**:251–262.

33 Alberti KGMM (1979) Metabolic comas and confusions. *Med Aust* **1**:612–628.

34 Gupta MM and Grover DN (1977) Hypocalcaemia and convulsions. *Postgrad Med J* **53**:330–333.

35 Schweitzer VG Thompson NW, Harness JK and Nishiyama RH (1978) Management of severe hypercalcaemia caused by primary hyperparathyroidism. *Arch Surg* **113**:373–381.

36 Chernow B, Smith J, Rainey T and Finton O (1982) Hypomagnesemia. Implications for the critical care specialist. *Crit Care Med* **10**:193–196.

Part VIII

Obstetrical emergencies

55 | Pre-eclampsia and eclampsia

WD Ngan Kee and T Gin

Pre-eclampsia is diagnosed when hypertension, proteinuria and generalized oedema (Table 55.1) occur during the second half of pregnancy, while eclampsia describes those patients with associated grand mal convulsions not caused by other cerebral pathology. Pre-eclampsia complicates 2–10% of all pregnancies, and it is the leading direct cause of maternal death in the UK[1] The incidence of eclampsia is 2–6/10 000 deliveries[2-4] with a maternal mortality in the UK of 1.8% and fetal/neonatal mortality of around 7%.[4] Although pre-eclampsia is typically a disease afflicting young women during their first pregnancy, mortality is greater in older multiparous women.[2] The main indications for admission to the ICU, particularly in the immediate postpartum period, are uncontrolled hypertension, eclampsia and problems with fluid balance, such as pulmonary oedema or persistent oliguria. Provided complications are avoided, the disease normally resolves completely.

Pathogenesis

The precise aetiology of pre-eclampsia remains undefined but may involve genetic[5] and immunological[6] factors. The primary defect occurs in the placenta, where inadequate trophoblastic invasion of the spiral arteries is thought to lead to placental hypoperfusion, with consequent injury or activation of placental endothelial cells. These cells release cytotoxic factors[7] which cause widespread systemic endothelial damage, with glomeruloendotheliosis in the kidney[8] and increased fibronectin and factor VIII antigen.[9] Systemic endothelial cell dysfunction causes manifestations in virtually every organ system.[9] There is widespread vasospasm associated with increased levels of circulating vasoconstrictors (e.g. endothelin and thromboxane), increased sensitivity to angiotensin II, and decreased levels of vasodilators (e.g. prostacyclin). Increased vascular permeability leads to oedema and proteinuria.

Activation of the coagulation system leads to

Table 55.1 Diagnostic criteria for pre-eclampsia

Hypertension
Diastolic arterial pressure 90 mmHg (12 kPa)
or Systolic arterial pressure $\geqslant 140$ mmHg (18.6 kPa)
or Relative rise in diastolic arterial pressure $\geqslant 15$ mmHg (2.0 kPa)
or Relative rise in systolic arterial pressure $\geqslant 25$ mmHg (3.3 kPa)

Proteinuria
$\geqslant 300$ mg protein during 24-h collection
or Urine protein concentration $\geqslant 1$ g/l or 1 + on dipstick

Generalized oedema

disseminated intravascular coagulation with platelet aggregation and destruction, decreased levels of procoagulants, intravascular appearance of fibrin degradation products and end-organ damage from microthrombi. Further injury to placental endothelial cells causes more release of cytotoxic factors, accelerating placental ischaemia and progressive worsening of pre-eclampsia. A decrease in the prostacyclin:thromboxane A_2 ratio is also thought to be important in pathogenesis.[10] This has led to investigation into the use of low-dose aspirin, which may have a prophylactic role in women at high risk of early-onset pre-eclampsia.[11] Other factors implicated in the pathogenesis are an imbalance between lipid peroxides and antioxidants,[12] reduction in endothelium-derived relaxing factor (nitric oxide),[13] and the presence of antiendothelial cell autoantibodies.[14]

Clinical presentation

Pre-eclampsia may be classified as either mild (Table 55.1), or severe (Table 55.2). Since pathological changes are not secondary to hypertension itself, severity does not necessarily correlate with blood

Table 55.2 Diagnostic features of severe pre-eclampsia

Features of pre-eclampsia plus one of the following:

Arterial pressure
Diastolic arterial pressure $\geqslant$ 110 mmHg (14.6 kPa)
Systolic arterial pressure $\geqslant$ 160 mmHg (21.3 kPa)

Renal
Proteinuria $\geqslant$ 5 g/24 h or 3 + on dipstick
Oliguria < 500 ml/24 h
Serum creatinine $\geqslant$ 0.09 mmol/l

Hepatic
Epigastric or right upper quadrant pain
Elevated bilirubin and/or transaminases

Neurological
Persistent headaches
Visual disturbances
Hyperreflexia and/or clonus

Haematological
Thrombocytopenia
Disseminated intravascular coagulation
Haemolysis

Cardiac/respiratory
Pulmonary oedema
Cyanosis

pressure, and systemic features of the disease are important indicators (Table 55.2). Eclampsia may occur without marked hypertension or without proteinuria.[4,15] Traditionally, hypertension was thought to be associated with increased vascular resistance and reduced plasma volume, but many patients have a hyperdynamic circulation, and increased cardiac output may be an important cause for hypertension.[16,17] Sudden ventricular tachycardia may occur during hypertensive crises.[18] Pulmonary oedema may occur because of iatrogenic fluid overload, decreased left ventricular function, increased capillary permeability, and narrowing of the colloid osmotic–pulmonary capillary wedge pressure (PCWP) gradient.[19] Pulmonary oedema is more common postpartum, when fluid is redistributed into the circulation faster than it can be excreted. Renal changes include reduced glomerular filtration rate and renal plasma flow, and increased serum uric acid. Oliguria is not uncommon, although acute renal failure is rare.[20] Neurological complications include eclamptic convulsions, cerebral oedema, and raised intracranial pressure. The most common haemostatic abnormality is a reduced platelet count in up to 50% of patients, which may be associated with decreased platelet function.[21] Clinically significant coagulopathy occurs in about 15% of severe cases.[22] Some patients with severe disease present with haemolysis, elevated liver enzymes, and low platelets (HELLP syndrome).[23] This is associated with hepatic parenchymal necrosis,

and patients are at risk of intrahepatic haemorrhage, subcapsular haematoma formation and liver rupture. Symptoms include epigastric or right upper quadrant pain, nausea or vomiting, and malaise.[24] The leading causes of maternal death in pre-eclampsia/eclampsia are intracranial haemorrhage and respiratory failure.[1,2] Fetal morbidity results from chronically decreased uteroplacental blood flow or acute maternal deterioration, and there is an increased risk of placental abruption.

Management

The principles of management include:

1 maintenance of placental perfusion with timely termination of pregnancy;
2 control of arterial pressure;
3 prevention of seizures;
4 control of fluid balance

The definitive treatment of pre-eclampsia is delivery of the fetus and placenta. In milder cases, the disease may be controlled while allowing fetal maturation.[25] Transfer of the mother to a tertiary centre before delivery should be considered, if a level III neonatal unit is not available (see Chapter 1). In more severe cases, the mother should be stabilized and the fetus delivered regardless of gestation. Delay in delivery in the hope of obtaining a more mature fetus has been a contributing factor to maternal and fetal mortality.[1,26] Admission into an ICU before delivery may be appropriate in severe cases, or when the labour ward lacks the expertise or equipment for intensive monitoring. After delivery, severe cases should preferably be managed in an ICU for 24–72 h. About 40% of patients who develop eclampsia have the first seizure after delivery,[4,15] and the risk of pulmonary oedema is greatest after delivery.[27]

General measures

Before delivery, patients should be rested in the lateral decubitus position, and have continuous fetal heart rate monitoring. Regular oral or IV ranitidine should be given to decrease gastric acidity and volume. Routine monitoring includes frequent clinical assessment and arterial pressure recordings, and accurate fluid balance with a urinary catheter. An arterial line is useful for frequent blood gas analysis and during infusions of antihypertensives. The electrocardiogram (ECG) should be monitored, especially during administration of phenytoin and magnesium. Pulse oximetry aids the detection of incipient pulmonary oedema. Central venous pressure (CVP) monitoring, preferably via an antecubital vein, and/or pulmonary artery catheterization may assist in fluid balance (see below). Essential investigations include full blood count, coagulation screen, electrolytes, uric acid, renal function, liver function and urinalysis. Serial investigations should be performed to monitor disease progression. Clotting factors and platelets are given to correct coagulopathy. Patients who have been receiving aspirin may have an increased transfusion requirement after delivery.[11]

Antihypertensive therapy

The aim of antihypertensive therapy is to prevent maternal complications (intracerebral haemorrhage, cardiac failure or placental abruption) while maintaining placental blood flow. Acute treatment is indicated when arterial pressure is greater than 160–170 mmHg (21.3–22.6 kPa) systolic or 110 mmHg (14.6 kPa) diastolic. Initially, systolic arterial pressure is reduced by only 20–30 mmHg (2.7–4.0 kPa) and diastolic by 10–15 mmHg (1.3–2.0 kPa).[28] Continuous fetal monitoring should be used during drug titration. Intravenous volume loading may be necessary when vasodilators are used. The vasodilators used are described below.

Hydralazine

Hydralazine causes direct arteriolar vasodilatation while improving renal and uteroplacental blood flow.[29] Usual dose is 5 mg IV initially, followed by 5–10 mg every 20 min to a maximum of 40 mg.[20] Onset time is 10–20 min and the duration of action is 6–8 h. Infusions of hydralazine may be difficult to titrate, and may be associated with a higher incidence of fetal distress.[30] In the presence of hypovolaemia, use of hydralazine without volume replacement may result in hypotension and fetal distress.[31] Other adverse effects include headache, tachycardia, tremor, nausea, and rare cases of neonatal thrombocytopenia.[32]

Labetalol

Labetalol is a non-selective β-adrenergic receptor blocker with some α_1-blocking effect. It rapidly reduces arterial pressure without decreasing uteroplacental blood flow,[33] and does not cause reflex tachycardia, headache or nausea. Although labetalol crosses the placenta, neonatal bradycardia and hypoglycaemia are rarely seen.[34] The initial IV dose is 10 mg, with doubling of the dose every 10 min as necessary, to a maximum of 300 mg. Alternatively, it can be given by continuous infusion, starting at 1–2 mg/min, reducing to 0.5 mg/min or less after arterial pressure is controlled.[20] Disadvantages of labetalol include interpatient variability in dose requirement and a variable duration of action. It should not be given to patients with asthma or myocardial dysfunction.

Nifedipine

Nifedipine is a calcium-channel blocker that causes direct relaxation of arterial smooth muscle. It does not produce reflex tachycardia, decreased uterine perfusion or fetal deterioration.[35] Dosage is 10 mg orally or sublingually, repeated if necessary after 30 min. Blood pressure is usually reduced after 10–20 min and the duration of action is 3–4 h. Mild side-effects include headache, flushing and nausea. Nifedipine causes relaxation of uterine muscle which may increase the risk of postpartum haemorrhage. An exaggerated hypotensive response may occur when it is used concurrently with magnesium (which is also a calcium antagonist).

Sodium nitroprusside

Sodium nitroprusside is a potent arterial and venous vasodilator that rapidly reduces arterial pressure in emergencies. Administration is by IV infusion, starting at 0.25 µg/kg per min and increased as necessary by 0.25 µg/kg per min every 5 min.[20] Direct arterial pressure monitoring should be used. Patients with depleted intravascular volume may be particularly sensitive to its effects. The risk of fetal cyanide toxicity may be minimized by limiting the dosage to < 4 µg/kg per min[30] or the duration of infusion to 30 min.[36]

Diazoxide

Diazoxide is a potent arteriolar vasodilator that may be effective in refractory cases. It should be given as frequent small boluses of 30 mg to avoid hypotension associated with larger doses.[37] Potential adverse effects include maternal and neonatal hypoglycaemia and displacement of protein-bound drugs such as phenytoin.[32]

Other vasodilators

Nitroglycerin given by infusion is easily titratable, and may be useful in cases complicated by pulmonary oedema.[30] *Methyldopa*, a central α_2-adrenergic agonist, has a long history of use in pregnancy, but its slow onset time makes it unsuitable for acute treatment. *Clonidine* has a similar mechanism of action, but rebound hypertension on cessation may be a problem. There is controversy over the use of *β-blockers* other than labetalol for acute blood pressure control. Concerns include risk of hepatotoxicity, decreased uteroplacental perfusion, fetal bradycardia and decreased fetal tolerance to hypoxia. *Trimethaphan* has been used, but may interact with suxamethonium, leading to prolonged neuromuscular block.[38] *Ketanserin*, a serotonin antagonist, has been shown to be effective without serious side-effects when given by IV bolus.[39] *Angiotensin-converting enzyme inhibitors* have been associated with a high incidence of intrauterine death in animals, and should not be used in patients before delivery.[40] *Diuretics* should be avoided since most pre-eclamptic patients have reduced plasma volume.

Anticonvulsant therapy

Severe pre-eclamptics should be started on anticonvulsants but there is controversy surrounding currently used agents.

Magnesium sulphate

In North America, magnesium is the drug of choice for the prevention and treatment of eclamptic convulsions,[41,42] although it is less popular in other parts of the world. Although it has been suggested that magnesium may not function as a true anticonvulsant because it is ineffective in the treatment of epilepsy[43] and fails to terminate seizure activity in laboratory models,[44] magnesium may be superior to phenytoin when used as an anticonvulsant in pre-eclampsia.[45] Magnesium may prevent the underlying pathological causes leading to eclamptic seizures.[46] By antagonism of calcium at membrane channels or intracellular sites, it may reduce systemic and cerebral vasospasm.[47] Magnesium amplifies endothelial release of prostacyclin by vascular endothelium, and this may inhibit platelet aggregation and vasoconstriction.[48] Doppler ultrasonography suggests that magnesium vasodilates smaller-diameter intracranial blood vessels, and may exert its main effect by relieving cerebral ischaemia.[49] Other effects of magnesium include tocolysis and reduction of catecholamine release.[50] As a mild general vasodilator, it has a mild antihypertensive action and increases renal and uterine blood flow.

Magnesium is administered by initial IV loading dose of 4–6 g over 20 min, followed by continuous infusion of 1–3 g/h (1g magnesium sulphate = 98 mg = 4.06 mmol = 8.12 mEq elemental magnesium). Intramuscular injections are painful. Magnesium is excreted by the kidney, and reduced dosage is indicated in renal impairment or reduced urine output. The therapeutic concentration is 2–4 mmol/l (normal 0.7–1.1 mmol/l) and should be monitored. Greater concentrations are associated with maternal and neonatal toxicity. Muscle weakness may lead to respiratory paralysis (>7.5 mmol/l). Increased conduction time with increased PR and QT intervals and QRS duration can lead to sinoatrial and atrioventricular block (>7.5 mmol/l) and cardiac arrest in diastole (>12.5 mmol/l). Depression of deep tendon reflexes is an early sign of toxicity, and the reflexes should be checked regularly. Toxicity is treated by small IV doses of calcium. Magnesium crosses the placenta and can cause neonatal flaccidity and respiratory depression. If repeated seizures occur despite therapeutic levels of magnesium, conventional anticonvulsants should be added.[51]

Phenytoin

Phenytoin is an effective anticonvulsant in pre-eclampsia.[52–54] Advantages include known central anticonvulsant action without effects on uterine tone, fetal heart rate variability or neonatal tone. A suggested regimen for IV administration in pre-eclampsia is 10 mg/kg initially, followed by 2 h later by 5 mg/kg. Doses are diluted in normal saline and administered no faster than 50 mg/min. ECG and arterial pressure should be monitored. Maintenance doses of 200 mg orally or IV are started 12 h after the second bolus and given 8-hourly. This protocol produces predictable and prolonged therapeutic levels in pre-eclamptic patients with minimal side-effects.[53] Plasma concentrations should be checked 6 and 12 h after the second bolus dose, then daily. Therapeutic range is 8–20 mg/l. As phenytoin is highly protein-bound, a low serum albumin will increase the unbound fraction, and may necessitate adjustment of the target therapeutic range.[53] Adverse effects include pain on injection, nystagmus, ataxia and lethargy at high plasma concentrations, and cardiotoxicity if given rapidly.

Other anticonvulsants

Diazepam is an effective agent for termination of seizures, but concerns about fetal heart rate changes, and neonatal respiratory depression, hypotonia, poor sucking and decreased body temperature make it less popular for seizure prophylaxis.[42,55] *Chlormethiazole* is not recommended because it requires relatively large volumes of fluid and may depress maternal respiration and laryngeal reflexes.

Eclampsia

The priorities in the management of eclamptic seizures are airway protection, oxygenation, control of seizures and delivery of the fetus after maternal stabilization. Patients should be placed in the left lateral position and given oxygen. Seizures can be terminated by IV diazepam 5–10 mg. A loading dose of phenytoin is administered if not already given. Alternatively, IV magnesium 4 g may be given no faster than 1 g/min, followed by a continuous infusion at 1 g/h. This is effective in terminating seizures and may be more effective than diazepam or phenytoin at preventing recurrent seizures.[56] Further boluses to a maximum of 8 g total are given for repeated seizures. If seizures are not controlled, thiopentone 3–4 mg/kg and suxamethonium 1 mg/kg should be given and the airway secured. Continued convulsions despite therapeutic concentrations of phenytoin or magnesium, may indicate additional cerebral pathology (e.g. cerebral oedema, intracerebral haemorrhage, venous thrombosis)[57] and a computed tomography (CT) scan should be done. Prolonged unconsciousness after seizures is associated with cerebral oedema in the majority of cases, and intracerebral haemorrhage in a lower proportion. Intensive neurological management, aimed at controlling intracranial pressure and optimizing cerebral perfusion, significantly reduces mortality.[58]

Fluid balance

Fluid management in pre-eclampsia is controversial. Volume expansion with crystalloid or colloid solution has been advocated to decrease arterial pressure, reduce systemic vascular resistance, increase cardiac output and avoid hypotension with vasodilator therapy.[59,60] However, injudicious fluid administration may cause acute or postpartum pulmonary oedema[19,27] and cerebral oedema.[61] Initial maintenance fluid should considt of IV crystalloid at 75–125 ml/h, aiming for urine output >0.5 ml/kg per h, averaged over 3–4 h. When there is oliguria or other signs of poor perfusion, repeated fluid challenge with 250–500 ml crystalloid or 100–200 ml colloid may be given, while monitoring oxygenation and examining for fluid overload.

Urinalysis is useful; sodium <20 mmol/l, osmolality >500 mosmol/kg or functional excretion of sodium <1 support a prerenal cause for oliguria. Persistent oliguria should be treated according to assessment with invasive monitoring. Although there is considerable controversy over the reliability of CVP and PCWP, and optimal CVP and PCWP values are unknown, progressive changes in response to fluid challenge are useful. There is poor correlation between CVP and PCWP, especially when CVP is greater than 6 mmHg (0.8 kPa).[19,62] Pulmonary artery catheterization may be useful to differentiate patients with predominantly high systemic resistance from those with high cardiac output. However, it has caused severe maternal morbidity and death,[22] and should only be used when clearly indicated (e.g. unresponsive hypertension, pulmonary oedema and refractory oliguria).[62] Pulmonary oedema is unlikely with a CVP less than 6 mmHg (0.8 kPa), but when it occurs, should be managed by oxygen therapy, positive-pressure ventilation, inotropes, vasodilators or diuretics as indicated.

Analgesia and anaesthesia

Regional anaesthesia in pre-eclampsia remains controversial. The main concern is the potential for hypotension from sympathetic block in patients who generally have reduced intravascular volume. However, epidural anaesthesia prevents arterial pressure fluctuations with labour pain, and avoids the hypertensive effects of rapid-sequence induction of general anaesthesia. With modest volume-loading and avoidance of aortocaval compression, significant hypotension can be avoided[63], uteroplacental blood flow may increase[64], circulating catecholamines are decreased,[65] and there may be protection against the risk of eclampsia.[66] Epidural anaesthesia is contraindicated in the presence of sepsis or coagulopathy.

Potential problems of general anaesthesia include risk of aspiration, difficult intubation from airway oedema, exaggerated hypertensive response to intubation, and increased sensitivity to muscle relaxants in patients on magnesium. Smaller-size endotracheal tubes may be required for intubation, and awake intubation under topical anaesthesia may be necessary when there is severe airway obstruction.[67] A number of different methods have been advocated for obtunding the hypertensive response to intubation, including pretreatment with labetalol (up to 1 mg/kg),[68] fentanyl (2.5 μg/kg),[69] alfentanil (10 μg/kg),[69,70] and magnesium sulphate (40 mg/kg).[70] A combination of alfentanil (7.5 μg/ml) with magnesium sulphate (30 mg/kg), given 60 seconds before intubation, is more effective than either drug given alone.[71]

Liver rupture

Liver rupture can be diagnosed by ultrasound, CT, peritoneal lavage or hepatic arteriography. Treatment is resuscitation with blood, fresh frozen plasma and platelets, and urgent laparotomy. Hepatic haemorrhage without rupture has been managed conservatively.[72]

References

1 Hibbard BM, Anderson MM, Drife JO *et al.* (1994) *Report on Confidential Enquiries into Maternal Deaths in the United Kingdom 1988–1990.* London: HM Stationery Office.

2 Porapakkham S (1979) An epidemiologic study of eclampsia. *Obstet Gynecol* **54:**26–30.

3 Saftlas AF, Olson DR, Franks AL, Atrash HK and Pokras R (1990) Epidemiology of preeclampsia and eclampsia in the United States, 1979–1986. *Am J Obstet Gynecol* **163:**460–465.

4 Douglas KA and Redman CWG (1994) Eclampsia in the United Kingdom. *Br Med J* **309:**1395–1400.

5 Kilpatrick DC, Liston WA, Gibson F and Livingstone J (1989) Association between susceptibility to pre-eclampsia within families and HLA DR4. *Lancet* **2:**1063–1065.

6 Klonoff-Cohen HS, Savitz DA, Cefalo RC and McCann MF (1989) An epidemiologic study of contraception and preclampsia. *JAMA* **262:**3143–3147.

7 Roberts JM, Taylor RN, Musci TJ, Rodgers GM, Hubel CA and McLaughlin MK (1989) Preeclampsia: an endothelial cell disorder. *Am J Obstet Gynecol* **161:**1200–1204.

8 Spargo B, McCartney CP and Winemiller R (1959)

Glomerular capillary endotheliosis in toxemia of pregnancy. *Arch Pathol* **68**:593–599.

9 De Groot CJM and Taylor RN (1993) New insights into the etiology of pre-eclampsia. *Ann Med* **25**:243–249.

into the etiology of pre–eclampsia. *Ann Med* **25**:243–249.

10 Walsh SW (1985) Preeclampsia: an imbalance in placental prostacyclin and thromboxane production. *Am J Obstet Gynecol* **152**:335–340.

11 CLASP (Collaborative Low-dose Aspirin Study in Pregnancy) Collabortative Group (1993) CLASP: a randomised trial of low-dose aspirin for the prevention and treatment of preeclampsia among 9364 pregnant women. *Lancet* **343**:619–629.

12 Wang Y, Walsh SW, Guo J and Zhang J (1991) The imbalance between thromboxane and prostacyclin in preeclampsia is associated with an imbalance between lipid peroxides and vitamin E in maternal blood. *Am J Obstet Gynecol* **165**:1695–1700.

13 Pinto A, Sorrentino R, Sorrentino P *et al.* (1991) Endothelial-derived relaxing factor released by endothelial cells of human umbilical vessels and its impairment in pregnancy-induced hypertension. *Am J Obstet Gynecol* **164**:507–513.

14 Rappaport VJ, Hirata G, Yap HK and Jordan SC (1990) Anti-vascular endothelial cell antibodies in severe preeclampsia. *Am J Obstet Gynecol* **162**:138–146.

15 Sibai BM, McCubbin JH, Anderson GD, Lipshitz J and Dilts PV Jr (1981) Eclampsia. I. Observations from 67 recent cases. *Obstet Gynecol* **58**:609–6013.

16 Cotton DB, Lee W, Huhta JC and Dorman KF (1988) Hemodynamic profile of severe pregnancy-induced hypertension. *Am J Obstet Gynecol* **158**:523–529.

17 Easterling TR (1992) The maternal hemodynamics of preeclampsia. *Clin Obstet Gynecol* **35**:375–386.

18 Naidoo DP, Bhorat I, Moodley J, Naidoo JK and Mitha AS (1991) Continuous electrocardiographic monitoring in hypertensive crises in pregnancy. *Am J Obstet Gynecol* **164**:530–533.

19 Benedetti TJ, Kates R and Williams V (1985) Hemodynamic observations in severe preeclampsia complicated by pulmonary edema. *Am J Obstet Gynecol* **152**:330–334.

20 Dildy GA III and Cotton DB (1991) Management of severe preeclampsia and eclampsia. *Crit Care Clin* **7**:829–850.

21 Burrows RF, Hunter DJS, Andrew M and Kelton JG (1987) A prospective study investigating the mechanism of thrombocytopenia in preeclampsia. *Obstet Gynecol* **70**:334–338.

22 Cheek TG and Samuels P (1991) Pregnancy-induced hypertension. In; Data S (ed.) *Anesthetic and Obstetric Management of High-Risk Pregnancy.* St Louis: Mosby–Year Book, pp. 423–456.

23 Weinstein L (1982) Syndrome of hemolysis, elevated liver enzymes, and low platelet count: a severe consequence of hypertension in pregnancy. *Am J Obstet Gynecol* **142**:159–167.

24 Sibai BM (1990) The HELLP syndrome (hemolysis, elevated liver enzymes, and low platelets):Much ado about nothing? *Am J Obstet Gynecol* **162**:311–316.

25 Odendaal HJ, Pattinson RC, Bam R, Grove D and Kotze TJvW (1990) Aggressive or expectant management for patients with severe preeclampsia between 28–34 weeks' gestation: a randomized controlled trial. *Obstet Gynecol* **76**:1070–1075.

26 Sibai BM, Taslimi M, Abdella TN, Brooks TF, Spinnato JA and Anderson GD (1985) Maternal and perinatal outcome of conservative management of severe preeclampsia in midtrimester. *Am J Obstet Gynecol* **152**:32–37.

27 Sibai BM, Mabie BC, Harvey CJ and Gonzalez AR (1987) Pulmonary edema in severe preeclampsia-eclampsia: analysis of thirty seven consecutive cases. *Am J Obstet Gynecol* **1156**:1174–1179.

28 Australasian Society for the Study of Hypertension in Pregnancy (1993) Management of hypertension in pregnancy: executive summary. *Med J Aust* **158**:700–702.

29 Ring G, Krames E, Shnider SM, Wallis KL and Levinson G (1977) Comparison of nitroprusside and hydralazine in hypertensive pregnant ewes. *Obstet Gynecol* **50**:598–602.

30 Silver HM (1989) Acute hypertensive crisis in pregnancy. *Med Clin North Am* **73**:623–638.

31 Vink GJ and Moodley J (1982) The effect of low–dose dihydrallazine on the fetus in the emergency treatment of hypertension in pregnancy. *S Afr Med J* **62**:475–477.

32 Probst BD (1994) Hypertensive disorders of pregnancy. *Emerg Med Clin North Am* **12**:73–89.

33 Jouppila P, Kirkinen P, Koivula A and Ylikorkala O (1986) Labetalol does not alter the placental and fetal blood flow or maternal prostanoids in pre-eclampsia. *Br J Obstet Gynaecol* **93**:543–547.

34 Mabie WC, Gonzalez AR, Sibai BM and Amon E (1987) A comparative trial of labetalol and hydralazine in the acute management of severe hypertension complicating pregnancy. *Obstet Gynecol* **70**:328–333.

35 Moretti MM, Fairlie FM, Akl S, Khoury AD and Sibai BM (1990) The effect of nifedipine therapy on fetal and placental Doppler waveforms in preeclampsia remote from term. *Am J Obstet Gynecol* **163**:1844–1848.

36 Strauss RG, Keefer JR, Burke T and Civetta JM (1980) Hemodynamic monitoring of cardiogenic pulmonary edema complicating toxemia of pregnancy. *Obstet Gynecol* **55**:170–174.

37 Dudley DKL (1985) Minibolus diazoxide in the management of severe hypertension in pregnancy. *Am J Obstet Gynecol* **151**:196–200.

38 Poulton TJ, James FM III and Lockridge O (1979) Prolonged apnea following trimethaphan and succinylcholine. *Anesthesiology* **50**:54–56.

39 Hulme VA and Odendaal HJ (1986) Intrapartum treatment of preeclamptic hypertension by ketanserin. *Am J Obstet Gynecol* **155**:260–263.

40 Ferris TF and Weir EK (1983) Effect of captopril

on uterine blood flow and prostaglandin E synthesis in the pregnant rabbit. *J Clin Invest* **71**:809–815.

41 Pritchard JA, Cunningham FG and Pritchard SA (1984) The Parkland Memorial Hospital protocol for treatment of eclampsia: evaluation of 245 cases. *Am J Obstet Gynecol* **148**:951–963.

42 Sibai BM (1990) Magnesium sulfate is the ideal anticonvulsant in preeclampsia–eclampsia. *Am J Obstet Gynecol* **162**:1141–1145.

43 Fisher RS, Kaplan PW, Krumholz A, Lesser RP, Rosen SA and Wolff MR (1968) Failure of high-dose intravenous magnesium sulfate to control myoclonic status epilepticus. *Clin Neuropharmacol* **11**:537–544.

44 Krauss GL, Kaplan P and Fisher RS (1988) Parenteral magnesium sulfate fails to control electroshock and pentylenetetrazol seizures in mice. *Epilepsy Res* **4**:201–206.

45 Lucas MJ, Leveno KJ and Cunningham FG (1995) A comparison of magnesium sulfate with phenytoin for the prevention of eclampsia. *N Engl J Med* **333**:201–205.

46 Kaplan PW, Lesser RP, Fisher RS, Repke JT and Hanley DF (1990) A continuing controversy: magnesium sulfate in the treatment of eclamptic seizures. *Arch Neurol* **47**:1031–1032.

47 Sadeh M (1989) Action of magnesium sulfate in the treatment of preeclampsia–eclampsia. *Stroke* **20**:1273–1275.

48 Watson KV, Moldow CF, Ogburn PL and Jacob HS (1986) Magnesium sulfate: rationale for its use in preeclampsia. *Proc Natl Acad Sci* **83**:1075–1078.

49 Belfort MA and Moise KJ Jr (1992) Effect of magnesium sulfate on maternal brain blood flow in preeclampsia: a randomized, placebo-controlled study. *Am J Obstet Gynecol* **167**:661–666.

50 James MFM, Beer RE and Esser JD (1989) Intravenous magnesium sulfate inhibits catecholamine release associated with tracheal intubation. *Anesth Analg* **68**:772–776.

51 Repke JT, Friedman SA and Kaplan PW (1992) Prophylaxis of eclamptic seizures: current controversies. *Clin Obstet Gynecol* **35**:365–374.

52 Slater RM, Wilcox FL, Smith WD *et al.* (1987) Phenytoin infusion in severe pre-clampsia. *Lancet* **1**:1417–1421.

53 Ryan G, Lange IR and Naugler MA (1989) Clinical experience with phenytoin prophylaxis in severe preeclampsia. *Am J Obstet Gynecol* **161**:1297–1304.

54 Appleton MP, Kuehl TJ, Raebel MA, Adams HR, Knight AB and Gold WR (1991) Magnesium sulfate versus phenytoin for seizure prophylaxis in pregnancy-induced hypertension. *Am J Obstet Gynecol* **165**:907–913.

55 Rowlatt RJ (1978) Effect of maternal diazepam on the newborn. *Br Med J* **i**:985.

56 The Eclampsia Trial Collaborative Group (1995) Which anticonvulsant for women with eclampsia? Evidence from the Collaborative Eclampsia Trial. *Lancet* **345**:1455–1463.

57 Dunn R, Lee W and Cotton DB (1986) Evaluation by computerized axial tomography of eclamptic women with seizures refractory to magnesium sulfate therapy. *Am J Obstet Gynecol* **155**:267–268.

58 Richards AM, Moodley J, Graham DI and Bullock MRR (1986) Active management of the unconscious eclamptic patient. *Br J Obstet Gynaecol* **93**:554–562.

59 Gallery EDM, Delprado W and Gyory AZ (1981) Antihypertensive effect of plasma volume expansion in pregnancy-induced hypertension. *Aust NZ J Med* **11**:20–24.

60 Sehgal NN and Hitt JR (1980) Plasma volume expansion in the treatment of pre-eclampsia. *Am J Obstet Gynecol* **138**:165–168.

61 Benedetti TJ and Quilligan EJ (1980) Cerebral edema in severe pregnancy-induced hypertension. *Am J Obstet Gynecol* **137**:860–862.

62 Clark SL and Cotton DB (1988) Clinical indications for pulmonary artery catheterization in the patient with severe preeclampsia. *Am J Obstet Gynecol* **158**:453–458.

63 Moore TR, Key TC, Reisner LS and Resnik R (1985) Evaluation of the use of continuous lumbar epidural anesthesia for hypertensive pregnant women in labor. *Am J Obstet Gynecol* **152**:404–412.

64 Jouppila P, Jouppila R, Hollmn A and Koivula A (1982) Lumbar epidural analgesia to improve intervillous blood flow during labor in severe preeclampsia. *Obstet Gynecol* **59**:158–161.

65 Abboud T, Artal R, Sarkis F, Henriksen EH and Kammula RK (1982) Sympathoadrenal activity, maternal, fetal, and neonatal responses after epidural anesthesia in the preeclamptic patient. *Am J Obstet Gynecol* **144**:915–918.

66 Merrell DA and Koch MAT (1980) Epidural anaesthesia as an anticonvulsant in the management of hypertensive and eclamptic patients in labour. *S Afr Med J* **58**:875–877.

67 Heller PJ, Scheider EP and Marx GF (1983) Pharyngolaryngeal edema as a presenting symptom in preeclampsia. *Obstet Gynecol* **62**:523–524.

68 Ramanathan J, Sibai BM, Mabie WC, Chauhan D and Ruiz AG (1988) The use of labetalol for attenuation of the hypertensive response to endotracheal intubation in preeclampsia. *Am J Obstet Gynecol* **159**:650–654.

69 Rout CC and Rocke DA (1990) Effects of alfentanil and fentanyl on induction of anaesthesia in patients with severe pregnancy-induced hypertension. *Br J Anaesth* **65**:468–474.

70 Allen RW, James MFM and Uys PC (1991) Attenuation of the pressor response to tracheal intubation in hypertensive proteinuric pregnant patients by lignocaine, alfentanil and magnesium sulphate. *Br J Anaesth* **66**:216–223.

71 Ashton WB, James MFM, Janicki P and Uys PC (1991) Attenuation of the pressor response to tracheal intubation by magnesium sulphate with and without alfentanil in hypertensive proteinuric patients undergoing Caesarean section. *Br J Anaesth* **67**:741–747.

72 Manas KJ, Welsh JD, Rankin RA and Miller DD (1985) Hepatic hemorrhage without rupture in pre-eclampsia. *N Engl J Med* **312**:424–426.

56 | Obstetric emergencies

T Gin and WD Ngan Kee

The ICU will encounter obstetric patients who present with the usual range of medical and surgical emergencies, and also provide supportive care for patients who suffer specific obstetric complications. Important points to recognize in treating emergencies in obstetric patients are:

1 Physiological changes in pregnancy may modify the presentation of the problem, the normal physiological variables used to guide treatment, and also the response to treatment; and
2 Both mother and fetus are affected by the pathology and subsequent treatment.

During pregnancy, the normal ranges for physiological variables change[1] so that therapy is guided by different end-points (Table 56.1). Specific maternal problems include aortocaval compression and difficult tracheal intubation. After 20 weeks' gestation, aortocaval compression by the gravid uterus can decrease uterine perfusion and venous return to the heart. This is best prevented by using the full left lateral position but a 15° left lateral tilt or manual displacement of the uterus may be more practicable. Oedematous tissues, delayed gastric emptying and increased oxygen consumption complicate tracheal intubation. Precautions should be taken against acid aspiration and supplemental oxygen is essential. The majority of physiological changes revert to normal several days after delivery. Perineal and breast nursing care should not be neglected.

The mother's welfare usually takes precedence over fetal concerns, especially as fetal survival is dependent on optimal maternal management. Nevertheless, it is important to monitor the fetus because of the problems associated with premature labour, placental transfer of drugs, and maintenance of placental perfusion and oxygenation. The uterine vascular bed is considered maximally dilated but still responsive to stimuli that cause vasoconstriction, such as circulating catecholamines.[2] An obstetric opinion should be sought regarding cardiotocography, ultrasound ex-

Table 56.1 Changes in physiological variables during late pregnancy

Systolic arterial pressure	-5 mmHg (-0.7 kPa)
Mean arterial pressure	-15 mmHg (-2.0 kPa)
Diastolic arterial pressure	-15 mmHg (-2.0 kPa)
Central venous pressure	No change
Pulmonary capillary wedge pressure	No change
Heart rate	$+15\%$
Stroke volume	$+30\%$
Cardiac output	$+45\%$
Systemic vascular resistance	-15%
Tidal volume	$+40\%$
Respiratory rate	$+10\%$
Minute volume	$+50\%$
Oxygen consumption	$+20\%$
pH	No change
Pa_{O_2}	$+10$ mmHg ($+1.3$ kPa)
Pa_{CO_2}	-10 mmHg (-1.3 kPa)
HCO_3^-	-4 mmol/l
Total blood volume	$+40\%$
Haematocrit	-0.06
Plasma albumin	-5 g/l
Oncotic pressure	-3 mmHg (-0.4 kPa)

amination and timing of delivery, especially during a prolonged stay in the ICU. The question of fetal viability also creates ethical dilemmas.

Trauma

Trauma is the leading non-obstetric cause of maternal mortality.[3,4] Head injuries and haemorrhagic shock account for most maternal deaths, while placental abruption and maternal death are the most frequent causes of fetal death.

Initial resuscitation should follow the normal plan of attention to airway, breathing and circulation.[5,6] Oxygen 100% should be given and cricoid pressure applied during tracheal intubation. Blood volume is increased during pregnancy and hypotension may not be evident until 35% or more of total blood volume is lost. Uterine blood flow is not autoregulated and may be decreased despite normal maternal haemodynamics, so that slight overhydration is preferred to underhydration. Femoral and lower limb venous catheters may not be appropriate because of pelvic injury. Treatment of hypotension includes positioning or manual uterine displacement to avoid aortocaval compression. Drug treatment of modest hypotension is often started with ephedrine, because it preserves uterine blood flow, but there should be no hesitation in using other vasopressors when necessary.

Necessary radiological investigations should be performed as indicated because radiation hazard to the fetus is very unlikely. Assessment of trauma should note the increased significance of pelvic fractures for uterine injury and retroperitoneal haemorrhage. Diagnostic peritoneal lavage should be performed through a surgical incision above the fundus. Chest drains are placed slightly higher than normal, in the third or fourth intercostal space. It is important to exclude herniation of abdominal contents through a ruptured diaphragm.

Fetal monitoring includes external cardiotocography, ultrasound and the Kleihauer–Betke test for fetal maternal haemorrhage.[7,8] Rh immune globulin 300 μg within 72 h of injury should be considered for all Rh D-negative women. Premature labour and placental abruption may not be diagnosed unless regular monitoring is continued for at least 4 h.

Cardiopulmonary resuscitation[9]

Defibrillation and cardioversion are performed with the usual technique. Normally, external cardiac massage produces only 30% of cardiac output and this is reduced further if there is vena caval compression. Left lateral tilt decreases the efficiency of closed chest compression,[10] and manual lateral displacement of the uterus may be preferable. However, many reports indicate that both maternal and fetal survival from cardiac arrest depend on prompt caesarean delivery. Certainly, in the third trimester, fetal survival is very likely and caesarean section will relieve the effects of aortocaval compression.

The decision to perform perimortem caesarean section must be made quickly, because the operation should be started within 4 min of cardiac arrest and delivery of the infant achieved by 5 min.[11] This timing is supported by reported case series and the fact that both maternal and fetal cerebral oxygen reserves are depleted in several minutes if there is no cardiac output.

Severe obstetric haemorrhage

Peripartum haemorrhage contributed to 15% of maternal deaths in the UK from 1988 to 1990 and

prompted publication of revised guidelines for the management of major haemorrhage.[12] The most common causes of peripartum haemorrhage are placenta praevia, placental abruption, placenta accreta, cervical or vaginal lacerations and uterine atony. Including ectopic pregnancy, 25% of maternal deaths were a result of haemorrhage. Unfortunately, many deaths reflected a failure of management because blood loss was often underestimated and volume replacement delayed. The treatment of massive haemorrhage requires sufficient IV access and the logistic capability quickly to replace circulating volume with warmed fluids, blood and clotting factors. More specific measures include aortal compression and the treatment of uterine atony with uterine massage and oxytocics given IV, IM or intramyometrially. The aorta can be compressed against the vertebral column by a fist pressed on the abdomen above the umbilicus. Control of haemorrhage allows time for resuscitation and more definitive treatment. Oxytocin (10 units) and ergonovine (0.2 mg) are less effective than prostaglandins, especially 15-methyl-prostaglandin $F_{2\alpha}$ (250 μg).[13]

If bleeding persists, specific invasive procedures to be considered are:

1 *angiographic arterial embolization.*[14] This requires a pre-existing radiological service and facility for continued resuscitation in the radiology suite. Logistic problems are thus responsible for the infrequent use of this technique, although prophylactic placement of catheters has been recommended;[15]
2 *surgical ligation* of the uterine, ovarian or internal iliac arteries;[16]
3 *hysterectomy.*

Septic shock[17]

Septic shock may occur following chorioamnionitis, postpartum endometritis, urinary tract infections, pyelonephritis and septic abortion. Gram-negative coliforms are the frequent causative organisms but streptococci and *Bacteroides* may also be present. The physiological changes of pregnancy may influence the course and presentation of septic shock. Animal studies suggest that pregnancy increases the susceptibility to endotoxin and that metabolic acidosis and cardiovascular collapse occur earlier. Management of septic shock follows normal guidelines (see Chapter 61), although the normal range for haemodynamic variables may be different. Mortality is low because these patients are young and in good health.

Venous thrombosis

Pulmonary thromboembolism is a common cause of maternal death, accounting for 15–25% of maternal mortality. Pregnancy is associated with a sixfold increase in thromboembolism because of venous stasis, a hypercoagulable state and vascular injury associated with delivery.

Symptoms of dyspnoea or pain in the leg or chest require accurate diagnosis, especially in the immediate postpartum period. Compression ultrasonography is non-invasive, but venography after the first trimester and ventilation–perfusion isotope lung scans should not be avoided if indicated. Pregnant patients with suspected or proven deep vein thrombosis or pulmonary embolus should be given full anticoagulant and thrombolytic therapy is indicated (see Chapter 30). Warfarin should not be used before delivery. Heparin is continued until labour begins, and restarted in the postpartum patient when bleeding has stopped.

Amniotic fluid embolism

Incidence

Amniotic fluid embolism (AFE) is the cause of 5–10% of maternal deaths. The incidence of AFE varies between 1 in 20 000 and 1 in 80 000 deliveries, although there must be undetected and unsuspected cases where minimal amounts of amniotic fluid produce few symptoms. Between 25 and 50% of patients with suspected or proven AFE die within the first hour and the overall maternal mortality may be as high as 86%,[18] with a perinatal and neonatal mortality of 40%.

Pathophysiology

The exact pathogenic factors for the syndrome of AFE remain an enigma.[19] Amniotic fluid is thought to enter the maternal circulation through endocervical or uterine lacerations, or uterine veins at the site of placental separation. Placental abruption may be a significant factor in the development of AFE. Amniotic fluid normally contains prostaglandins, leukotrienes and fetal debris which can cause complement activation, pulmonary vasoconstriction and physical blockage of pulmonary capillaries with resultant damage and release of further mediators. However, experimental clear amniotic fluid infusion in primates is relatively benign.[20] The degree of complement activation by amniotic fluid varies considerably among patients, and the development of AFE syndrome may be a result of abnormal amniotic fluid.[21] Leukotrienes contribute to the pathogenesis and 5-lipoxygenase inhibitors can prevent acute death.[22] Coagulopathy may develop and is probably related to tissue factor[23] or trophoblasts in the amniotic fluid.

Clinical presentation

AFE was thought to be associated with vigorous labour and the use of oxytocics, but it may occur in any parturient. The initial diagnosis of AFE is made on clinical grounds and is often one of exclusion. Classically, patients may present with severe dyspnoea, cyanosis, sudden cardiovascular collapse, coma or convulsions during labour, but AFE may occur earlier during pregnancy, during delivery or in the early puerperium. Differential diagnoses include thromboembolism, air embolism, aspiration pneumonitis, eclamptic convulsions and coma, local anaesthetic toxicity, placental abruption, haemorrhagic shock, anaphylaxis, intracranial haemorrhage and acute heart failure.

Animal studies indicate that AFE causes a biphasic response. The early phase probably lasts less than 30 min, and is characterized by severe hypoxia and right heart failure as a result of pulmonary hypertension from vasoconstriction or vessel damage. Half of the patients may die within the first hour. Patients who survive this first phase develop left ventricular failure with return of normal right ventricular function. Left ventricular failure may be a result of the initial hypoxia or the depressant effects of mediators. Hypoxia persists because of the acute lung injury and pulmonary oedema. Uterine atony may occur and a coagulopathy develops in 40% of patients.

Traditionally, AFE was confirmed by detection of fetal squamous cells and debris in the pulmonary circulation either at autopsy or in blood samples from a pulmonary artery catheter.[24] However, fetal squames have been detected in women without AFE and a recently described monoclonal antibody test should be more specific.[25]

Management

No specific therapy is available. Immediate cardiopulmonary resuscitation and 100% oxygen are necessary. Oxygen therapy often requires endotracheal intubation and positive-pressure ventilation. Assessment of CVP may be misleading, and early pulmonary artery catheterization has been advocated in a series reporting 100% survival[26] in 5 patients by treating left ventricular failure aggressively. The differential diagnoses must be evaluated quickly because urgent delivery of the fetus by caesarean section may improve resuscitation and prevent further AFE. Patients who survive the first few hours will continue to require supportive treatment for their acute lung injury.

Hydrocortisone 1 g 6-hourly for 48 h has been strongly recommended,[27] but its efficacy has not been proved. Clotting factors are given as necessary to manage the coagulopathy, although the use of fibrinogen and heparin remains controversial.

Outcome

AFE is rare but carries a high mortality. Survivors regain normal cardiorespiratory function but may have neurological sequelae.[28,29] There are two case reports of subsequent pregnancies, both with uncomplicated deliveries.[30]

Acid aspiration (Mendelson's) syndrome

Obstetric patients are at increased risk of acid aspiration because of decreased gastric emptying, increased gastric acidity and volume and increased intra-abdominal pressure. Tracheal intubation is a particularly hazardous event because anatomical changes can make intubation difficult. Despite the notoriety of acid aspiration in obstetric patients, it is not known if pregnant patients' lungs are more susceptible to injury. Aspiration of acidic material will cause acute lung injury, the severity being related to the amount, content and acidity of the aspirate. The initial presentation is hypoxaemia and bronchospasm and the chest X-ray may appear normal. Chemical pneumonitis and increased permeability pulmonary oedema develop over several hours. Treatment includes standard respiratory support (see Chapter 34). Rigid bronchoscopy may be required to remove large food particles. Bronchoalveolar lavage and steroids are not useful and antibiotics should only be given for proven infection.

Tocolytic therapy and pulmonary oedema[31]

Pulmonary oedema is an uncommon but serious complication of tocolytic therapy with β-adrenergic agonists. The underlying mechanism for pulmonary oedema is probably fluid overload and increased hydrostatic pressure, rather than increased pulmonary capillary permeability or left ventricular dysfunction. The initial management of pulmonary oedema is discontinuation of the β-adrenergic agonist and oxygen therapy, with further monitoring, diuretics and respiratory support as necessary.

Cocaine toxicity

Cocaine abuse during pregnancy has become a significant problem in the USA, where maternal cocaine use may be as high as 30% in some populations.[32,33] Cocaine causes maternal hypertension, tachycardia and increased cardiac output, but decreases uterine blood flow.[34] There is increased risk of placental bleeding, and acute toxicity may mimic pre-eclampsia by presenting with cerebral haemorrhage or convulsions. The drug of choice for the treatment of hypertension is controversial. Although hydralazine is often used to treat maternal hypertension, it is not the drug of choice for cocaine-induced hypertension[35] and labetalol is preferred.

Other severe acute disorders

Cardiac disease in pregnancy is discussed in Chapter 57 and other acute severe conditions which may be encountered in the obstetric patient such as acute fatty liver, asthma, and haemolytic–uraemic syndrome are discussed in their respective chapters.

References

1 Hytten F and Chamberlain G (1991) *Clinical Physiology in Obstetrics*, 2nd edn. Oxford: Blackwell.

2 Greiss FC Jr (1967) A clinical concept of uterine blood flow during pregnancy. *Obstet Gynecol* 30:595–604.

3 Esposito TJ (1994) Trauma during pregnancy. *Emerg Med Clin North Am* 12:167–199.

4 Kuhlmann RS and Cruikshank DP (1994) Maternal trauma during pregnancy. *Clin Obstet Gynecol* 37: 274–293.

5 Neufeld JDG (1993) Trauma in pregnancy, what if...? *Emerg Med Clin North Am* 11:207–224.

6 ACOG Technical Bulletin Number 161 (1993) Trauma during pregnancy. *Int J Gynecol Obstet* 40:165–170.

7 Pearlman MD and Tintinalli JE (1991) Evaluation and treatment of the gravida and fetus following trauma during pregnancy. *Obstet Gynecol Clin North Am* 18:371–381.

8 Towery R, English TP and Wisner D (1993) Evaluation of pregnant women after blunt injury. *J Trauma* 35:731–736.

9 Lee RV, Rodgers BD, White LM and Harvey RC (1986) Cardiopulmonary resuscitation of pregnant women. *Am J Med* 81:311–318.

10 Rees GAD and Willis BA (1988) Resuscitation in late pregnancy. *Anaesthesia* 43:347–349.

11 Katz VL, Dotters DJ and Droegemueller W (1986) Perimortem cesarean delivery. *Obstet Gynecol* 68: 571–576.

12 Hibbard BM, Anderson MM, Drife JO *et al.* (1988) *Report on Confidential Enquiries into Maternal Deaths in the United Kingdom 1988–1990*. London: Her Majesty's Stationery Office.

13 Hayashi RH (1990) The role of prostaglandins in the treatment of postpartum haemorrhage. *J Obstet Gynaecol* 10 (suppl 2), S21–S24.

14 Yamashita Y, Harada M, Yamamoto H *et al.* (1994) Transcatheter arterial embolization of obstetric and gynaecological bleeding: efficacy and clinical outcome. *Br J Radiol* 67:530–534.

15 Mitty HA, Sterling KM, Alvarez M and Gendler R (1993) Obstetric hemorrhage: prophylactic and emergency arterial catheterization and embolotherapy. *Radiology* 188:183–187.

16 Likeman RK (1992) The boldest procedure possible for checking the bleeding. *Aust NZ J Obstet Gynaecol* 32:256–262.

17 Gonik B (1986) Septic shock in obstetrics. *Clin Perinatol* 13:741–754.

18 Morgan M (1979) Amniotic fluid embolism. *Anaesthesia* **34**:20–32.

19 Clark SL (1990) New concepts of amniotic fluid embolism: a review. *Obstet Gynecol Surv* **45**:360–368.

20 Adamsons K, Mueller-Heubach E and Myers RE (1971) The innocousness of amniotic fluid infusion in the pregnant rhesus monkey. *Am J Obstet Gynecol* **109**:977–984.

21 Hammerschmidt DE, Ogburn PL and Williams JE (1984) Amniotic fluid activates complement: a role in amniotic fluid embolism syndrome? *J Lab Clin Med* **104**:901–907.

22 Azegami M and Mori N (1986) Amniotic fluid embolism and leukotrienes. *Am J Obstet Gynecol* **155**:1119–1124.

23 Lockwood CJ, Bach R, Guha A, Zhou XZ, Miller WA and Nemerson Y (1991) Amniotic fluid contains tissue factor, a potent initiator of coagulation. *Am J Obstet Gynecol* **165**:1335–1341.

24 Masson RG (1992) Amniotic fluid embolism. *Clin Chest Med* **13**:657–665.

25 Kobayashi H, Ohi H and Terao T (1993) A simple noninvasive, sensitive method for diagnosis of amniotic fluid embolism by monoclonal antibody TKH-2 that recognises NeuAcα2-6GalNAc. *Am J Obstet Gynecol* **168**:848–853.

26 Clark SL, Cotton DB, Gonik B *et al.* (1988) Central hemodynamic alterations in amniotic fluid embolism. *Am J Obstet Gynecol* **158**:1124–1126.

27 Kotelko DM (1993) Amniotic fluid embolism. In: Shnider SM and Levinson G (eds) *Anesthesia for Obstetrics*, 3rd edn. Baltimore: Williams & Wilkins, pp. 377–384.

28 Alon E and Atanassoff PG (1992) Successful cardio-pulmonary resuscitation of a parturient with amniotic fluid embolism. *Int J Obstet Anaesth* **1**:205–207.

29 Noble WH and St-Amand J (1993) Amniotic fluid embolus. *Can J Anaesth* **40**:971–980.

30 Clark SL (1992) Successful pregnancy outcomes after amniotic fluid embolism. *Am J Obstet Gynecol* **167**:512–513.

31 Pisani RJ and Rosenow EC III (1989) Pulmonary edema associated with tocolytic therapy. *Ann Intern Med* **110**:714–718.

32 Newman LM (1992) The chemically dependent parturient. *Semin Anesth* **11**:66–75.

33 Slutsker L (1992) Risks associated with cocaine use during pregnancy. *Obstet Gynecol* **79**:778–779.

34 Plessinger MA and Woods JR Jr (1991) The cardio-vascular effects of cocaine use in pregnancy. *Reprod Toxicol* **5**:99–113.

35 Vertommen JD, Hughes SC, Rosen MA *et al.* (1992) Hydralazine does not restore uterine blood flow during cocaine-induced hypertension in the pregnant ewe. *Anesthesiology* **76**:580–587.

57 | Severe cardiac disease in pregnancy

G Yau and TE Oh

The incidence of severe heart disease in pregnancy is rare (0.5–2.0%).[1-3] However, congenital heart disease in pregnancy is increasing, as improved care has resulted in more patients surviving to reproductive age.[4] This contrasts with the decline of rheumatic fever and rheumatic heart disease in pregnancy.[5,6] Pregnancy significantly worsens heart disease. ICU management is necessary to minimize or treat cardiac decompensation and complications.

Mortality and counselling[7,8]

Despite a low incidence, cardiac disease can account for up to 30% maternal mortality in pregnancy.[7] Mortality varies from under 1% in uncomplicated mitral stenosis to 40% in Eisenmenger's syndrome with pulmonary hypertension. The New York Heart Association (NYHA) grade of cardiac diseases is not a useful prognostic guide. Up to 40% of patients who developed heart failure during pregnancy started as class 1 or 2 (i.e. uncompromised or only slightly compromised cardiac status).[9] Young women with severe heart disease should be counselled on the risks that pregnancy presents to themselves and their intended or unborn babies.

Physiology[10]

Pregnancy causes profound haemodynamic changes which can be hazardous for those with cardiac disease. An understanding of these changes and their interaction with the underlying cardiac condition is important for successful management.

Blood volume

Increase in blood volume begins in the 12th week, and may reach 50% above non-pregnant levels at term. This volume increase is poorly tolerated by those with valvular lesions or myocardial dysfunction.

Cardiac output

Stroke volume and cardiac output progressively increase in the first and second trimesters, and remain increased through the third trimester. Further fluctuations occur during labour, delivery and immediately afterwards (see below) which may precipitate heart failure.

Systemic vascular resistance

Systemic vascular resistance (SVR) is decreased due to hormonal effects. This may worsen shunt flow in right-to-left shunts.

Heart rate

Heart rate also tends to increase progressively by up to 20%. Further increase during labour and delivery is poorly tolerated by those with mitral stenosis, ischaemic heart disease or obstructive cardiomyopathy.

Cardiovascular changes during labour

First stage

At the onset of labour, pain and anxiety increase circulating catecholamines, which cause further rises in stroke volume and cardiac output (up to 45% above pre-pregnancy levels). Also, uterine contractions effectively cause an autotransfusion, which may increase cardiac output by 25%. This normally tolerated stress can precipitate heart failure in pre-existing cardiac disease.

Second stage

Bearing down in the second stage of labour is a modified Valsalva manoeuvre, with high intra-abdominal and intra-thoracic pressures that decrease venous return and cardiac output.

Third stage

After delivery, autotransfusion of 500 ml blood from uterine contraction and relief of aortocaval obstruction increase blood volume, which may precipitate heart failure. Stroke volume and cardiac output gradually return to pre-pregnant levels by the second postpartum week.

Pathophysiology[11,12]

Acquired heart disease

Although rheumatic fever has declined, most acquired cardiac lesions are still rheumatic in origin. The dominant valve lesion is mitral stenosis (90%), followed by mitral regurgitation (6.6%), aortic regurgitation (2.5%) and aortic stenosis (1%). Right-sided lesions secondary to infective endocarditis from intravenous drug abuse are seen occasionally.

Mitral stenosis

Decreased mitral valve area causes a ventricular diastolic filling obstruction, which leads to a relatively fixed cardiac output state. Increase in pulmonary capillary wedge pressure (PCWP) follows the rise in left atrial (LA) pressure, which eventually results in pulmonary artery (PA) hypertension. Any tachy-dysrhythmia may exacerbate this process.

Mitral regurgitation

The left atrium dilates to accommodate regurgitant blood through the incompetent mitral valve. LA pressure, however, does not rise until late in the disease. Increased preload from the hypervolaemic left atrium leads to left ventricular (LV) dilatation. Ejection fraction may be only 50–60% normal. Decreased SVR and increasing heart rate may help to increase the ejection fraction. This condition is usually well-tolerated in pregnancy, although decompensation due to LV failure may occur.

Aortic valve lesions

Aortic regurgitation due to rheumatic fever is often associated with mitral valve disease. Due to valvular incompetence, part of the LV output returns to the ventricle during diastole, and LV dilatation results. However, reduced SVR may help to increase ejection fraction. Hence, this condition is generally well-tolerated in pregnancy. *Aortic stenosis* is uncommon. Obstruction to LV outflow leads to hypertrophy and myocardial ischaemia. Cardiac output eventually becomes relatively fixed. Thus any preload reduction (e.g. from blood loss) will have severe consequences.

Congenital heart disease[13]

Left-to-right shunt

Atrial septal defect (ASD)

This is the most common congenital cardiac lesion in pregnancy. Most women with uncomplicated ostium secundum ASD tolerate pregnancy well, although there is a risk of right ventricular (RV) failure. The left-to-right shunt increases RV preload and pulmonary flow. There is a compensatory decrease in pulmonary vascular resistance (PVR), such that PA pressures are usually normal until the fourth or fifth decade. Increase in right and left atrial blood volume leads to distension and dysrhythmias, particularly atrial fibrillation.

Ventricular septal defect (VSD)

This may occur in isolation or in conjunction with other congenital cardiac lesions, e.g. Fallot's tetralogy. Small defects are usually well-tolerated, but with large defects, increased pulmonary flow leads to a rise in PA pressure, which eventually becomes fixed Increased LV work leads to LV dysfunction, and then increased pulmonary venous pressure and worsening pulmonary hypertension. Eventually, there is equalization of pressures and bidirectional or reversed flow (i.e. Eisenmenger's syndrome). Any increase in heart rate, cardiac output and intravascular volume may increase left-to-right flow, exacerbate pulmonary hypertension or induce failure of one or both ventricles.

Patent ductus arteriosus (PDA)

Surgical treatment of PDA in childhood makes it a rare problem in pregnancy. Most patients are asymptomatic and tolerate pregnancy well.

Right-to-left shunt

Tetralogy of Fallot

This is characterized by the cyanotic complex of RV hypertrophy, RV outflow obstruction, VSD and an overriding aorta. Obstruction to RV outflow leads to right-to-left shunting through the VSD. The degree of shunting and consequent cyanosis depend on the size of VSD. Stresses of pregnancy and labour increase PVR, and thus increase size of shunt. Decrease in SVR in pregnancy and postpartum may also increase the shunt. Most cases of corrected Fallot's tetralogy tolerate pregnancy well, but in those with uncorrected lesions, maternal mortality ranges from 5 to 15%. A poor prognosis is associated with maternal haematocrit exceeding 0.65, RV pressure exceeding 120 mmHg (20 kPa) and Sao_2 below 80%.

Eisenmenger's syndrome

As in Fallot's tetralogy, the severity of right-to-left shunting depends on pulmonary hypertension and the size of the right-to-left communication. The relationship between PVR and SVR is also important.

Increases in PVR or decreases in SVR, which occur in pregnancy, will increase right-to-left shunting. Pulmonary flow will decrease and lead to hypoxaemia. Any decrease in RV preload (as in blood loss) will further reduce pulmonary flow, worsen hypoxaemia, and may cause sudden death. Moreover, a high percentage of maternal deaths in Eisenmenger's syndrome, particularly in the immediate postpartum, is associated with thromboembolism. Estimated risks may be as high as 30–70%. Association with VSD appears to carry a higher mortality than with ASD or PDA.

Other congenital heart diseases

Coarctation of aorta
This presents an obstruction to LV output, similar to aortic stenosis. The most common coarctation site is the origin of the left subclavian artery. Associated anomalies include PDA, VSD and intracranial aneurysms in the circle of Willis. In addition, changes in the aortic wall may lead to dissection or aneurysmal dilatation. Prognosis is good in uncomplicated cases.

Congenital aortic stenosis
This may be supravalvular, valvular or subvalvular. The most common valvular abnormality is bicuspid aortic valve; 20–30% eventually develop aortic stenosis secondary to turbulent flow and fibrin deposition. Pathophysiology is similar to rheumatic aortic stenosis. Susceptibility to infective endocarditis is high.

Congenital pulmonary stenosis
This accounts for 13% of all congenital heart disease, and may be valvular or subvalvular (infundibular). Prognosis is determined by degree of obstruction rather than site. RV outflow obstruction leads to concentric RV hypertrophy. Decompensation occurs late. RV output decreases, leading to reduced LV preload and cardiac output. Sudden increases in RV preload during labour and immediately postpartum may precipitate RV failure.

Congenital mitral valve prolapse (MVP)
This is more common during pregnancy than rheumatic mitral regurgitation, and occurs in up to 17% of healthy young women. It is generally well-tolerated during pregnancy, although prophylaxis against infective endocarditis is advised.

Ebstein anomaly[14]
A malformed tricuspid valve is displaced into a poorly developed right ventricle, which copes inadequately with increases in blood volume during pregnancy and labour. Tricuspid regurgitation and dysrhythmias are frequently encountered, which will further compromise RV output. Other associated anomalies include ASD or PDA, which may cause right-to-left shunting and cyanosis.

Other heart diseases

Primary pulmonary hypertension
This is mainly a condition of young women and is associated with a maternal mortality over 50%. Fetal mortality exceeds 40% and therapeutic abortion is usually advised. Pulmonary hypertension (mean PA pressure over 25 mmHg or 3.3 kPa) leads to RV hypertrophy and failure.

Cardiomyopathy

Peripartum cardiomyopathy[15]
This is usually a diagnosis by exclusion. It presents in the last month of pregnancy, or the first 6 months postpartum in women without previous cardiac diseases. There is progressive dyspnoea, fatigue and peripheral and pulmonary oedema. Echocardiogram reveals gross LV dilatation with global hypokinesia. Some patients (50%) may develop pulmonary or systemic embolism. Recurrence in subsequent pregnancies is common, especially if heart size does not return to normal within 6–12 months. Aetiology is unknown, although viral, immunological and nutritional mechanisms are postulated.

Hypertrophic obstructive cardiomyopathy[16]
LV hypertrophy, especially involving the interventricular septum, reduces ventricular cavity. There is also myocardial fibrosis, resulting in a stiff and inelastic ventricle resistant to filling. During diastole, the septum bulges up and obstructs the outflow tract. LV failure eventually results. The increase in intravascular volume in pregnancy may help by causing ventricular dilatation to decrease obstruction. However, increases in heart rate and myocardial contractility during labour may worsen outflow obstruction. Despite the potential hazards, maternal and fetal outcome are generally good.

Myocardial infarction[17]
Coronary artery disease and myocardial infarction are rare in women of reproductive age. However, when it occurs, mortality may reach 35%. Most reported cases occurred during the third trimester. Delivery within 2 weeks of infarction is associated with high mortality.

Cardiac surgery and pregnancy[18]
Mortality of cardiac surgery during pregnancy relates to the procedure, and is no different to that in non-pregnant women. Fetal mortality was previously high, but with advances in fetal monitoring and placental perfusion, is now under 10%. Women with good recovery of cardiac function after cardiac surgery should cope well with pregnancy.

Prosthetic valves[19]
Choice of anticoagulation for pregnant patients with prosthetic heart valves remains controversial. The risk

of teratogenicity with warfarin is weighed against thromboembolism from heparin. The American recommendation is to use subcutaneous heparin from conception to delivery.[20] Heparin is injected 8–12 hourly to achieve an activated partial thromboplastin time of 1.5–2.0 times control, 6 h after injection.[20] Patients with bioprosthetic valves or xenograft valves do not require anticoagulation unless they are in atrial fibrillation.

Prenatal management

The obstetrician, cardiologist, anaesthetist, intensivist and paediatrician should be informed well before the anticipated delivery date. Labour and delivery should be planned during normal working hours. Prenatal management aims to limit heart strain (e.g. to restrict activity, reduce obesity, correct anaemia, and prevent infection, hypotension and dysrhythmia). Patients with severe disease may require prolonged bed rest. The risk of thromboembolism makes it prudent to consider anticoagulation.[20] Atrial fibrillation with cardiomegaly, valvular disease and previous thromboembolism warrants anticoagulation. Patients with valvular abnormalities or prostheses and certain congenital diseases (e.g. VSD, PDA, coarctation and MVP) should receive antibiotic prophylaxis for dental and surgical procedures (see below). Tocolytic therapy such as β_2-adrenergic agonists for premature labour is inadvisable, because of the propensity to precipitate pulmonary oedema.[21] They are contraindicated in patients with fixed cardiac output states (e.g. hypertrophic obstructive cardiomyopathy and aortic stenosis).

Management during labour

Supportive management

These patients should be managed in an ICU with facilities for invasive monitoring and close supervision by midwives and ICU nurses. An operating room should be close by.

Delivery

No data are available on the best mode of delivery for women with heart disease, but current practice favours vaginal delivery. Caesarean section is undertaken if there are obstetric indications.[22] In patients with marked exercise intolerance, the second stage should be shortened by forceps delivery. Effective analgesia is important to minimize stress on the heart. Epidural analgesia is the technique of choice, but must be used cautiously in those who cannot tolerate a sudden decrease in SVR (e.g. patients with aortic stenosis, pulmonary hypertension and intracardiac shunts).[23] However, epidural opioids, relatively

risk-free from systemic hypotension, may be beneficial.[24]

Haemodynamic monitoring[25]

The risks and benefits of invasive monitoring should be considered on an individual basis. Generally, asymtomatic NYHA class 1 and 2 patients without progressive disease or heart failure require noninvasive blood pressure, heart rate, electrocardiogram (ECG) and pulse oximetry monitoring. Symptomatic NYHA class 3 and 4 patients justify invasive monitoring, i.e. arterial line and PA catheter.

Haemodynamic therapy[26]

The same principles of managing non-pregnant patients with heart failure are followed:

1 *Preload* may be increased with fluids if indicated. Preload may be decreased by diuretics or venodilators (e.g. nitroglycerin).
2 *Afterload* may be increased by volume replacement or inotropic drugs (e.g. dopamine). Vasopressors may impair placental flow. Ephedrine appears to be the drug of choice.[27] Reduction of afterload may be achieved cautiously with vasodilators (e.g. hydralazine, sodium nitroprusside or nitroglycerin).
3 *Contractility* may be increased by inotropic agents (e.g. dopamine or adrenaline). Therapy should aim to return the haemodynamic state to what is normal for pregnancy (i.e. raised cardiac output and decreased SVR) as far as the patient's disease allows.

Antibiotics

Antibiotics should be given to those at risk of infective endocarditis. The prophylactic regimen is ampicillin 2.0 g plus gentamicin 1.3 mg/kg IV, 30 min before delivery, and 8 h later. In patients allergic to penicillin, vancomycin 1.0 g is given instead.

Positioning

Aortocaval compression should be avoided by placing the patient in a left lateral tilt of 15–20°.

Specific conditions
Mitral stenosis

Cardiac output in these patients depends on adequate diastolic filling time. Hence prevention of rapid ventricular rates is important. The most hazardous time is the immediate postpartum period, when sudden rises in blood volume can precipitate pulmonary oedema. However, a high normal PCWP is required to maintain adequate ventricular filling pressure. A PCWP up to 14 mmHg (1.9 kPa) appears optimal in the pre-delivery period.[23] Any preload manipulation should be undertaken with extreme caution. Caesarean sections under general anaesthesia were previously undertaken for these patients, but with effective epidural anaesthesia and careful management, vaginal delivery can be safe.

Mitral regurgitation

Although generally well-tolerated in pregnancy, there is a risk of developing atrial enlargement and fibrillation. Digitalization is recommended.[28]

Aortic stenosis[29]

Due to the increase in blood volume during pregnancy, mild disease is usually well-tolerated. In severe disease, cardiac output is relatively fixed, and may be inadequate for coronary perfusion during periods of stress. Bed rest is thus advisable. Any reduction in preload (e.g. blood loss or aortocaval compression) is extremely detrimental. In congenital aortic stenosis with a gradient over 50 mmHg (6.7 kPa), balloon dilatation may improve response to pregnancy.[30] Epidural anaesthesia in these patients has been successfully used, but hypotension must be avoided.[31] Use of a PA catheter is recommended and PCWP should be maintained on the high normal side (14–16 mmHg, 1.9–2.1 kPa). A shortened second stage is also recommended.

Hypertrophic obstructive cardiomyopathy[32]

Tachycardia must be avoided. Excessive expulsive efforts will also decrease cardiac output. Epidural anaesthesia for normal delivery with a shortened second stage is recommended; hypotension is especially hazardous. Antibiotic prophylaxis is also recommended.

Peripartum cardiomyopathy[15]

Management is supportive: to optimize circulatory volume, minimize myocardial oxygen consumption and avoid cardiodepressant drugs. Digitalization, diuretics, salt restriction and bed rest are advisable. In refractory cases, afterload reduction with nitrates may be used.

Eisenmenger's syndrome and other right-to-left shunts[33]

These conditions are associated with high mortality, and therapeutic abortion is advisable. Any decrease in SVR will increase right-to-left shunting. Hypotension must be avoided, as sudden death may result (see above). Oxygen is a good pulmonary vasodilator and increasing inspired oxygen concentration is recommended. A PA catheter helps haemodynamic management, but incurs risks of complications in

patients with pulmonary hypertension.[34] PCWP is maintained on the high side (16–18 mmHg, 2.1–2.4 kPa) to 'cushion' against acute hypotension. As blood pressure fluctuates during labour, caesarean section may be preferred. Epidural anaesthesia has been successfully used, but great care must be taken to avoid hypotension.[35]

Management of third stage of labour

Oxytocic drugs should be used with great care in the third stage, because of profound haemodynamic changes. Ergometrine increases SVR and worsens cardiac output in regurgitant lesions. It is also emetogenic. Syntocinon in bolus doses decreases SVR, with resultant problems in those with shunts and fixed-output states. If indicated on obstetric grounds, it should be given as an infusion.

Cardiac arrhythmias in pregnancy[36]

The incidence of arrhythmias during pregnancy is reported to be increased, and haemodynamic, autonomic and hormonal changes are implicated.[37] Most arrhythmias are benign, and precipitating causes, e.g. smoking, alcohol and caffeine should be sought. Antiarrhythmic drugs should be reserved for those with significant haemodynamic disturbances. Most antiarrhythmic drugs cross the placenta. Use of known safe agents and monitoring of blood drug concentrations are recommended.

Atrial fibrillation

This is usually associated with underlying heart disease, especially mitral stenosis or thyrotoxicosis. Rate control may be achieved with digoxin. Serum concentrations during pregnancy may be lower (possibly due to increased glomerular filtration) but doses should only be increased if therapeutic effect is not achieved. Although digoxin transfers freely across the placenta, it has been extensively used in pregnancy without adverse effects on the neonate.[38]

Atrial flutter

An atrial rate of 300 beats/min or more is usually found, with a 2:1 conduction block. Carotid sinus massage may prolong the block, but is unlikely to terminate the dysrhythmia. Digoxin or β-adrenergic blockers may be used to control ventricular rate. The latter can cross the placenta readily, and fetal bradycardia, hypoglycaemia, hyperbilirubinaemia and intrauterine growth retardation are concerns. However, most reports have not shown significant adverse fetal effects,[39–41] but β-blockers should probably be avoided in known intrauterine growth retardation.

Supraventricular tachycardia (SVT)

This is characterized by a rapid atrial rate of 160–200 beats/min, usually with 1:1 ventricular conduction. In general, vagal manoeuvres should be attempted before drug therapy.

Quinidine[42]

Obstetric use over six decades has shown it to be safe. An oral dose acts within 1 h and lasts 6–8 h.

Disopyramide[43]

This is effective for SVT and ventricular arrhythmias. Inducing premature labour is a possible concern. Experience of this drug in pregnancy is limited, and its negative inotropic effects mandate cautious use.

Calcium-channel blockers[44]

Reports on their use in pregnancy have been favourable, although experience remains limited. Intravenous bolus doses (e.g. with verapamil) can precipitate acute maternal hypotension.

β-Adrenergic blockers

See Atrial flutter above.

Adenosine[45,46]

A rapidly metabolized endogenous purine nucleotide, adenosine has been used successfully to treat SVT and Wolff–Parkinson–White syndrome in pregnancy. Its rapid onset of action (within 1 min), lower risk of hypotension, short half-life (1.5 s) and minimal placenta transfer make it suitable for use in pregnancy. It has been associated with bronchospasm, and should be avoided in asthmatics.

Ventricular arrhythmias[47]

Ventricular arrhythmias, including ventricular tachycardia, are less common and are usually associated with underlying heart disease. Therapeutic agents which may be used include the following.

Lignocaine[48]

It crosses the placenta rapidly, but information on its use in pregnancy is limited. There are no reports of teratogenicity, but possible neonatal neurobehavioural effects are concerns.

Flecainide[49]

There have been a few reports of its safe and effective use in pregnancy. It crosses the placenta readily. Lack of fetal toxic effects is possibly due to a lower sensitivity of immature cardiac tissue to its electrophysiological effects.

Amiodarone[50]

This agent carries risks of neonatal hypothyroidism. Although highly effective, it should be reserved to treat refractory, life-threatening ventricular and supraventricular arrhythmias.

Cardioversion[51]

Cardioversion has been performed safely during all stages of pregnancy. Nevertheless, transient fetal dysrhythmia has been described, and fetal heart monitoring is advised.

References

1 Oakley GDG (1989) Pregnancy and heart disease. In: Julian DG, Camm AJ, Fox KM, Hall RJC and Poole-Wilson PA (eds). *Diseases of the Heart.* London: Baillière Tindall, pp. 1363–1371.

2 Oakley CM (1989) Pregnancy in heart disease: pre-existing heart disease. In: Douglas PS (ed.) *Cardiovascular Clinics*, Vol. 19. *Heart Disease in Women.* Philadelphia: FA Davis, pp. 57–80.

3 Ueland K (1978) Cardiovascular disease complicating pregnancy. *Clin Obstet Gynecol* **21**:429–442.

4 Hoffman JI and Christianson R (1978) Congenital heart disease in a cohort of 19502 births with long term follow up. *Am J Cardiol* **42**:641–647.

5 Gordis L (1985) The virtual disappearance of rheumatic fever in the United States: lessons in the rise and fall of disease. *Circulation* **72**:1155–1162.

6 Shime J, Mocarski EJM, Hastings D, Webb GD and McLaughlin VR (1987) Congenital heart disease in pregnancy. Short and long term implications. *Am J Obstet Gynaecol* **156**:313–322.

7 Steinberg WM and Farine D (1985) Maternal mortality in Ontario from 1970–1980. *Obstet Gynecol* **66**:510–512.

8 Clark SL, Cotton DB, Hankins GD and Phelan JP (1991) Cardiac disease in pregnancy. In: Cotton DB (ed.) *Obstetrics and Gynecology Clinics of North America*, Philadelphia: WB Saunders, **18**:237–256.

9 Criteria Committee of the New York Heart Association (1979) *Nomenclature and Criteria for the Diagnosis of Diseases of the Heart and Great Vessels,* 8th edn. New York: New York Heart Association.

10 Elkayam U and Gleicher N (1990) Changes in cardiac findings during normal pregnancy. In: Elkayam U and Gleicher N (eds) *Cardiac Problems in Pregnancy*, 2nd edn. New York: Alan R Liss, pp. 31–38.

11 Metcalfe J, McAnulty JH and Ueland K (1986) *Burwell and Metcalfe's Heart Disease and Pregnancy: Physiology and Management* 2nd edn. Boston: Little, Brown, pp. 11–54.

12 Mangano DT (1993) Anaesthesia for pregnant cardiac patient. In: Schnider S and Levinson C (eds) *Anesthesia for Obstetrics*, 3rd edn, Baltimore: Williams & Wilkins, pp. 485–524.

13 Pitkin RM, Perloff JK, Koos BJ and Beall MH

(1990) Pregnancy and congenital heart disease. *Ann Intern Med* 112:445–454.

14 Donnelly JE, Brown JM and Radford DJ (1991) Pregnancy outcome and Ebstein anomaly. *Br Heart J* 66:368–371.

15 Hsieh CC, Chiang CW, Hsieh TT and Soong YK (1992) Peripartum cardiomyopathy. *Jpn Heart J.* 33:343–349.

16 Oakley GDG, McGarry K and Limb DG (1979) Management of pregnancy in patients with hypertrophic cardiomyopathy. *Br Med J* 1:1749–1750.

17 Hands ME, Johnson MD, Saltzman DH and Rutherford JD (1990) The cardiac, obstetric and anesthetic management of pregnancy complicated by acute myocardial infarction. *J Clin Anesth* 2:258–268.

18 Bernal JM and Miralles PJ (1986) Cardiac surgery with cardiopulmonary bypass during pregnancy. *Obstet Gynecol Surv* 41:1–6.

19 Greenspoon J (1987) Prosthetic valves, asthma and anticoagulation in pregnancy. In: Clark SL (ed.) *Critical Care Obstetrics*. Oradell, NJ: Medical Economics Books, pp. 114–125.

20 Dalen E and Hirsh J (1986) American College of Chest Physicians and the National Heart, Lung and Blood Institute national conference on antithrombotic therapy. *Chest* 89:1S-106S.

21 Pisani RJ and Rosenow EC (1989) Pulmonary oedema associated with tocolytic therapy. *Ann Intern Med* 110:714–718.

22 Clark SL (1986) Labour and delivery in the patient with structural cardiac disease. *Clin Perinatol* 13:695–703.

23 Clark SL, Phelan JP and Greenspoon J (1985) Labour and delivery in the presence of mitral stenosis: central haemodynamic observations. *Am J Obstet Gynecol* 152:984–988.

24 Abboud JK, Raya, J, Noueihed R (1983) Intrathecal morphine for relief of labour pain in a parturient with severe pulmonary hypertension. *Anesthesiology* 59:477–479.

25 Jones MM and Joyce TH (1987) Anesthesia for the patient with pregnancy induced hypertension and the pregnant cardiac patient. In: Clark SL (ed.) *Critical Care Obstetrics*. Oradell, NJ: Medical Economics Books, pp. 415–433.

26 Burlew BS (1990) Managing the pregnant patient with heart disease. *Clin Cardiol* 13:757–762.

27 Alahuta S, Rasanen J, Joupilla P, Joupilla R and Hollmen AI (1992) Ephedrine and phenylephedrine for avoiding maternal hypotension due to subarachnoid block for caesarean section. *Int J Obstet Anesth* 1:129–134.

28 Wlody D (1993) The pregnant patient with cardiac disease. In: Simpson JI (ed.) *Anesthesia and the Patient with Coexisting Heart Disease*. Boston: Little, Brown, pp. 293–314.

29 Easterling TR, Chadwick HS and Otto CM (1988) Aortic stenosis in pregnancy. *Obstet Gynecol* 72:113–118.

30 Banning AP, Pearson JF and Hall RJC (1993) Role of balloon dilatation of aortic valve in pregnant patients with severe aortic stenosis. *Br Heart J* 170:544–545.

31 Shin YK and King JC (1993) Combined mitral and aortic stenosis in a parturient: epidural anaesthesia for labour and delivery. *Anesth Analg* 76:682–683.

32 Lang RM and Borow KM (1991) Heart disease. In: Barron WM and Lindheimer MD (eds) *Medical Disorders During Pregnancy*. St Louis: Mosby Year Book, pp. 148–196.

33 Gleicher N, Midwall J, Hochberger D and Jaffin H (1979) Eisenmenger syndrome and pregnancy. *Obstet Gynecol Surv* 34:721–741.

34 Devitt JH, Noble WH and Byrick RJ (1982) A Swan-Ganz catheter related complication in a patient with Eisenmenger syndrome. *Anesthesiology* 57:335.

35 Spinnato JA, Karaynack BJ and Cooper MW (1981) Eisenmenger's syndrome in pregnancy: epidural anesthesia for elective caesarean section. *N Engl J Med* 304:1215–1217.

36 Cox JI and Gardner MJ (1993) Treatment of cardiac arrhythmias during pregnancy. *Prog Cardiovasc Dis* 36:137–178.

37 Widerhorn J, Widerhorn ALM, Rahimtoola SH. (1992) Wolff–Parkinson–White syndrome during pregnancy: increased incidence of supraventricular arrhythmias. *Am Heart J.* 123:796–798.

38 Soyka LF (1975) Digoxin: placental transfer, effects on the fetus and therapeutic use in the newborn. *Clin Perinatol* 2:23–35.

39 Frishman WH and Chesner M (1988) Beta adrenergic blockers in pregnancy. *Am Heart J* 115:147–152.

40 Taylor EA and Turner P (1981) Antihypertensive therapy with propranolol during pregnancy and lactation. *Postgrad Med J* 57:427–430.

41 Livingstone I, Craswell PW and Beran EB (1983) Propranolol in pregnancy: three year prospective study. *Clin Exp Hypertens* 2:341–350.

42 Hill LM and Malkasian GD (1979) The use of quinidine sulfate throughout pregnancy. *Obstet Gynecol* 54:366–368.

43 Tadmor OP, Keren A and Rosenak D (1990) The effect of diisopyramide on uterine contractions during pregnancy. *Am J Obstet Gynecol* 162:482–486.

44 Byerly WC, Hartmann A and Foster DE (1991) Verapamil in the treatment of maternal paroxysmal supraventricular tachycardia. *Ann Emerg Med* 20:552–554.

45 Mason BA, Goodman JR and Koos B (1992) Adenosine in the treatment of maternal paroxysmal supraventricular tachycardia. *Obstet Gynecol* 80:478–480.

46 Afridi I, Moise KJ and Rokey R (1992) Termination of supraventricular tachycardia with adenosine in a pregnant woman with Wolff Parkinson White syndrome. *Obstet Gynecol* 80:481–483.

47 Braverman AC, Bromley BS and Rutherford JD (1991) New onset ventricular tachycardia during pregnancy. *Int J Cardiol* 33:409–412.

48 Rotmensch HH, Pines A and Donchin Y (1990) Antiarrhythmic drugs in pregancy. In: Elkayam U and Gleicher N (eds) *Cardiac Problems in Pregnancy: Diagnosis and*

Management of Maternal and Fetal Disease, 2nd edn. New York: Liss, pp. 361–379.

49 Doig JC, McComb JM and Reid DS (1992) Incessant atrial tachycardia accelerated by pregnancy. *Br Heart J* **67**:266–268.

50 Plomp TA, Valsma T and de-Viljhder JJ (1992) Use of amiodarone during pregnancy. *Eur J Obstet Gynaecol Reprod Biol* **43**:201–207.

51 Rosemond RL (1993) Cardioversion during pregnancy. *J Am Med Assoc* **269**:3167.

Part IX

Infections and immune disorders

58 | Anaphylaxis

MM Fisher

Anaphylaxis is the symptom complex accompanying the acute reaction to a foreign substance to which a patient has been previously sensitized (immediate hypersensitivity or type 1 hypersensitivity).[1] The term anaphylactoid reaction is used to describe reactions clinically indiscernible from anaphylaxis in which the mechanism is non-immunological, or has not been determined.[2] Both conditions can be incorporated under the title 'clinical anaphylaxis'. The symptom complex may be produced by direct drug effects, physical factors or exercise, and a causative agent cannot always be determined. Anaphylaxis is an example of a host defence mechanism producing a hostile response, and the mediators involved are the same as those in other acute inflammatory responses.

Aetiology and pathophysiology[1]

Clinical anaphylaxis commonly follows injection of drugs, blood products, plasma substitutes or contrast media, ingestion of foods or food additives or insect stings.

In anaphylaxis, sensitization occurs following exposure to an allergenic substance, which either alone, or by combination with a hapten, stimulates the synthesis of immunoglobulin E (IgE) which binds to the surface of mast cells and basophils. Later, re-exposure to antigen produces an antigen–cell surface IgE antibody interaction, resulting in mast cell degranulation and the release of histamine and other mediators, including interleukin, prostaglandins and platelet-activating factor. Histamine is responsible for the early signs and symptoms, but is rapidly cleared from plasma. The overall effects of the mediators are to produce vasodilators, smooth muscle contraction, increased glandular secretion and increased capillary permeability.

In an anaphylactoid reaction, the clinical expression is identical to anaphylaxis, but the mechanism of its initiation is uncertain. Intravenous hypnotic drugs and X-ray contrast media may activate the complement system. Plasma protein and human serum albumin reactions are thought to be induced by either albumin aggregates or stabilizing agent-modified albumin molecules. Other reactions, including those to dextrans and gelatin preparations, may be activated by non IgE antibody already present in the plasma.[3]

The direct histamine-releasing effects of some drugs may produce reactions due to the effect of histamine alone, and such reactions are related to volume, rate and amount of infusion. Recent work suggests that the site of release of histamine may be important in its clinical effects. Drugs such as morphine release histamine from skin alone,[4] and are unlikely to produce symptoms such as asthma, whereas drugs which produce release from lung mast cells (e.g. atracurium, vecuronium and propofol) may be more likely to produce bronchospasm.[5] Direct histamine release is usually a transient phenomenon, but in some patients severe manifestations may occur, particularly with Haemaccel.

Anaphylactic reactions are usually seen in fit patients. It is likely that the adrenal response to stress 'pretreats' sick patients, and blocks the release and effects of anaphylactic mediators. The exception to this appears to be patients with asthma, in whom reactions to the additives in steroid and aminophylline preparations may occur, and this may be related to the reduced catecholamine response in asthma.[6]

Clinical presentation[7]

The latent period between exposure and development of symptoms is variable, but usually occurs within 10 min if the provoking agent is given parenterally. Reactions may be transient or protracted, lasting days, and may vary in severity from mild to fatal. Cutaneous, cardiovascular, respiratory or gastrointestinal manifestations may occur singly or in combination. The incidence of clinical features is shown in Table 58.1.

Cutaneous features include erythmatous flush, generalized urticaria, angioneurotic oedema, con-

Table 58.1 Clinical features of anaphylaxis in 500 patients

	Number	Sole feature	Worst feature
Cardiovascular collapse	445	52	399
Bronchospasm	191	18	91
Transient	76		
Asthmatics	85		
Cutaneous			
Rash	65		
Erythema		232	
Urticaria	42		
More than 1	30		
Angioedema	124	6	17
Generalized oedema	36		
Pulmonary oedema	13	2	3
Gastrointestinal	36		

junctival injection, pallor and cyanosis. Cardiovascular system involvement is the most common and may occur as a sole clinical manifestation. It is evidenced by tachycardia, hypotension and the development of shock. Respiratory manifestations include rhinitis, bronchospasm and laryngeal obstruction. Gastrointestinal symptoms of nausea, vomiting, abdominal cramps and diarrhoea may be present. Other features include apprehension, metallic taste, choking sensation, coughing, paraesthesiae, arthralgia, convulsions, clotting abnormalities and loss of consciousness. Pulmonary oedema is a common postmortem finding, and rarely, a massive high-protein pulmonary oedema may occur.

Anaphylaxis is rare in the ICU, possibly because of the protective effects of the adrenal response to stress. Recently, use of the mast cell tryptase assay (see below) has detected anaphylaxis as an unsuspected cause of shock in intensive care.

Pathophysiology of cardiovascular changes

The traditional concept of the cardiovascular changes in clinical anaphylaxis is that of an initial vasodilatation, followed by capillary leak of plasma which produces endogenous hypovolaemia, reduced venous return and lowered cardiac output.

Whether or not cardiac function is impaired has been controversial. Although most anaphylactic mediators adversely affect myocardial function *in vitro*, most case reports of anaphylaxis in which invasive cardiovascular monitoring has been used suggest minimal impairment of cardiac function. Patients with normal cardiac function before the reaction rarely show evidence of cardiac failure or arrhythmias other than supraventricular tachycardia, but the incidence of serious arrhythmias and cardiac failure increases in those with prior cardiac disease.[8]

Recently, two reactions in patients with no previous cardiac disease were reported.[9] The major feature was prolonged global myocardial dysfunction, and the use of a balloon counterpulsator was life-saving. The myocardial dysfunction may have been related to adrenaline infusion.

Management[8-10]

Oxygen

Oxygen is given by facemask. Endotracheal intubation may be required to facilitate ventilation, especially if angioneurotic oedema or laryngeal oedema is present. Mechanical ventilation is indicated for severe bronchospasm, apnoea or cardiac arrest.

Adrenaline

Adrenaline is the drug of choice for severe reactions.[10] A dose of 0.3–1.0 mg is given intramuscularly (IM) and 0.5 mg is often sufficient. If muscle blood flow is thought to be compromised by shock, or as a chosen alternative, an intravenous infusion of 1–2 mg in 100 ml saline is started with electrocardiographic (ECG) monitoring. Adrenaline should be used with caution in patients who have received volatile anaesthetics. In such patients, a trial of metaraminol may avoid ventricular arrhythmias. Adrenaline, by increasing intracellular levels of cyclic adenosine monophosphate (cAMP) in leukocytes and mast cells, inhibits further release of histamine. It has beneficial effects on myocardial contractility, peripheral vascular tone and bronchial smooth muscle. A common management error is not to institute external cardiac massage (ECM) as the arrhythmia is benign. If the patient is pulseless, ECM should be instituted irrespective of rhythm.

Colloids

Plasma or plasma expanders are given rapidly to correct the hypovolaemia consequent to acute vasodilatation and leakage of fluid from the intravascular space.[11] Plasma protein solution, dextran 70 and gelatin preparations are favoured above crystalloids, as they remain longer within the vascular compartment. Very large volumes of fluid may be required and central venous pressure (CVP) monitoring and measurement of haematocrit are helpful.

Noradrenaline

If hypotension persists in spite of adrenaline and colloids, noradrenaline may be life-saving[8] and the heart should be imaged.

Bronchodilators

Nebulized salbutamol should be given for severe asthma. Aminophylline 5.6 mg/kg IV may be given over 30 min, if bronchospasm is unresponsive to adrenaline alone. Aminophylline increases intracellular cAMP by phosphodiesterase inhibition, and its effect on inhibiting histamine and interleukin release is theoretically additive to that of adrenaline. Volatile anaesthesia, ketamine and magnesium sulphate may produce improvement in some patients with severe asthma.

Corticosteroids

Steroids have no proven benefit and should be reserved for refractory bronchospasm.

Antihistamines

Antihistamines are only indicated in protracted cases or in those with angioneurotic oedema which may recur. The data on antihistamines are not conclusive, but in protracted anaphylaxis, improvement is often reported with H_2 blockers.

Ideally, patients are managed in the ICU. Continuous ECG monitoring enables detection of arrhythmias secondary to hypoxia, hypotension or exogenous adrenaline. Close monitoring of arterial blood pressure, CVP and arterial blood gases is mandatory during the acute phase.

Diagnosis

The most important advance in the diagnosis of anaphylaxis has been the introduction of an assay for mast cell tryptase.[11] The mast cell enzyme is elevated 1 h after a reaction begins, and the elevation may persist for up to 4 h. It can also be used to diagnose anaphylaxis from post mortem specimens[12,13] The assay is highly specific and sensitive for anaphylaxis.

Follow-up

Following successful acute management, the drug or agent responsible should be determined by *in vitro* or *in vivo* testing if possible. Hyposensitization should be considered for food, pollen and bee-sting allergy. A medicalert bracelet should be worn, and the patient given a letter stating the nature of the reaction to the particular causative agent.

If re-exposure to the allergen is likely at home, patients or their relatives should be instructed in the use of adrenaline, salbutamol inhalation and antihistamines. Clinical anaphylaxis may be modified by pretreatment with disodium cromoglycate, corticosteroids, antihistamines, salbutamol and isoprenaline.[1]

References

1 Fisher MM (1987) Anaphylaxis. *Disease Month* **33:** 435–479.

2 Watkins J and Clarke RSJ (1978) Report of a symposium: adverse responses to intravenous agents. *Br J Anaesth* **50:**1159–1164.

3 Ring J, Stephan W and Brendel W (1979) Anaphylactoid reactions to infusions of plasma protein and human serum albumin. *Clin Allergy* **9:**87–97.

4 Tharp M D, Kagey–Sobotka A, Fox CC *et al.* (1987) Functional heterogeneity of human mast cells from different anatomic sites: *in vitro* responses to morphine sulphate. *J Allergy Clin Immunol* **79:** 646–653.

5 Stellato C, de Paulis A, Cirillo R *et al.* (1991) Heterogeneity of human mast cells and basophils in response to muscle relaxants. *Anesthesiology* **74:** 1078–1086.

6 Ind PW, Causon RC, Brown MJ *et al.* (1985) Circulating catecholamines in acute asthma. *Br Med J* **290:**267–269.

7 Fisher MM and More DG (1981) The epidemiology and clinical features of anaesthetic anaphylactic reactions. *Anaesth Intens Care* **9:**226–234.

8 Fisher MM (1986) Clinical observations on the pathophysiology and treatment of anaphylactic cardiovascular collapse. *Anaesth Intens Care* **14:**17–21.

9 Raper RF and Fisher MM. (1988) Profound reversible myocardial depression following human anaphylaxis. *Lancet* **ii:**386.

10 Fisher MM (1992) Treating anaphylaxis with sympathomimetic drugs. *Br Med J* **305:**1107–1108.

11 Fisher MM (1977) Blood volume replacement in acute anaphylactic cardiovascular collapse related to anaesthesia. *Br J Anaesth* **49:**1023–1026.

12 Yunginger JW, Nelson DR, Squilace DL *et al.* (1991) Laboratory investigation of deaths due to anaphylaxis. *J Forensic Sci* **36:**857–865.

13 Fisher MM and Baldo BA (1993) The diagnosis of fatal anaphylactic reactions during anaesthesia: employment of immunoassays for mast cell tryptase and drug-reactive IgE antibodies. *Anaesth Intens Care* **21:**353–357.

MAH French

Host defence mechanisms

The body is normally protected from the effects of a multitude of pathogenic microorganisms by many host defence mechanisms (Table 59.1). Arguably, the most important is the immune system, a complex system of interacting plasma proteins and cells of predominantly bone marrow origin. Higher mammals have very diverse immune responses to protect the different anatomical compartments of the body from a great variety of microorganisms. Consequently, there are many ways in which the immune system can be defective. The result of such defects may be an increased propensity to infections, resulting in an immunodeficiency disease.

The immune system

The immune system is capable of reacting to microorganisms without having been previously exposed to antigens from those microorganisms. This innate immune system consists of some types of antibody (natural antibodies), components of the complement system (the alternative pathway), a subset of lymphocytes with cytotoxic activity (natural killer or NK cells), and some macrophage functions. Innate immune responses provide a first line of defence against many pathogenic microorganisms. It is, however, the adaptive immune system which provides the most effective response against most microorganisms.

Adaptive immune responses are particularly effective because they are characterized by specificity, memory, amplification and diversity. The specificity of an immune response against a particular antigenic component of a micro-organism, and the memory which results in a prompt response on subsequent exposures, is determined by lymphocytes and antigen receptors on their surface. Amplification and diversity of immune responses is regulated by molecules known as cytokines, which are secreted by lymphocytes and

Table 59.1 Host defence mechanisms

Physical barriers
   Skin and mucosal surfaces
   Cilia
Fever
Acute-phase proteins, e.g. C-reactive protein
Lysozyme
Lactoferrin
Fibronectin
Immune system, including secondary mediators
Other mediators of inflammation
   Kinins
   Vasoactive amines
   Coagulation system

other cells, and through the effects of various lymphocyte surface molecules, including adhesion molecules and activation proteins. Cytokines which have immunoregulatory actions include the interleukins (of which there are at least 13), tumour necrosis factor (TNF), lymphotoxins and interferon-γ (IFN-γ).

The most important events in the initiation of an immune response are the processing and presentation of fragments of the microorganism in a form which makes the fragments antigenic to lymphocytes. Major histocompatibility complex (MHC) class I (human leukocyte antigen (HLA)-A, B, C) and class II (HLA-DR, DP, DQ) molecules are the major cell-surface antigen presentation molecules. These molecules also determine the nature of the subsequent response against the antigen. Class I MHC molecules are present on most nucleated cells, and present processed endogenous peptides (such as fragments of viruses) to the antigen receptor (T-cell receptor; TcR) of T-cells expressing CD8 molecules. Class II MHC molecules present antigenic fragments of microorganisms which are exogenous to cells and have been taken into the cell by phagocytosis, in the case of macrophages and monocytes, or by binding to antigen-specific surface immunoglobulins (the B-cell antigen receptor), in the case of B-cells. Antigens presented on class II MHC molecules bind to TcRs on CD4+ T-cells.

CD8+ T-cells have a cytotoxic effect on cells expressing class I MHC-associated viral antigens, resulting in the death of the cell and inhibition of viral replication. Antigen-induced stimulation of CD4+ T-cells results in activation of the T-cell, and the expression of cell-surface molecules and secretion of cytokines with immunoregulatory effects. These immunoregulatory molecules augment the functions of many other cells, including B-cells, T-cells and macrophages (T-cell help). A response to an antigen mediated by CD4+ T-cells may also elicit macrophage activation and killing of the microorganism express-ing that antigen. Activation of macrophages by CD4+ T-cells is critically dependent on the production of IFN-γ.

The activation and proliferation of T-cells occurs under the influence of cytokines and other regulatory molecules, including T-cell membrane activation molecules such as the ligand of the B-cell membrane molecule CD40 (CD40L). Proliferating B-cells dif-ferentiate into plasma cells, which secrete immuno-globulins with antibody activity against the initiating antigen. Nine isotypes of immunoglobulin can be produced each of which has a different function.

Immunoglobulin M (IgM) is a large pentameric molecule which is particularly effective as a bacterial agglutinator and activator of the complement system, and has its major effect within the circulation. IgA1 and IgA2 are produced at secretory surfaces, such as the mucosa of the gut and respiratory tract, and also in the breast, where IgA is a major constituent of the colostrum and provides secretory antibody to the gut of the neonate. IgE antibodies are also produced at mucosal surfaces where they form an important part

of the immune response against parasitic infections. IgG antibodies are able to move from the circulation to interstitial spaces and across the placenta. Antibodies of the IgG1 and IgG3 subclass are particularly effective at activating the complement system and binding to Fc receptors on phagocytic cells, whereas IgG2 antibodies are mainly active against polysaccharide antigens, such as those present in bacterial cell walls. The functions of IgG4 antibodies are unclear.

The elimination of a microorganism by antibodies usually requires the activation of a secondary effector mechanism, of which there are several. The complement system is a system of plasma proteins which are sequentially activated by either antigen–antibody complexes through the classical pathway, or directly by components of microorganisms through the alternative pathway (Fig. 59.1). Activation of the complement system results in the generation of biologically active molecules, such as C3b, which is an important opsonin, and the activation of the membrane attack complex (MAC) which lyses bacterial cell walls. Like C3b, antibodies of the IgM, IgG1 and IgG3 isotype are also important opsonins. These molecules, when bound to the surface of a microorganism, facilitate their opsonization and phagocytosis. These effects of complement and antibody are mediated through complement receptors (CRs) and receptors for the Fc portion of the immunoglobulin molecules (Fc receptors) on the phagocytic cell surface. The most important phago-cytic cells are neutrophils and macrophages.

The type of immune response produced against a microorganism varies according to the nature of the infecting organism. Thus virus-infected cells elicit a cytotoxic CD8 + T-cell response; intracellular patho-gens such as mycobacteria and protozoa elicit a CD4 + T-cell response which results in macrophage activation; encapsulated bacteria elicit an opsonizing

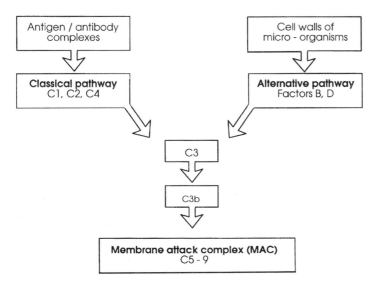

Fig. 59.1 The complement system.

antibody response; and some bacteria such as *Neisseria* spp. elicit a component-activating antibody response. The nature of the immune response is regulated by cytokines. Thus, Interleukein-2 (IL-2), IL-12 and IFN-γ production induces a predominantly cellular immune response (type I help), whereas the production of IL-4, IL-6 and IL-10 induces a predominantly antibody-mediated immune response (type II help).

Immune defects underlying immunodeficiency diseases

Defects of the immune system which give rise to an immunodeficiency disease are generally of four types – antibody deficiency, cellular immuno-deficiency, complement deficiency and phagocyte defects.

Antibody deficiency

A deficient systemic antibody response must commonly results in a lack of opsonizing antibody, and a propensity to infections with encapsulated bacteria such as pneumococci and *Haemophilus influenzae*. Recurrent respiratory tract infections are therefore the most common complication of this type of immune defect. Much less commonly, patients may develop echovirus infections of the nervous system and infections with some mycoplasmas.

Deficient secretory antibody responses are common in patients with IgA deficiency, but most affected individuals are able to produce compensatory secretory IgM or IgG responses and do not suffer from infections.

Cellular immunodeficiency

Impairment of cell-mediated immune responses leads to an increased propensity to infection with microorganisms which are normally controlled by cellular immunity (Table 59.2). In general, these microorganisms are intracellular pathogens, which cause persistent (latent) infections that reactivate when the cellular immune response against them becomes ineffective. Fungal and yeast infections are virtually always mucocutaneous and not systemic, implying that cellular immunity is not important in the control of systemic fungal infections.

Complement deficiency

Complement-mediated lysis of bacterial cell walls is a critical mechanism in the immune response against certain bacteria, especially *Neisseria* spp. and related bacteria such as *Moraxella* spp. and *Acinetobacter* spp. Deficiency of complement components, particularly MAC components, may therefore result in infection with these bacteria. C3b is an important opsonin and C3 deficiency will often impair

Table 59.2 Common microorganisms infecting patients with cellular immunodeficiency

Protozoa	*Pneumocystis carinii*
	Toxoplasma gondii
	Cryptosporidia
Mycobacteria	*Mycobacterium tuberculosis*
	Non-tuberculous (atypical) mycobacteria
Bacteria	*Salmonella* spp.
	Shigella spp.
	Listeria monocytogenes
Fungi and yeasts	*Candida* spp. (mucosal infections)
	Cryptococci
	Aspergillus spp.
	Dermatophytes
	Pityrosporon spp.
Viruses	Herpes viruses
	Cytomegalovirus
	Varicella-zoster
	Herpes simplex
	Epstein–Barr virus
	Molluscum contagiosum virus
	JC virus (progressive multifocal leukoencephalopathy)

phagocytosis of bacteria. Deficiency of classical pathway components may also result in impaired antibody responses.

Phagocyte defects

Depletion or functional impairment of phagocytes results in an increased propensity to bacterial and fungal infections, particularly infection with *Staphylococcus aureus*, Gram-negative enteric bacteria *Candida* spp. and *Aspergillus* spp. Fungal and yeast infections are often systemic, indicating the importance of phagocytes in the systemic immune response against these microrganisms.

Phagocytosis of a bacterium or fungus by a neutrophil leukocyte or macrophage is dependent on chemotactic attraction of phagocytes to the site of infection, their adhesion to endothelial cells via adhesion molecules such as integrins, binding to opsonins on the microorganism, ingestion and intracellular killing. Intracellular killing involves both oxidative and non-oxidative mechanisms. Primary or acquired defects of phagocytes may result in localized pyogenic infections or pneumonia. However, in the neutropenic patient, localized infections may show little inflammatory reaction and overwhelming systemic infections are common.

Immunodeficiency diseases

Immunodeficiency diseases are classified as primary or acquired. Primary immunodeficiency diseases are the result of a developmental anomaly or a genetically-determined defect of the immune system. Genetically-determined defects are usually of two types:

1 first, the consequence of an absent or non-functional gene product, which is critical for the normal development or function of a component of the immune system.
2 second, aberrant regulation of lymphocyte maturation and differentiation, which is probably determined by the products of several genes and possibly by environmental factors.

Immunodeficiency diseases caused by the latter type of defect usually present later in life than congenital immunodeficiency caused by a non-functioning gene product. Acquired immunodeficiency diseases are more common than primary immunodeficiency diseases, and may present at any time after early childhood. Most result from an immune defect which is a consequence of a disease process (disease-related immunodeficiency) or therapy for a disease (therapy-related immunodeficiency).

Diagnosis of an immunodeficiency disease in a patient with an abnormal propensity to infections is dependent on the demonstration of an immune defect, as indicated in Table 59.3.

Antibody deficiency diseases

Primary antibody deficiency diseases

Failure of B-cell production or the presence of 'immature' B-cells due to a defect of differentiation are the cause of most primary antibody deficiency diseases. B-cells are absent from blood and secondary lymphoid tissues in patients with X-linked agammaglobulinaemia (XLA), because mutations of the *Btk* gene on the X-chromosome result in the absence of a B-cell tyrosine kinase necessary for the maturation of pre-B-cells to B-cells in the bone marrow.[1] In the *hyper-IgM immunodeficiency syndrome*, B-cells are able to differentiate into plasma cells secreting IgM, but not IgG or IgA. The X-linked form of this condition results from mutations in the gene of CD40L which is critical in delivering a T-cell signal to differentiating B-cells.[1]

Common variable immunodeficiency (CVID) and *IgA deficiency* appear to be the consequence of an immunoregulatory defect which results in impaired B-cell differentiation. Hypogammaglobulinaemia and systemic antibody deficiency are characteristic of CVID, whereas most individuals with IgA deficiency are asymptomatic. Those IgA-deficient patients who suffer from recurrent infections often have a defect of systemic antibody responses, which commonly

Table 59.3 Tests of immunocompetence

Antibody-mediated immunity
Serum immunoglobulins, including IgG subclasses
Systemic antibody responses (after vaccination if necessary)
   Polysaccharide antigens, e.g. pneumococcal
   Protein antigen, e.g. tetanus toxoid
Blood B-cell (CD19 +, CD20 +) numbers

Cell-mediated immunity
Delayed-type hypersensitivity (DTH) skin test responses
   Multitest CMI method
   Mantoux method
Blood T-cell (CD3 +) and T-cell subset (CD4 + or CD8 +) numbers

Phagocyte function
Blood neutrophil numbers
Tests of oxidative killing mechanisms, e.g. NBT test
Leukocyte expression of CR3 (a CD18 integrin)
Neutrophil migration assays
Bacteria or *Candida* killing assays

Complement system
Immunochemical quantitation of individual components
Functional assays of the whole system (CH50) or part of it

IgG = Immunoglobulin G; DTH = delayed-type hypersensitivity; CMI = cell-mediated immunity; NRT = nitrobule tetrazolium.

manifests as deficiency of an IgG subclass and/or impairment of antibody responses to polysaccharide antigens.[2] Antibody deficiency is occasionally associated with other patterns of immunoglobulin deficiency, such as IgG deficiency, or even with normal serum immunoglobulin concentrations in some patients with deficient antibody responses against polysaccharide antigens.[3]

The immunoregulatory defect underlying CVID and IgA deficiency sometimes results in an increased propensity to autoimmunity, which can include the production of anti-IgA antibodies. These antibodies may be the cause of anaphylactoid reactions to blood products.[4]

Acquired antibody deficiency diseases

Disease-related

B-cell chronic lymphocytic leukaemia or *lymphoma* and *myeloma* are commonly associated with reduced synthesis of normal immunoglobulins, which may result in antibody deficiency and bacterial infections. A thymoma is also sometimes associated with hypogammaglobulinaemia, and should always be considered in a patient presenting with primary hypogammaglobulinaemia after the age of 40.

Impaired production of antibodies against polysaccharide antigens contributes to the susceptibility which *postsplenectomy* patients have to infection with encapsulated bacteria, such as pneumococci and meningococci.[5]

Therapy-related

Several drugs affect B-cell differentiation and cause immunoglobulin deficiency, particularly IgA deficiency. The most common offenders are phenytoin and penicillamine. Most patients do not have antibody deficiency severe enough to cause infections. Intensive plasmapheresis may also cause severe immunoglobulin deficiency if immunoglobulin replacement is not used.

Treatment of antibody deficiency disease

Infections can be prevented by regular infusions of IV immunoglobulin (IVIG) in patients with primary and acquired antibody deficiency.[4,6] The usual dose is 300–500 mg/kg given monthly. Acute infections should be treated with appropriate antibiotics.

Cellular immunodeficiency

Primary cellular immunodeficiency diseases

Complete or partial absence of the thymus gland resulting in depletion of T-cells from blood and lymphoid tissue is the characteristic immunological abnormality in children with the *Di George syndrome*.[7] Infections of the type listed in Table 59.2 occur from birth onwards. A less severe defect of cellular immunity is present in patients with chronic mucocutaneous candidiasis. This syndrome is the result of several poorly defined immune defects, which result in an abnormal propensity to mucocutaneous infections with *Candida* spp. and some fungi.[8]

Acquired cellular immunodeficiency diseases

Acquired defects of cellular immunity are by far the most common cause of cellular immunodeficiency.

Disease-related
Cellular immunodeficiency resulting from infection of the immune system by human immunodeficiency viruses (HIVs) 1 and 2 is common (see Chapter 60). Less commonly, *Hodgkin's disease, T-cell lymphomas* and *sarcoidosis* may also be complicated by opportunistic infections occurring as a consequence of cellular immunodeficiency. A *thymoma* may be associated with a chronic mucocutaneous candidiasis syndrome which, like thymoma and hypogammaglobulinaemia, occurs later in life.

Therapy-related
Suppression of cellular immune responses is an intended effect of many *immunosuppressant* drugs used to treat allograft rejection, graft-versus-host disease (GVHD), autoimmune diseases and vasculitis. Opportunistic infections are a complication of this type of immunodeficiency, and often cause severe morbidity and sometimes death.[9]

Treatment of cellular immunodeficiency diseases

Since most infections complicating cellular immunodeficiency are reactivated latent infections, an important aspect of management is prevention of symptomatic infection by the use of prophylactic antimicrobial drugs, as exemplified by HIV-induced immunodeficiency.[10] Acquired cellular immunodeficiency may be corrected, at least temporarily, by removing its cause (e.g. by suppressing HIV infection or ceasing immunosuppressive therapy). Thymus transplantation may be effective in children with thymus aplasia.[7]

Complement deficiency

Deficiency of complement components is an uncommon but often overlooked cause of recurrent bacterial infections.[11]

Primary complement deficiency

Congenital deficiency of *C3* is extremely rare, and usually causes a propensity to severe pyogenic infections. Deficiency of *MAC components* (C5–9) is more common, and should be considered in patients with meningococcal infections, particularly when the infections are recurrent. Deficiency of *classical pathway components* (C1,C2,C4) may also result in an increased propensity to infection with meningococci and some other bacteria, but many affected individuals do not experience recurrent infections.

Acquired complement deficiency

Disease-related
Disease processes which cause persistent activation of the complement system may cause depletion of complement components, particularly classical pathway components. This can result in infections with *Neisseria* spp. or related bacteria, and sometimes overwhelming septicaemia when the complement deficiency is severe. Systemic lupus erythematosus, myeloma and chronic atrioventricular shunt infections are the commonest causes.[12]

Phagocyte defects

Primary phagocyte defects

Congenital neutropenias are rare. Defects of phagocyte function usually affect chemotaxis, adhesion or intracellular killing, either alone or in combination. The best characterized defect of phagocyte adherence results from a congenital absence of the β-subunit of

CD18 integrins in patients with the leukocyte adhesion deficiency syndrome.[13] Defects of intracellular killing are usually caused by a deficiency of an enzyme critical for the functioning of killing mechanisms. In chronic granulomatous disease (CGD), deficiency of a phagosome enzyme (NADPH oxidase) results in ineffective oxidative killing mechanisms.[14] CGD usually presents in childhood but may present in adults, even as late as the seventh decade.[15] It should be considered in patients with recurrent abcesses or suppurative lymphadenitis, and in patients with pneumonia caused by *Staphylococcus aureus* or *Aspergillus* spp. infection.

Acquired phagocyte defects

Disease-associated
Severe *neutropenia* may be complicated by bacterial or fungal infections. There are many causes of neutropenia, including autoimmune neutropenia, drug therapy and haematological diseases such as cyclic neutropenia, myelodysplastic syndromes and aplastic anaemia.

Therapy-related
Cytotoxic chemotherapy, used to treat various malignancies, commonly causes neutropenia, which can be complicated by severe bacterial and fungal infections.

Treatment of phagocyte defects

Acquired neutropenia may be corrected by removing the underlying cause and/or use of granulocyte colony stimulating factor (G-CSF).[16,17] The frequency of infections in patients with phagocyte dysfunction can be reduced by the use of prophylactic co-trimoxazole. In addition, INF-γ therapy is effective in patients with CGD.[18]

Combined immunodeficiency diseases

Several immunodeficiency diseases result from a combination of immune defects. Some combinations of congenital immune defects are so severe that death is a common occurrence, unless the defect can be corrected. Such diseases are classified as severe combined immune deficiency (SCID) diseases.

Primary combined immunodeficiency diseases

There are many primary combined immunodeficiency diseases which present in early childhood. Most are classified descriptively, but the molecular defects have now been demonstrated for some of them. Defective expression of MHC class II molecules,[19] adenosine deaminase (ADA) deficiency,[20] IL-2 deficiency[21] and deficiency of the γ-chain of the IL-2R all result in a deficiency and/or functional impairment of B cells and

T-cells and a SCID. Deficiency of the IL-2R γ-chain results from mutations of its gene on the X-chromosome and is the underlying defect of X-linked SCID.[1]

Acquired combined immunodeficiency diseases

Combined immune defects can result in severe infections in patients who have received a bone marrow transplantation.[22] Following transplantation, the recipient's immune system is reconstituted with donor cells. A degree of immunocompetence is passively transferred from the donor to recipient by antigen-specific lymphocytes, but as this and any residual immunocompetence of the recipient declines, an immunodeficient state exists until the donor immune system is established. Consequently, both antibody-mediated and cell-mediated immunity are deficient in the first 3–4 months after transplantation, and may remain deficient for a longer period of time in patients with GvHD. This combined immune defect is often compounded by neutropenia and/or the effects of steroid or immunosuppressant therapy for GvHD. Defective antibody responses may persist for 1–2 years after transplantation, particularly antibody responses against polysaccharide antigens.

Many patients who are critically ill as a result of surgery, trauma or thermal injury also have acquired immune defects.[23] These defects include abnormalities of cellular immunity, immunoglobulin deficiency and impaired neutrophil function. They appear to be associated with an increased propensity to infections and arise from abnormalities which are complex and multifactorial.

Impairment of cell-mediated immune responses usually manifests as decreased T-cell proliferation and impaired delayed-type hypersensitivity responses, and probably results from a combination of factors, including the effects of anaesthetic drugs, blood transfusion, negative nitrogen balance and serum suppressor factors, including cytokines such as TNF-α. Phagocyte defects are mostly due to impairment of neutrophil chemotaxis by serum factors, and impaired intracellular killing. Deficiency of serum immunoglobulins also occurs, especially IgG deficiency, and may be associated with antibody deficiency. Serum leakage is a factor in patients with thermal injuries, and reduced synthesis and increased catabolism of immunoglobulins occur in many critically ill patients.

Treatment of combined immunodeficiency diseases

Bone marrow transplantation is the treatment of choice for many types of primary SCID, though enzyme replacement therapy or gene replacement therapy can be effective in ADA deficiency. Antibody replacement with IVIG therapy and prophylaxis for opportunistic infections are important in primary SCID and also in SCID secondary to bone marrow transplantation.

The correction of immune defects in critically ill patients has been intensely investigated, but no effective treatment regimen has been defined.[23] General measures such as adequate nutrition, achieving a positive nitrogen balance and excision of thermally injured tissue are effective. Biological response modifiers, cytokine and mediator inhibitors, and IVIG therapy have all been evaluated, The number of acute infections, particularly pneumonia, can be reduced by the use of IVIG therapy, but patient survival is not increased.[24,25]

References

1 Ochs HD and Aruffo A (1993) Advances in X-linked immunodeficiency disease. *Curr Opin Paediatr* 5:684–691.

2 French MAH, Denis K, Dawkins RL and Peter JB (1995) Infection susceptibility in IgA deficiency: correlation with low polysaccharide antibodies and deficiency of IgG2 and/or IgG4. *Clin Exp Immunol* 100:47–53.

3 Rijkers GT, Sanders LAM and Zegers BJM (1993) Anti-capsular polysaccharide antibody deficiency states. *Immunodeficiency* 5:1–21.

4 Buckley RH and Schiff RI (1991) The use of intravenous immune globulin in immunodeficiency diseases. *N Engl J Med* 325:110–117.

5 Di Padova F, Durig M, Wadstrom J and Harder F (1993) Role of spleen in immune response to polyvalent pneumococcal vaccine. *Br Med J* 287: 1829–1833.

6 Stiehm ER (1991) Use of immunoglobulin therapy in secondary antibody deficiencies. In: Imbach P (ed.) *Immunotherapy with Intravenous Immunoglobulins.* London: Academic Press, pp. 115–126.

7 Hong R (1991) The Di George anomaly. *Immunodeficiency Rev* 31–14.

8 Dwyer JM (1981) Chronic mucocutaneous candidiasis. *Annu Rev Med* 32:491–497.

9 Revillard JP (1990) Iatrogenic immunodeficiencies. *Curr Opin Immunol* 2:445–450.

10 Gallant JE, Moore RD and Chaisson RE (1994) Prophylaxis for opportunistic infections in patients with HIV infection. *Ann Intern Med* 120:932–944.

11 Figueroa JE and Densen P (1991) Infectious diseases associated with complement deficiencies. *Clin Microbiol Rev* 4:359–395.

12 Ellison RT, Kohler PF, Curd JG, Judson FN and Reller LB (1983) Prevalence of congenital or acquired complement deficiency in patients ˙with sporadic meningococcal disease. *N Engl J Med* 308:913–916.

13 Arnaout MA (1990) Leukocyte adhesion molecule deficiency: its structural basis, pathophysiology and implications for modulating the inflammatory response. *Immunol Rev* 114:145–180.

14 Forrest CB, Forehand JR, Axtell RA, Roberts RL and Johnson RB (1988) Clinical features and current management of chronic granulomatous disease. *Haematol Oncol Clin North Am* 2:253–266.

15 Schapiro BL, Newburger PE, Klempner MS and Dinauer MC (1991) Chronic granulomatous disease presenting in a 69 year-old man. *N Engl J Med* 325:1786–1790.

16 Lieschke GJ and Burgess AW (1992) Granulocyte colony-stimulating factor and granulocyte-macrophage colony-stimulating factor (part 1). *N Engl J Med* 327:28–35.

17 Lieschke GJ and Burgess AW (1992) Granulocyte colony-stimulating factor and granulocyte-macrophage colony-stimulating factor (part 2). *N Engl J Med* 327:99–106.

18 Alan R, Ezekowitz B, Dinauer MC, Jaffe HS, Orkin SH and Newburger PE (1988) Partial correction of the phagocyte defect in patients with X-linked chronic granulomatous disease by subcutaneous interferon gamma. *N Engl J Med* 319:146–151.

19 Griscelli C and Lisowska-Grospierre B (1993) Combined immunodeficiency with defective expression in MHC class II genes. In: Gupta S and Griscelli C (eds) *New Concepts in Immunodeficiency Diseases.* Chichester: John Wiley, pp. 177–190.

20 Hirschhorn R (1990) Adenosine deaminase deficiency. *Immunodeficiency Rev* 2:175–198.

21 Weinberg K and Parkman R (1990) Combined immunodeficiency due to a specific defect in the production of interleukin-2 *N Engl J Med* 322: 1718–1723.

22 Sable CA and Donowitz GR (1994) Infections in bone marrow transplant recipients. *Clin Infect Dis* 18:273–284.

23 Munster AM (1991) Control of infection following major burns: the immunological approach. In: Imbach P (ed.). *Immunotherapy with Intravenous Immunoglobulins.* London: Academic Press, 149–163.

24 Glinz W, Grob PJ, Nydegger UE *et al.* (1985) Polyvalent immunoglobulins for prophylaxis of bacterial infections in patients following multiple trauma: a randomized, placebo-controlled study. *Intensive Care Med* 11:288–294.

25 The Intravenous Immunoglobulin Collaborative Study Group (1992) Prophylactic intravenous administration of standard immune globulin as compared with core-lipopolysaccharide immune globulin in patients at high risk of postsurgical infection. *N Engl J Med* 327:234–240.

HIV infection and the acquired immunodeficiency syndrome

MAH French

Human immunodeficiency viruses

Human immunodeficiency viruses (HIVs) 1 and 2 are retroviruses of the Lentivirus group. Like other lentiviruses, they have a tropism for cells of the immune system, and cause immunological and neurological disease. Entry of HIV into cells is via cell-surface receptors, particularly the CD4 molecule, but also Fc and complement receptors. Inside the cell, the viral RNA is reverse transcribed into DNA by a viral reverse transcriptase enzyme, and the DNA is incorporated into the DNA of the host cell as proviral DNA. The proviral DNA remains there until the cell is activated, when it is transcribed into RNA which provides the template for assembly of new HIVs under the control of viral enzymes such as proteases. Budding of new virus from the cell is followed by infection of new cells and a repeat of the replication cycle.

Acute HIV infection

Initial infection by HIV-1 is associated with an acute HIV infection syndrome (seroconversion illness) in 50–70% of patients. This syndrome is similar to infectious mononucleosis, being characterized by fever, lymphadenopathy, headache, photophobia, fatigue and myalgia. However, mucocutaneous lesions, neurological disease and even transient immunodeficiency may also occur which, when present, differentiates it from infectious mononucleosis.[1]

Chronic HIV infection

The viraemia associated with acute HIV infection is controlled by a cellular and antibody-mediated immune response, which results in resolution of symptoms. However, even though the great majority of people become asymptomatic, HIV replication continues to take place. This results in activation of the immune system, depletion of CD4+ T-cells, and immunodeficiency, especially cellular immunodeficiency. These abnormalities develop at different rates in different individuals. The median time to develop the acquired immunodeficiency syndrome (AIDS) after acquiring HIV infection is 9 years, and about 5% of HIV-infected individuals have no abnormalities even after 15 years.

Early in the course of chronic HIV infection, virus is present in lymphoid tissues where it is bound to follicular dendritic cells. Viral replication in lymphoid tissue and the resulting immune response often give rise to persistent generalized lymphadenopathy (PGL). There is a persistent immune response against the HIV but, as this fails, viral replication increases, and the viral load becomes larger and other cells become infected, including macrophages, microglial cells of the nervous system and CD4+ T-cells.

Chronic HIV infection may cause weight loss, fevers and diarrhoea, though such symptoms are more likely to be caused by an opportunistic infection in immunodeficient patients. Effects of worsening HIV infection are an immunodeficiency syndrome, which results in the development of opportunistic infections and tumours, and neurological disease. Neurological disease is a consequence of HIV infection of macrophages and microglial cells in the central and peripheral nervous system.

Diagnosis of HIV infection

A diagnosis of HIV infection can usually be made by demonstrating anti-HIV antibodies in the patient's serum. However, the serological diagnosis of HIV infection can sometimes be problematic.

A small minority of individuals who are not infected by HIV have serum antibodies which are reactive with some HIV proteins, and give false-positive results with some enzyme-linked immunosorbent assays (ELISAs). Many laboratories use two different types of ELISA to identify such sera. To ensure that HIV infection is not incorrectly diagnosed, an antibody test should only be considered positive if antibody is also detected according to defined criteria, using a confirmatory antibody test such as a Western blot immunoassay.[2]

Anti-HIV antibodies may be absent from the serum of patients with acute HIV infection. They are usually detectable by 2–6 weeks after infection, and almost always detectable by 12 weeks. After this time, absence of HIV antibodies excludes HIV infection in all but the most advanced cases of AIDS, or in a patient with an antibody deficiency disease. Sera from patients with acute HIV infection which do not contain anti-HIV antibodies may be positive for p24 antigen (a component of the HIV core proteins) or HIV RNA.

The serological diagnosis of infection with HIVs originating from West Africa can be particularly problematic. Antibodies against HIV-2 may not be detected by assays for HIV-1 antibodies, and it is therefore essential to use an HIV-2-specific antibody assay if HIV-2 infection is a possibility.[3] Furthermore, a subtype of HIV-1, known as subtype O, which is also present in West Africa, may not be detected by ELISAs for HIV-1 or HIV-2 antibodies.[4] Such situations are very uncommon in Australia, Europe and the USA, but infection with HIV-2 or HIV-1 subtype O must be considered in patients from West Africa and their sexual partners.

If HIV-induced immunodeficiency is suspected in a patient with a negative HIV antibody test, or in a patient in whom an HIV antibody test cannot be performed, demonstration of a low blood CD4+ T-cell count is highly suggestive of HIV infection. However, a rare acquired cellular immunodeficiency syndrome characterized by very low CD4+ T-cell counts may also occur in patients without HIV infection.[5]

Monitoring of HIV disease

Immunodeficiency and neurological disease caused by HIV infection usually develop gradually over months to years. It is important to monitor their severity to determine when to commence therapy, and when the patient is susceptible to various disease manifestations.

Measurement of the blood 'HIV load' is a means of demonstrating the severity of HIV infection. This can be done most practically by quantitating HIV RNA in plasma. The blood CD4+ T-cell count or percentage is the best indicator of the severity of HIV-induced immunodeficiency, and the type of infection which is likely to develop, even though the immunodeficiency is not solely caused by CD4+ T-cell depletion. Measurement of the blood CD4+ T-cell count or percentage is therefore very valuable in determining

if the symptoms of an HIV-infected patient are likely to be caused by an opportunistic infection, and if so, what type of infection (see below).

Other investigations provide additional information about the severity of HIV-induced immunopathology. HIV infection causes activation of the immune system, the severity of which can be assessed by measuring serum concentrations of β_2-microglobulin (lymphocyte activation), immunoglobulin A (IgA; B-cell activation), and neopterin (macrophage activation).[6] Measurement of cutaneous delayed-type hypersensitivity (DTH) responses is a means of measuring cellular immune function, and also has clinical utility in some circumstances.[7]

Treatment of HIV infection

Suppression of HIV replication is currently the most effective way of preventing or reversing HIV disease. Whilst augmentation of anti-HIV immunity by vaccination holds promise for the future, the most effective way of doing this at present is to use drugs which impede HIV replication. Two classes of antiretroviral drugs are currently in use – reverse transcriptase inhibitors and protease inhibitors. Reverse transcriptase inhibitors are of two types (Table 60.1). Nucleoside analogues act by substituting for natural nucleosides during HIV replication, thereby inhibiting DNA chain elongation and the effects of the reverse transcriptase enzyme. Non-nucleoside reverse transcriptase inhibitors (NNRTIs) inhibit the reverse transcriptase enzyme by a different mechanism.

All antiretroviral drugs have a limited time of efficacy because the HIV eventually develops resistance to them. The use of drug combinations appears to be more effective than single drugs, partly because drug resistance develops more slowly.

Table 60.1 Antiretroviral drugs used to treat human immunodeficiency virus (HIV) infection

Reverse transcriptase inhibitors
Nucleoside analogues
   Zidovudine (azidothymidine, AZT)
   Didanosine (dideoxyinosine, ddI)
   Zalcitabine (dideoxycytidine, ddC)
   Stavudine (2,3,didehydro-3′-deoxythymidine, d4T)
   Lamivudine (2′-deoxy-3′-thiacytidine, 3TC)
Non-nucleoside reverse transcriptase inhibitors
   Nevirapine
   Loviride
   Delavirdine
Protease inhibitors
   Saquinavir
   Indinavir
   Ritonavir

Adverse effects of antiretroviral drugs are common, and are a cause of morbidity and even mortality. Zidovudine may cause myelosuppression, particularly in severely immunodeficient patients, and a mitochondrial myopathy in patients who have taken therapy for long periods of time.[8] Didanosine may cause pancreatitis which can be fatal, though this is uncommon with the doses which are now used. Both zalcitabine and didanosine may cause a sensorimotor neuropathy which can be severe. Hepatic steatosis with or without lactic acidosis is a rare but potentially fatal complication of treatment with all nucleoside analogues.[9] It probably results from inhibition of mitochondrial DNA function. The most common adverse effect of NNRTIs is a skin rash.

HIV-induced immunodeficiency

Both CD4+ T-cell depletion and the effects of other poorly defined immune defects lead to the development of an immunodeficiency syndrome. This syndrome is characterized by impaired cellular immunity and an increased propensity to opportunistic infection (Table 60.2 and see Chapter 59). In addition, some patients have impaired antibody responses and phagocyte function, which results in infections with encapsulated bacteria and systemic fungal infections.

Mild cellular immunodeficiency

Infectious complications of cellular immunodeficiency may occur when there is relatively mild impairment of cellular immune responses (CD4+ T-cell counts of 200–500/μl). Mucocutaneous infections occur most commonly (Table 60.2) but infections with bacteria such as *Campylobacter jejuni*, *Salmonella* spp. or *Shigella* spp. are a cause of diarrhoea, and occasionally bacteraemia. Most of these infections are not restricted to patients with HIV infection, and are therefore not considered to be AIDS-defining opportunistic infections. However, when they present atypically, are severe or are

Table 60.2 Mucocutaneous opportunistic infections in patients with human immunodeficiency virus (HIV) induced immunodeficiency

Herpes zoster (varicella-zoster virus infection)
Mucosal candidiasis
Oral hairy leukoplakia (Epstein–Barr virus infection)
Seborrhoeic dermatitis (*Pityrosporon* spp. yeast infection)
Molluscum contagiosum (poxvirus infection)
Genital and cutaneous warts (human papillomavirus infection)
Fungal infections of the skin and nails
Recurrent mucocutaneous herpes simplex virus infections
Folliculitis (*Staphylococcus aureus*, *Pityrosporon* spp.)

recurrent, they may be the first indication of underlying HIV-induced immunodeficiency. In contrast to the other infections, oral hairy leukoplakia is almost always indicative of HIV infection.

Infection with *Mycobacterium tuberculosis* may also occur when there is mild immunodeficiency, because of the virulence of this microorganism. Most cases of tuberculosis are the result of reactivation of latent *M. tuberculosis* infection and, therefore, the incidence of tuberculosis in HIV-infected patients is proportional to the rate of endemic infection. For this reason, tuberculosis is particularly common in Africans, Asians and individuals from underprivileged groups in Europe and the USA. In patients with HIV-induced immunodeficiency, tuberculosis often has an atypical presentation which includes extrapulmonary disease.[10]

Severe cellular immunodeficiency

Cellular immunodeficiency which is severe enough to result in an increased propensity to systemic opportunistic infections is often present in patients with a CD4+ T-cell count of <200/μl. Such infections are considered to be indicative of the presence of AIDS.[11] Infection with many different microorganisms may occur, including infection with unusual microorganisms.[12] Only the most common are described here.

Pneumocystis carinii pneumonia (PCP)

Infection of the lungs by *Pneumocystis carinii* causes an interstitial pneumonitis. Patients with this condition usually have a history of dyspnoea, cough, fever and weight loss. Examination often reveals basal pulmonary crackles. The chest X-ray usually shows interstitial infiltrates but is occasionally normal. Other findings which would support a diagnosis of PCP are hypoxaemia, an increased serum lactic dehydrogenase (LDH) concentration, and diffuse uptake of radiolabelled gallium into the lungs on a gallium scan. A definitive diagnosis can be made by demonstrating *Pneumocystis* cysts in an induced sputum specimen, bronchoalveolar lavage fluid or a transbronchial biopsy.[13]

PCP is treated with co-trimoxazole (trimethoprim–sulphamethoxazole), given orally or IV depending on severity. However, many patients develop a hypersensitivity reaction, and alternative medications, including oral dapsone and trimethoprim, or IV pentamidine have to be used.[14] Steroid therapy should also be used if the Pao_2 is < 70 mmHg (9.3 kPa).[15]

Respiratory failure complicating PCP is the most common reason for admitting an HIV-infected patient to an ICU. Survival following ventilation for PCP was poor in the early 1980s, but improved later in the decade, probably as a result of improved treatment and selection of patients.[16,17] In recent years, survival has worsened again, particularly for patients with a CD4+ T-cell count of <50/μl and for those who develop pneumothorax as a result of barotrauma.[17] The poor outcome in recent years may reflect the fact that patients are living longer because of improved therapy, and are hence often more immunodeficient when PCP develops. Whatever the cause, the cost-effectiveness of treating patients with PCP is now being scrutinized,[17] and it is important to select patients for ventilation carefully. A first episode of PCP, a CD4+ T-cell count of $> 50/\mu l$, and no previous antiretroviral therapy are all favourable factors. Furthermore, ventilation may be avoided by the use of continuous positive airways pressure (CPAP) or bi-level positive airways pressure, thereby reducing the risks of a pneumothorax, airway obstruction and nosocomial infection.[18,19]

Pneumocystis infection can be prevented by prophylactic medications. All patients with a CD4+ T-cell count of $< 200/\mu l$ should be offered prophylaxis. The most effective drug is co-trimoxazole. Alternatives for patients who are sensitive to co-trimoxazole include dapsone with trimethoprim or pyrimethamine, or inhaled pentamidine.[20]

Oesophageal candidiasis

Candida infection of the oesophageal mucosa presents with odynophagia and dysphagia. The occurrence of such symptoms in association with oral candidiasis is usually sufficient to make a presumptive diagnosis of oesophageal candidiasis and to start treatment. An azole such as ketoconazole or fluconazole is usually used.[21] If there is no response to treatment, endoscopy should be performed to exclude other causes of odynophagia.

Cryptococcal meningitis

Meningitis is the most common manifestation of infection with *Cryptococcus neoformans* in patients with AIDS.[22] It usually presents with headache and fever, but sometimes confusion or behavioural abnormalities are predominant abnormalities. Neck stiffness is often minimal or absent. Cerebrospinal fluid examination may reveal little evidence of inflammation, particularly in the most severe cases, but cryptococcal antigen is virtually always present and cultures for cryptococci are positive. Most patients also have cryptococcal antigen in their serum. Intravenous amphotericin is the treatment of choice, and must be followed by permanent suppressive therapy to prevent relapses. Oral fluconazole or, if that fails, intermittent IV amphotericin are the most effective suppressive therapies.[23]

Toxoplasma encephalitis

Reactivation of *Toxoplasma gondii* infection most commonly presents as a focal encephalitis.[24] This may cause headaches, fever, focal neurological deficits, convulsions and even coma. One or more brain lesions may be present. They usually produce ring-enhancing lesions with surrounding oedema on a brain computed tomography (CT) scan, and can occur in many sites, with a predilection for the basal ganglia. Evidence of previous *Toxoplasma* infection is present in virtually all patients, and absence of serum *Toxoplasma* antibody essentially excludes the diagnosis. Treatment is with IV sulphadiazine or clindamycin and oral pyrimethamine. Hypersensitivity reactions to sulphadiazine and clindamycin are common, and an alternative drug regimen may be necessary.[14] A brain CT scan should be repeated after 2–3 weeks of therapy, and an alternative diagnosis considered if there has been no resolution of the lesions. Cerebral lymphoma can produce very similar lesions to *Toxoplasma* encephalitis. A brain biopsy may be necessary to make the diagnosis.

Very severe cellular immunodeficiency

Other systemic infections occur in patients with very severe immunodeficiency (CD4+ T-cell count $< 50/\mu l$).

Cytomegalovirus (CMV) infection

The most common site for reactivation of CMV infection is the retina. CMV retinitis usually presents with blurred vision, visual field loss or 'floaters'. Diagnosis is by fundoscopy and confirmation by an ophthalmologist should be undertaken. Treatment is with IV ganciclovir or foscarnet, followed by lifelong suppressive therapy to prevent relapses.[25]

CMV infection less commonly presents with infection of other organs, particularly the oesophagus, bile ducts, colon or lungs. Biopsy of affected tissue is necessary to make a definitive diagnosis, but presence of CMV antigens in blood leukocytes provides support for a diagnosis, whereas failure to culture CMV from urine argues against it.

Cryptosporidiosis

Infection of the gastrointestinal tract by *Cryptosporidium parvum* causes a severe and intractable secretory diarrhoea, which is often associated with a malabsorbtion syndrome.[26] It can also cause cholangitis. Diagnosis is by demonstrating *Cryptosporidium* oocysts in faeces and/or a rectal or duodenal biopsy. There is no satisfactory treatment, but paromomycin is of use in some patients.

Mycobacterium avium complex infection

Infection with *Mycobacterium avium* complex (MAC) is usually disseminated and affects blood leukocytes, liver, spleen and lymph nodes, and the gastrointestinal tract.[27] This infection often results in weight loss, fatigue, fevers, anaemia and diarrhoea. The diagnosis is usually made by culturing MAC from blood, but sometimes stool microscopy and culture or biopsy of affected tissues are necessary. Treatment with multiple drug therapy is often successful. Commonly used drugs are clarithromycin, rifabutin, ethambutol.

Infectious complications of other immune defects

Some infections appear to develop as a consequence of impaired antibody-mediated immunity or phagocyte defects. Acute infection of the respiratory tract by *Haemophilus influenzae* and *Streptococcus pneumoniae* occurs particularly in injecting drug users, the elderly and children.[28,29] These infections may occur long before the onset of symptomatic cellular immunodeficiency. In contrast, infections with *Pseudomonas aeruginosa* are most common in patients with advanced HIV disease, particularly those with neutropenia.[30] Infection of the respiratory tract by *Aspergillus* spp. and some other uncommon fungi may also occur in patients who are neutropenic.[31]

Chronic infections of the respiratory tract are a common and often difficult problem to manage in patients with advanced HIV disease. Nasal sinusitis causes headaches and fever, and may be associated with chronic suppurative bronchitis or bronchiectasis.[32] Infection of the sinuses by *H. influenzae*, pneumococci or *Pseudomonas* is the most common cause, but infection with *Aspergillus* or other fungi also occurs. A CT scan of the sinuses is the most sensitive radiological investigation. Treatment is with antibiotics or antifungal drugs and nasal decongestants. Drainage of the sinuses and microbiological examination of the sinus contents may be necessary if there is no response to therapy.

HIV-associated neoplasms

Certain neoplasms are a characteristic complication of cellular immunodeficiency diseases, including HIV-induced immunodeficiency. Uncontrolled replication of an additional microorganism resulting from the immunodeficiency is probably involved in the pathogenesis of all of these neoplasms.

Kaposi's sarcoma (KS) is an angioproliferative tumour which originates from vascular endothelium.[33] There is much evidence implicating an infectious agent in the pathogenesis of KS. This has recently been identified as a herpesvirus (Human Herpesvirus 8; HHV8). KS usually presents as skin lesions which have a reddish-brown colour. They vary in extent from one or two small papules to numerous bulbous lesions. The mucosal surface of the gastrointestinal tract, lymph nodes and, rarely, internal organs may also be involved. A clinical diagnosis of KS can be confirmed by biopsy of a lesion. KS may be a complication of any degree of immunodeficiency (CD4+ T-cell count $< 500 \times 10^6/\mu l$) but occurs most often in patients with moderate to severe immunodeficiency.

Lymphomas are also a complication of HIV-induced immunodeficiency.[34] The great majority are B-cell lymphomas, and reactivation of Epstein–Barr virus infection is implicated in the pathogenesis of many cases. Primary cerebral lymphoma or extracerebral lymphoma with frequent extranodal involvement are common in patients with severe immunodeficiency. These lymphomas are usually high-grade with poor prognosis. Low-grade lymphomas occur less commonly in patients with mild immunodeficiency, and are associated with a better prognosis.

Cervical intraepithelial neoplasia (CIN) is more common than normal in women with HIV infection. This is presumably because human papillomavirus (HPV) infection is more likely to be present in women with HIV infection, and the cellular immunodeficiency permits HPV replication. As a consequence, the incidence of cervical carcinoma appears to be increased in HIV-infected women.

HIV-associated neurological disease

In addition to opportunistic infections of the nervous system in patients with AIDS, HIV infection of macrophages and microglial cells in the nervous system often results in neurological disease by incompletely understood mechanisms.[35] Encephalopathy, myelopathy, peripheral neuropathy or myopathy are all possible, and in a small number of patients, the neurological disease is more problematical than the immunodeficiency. The encephalopathy usually develops insidiously and eventually results in cognitive, motor and behavioural abnormalities. Myelopathy results in an ataxic spastic paraparesis, which is often associated with bladder dysfunction.

HIV infection and AIDS in the ICU

Although AIDS remains an incurable disease, the admission of a patient with AIDS to an ICU is indicated in some circumstances.[16] The most common indications are:

1 respiratory failure complicating PCP;
2 coma or convulsions complicating opportunistic infections or tumours of the brain;
3 non-HIV-related conditions such as a self-poisoning.

Selection of patients for intensive care is important.[16,17] In the case of PCP and respiratory failure, the blood CD4+ T-cell count is valuable in predicting outcome (see above[17]). However, the only indicator of outcome of coma or convulsions apears to be the severity of the neurological deficit.[36]

Patients with unrecognized HIV infection or AIDS may also be admitted to an ICU with the first manifestation of HIV disease. It is therefore important for all ICU staff to practise stringent infection control procedures at all times.

References

1. Tindall B and Cooper DA (1991) Primary HIV infection: host responses and intervention strategies. *AIDS* **5**:1–14.
2. Robertson P and Dwyer D (1993) Western blot assay. In: Lee N (ed.) *Clinical Microbiology Update No. 35*. Sydney: University of New South Wales, pp. 9–16.
3. O'Brien TR, George JR and Holmberg D (1992) Human immunodeficiency virus type 2 infection in the United States: epidemiology, diagnosis, and public health implications. *J Am Med Assoc* **20**:2775–2776.
4. Loussert-Ajaka I, Ly TD, Chaix ML *et al.* (1994) HIV-1/HIV-2 seronegativity in HIV-1 subtype O infected patients. *Lancet* **343**:1393–1394.
5. Smith DK, Joyce JN, Holmberg SC and the Centers for Disease Control idiopathic CD4 + T-lymphocytopenia task force (1993) Unexplained opportunistic infections and CD4+ T-lymphocytopenia without HIV infection. *N Engl J Med* **328**:373–379.
6. Fahey JL, Taylor JMG, Detels R *et al.* (1990) The prognostic value of cellular and serologic markers in infection with human immunodeficiency virus type 1. *N Engl J Med* **322**:166–172.
7. Gordin FM, Hartigan PM, Klimas NG *et al.* (1994) Delayed-type hypersensitivity skin tests are an independent predictor of human immunodeficiency virus disease progression. *J Infect Dis* **169**:893–897.
8. Peters BS, Winer DN, Landon DN *et al.* (1993) Mitochondrial myopathy associated with chronic zidovudine therapy in AIDS. *Q J Med* **86**:5–15.
9. Freiman JP, Helfert KE, Hamrell MR and Stein DS (1993) Hepatomegaly with severe steatosis in HIV-seropositive patients. *AIDS* **7**:379–385.
10. Dupon M and Ragnaud JM (1992) Tuberculosis in patients infected with human immunodeficiency virus 1: a retrospective multicentre study in 123 cases in France. *Q J Med* **306**:719–730.
11. Centers for Disease Control and Prevention (CDC) (1992) 1993 revised classification system for HIV infection and expanded surveillance case definition for AIDS among adolescents and adults. *MMWR* **41**:1–18.
12. Gradon JD, Timpone JG and Schnittman SM (1992) Emergence of unusual opportunistic pathogens in AIDS: a review. *Clin Infect Dis* **15**:134–157.
13. Miller RF, Leigh TR, Collins JV and Mitchell DM (1990) Tests giving an aetiological diagnosis in pulmonary disease in patients infected with HIV. In: Mitchell D and Woodcock A (eds) *AIDS and the Lung*. London: British Medical Journal, pp. 26–36.
14. Lane HC, Laughon BE, Falloon J *et al.* Recent advances in the management of AIDS-related opportunistic infections. *Ann Intern Med* **120**:945–955.
15. The National Institutes of Health–University of California expert panel for corticosteroids as adjunctive therapy for *Pneumocystis* pneumonia (1990) Consensus statement on the use of corticosteroids as adjunctive therapy for *Pneumocystis* pneumonia in the acquired immunodeficiency syndrome. *N Engl J Med* **323** 1500–1504.
16. Wachter RM, Luce JM and Hopewell PC (1992) Critical care of patients with AIDS. *J Am Med Assoc* **267**:541–547.
17. Wachter RM, Luce JM, Safrin S *et al.* (1995) Cost and outcome of intensive care for patients with AIDS, *Pneumocystis carinii* pneumonia, and severe respiratory failure. *J Am Med Assoc* **273**:230–235.
18. Gachot R, Clair B, Wolff M *et al.* (1992) Continuous positive airway pressure by face mask or mechanical ventilation in patients with human immunodeficiency virus infection and severe *Pneumocystis carinii* pneumonia. *Intensive Care Med* **18**:55–159.
19. DeVita MA, Friedman Y and Petrella V (1993) Mask continuous positive airway pressure in AIDS. *Crit Care Clin* **9**:137–151.
20. Gallant JE, Moore RD and Chaisson RE (1994) Prophylaxis for opportunistic infections in patients with HIV infection. *Ann Intern Med* **120**:932–944.
21. Laine L, Dretler RH, Conteas CN *et al.* (1992) Fluconazole compared with ketoconazole for the treatment of *Candida* esophagitis in AIDS: a randomized trial. *Ann Intern Med* **117**:655–660.
22. Dismukes WE (1988) Cryptococcal meningitis in patients with AIDS. *J Infect Dis* **157**:624–628.
23. Powderly WG, Sagg MS, Cloud GA *et al.* (1992) A controlled trial of fluconazole or amphotericin B to prevent relapse of cryptococcal meningitis in patients with the acquired immunodeficiency syndrome. *N Engl J Med* **326**:793–798.
24. Porter SB and Sande M (1992) Toxoplasmosis of the central nervous system in the acquired immunodeficiency syndrome. *N Engl J Med* **327**:1643–1648.
25. Drew WL (1992) Cytomegalovirus infection in patients with AIDS. *Clin Infect Dis* **14**:608–615.
26. Peterson C (1992) Cryptosporidiosis in patients infected with the human immunodeficiency virus. *Clin Infect Dis* **15**:903–909.
27. Benson CA and Ellner JJ (1993) *Mycobacterium avium* complex infection and AIDS: advances in theory and practice. *Clin Infect Dis* **17**:7–20.
28. Casadevall A, Dobroszycki J, Small C and Pirofski LA (1992) *Haemophilus influenzae* type b bacteremia in adults with AIDS and at risk for AIDS. *Am J Med* **92**:587–590.
29. Janoff EN, Breiman RF, Daley CL and Hopewell PC (1992) Pneumococcal disease during HIV infection: epidemiologic, clinical, and immunologic perspectives. *Ann Intern Med* **117**:314–334.
30. Mendelson MH, Gurtman A, Szabo S *et al.* (1994) *Pseudomonas aeruginosa* bacteremia in patients with AIDS. *Clin Infect Dis* **18**:886–895.
31. Pursell KJ, Telzak E and Armstrong D (1992) *Aspergillus* species colonization and invasive disease in patients with AIDS. *Clin Infect Dis* **14**:141–148.
32. Zurlo JJ, Irwin MF, Lebovics R and Lane HC (1992) Sinusitis in HIV-1 infection. *Am J Med* **93**:157–159.
33. Lilenbaum RC and Ratner L (1994) Systemic treatment of Kaposi's sarcoma: current status and future directions. *AIDS* **8**:141–151.
34. Shibata D (1994) Biologic aspects of AIDS-related lymphoma. *Curr Opin Oncol* **6**:503–507.
35. McArthur JC (1987) Neurologic manifestations of AIDS. *Medicine* **66**:407–437.
36. Bedos JP, Chastang C, Lucet JC *et al.* (1995) Early predictors of outcome for HIV patients with neurological failure. *J Am Med Assoc* **273**:35–40.

61   Severe sepsis

GM Clarke

Sepsis has traditionally implied infection accompanied by systemic inflammatory manifestations. However, the systemic changes are indistinguishable from those of non-infective inflammatory conditions (e.g. pancreatitis, acute hepatic failure, immunological reactions and gross trauma including burns). Consequently, much confusion arose when terms such as sepsis and septic syndrome were applied to these conditions.[1] This led to a consensus conference of the American College of Chest Physicians and Society of Critical Care Medicine to define terms related to infection and the systemic response (Table 61.1; Fig. 61.1).[2] Thus, sepsis is the systemic inflammatory response to infection. It is the commonest contributor to death in the ICU.[3]

Aetiology and epidemiology

Sepsis may be caused by Gram-negative and Gram-positive bacteria, fungi, *Rickettsia*, viruses and spirochaetes. In the ICU, common infective Gram-negative organisms include *Escherichia coli*, *Pseudomonas*, *Klebsiella*, *Proteus*, *Enterobacter* and *Bacteroides*; Gram-positive organisms include staphylococci, streptococci and *Clostridium*. Systemic infection with fungi, especially *Candida*, is a risk in immunodeficient patients receiving broad-spectrum antibiotics. The EPIC study reported that 17% of ICU patients had fungal and/or protozoal infection.[4]

Nosocomial infection rates in ICU patients are 5–10 times higher than among general ward patients. Organisms posing serious resistance problems in the ICU setting include methicillin-resistant staphylococci, enterococci, certain Enterobacteriaceae, *Pseudomonas aeruginosa*, *P. cepacia*, *Xanthomonas maltophilia*, *Acinetobacter* and *Candida* species.[5]

Many infections acquired in the ICU are endogenous and follow colonization of the alimentary tract by organisms usually insignificant in healthy individuals (e.g. *E. coli*, *Klebsiella*, *Proteus* and *Pseudomonas*).[6] Sepsis related to intravascular catheters is commonly due to *Staphylococcus epidermidis*, a normal skin commensal.

Pathogenesis

The host response, rather than the infecting organism, predominantly determines the severity of an infection.[7] Pathogenesis of the extremely complex systemic inflammatory response involves host defence mechanisms, products of infecting organisms (e.g. exotoxins and endotoxins) and a multitude of mediators (Fig. 61.2).

Host defence mechanisms

Local organ defences

These may be impaired by critical illness or therapeutic interventions.

Respiratory system
Coughing may be impaired by pain, illness or drugs. The mucociliary escalator system may be depressed by opioids, aspirin, inspired oxygen, inadequate humidification or endotracheal suctioning. Laryngeal dysfunction, from neurological dysfunction, drugs or nasogastric or endotracheal tubes, can lead to aspiration.

Alimentary tract
Gastrointestinal tract (GIT) mucosa and motility, secretion of mucus and immunoglobulin A, and indigenous anaerobes resist gut colonization by aerobic bacteria.[6] GIT flora may rapidly alter in the ICU patient. Following hospitalization, mouth flora changes from predominantly anaerobic to Gram-negative organisms such as *E. coli*, *Klebsiella* and *Pseudomonas*. *Staphylococcus aureus* and *Candida albicans* may become part of the flora. The stomach, which is normally sterile, becomes colonized with similar organisms if the gastric pH is above 4.0 –

Table 61.1 Definitions of sepsis[2]

Infection
Microbial phenomenon characterized by an inflammatory response to the presence of microorganisms or the invasion of normally sterile host tissue by those organisms

Bacteraemia
The presence of viable bacteria in the blood

Systemic inflammatory response syndrome SIRS
The systemic inflammatory response to a variety of severe clinical insults. The response is manifested by two or more of the following conditions:
   Temperature >38°C or <36°C
   Heart rate >90 beats/min
   Respiratory rate >20 breaths/min or $Paco_2$ <4.3 kPa (<32 Torr)
   White blood cell count >12 000 cells/mm^3, or >10% immature (band) forms

Sepsis
The systemic response to infection. This systemic response is manifested by two or more of the following conditions as a result of infection:
   Temperature >38°C or <36°C
   Heart rate >90 beats/min
   Respiratory rate >20 breaths/min or $Paco_2$ <4.3 kPa (<32 Torr)
   White blood cell count >12 000 cells/mm^3, or >10% immature (band) forms

Severe sepsis
Sepsis associated with organ dysfunction, hypoperfusion or hypotension. Hypoperfusion and perfusion abnormalities may include, but are not limited to, lactic acidosis, oliguria or an acute alteration in mental status

Septic shock
Sepsis with hypotension, despite adequate fluid resuscitation, along with the presence of perfusion abnormalities that may include, but are not limited to, lactic acidosis, oliguria or an acute alteration in mental status. Patients who are on inotropic or vasopressor agents may not be hypotensive at the time when perfusion abnormalities are measured

Hypotension
A systolic blood pressure of <90 mmHg or a reduction of >40 mmHg from baseline in the absence of other causes for hypotension

Multiple organ dysfunction syndrome MODS
Presence of altered organ function in an acutely ill patient such that homeostasis cannot be maintained without intervention.

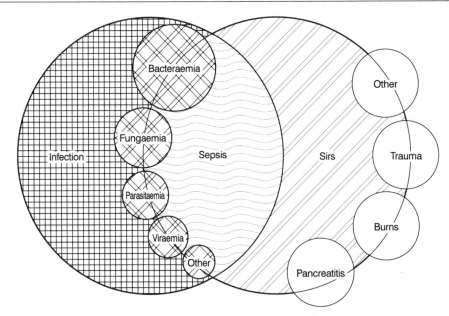

Fig. 61.1 Interrelationship of systemic inflammatory response syndrome (SIRS), sepsis and infection. From American College of Chest Physicians/Society of Critical Care Medicine,[2] with permission.

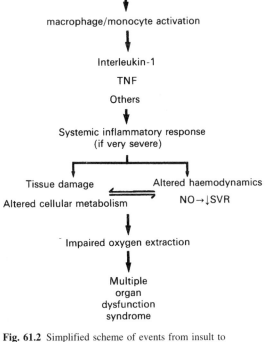

Insult

↓

macrophage/monocyte activation

↓

Interleukin-1

TNF

Others

↓

Systemic inflammatory response
(if very severe)

Tissue damage   Altered haemodynamics

Altered cellular metabolism   NO→↓SVR

↓

Impaired oxygen extraction

↓

Multiple
organ
dysfunction
syndrome

Fig. 61.2 Simplified scheme of events from insult to systemic inflammatory response to multiple organ dysfunction syndrome. TNF = Tumour necrosis factor; NO = nitric oxide; SVR = systemic vascular resistance.

likely if antacids or H_2-blockers are prescribed. Antibiotics rapidly alter normal gut flora. Overgrowth of *Candida* is common; overgrowth with *Clostridium difficile* in the large bowel, though uncommon, may cause pseudomembranous colitis due to its toxins.

Eyes
Impaired blinking results in drying of cornea and conjunctiva. Loss of the irrigating and antibacterial properties of tears predisposes to infection.

Genitourinary tract
The urethral catheter is a common route of urinary tract infection, especially by perineal faecal bacteria.

Skin
This may be breached by invasive catheters, all of which increase the risk of infection from skin organisms.

General body defence mechanisms

Defects in immune competence are frequently seen in the critically ill (see Chapters 59 and 90). Some defects are set out below, but considerable overlap and interaction occur.

Reticuloendothelial system
Reticuloendothelial blockade results in defective phagocytic activity. This is partly related to lowered opsonic activity (i.e. promotion of phagocytosis is decreased). Sepsis itself can result in consumption of opsonic proteins, termed consumptive opsoninopathy. Apart from diminished phagocytic activity, defects in polymorph chemotaxis and intracellular killing may be present.

Cell-mediated immunity
Anergy (failure of delayed hypersensitivity), possibly reflecting defective T-helper cell function, has proven to be a marker for altered host resistance, sepsis and mortality in surgical patients.[8] Age, cancer, sepsis, major trauma, malnutrition and increased T-suppressor cell activity have been implicated.[8] The presence of a T-cell suppressive factor (possibly a peptide) has been demonstrated in sera of trauma and cancer patients.[9] Steroids, immunosuppressive agents, halothane and antibiotics (e.g. tetracycline, chloramphenicol and clindamycin) may impair cellular immunity. Protein-calorie malnutrition may be associated with anergy, diminished complement levels and impaired immunoglobulin synthesis.[10]

Infections by well-encapsulated bacteria (e.g. staphylococci and streptococci) are generally handled by humoral defence mechanisms. Cell-mediated immunity is important in infections by poorly encapsulated Gram-negative organisms, such as *Pseudomonas* and intestinal anaerobes – common causes of severe sepsis in the critically ill.

Humoral immunity
Defects in humoral immunity are seen in postsplenectomy patients.[11] Immunoglobulin (especially immunoglobulin M; IgM) and complement deficiencies and diminished properdin activity have been reported in these patients. The latter alternative complement pathway factor is important, as pneumococci are more efficiently opsonized via the alternative pathway in the immunedeficient host. The asplenic patient is thus predisposed to overwhelming bacterial sepsis, with pneumococci, *Neisseria meningitidis*, *E. coli*, *Haemophilus influenzae* and *Staphylococcus aureus* having been reported. The risk of splenectomy-associated sepsis is considerably higher in trauma than in Hodgkin's disease, idiopathic thrombocytopenia and acquired haemolytic anaemic.

Exotoxins

Exotoxins are products of microorganisms harmful to the host, usually being high-molecular-weight, heat-labile and antigenic proteins. (The toxins of *Staphylococcus* are poorly antigenic; fungal toxins are non-antigenic of low molecular weight.[12])

Some bacteria produce only one significant toxin to cause disease (e.g. tetanus, diphtheria, cholera and botulism). Other bacteria may produce an array of toxins, the significance and action of many being ill understood (e.g. *Staphylococcus, Streptococcus* and *Clostridiun perfringens*). A group may harm the host through the actions of both exotoxins and endotoxins (e.g. *Pseudomonas*).

Endotoxin

Endotoxin is part of the outer membrane of Gram-negative bacteria. Whereas exotoxins are heat-labile proteins, endotoxin is a lipopolysaccharide (LPS) and is much more heat-stable. LPS is known to consist of:

1 a lipid moiety (lipid A) which is responsible for most, if not all of the biological activity of bacterial endotoxin;
2 a core polysaccharide;
3 oligosaccharide side chains which confer O-antigen specificity to the molecule and differ widely from strain to strain.

However, core polysaccharide–lipid A complexes of most Gram-negative bacteria are very similar in structure. Reasons given for implicating LPS in the pathophysiology of Gram-negative sepsis include the following:

1 Endotoxins on the surface of circulating bacteria are in a position to activate biological mediators of shock, even if endotoxin is below detectable levels.
2 Clinical features of Gram-negative bacteraemia are identical to the effects of endotoxin administered IV.
3 Antibiotics cannot reverse, and may possibly even aggravate, these features when bacteria are killed.[13]

Mediators[14]

There are over 100 known mediators which may be involved in the systemic inflammatory response. Known important ones are listed in Table 61.2. Some cytokines exist in both circulatory and cell-associated forms (e.g. interleukin-1 (IL-1), tumour necrosis factor (TNF)). Actions and interactions are complex, with some mediators inducing the release of others. A variety of feedback systems moderate the whole response. Primary mediators such as TNF can induce toxic responses by activating neutrophils and the coagulation system, and endothelial cells to produce nitric oxide (NO; see below). Natural inhibitors also exist, e.g. C1-esterase inhibitors, soluble TNF receptors and IL-1 receptor antagonists (IL-1ra). IL-10 is a potent macrophage-deactivating factor inhibiting the production of TNF and interferon-γ (IFN-γ). IL-4, being a primary B-cell stimulant, reduces IL-1 and TNF production, and is thus anti-inflammatory.

Table 61.2 Important mediators in severe sepsis

Cytokines (e.g. tumour necrosis factor, interleukins, interferon-γ)

Complement system

Contact system and extrinsic pathways of coagulation

Fibrinolytic system

Cells such as mononuclears, macrophages, microphages (predominantly neutrophils), endothelial cells and platelets

Prostaglandin

Leukotrienes

Platelet-activating factor

Oxygen free radicals

Proteases

Nitric oxide

Cardiovascular pathophysiology

The systemic response of sepsis has significant cardiovascular effects which reflect some of the pathogenetic mechanisms.

Systemic vascular resistance

Severe sepsis is commonly associated with a decreased systemic vascular resistance index (SVRI), which results in hypotension despite a normal or increased cardiac index (CI).[15] This is now believed to be due principally to NO production in endothelial and vascular smooth muscle cells, via NO synthase, an enzyme that can be induced by endotoxin and certain cytokines (e.g. IFN-γ, TNF and some interleukins).[16] Other mediators implicated include histamine, β-endorphins, decreased C3 complement, C3 proactivator and decreased prekallikrein.[17] Most non-survivors of severe sepsis show persistent vasodilation with refractory hypotension.

Venous capacitance

Increased venous capacitance, due to decreased venous tone (probably due to increased NO production), results in relative hypovolaemia.

Pulmonary vascular resistance (PVR)

PVR may be normal initially, but frequently rises at a later stage of sepsis.[18] The mechanisms of increased PVR are ill understood; PVR may still be increased in the absence of hypoxaemia or acidosis. Postulated causative factors include microthrombi, vasoactive amine, endotoxin, angiotensin, platelet-activating factor (PAF), thromboxane A_2 and endothelin-1. Increased PVR has been associated with increased mortality.[18]

Capillary permeability

Capillary permeability of both systemic and pulmonary capillary beds may increase rapidly so that fluid is lost from the circulation. Clearance of radio-iodinated serum albumin has been shown to increase from a normal of 5–10%/h to 20–35%/h in severe sepsis.[19]

Myocardial function

Myocardial dysfunction is common with severe sepsis and is usually associated with high mortality. Radionuclide scans showed that survivors had an initially depressed biventricular ejection fraction with biventricular dilatation.[20] These changes returned towards normal over 7–10 days with recovery. Non-survivors had minimally increased biventricular ejection fraction and ventricular size, without significant change over time, and most died of refractory hypotension. Why functionally worse patients paradoxically survived is not clear; ventricular dilatation may be a beneficial compensatory mechanism to improve stroke volume.

Possible causes of myocardial dysfunction include a myocardial depressant factor (MDF) and dimin-ished coronary blood flow.[17] The latter is not supported by coronary sinus catheter studies reporting normal myocardial blood flow and increased myocardial lactate uptake.[21,22] Systemic acidosis and hypoxaemia will have added deleterious effects on myocardial function. Some mediators (e.g. TNF and PAF) directly or indirectly depress the myocardium. TNF and IL-1 inhibit myocardial responses to β-adrenergic stimulation.[14] *In vitro* studies have also implicated NO.[23]

Global oxygen transport and consumption

In severe sepsis, and especially in septic shock, there are major disturbances in oxygen transport and consumption. Correction of hypovolaemia usually results in a hyperdynamic circulation – high CI and low SVRI. Oxygen consumption (Vo_2) is frequently normal or decreased relative to metabolic demands.[24]

None the less, the presence of hyperlactic acidaemia suggests inadequate oxygen delivery (Do_2) and utilization in some regional vascular beds.[25,26] Decreased oxygen extraction (i.e. increased mixed venous oxygen saturation with decreased arterio-venous oxygen difference) is a common finding. This may result from peripheral arteriovenous shunts (due to maldistribution of blood flow secondary to impaired vasoregulation and interstitial oedema), and cellular metabolic defects limiting the cell's ability to utilize oxygen.

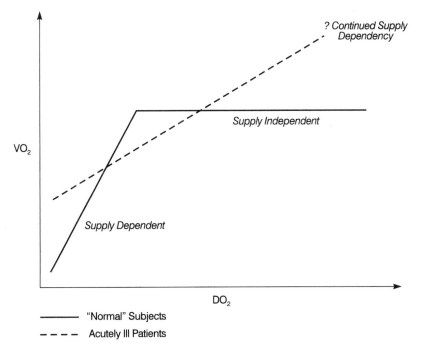

Fig. 61.3 Relationship of oxygen consumption (Vo_2) to oxygen delivery (Do_2).

The concept of pathological supply dependency of oxygen uptake (reflected by V_{O_2}) on oxygen delivery has been proposed in sepsis (Fig. 61.3).[27,28] V_{O_2} is dependent on D_{O_2}, denoting inadequate oxygen supply to tissue. Thus, the implication is to use high (supranormal) D_{O_2} and haemodynamic values as therapeutic targets (see below). However, this supply dependency concept has not been demonstrated in more recent studies (see below and Chapter 22). Also, should oxygen demand vary (as it does in a febrile, septic, restless patient) then oxygen supply is expected to co-vary, i.e. D_{O_2} would follow or be dependent upon V_{O_2} (as in exercise), and not the other way around.[29]

Regional perfusion and oxygen consumption

Regional changes in oxygen transport in septic shock cannot be predicted from whole-body changes. Splanchnic blood flow, oxygen extraction and V_{O_2} can increase during the acute phase of septic shock, despite reduced whole-body oxygen extraction.[30] This marked splanchnic hypermetabolism may contribute to a regional mismatch between oxygen demand and supply. Noradrenaline produces a more favourable splanchnic haemodynamic profile than dopamine,[31] with increased gastric intramucosal pH (pHi), indicating improved regional oxygen utilization. Dopamine, while increasing splanchnic blood flow, decreases pHi, indicating an uncompensated increase in regional oxygen requirements.[31]

Clinical presentation

Sepsis, severe sepsis and septic shock (Table 61.1) are stages in a spectrum of pathophysiological disturbances in the infected patient. Sepsis is common and can present many faces. Many septic patients are referred to the ICU with such labels as cardiogenic shock, pulmonary embolism, hypovolaemic shock, profound hypothermia and haemolytic–uraemic syndrome. Conversely, there are many causes of systemic inflammatory response syndrome (SIRS) and multiple organ dysfunction syndrome (MODS) other than sepsis. However, as sepsis requires specific therapy, the patient with signs consistent with sepsis should be considered as being infected until proven otherwise.

Sepsis may present with a wide spectrum of manifestations. Body temperature may be normal, increased or decreased. Tachycardia and tachypnoea are common. A leukocytosis and increased numbers of immature (band) forms is usual, although leukopenia may be seen. Other signs and symptoms may relate to the site of infection (e.g. productive cough, dyspnoea, cyanosis and pleuritic pain with pneumonia). Other features often relate to organ dysfunction (MODS), e.g. encephalopathy, renal impairment and gut dysfunction. Coagulopathy is occasionally present. Glucose intolerance is common, although if hepatic dysfunction is present, hypoglycaemia may occasionally occur.

The picture of a septic patient with warm skin, bounding pulses and a hyperdynamic circulation is not always present. Hypotension, vasoconstriction and peripheral cyanosis (i.e. cold shock) may present if the patient is hypovolaemic, has pre-existing myocardial dysfunction, or has been referred late.

Management

Septic shock has a high mortality rate and efforts should be made to diagnose and treat sepsis before shock occurs. As with any critically ill patient, these management principles are important:

1 initial assessment with resuscitation;
2 steps to ensure adequate oxygen delivery to meet oxygen demands (Table 61.3);
3 attempts to diagnose and eradicate the cause of illness.

General measures

Oxygenation and ventilation

Hypoxaemia is common. If oxygen by mask is inadequate, then continuous positive airway pressure (CPAP) by mask may be employed. Where respiratory failure is severe, endotracheal intubation and either CPAP or mechanical ventilatory support is necessary. An adequate haemoglobin level must also be maintained.

Table 61.3 General measures in septic shock

Administer oxygen, ventilatory support if indicated
Basic clinical monitoring
    ECG, systemic arterial pressure (SAP)
    Central venous pressure (CVP)
    Pulmonary artery pressure (PAP)
    Pulmonary capillary wedge pressure (PCWP)
    Cardiac output (CO)
    Oxygen delivery (D_{O_2})
    Temperature, urine output
Chest X-ray
Basic laboratory monitoring
    Arterial blood gas/acid–base
    Lactate
    Electrolytes, creatinine
    Blood sugar, haemoglobin
    Platelet and white blood cell count
    INR
    Liver function tests

ECG = Electrocardiogram; INR = international normalized ratio.

Clinical monitoring and intervention

A central venous (preferably multi-lumen) and arterial line and a urethral catheter are inserted. Heart rate, rhythm, mean arterial pressure (MAP), central venous pressure (CVP) and urine output are continuously monitored.

Haemodynamic manipulation

There is no consensus view on the correct haemodynamic goals in septic shock, but a plan of haemodynamic management is needed. Tachycardia is common in sepsis, so increasing heart rate is usually not an issue. Volume loading is usually with colloids, such as 5% albumin or Haemaccel (1–2 l) followed by normal saline. If MAP is inadequate (i.e. <65–80 mmHg or 8.6–10.6 kPa) despite attaining a CVP of 15 cm H_2O (10–12 mmHg or 1.3–1.6 kPa), an inotrope infusion should be started – usually adrenaline initially, at 5 μg/kg per min and varying the dose as necessary. A pulmonary artery catheter should be inserted to monitor pulmonary capillary wedge pressure (PCWP), CI and SVRI, if inotropes are started. Volume loading is continued if necessary, to a PCWP of 12 mmHg (1.6 kPa). A PCWP of 10–12 mmHg (1.3–1.6 kPa) is associated with peak left ventricular stroke work and CI in septic patients.[32] Sustained PCWP over 12 mmHg (1.6 kPa) may lead to pulmonary oedema due to increased pulmonary capillary leak.

An adequate MAP (i.e. 65–80 mmHg or 8.6–10.6 kPa) and CI (>4.0) should be aimed for. Blood pressure is important; blood flow to most organs is pressure-dependent, and autoregulation is probably lost with the profound vasodilatation in septic shock. Arterial pressure and SVRI have been shown to correlate directly with survival in septic shock.[33,34] Noradrenaline vasopressor is reported to improve SVRI, blood pressure, regional blood flow, oxygen extraction and urine output.[30,31,35] Haemoglobin concentration should be maintained above 10 g/dl for adequate Do_2. Haemodynamic interventions should avoid:

1 overdriving the heart with excessive catecholamines which are cardiotoxic, arrhythmogenic and increase oxygen requirements;
2 using inappropriate agents, e.g. dobutamine (an inodilator) instead of noradrenaline in a patient with profoundly low SVRI.

Afterload reduction to improve right ventricular function is a consideration in pulmonary hypertension, which is associated with a high mortality.[18] Vasodilators such as hydralazine, sodium nitroprusside and prostacyclin lower PVR and also SVRI, and are prone to cause hypotension and increase pulmonary shunt. NO, by inhalation, is a selective pulmonary vasodilator,[36] but its use is still experimental.

Urine output

A urine output over 0.7 ml/kg per h should be maintained. If severe oliguria persists despite the above measures, IV mannitol (0.3 g/kg) and/or IV frusemide 250–500 mg is commonly given. These agents may increase renal blood flow and promote diuresis. However, frusemide can precipitate hypotension (by causing vasodilatation) and may worsen toxic nephropathy.

Chest X-ray

An early erect chest X-ray may show evidence of raised pulmonary venous pressure. In severe sepsis, considerable tachypnoea and hypoxaemia may exist despite a deceptively normal-looking chest film.

Laboratory monitoring

Increases in blood lactate suggest severe tissue hypoxaemia, and may indicate an advanced stage of decompensation. However, in severe sepsis, lactate may be increased by other mechanisms. For example, increased circulating catecholamines promote glycolysis (by stimulating cyclic adenosine monophosphate to augment glycogen phosphorylase). The increased concentration of pyruvate so produced leads to increased production of lactate. Conversely, in malnourished patients with low glycogen stores, the increase in lactate for a given level of hypoxia may be less. Hence, lactate may be an insensitive marker of tissue hypoxia.[37]

Controversies in haemodynamic management

It has been suggested that the optimal goals of therapy in septic patients may be supranormal values (Table 61.4).[38,39] Using these goals, better survival has been reported, and pathological supply dependency was demonstrated (i.e. increases in Do_2 were reflected by increases in Vo_2).[40,41] However, these recommendations have been challenged. Other workers have shown no differences in outcome.[42–47] In one study, target Vo_2 values could not be attained in some patients despite achieving target CI and Do_2,[48]

Table 61.4 Supranormal values[38] (normal values in brackets)

Cardiac index > 4.5 l/min per m^2 (2.5–3.5)
Do_2 > 600 ml/min per m^2 (400–700)
Vo_2 > 170 ml/min per m^2 (130–150)
PCWP = 18 mmHg; 2.4 kPa (15 mmHg; 2.0 kPa)
Severe trauma and septic patients may require greater increases[39]

Do_2 = Oxygen delivery; Vo_2 = oxygen consumption; PCWP = pulmonary capillary wedge pressure.

suggesting that increasing D_{O_2} does not affect the inability of tissues to extract or utilize oxygen. Future efforts should be directed away from global values of CI, D_{O_2} and V_{O_2} towards monitors and markers of individual organ oxygenation and function. Currently, pHi is of much interest. It is more likely to benefit patients at risk of developing shock rather than those already in shock,[49] but further evaluation of its role is necessary.

Dobutamine has been the most common inotropic agent used in reported studies. The possibility exists that dobutamine may have worsened peripheral maldistribution of blood in those patients. Also, aggressive use of dobutamine to achieve supranormal goals may have been detrimental.[47] In clinical practice, the choice of inotrope should be influenced by the initial MAP, CI and SVRI following volume loading, and by the clinical response.

Specific measures

Blood cultures

Blood cultures are taken repeatedly before antibiotics are given. A set of cultures consists of six bottles – three aerobic and three anaerobic – each bottle receiving 5 ml of blood.

Gram stain and culture

Appropriate specimens of sputum, urine, peritoneal dialysis fluid, cerebrospinal fluid (CSF) and pus should be examined microscopically, Gram-stained and cultured.

Specimens for specific antigens and serology

Specific serological tests should be requested if appropriate. Similarly, a search for specific antigens (e.g. pneumococcal and meningococcal) may be relevant, especially in CSF specimens of patients with suspected bacterial meningitis who were previously given antibiotics.

Antibiotics

Adequate antibiotics are given following collection of blood and specimens for cultures. The regimen is initially a best guess based on:

1 the possible site of infection;
2 whether the infection was acquired outside or within the hospital;
3 the age of the patient;
4 any history of hypersensitivity;
5 renal function;
6 whether previous antibiotics have been given.

The regimen may need to be changed once the organism and sensitivities are known (see Chapter 64).

Surgical drainage

Surgical debridement or drainage of infection source is vital. If intra-abdominal abscesses are left undrained, mortality approaches 100%.[50] Locating sources of infection can prove difficult and frustrating. In suspected intra-abdominal sepsis, plain abdominal X-rays, ultrasonography, computed tomography (CT) scan, gallium 67 citrate scan and indium 111-labelled leukocytes may be helpful,[51] but may also be misleading. The choice of investigation is guided by availability, expertise and the clinical situation. If intra-abdominal sepsis is strongly suspected despite negative clinical findings, exploratory laparotomy should be undertaken.[52] Direct percutaneous drainage may be attempted in selected cases, when a definite abscess is located by ultrasonography or CT scan.

Severe diffuse peritonitis has a high mortality, and aggressive forms of therapy have been tried. However, radical peritoneal debridement or postoperative continuous peritoneal lavage offers no benefit. Repeated laparotomies also confer poor results.[53] Electively staged laparotomies and open management of the abdomen (possibly with use of a mesh zipper)[54] are also proposed.[55,56] Advantages claimed for open management include maximal drainage, ease of repeated debridement and lowered intra-abdominal pressure.[55] This method should be reserved for severe cases; mortality remains high and its superiority remains unestablished.[56]

Measures for specific infections

Additional measures are relevant to the following infections.

Gas gangrene
Massive doses of crystalline penicillin are given with clindamycin, and urgent radical debridement or amputation is undertaken. Hyperbaric oxygen may be beneficial, but prospective evidence to support its use is lacking (see Chapter 63).

Systemic candidiasis
This is usually seen in immunodepressed patients receiving antibiotics. As fungaemia may arise by translocation from the bowel,[57] ICU patients on broad-spectrum antibiotics should be given prophylactic oral or nasogastric nystatin suspension or amphotericin B. In suspected systemic candidiasis, ophthalmitis, osteomyelitis, arthritis, myocarditis, meningitis and macronodular skin lesions must be excluded. Established agents for treating *Candida* infections are amphotericin B, flucytosine and fluconazole[58] (see Chapter 64).

Necrotizing fasciitis
Necrotizing fasciitis is a fulminant infection of subcutaneous tissues with extensive undermining of

skin, usually occurring on the extremities, perineum and abdominal wall. Patients with cirrhosis, diabetes and immunocompromised conditions are more likely victims. Infecting organisms are usually enteric bowel organisms, *Vibrio* spp., group A streptococci, and occasionally *Staphylococcus aureus*. Extensive early debridement and antibiotic therapy are the essential components of therapy (see Chapter 63).

Meningococcal meningitis and meningococcaemia

These fulminant conditions have a high mortality. Antibiotics must be given immediately; ceftriaxone 1–2 g 12-hourly or cefotaxime 1–2 g 6–8-hourly is usually appropriate. Dexamethasone 0.15 mg/kg 6-hourly for 2 days should be started before antibiotics in children, but not for adults. Lumbar puncture will be unsafe if coagulopathy is present (see Chapter 46).

Complications of sepsis

Metabolic acidosis

This is commonly present because of lactic acidaemia from anaerobic metabolism. Measures to improve Do_2 will usually reverse this. However, severe metabolic acidosis worsens myocardial depression and increases PVR and venoconstriction. Use of bicarbonate remains controversial.[59]

Hyperglycaemia

Glucose intolerance is commonly precipitated by severe sepsis, and aggravated by steroids and hypertonic glucose infusions. A low-dose insulin infusion may be necessary. Hypoglycaemia may occasionally be seen, especially in the very young and those with severe hepatic dysfunction.

Coagulopathy

Mild to severe disseminated intravascular coagulation may occur in septic shock. Platelets, fresh frozen plasma and other factors are given if necessary (see Chapter 89). Vitamin K and folate are routinely given if no contraindication exists.

Gastrointestinal bleeding

Antacids, H_2-receptor blockers and sucralfate are effective in reducing GIT bleeding in sepsis (see Chapter 35). Sucralfate has a minimal effect on intragastric pH and has antimicrobial properties. Whether it is associated with less gastric colonization and nosocomial pneumonia in ventilated patients is debatable.[60,61]

Hypercatabolism

Severe sepsis is associated with a hypercatabolic state. Muscle wasting can be profound. Negative nitrogen balance can be minimized by providing adequate nutritional support.

Multiple organ dysfunction and failure

Multiple organ dysfunction and/or failure is a feature of severe sepsis and septic shock. Virtually any organ may be involved (see Chapter 85).

Novel, experimental and controversial therapies

Antiendotoxin antibodies

Antiendotoxin antibodies have not improved survival in several clinical trials.[62] These included polyclonal antiendotoxin anticore antibodies against *E. coli* J5,[62–68] and monoclonal antiendotoxin antibodies E5 (Xoma)[69,70] and HA-1A (Centocor).[71,72] The CHESS HA-1A study was stopped because mortality in the treated group exceeded that of patients given placebo.[73] At present, agents with a higher binding affinity with endotoxin than antibodies previously studied are being developed.[62]

Anticytokine therapies

Cytokines are small proteins produced by macrophages and other immune cells, and are primary mediators of inflammation with an important role in regulating host defences. Levels of TNF, IL-1 and IL-6 are increased in septic shock.[74] Anticytokine therapy is thus based on the assumption that suppression of an exaggerated inflammatory response is beneficial. However, anti-TNF antibodies and soluble TNF receptors did not affect 28-day mortality in a multicentre trial.[62] Although increasing doses of IL-1ra were reported to relate to improved survival,[75] no difference in mortality was shown in a larger IL-1ra trial.[76]

Modifying neutrophil function

Experimental studies of monoclonal antibodies to inhibit neutrophil adhesion have shown varying beneficial and adverse effects.[77,78] Granulocyte colony-stimulating factor (GCSF) has been shown to be beneficial in animal experiments.[79,80] However, evidence of clinical benefit is lacking.

Nitric oxide

NO has important roles in neurotransmission, regulation of vascular tone, platelet inhibition and leukocyte adhesion, with antitumour and bactericidal effects in higher concentrations. Blocking its production in sepsis is rationalized by its implications in myocardial depression[23] and vasoplegia.[81] NO synthase inhibitors have been used in sepsis to treat hypotension.[82–84] However, improved survival has yet to be shown convincingly. Indeed, anti-NO therapy could well be harmful.

Steroids

The use of high-dose steroids (e.g. methylprednisolone 30 mg/kg and dexamethasone 6 mg/kg) does not improve overall survival in septic shock.[85] Moreover, steroid treatment is associated with more deaths related to secondary infection.[86,87] Use of steroids cannot be recommended except for bacterial meningitis in children[88] and *Pneumocystis* pneumonia.[89]

Prostaglandins

Prostaglandins participate in the pathophysiology of septic shock. Indomethacin and ibuprofen, prostaglandin cyclooxygenase inhibitors, have not been shown to improve human survival in sepsis.[90,91] Prostacyclin (prostaglandin; PGI_2) is a vasodilator; it antagonizes thromboxane A_2 and inhibits platelet aggregation, and is reported to improve peripheral oxygen utilization in critically ill patients,[92] but evidence of benefits in sepsis is lacking. Alprostadil (prostaglandin E_1) produced no improvement in survival in patients with acute respiratory distress syndrome (ARDS).[93]

Naloxone

Endogenous opioid peptides derived from β-lipotropin are released in septic shock and other stress states. Despite earlier encouraging reports, naloxone, an opioid receptor blocker, offers no real therapeutic benefits in septic shock.[94]

Thyrotrophin-releasing hormone (TRH)

TRH, like naloxone, opposes many opioid-mediated actions. Although it has been studied in experimental shock, its clinical role is unknown.

Phospholipase A_2 inhibitors

Endotoxin and bacterial products activate cell phospholipases to liberate arachidonic acid (and initiate synthesis of leukotrienes, prostaglandins and thromboxanes) and, with phospholipase A_2, activate PAF. Drugs that inhibit phospholipase A_2 have been shown to prevent lung injury in animals,[95,96] but usefulness in human sepsis is unknown.

Antioxidants

Free radical production is increased in sepsis and produces a toxic effect by interacting with cell structure, processes or genetic activity. Endogenous protective antioxidants include vitamins C, E, B carotene, sulphydryl group donors (e.g. glutathione), proteins with sulphydryl group and enzymes (e.g. superoxide dismutase and catalase). Encouraging results have been reported in ARDS, and antioxidants may have potential benefits in sepsis,[97] but prospective clinical trials are required.

Ketoconazole

Ketoconazole, a thromboxane A_2 synthetase inhibitor, has been shown to reduce the incidence of ARDS[98,99] and mortality in septic patients.[98] Ketoconazole also inhibits the synthesis of leukotrienes and interacts with other mediators such as IL-1 and TNF.

Pentoxifylline

Pentoxifylline is a phosphodiesterase inhibitor, thus blocking chemotaxis and activation of neutrophils. It reduces the formation of TNF and increases survival in murine endotoxic shock,[100] and has been safely given to patients with ARDS.[101] Further investigation of this agent is needed.

Haemofiltration

Haemofiltration can remove certain circulating cytokines from septic patients,[102,103] and benefits have been suggested.[103–105] In particular, plasma exchange has been used in the treatment of meningococcal infection.[106] However, haemofiltration will not affect cytokines that are fixed to cells, and many mediators of sepsis are cell-associated. Prospective controlled clinical trials on dialytic therapies for sepsis are required.[107]

Prognosis

Mortality increases with increasing severity score (e.g. APACHE II), number of dysfunctional/failed organs and duration of such failure.[108,109] Several factors influence the prognosis in bacteraemia and fungaemia in adults:[110,111] source of infection, where acquired, blood pressure, organism isolated, body temperature, age and predisposing factors. Survival is improved by appropriate use of antibiotics and surgical drainage (where applicable).[111] The ability to maintain an increased CI, Do_2 and Vo_2 is associated with better prognosis.[33] Pulmonary hypertension is an adverse factor.[18] Peripheral vascular failure may be a major haemodynamic determinant of mortality, as survivors of septic shock are more able to augment SVRI.[34]

Prevention of sepsis in ICUs

Four main facets are important: reducing available routes of infection; preventing transfer of pathogenic organisms and development of resistant strains;

improving host defences; and reducing risk of endogenous infection from the gut.

Reducing available routes of infection

All invasive cannulae and tubes should be removed when no longer necessary. Subclavian central lines have lower rates of infection than femoral sites and are preferred.[112] Triple-lumen central venous catheters induce a higher sepsis rate than single-lumen catheters.[113]

Preventing transfer of pathogenic organisms and development of resistant strains

Hand-washing must be performed by staff members before and after attending each patient. All invasive procedures, including endotracheal suctioning, must be done aseptically. If prophylactic antibiotics are employed, narrow-spectrum agents should be used with a limited duration. Indiscriminate use of antibiotics leads to serious outbreaks of infection within the ICU (see Chapter 64).

Improving host defences

Potentially valuable measures include:

1 *nutritional repletion*;
2 *surgery*, e.g. drainage, control of haemorrhage and resection of colonic cancer;
3 *active immunization*, e.g. pneumococcal,[114] *Haemophilus influenzae* type B,[115] and meningococcal[116] vaccination of splenectomized patients; tetanus and hepatitis B vaccines;
4 *passive immunization* (e.g. human antitetanus, and pneumococcal and hepatitis B globulin);
5 *granulocyte transfusion* in the profoundly leukopenic patient.

Immunostimulation with agents such as levamisole, bacillus Calmette-Guérin (BCG) and *Corynebacterium parvum* may be useless or even dangerous.[9] Infusions of fibronectin, cryoprecipitate, fresh frozen plasma, γ-globulin and transfer factor are of unproven benefit.

Reducing risk of endogenous infection from the gut

Early enteral feeding

Early enteral feeding can reduce bacterial and endotoxin translocation from the gut, and infection rates in animals and humans.[117] Larger studies are needed on outcome and influence of food composition.

Improving gut blood flow

Bacteraemia commonly occurs in patients with haemorrhagic shock.[118] Decreased intestinal blood flow may be important in bacterial gut translocation. Early adequate resuscitation aims to improve gut blood flow.

Selective oropharyngeal and gastrointestinal decontamination

Organisms commonly causing infections in the compromised patient may be community-acquired (e.g. *Streptococcus pneumoniae*, *Haemophilus influenzae*, *Branhamella catarrhalis*, *E. coli*, *Staphylococcus aureus* and *Candida albicans*) or nosocomial (hospital/ICU-acquired, e.g. *Klebsiella*, *Proteus*, *Morganella*, *Enterobacter*, *Citrobacter*, *Serratia*, *Acinetobacter* and *Pseudomonas*).[119] Normal indigenous flora of the throat and alimentary tract are anaerobic (> 99%), and are rarely involved in infection. Selective decontamination aims to prevent or eradicate colonization by community/hospital-acquired pathogens, and preserve protective normal flora.

Community flora are eradicated by short-term parenteral antibiotics. Therapy against hospital-acquired flora is by topical application of non-absorbable antimicrobial agents (Table 61.5).[120] Initial reports[120–122] and meta-analysis of available studies[123,124] are favourable, but outcome has remained unchanged.[125]

Table 61.5 A regimen for oropharyngeal and gastrointestinal decontamination

Systemic antibiotic (first 4 days) cefotaxime IV
50–100 mg/kg per day in four divided doses
Topical antimicrobial (whole of ICU stay)
  Oropharyngeal:
    Cleanse mouth with 0.1% chlorhexidine aqueous
      solution
    Apply carboxymethylcellulose (Orabase) containing:
    2% polymyxin E
    2% tobramycin
    2% amphotericin B
    A small quantity on a gloved finger is applied to buccal
      mucosa four times a day.
  Gastrointestinal:
    100 mg polymyxin E
    80 mg tobramycin
    500 mg amphotericin B
    as a 10-ml mixture, delivered four times a day via a
      nasogastric tube

References

1. Sibbald WJ, Marshall J, Christou N *et al.* (1991) 'Sepsis' – clarity of existing terminology – or more confusion? *Crit Care Med* **19**:996–998.

2. American College of Chest Physicians/Society of Critical Care Medicine consensus conference (1992) Definitions for sepsis and organ failure and guidelines for the use of innovative therapies in sepsis. *Crit Care Med* **20**:864–874.

3. Parrillo JE, Parker MM, Natanson C *et al.* (1990) Septic shock: advances in the understanding of pathogenesis, cardiovascular dysfunction, and therapy. *Ann Intern Med* **113**:227–242.

4. EPIC study group (1992) The Epic study – preliminary results. *HOST*; **9**:12–13.

5. Trilla A (1994) Epidemiology of nosocomial infections in adult intensive care units. *Intensive Care Med* **20**:S1–S4.

6. Ledingham I MCA and Bradley JA (1988) Update in host defence mechanisms. In: Vincent JL (ed.) *Update in Intensive Care and Emergency Medicine*, vol. 5. Berlin: Springer-Verlag, pp. 65–67.

7. Wiles JB, Cerra FB, Siegel JH and Border JR (1980) The systemic septic response: does the organism matter? *Crit Care Med* **8**:55–60.

8. Pietsch JB, Meakins JL and Maclean LD (1977) Delayed hypersensitivity response: application in clinical surgery. *Surgery* **82**:349–355.

9. McIrvine AJ and Mannick JA (1983) Lymphocyte function in the critically ill surgical patient. *Surg Clin North Am* **63**:245–261.

10. Sirisinha S, Suskind R, Edelman R, Charupatana C and Olsen RE (1973) Complement and C3 proactivator levels in children with protein-calorie malnutrition and effect of dietary treatment. *Lancet* **i**:1016–1020.

11. Krivit W, Giebink GS and Leonard A (1979) Overwhelming postsplenectomy infection. *Surg Clin North Am* **59**:223–231.

12. Stephen J and Pietrowski RA (1981) *Bacterial Toxins.* Walton-on-Thames: Nelson, p. 7.

13. Buxton Hopkin DA (1977) Too rapid destruction of Gram-negative organisms. *Lancet* **2**:603–604.

14. Lamy M and Thijs LG (1994) Round table conference on mediators in sepsis. *Intensive Care Med* **20**:238–241.

15. Parker MM, Shelhamer JH, Natanson C *et al.* (1983) Serial haemodynamic patterns in survivors and non-survivors of septic shock in humans. *Clin Res* **31**:671A.

16. Moncada S, Palmer R and Higgs E (1991) Nitric oxide: physiology, pathophysiology and pharmacology. *Pharmacol Rev* **43**:109–142.

17. Hess ML, Hastillo A and Greenfield LJ (1981) Spectrum of cardiovascular function during Gram-negative sepsis. *Prog Cardiovasc Dis* **23**:279–298.

18. Sibbald WJ, Paterson NAM, Holiday RL, Anderson RA, Lobb TR and Duff JH (1978) Pulmonary hypertension in sepsis. Measurement by pulmonary arterial diastolic–pulmonary wedge pressure gradient and the influence of passive and active factors. *Chest* **73**:583–591.

19. Wilson RF (1976) The diagnosis and management of severe sepsis and septic shock. *Heart Lung* **5**:422–429.

20. Parker MM, Shelhamer JH, Bacharach SL *et al.* (1984) Profound but reversible myocardial depression in patients with septic shock. *Ann Intern Med* **100**:483–490.

21. Cunnion RE, Schaer GL, Parker MM *et al.* (1986) The coronary circulation in human septic shock. *Circulation* **73**:637–644.

22. Dhainault JF, Huyghebaert MF, Monsallier JF *et al.* (1987) Coronary hemodynamics and myocardial metabolism of lactate, free fatty acids, glucose and ketones in patients with septic shock. *Circulation* **75**:533–541.

23. Finkel MS, Oddis CV, Jacob TD, Watkins SC, Hattler BG and Simmons RL (1992) Negative inotropic effects of cytokines on the heart mediated by nitric oxide. *Science* **257**:387–389.

24. Shoemaker WC (1987) Relation of oxygen transport patterns to the pathophysiology and therapy of shock states. *Intensive Care Med* **13**:230–243.

25. Abraham E, Shoemaker WC, Bland RD and Cobo JC (1983) Sequential cardiorespiratory patterns in septic shock. *Crit Care Med* **11**:799–803.

26. Gilbert EM, Haupt MT, Mandanas RY, Huaringa AJ and Carlson RW (1986) The effect of fluid loading, blood transfusion and catecholamine infusion on oxygen delivery and consumption in patients with sepsis. *Am Rev Respir Dis* **134**:873–878.

27. Mohensifar Z, Goldbach P, Tashkin DP *et al.* (1983) Relationship between O_2 delivery and O_2 consumption in the adult respiratory distress syndrome. *Chest* **84**:267–271.

28. Danek SJ, Lynch JP, Weg JG and Dantzker DR (1980) The dependence of oxygen uptake on oxygen delivery in the adult respiratory distress syndrome. *Am Rev Respir Dis* **122**:387–395.

29. Pinsky MR (1994) Beyond global oxygen supply–demand relations: in search of measures of dysoxia. *Intensive Care Med* **20**:1–3.

30. Ruokonen E, Takala J, Kari A, Saxen H, Mertsola J and Hansen EJ (1993) Regional blood flow and oxygen transport in septic shock. *Crit Care Med* **21**:1296–1303.

31. Marik P and Mohedin M (1994) The contrasting effects of dopamine and norepinephrine on systemic and splanchnic oxygen utilization in hyperdynamic sepsis. *J Am Med Assoc* **272**:1354–1357.

32. Packman MI and Racklow EC (1983) Optimum left heart filling pressure during fluid resuscitation of patients with hypovolemic and septic shock. *Crit Care Med* **11**:165–169.

33. Parker MM, Shelhamer JH, Natanson C *et al.* (1987) Serial cardiovascular variables in survivors and non-survivors of human septic shock. *Crit Care Med* **15**:923–929.

34. Groeneveld ABJ, Nauta JJP and Thijs LG (1988) Peripheral vascular resistance in septic shock: its relation to outcome. *Intensive Care Med* **14**:141–147.

35. Schreuder WO, Schneider AJ, Groeneveld AB and Thijs LG (1989) Effect of dopamine vs norepinephrine on hemodynamics in septic shock. Emphasis on right ventricular performance. *Chest* **95**:1282–1288.

36. Rossaint R, Falke KJ, Lopez F, Slama K, Pison U and Zapol WM (1993) Inhaled nitric oxide for the adult respiratory distress syndrome. *N Engl J Med* **328**:399–405.

37. Dantzker DR (1987) Interpretation of data in the hypoxic patient. In: Bryan-Brown CW and Ayres SM (eds) *Oxygen Transport and Utilisation. New Horizons.* Fullerton, Ca: SCCM, pp. 93–108.

38. Shoemaker WC, Bland RD and Appel PL (1985) Therapy of critically ill postoperative patients based on outcome prediction and prospective clinical trials. *Surg Clin North Am* **65**:811–833.

39. Shoemaker WC, Appel PL and Kram HB (1987) Role of oxygen transport patterns in the pathophysiology, prediction of outcome and therapy of shock. In: Bryan-Brown CW and Ayres SM (eds) *Oxygen Transport and Utilisation, New Horizons,* Fullerton, Ca: SCCM, pp. 65–92.

40. Edwards JD, Ceri G, Brown S, Nightingale P, Slater RM and Faragher EB (1989) Use of survivors' cardiorespiratory values as therapeutic goals in septic shock. *Crit Care Med* **17**:1098–1103.

41. Tuchsmidt J, Fried J, Astiz M and Rackow E (1992) Elevation of cardiac output and oxygen delivery improves outcome in septic shock. *Chest* **102**:216–220.

42. Vermeij CG, Feenstra BWA and Bruining HA (1990) Oxygen delivery and oxygen uptake in postoperative and septic patients. *Chest* **98**:415–420.

43. Ronco JJ, Phang PT, Wiggs B, Whalley KR, Fenwick JC and Russell JA (1991) Oxygen consumption is independent of increases in oxygen delivery in severe adult respiratory distress syndrome. *Am Rev Respir Dis* **143**:1267–1273.

44. Wysocki M, Bebes M, Roupie E and Brun-Buisson C (1992) Modification of oxygen extraction ratio by change in oxygen transport in septic shock. *Chest* **102**: 221–226.

45. Ronco JJ, Fenwick JC, Wiggs B, Phang PT, Russell JA and Tweedale MG (1993) Oxygen consumption is independent of increases in oxygen delivery by dobutamine in septic patients who have normal or increased plasma lactate. *Rev Respir Dis* **147**:25–31.

46. Hanique G, Dugernier T, Laterre PF, Dougnac A, Roeseler J and Reynaert MS (1993) Significance of pathologic oxygen supply dependency in critically ill patients: comparison between measured and calculated methods. *Intensive Care Med* **20**:12–18.

47. Hayes MA, Timmins AC, Yau EH, Palazzo M, Hinds CJ and Watson D (1994) Elevation of systemic oxygen delivery in the treatment of critically ill patients. *N Engl J Med* **330**:1717–1722.

48. Hayes MA, Yau EHS, Timmins AC, Hinds CJ and Watson D (1993) Response of critically ill patients to treatment aimed at achieving supranormal oxygen delivery and consumption. Relationship to outcome. *Chest* **103**:887–895.

49. Arnold J, Hendriks J, Ince C and Bruining H (1994) Tonometry to assess the adequacy of splanchnic oxygention in the critically ill patient. *Intensive Care Med* **20**:452–456.

50. Altemeier WA, Culbertson WR, Fullen WD *et al.* (1973) Intra-abdominal abscesses. *Am J Surg* **125**:70.

51. Snyder SK and Hahn HH (1982) Diagnosis and treatment of intra-abdominal abscess in critically ill patients. *Surg Clin North Am* **62**:229–239.

52. Polk HC and Shields C (1977) Remote organ failure: a valid sign of occult intra-abdominal infection. *Surgery* **81**:310–313.

53. Harbrecht PJ, Garrison RN and Fry DE (1984) Early urgent relaparotomy. *Arch Surg* **119**:369–374.

54. Hedderick GS, Wexler MJ, McLean APH and Meakins JL (1986) The septic abdomen: open management with Marlex mesh with a zipper. *Surgery* **99**:399–407.

55. Schein M, Saadia R and Decker GGA (1986) The open management of the septic abdomen. *Surg Gynecol Obstet* **163**:587–592.

56. Saadia MS, Freinkel Z and Decker G (1988) Aggressive treatment of severe diffuse peritonitis: a prospective study. *Br J Surg* **75**:173–176.

57. Krause W, Matheis H and Wulf K (1969) Fungemia and funguria after oral administration of *Candida albicans. Lancet* **i**:598–599.

58. British Society for Antimicrobial Chemotherapy working party (1994) Management of deep *Candida* infection in surgical and intensive care unit patients. *Intensive Care Med* **20**:522–528.

59. Hindman BJ (1990) Sodium bicarbonate in the treatment of subtypes of acute lactic acidosis: physiologic considerations. *Anesthesiology* **72**:1064–1076.

60. Tryba M (1987) Risk of acute stress bleeding and nosocomial pneumonia in ventilated intensive care unit patients – sulcralfate versus antacids. *Am J Med* **83**(suppl 3B):117–124.

61. Ben-Menachem T, Fogel R, Patel RV *et al.* (1994) Prophylaxis for stress related gastric hemorrhage in the medical intensive care unit. A randomized, controlled, single-blind study. *Ann Intern Med* **121**:568–575.

62. Natanson C, Hoffman WD, Suffredini AF, Eichacker PQ and Danner RL (1994) Selected treatment strategies for septic shock based on proposed mechanisms of pathogenesis. NIH conference. *Ann Intern Med* **120**:771–783.

63. Ziegler EJ, McCutchan JA, Fierer J *et al.* (1982) Treatment of Gram-negative bacteremia and shock with human antiserum to a mutant *Escherichia coli. N Engl J Med* **307**:1225–1230.

64. McCutchan JA, Wolf JL, Ziegler EJ and Braude AI (1983) Ineffectiveness of single dose human antiserum to core glycolipid (*E. coli* J5) for prophylaxis of bacteremic, Gram negative infection in patients with prolonged neutropenia. *Schweiz Med Wochenschr* **113**(suppl 14):40–45.

65. Baumgartner JD, Glauser MP, McCutchan JA *et al.* (1985) Prevention of Gram negative shock and death in surgical patients by antibody to endotoxin core glycolipid. *Lancet* **2**:59–63.

66. J5 study group (1992) Treatment of severe infectious purpura in children with human plasma from donors immunised with *Escherichia coli* J5: a prospective double-blind study. *J Infect Dis* **165**:695–701.

67. Calandra T, Glauser MP, Schellekens J and Verhoef J

(1988) Treatment of Gram negative septic shock with human IgG antibody to *Escherichia coli* J5: a prospective, double-blind randomised trial. *J Infect Dis* **158**:312–319.

68. The intravenous immunoglobulin collaborative study group (1992) Prophylactic intravenous administration of standard immune globulin as compared with core lipo-polysaccharide immune globulin in patients at high risk of post surgical infection. *N Engl J Med* **327**:234–240.

69. Greenman RL, Schein RM, Martin MA *et al.* (1991) A controlled clinical trial of E5 murine monoclonal IgM antibody to endotoxin in the treatment of Gram negative sepsis. The XOMA sepsis study group. *J Am Med Assoc* **266**:1097–1102.

70. Wenzel R, Bone RC, Fein A *et al.* (1991) Results of a second double-blind randomised, controlled trial of anti-endotoxin antibody E5 in Gram negative sepsis (abstract). Program and Abstracts of the Thirty-first Interscience Conference of Antimicrobial Agents and Chemotherapy 1991:294.

71. Ziegler EJ, Fisher CJ Jr, Sprung CL *et al.* (1991) Treatment of Gram negative bacteremia and septic shock with HA-1A human monoclonal antibody against endotoxin. A randomised, double-blind, placebo controlled trial. *N Engl J Med* **324**:429–436.

72. Luce JM (1993) Introduction of new technology into critical care practice: a history of HA-1A human mono-cloal antibody against endotoxin. *Crit Care Med* **21**:1233–1241.

73. McCloskey RV, Straube RC, Sanders C, Smith SM, Smith CR, CHESS Trial Study Group (1994) Treatment of septic shock with human monoclonal antibody HA-1A. A randomized, double-blind, placebo controlled trial. *Ann Intern Med* **121**:1–5.

74. Calandra T, Baumgartner JD, Grau G *et al.* (1990) Prognostic values of tumour necrosis factor/cachectin, interleukin 1, interferon-α and interferon-γ in the serum of patients with septic shock. *J Infect Dis* **161**:982–987.

75. Fisher CJ Jr, Slotman GJ, Opal SM *et al.* (1994) Initial evaluation of human recombinant interleukin-1 receptor antagonist in the treatment of sepsis syndrome: a rando-mised, open-label, placebo controlled multicenter trial. *Crit Care Med* **22**:12–21.

76. Fisher CJ Jr, Dhainaut J-F, Pribble JP, Knaus WA, IL-1 Receptor Antagonist Study Group (1993) A study evaluat-ing the safety and efficacy of human recombinant interleukin-1 receptor antagonist in the treatment of patients with sepsis syndrome: preliminary results from a phase III multicenter trial (abstract). *Clin Intensive Care* **4**:8S.

77. Walsh CJ, Carey PD, Cook DJ, Bechard DE, Fowler AA and Sugerman HJ (1991) Anti-CD18 antibody attenuates neutropenia and alveolar capillary membrane injury during Gram negative sepsis. *Surgery* **110**:205–212.

78. Eichacker PQ, Hoffman WD, Farese A *et al.* (1993) Leukocyte CD18 monoclonal antibody worsens endotox-emia and cardiovascular injury in canines with septic shock. *J Appl Physiol* **74**:1885–1892.

79. Cairo MS, Plunkett JM, Mauss D and Van de ven C (1990) Seven day administration of recombinant human granulocyte colony stimulating factor to newborn rats: modulation of neonatal neutrophilia, myelopoieses, and group B streptococcus sepsis. *Blood* **76**:1788–1794.

80. Eichacker PQ, Waisman Y, Natanson C *et al.* (1993) Recombinant granulocyte colony stimulating factor redu-ces endotoxemia and improves cardiovascular function and survival during bacterial sepsis in non-neutropenic canines (abstract). *Clin Res* **41**:240.

81. Nava E, Palmer RM and Moncada S (1991) Inhibition of nitric oxide synthesis in septic shock: how much is beneficial? *Lancet* **338**:1555–1557.

82. Petros A, Bennett D and Vallance P (1991) Effect of nitric oxide synthase inhibitors on hypotension in patients with septic shock. *Lancet* **338**:1557–1558.

83. Lorente JA, Landin L, de Pablo R, Renes E and Liste D (1993) L-arginine pathway in the sepsis syndrome. *Crit Care Med* **21**:1287–1295.

84. Schilling J, Cakmakci M, Battig U and Geroulanos S (1993) A new approach in the treatment of hypotension in human septic shock by N^G-monomethyl-L-arginine, an inhibitor of the nitric oxide synthetase. *Intensive Care Med* **19**:227–231.

85. Sprung CL, Caralis PV, Marcial EH *et al.* (1984) The effects of high dose corticosteroids in patients with septic shock. *N Engl J Med* **311**:1137–1143.

86. Bone RC, Fisher CJ, Clemmer TP, Slotman GJ, Metz CA and Balk RA (1987) A controlled clinical trial of high dose methylprednisolone in the treatment of severe sepsis and septic shock. *N Engl J Med* **317**:653–658.

87. The Veterans Administration Systemic Sepsis Co-oper-ative Study Group (1987) Effect of high dose glucocortoid therapy on mortality in patients with clinical signs of systemic sepsis. *N Engl J Med* **317**:659–665.

88. Odio CM, Faingezicht I, Paris M *et al.* (1991) The beneficial effects of early dexamethasone administration in infants and children with bacterial meningitis. *N Engl J Med* **324**:1525–1531.

89. The National Institutes of Health–University of California expert panel for corticosteroids as adjunctive therapy for *Pneumocystis* pneumonia (1990) Consensus statement on the use of corticosteroids as adjunctive therapy for *Pneumocystis* pneumonia in the acquired immunodefi-ciency syndrome. *N Engl J Med* **323**:1500–1504.

90. Bernard GR, Reines HD, Halushka PV *et al.* (1991) Prostacyclin and thromboxane A_2 formation is increased in human sepsis syndrome: effects of cyclo-oxygenase inhibition. *Am Rev Respir Dis* **144**:1095–1101.

91. Haupt MT, Jastremski MS, Clemmer TP, Metz CA and Goris GB (1991) Effect of ibuprofen in patients with severe sepsis: a randomised, double blind multicentre study. *Crit Care Med* **19**:1339–1347.

92. Bihari D, Smithers M, Gimson A and Tinker J (1987) The effects of vasodilation with prostacyclin on oxygen delivery and uptake in critically ill patients. *N Engl J Med* **317**:397–403.

93. Bone RC, Slotman G, Maunder R *et al.* (1989) Random-ized double blind, multicenter study of prostaglandin E_1 in patients with the adult respiratory distress syndrome. *Chest* **96**:114–119.

94. Hackshaw KV, Parker GA and Roberts JW (1990) Naloxone in septic shock. *Crit Care Med* **18**:47–51.

95. Tighe D, Moss R, Parker-Williams J *et al.* (1987) A phospholipase inhibitor modifies the pulmonary damage associated with peritonitis in rabbits. *Intensive Care Med* **13**:284–290.

96. Koike K, Moore EE, Moore FA *et al.* (1992) Phospholipase A_2 inhibition decouples lung injury from gut ischemia reperfusion. *Surgery* **112**:173–180.

97. Goode HF and Webster NR (1993) Free radicals and antioxidants in sepsis. *Crit Care Med* **21**:1770–1776.

98. Yu M and Tomasa G (1993) A double blind, prospective, randomized trial of ketoconazole, a thromboxane synthetase inhibitor, in the prophylaxis of the adult respiratory distress syndrome. *Crit Care Med* **21**:1635–1642.

99. Slotman GJ, Burchard KW, D'Arezzo A *et al.* (1988) Ketoconazole prevents acute respiratory failure in critically ill surgical patients. *J Trauma* **28**:648–654.

100. Schade UF (1990) Pentoxifylline increases survival in murine endotoxin shock and decreases formation of tumor necrosis factor. *Circ Shock* **31**:171–181.

101. Montravers P, Fagon JY, Gilbert C, Blanchet F, Novara A and Chastre J (1993) Pilot study of cardiopulmonary risk from pentoxifylline in adult respiratory distress syndrome. *Chest* **103**:1017–1022.

102. Bellomo R, Tipping P and Boyce N (1993) Continuous veno-venous haemofiltration with dialysis removes cytokines from the circulation of septic patients. *Crit Care Med* **21**:522–526.

103. Gotloib L, Barzilay E, Shustak A, Wais Z, Jaickenko L and Lev A (1986) Hemofiltration in septic ARDS. The artificial kidney as an artificial endocrine lung. *Resuscitation* **13**:123–132.

104. Garzia F, Todor R and Scalea T (1991) Continuous arteriovenous hemofiltration countercurrent dialysis (CAVH-D) in acute respiratory failure (ARDS). *J Trauma* **31**:1277–1285.

105. DiCarlo JV, Dudley TE, Sherbotie JR, Kaplan BS and Costarino AT (1990) Continuous arteriovenous hemofiltration/dialysis improves pulmonary gas exchange in children with multiple organ system failure. *Crit Care Med* **18**:822–826.

106. Drapkin MS, Wisch JS, Gelfand JA *et al.* (1989) Plasmapheresis for fulminant meningococcemia. *Pediatr Infect Dis J* **8**:399–400.

107. Schetz M, Ferdinande P, Van den Berghe G, Verwaest C and Lauwers P (1995) Removal of proinflammatory cytokines with renal replacement therapy: sense or nonsense? *Intensive Care Med* **21**:169–176.

108. Knaus WA, Draper EA, Wagner DP and Zimmerman JE (1985) Prognosis in acute organ system failure. *Ann Surg* **202**:685–693.

109. Chang RWS, Jacobs S and Lee B (1988) Predicting outcome among intensive care unit patients using computerised trend analysis of daily APACHE II scores corrected for organ system failure. *Intensive Care Med* **14**:558–566.

110. An expert report of the European Society of Intensive Care Medicine (1994) The problem of sepsis. *Intensive Care Med* **20**:300–304.

111. Weinstein MP, Murphy JR, Reller LB and Lichtenstein KA (1983) The clinical significance of positive blood cultures: comprehensive analysis of 500 episodes of bacteremia and fungemia in adults. Clinical observations, with special reference to factors influencing prognosis. *Rev Infect Dis* **5**:54–70.

112. Collignon P, Soni N, Pearson I, Sorrell T and Woods P (1988) Sepsis associated with central vein catheters in critically ill patients. *Intensive Care Med* **14**:227–231.

113. Hilton E, Haslett TM, Borenstein MT, Tucci V, Isenberg HD and Singer C (1988) Central catheter infections: single versus triple lumen catheters. *Am J Med* **84**:667–671.

114. Di Padova F, Durig M, Wadstrom J and Harder F (1983) Role of spleen in immune response to polyvalent pneumococcal vaccine. *Br Med J* **287**:1829–1832.

115. Cooke R, Gover P and Grace R (1994) Americans recommend additional immunisation (letter). *Br Med J* **308**:132.

116. Condon R (1992) Quadrivalent meningococcal vaccine for use after splenectomy (letter). *Med J Aust* **156**:294.

117. Alexander JW (1993) Prevention of bacterial translocation with early enteral feeding – a feasible approach? In: Faist E, Meakins JL and Schildberg FW (eds) *Host Defense and Dysfunction in Trauma, Shock and Sepsis.* Berlin: Springer-Verlag, pp.903–909.

118. Rush BF, Sori AJ, Murphy TF, Smith S, Flanagan JJ and Machiedo GW (1988) Endotoxemia and bacteremia during hemorrhagic shock. The link between trauma and sepsis? *Ann Surg* **207**:549–554.

119. Van Saene JKF, Stoutenbeek CP and Zandstra DF (1988) Selective elimination of oropharyngeal and gastrointestinal flora: a step forward in the control of infection in ICU? In: Vincent JL (ed.) *Update in Intensive Care and Emergence Medicine*, vol. 5. Berlin: Springer-Verlag, pp. 68–76.

120. Van Uffelen R, Rommes JH and Van Saene HKF (1987) Preventing lower airway colonisation and infection in mechanically ventilated patients. *Crit Care Med* **15**:99–102.

121. Stoutenbeek CP, Van Saene HKF, Miranda DR and Zandstra DF (1984) The effect of selective decontamination of the digestive tract on colonisation and infection in multiple trauma patients. *Intensive Care Med* **10**:185–192.

122. Van Saene HKF, Stoutenbeek CP, Miranda DR, Zandstra DF and Langrehr D (1986) Recent advances in the control of infection in patients with thoracic injury. *Injury* **17**:332–335.

123. Selective decontamination of the digestive tract trialists collaborative group (1993) Metanalysis of randomised controlled trials of selective decontamination of the digestive tract. *Br Med J* **307**:525–532.

124. Heyland DK, Cook DJ, Jaeschke R *et al.* Selective decontamination of the digestive tract: an overview. *Chest* **105**:1221–1229.

125. Cook D (1993) Selective digestive decontamination: a critical appraisal. In: Vincent J-L (ed.) *Yearbook of Intensive Care and Emergency Medicine.* Berlin: Springer-Verlag, pp. 281–286.

62 | Nosocomial infections

JD Santamaria

Nosocomial or hospital-acquired infections[1,2] develop as a result of a patient's admission to hospital. They are associated with significant mortality and morbidity, and add to increasing health costs. Infections are often due to organisms which are, or become, resistant to antibiotics. The Centers for Disease control (CDC) definitions for nosocomial infections are shown in Table 62.1.[3]

General overview

Approximately 5–10% of patients admitted to hospital develop a nosocomial infection; an Australian survey showed that 6.2% of patients in 269 hospitals had a hospital-acquired infection.[4] Nosocomial infections can involve any organ, but those of the urinary tract, surgical wounds and lower respiratory tract account for the majority. The relative incidences (Table 62.2) have remained constant over the years.

Table 62.1 Principles for the diagnosis of nosocomial infections[3]

Finding the presence and location of an infection involves combinations of clinical findings and results of laboratory and other diagnostic tests

The clinician's diagnosis of infection derived from direct observation at surgery, endoscopy or other diagnostic procedure is an acceptable criterion for an infection

There must be no evidence that the infection was present or incubating at the time of hospital admission. Infection acquired in hospital but only evident after hospital discharge fulfils the criteria

No specific time during or after hospitalization is given to determine *whether* an infection is nosocomial or community-acquired. Each infection is examined for evidence that links it to hospitalization.

Three per cent of patients die from such infections, although mortality rates vary with the site of sepsis. The economic impact is staggering; US studies have estimated that an infection extends hospital stay by 4 days, with an added cost of 5–10 billion dollars! ICUs represent 2–7% of hospital beds, but are responsible for 25% of all nosocomial blood stream and pulmonary infections.[5]

Infecting organisms may originate from exogenous sources (e.g. contaminated IV fluids and respiratory equipment) or, more commonly, from the patient's own endogenous flora in the oropharynx, bowel, genital tract and skin surface (Table 62.3).

The organisms responsible for most nosocomial infections have changed over the past 30 years. During the 1950s, *Staphylococcus aureus* was the predominant infecting organism. Gram-negative organisms rose to prominence during the 1970s, but Gram-positive cocci demonstrating resistance to multiple antibiotics have emerged as major pathogens during the 1980s.[6,7] Other bacteria of usually low virulence as well as viruses, fungi and parasites continue to affect immunocompromised patients; these problems have increased with the current epidemic of acquired immunodeficieny syndrome (AIDS). Blood-borne infections such as hepatitis B, hepatitis C and human immunodeficiency virus (HIV), for which treatment is limited, pose problems for staff as well as patients, but

Table 62.2 Relative incidences of nosocomial infection by site[79]

Location	Percentage
Urinary tract	42%
Surgical wound	20%
Lower respiratory tract	14%
Blood stream	8%
All other	16%

Table 62.3 Organisms responsible for nosocomial infections[79]

Organism	Percentage
Escherichia coli	18.6%
Staphylococcus aureus	10.8%
Enterococcus spp.	10.7%
Pseudomonas aeruginosa	10.6%
Klebsiella spp.	7.4%
Proteus spp.	5.4%
Enterobacter spp.	5.8%
Coagulase-negative staphylococci	6.1%
Candida spp.	5.1%
All others	19.5%

fortunately contribute little to the overall incidence of nosocomial infections.

Predisposing factors

Many clinical studies have defined factors which contribute to specific infections (see below). Four basic concepts emerge from these reports – endogenous flora, hospital factors, patient factors and antibiotic resistance.

Endogenous flora

Organisms which constitute the normal flora of various organs may cause infections when usual barriers are compromised, e.g. patients with endotracheal tubes, intravascular devices or urinary catheters. In these instances, the antibacterial properties of the mucosa or skin are effectively bypassed, and organisms gain direct access to usually sterile tissues (e.g. lung, blood or urine).

Hospital factors

Hospitals become reservoirs of pathogenic organisms. Reasons include the presence of very sick patients, attending staff who transfer organisms between patients, widespread use of antibiotics and equipment used to monitor or treat patients. All these factors promote the growth and spread of organisms within a hospital and their transfer from patient to patient.

Patient factors

Several factors intrinsic to the patient interact with the above to increase the chances of infection. Some are specific to individual infection sites but others apply generally. Infections are more common in the elderly, those with underlying chronic disorders, in contaminated wounds, during steroid or immunosuppressive therapies and during prolonged hospital admissions.

Antibiotic resistance

Resistance to one or more antibiotics is often a feature of organisms responsible for these infections. Widespread use of broad-spectrum antibiotics contributes to the problem. These drugs eradicate the normal flora within the gastrointestinal tract, the pharynx and the genitourinary tract, allowing overgrowth of more resistant strains.

While there are several mechanisms by which organisms become resistant to antibiotics,[8] the production of enzymes such as β-lactamase remains a major problem. These enzymes are either chromosomally coded within the organism's genetic structure, or are passed from one organism to another by extrachromosomal material such as plasmids, bacteriophages or transposons. Thus, as one species of organism develops resistance, the information can be passed to other species very rapidly. The rate at which some enzymes are produced is influenced by the presence of the antibiotic – a process called induction. An organism initially sensitive to an antibiotic (e.g. a third-generation cephalosporin) may, over several days, become resistant as the enzyme levels increase.

Strategies for control of nosocomial infections

Many measures exist to reduce the incidence and impact of nosocomial infections. Most are specific to the infection involved (e.g. pneumonia or cystitis) but the following can be considered of general value.

Hand-washing

The importance of hand-washing to reduce infection was promoted by Semmelweis almost 150 years ago. Despite its known value, compliance rates are low.[9–12] It has been suggested that better handwashing by staff can lead to a 25–50% reduction in nosocomial infections.[13]

Infection control teams

Hospital infection control teams aim to minimize the risk of infection for patients and staff by a series of functions (Table 62.4). Such teams provide valuable feedback to other members of staff, and they act as

Table 62.4 Roles of infection control teams

Surveillance and investigation of infection outbreaks
Education of staff
Review of antibiotic utilization
Review of antibiotic resistance patterns
Review of infection control procedures and policies

educators on infection control measures. More recently, infection control teams have become involved in the issues of staff health, particularly with the increase in blood-borne infections transmitted by needlestick injuries (i.e. HIV, hepatitis B, hepatitis C). There is now evidence that infection control programmes work. Results from the large SENIC multicentre trial[14] show that, over several years, infections increased in hospitals without an effective programme while centres with effective programmes showed a reduction in all types of nosocomial infections.

Selective decontamination of the digestive tract (SDD)

As bacterial overgrowth of the gastrointestinal tract (GIT) is considered to lead to nosocomial pneumonia and multiple organ dysfunction syndrome, numerous studies have examined whether SDD can break the colonization–infection cycle. Thus patients have been commenced on oral non-absorbable antibiotics directed to the usual pathogens; these preparations include polymyxin, tobramycin, gentamicin, neomycin, nystatin and amphotericin, which are active against Gram-negative organisms and fungi. These antibiotics are made into pastes which are applied to the oropharynx and administered through nasogastric tubes. Some studies have included a course of parenteral antibiotic to eradicate infections present at the time of admission.

Since the original study of Stoutenbeek *et al.*,[15] many papers have been published, with some showing benefit, others concluding no advantage, and a few pointing to problems of antibiotic resistance. Some studies examined the cost-effectiveness of such treatment. Difficulties exist when evaluating these studies, particularly the different outcome measures

used, the statistical power of the studies and the methods employed to make a positive diagnosis of infection. For example, pneumonia can be diagnosed by clinical signs, results of expectorated sputum or cultures obtained from sterile protected brushes during bronchoscopy. As a result, different incidences and prevalences of infection are reported. Furthermore, reduction in infection rates may not alter mortality when underlying diseases play the major role.

To overcome some of these problems, several authors have used meta-analysis – a statistical technique which combines data from many trials to provide larger numbers for testing hypotheses.[16] While useful, meta-analyses do not supplant carefully designed clinical studies. Two meta-analyses of SDD were published recently (Table 62.5)[17,18] and are summarized below:

1 Compared to no treatment or placebo, SDD reduces the incidence of nosocomial infection. Effectiveness is related to baseline risk of nosocomial pneumonia, and is less when more rigorous definitions of pneumonia are used.
2 Infection rates for Gram-negative organisms are lower than rates for Gram-positive organisms. Given the antibiotics included in the protocols, this result is expected.
3 Subset analysis has not shown that certain groups (e.g. trauma victims) respond better to SDD than other groups.
4 SDD involves additional costs which may be offset by reduced infection rates.
5 The effect on mortality is marginal but favours active treatment. Subgroup analysis reveals no benefit, but a larger effect is seen when systemic antibiotics are included in the protocols.
6 Length of hospital stay is unaffected by treatment.

Table 62.5 Summary of meta-analyses of selective decontamination of the digestive tract (SDD)

Measure	Heyland et al.[18] Relative risk (96% CI), SDD vs control	Kollef[17] Rates of infection control vs SDD
Acquired infection rate		
Gram-positive infections		0.206, 0.171*
Gram-negative infections		0.355, 0.087***
Mixed infections		0.081, 0.022***
Pneumonia	0.46 (0.39, 0.56)	0.219, 0.074***
Pneumonia, Gram-negative		0.138, 0.019***
Mortality	0.87 (0.79, 0.97)	0.262, 0.243 NS
Length of stay (days)	15.5 (SDD) vs 17.0 (control)	

The results in each study have been expressed differently. Heyland *et al.* use the relative risk (with 95% confidence intervals; CI) where a value less than 1 indicates reduced infection rates for those receiving SDD. Kollef quotes the incidence of infection in both groups. *$P < 0.05$; ***$P < 0.001$; NS = not significant.

7 SDD is usually without side-effects, although the possibility of drug allergy exists. The emergence of resistant strains has been documented.[19-21]

It thus appears that SDD will reduce the incidence of infection in critically ill patients, but improvements in outcome, such as mortality and length of stay, remain unproven.

Urinary tract infections[22]

Urinary tract infections are the most common nosocomial infection reported. Although mortality rates for these infections are low, patients can die from urinary tract sepsis.

Pathogenesis

Nosocomial urinary tract infections are almost always due to the presence of a urinary catheter. Organisms gain access to the bladder by migration along the catheter lumen (intraluminal) or alongside the catheter from the urethral meatus (extraluminal). Pyuria and bacteriuria can be found in most patients in whom a catheter has been present for over 5 days – the risk of infection increases by 5% for each catheterized day. Hence the infection risk is enormous as 15% of hospital patients are catheterized.

Complications of bacteriuria include symptomatic urinary tract infections, bacteraemia in 1–5% (more common in men), pyelonephritis, urinary stones and perinephric abscess. Mortality is related to bacteraemia. It is reported that the urinary tract is responsible for 13% of all bacteraemic deaths.[23]

Microbiology

Gram-negative organisms are the most frequent cause of infections (Table 62.6). The GIT is the usual reservoir of these organisms, but outbreaks have occurred with contamination of antiseptic solutions, irrigation fluids and urine containers.

Table 62.6 Organisms responsible for nosocomial urinary tract infections[79]

Organism	Percentage
Escherichia coli	30.0%
Enterococcus spp.	15.0%
Pseudomonas aeruginosa	12.5%
Klebsiella spp.	7.6%
Proteus spp.	7.3%

Risk factors

Nine independent risk factors for bacteriuria were defined in a study of 1474 catheterizations.[24] These included duration of catheterization, open systems, diabetes, female patient and abnormal creatinine.

Treatment

As a general rule, the catheter should be removed or replaced as soon as possible. Antibiotics are recommended if there are signs of systemic infection such as fever or loin pain. This may be difficult in critically ill patients where catheter removal is impractical, and any infection requires treatment. Antibiotic choice is determined by urine cultures and sensitivity testing, but empirical therapy often includes a broad-spectrum cephalosporin or aminoglycoside. Quinolones (e.g. norfloxacin and ciprofloxacin) may be useful.

Prevention

The most important consideration should be the need for catheterization. Catheters should not be inserted for convenience (e.g. an incontinent patient) and should be removed as soon as possible. Even short-term catheterization, such as 'in–out' techniques practised in emergency or obstetric departments, carries a risk of infection. Catheters should be inserted aseptically and a closed drainage system used to collect the urine; samples for laboratory analyses must be taken in a sterile manner. Care should be taken to secure the catheter and provide continuous unobstructed drainage. Other recommendations of uncertain efficacy include the use of meatal antiseptics, antibiotic-impregnated catheters and periodic bladder irrigations.

Nosocomial pneumonia[25,26]

Pneumonia is the third commonest nosocomial infection after urinary tract and surgical wounds. Its incidence varies depending upon the type of patient and severity of illness. Estimates from surveys range from 0.6 to 1.1%;[27,28] advancing age increases the risk. Mortality rates vary from 25 to 40%[29] and nosocomial pneumonia may directly cause or contribute to 16% of all infection-related deaths.

Predisposing factors

Several factors are known to increase the chance of nosocomial pneumonia:

1 *Intubation*: Intubated patients have four times the number of infections than non-intubated patients. Tracheostomies may further increase the risk.
2 *ICUs*: Patients admitted to an ICU, even if they do not require intubation, are at greater risk than patients in general ward areas.

3 *Antibiotics*: May assist in the colonization of the oropharynx by selectively eradicating the normal flora.

4 *Recent surgery*: Patients who are obese, of advanced age, or who are acutely ill, or following surgery to the thorax or abdomen have more respiratory infections; incidences of 20–50% have been reported.

5 *Advanced age.*

6 *Immunosuppression.*

7 *Chronic lung disease.*

Diagnosis

The recent CDC guidelines for the diagnosis of nosocomial pneumonia are shown in Table 62.7. While useful for hospital-wide surveys, they are less useful in critically ill patients where fever is common,

Table 62.7 Principles for the diagnosis of nosocomial pneumonia[3]

Crackles on auscultation or dullness to percussion on physical examination of the chest and any of the following:

New onset of purulent sputum

Organism isolated from blood cultures

Isolation of pathogen from specimen obtained by transtracheal aspirate, bronchial brushing or biopsy

Chest radiographic examination shows new or progressive infiltration, consolidation, cavitation or pleural effusion

Isolation of virus or detection of virus antigen in respiratory secretions

Diagnostic single antibody titre (IgM) or fourfold increase in paired serum samples (IgG) for pathogen

Histopathological evidence of pneumonia

IgM = Immunoglobulin M.

and chest signs and radiographic appearances may be due to non-infectious conditions such as acute respiratory distress syndrome.[30] Routine samples collected during endotracheal suctioning of intubated patients are rarely free of organisms, despite the absence of lower respiratory tract infections. The recognized gold standard for diagnosis of infection – histopathological examination of lung tissue – is impractical for routine use and is reserved for patients with unusual infections or immunosuppression.

Diagnostic tests include examination and culture of expectorated sputum, endotracheal aspirates, samples obtained during bronchoscopy (i.e. aspiration, lavage and protected specimen brushes) and trans-

thoracic needle aspiration.[31] Results from *expectorated sputum* must be viewed critically. Satisfactory specimens should contain <25 polymorphs and >10 squamous epithelial cells per low-power field. Samples obtained by *endotracheal suctioning* of intubated patients are frequently sent for culture. They are rarely negative and organisms obtained may differ from the true pathogen in 40% of patients with proven pneumonia.[32] For this reason, samples from distal airways, obtained without oropharyngeal contamination (e.g. using protected brushes or bronchoalveolar lavage during fibreoptic bronchoscopy) are often preferred and strongly recommended in research studies.

Pathogenesis

Nosocomial pneumonias may develop from aspiration of organisms, by direct extension from adjacent infections, or by blood-borne spread. Aspiration remains the major factor, and it occurs in normal subjects as well as in those with impaired conscious state;[33] endotracheal and nasogastric tubes increase the risk of aspiration. Under normal circumstances, the oropharynx resists colonization with Gram-negative bacteria. Sick people, on the other hand, become colonized within days of admission to hospital; an estimated 70% of ICU patients undergo this change in flora.[34] Pneumonia will develop in up to 25% of patients colonized, compared to a 3% incidence in non-colonized patients. Risks for colonization include severity of illness, duration of hospitalization, prior or concomitant use of antibiotics, intubation, renal failure and underlying respiratory disease.

Most bacteria colonizing the oropharynx originate in the gastrointestinal tract. Several studies have shown that organisms responsible for pneumonia can be grown from the stomach before pneumonia is evident.[35,36] Contaminated respiratory equipment such as nebulizers, respiratory circuits and blood-gas analysers have featured in some epidemics.

Microbiology

The organisms responsible for nosocomial pneumonias vary depending upon the type of sample cultured. Enterobacteriaceae (*Enterobacter* spp., *Klebsiella* spp., *Escherichia coli*, *Serratia* spp., *Proteus* spp.) comprise the majority.[37–40] *Pseudomonas* spp., *Staphylococcus aureus*, *Haemophilus* spp. and *Streptococcus pneumoniae* are relatively common, as are polymicrobial infections. Fungi and viruses have featured in some reports, and minor epidemics of *Legionella* spp. have been described. Enterobacteriaceae spp. probably arise from the endogenous flora while *Pseudomonas* spp. is an environmental contaminant spread by hands and objects. It is this profile of organisms which determines the best empirical choice of antibiotics.

Treatment

While some studies have suggested that antibiotics may not alter the outcome of nosocomial pneumonia, there is increasing evidence that the correct choice of antibiotics does reduce mortality.[39,41] Certain factors should be taken into consideration – severity of infection, duration of hospitalization, prior antibiotics and prevalence of organisms (and resistance patterns) within the hospital.

Infections early in the course of an admission are more likely to be sensitive to antibiotics than subsequent infections. This is partly due to the ability of some organisms to produce antibiotic neutralizing enzymes such as β-lactamase. The duration of antibiotic therapy remains contentious and must be modified for each individual patient; penetration of most antibiotics into lung tissue and sputum is poor.[42]

The recent *Antibiotic Guidelines*[43] recommend empirical therapy with a broad-spectrum third-generation cephalosporin (e.g. cefotaxime and ceftriaxone), to which erythromycin is added if *Legionella* is suspected. Subsequent infections often exhibit resistance to these antibiotics; the addition of an aminoglycoside or change to a carbapenem (e.g. imipenem) has been suggested. Cloxacillin or flucloxacillin can be added if *Staphylococcus aureus* is suspected, or vancomycin if methicillin-resistant *S. aureus* is prevalent. In units caring for patients with chronic lung diseases (e.g. bronchiectasis and cystic fibrosis), antibiotic regimens should include drugs with proven activity against *Pseudomonas* spp. (e.g. ticarcillin/piperacillin plus gentamicin/tobramycin; see Chapter 33).

Interventions to reduce nosocomial pneumonia

General measures (Table 62.8)

Endotracheal and nasogastric tubes should be removed as soon as possible and antibiotic usage limited to treating documented infections and for established prophylactic regimens.

Respiratory circuits can become contaminated and should be changed every 48 h, especially when in-line heated humidifiers are used. Heat and moisture exchangers with antibacterial properties reduce bacte-

Table 62.8 General measures to reduce nosocomial pneumonia[26]

Hand-washing by staff
Evaluate swallowing mechanisms
Limit antibiotic administration
Remove nasogastric tubes and endotracheal tubes
Elevate head of bed 30°
Implement preoperative and postoperative respiratory care

rial aerosols from ventilator circuits,[44] and may reduce infections in selected patients and reduce the frequency of circuit changes. Correct methods of suctioning of endotracheal tubes are taught to, and reinforced with, all attending staff. Nebulized, prophylactic antibiotics are no longer recommended.[45]

Reduction in gastrointestinal colonization

SDD is discussed above. The role of gastric pH and its modification in the pathogenesis of infections remain controversial. A long-standing feature of critical illness has been the tendency to gastrointestinal haemorrhage from peptic ulceration. Antacids and, later, H_2-antagonists such as cimetidine and ranitidine have reduced the number of critically ill patients who have a major gastrointestinal haemorrhage during their admission; the presumed mechanism is elevation of gastric pH, although improved resuscitation has also contributed. However, an acid environment within the stomach inhibits the growth of organisms, while gastric colonization is promoted by an alkaline pH. Several authors have shown an increased incidence of nosocomial pneumonia when gastric pH has been raised to 5.0 or above.[46,47]

Attention has turned to the usefulness of sucralfate, which exerts a cytoprotective effect upon the gastric mucosa but does not alter pH. Several controlled trials have compared antacids/H_2-antagonists with sucralfate, and used gastrointestinal bleeding and nosocomial pneumonia as measures of outcome.[35,48–51] Although results have been variable, two meta-analyses of randomized controlled trials have been reported and are summarized below.[52,53]

1 With respect to gastrointestinal haemorrhage, sucralfate is no less effective than high-dose antacids or H_2-antagonists.[53]
2 Increasing pH did not appear to increase the risk of pneumonia in one analysis,[52] while infection rates were consistently higher in patients with antacids/H_2-antagonists in the other.[53] A major difficulty of the meta-analyses is that criteria to diagnose pneumonia varied from study to study. A recent study found that early-onset pneumonia (<4 days) did not differ between the groups, but late-onset pneumonia was lower in patients receiving sucralfate (5%) than those receiving high-dose antacids (16%) or ranitidine (21%).[35] Further studies are required which take into account patient profiles, severity of illness, timing of infection and more precise methods to diagnose nosocomial pneumonia.

Sepsis and intravascular devices

Intravascular devices are responsible for a significant number of infections, both local (phlebitis and abscess) and systemic (e.g. bacteraemia and endocarditis). The majority of primary nosocomial bacteraemias are due to such devices.

Pathogenesis

A catheter traverses the skin for siting within a vessel, and a giving set connects the fluid (infusate) to the catheter at the hub. Contamination and infection can occur at all these sites. Contamination of infusates is uncommon, but has been described in the manufacturing process and during addition of medications. In a study of over 2000 catheters, cutaneous colonization of the insertion site and contamination of the hub were major risk factors for infection.[54] Other factors, e.g. catheter material, number of lumens, experience of staff inserting the device, concomitant sepsis and the nature of the fluid infused may contribute.

Microbiology

Staphylococcus aureus and *S. epidermidis* remain the most common organisms isolated. *S. epidermidis* can produce a 'slime' which allows better adherence to catheters.[55] Other organisms include Gram-negative bacteria, *Candida* spp., and JK diphtheroids. *Candida* infections remain troublesome, and have been linked to administration of parenteral nutrition and, more recently, to the administration of antibiotics.[56]

Diagnosis

It is sometimes difficult to diagnose a catheter-related infection as signs of local inflammation are present in under 50% of cases. A high index of suspicion that any new fever or sepsis may be due to an infected intravascular device is necessary. Culture of the removed device using semiquantitative methods is considered the current diagnostic gold standard;[57] colony counts >15 are used to define an infected catheter. Blood cultures may be necessary and provide confirmatory evidence.

Peripheral intravenous catheters

Most hospital patients receive a peripheral IV line at some stage. Infections are more likely with lines placed distally (hands versus arms), in the lower limbs, and by cut-down techniques. Risk factors include colonization of the skin, contamination of the hub, moisture under the dressing and prolonged catheterization.[54] Changing cannulae every 48–72 h is commonly recommended. The materials contained within the catheter may also influence infection rates.[58] Variable results have been reported with occlusive dressings;[54,59] a recent meta-analysis of seven studies demonstrated an increased risk for catheter tip infection when transparent dressings were applied.[60]

Central venous catheters (CVC)

In CVC-related infections, the risk of infection rises with increased duration of insertion. Hence some ICUs define weekly changes for all CVCs. Catheters exchanged over a guide wire have fewer local complications (e.g. pneumothorax and arterial puncture) but may result in more infections.[61,62] Local infection remains the major risk factor. Cercenado *et al.*[63] found that, in 56.6% of catheter infections, the same organism was isolated from the catheter tip and the surrounding skin; in 22%, the same organisms were grown from the hub. Increased infection rates have been found with multi-lumen catheters,[61] while other studies have found no increase.[64] In recent years, reduced infection rates have been reported with an attachable silver impregnated cuff,[65,66] and by bonding of antibiotics to the catheter.[67] A catheter impregnated with silver sulfadiazine and chlorhexidine has been marketed in recent years.[68] Location of the CVC affects infection rates. The lowest rates are seen with subclavian lines, followed by jugular and then by femoral lines.

For patients requiring long-term central venous access, Silastic catheters have been associated with very low infection rates.[69,70] These catheters were originally tunnelled surgically, but can be placed percutaneously while maintaining low infection rates.[71]

Pulmonary artery catheters

Pulmonary artery (PA) catheters are commonly used with little consideration for infective complications. Infections are related to the introducer, the hubs and the portion of the PA catheter within the introducer. In a prospective study of 71 PA catheters, local infections were seen in 17% and bacteraemias in 5.6%. The risk for infection rose from 9% for catheters of <4 days' duration to 18% for catheters >4 days.[71] In another study, septicaemias were observed with colonization of the sheath, the skin or the extravascular component of the catheter.[72] This has led to recommendations that PA catheters be replaced between 4 and 7 days.

Arterial lines

General recommendations have included routine replacement of arterial lines every 3–4 days. Several recent studies provide additional information. Leroy *et al.*[73] reported positive tip cultures in 22.5% and positive cultures of infusates in 23.5% of cannulations, but no episodes of bacteraemia were observed. Norwood *et al.*[74] reported no infections or skin contamination with catheters which were changed within 96 h; 9.5% of radial/femoral sites and 44% of axillary sites were associated with catheter-related infections, all associated with positive skin sites. Raad *et al.*[71] found local infection in 15% and septicaemias in 5.5% of cannulations, all with catheters longer than 4 days' duration.

Treatment of infections

In general, patients with bacteraemia and fever require appropriate antibiotics. Any catheter with sepsis at the puncture site must be removed. If the cause of a bacteraemia remains obscure, all intravascular devices, particularly CVCs, should be removed and cultured. Insertion of another CVC is best avoided for several days, as it could become colonized by the resolving bacteraemia. It is questionable whether railroading (removing an infected catheter over a guide wire and inserting a new one over the same wire) should be used.

The final choice of antibiotic depends upon results of cultures and sensitivity testing. Flucloxacillin with gentamicin is recommended as empirical therapy. For patients allergic to penicillin, immunocompromised patients and those in hospitals with significant methicillin-resistant *Staphylococcus* spp., vancomycin is used instead of flucloxacillin.

Broviac or Hickman catheters may also become colonized, but antibiotics administered through the infected catheter may eradicate the infection, thus avoiding removal of the catheter.[75,76] This seems a reasonable approach, as these catheters are difficult to insert and remove, often requiring a general anaesthetic. Although antibiotic therapy alone has been extensively documented in paediatric oncological literature, there is a recent report of an antibiotic-lock technique for patients on home parenteral nutrition.[77]

Prevention of infections related to intravascular devices

General and specific guidelines have been suggested to diminish infections related to intravascular devices. Some suggestions, however, require confirmation by appropriate clinical studies.

General

1 adequate hand-washing;
2 adequate skin disinfection;
3 insertion under aseptic conditions;
4 intravenous team to insert and manage lines;
5 anchoring of lines to prevent excessive movement;
6 closed systems with limited interruptions to the lines;
7 application of sterile dressings to the insertion site;
8 daily inspection of catheter site.

Peripheral venous

Frequent rotation of sites at 48–72-hourly intervals.

Central venous

1 adequate preparation of site;
2 aseptic insertion technique;
3 frequent inspection of insertion site.

Parenteral nutrition lines

1 lines dedicated to parenteral nutrition;
2 management of catheters and lines by a parenteral nutrition team.

Arterial

1 replacement of lines after 96 h;
2 aseptic techniques to fill domes and lines;
3 avoidance of unnecessary stopcocks.

Techniques of unproven benefit

1 antiseptic cream at insertion site;
2 routine changes of dressings at frequent intervals;
3 occlusive antimicrobial dressings;
4 in-line filters;
5 tunnelling of central venous catheters;
6 routine flushing of long-term central venous catheters.

Wound infections[78]

Wound infections represent 20–25% of all nosocomial infections. They are a major problem in all hospitals, and are capable of inflicting considerable pain and suffering. In an Australian survey, 4.6% of hospital inpatients had a postoperative wound infection.[4]

Pathogenesis

Most surgical wound infections result from organisms introduced at the time of surgery, usually from the patient's own flora. Occasionally, infections may result from contamination of equipment or solutions used in the procedure, or from attendant staff.

Risk factors

A major determinant of infection is the nature of the procedure itself.

1 *Clean* procedures do not involve entry of the respiratory, gastrointestinal or genitourinary tracts; such procedures include plastic and most orthopaedic surgery. Infection rates are usually less than 10%.
2 *Clean-contaminated* procedures involve entry of respiratory, gastrointestinal or genitourinary tracts, but without major contamination of the surgical field. Infection rates are higher than clean procedures and estimated at 10–15%.

3 *Contaminated* procedures include traumatic wounds, situations where a major break in technique occurs or where there is spillage of gastrointestinal contents. Infections are more common again with rates around 20%.

4 *Dirty* procedures are those in which an infected process already exists; wound infections occur in 30–40% of such instances.

Other factors contributing to increased infection rates include operations of long duration, advanced age, poor nutritional status, diabetes, renal failure and steroid therapy. In Australia, infections are more common in large public hospitals (5.4%) compared to private hospitals (2.5%) and in males (6.5%) compared to females (3.4%).

Microbiology

Common infecting organisms are listed by occurrence in Table 62.9. Early infections (24–48 h) are usually due to β-haemolytic streptococci or to clostridial species; the latter are rarely seen in practice. These infections cause fever and intense

Table 62.9 Organisms responsible for postoperative wound infections[79]

Organism	Percentage
Staphylococcus aureus	19.0%
Enterococcus spp.	11.4%
Escherichia coli	11.4%
Staphylococci, coagulase-negative	8.4%
Pseudomonas aeruginosa	8.1%
Enterobacter spp.	6.9%
Proteus spp.	5.0%

wound pain and must be treated early and adequately. Staphylococcal infections usually occur within 3–6 days of surgery. These wounds tend to be oedematous and inflamed, but respond quickly to adequate drainage. On the other hand, wound infections from Gram-negative organisms may not appear for 7–10 days, and local signs are less intense. However, fever, tachycardia and bacteraemias are more common.

Prevention[43,78]

General

The importance of simple measures cannot be overstressed; operative technique, removal of devitalized tissue, maintenance of sterility and removal of staff with active infections from operating theatres are important in reducing infection rates.

Antibiotic prophylaxis

Antibiotics have often been used to prevent wound infections, but use and effectiveness depend upon the surgery undertaken. Antibiotics are essential for dirty procedures, when their use should be considered therapeutic rather than prophylactic. At the other extreme, most clean procedures require no therapy.

Prophylactic antibiotics are indicated where there is a significant risk of infection or where a postoperative infection would have severe complications. To be effective, prophylactic antibiotics should be administered at the time of surgery to ensure maximal concentrations during the procedure. They should also cover the potential pathogens. A single dose should suffice, although a second dose is recommended if the procedure extends beyond 3 h; prolonged administration increases the chance of antibiotic resistance and unnecessarily exposes the patient to adverse effects from the drugs (see Chapter 64).

Cardiac surgery
Prophylaxis for coronary artery bypass grafts and valve replacements is well-established, although unproven. A single agent such as cephalothin, cefamandole or cephazolin is often used, although a combination of flucloxacillin with gentamicin is a suitable alternative.

Vascular surgery
Similar recommendations have been made for major aortic repairs or for surgery involving the lower limbs, especially if groin incisions are made. A first-generation cephalosporin or a combination of flucloxacillin and gentamicin is recommended.

Orthopaedic surgery
Another indication for prophylactic antibiotics is the insertion of orthopaedic prostheses such as prosthetic joint replacements and internal fixation of some fractures. As staphylococcal infections represent the major risk, single antibiotic regimens such as cephalothin or flucloxacillin are used.

Biliary tract and upper gastrointestinal tract surgery
Bile in health is usually sterile, but organisms can be cultured from bile of patients with chronic calculus disease, acute cholecysititis, obstructive jaundice and common duct stones. Furthermore, postoperative infections are commoner in patients over 70 years of age and in patients with a history of fever prior to surgery; enterococci are often encountered. Recommended antibiotics for prophylaxis include metronidazole with a cephalosporin such as cephalothin; gentamicin; or a broader-spectrum cephalosporin such as cefoxitin.

Colorectal surgery

The human bowel contains many organisms which are potentially harmful outside their normal environment. The organisms increase in quantity from the sparsely colonized small bowel to the densely inhabited colon. As preoperative mechanical preparation is not sufficient to prevent infection, various antibiotic regimens have been proposed, including a combination of oral erythromycin and neomycin. However, many regimens combine metronidazole and a first-generation cephalosporin; recommend gentamicin alone; or suggest a broader-spectrum cephalosporin such as cefoxitin.

Gynaecological surgery

Infections following hysterectomies are more common in younger premenopausal women, following prolonged procedures and after abdominal as well as vaginal approaches. Antibiotics such as tinidazole alone or metronidazole combined with cephalothin are recommended.

Urological surgery

In general, antibiotic prophylaxis for urological procedures does not confer any benefit. Patients with urinary tract infections should be treated before surgery. If the operation cannot be delayed, appropriate antibiotics should be continued during and following the procedure.

References

1. Mandell G, Douglas R and Bennett J (1990) *Principles and Practice of Infectious Diseases.* New York: Churchill Livingstone.
2. Wenzel R (1986) The evolving art and science of hospital epidemiology. *J Infect Dis* **153**:462–470.
3. Centers for Disease Control (1989) CDC definitions for nosocomial infections, 1988. *Am Rev Respir Dis* **139**:1058–1059.
4. Department of Health (1987) The Australian nosocomial infection prevalence survey. First report, March 1987. Sydney: University of Sydney.
5. Trilla A (1994) Epidemiology of nosocomial infections in adult intensive care units. *Intensive Care Med* **20**(suppl):S1–4.
6. Pavillard R, Harvey K, Douglas D *et al.* (1982) Epidemic of hospital-acquired infection due to methicillin-resistant *Staphylococcus aureus* in major Victorian hospitals. *Med J Aust* **1**:451–454.
7. King K, Brady L, Thomson M *et al.* (1982) Antibiotic-resistant staphylococci in a teaching hospital. *Med J Aust* **2**:461–465.
8. Mayer K, Opal S and Medeiros A (1990) Mechanisms of antibiotic resistance. In: Mandell G, Douglas R and Bennett J (eds) *Principles and Practice of Infectious Diseases.* London: Churchill Livingstone, pp. 218–228.
9. Albert RK and Condie F (1981) Hand-washing patterns in medical intensive-care units. *N Engl J Med* **304**:1465–1466.
10. Graham M (1990) Frequency and duration of handwashing in an intensive care unit. *Am J Infect Control* **18**:77–81.
11. Quraishi ZA, McGuckin M and Blais FX (1984) Duration of handwashing in intensive care units: a descriptive study. *Am J Infect Control* **12**:83–87.
12. Jarvis W (1994) Handwashing – the Semmelweis lesson forgotten? *Lancet* **344**:1311–1312.
13. Doebbeling B, Stanley G, Sheetz C *et al.* (1992) Comparative efficacy of alternative hand-washing agents in reducing nosocomial infections in intensive care units. *N Engl J Med* **327**:88–93.
14. Haley RW, Culver DH, White JW *et al.* (1985) The efficacy of infection surveillance and control programs in preventing nosocomial infections in US hospitals. *Am J Epidemiol* **121**:182–205.
15. Stoutenbeek C, van Saene H, Miranda D *et al.* (1984) The effects of selective decontamination of the digestive tract on colonisation and infection rate in multiple trauma patients. *Intensive Care Med* **10**:185–192.
16. L'Abbe KA, Detsky AS and O'Rourke K (1987) Meta-analysis in clinical research. *Ann Intern Med* **107**:224–233.
17. Kollef M (1994) The role of selective digestive tract decontamination on mortality and respiratory tract infections. A meta-analysis. *Chest* **105**:1101–1108.
18. Heyland D, Cook D, Jaeschke R *et al.* (1994) Selective decontamination of the digestive tract. An overview. *Chest* **105**:1221–1229.
19. Konrad F, Schwalbe B, Heeg K *et al.* (1989) Frequency of colonization and pneumonia and development of resistance in long-term ventilated intensive-care patients subjected to selective decontamination of the digestive tract. *Anaesthesist* **38**:99–109.
20. Brun-Buisson C, Legrand P, Rauss A *et al.* (1989) Intestinal decontamination for control of nosocomial multiresistant Gram-negative bacilli. Study of an outbreak in an intensive care unit. *Ann Intern Med* **110**:873–881.
21. Bonten MJ, van Tiel FH, van der Geest S *et al.* (1993) *Enterococcus faecalis* pneumonia complicating topical antimicrobial prophylaxis. *N Engl J Med* **328**:209–210.
22. Warren J (1990) Nosocomial urinary tract infections. In: Mandell G, Douglas R and Bennett J (eds) *Principles and Practice of Infectious Diseases.* London: Churchill Livingstone, pp. 2205–2215.
23. Bryan CS and Reynolds KL (1984) Hospital-acquired bacteremic urinary tract infection: epidemiology and outcome. *J Urol* **132**:494–498.
24. Platt R, Polk BF, Murdock B *et al.* (1986) Risk factors for nosocomial urinary tract infection. *Am J Epidemiol* **124**:977–985.
25. Pennington J (1990) Nosocomial respiratory infection. In: Mandell G, Douglas R and Bennett J (eds) *Principles and Practice of Infectious Diseases.* London: Churchill Livingstone, pp. 2199–2205.
26. Dal Nogare AR (1994) Nosocomial pneumonia in the medical and surgical patient. Risk factors and primary management. *Med Clin North Am* **78**:1081–1090.

27. Haley RW, Hooton TM, Culver DH *et al.* (1981) Nosocomial infections in US hospitals, 1975–1976: estimated frequency by selected characteristics of patients. *Am J Med* **70**:947–959.

28. Hughes JM, Culver DH, White JW *et al.* (1983) Nosocomial infection surveillance, 1980–1982. *MMWR CDC Surveill Summ* **32**:1SS–16SS.

29. Wenzel R (1989) Hospital-acquired pneumonia: overview of the current state of the art for prevention and control. *J Clin Microbiol Infect Dis* **8**:56–60.

30. Niederman M, Craven D, Fein A *et al.* (1990) Pneumonia in the critically ill hospitalized patient. *Chest* **97**:170–181.

31. Griffin JJ and Meduri GU (1994) New approaches in the diagnosis of nosocomial pneumonia. *Med Clin North Am* **78**:1091–1122.

32. Hill JD, Ratliff JL, Parrott JC *et al.* (1976) Pulmonary pathology in acute respiratory insufficiency: lung biopsy as a diagnostic tool. *J Thorac Cardiovasc Surg* **71**:64–71.

33. Huxley EJ, Viroslav J, Gray WR *et al.* (1978) Pharyngeal aspiration in normal adults and patients with depressed consciousness. *Am J Med* **64**:564–568.

34. Johanson WG Jr, Pierce AK, Sanford JP *et al.* (1972) Nosocomial respiratory infections with Gram-negative bacilli. The significance of colonization of the respiratory tract. *Ann Intern Med* **77**:701–706.

35. Prod'hom G, Leuenberger P, Koerfer J *et al.* (1994) Nosocomial pneumonia in mechanically ventilated patients receiving antacid, ranitidine, or sucralfate as prophylaxis for stress ulcer. A randomized controlled trial. *Ann Intern Med* **120**:653–662.

36. Garvey BM, McCambley JA and Tuxen DV (1989) Effects of gastric alkalization on bacterial colonization in critically ill patients. *Crit Care Med* **17**:211–216.

37. Bartlett JG, O'Keefe P, Tally FP *et al.* (1986) Bacteriology of hospital-acquired pneumonia. *Arch Intern Med* **146**:868–871.

38. Bryan CS and Reynolds KL (1984) Bacteremic nosocomial pneumonia. Analysis of 172 episodes from a single metropolitan area. *Am Rev Respir Dis* **129**:668–671.

39. Celis R, Torres A, Gatell JM *et al.* (1988) Nosocomial pneumonia. A multivariate analysis of risk and prognosis. *Chest* **93**:318–324.

40. Centers for Disease Control (1983) National nosocomial infections study. *Morb Mort Week Rep* **33**.

41. Hilf M, Yu VL, Sharp J *et al.* (1989) Antibiotic therapy for *Pseudomonas aeruginosa* bacteremia: outcome correlations in a prospective study of 200 patients. *Am J Med* **87**:540–546.

42. Niederman MS (1994) An approach to empiric therapy of nosocomial pneumonia. *Med Clin North Am* **78**:1123–1141.

43. Victorian Drug Usage Advisory Committee (1994) *Antibiotic Guidelines*. Melbourne: Victorian Medical Postgraduate Foundation.

44. Saravolatz L, Pohlod D, Conway W *et al.* (1986) Lack of bacterial aerosols associated with heat and moisture exchangers. *Am Rev Respir Dis* **134**:214–216.

45. Feeley TW, Du Moulin GC, Hedley-Whyte J *et al.* (1975) Aerosol polymyxin and pneumonia in seriously ill patients. *N Engl J Med* **293**:471–475.

46. du Moulin GC, Paterson DG, Hedley-Whyte J *et al.* (1982) Aspiration of gastric bacteria in antacid-treated patients: a frequent cause of postoperative colonisation of the airway. *Lancet* **1**:242–245.

47. Donowitz LG, Page MC, Mileur BL *et al.* (1986) Alteration of normal gastric flora in critical care patients receiving antacid and cimetidine therapy. *Infect Control* **7**:23–26.

48. Driks MR, Craven DE, Celli BR *et al.* Nosocomial pneumonia in intubated patients given sucralfate as compared with antacids or histamine type 2 blockers. The role of gastric colonization. *N Engl J Med* **317**:1376–1382.

49. Tryba M (1987) Risk of acute stress bleeding and nosocomial pneumonia in ventilated intensive care unit patients: sucralfate versus antacids. *Am J Med* **83**:117–124.

50. Kappstein I, Schulgen G, Friedrich T *et al.* (1991) Incidence of pneumonia in mechanically ventilated patients treated with sucralfate or cimetidine as prophylaxis for stress bleeding: bacterial colonization of the stomach. *Am J Med* **91**:125S–131S.

51. Simms HH, DeMaria E, McDonald L *et al.* (1991) Role of gastric colonization in the development of pneumonia in critically ill trauma patients: results of a prospective randomized trial. *J Trauma* **31**:531–536.

52. Cook DJ, Laine LA, Guyatt GH *et al.* (1991) Nosocomial pneumonia and the role of gastric pH. A meta-analysis. *Chest* **100**:7–13.

53. Tryba M (1991) Sucralfate versus antacids or H$_2$-antagonists for stress ulcer prophylaxis: a meta-analysis on efficacy and pneumonia rate. *Crit Care Med* **19**:942–949.

54. Maki DG and Ringer M (1987) Evaluation of dressing regimens for prevention of infection with peripheral intravenous catheters. Gauze, a transparent polyurethane dressing, and an iodophor-transparent dressing. *J Am Med Assoc* **258**:2396–2403.

55. Peters G, Locci R, Pulverer G *et al.* (1982) Adherence and growth of coagulase-negative staphylococci on surfaces of intravenous catheters. Comparison of the sterility of long-term central venous catheterization using single lumen, triple lumen, and pulmonary artery catheters. *J Infect Dis* **146**:479–482.

56. Wey SB, Mori M, Pfaller MA *et al.* (1989) Risk factors for hospital-acquired candidemia. A matched case-control study. *Arch Intern Med* **149**:2349–2353.

57. Maki DG, Weise CE and Sarafin HW (1977) A semi-quantitative culture method for identifying intravenous-catheter-related infection. *N Engl J Med* **296**:1305–1309.

58. Maki DG and Ringer M (1991) Risk factors for infusion-related phlebitis with small peripheral venous catheters. A randomized controlled trial. *Ann Intern Med* **114**:845–854.

59. Conly JM, Grieves K and Peters B (1989) A prospective, randomized study comparing transparent and dry gauze dressings for central venous catheters. *J Infect Dis* **159**:310–319.

60. Hoffmann KK, Weber DJ, Samsa GP *et al.* (1992) Transparent polyurethane film as an intravenous catheter dressing. A meta-analysis of the infection risks. *J Am Med Assoc* **267**:2072–2076.

61. Hilton E, Haslett TM, Borenstein MT *et al.* (1988) Central catheter infections: single- versus triple-lumen catheters. Influence of guide wires on infection rates when used for replacement of catheters. *Am J Med* **84**:667–672.

62. Cobb DK, High KP, Sawyer RG *et al.* (1992) A controlled trial of scheduled replacement of central venous and pulmonary-artery catheters. *N Engl J Med* **327**: 1062–1068.

63. Cercenado E, Ena J, Rodriguez Creixems M *et al.* (1990) A conservative procedure for the diagnosis of catheter-related infections. *Arch Intern Med* **150**:1417–1420.

64. Farkas JC, Liu N, Bleriot JP *et al.* (1992) Single- versus triple-lumen central catheter-related sepsis: a prospective randomized study in a critically ill population. *Am J Med* **93**:277–282.

65. Maki DG, Cobb L, Garman JK *et al.* (1988) An attachable silver-impregnated cuff for prevention of infection with central venous catheters: a prospective randomized multi-center trial. *Am J Med* **85**:307–314.

66. Flowers RHD, Schwenzer KJ, Kopel RF *et al.* (1989) Efficacy of an attachable subcutaneous cuff for the prevention of intravascular catheter-related infection. A randomized, controlled trial. *J Am Med Assoc* **261**:878–883.

67. Kamal GD, Pfaller MA, Rempe LE *et al.* (1991) Reduced intravascular catheter infection by antibiotic bonding. A prospective, randomized, controlled trial *J Am Med Assoc* **265**:2364–2368.

68. Mermel LA, Stolz SM and Maki DG (1993) Surface antimicrobial activity of heparin-bonded and antiseptic-impregnated vascular catheters. *J Infect Dis* **167**: 920–924.

69. Broviac JW, Cole JJ, Scribner BH *et al.* (1973) A silicone rubber atrial catheter for prolonged parenteral alimentation. *Surg Gynecol Obstet* **136**:602–606.

70. Hickman RO, Buckner CD, Clift RA *et al.* (1979) A modified right atrial catheter for access to the venous system in marrow transplant recipients. *Surg Gynecol Obstet* **148**:871–875.

71. Raad I, Davis S, Becker M *et al.* (1993) Low infection rate and long durability of nontunneled Silastic catheters. A safe and cost-effective alternative for long-term venous access. *Arch Intern Med* **153**:1791–1796.

72. Maki DG, Stolz SS, Wheeler S *et al.* (1994) A prospective, randomized trial of gauze and two polyurethane dressings for site care of pulmonary artery catheters: implications for catheter management. *Crit Care Med* **22**:1729–1737.

73. Leroy O, Billiau V, Beuscart C *et al.* (1989) Nosocomial infections associated with long-term radial artery cannulation. *Intensive Care Med* **15**:241–246.

74. Norwood SH, Cormier B, McMahon NG *et al.* (1988) Prospective study of catheter-related infection during prolonged arterial catheterization. *Crit Care Med* **16**:836–839.

75. Hiemenz J, Skelton J and Pizzo PA (1986) Perspective on the management of catheter-related infections in cancer patients. *Pediatr Infect Dis* **5**:6–11.

76. Hartman GE and Shochat SJ (1987) Management of septic complications associated with Silastic catheters in childhood malignancy. *Pediatr Infect Dis J* **6**:1042–1047.

77. Messing B, Peitra-Cohen S, Debure A *et al.* (1988) Antibiotic-lock technique: a new approach to optimal therapy for catheter-related sepsis in home-parenteral nutrition patients. *J Parenter Enteral Nutr* **12**:185–189.

78. Kaiser A (1990) Postoperative infections and antimicrobial prophylaxis. In: Mandell G, Douglas R and Bennett J (eds) *Principles and Practice of Infectious Diseases*. London: Churchill Livingstone, pp. 2245–2257.

79. Jarvis WR, White JW, Munn VP *et al.* (1984) Nosocomial infection surveillance, 1983. *MMWR CDC Surveill Summ* **33**:9SS–21SS.

J Lipman

The skin is the largest organ and acts as an excellent barrier against infection. It consists of the epidermis and dermis, and resides on fibrous connective tissue, the superficial and deep fasciae (Fig. 63.1). The fascial cleft, with nerves, arteries, veins, lymphatics and adipose tissue, lies between these fascial planes. Normal skin flora includes *Corynebacterium* spp., coagulase-negative staphylococci, *Micrococcus* spp., *Lactobacillus* and sometimes *Staphylococcus aureus*. Colonization by Gram-negative bacteria occurs in hospital patients, and there are more *S. aureus* in the altered flora.

Microorganisms seldom cause skin and soft-tissue infections. Serious infections can occur if:

1 there is a break in the skin;
2 soft tissues are ischaemic and non-viable;

3 colonizing bacteria are particularly virulent;
4 the patient is immunocompromised (Fig. 63.2).[1-9]

Infection is more likely to be found in patients with diabetes mellitus, cirrhosis, malnutrition, major trauma, advanced age, renal failure, steroid use, collagen vascular diseases and malignancies.[1-10] Differentiation between soft-tissue infections can be difficult, and one unified management approach to severe forms is appropriate.[11,12]

Classification

The bacteriology and subtypes of severe soft-tissue infections have not changed significantly over the last century.[13-15] Many organisms can cause different

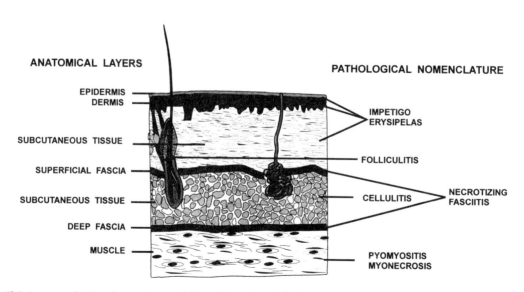

Fig. 63.1 Anatomy of skin and nomenclature of skin and deep tissue infections.

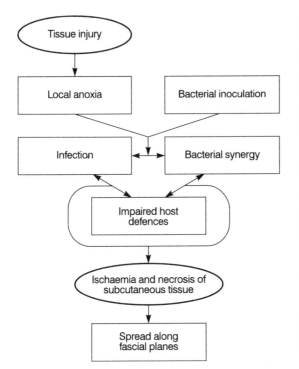

Fig. 63.2 Pathogenesis of severe soft-tissue infections.

clinical syndromes and classification of soft-tissue infections can be confusing. A wealth of terms have been used, but many refer to the same diseases (e.g. Meleney's gangrene, haemolytic streptococcal gangrene and progressive bacterial synergistic gangrene).[13] Classification according to the anatomical site of infection is more logical (Fig. 63.1).

Impetigo[1-3]

Impetigo is a superficial skin infection more common in children, caused by group A streptococci, *Staphylococcus aureus* or both. Mild infections can be managed with topical antibiotics; more serious infections need parenteral penicillin.

Folliculitis[2,3]

This is an infection arising in hair follicles and apocrine glands. *S. aureus* is the usual causative organism. Topical antibiotic treatment is usually all that is required.

Erysipelas[1,2]

This superficial dermal infection is caused largely by group A streptococci, and also by other strepto-

cocci and *S. aureus*. The prominent lymphatic blockade results in a painful, bright, red patch (*peau d'orange*). A raised sharp border clearly demarcates the infection from normal surrounding skin. Fever and chills often precede the skin eruption. Predisposing conditions include ulcers, venostasis, diabetes, alcoholism and paraparesis. Treatment is penicillin (by the parenteral route in severe cases) or erythromycin.

Cellulitis[1-3,6-9]

Cellulitis is an acute spreading infection of the skin, extending below the superficial fascia usually to involve only the upper part of the subcutaneous tissue. As lymphatic involvement is less prominent, the borders of the infection are often not well-defined. None the less, differentiation between cellulitis and erysipelas is sometimes difficult. Fever, malaise and rigors are common.

Streptococcus pyogenes is the most common pathogen, but other Gram-positive and negative organisms can also cause cellulitis. A severe and fulminant form of cellulitis can be caused by marine bacteria of the *Vibrio* spp. Any of these organisms may produce gas, hence crepitus is sometimes present (Table 63.1).

Appropriate microbiological tests are undertaken prior to starting antibiotics. Any skin abrasion or sites of drains are swabbed for Gram stain and culture. Needle aspiration, skin biopsy and blood cultures produce only a 25% positive yield.[1] Treatment involves site elevation and cloxacillin 2 g IV 4-hourly or a first-generation cephalosporin (e.g. cefazolin 2.0 g IV 6-hourly). Vancomycin 1.0 g IV 12-hourly or clindamycin 600 mg IV 6-hourly are alternative antibiotics. An aminoglycoside is added if Gram-negative organisms are suspected (e.g. an immunocompromised patient) or isolated. If *Vibrio* spp. is suspected or isolated, and oral tetracycline can be tolerated, doxycycline 100 mg b.d. may be added, since in murine sepsis, activity of tetracyclines against *V. vulnificus* is better than third-generation cephalosporins.[16]

Table 63.1 Infective causes of soft-tissue crepitus

Cellulitis	Usually anaerobic organisms, clostridial and non-clostridial
Bursitis	Gram-negative organisms
Necrotizing fasciitis	Usually type I (mixed infections, Gram-negative organisms)
Myonecrosis	Clostridial organisms
Infected vascular gangrene	Any organism

Necrotizing fasciitis[1,2,4,6–12,17–21]

Necrotizing fasciitis is a deeper infection of the skin with extensive undermining of surrounding tissues. Interest in this fulminant infection has recently increased.[13,17,22] The World Health Organization reports 160 cases since 1989, but the incidence in the USA is about 100 cases annually.[13] Necrotizing fasciitis usually occurs on the extremities, perineum and abdominal wall. Involvement of male genitalia is known as Fournier's gangrene.[14] Two types are described, depending on causative organisms.[20] Type I are mixed infections usually caused by enteric bowel organisms or *Vibrio* spp. Type II infections are caused by group A streptococci (occasionally by *Staphylococcus aureus*), and has a recent increased incidence in Europe.[17] Secondary infections with zygomycetes may occur.[19,21] There is no difference in the clinical course, morbidity and mortality between the two types in any of these infections.

Clinical presentation

A history of minor trauma is common, and necrotizing fasciitis can complicate surgery and varicella infections.[17,23] Patients with cirrhosis, diabetes and other immunocompromised conditions are more likely victims. Necrotizing fasciitis begins as an area of cellulitis that typically fails to improve on antibiotics and quickly spreads. Pathophysiological sequelae of sepsis result in microthrombi and impaired perfusion, leading to gangrene. Pain is out of keeping with other presenting symptoms and signs. Fever, rigors and shock are common.[17] Manifestations of the systemic inflammatory response syndrome are evident (i.e. multiple organ failure). Bullae may form, and late lesions may resemble deep burns that are pain free, because of the necrosis of nerve fibres. Crepitus may be present (Table 63.1). The normally adherent fascia may be easily peeled off the underlying muscle bed.

Management

A complete microbiological investigation is of utmost importance. This includes sampling for culture by aseptic needle aspiration of any crepitant area. Treatment with antibiotics alone is usually unsuccessful. Urgent and extensive surgical removal of necrotic and damaged tissues is essential.[11,12,17–19,21] Planned surgery at 24-h intervals to debride spreading necrotic tissue is necessary, until the necrotic process stops. If extremities are involved, amputation may be life-saving.

Initial antibiotic therapy includes penicillin 2–4 g 4-hourly IV plus gentamicin 5 mg/kg per day IV. Clindamycin 600 mg 6-hourly IV is an alternative to penicillin. Third-generation cephalosporins could also be used. Metronidazole and chloramphenicol

have also been successfully used.[21] If fungi (e.g. *Mucormycosis*) are isolated, amphotericin B 0.5 mg/ kg per day IV should be given for at least 2 weeks.[19,21] As in cellulitis, *Vibrio* spp. may respond better to tetracyclines.[16]

Supportive care, especially organ support, is also fundamental treatment, and is discussed in other chapters. Hyperbaric oxygen therapy has no proven benefit, and is likely to delay surgical intervention. Mortality from necrotizing fasciitis is high, and survival appears better when surgery is undertaken early.

Pyomyositis and myonecrosis[1,2,5,6–9,11,12,18,19,24,25]

Muscles are remarkably resistant to infection, so bacterial infections are rare. Infections of muscles are termed myonecrosis when *Clostridium* spp. is the causative organism, and pyomyositis when infection is from other bacteria. Often, more than one bacterial species is isolated from infected muscles. In such conditions, bacteria act synergistically, and often produce various toxins (Fig. 63.2).[5,26] As infection is likely to be mixed, differentiation of pyomyositis and myonecrosis is bacteriological, and important only for antibiotic choices.

Pyomyositis

Pyomyositis is more common in the tropics. The causative organism in over 90% of cases is *Staphylococcus aureus*, with others being *Streptococcus pyogenes*, *E. coli* and *S. pneumoniae*. Pyomyositis often follows blunt trauma to torso, thigh or buttock muscles, or from physical overexertion of these muscles. Spontaneous staphylococcal muscle abscesses may occasionally occur.[2]

Initial presentation is with aching muscles, which feel indurated on examination. If untreated, the muscles become erythematous and boggy, and are eventually destroyed. Spontaneous drainage of debris and pus does not occur. Instead, there is contagious spread to surrounding tissues and metastatic spread to the chest (e.g. empyemas) and heart (e.g. endocarditis and pericarditis).

Investigations include needle biopsy (for Gram stain of the aspirate), ultrasound (for localized muscle oedema) and, more recently, magnetic resonance imaging.[2] Large increases in serum creatine phosphokinase may be indicative of the muscle condition.[25]

Antibiotic therapy with penicillin or a third-generation cephalosporin may be successful in the early stages. More often, though, the condition is not recognized early because of diagnostic difficulties, and extensive surgical drainage is mandatory for a favourable outcome.[25] Even after disfiguring muscle destruction, functional prognosis is good.

Myonecrosis

The bacterial infection of muscles by clostridial organisms (usually *Clostridium perfringens* or *C. septicum*) has been called gas gangrene as crepitus may occur. However, other causes of skin crepitus are just as common (Table 63.1). Predisposing causes are contaminated wounds (e.g. in trauma and septic abortions) and surgery in immunocompromised patients.

Onset is often abrupt, with involved areas being very painful and swollen. The patient presents with signs of severe sepsis. If a wound is present, there is usually a profuse serosanguineous discharge of sweet odour. Later, the skin becomes red, yellow, green or black. Bullae and crepitus may form.

A Gram stain revealing Gram-positive rods of *Clostridium* is diagnostic. Treatment of myonecrosis involves prompt, extensive surgical debridement of all infected tissue and antibiotics (i.e. penicillin plus clindamycin).[2] At surgery, the muscle is pale or brick-coloured and does not bleed. Hyperbaric oxygen has its proponents[27,28] and may be beneficial in conjunction with good supportive care. However, there is no prospective evidence to support use of hyperbaric oxygen.[29]

Special areas of soft-tissue infections

Neck infections[30-32]

Since the advent of antibiotics, oropharyngeal infections are no longer major causes of neck infections. Dental infection and regional trauma are now more common causes. Neck infections include Ludwig's angina, retropharyngeal abscesses, parapharyngeal abscesses and necrotizing cervical fasciitis. Ludwig's angina is a submandibular space infection. There is deep and tender swelling of the submandibular and submaxillary area, with swelling of the floor of the mouth and elevation of the tongue.

Causative organisms are the usual mouth commensals, Gram-negative rods and *Staphylococcus aureus*. Pain and odynophagia are almost always the presenting symptoms. Local swelling is usually present. Trismus and dental pathology are common. Systemic inflammatory signs occur in about two-thirds of patients.

Neck X-rays usually demonstrate some abnormality. Computerized tomography will define anatomy and may help to decide on a course of conservative, expectant therapy.[32] Oesophagoscopy should be performed on all retropharyngeal abscesses, as foreign-body ingestion is a common predisposing event.

Airway control must take top priority in any neck swelling. Antibiotics, in doses similar to necrotizing fasciitis, should incorporate cover for Gram-positive cocci and Gram-negative rods. Penicillin or clindamycin plus gentamicin, or a third-generation cephalosporin plus metronidazole are suitable. Some abscesses may be treated conservatively, especially those in children.[32] However, early surgical drainage remains the mainstay of management for large neck abscesses that impinge on airway patency, or deep neck infections that pursue a fulminant course.

Retroperitoneal space infections[33]

Retroperitoneal necrotizing fasciitis is particularly vicious, with a high mortality due partly to the difficulty in diagnosis. Abdominal or perineal trauma or sepsis is always the predisposing event. Diagnosis can only be made at laparotomy for the presenting acute abdomen. Broad-spectrum antibiotic therapy and aggressive surgery (repeated debridement of all necrotic tissue) with planned 'relook' laparotomies is strongly suggested.

References

1. Conly J (1992) Soft tissue infections. In: Hall JB, Schmidt GA and Wood LDH (eds) *Principles of Critical Care*. New York: McGraw-Hill, pp. 1325–1334.
2. Canoso JJ and Barza M (1993) Soft tissue infections. *Rheum Dis Clin North Am* **19**:293–309.
3. Swartz MN (1990) Cellulitis and superficial infections. In: Mandell GL, Douglas RG and Bennett JE (eds) *Principles and Practice on Infectious Diseases*, 3rd edn. New York: Churchill Livingstone, pp. 796–807.
4. Swartz MN (1990) Subcutaneous tissue infections and abscesses. In: Mandell GL, Douglas RG and Bennett JE (eds) *Principles and Practice on Infectious Diseases*, 3rd edn. New York: Churchill Livingstone, pp. 808–812.
5. Swartz MN (1990) Myositis. In: Mandell GL, Douglas RG and Bennett JE (eds) *Principles and Practice on Infectious Diseases*, 3rd edn. New York: Churchill Livingstone, pp. 812–818.
6. Ahrenholz DH (1991) Necrotizing fasciitis and other soft tissue infections. In: Rippe JM, Irwin RS, Alpert JS and Fink MP (eds) *Intensive Care Medicine*, 2nd edn. Boston: Little, Brown, pp. 1334–1342.
7. Cha JY, Releford BJ and Marcarelli P (1994) Necrotizing fasciitis: a classification of necrotizing soft tissue infections. *J Foot Ankle Surg* **33**:148–155.
8. Sutherland ME and Meyer AA (1994) Necrotizing soft-tissue infections. *Surg Clin North Am* **74**:591–607.
9. Ahrenholz DH (1988) Necrotizing soft-tissue infections. *Surg Clin North Am* **68**:199–214.
10. Ward RG and Walsh MS (1991) Necrotizing fasciitis: 10 years' experience in a district general hospital. *Br J Surg* **78**:488–489.
11. Kaiser RE and Cerra FB (1981) Progresive surgical infections – a unified approach. *J Trauma* **21**:349–355.
12. Freischlag JA, Ajalat G and Busuttil RW (1985) Treatment of necrotizing soft tissue infections: the need for a new approach. *Am J Surg* **149**:751–755.
13. Loudon I (1994) Necrotising fasciitis, hospital gangrene, and phagedena. *Lancet* **344**:1416–1419.
14. Fournier AJ (1884) Clinical study of fulminating gangrene of the penis. *Sem Med* **4**:69.

15. Meleney FL (1924) Hemolytic streptococcus gangrene. *Arch Surg* **9**:317–319.

16. Bowdre JH, Hull JH and Cocchetto DM (1983) Antibiotic efficacy against *Vibrio vulnificus* in the mouse: superiority of tetracycline. *J Pharmacol Exp Ther* **225**:595–598.

17. Chelsom J, Halstensen A, Haga T and Holby EA (1994) Necrotising fasciitis due to group A streptococci in western Norway: incidence and clinical features. *Lancet* **344**:1111–1115.

18. Baxter CR (1972) Surgical management of soft tissue infections. *Surg Clin North Am* **52**:1483–1499.

19. Patino JF and Castro D (1991) Necrotizing lesions of soft tissues: a review. *World J Surg* **15**:235–239.

20. Guiliano A, Lewis F, Hadley K and Blaisdell FW (1977) Bacteriology of necrotising fasciitis. *Am J Surg* **134**:52–57.

21. Patino JF, Castro D, Valencia A and Morales P (1991) Necrotizing soft tissue lesions after a volcanic cataclysm. *World J Surg* **15**:240–247.

22. Burge TS and Watson JD (1994) Necrotising fasciitis. *Br Med J* **308**:1453–1454.

23. Falcone PA, Pricolo VE and Edstrom LE (1988) Necrotizing fasciitis as a complication of chickenpox. *Clin Pediatr* **27**:339–343.

24. Stone HH and Martin JD (1972) Synergistic necrotizing cellulitis. *Ann Surg* **175**:702–710.

25. Hird B and Byne K (1994) Gangrenous streptococcal myositis: case report. *J Trauma* **36**:589–591.

26. Kingston D and Seal DV (1990) Current hypothesis on synergistic microbial gangrene. *Br J Surg* **77**:260–264.

27. Thom S (1993) A role for hyperbaric oxygen in clostridial myonecrosis. *Clin Infect Dis* **17**:238.

28. Brown DR, Davis NL, Lepawsky M, Cunningham J and Kortbeek J (1994) A multicenter review of the treatment of major truncal necrotizing infections with and without hyperbaric oxygen therapy. *Am J Surg* **167**:485–489.

29. Heimbach D (1993) Use of hyperbaric oxygen. *Clin Infect Dis* **17**:239–240.

30. Sethi DS and Stanley RE (1994) Deep neck abscesses -- changing trends. *J Laryngol Otol* **108**:138–143.

31. Linder HH (1986) The anatomy of the fasciae of the face and neck with particular reference to the spread and treatment of intraoral infections (Ludwig's) that have progressed into adjacent fascial spaces. *Ann Surg* **204**:705–714.

32. Broughton RA (1992) Nonsurgical management of deep neck infections in children. *Pediatr Infect Dis J* **11**:14–18.

33. Mokoena T, Luvuno FM and Marivate M (1993) Surgical management of retroperitoneal necrotising fasciitis by planned repeat laparotomy and debridement. *S Afr J Surg* **31**:65–70.

64 Antibiotic guidelines

IKS Tan, J Lipman, K Klugman and TE Oh

ICU patients account for 5–10% of all hospital patients, but for approximately 25% of all hospital infections, and 90% of outbreaks.[1] The ICU is associated with extensive antibiotic use, and bacterial resistance to antibiotics is a consequence. Rational use of antibiotics minimizes the emergence of resistant strains and increases the cost-effectiveness of therapy.

General principles

1 All appropriate microbiological specimens, including blood cultures, must be obtained before antibiotic therapy is started. An immediate Gram stain may indicate the antibiotic to use.
2 The choice of antibiotic considers factors such as the system infected, origin of infection (nosocomial or community-acquired), history of recent antibiotic usage, clinical response and host immune status. These factors determine the likely infecting organisms and their likely sensitivities.
3 A narrow-spectrum antibiotic is used whenever possible. For example, cephalosporins should not normally be used against *Staphylococcus aureus*, *Streptococcus pyogenes* and *S. pneumoniae*.
4 Monotherapy with a single agent effective against the expected organisms aims to decrease the risk of drug antagonism, reaction or toxicity. Monotherapy often costs less than multiple antibiotic usage. However, prolonged use of a single broad-spectrum antibiotic may lead to resistant organisms.
5 Sensitivity tests should be interpreted carefully.[2] *In vitro* sensitivity does not equate with clinical effectiveness; *in vitro* resistance generally predicts clinical ineffectiveness. The pharmacodynamics, pharmacokinetics (e.g. penetration into relevant tissues) as well as the spectrum of activity of the antibiotic must be considered.
6 Tests such as minimal inhibitory concentration (MIC), minimal bactericidal concentration (MBC), antibiotic assay, serum bactericidal activity and tests of antibiotic synergy may be useful in serious infections (e.g. endocarditis). Antibiotic peak serum concentrations 4–10 times the MIC are usually effective against the sensitive organism (although peak aminoglycoside concentrations should be higher). An MBC significantly greater (e.g. more than 15 times) than the MIC suggests tolerance to the antibiotic, and *in vivo* antibiotic concentrations above MBC may be required for successful therapy.
7 Adequate drug doses must be given. The intravenous route is preferable in critically ill patients, but other routes should also be considered. A loading dose should be given when appropriate.
8 Serum concentrations of toxic antibiotics should be measured, especially if hepatic or renal dysfunction is present. However, there is no conclusive evidence that maintaining aminoglycoside levels within the therapeutic range is better than clinical judgement alone, in improving outcome or reducing toxicity.[3,4] Also, the therapeutic range for once-daily aminoglycoside dosing has not been established.
9 Certain antibiotics, such as quinolones and imipenem/cilastatin, are not recommended for routine use. They are best held in reserve for organisms resistant to commonly used agents.
10 Consultations with infectious disease specialists are always useful. Surgical or radiological intervention is required for many infections, and appropriate consultations should be obtained.
11 General signs of infection are signs of systemic inflammation. Although bacterial infection is likely, non-bacterial infection and non-infective causes should also be considered.
12 Antibiotic guidelines are only one aspect of infection control. Identification and elimination of reservoirs of infection, blocking transmission of infection, interrupting progression from colonization to infection, and eliminating risk factors such as invasive devices are also important.

Common errors when using antibiotics

1 administration of antibiotics before microbiological specimens are obtained;
2 extended use of antibiotics after eradication of infection;
3 inadequate dosing of antibiotics (e.g. a loading dose is not given or given incorrectly and serum concentrations are not monitored);
4 failure to recognize toxic effects of antibiotics, particularly when polypharmacy is used;
5 failure to use oral therapy when appropriate (i.e. if the oral route yields adequate plasma or tissue concentrations);
6 use of combination therapy, irrespective of infection.

Empirical antibiotic guidelines in intensive care[5-7]

The following antibiotic guidelines refer to infections from a presumed site caused by unknown organisms. Suggested dosages apply to an average-sized adult without liver or renal dysfunction, and may need adjustment. Antibiotics should not be used in a pregnant patient until deemed safe. Regimens are intravenous unless stated otherwise. The aminoglycoside suggested below is gentamicin, but netilmicin or tobramycin (identical dosages to gentamicin) may be substituted. Aminoglycosides are given once daily.[8] In all situations, adjunct management, including removal of infecting devices, surgical or radiological intervention, and other drugs must also be considered.

Cardiovascular infections

Endocarditis (see Chapter 18)

Empirical therapy should use bactericidal antibiotics to cover *Staphylococcus aureus*, streptococci including enterococci and Gram-negative bacillus. Cloxacillin 2 g 4-hourly plus ampicillin 2 g 4-hourly plus gentamicin 5 mg/kg daily is a reasonable regimen. Specific treatment and antibiotic prophylaxis are discussed in Chapter 18.

Bacteraemia

Efforts are made to ascertain the likely sites of infection. Antibiotic choice is made as detailed below. Bacteraemia is of prognostic value, and allows identification of the organism.[9] Despite low positive recovery rates,[10] anaerobic blood cultures are commonly undertaken, as anaerobes are important in many infections. Fungaemia is more common and can be isolated from aerobic bottles, though the media is often suboptimal.

Respiratory infections

Community and hospital-acquired pneumonias (see Chapter 33)

Severe community-acquired pneumonias that require ICU admission have a different spectrum of causative organisms from mild forms.[11] There is a higher incidence of *Legionella* spp. and aerobic Gram-negative bacilli.[11,12] *Mycobacterium tuberculosis* is common in many parts of the world.[12,13] Clinical features are often inadequate to direct specific treatment against a particular organism.[11,14]

Community-acquired pneumonia in an immunocompetent adult may be treated with cefuroxime 1.5 g 8-hourly and erythromycin 500 mg 6-hourly. Gentamicin 5 mg/kg daily may be added. If Gram-negative bacilli are important (e.g. patients with bronchiectasis or chronic bronchitis, and from old-age homes), ceftazidime 1 g 8-hourly, instead of cefuroxime, is required. In patients hypersensitive to penicillin, ciprofloxacin or imipenem/cilastatin may be used.

Coverage is specific when the bacteriological agent is confirmed.

1 *Streptococcus pneumoniae* is treated with penicillin G 2 M units 4-hourly.
2 *Haemophilus influenzae* requires cefuroxime, as there is a high incidence of amoxicillin resistance.
3 *Staphylococcus aureus* pneumonia is treated with cloxacillin 1 g 4-hourly. If methicillin-resistant *Staphylococcus aureus* (MRSA) is prevalent (e.g. patient from an old-age nursing home), vancomycin 1 g q. 12 h is given.
4 *Mycoplasma pneumoniae* or *Legionella pneumophila* requires erythromycin 1 g 6-hourly.
5 Psittacosis or Q fever should be treated with doxycycline 100 mg 12-hourly.
6 *Pneumocystis carinii* is treated with co-trimoxazole 25/5 mg/kg 6-hourly, and steroids may be indicated.

The use of aminoglycosides is debatable. There is only 30% penetration into lung followed by inactivation in the acidic environment. If given IV, useful levels are toxic. Nebulized aminoglycosides are under research. *Pseudomonas* and *Acinetobacter* spp. infections and bacteraemia would favour the addition of an aminoglycoside.

Nosocomial pneumonia (see Chapters 33 and 62)

Nosocomial pneumonias are hospital-acquired. Bacterial colonization of the oropharynx, predominantly with Gram-negative organisms, is the major factor responsible for nosocomial pneumonia. Treatment is usually an anti-pseudomonal β-lactam (e.g. ceftazidime) plus gentamicin. Metronidazole is added if aspiration is a concern, and vancomycin if MRSA is likely. Diagnostic techniques such as bronchoalveolar lavage or protected brush specimens may be needed. Piperacillin/tazobactam plus amikacin, quinolones, or imipenem/cilastatin may have to be used.

Aspiration pneumonia (see Chapter 34)

In hospitalized patients, anaerobic and aerobic organisms commonly reflect the oropharyngeal flora, whereas in non-hospitalized patients, anaerobic organisms predominate. If antibiotics are deemed necessary, penicillin G may be used for new admissions. For hospitalized patients, ceftazidime plus gentamicin plus metronidazole is acceptable.

Upper respiratory tract infections

Epiglottitis is usually due to *Haemophilus influenzae* and is treated with cefuroxime 25 mg/kg 8-hourly. Sinusitis in the ICU has a spectrum of organisms similar to nosocomial pneumonia, and similar antibiotics are employed. Soft-tissue infections (e.g. Ludwig's angina, retropharyngeal or lateral pharyngeal space infections) require penicillin G 2 M units 4-hourly plus gentamicin 5 mg/kg daily plus metronidazole 500 mg 8-hourly (see Chapter 63).

Intra-abdominal infections

Acute peritonitis

1 *Primary peritonitis* or spontaneous bacterial peritonitis occurs in patients with ascites. Cefotaxime 1 g 6-hourly is the drug of choice for cirrhotic patients.[15] Ampicillin/sulbactam 1000/500 mg 8-hourly or co-amoxiclav 1.2 g (amoxycillin 1 g/ clavulanate 200 mg) IV 6–8-hourly (maximum 6 g) is effective for nephrotic patients.
2 *Secondary peritonitis*[16] arises from loss of integrity of the gastrointestinal tract. Causative organisms are aerobic and anaerobic faecal flora. Critically ill patients (e.g. APACHE II score > 14) may have a different spectrum of organisms,[17] with increased frequency of *Candida*, *Enterococcus* spp. and *Staphylococcus epidermidis*.

   Clindamycin-resistant *Bacteroides fragilis* is now seen in 20–38% of cases, while metronidazole resistance remains rare. The accepted regimen has been gentamicin plus metronidazole 500 mg 8-hourly, with or without ampicillin. The aminoglycoside component is notoriously toxic, and has been associated with treatment failure.[18] Substitutes for the aminoglycoside include second-generation cephalosporins such as cefuroxime 1.5 g 8-hourly. Aztreonam plus metronidazole is not acceptable as there is no Gram-positive cover.[19] Cefoxitin may be unsuitable, as its *in vitro* resistance is increasing (26% in Canada).[20] Piperacillin/tazobactam[21] and imipenem/cilastin[22] are good, but are better reserved for difficult-to-treat infections.

3 *Tertiary peritonitis*, or persistent generalized peritonitis, occurs when secondary peritonitis fails to resolve. Predominant pathogens are fungi, *S. epidermidis*, *Pseudomonas* and *Enterococcus* spp. Ampicillin plus gentamicin plus metronidazole may be used initially, while awaiting identification of organisms and sensitivities.

Pseudomembranous colitis

Pseudomembranous colitis is caused by toxins produced by *Clostridium difficile*, and is usually associated with antibiotic use (classically clindamycin). Therapy is with vancomycin, giving the parenteral preparation via the nasogastric tube as 125 mg 6-hourly for 10 days. Oral/nasogastric metronidazole 500 mg 8-hourly is preferred in many centres. If oral medication cannot be tolerated, IV metronidazole 500 mg 8-hourly is given.

Pelvic abscess/pelvic inflammatory disease

Causative organisms include *Neisseria gonorrhoeae*, *Bacteroides*, Enterobactericeae, *Chlamydia* and *Mycoplasma*. Cefoxitin 2 g 6-hourly plus doxycycline 100 mg 12-hourly is effective.

Pancreatitis

Prophylactic antibiotics in pancreatitis are generally not recommended. However, prophylactic cefuroxime 1.5 g 8-hourly may reduce mortality in severe necrotizing pancreatitis.[23]

Hepatobiliary infections

Cholecystitis requires antibiotic treatment as for cholangitis. Causative organisms are usually aerobic Gram-negative bacilli. Antibiotics for cholangitis are used in conjunction with drainage of the obstructed biliary tree.[24] Mezlocillin (which undergoes biliary excretion) as a sole agent is better than ampicillin plus gentamicin.[25] However, in biliary obstruction, biliary concentrations of drugs excreted by the biliary route, including cefoperazone, are minimal.[26] A regimen comprising ampicillin 500 mg 6-hourly, ceftazidime 1 g 8-hourly and metronidazole 500 mg 8-hourly is acceptable.[27] Cefoperazone 2 g 12-hourly may be substituted for ceftazidime. Ciprofloxacin for cholangitis requires more evaluation.[28]

Liver abscesses may be treated with a combination of ampicillin/ceftazidime/metronidazole as for cholangitis above.

Neurological infections

Meningitis (see Chapter 46)

Treatment delay results in a poorer outcome.[29] Aetiology and thus antibiotic choice[30] vary with age:

1 0–3 months: Ampicillin (50 mg/kg 6-hourly) and cefotaxime (50 mg/kg 8-hourly), or ampicillin plus an aminoglycoside.

2 3 months–50 years: Pathogens are *Streptococcus pneumoniae*, *Neisseria meningitidis* (meningococci) and *Haemophilus influenzae*. Ceftriaxone 100 mg/kg in divided doses for infants and children, 1–2 g 12-hourly for adults, or cefotaxime 50–180 mg/kg daily in divided doses for infants and children, 1–2 g 6–8-hourly for adults are appropriate. Dexamethasone 0.15 mg/kg 6-hourly for 2 days[31] should be started before antibiotics in children.

3 >50 years: Enterobacticeae becomes common, and *Listeria monocytogenes* is a concern in diabetics, alcoholics and the immunosuppressed. Ampicillin 2 g 4-hourly plus ceftriaxone 1–2 g 12-hourly is required.

With bacteriological confirmation, the coverage is optimized.

1 *S. pneumoniae* (non-penicillin-resistant) and *N. meningitidis* are treated with penicillin G 4 M units 4-hourly.

2 *S. pneumoniae* (penicillin-resistant) and *H. influenzae* are treated with ceftriaxone 1–2 g 12-hourly.

3 *L. monocytogenes* is treated with ampicillin 2 g 4-hourly plus gentamicin 5 mg/kg daily.

4 Enterobactericeae is treated with ceftazidime 2 g 8-hourly plus gentamicin 5 mg/kg daily.

Prophylaxis for intimate but not all contacts (e.g. family, roommate and staff involved in resuscitation) is indicated.[1,2,5,9] The accepted regimen is rifampicin 20 mg/kg daily for 4 days for *H. influenzae* and 10 mg/kg 12-hourly for 2 days for *N. meningitidis*, with doses not exceeding 600 mg/day. Ciprofloxacin as a single 500–750 mg dose or 250 mg b.d. for 2 days is also effective for *N. meningitidis*.

Shunt infections require removal of the shunt. Vancomycin 1 g 12-hourly plus ceftazidime 2 g 8-hourly are used, as organisms are often nosocomial.

Brain abscess (see Chapter 46)

Empirical penicillin G 4 M units 4-hourly plus metronidazole 500 mg IV 8-hourly plus a third-generation cephalosporin can be used if infecting organisms are not isolated.

Urinary tract

Treatment for pyelonephritis is ampicillin plus gentamicin, as aetiological agents are *E. coli* and other Gram-negative enteric organisms. However, patients admitted to the ICU generally have failed to respond to the above treatment. The urosepsis may be complicated by obstruction or abscesses, which require urgent imaging. Of the alternatives, a third-generation cephalosporin (e.g. ceftriaxone 2 g daily) may be used. Since critically ill patients with urosepsis are generally in renal failure, it is advisable to avoid nephrotoxic agents such as aminoglycosides. *Staphylococcus* is a common organism in perinephric abscesses, and requires the addition of cloxacillin.

Patients with long-term indwelling urinary catheters may develop bacteriuria. Bacteriuria does not need antibiotic treatment unless signs of infection are present. Funguria is also common, and may require intravesical amphotericin B or IV fluconazole.

Soft-tissue infections (see Chapter 63)

Necrotizing fasciitis is a polymicrobial infection, and may be treated with cloxacillin 1 g 4-hourly plus gentamicin 5 mg/kg daily plus metronidazole 500 mg 8-hourly, along with debridement with or without hyperbaric oxygen therapy. Tetanus prophylaxis is given as indicated. Severe group A *Streptococcus* infections[32] are treated with penicillin G 3 M units 4-hourly. Toxic shock syndrome cases need cloxacillin 2 g 6-hourly.

Vascular catheter-related infections

Common infecting organisms of vascular catheters include *Streptococcus epidermidis*, *Candida albicans* and *Staphylococcus aureus*. Before starting antibiotics, blood is sampled for culture through the catheter and from a different site, and the catheter tip sent for quantitative culture. Treatment[33] depends on the host status, causative organisms and extent of infection. The decision to remove a long-term implanted catheter can be difficult. Generally, an exit-site infection does not require removal, while a tunnel infection always requires catheter removal. Removal of the implanted catheter is required in systemic infections by *S. aureus* or *Pseudomonas*, or if there is no response to antibiotics.

Cloxacillin 2 g 6-hourly is used for *S. aureus* infections, with vancomycin 1 g 12-hourly for *Streptococcus epidermidis*, MRSA, *Corynebacterium* JK strains and *Bacillus* spp. If the catheter is left *in situ*, antibiotics are administered through the catheter.

Other antimicrobial agents

Amphotericin B[34] is given as a test dose of 1 mg over 15 min. If there is no reaction, a maintenance dose of 0.5 mg/kg in 5% dextrose is given over 4 h. Intravesical amphotericin B may be given as 2 mg in 200 ml sterile water, *in situ* for 2 h, twice daily for 2 days. Flucytosine is required besides amphotericin B for *Candida* meningitis and endocarditis.[35] Dosage is

25 mg/kg 8-hourly orally, maintaining serum concentrations at 30–80 mg/l. Fluconazole 200 mg 12-hourly is as effective as amphotericin B for candidiasis,[36] and may be used in patients with amphotericin B toxicity or failure of therapy, and for cryptococcal meningitis. *C. krusei* and *C. glabrata* are resistant to fluconazole. Itraconazole 200 mg 12-hourly orally may be used for aspergillosis; experience is limited.

Antituberculous agents include isoniazid 5 mg/kg, rifampicin 10 mg/kg, pyrazinamide 15 mg/kg and ethambutol 20 mg/kg orally daily. Ciprofloxacin 750 mg 12-hourly and amikacin 15 mg/kg daily are also used for *Mycobacterium avium-intracellulare* complex. Clarithromycin for disseminated *Mycobacterium avium* complex infection requires further evaluation.

Severe bronchiolitis in infants is commonly due to respiratory syncytial virus. Aerosolized ribavirin (20 mg/ml) decreases the duration of mechanical ventilation, oxygen treatment and the hospital stay.[37] Ganciclovir is used for treatment of cytomegalovirus infections. Induction dose is 5 mg/kg 12-hourly.

Severe malaria is treated with IV quinine loading dose 20 mg/kg (maximum of 600 mg) diluted in 10 ml/kg 5% dextrose over 4 h, followed by 10 mg/kg over 4 h 8-hourly, till oral therapy is tolerated. In addition, doxycycline 100 mg 12-hourly is required for *Plasmodium falciparum*, and primaquine 0.3 mg/kg daily for *P. ovale* and *P. vivax*. Exchange transfusions and desferoxamine may be required.[38]

Strongyloides hyperinfection may occur in the immunosuppressed host. Treatment is with oral thiabendazole 25 mg/kg 12-hourly.

Infections in the immunocompromised host

The ICU is increasingly concerned with patients immunosuppressed by drug treatment or by underlying pathology. Treatment requires an understanding of likely infecting organisms due to specific immune deficits (see Chapter 59).

For the febrile neutropenic patient[39] the EORTC regimen[40] may be used: ceftriaxone 30 mg/kg plus amikacin 20 mg/kg IV daily. Re-evaluation is done after 72 h. If fever resolves, antibiotics are maintained for 7 days and when the neutrophil count exceeds 500/mm³. If fever persists, but the patient is improving, antibiotics are continued till day 7 and amphotericin B is added if the patient is still febrile on that day. If the patient deteriorates, vancomycin may be added, with amphotericin B on day 7. Addition of vancomycin 1 g 12-hourly to the initial regimen is indicated in centres where MRSA is a problem, or if coagulase-negative *Staphylococcus* is probable (e.g. patients with indwelling central venous catheters). Ceftazidime 33 mg/kg 8-hourly is substituted for ceftriaxone if *Pseudomonas* spp. are a concern. Monotherapy

ceftazadime has recently been shown to be as effective as, and safer than, a standard piperacillin/tobramycin combination empirical therapy in febrile neutropenic patients.[41] If a diffuse chest infiltrate is present, co-trimoxazole plus erythromycin is added. Necrotizing enterocolitis (typhlitis) may be a cause of abdominal pain, and requires addition of metronidazole. Colony-stimulating factors may be used to reduce the duration of neutropenia. Infection in acquired immunodeficiency syndrome (AIDS) patients is discussed in Chapter 60.

Trauma surgery

Traumatized patients should be considered as infected. In surgery for severe skeletal and soft-tissue trauma, cloxacillin 1 g 4-hourly plus gentamicin 5 mg/kg daily plus metronidazole 500 mg 8-hourly is given for 48 h, and then guided by culture results. Tetanus prophylaxis is also given when indicated. Prophylactic antibiotics are not recommended for skull fractures and any resulting cerebrospinal fluid leak.[42]

Surgical antibiotic prophylaxis[43,44]

Indications for prophylaxis are shown in Table 64.1. Achieving effective tissue concentrations prior to contamination and for the duration of the procedure is vital. Hence antibiotic prophylaxis must be given parenterally 30–60 min before the incision or at induction of anaesthesia. A single dose is sufficient,

Table 64.1 Indications for antibiotic prophylaxis in surgery[42]

Clean surgery	Clean-contaminated surgery
Prosthesis (valvular, vascular, orthopaedic)	Gastric surgery with hypochlorhydria
Remote infection before surgery	Colorectal surgery
Carrier of pathogenic organisms	Pulmonary surgery*
Neurosurgery	Compromised vascular circulation
Immunosuppressed patients*	Obstructed urinary tract surgery
Patients receiving corticosteroids*	Vaginal hysterectomy
Advanced age over 85 years*	Ear, nose and throat cancer surgery
Uncontrolled diabetes*	Arthroplasty, closed fracture surgery
Morbid obesity*	Oro/nasopharynx access in neurosurgery*
Cancer surgery	Opened air sinuses in neurosurgery*

*Absent or too few controlled studies.

but in long procedures, reinjection of agents with short half-lives may be necessary after 2–3 h. Antibiotic prophylaxis is commonly recommended for a duration of 24 h, but there is no evidence to support this over a single-dose regimen. Appropriate antibiotics are continued if there is *established* infection. Surgical prophylaxis must not be confused with infected patients undergoing surgery. Chosen antibiotics should be active against pathogens commonly associated with wound infections and those endogenous to the operative site. Vancomycin is added if MRSA is common in the hospital. Commonly recommended regimens in the UK and the USA are described below:[43,44]

Cardiothoracic surgery

Valve and coronary artery bypass surgery

1 Cefamandole *or* cefuroxime *or* cefazolin 1–2 g IV *or*
2 Cloxacillin 2 g IV plus gentamicin 1.3 mg/kg IV *or*
3 Clindamycin 600 mg IV *or* vancomycin 1 g IV if allergic to β-lactams.

Lung surgery

1 Cefuroxime *or* cefazolin 1–2 g IV *or*
2 Doxycycline 200 mg IV if allergic to β-lactams.

Gastrointestinal surgery

Upper gastrointestinal tract surgery

1 Cefazolin 1–2 g IV *or*
2 Gentamicin 1.3 mg/kg IV plus metronidazole 500 mg IV if allergic to β-lactams.

Lower gastrointestinal tract surgery

1 Cefoxitin 1–2 g IV *or*
2 Cefuroxime 1–2 g IV plus metronidazole 500 mg IV.

Gentamicin 1.3 mg/kg replaces cefuroxime if the patient is allergic to β-lactams.

Biliary surgery

1 Cefazolin 1–2 g IV *or*
2 Gentamicin 1.3 mg/kg if the patient is allergic to β-lactams.

Neurosurgery[42]

Clean-non-implant procedures

First- or second-generation cephalosporin, e.g. cefuroxime 1–2 g IV.

Clean-contaminated procedures

1 Co-amoxiclav 1.2 g (amoxycillin 1 g/clavulanate 200 mg) IV *or*
2 Cefuroxime 1–2 g IV plus metronidazole 500 mg IV if allergic to β-lactams.

Cerebrospinal fluid shunt surgery

No evidence is available to support prophylactic antibiotics against ventriculitis. If used, intraventricular instillation of vancomycin plus gentamicin is a logical regimen.

Vascular surgery

Abdominal aorta and lower limb surgery

1 Cefamandole *or* cefuroxime *or* cefazolin 1–2 g IV *or*
2 Cloxacillin 2 g IV plus gentamicin 1.3 mg/kg IV *or*
3 Clindamycin 600 mg IV *or* vancomycin 1 g IV if allergic to β-lactams.

Head and neck and ear, nose and throat cancer surgery

1 Cefazolin 1–2 g IV plus metronidazole 500 mg IV *or*
2 Clindamycin 600 mg IV if allergic to β-lactams *or*
3 Gentamicin 1.3 mg/kg IV plus metronidazole 500 mg IV.

Orthopaedic surgery

Arthroplasty and closed uncontaminated fractures

Cefazolin 1–2 g IV.

References

1. Trilla A (1994) Epidemiology of nosocomial infections in adult intensive care units. *Intensive Care Med* **20**:S1–S4.
2. A guide to sensitivity testing. Report of the Working Party on Antibiotic Sensitivity Testing of the British Society for Antimicrobial Chemotherapy. *J Antimicrob Chemother* **27**(suppl D):1–50.
3. McInnes GT (1989) The value of therapeutic drug monitoring to the practising physician – an hypothesis in need of testing. *Br J Clin Pharmacol* **27**:281–284.
4. McCormack JP and Jewesson PJ (1992) A critical reevaluation of the 'therapeutic range' of aminoglycosides. *Clin Infect Dis* **14**:320–339.
5. Sanford JP (1993) *Guide to Antimicrobial Therapy.* West Bethesda, MD; Antimicrobial Therapy.

6. Mandell GL, Douglas RG and Bennett JE (1994) *Principles and Practice of Infectious Diseases*, 4th edn. New York: Churchill Livingstone.

7. McLean AS (1988) A review of antibiotic agents in acute sepsis. In: Oh TE (ed.) *Therapeutics in Emergency Medicine. Med J Aust* 1988 **149**:43–8.

8. Parker SE and Davey PG (1993) Once-daily aminoglycoside dosing. *Lancet* **341**:346–347.

9. Niederman MS and Fein AM (1994) Predicting bacteremia in critically ill patients: a clinically relevant effort? *Intensive Care Med* **20**:405–406.

10. Murray PR, Traynor P and Hopson D (1992) Critical assessment of blood culture techniques: analysis of recovery of obligate and facultative anaerobes, strict aerobic bacteria, and fungi in aerobic and anaerobic blood culture bottles. *J Clin Microbiol* **30**:1462–1468.

11. Niederman MS, Bass JB Jr, Campbell GD *et al.* (1993) Guidelines for the initial management of adults with community-acquired pneumonia: diagnosis, assessment of severity, and initial antimicrobial therapy. *Am Rev Respir Dis* **148**:1418–1426.

12. Dahmash NS and Choedhury MNH (1994) Re-evaluation of pneumonia requiring admission to an intensive care unit – a prospective study. *Thorax* **49**:71–76.

13. Chan CH, Cohen M and Pang J (1992) A prospective study of community-acquired pneumonia in Hong Kong. *Chest* **101**:442–446.

14. Moine P, Vercken JB, Chevret S *et al.* (1994) Severe community-acquired pneumonia – etiology, epidemiology, and prognostic factors. *Chest* **105**:1487–1495.

15. Ariza J, Xiol X, Esteve M *et al.* (1991) Aztreonam vs. cefotaxime in the treatment of Gram-negative spontaneous peritonitis in cirrhotic patients. *Hepatology* **14**:91–98.

16. McClean KL, Sheehan GJ and Harding GKM (1994) Intraabdominal infection: a review. *Clin Infect Dis* **19**: 100–116.

17. Sawyer RG, Rosenlof LK, Adams RB, May AK, Spengler MD and Pruett TL (1992) Peritonitis into the 1990s: changing pathogens and changing strategies in the critically ill. *Am Surg* **58**:82–87.

18. Gorbach SL (1993) Intraabdominal infections. *Clin Infect Dis* **17**:961–967.

19. Sawyer MD and Dunn DL (1992) Antimicrobial therapy of intra-abdominal sepsis. *Infect Dis Clin North Am* **6**:545–570.

20. Bourgault AM, Harding GK, Smith JA, Horsman GB, Marrie TJ and Lamothe F (1992) Survey of *Bacteroides fragilis* group susceptibility patterns in Canada. *Antimicrob Agents Chemother* **36**:343–347.

21. Polk HC Jr, Fink MP, Laverdiere M *et al.* (1993) Prospective randomized study of piperacillin/tazobactam therapy of surgically treated intra-abdominal infection. *Am Surg* **59**:598–605.

22. Solomkin JS, Dellinger EP, Christou NV and Bussutil RW (1990) Results of a multicenter trial comparing imipenem/cilastatin to tobramycin/clindamycin for intra-abdominal infections. *Ann Surg* **212**: 581–591.

23. Saino V, Kemppainen E, Puolakkainen P *et al.* (1995) Early antibiotic treatment in acute necrotising pancreatitis. *Lancet* **346**:663–667.

24. Lai ECS, Mok FPT, Tan ESY *et al.* (1992) Endoscopic biliary drainage for severe acute cholangitis. *N Engl J Med* **326**:1582–1586.

25. Gerecht WB, Henry NK, Hoffmann WW *et al.* (1989) Prospective randomized comparison of mezlocillin therapy alone with combined ampicillin and gentamicin therapy for patients with cholangitis. *Arch Intern Med* **149**: 1279–1284.

26. Leung JWC, Chan RCY, Cheung SW, Sung JY, Chung SCS and French GL (1990) The effect of obstruction on the biliary excretion of cefoperazone and ceftazidime. *J. Antimicrob Chemother* **25**:399–406.

27. French GL, Chan RCY, Chung SCS and Leung JWC (1989) Antibiotics for cholangitis. *Lancet* **11**:1271–1272.

28. Leung JWC, Lee JG, Ling TKW *et al.* (1993) Antibiotics for biliary sepsis associated with CBD stones. *Gastrointest Endosc* **39**:323.

29. Strang JR and Pugh EJ (1992) Menigococcal infections: reducing the case fatality rate by giving penicillin before admission to hospital. *Br Med J* **305**:141–143.

30. Tunkel AR, Wispelwey B and Scheld WM (1990) Bacterial meningitis: recent advances in pathophysiology and treatment. *Ann Intern Med* **112**:610–623.

31. Syrogiannopoulos GA, Lourida AN, Theodoridou MC *et al.* (1994) Dexamethasone therapy for bacterial meningitis in children: 2-versus 4-day regimen. *J Infect Dis* **169**:853–858.

32. Stevens DL (1992) Invasive group A streptococcus infections. *Clin Infect Dis* **14**:2–11.

33. Raad II and Bodey GP (1992) Infectious complications of indwelling vascular catheters. *Clin Infect Dis* **15**: 197–208.

34. Terrell CL and Hughes CE (1992) Antifungal agents used for deep-seated mycotic infections. *Mayo Clin Proc* **67**:69–91.

35. British Society for Antimicrobial Chemotherapy working party (1994) Mangement of deep *Candida* infection in surgical and intensive care unit patients. *Intensive Care Med* **20**:522–528.

36. Rex JH, Bennett JE, Sugar AM *et al.* (1994) A randomized trial comparing fluconazole with amphotericin B for the treatment of candidemia in patients without neutropenia. *N Engl J Med* **331**:1325–1330.

37. Smith DW, Frankel LR, Mathers LH, Tang AT, Ariagno RL and Prober CG (1991) A controlled trial of aerosolized ribavirin in infants receiving mechanical ventilation for severe respiratory syncytial virus infection. *N Engl J Med* **325**:24–29.

38. Gordeuk VR, Thuma PE, Brittenham GM *et al.* (1993) Iron chelation as a chemotherapeutic strategy for falciparum malaria. *Am J Trop Med Hyg* **48**:193–197.

39. Working Committee, Infectious Diseases Society of America (1990) Guidelines for the use of antimicrobial agents in neutropenic patients with unexplained fever. *J Infect Dis* **161**:381–396.

40. The International Antimicrobial Therapy Cooperative Group of the EORTC (1993) Efficacy and toxicity of single daily doses of amikacin and ceftriaxone versus multiple daily doses of amikacin and ceftazidime for infection in patients with cancer and granulocytopenia. *Ann Intern Med* **119**:584–593.

41. De Pauw BE, Deresinski SC, Feld R *et al.* (1944) Ceftazidime compared with piperacillin and tobramycin for the empiric treatment of fever in neutropenic patients with cancer: a multicenter randomized trial. *Ann Intern Med* **120**:834–844.

42. Infection in Neurosurgery Working Party of the British Society for Antimicrobial Chemotherapy. Antimicrobial prophylaxis in neurosurgery and after head injury. *Lancet* **344**:1547–1551.

43. Dellinger EP, Gross PA, Barrett TL *et al.* (1994) Quality standard for antibiotic prophylaxis in surgical procedures. *Clin Infect Dis* **18**:422–427.

44. Martin C, Auffray JP and Bantz P (1992) General concepts for antimicrobial prophylaxis in surgery. In: Vincent J-L (ed.) *Yearbook of Intensive Care and Emergency Medicine.* Berlin: Springer-Verlag, pp. 443–456.

Part X

Trauma

Severe and multiple trauma

JA Judson

Trauma can be defined as physical injury from mechanical energy. It is usually categorized as blunt or penetrating. In western countries, severe blunt trauma is common, caused by road crashes, falls and, less frequently, blows and assault. Severe penetrating trauma, usually from stabbings and gunshots, is less common except in larger cities of the USA,[1,2] South Africa and war zones. Blunt trauma is often more difficult to treat than penetrating trauma. Assessment is more difficult, because injuries are frequently internal, multiple and not obvious initially. The risk of missing serious injuries can only be lessened by a systematic approach and repeated assessments.[3,4]

Assessment and priorities

Triage

An important first step is triage – sorting patients with acute life-threatening injuries and complications from those whose lives are not in danger. The severity of total body injury is related to the number of separate injuries present, and to the severity of individual injuries. Assessment can be made either at the scene of injury or on arrival at hospital. As in any emergency, assessment, diagnosis and treatment need to be concurrent. There is limited time for detailed histories, examinations, investigations or well-considered diagnoses before starting emergency care. Most patients with severe injury can be distinguished early by the following:

1 *Depressed consciousness* in the trauma patient can be related to brain injury, hypoxaemia, shock, alcohol or other ingested drugs, or precipitating neurological or cardiac events. Frequently, a combination of factors is present, and the precise extent of physical brain injury is not known initially.
2 *Breathing difficulties* are common in patients with trauma to the head, face, neck and chest. If rapid or distressed breathing is present, airway obstruction, laryngeal injury, pulmonary aspiration and lung or

chest wall injury (especially pneumothorax and lung contusion) must be considered.
3 *Shock* is almost always hypovolaemic from blood loss, but cardiogenic shock occasionally occurs in trauma (see below).

Priorities

A trauma patient often has multiple problems requiring attention; determining priorities is not always easy. In general, the priorities are to:

1 *support life*: The patient is kept alive with resuscitative techniques, while the various injuries and complications are attended to;
2 *locate and control bleeding*, which may be varied (see below);
3 *prevent brainstem compression* and spinal cord damage;
4 *diagnose and treat all other injuries* and complications.

Basic treatment principles

A systematic approach to managing severe and multiple trauma is important. Effective programmes developed by the American and Australasian colleges of surgeons are now well-established.[5,6] A number of basic treatment principles apply to all severe trauma patients.

Emergency assessment (primary survey)

The following must be recognized and treated before anything else:

1 *A – Airway obstruction*: suggested by noisy (or silent) breathing, with paradoxical chest movements and breathing distress, and *inadequate airway protection* from impaired gag reflexes in patients with depressed consciousness.

2 *B – Breathing difficulty*: suggested by tachypnoea, abnormal pattern, cyanosis or mental confusion.

3 *C – Circulatory shock*: manifested by cold peripheries with delayed capillary refill, rapid weak pulse or low blood pressure (see below).

Oxygen and ventilatory therapy

High-flow oxygen by mask is given to all trauma patients. However, patients with severe trauma frequently require ventilatory support. A restless uncooperative patient should be intubated under a crash induction to facilitate resuscitation.

Blood cross-match

Six units of red cells should be cross-matched urgently, but it is impossible to predict the amount of blood that will be required. Blood is concurrently sent for baseline haematological and biochemical tests.

Fluid resuscitation

Resuscitation fluids are given (see below). If necessary, two or three large 14- or 16-gauge IV cannulas are inserted in upper limb or external jugular veins.

Analgesia

Analgesia is easily overlooked. Opioid agents should be titrated IV, and not given IM or subcutaneously. Large doses may be needed.

Urine output

A urinary catheter is inserted, unless a ruptured urethra is suspected (because of blood at the urinary meatus, severe fractured pelvis or abnormal prostate position on rectal examination). Urine output monitoring is an important guide to resuscitation.

Other injuries

All injuries should be evaluated (following section).

Clinical evaluation of injuries (secondary survey)

Injuries are easily missed in an emergency, especially when one injury is obvious. The back and the front of the patient should be examined. Special attention is paid to regions with external lacerations, contusions and abrasions. All body regions are examined systematically:

Head

Neurological observations are made (see below). The ears and nose are inspected for cerebrospinal fluid and blood, and the scalp is examined thoroughly.

Face

Bleeding into the airway should be excluded, and the face and jaws tested for abnormal mobility.

Spine

A cervical spine fracture or dislocation is assumed in all patients with depressed consciousness until proved otherwise. Signs of spinal cord injury should be sought (e.g. warm dilated peripheries from loss of vasomotor tone, diaphragmatic breathing, paralysis, priapism and loss of anal tone). The thoracic and lumbar spine should be inspected and palpated.

Thorax

Fractured ribs in themselves are not usually life-threatening, but haemothorax, pneumothorax, lung contusion and chest wall instability (flail chest) will require attention if present. Less common but very serious injuries can occur to the heart and great vessels (see Chapter 68).

Abdomen

The spleen, liver and mesenteries are often damaged. Retroperitoneal haemorrhage is common. Injuries to the pancreas, duodenum and other hollow viscera are less frequent, and may be missed until signs of peritonitis occur. Renal injury with retroperitoneal haemorrhage is suggested by haematuria and loin pain (see Chapter 70).

Pelvis

Pelvic fractures may be difficult to detect clinically, especially in the unconscious patient. Blood loss may be massive, particularly with posterior fractures involving sacroiliac dislocation. Ruptured bladder and ruptured urethra may occur with anterior fractures.

Extremities

A litre or more of blood may be lost into a fractured femur. Long bone fractures are more serious when they are open, comminuted or displaced, or if associated with nerve or arterial damage.

External

Contusions may be extensive and serious, especially in falls from heights, and may be overlooked if the victim's back is not examined. Road crash victims may sustain serious burns or abrasions.

Shock in the trauma patient

The earliest, most constant and reliable signs of shock are seen in the peripheral circulation. A patient with cold, pale peripheries has shock until proved otherwise. Tachycardia is not always present and hypotension is a late sign of shock.

Cardiogenic shock

If the trauma patient with shock has distended neck veins, possible causes are tension pneumothorax, concurrent myocardial infarction, cardiac tamponade or myocardial contusion.

Hypovolaemic shock

If the neck veins are empty, hypovolaemic shock should be inferred. Possible sites of blood loss causing shock are:

1 *External loss* which is obvious clinically from blood-soaked clothing and pooled blood.
2 *Major fractures*, which are obvious clinically by deformity, swelling, crepitus, pain and tenderness (e.g. femurs) or seen on a plain X-ray (e.g. pelvis).
3 *Pleural cavity*, detected on urgent chest X-ray. Intrapleural drains will reveal the amount and rate of blood loss.
4 *Peritoneal cavity*, detected by laparotomy, peritoneal lavage or computed tomography (CT) scan. Clinical examination of the abdomen can be misleading when the patient is intoxicated, has depressed consciousness or has multiple injuries. A single clinical examination is of limited value: changes over time are more important.
5 *Retroperitoneum*, detected at laparotomy or by CT scan, or inferred when all the above are negative, especially in the presence of pelvic or lumbar spine fracture.

Diagnostic peritoneal lavage

Peritoneal lavage using 1 l (or 10 ml/kg) of isotonic saline (after drainage of the stomach and bladder) is used to diagnose intra-abdominal bleeding, particularly when shock is present. It is also indicated when repeated clinical examination of the abdomen is not possible. Caution is needed with pregnancy, previous abdominal surgery or massive pelvic injury.

The presence of more than 10 ml frank blood on catheter aspiration necessitates immediate laparotomy; otherwise a lavage fluid specimen should be examined for red and white cell counts and amylase concentration. A red cell count over 100 000/mm³, white cell count over 500/mm³, or an increased amylase concentration suggests bleeding or viscus injury, and laparotomy should be undertaken immediately. These absolute figures are debatable, and lower values are accepted in penetrating trauma.[5–7] Peritoneal lavages inevitably result in some false-positive laparotomies. However, in severe trauma, morbidity of a non-therapeutic laparotomy (i.e. no

definitive surgery) is insignificant compared with the dire consequences of not treating intra-abdominal bleeding.

CT abdomen

Abdominal CT is not indicated in shock, but can be useful in the stable patient. Visualization of intra-abdominal and pelvic organs and haemorrhage is excellent,[8,9] but results can be misleading and disastrous with poor technique.[4]

Fluid resuscitation

Fluids

Almost all patients who are hypotensive or noticeably vasoconstricted will need blood transfusion. However, as cross-matched blood is not immediately available, other fluids are used first. Uncross-matched group O Rh-negative blood is occasionally indicated in the exsanguinating patient, but in general transfusion of large quantities of blood is wasteful while bleeding is uncontrolled. Extensive fluid resuscitation in penetrating trauma prior to haemostasis may be detrimental.[10] The place of hypertonic fluids in trauma resuscitation is unresolved.

Isotonic saline or a balanced salt solution should be the first fluids infused. Shocked patients may need 2–3 l in the first few minutes. One litre bags or bottles and giving sets with in-line pumps should be used on all IV lines. A colloid plasma expander can be the second fluid used, and by 20–30 min, cross-matched red cells should be available. Platelets and fresh frozen plasma are reserved for documented or suspected coagulopathy (i.e. dilutional coagulopathy with fluids deficient in haemostatic factors and disseminated intravascular coagulopathy (DIC) from prolonged shock).

All resuscitation fluids have a high sodium concentration, similar to that of extracellular fluid. Glucose 5% and glucose–saline solutions are not effective resuscitation fluids. Few trauma patients actually require them in the first day.

Urine output

Hourly urine output is a useful guide to resuscitation from shock. Minimal acceptable urine output is 0.5 ml/kg per h, but 1–2 ml/kg per h is more adequate. Frusemide has no place in initial resuscitation. Apart from adequate resuscitation, diuresis can be due to ethanol, mannitol, dopamine, nephrogenic or neurogenic diabetes insipidus, or non-oliguric renal failure. Polyuria may mask early recognition of acute renal failure.

Inadequate resuscitation

Patients in shock have depleted interstitial fluid as well as circulating blood volume, and need resuscitation fluid volumes greater than the actual volume of blood lost. With blunt injury, volume losses often continue for 24–48 h. Prolonged shock from delayed and inadequate resuscitation, leads to renal failure, acute respiratory distress syndrome (ARDS), sepsis, DIC and multiorgan dysfunction.[11,12]

Pulmonary oedema

Pulmonary oedema during resuscitation may be related to fluid overload, direct lung trauma, aspiration of gastric contents, pulmonary responses to non-thoracic trauma and reactions to resuscitation fluids. They can all cause leaky capillaries and produce non-cardiogenic pulmonary oedema.

Radiology for trauma patients

Patients with depressed consciousness, breathing difficulties or unstable circulation, should be X-rayed in the emergency department, and not sent to a radiology department remote from skilled resuscitation facilities. Conversely, extensive imaging examinations of shocked patients in the emergency department are unacceptable. Only three or four examinations should be requested in the emergency department:

Chest

This is the only X-ray ever justified in an unresuscitated patient. A supine film is usually sufficient. An erect film is better for showing intrapleural air or fluid, ruptured diaphragm, free abdominal gas and for defining an abnormal mediastinum, but is often impractical in shock or suspected spinal injury. It can be done later if feasible. An obvious pneumothorax does not require a chest X-ray before insertion of an intercostal drain.

Lateral cervical spine

This should be done in all patients with head injury or multiple injuries, as cervical spine fractures are often missed. With head or facial injuries, a cervical fracture should be assumed initially and a cervical collar applied. A lateral cervical spine X-ray can be taken after the patient has been resuscitated. In the comatose patient, adequate examination requires anteroposterior and odontoid views, and possibly a CT scan.[4]

Pelvis

Unexplained blood loss can be due to a missed pelvic fracture. A dislocated hip can be missed in multiple injuries. Pelvic X-ray are not needed in awake patients with no pelvic abnormalities.

'One-shot' intravenous urogram (IVU)

The value of this investigation before laparotomy is debatable.[13] It is more frequently performed in the operating room, avoiding a lengthy formal IVU in the radiology department.

Other radiological investigations

Other X-rays should be performed after adequate resuscitation in the radiology department, operating room or ICU:

1 *Skull*: Plain skull X-rays do not guide immediate treatment. A CT scan of the brain is a more useful urgent investigation (see below).
2 *Extremities*: X-rays of the extremities to assess bony injuries are not urgent unless there is vascular injury. Therefore, these films should not be taken in the emergency department for diagnosis, unless the patient is going directly to the operating room for fracture fixation.
3 *Spine*: X-rays of thoracic or lumbosacral spine are seldom indicated in the emergency department.
4 *Abdomen*: A plain abdominal X-ray is of limited value in the initial evaluation of trauma.
5 *CT abdomen*: This can be valuable to evaluate a patient who is haemodynamically stable (see above).
6 *CT head*: This is vital in the treatment of severe head injuries (see below).
7 *Aortography*: If aortic rupture is suspected, the duty radiologist should be consulted immediately. In general, diagnosis of ruptured aorta takes priority over other injuries, except those requiring immediate laparotomy or craniotomy. This approach is a calculated risk because the incidence of positive aortography is low (10–20%;[14] see Chapter 68).
8 *Interventional radiology*: Percutaneous transcatheter embolization is therapeutic rather than diagnostic. It can provide life-saving haemostasis in massive retroperitoneal haemorrhage associated with pelvic fracture.[15] The logistics of managing such haemodynamically unstable patients in the radiology department are formidable.

Head trauma (see Chapter 66)

Head injuries are common, but those requiring urgent cranial operations are less so. The head injury may initially be the most obvious in multiple injuries, but may not be the most important. Conversely, a severe head injury may seem unimportant initially. Head injury is a major determinant of outcome in critically injured patients.

Emergency treatment

Resuscitation measures in the primary survey above are undertaken. Victims with one or both dilated, unreactive pupils should be given mannitol 1 g/kg IV to relieve brainstem compression, until definitive diagnosis and treatment can be arranged.

Shocked trauma patients with or without head injuries require the same resuscitation fluids. Treatment of shock and maintenance of cerebral perfusion are vital, as hypotension is disastrous to an already damaged brain.[16,17] Contrary to common belief, sodium-containing fluids are not inherently dangerous in head trauma. However, after adequate resuscitation, further sodium administration is usually not indicated. Excessive (free) water is potentially dangerous, as it can lead to hypo-osmolar brain swelling.[18]

Neurological evaluation

Factors such as hypoxaemia, shock, alcohol, analgesics, anaesthetic agents, muscle relaxants and other drugs depress consciousness and confound neurological signs. Clinical neurological evaluation includes the Glasgow coma score (GCS)[19,20] and a search for lateralizing signs.

CT scanning is indicated in all patients who will not obey verbal commands, especially if they are rendered neurologically inaccessible by sedative and relaxant agents. Lateralizing motor or pupillary signs with a deteriorating level of consciousness are indications for immediate CT scanning (or, if unavailable, emergency burr holes).

In an unstable patient, a laparotomy for intraabdominal haemorrhage should take priority over a head CT scan.[21] Conversely, a stable patient with a positive peritoneal lavage and localizing neurological signs should have a head CT prior to laparotomy.

Severity and morbidity of trauma

Severity of injury is measured by the abbreviated injury scale (AIS),[22,23] which divides the body into six regions – head and neck, face, thorax, abdomen, pelvis and extremities, and external. Specific injuries in body region are coded on a scale of 1 (minor), 2 (moderate), 3 (serious, not life-threatening), 4 (severe, life-threatening, survival probable), 5 (critical, survival uncertain) and 6 (unsurvivable). The AIS was designed for motor vehicle injuries, but has been validated for blunt and penetrating trauma. It can provide a basis for research, education, audit and allocation of resources.

Severity of trauma is related not just to the severity of individual injuries, but also to the combined effects of multiple injuries. Multiple injuries are graded by the injury severity score (ISS), which is an empirical system based on the AIS grades for the three worst body regions.[24,25] ISS gives a score between 0 and 75 for total body injury; 16 or more indicates major trauma. Death with an ISS below 24 should be rare. Above an ISS of 25, there is a stepwise increase in mortality, with very high rates over 50.[26,27]

AIS and ISS study mostly the anatomy of injury. Other factors influence trauma mortality and morbidity, including age, pre-existing health, degree of physiological derangement, standard of pre-hospital and early hospital care and complications. Degree of physiological derangement can be measured by the revised trauma score,[28] which is computed from the coded values of GCS, systolic blood pressure and respiratory rate, usually at admission to the emergency department.[28] The TRISS severity index is based on the revised trauma score, ISS, and patient age.[29] It correlates well with outcome, and has been used to compile survival norms for blunt and penetrating trauma.[26,27] Physiological scoring systems like APACHE do not work well for trauma patients[30,31] (see Chapter 2). Preinjury illness (comorbidity) has a profound effect on trauma outcome.[32]

Shock influences trauma mortality and morbidity. Correcting shock in the first 'golden hour' is an important concept.[6] The longer a patient is in shock, the higher is the probability of immediate or delayed complications. Complications include renal failure, acute respiratory distress syndrome, sepsis, liver failure and multiorgan dysfunction.[11,12,33] Acute oliguric renal failure on the first day after trauma is now rare, but non-oliguric renal failure is often seen 2–4 days later, caused by the shock and delayed or inadequate resuscitation. It is often heralded by polyuria, which is misinterpreted as a sign of adequate resuscitation.

Epidemiology of injuries[34,35]

Of trauma deaths, the time interval between injury and death has three peaks.[1] The majority of deaths are immediate (within minutes) at the scene of injury. Some deaths are early (within hours) in the emergency department or the operating room, while some are late (after days or weeks) and occur in the ICU or

Table 65.1 Percentage of ICU trauma patients with grades of injury in different body regions

	AIS ≥ 4	*AIS = 3*	*AIS ≤ 2*	*AIS = 0*
Head and neck	63	9	11	17
Face	3	11	7	79
Thorax	9	17	5	69
Abdomen	15	4	1	80
Extremities	1	35	10	54
External	0	<1	67	33

Data on 1465 adult trauma patients in the DCCM, Auckland Hospital, 1988–93. Abbreviated injury scale (AIS) codes:[22] 0 = no injury; 1 = minor; 2 = moderate; 3 = serious; not life-threatening; 4 = severe, life-threatening, survival probable; 5 = critical, survival uncertain; 6 = unsurvivable.

ward. Those in the ICU are mostly from severe head injury within a few days and, less commonly, multiorgan dysfunction later.

Of trauma admissions to hospital, only a minority had severe or multiple trauma.[36] In order of frequency, life-threatening injuries involved the head, abdomen, and chest (Table 65.1), and were often multiple.[36] The hospital services which this small number of severely injured patients used out of proportion to their numbers were major surgery, intensive care, radiography and CT scanning.[36] Recent major trauma outcome studies in the USA[26] and the UK[27] offer valuable epidemiological data. The USA study found that mortality for direct admissions was strongly related to serious head injury.

Organization of trauma care

Many of the problems of trauma care are organizational. Problems faced by health authorities are the provision of advanced care at the scene of injury, rapid transportation to hospital, policies on which hospitals should receive trauma patients, systems for rapid evaluation and decision-making in hospitals, and rapid, safe patient transfer between hospitals. If survival from major trauma is to be maximized, prehospital and hospital care must be coordinated.

Regionalization of trauma care has become an accepted concept.[2,37] Trauma centres are designated hospitals which meet certain requirements. Main prerequisites are in-house experienced surgeons, anaesthetists and neurosurgeons, and a minimum number of patients seen annually for staff expertise. Regionalization involves the concept of ambulances bypassing non-designated hospitals.[2] Helicopters are used increasingly to speed patient transportation.[38] Trauma teams are teams of surgeons and intensivists or anaesthetists who immediately attend the trauma victim on arrival at hospital.[2-4,33]

Trauma registries and databases are important tools in organizing and improving trauma care. The UK major trauma outcome study[27] showed that the doctors in charge of resuscitation were often junior, delays in performing urgent operations were common, and the number of preventable deaths was significant. The hospital may not see enough trauma patients to justify a trauma team or supply adequate experience for its staff, and may not have all the facilities required by trauma patients. Transfer to a trauma hospital may be desirable, but geography and limited transport facilities may make such transfers hazardous.

In western countries trauma is a leading cause of death and disability under the age of 38.[26] Reduction of mortality and morbidity depends on public education, new legislations, on-site advanced care, rapid evacuation (see Chapter 3), hospital trauma expertise and coordination of services.[39,40]

References

1. Trunkey DD (1983) Trauma. *Sci Am* **249**:20–27.
2. Trunkey DD (1982) Overview of trauma. *Surg Clin North Am* **62**:3–7.
3. Trunkey DD (1991) Initial treatment of patients with extensive trauma. *N Engl J Med* **324**:1259–1263.
4. Enderson BL and Maull KI (1991) Missed injuries: the trauma surgeon's nemesis. *Surg Clin North Am* **71**:399–418.
5. Committee on Trauma, American College of Surgeons (1993) *Advanced Trauma Life Support (ATLS) Program for Physicians*, 5th edn. Chicago: American College of Surgeons.
6. Trauma Committee, Royal Australasian College of Surgeons (1992) *Early Management of Severe Trauma (EMST)*. Melbourne: Royal Australasian College of Surgeons.
7. Day AC, Rankin N and Charlesworth P (1992) Diagnostic peritoneal lavage: integration with clinical information to improve diagnostic performance. *J Trauma* **32**:52–57.
8. Trunkey DD and Federle MP (1986) Computed tomography in perspective (editorial). *J Trauma* **26**:660–661.
9. Padhani HR, Watson CJE, Clements L, Calne RY and Dixon AK (1992) Computed tomography in abdominal trauma: an audit of usage and image quality. *Br J Radiol* **65**:397–402.
10. Bickell WH, Wall MJ, Pepe PE *et al.* (1994) Immediate versus delayed fluid resuscitation for hypotensive patients with penetrating torso injuries. *N Engl J Med* **331**:1105–1109.
11. Cowley RA and Trump BF (1982) Editors' summary: Organ dysfunction in shock. In: Cowley RA and Trump BF (eds) *Pathophysiology of Shock, Anoxia, and Ischaemia*. Baltimore: Williams & Wilkins, pp. 281–284.
12. Faist E, Baue AE, Dittmer H and Heberer G (1983) Multiple organ failure in polytrauma patients. *J Trauma* **23**:775–787.
13. Stevenson J and Battistella FD (1994) The 'one-shot' intravenous pyelogram: is it indicated in unstable trauma patients before celiotomy? *J Trauma* **36**:828–834.
14. Lee RB, Stahlmann GC and Sharp KW (1992) Treatment priorities in patients with traumatic rupture of the thoracic aorta. *Am Surg* **58**:37–43.
15. Panetta T, Sclafari SJA, Goldstein AS, Phillips TF and Shaftan GW (1985) Percutaneous transcatheter embolisation for massive bleeding from pelvic fractures. *J Trauma* **26**:1021–1029.
16. Chestnut RM, Marshall LF, Klauber MR *et al.* (1993) The role of secondary brain injury in determining outcome from severe head injury. *J Trauma* **34**:216–222.
17. Wilden JN (1993) Rapid resuscitation in severe head injury (commentary). *Lancet* **342**:1378.
18. Fishman RA (1953) Effects of isotonic intravenous solutions on normal and increased intracranial pressure. *Arch Neurol Psychiatry* **70**:350–360.
19. Teasdale G and Jennett B (1974) Assessment of coma and impaired consciousness: a practical scale. *Lancet* **ii**:81–84.
20. Jennett B and Teasdale G (1977) Aspects of coma after severe head injury. *Lancet* **i**:878–881.

21. Thomason M, Messick J, Rutledge R *et al.* (1993) Head CT scanning versus urgent exploration in the hypotensive blunt trauma patient. *J Trauma* **34**:40–45.

22. Committee on Injury Scaling (1980) *The Abbreviated Injury Scale – 1980 Revision*. Morton Grove, Il: American Association for Automotive Medicine.

23. Committee on Injury Scaling (1990) *The Abbreviated Injury Scale – 1990 Revision*. Des Plaines, Il: American Association for Automotive Medicine.

24. Baker SP, O'Neill B, Haddon W and Long WB (1974) The injury severity score: a method for describing patients with multiple injuries and evaluating emergency care. *J Trauma* **14**:187–196.

25. Baker SP and O'Neill B (1976) The injury severity score: an update. *J Trauma* **16**:882–885.

26. Champion HR, Copes WS, Sacco WJ *et al.* (1990) The major trauma outcome study: establishing national norms for trauma care. *J Trauma* **30**:1356–1365.

27. Yates DW, Woodford M and Hollis S (1992) Preliminary analysis of the care of injured patients in 33 British hospitals: first report of the United Kingdom major trauma outcome study. *Br Med J* **305**:737–740.

28. Champion HR, Sacco WJ, Copes WS, Gann DS, Gennarelli TA and Flanagan ME (1989) A revision of the trauma score. *J Trauma* **29**:623–629.

29. Boyd CR, Tolson MA and Copes WS (1987) Evaluating trauma care: the TRISS method. *J Trauma* **27**:370–378.

30. McAnena OJ, Moore FA, Moore EE, Mattox KL, Marx JA and Pepe P (1992) Invalidation of the APACHE II scoring system for patients with acute trauma. *J Trauma* **33**:504–507.

31. Roumen RMH, Redl H, Schlag G, Sandtner W, Koller W and Goris RJA (1993) Scoring systems and blood lactate concentrations in relation to the development of adult respiratory distress syndrome and multiple organ failure in severely traumatized patients. *J Trauma* **35**:349–355.

32. Sacco WJ, Copes WS, Bain LW *et al.* (1993) Effect of preinjury illness on trauma patient survival outcome. *J Trauma* **35**:538–543.

33. Cowley RA, Dunham CM (eds) (1982) *Shock Trauma/ Critical Care Manual*. Baltimore: University Park Press.

34. Baker CC, Oppenheimer L, Stephens B, Lewis FR and Trunkey DD (1980) Epidemiology of trauma deaths. *Am J Surg* **140**:144–150.

35. Smeeton WMI, Judson JA, Synek BJ, Sage MD, Koelmeyer TD and Cairns FJ (1987) Deaths from trauma in Auckland: a one year study. *NZ Med J* **100**:337–340.

36. Streat SJ, Donaldson ML and Judson JA (1987) Trauma in Auckland: an overview. *NZ Med J* **100**:441–444.

37. Eggold R (1983) Trauma care regionalisation: a necessity (editorial). *J Trauma* **23**:260–262.

38. Freeark RJ (1983) The trauma center: its hospitals, head injuries, helicopters, and heroes (1982 AAST presidential address). *J Trauma* **23**:173–178.

39. Judson JA (1985) Trauma management: modern concepts (editorial). *NZ Med J* **98**:8–9.

40. Trunkey DD (1982) On the nature of things that go bang in the night. *Surgery* **92**:123–132.

66 | Severe head injuries

WR Thompson

Head injuries are a major medical and social problem in developed countries. Neurotrauma accounts for approximately a third of the trauma-related deaths and is the leading cause of mortality and morbidity in the 15–24-year-old age group. In addition to the loss of life (22–28 per 100 000 population),[1-3] there is the added social burden of hospital care, rehabilitation and chronic maintenance, which in 1980 was estimated at US$3.9 billion for the USA.

In the USA, some 410 000–430 000 patients per year are admitted to hospital with head injuries – an occurrence rate of 180–200 per 100 000 population[1,2] Approximately 72% are minor head injuries, most of which are admitted for observation for 12–48 h. However, some 11% are dead on admission and 8–11% are severe head injuries.[2,4,5]

In general, only patients with severe head injuries (Glasgow coma scale (GCS) ≤ 8)[6,7] plus head injuries associated with multiple trauma or complicated by other medical problems are admitted to the ICU. This group remains exposed to a mortality of 30–60%, dependent on the type of intracranial lesion. Aggressive ICU treatment has been shown to improve the outcome of patients with severe head injuries without increasing the number of severely disabled or vegetative survivors.[8-11]

Initial assessment

Initially, the severely head-injured patient must have a rapid but complete primary trauma survey followed by resuscitation (see Chapter 65). General measures must be instituted as necessary to reduce the incidence of secondary insults, particularly hypoxia, hypercarbia and hypotension.[7,12,13] These include:

1 *Establishment of a clear airway and adequate ventilation with added oxygen:* Intubation and intermittent positive-pressure ventilation are required if ventilation or gas exchange is inadequate, and/or if the patient is incapable of protecting the airway. Thirty per cent of patients with severe head injuries, particularly those associated with multiple trauma, are hypoxaemic and should be intubated promptly.[12,13] Adequate ventilation should produce a PCO_2 of 30–35 mmHg (4–4.7 kPa) and a PO_2 >80 mmHg (10.7 kPa). Until proven otherwise, with adequate X-rays of the cervical spines, all of these patients should be considered to have a cervical spine fracture and handled accordingly.

2 *Treatment of shock:* Hypovolaemia is a common finding in head injuries associated with multiple trauma. Prompt and effective resuscitation is required. However, in isolated head injuries shock is an uncommon finding, with the exception of cases involving young children, medullary injuries or large scalp lacerations.

Following the initial resuscitation the secondary trauma survey is undertaken in order to ascertain other injuries (particularly injuries to the head and neck, chest, abdomen and limbs) and to decide the priorities of treatment.

Emphasis will be placed on the determination of a detailed baseline neurological examination. The most important features are:

1 *Level of conscious state and assessment of GCS :*[6,14] Its use in all head injuries has been advocated[15] and it has some prognostic significance by itself[16-18] and also in conjunction with other clinical and laboratory findings.[19-21] It is useful in comparing head injuries and treatment regimens from different centres. It is not, however, a complete neurological assessment. Drug or alcohol intoxication will make the assessment of conscious state difficult (intoxicated patients often have an associated head injury).

2 *Pupils:* Pupil size and reactivity are especially important when the conscious state is impaired. Abnormalities of the pupil size and reactivity indicate compression and compromise of the third

cranial nerve. This may help in the localization of supratentorial lesions. Signs of third nerve compression, depression of conscious state, plus asymmetrical motor responses are the triad of signs for transtentorial herniation. Extraocular movements (doll's eye and response to aural caloric testing) are also important in the assessment of the midbrain and pons. The doll's-eye manoeuvre should not be performed until fractures of the cervical spine have been excluded. Papilloedema is uncommon in the acute phase of head injuries.[22]

3 *Motor function:* Evidence of motor dysfunction, especially decerebrate rigidity, hemiplegia or other localizing signs, should be sought for.

4 *Other examination features:* Should include assessment of the gag reflex, cough reflex, cardiac status (particularly arrhythmias), ventilatory patterns and examination of the remaining cranial nerves.

If the patient is responsive to commands or questions, then a more detailed neurological examination should be performed. A head injury is a dynamic process, which evolves with time. Therefore the neurological examination must be repeated at regular intervals in order to track changes in the patient's condition.

Further history should be obtained with particular reference to the circumstances of the injury and retrieval, seizures, intoxication, pre-existing medical problems and medication. It must be stressed that patients with severe head injuries should be seen early in the process by a neurosurgeon.[23] Patients with a GCS < 8 or those in whom there is evidence of progressive deterioration or neurological status should be seen immediately by a neurosurgeon. Early (following initial assessment, resuscitation and stabilization) computed tomography (CT) scanning should be performed. Intracranial mass lesions occur in only 6–7% of total head-injury admissions but in 40–60% of severe head injuries.[19–21,24]

Further diagnostic measures

Computed tomography[25]

Since its introduction in 1972, the CT scan has become the most informative radiological technique in the evaluation of the acute head injury. It is the procedure of choice for determining the presence or absence of mass lesions. It will also indicate areas of oedema, infarction, contusion and intracranial air plus the size of the ventricular system. In addition, the results of the CT scan may aid in the decision regarding intracranial pressure (ICP) monitoring[26] and may be of some prognostic value.[27–29]

It is important to plan for all the logistical problems involved in moving an acutely injured patient to the CT scanner. The patient is required to lie completely still during the performance of the scan. Any patient movement, due to pain, restlessness or obstructed breathing, will produce an inadequate scan.

Skull X-rays

The presence of a fracture indicates the likelihood of complications occurring (e.g. intracranial haematoma),[30] and may be a help in localization if there is loss of consciousness due to an extradural haemorrhage. If a calcified pineal gland can be seen, then its position relative to the midline may indicate the degree of shift of the intracranial contents. Fractures of the base of the skull may be seen on X-ray without a prior clinical indication of their presence. Skull X-rays may also be important in the assessment of skull fractures and the future planning of reconstructive surgery. However, skull X-rays are not generally as helpful as CT scanning and their routine use in the emergency evaluation of head-injured patients has been questioned.[30–32]

Mention has already been made of the importance of adequate cervical X-rays, if a fracture of the cervical spine is suspected.

Cerebral angiography

This is now rarely indicated when there is ready access to a CT scanner. However, if an isodense traumatic lesion is suspected on the CT scan, if the patient's clinical condition is not consistent with the CT findings or if a vascular lesion is suspected, then cerebral angiography should be performed. In the absence of a CT scanner, cerebral angiography can be used in the diagnosis of intracranial haematoma.

Ventriculography

Ventriculography has been to a large extent superseded by CT scanning. Ventriculography will provide information on the degree of midline shift and allow measurement of the intracranial pressure.

Echo encephalography

This has been superseded by the CT scanner.

Radioisotope scan

This is of little benefit unless a CT scan cannot be obtained, but it does give some information on cerebral vascularity. Newer imaging techniques, e.g. positron emission tomography (PET), will provide additional information on cerebral blood flow (CBF) and neuronal function.

Magnetic resonance imaging (MRI)

MRI[33] of head injuries may have some advantages over CT scanning in:

1 estimating the size of extracerebral fluid collections and diagnosing small collections;
2 distinguishing chronic subdural haematomas from hygromas;
3 displaying non-haemorrhagic contusions.

However, there are many logistical problems in supporting and monitoring injured patients during MRI[34] and CT scanning remains superior in the diagnosis of acute parenchymal haemorrhages and acute subarachnoid haemorrhages.[33] CT therefore remains the procedure of choice for acute head injuries and MRI has yet to find its place in the acute management of head injuries, particularly severe head injuries. It has been suggested that MRI may be of prognostic value in the management of mild and moderate head injuries.[35]

Monitoring

Routine physiological monitoring for head injuries includes electrocardiogram (ECG), arterial blood pressure, oxygen saturation end-tidal CO_2 and ventilatory parameters supplemented by arterial blood gases. Specific forms of monitoring for severe head injuries include the following:

Intracranial pressure monitoring

Surgically amenable intracranial mass lesions should be diagnosed and treated early in head-injured patients. The continuous measurement of ICP is of great value, particularly in a patient who is comatose or on a mechanical ventilator, when assessment of neurological function is difficult. The value of continuous ICP measurement has been established.[8,10,11,36-38] Prolonged levels of ICP greater than 25 mmHg (3.3 kPa) are associated with a very poor prognosis.[37] There is evidence that the results of head injury management could be improved if ICPs > 15–20 mmHg (2.0–2.7 kPa) were treated with aggressive therapy.[10,11,37,39] However, early evacuation of intracranial haematoma without ICP measurement can produce comparable results.[40] Analysis of ICP waveforms may assist in determining cerebral compliance and disturbances in autoregulation.[41]

Cerebral perfusion pressure (CPP)

For simplicity of measurement, the CPP is considered to be mean arterial pressure minus mean ICP. CPP should be measured in all severe head injuries,[42] and below 70 mmHg (9.3 kPa) the jugular venous oxygen saturation (Sjo_2) decreases and the cerebral arteriovenous oxygen difference $(AVDo_2)$ increases.[43]

Jugular venous oxygen saturation

Retrograde jugular vein catheterization with a fibreoptic catheter with the tip located between the base of the skull and C2 allows the continuous measurement of Sjo_2 and the calculation of $AVDo_2$.[41] These measurements enable the intensivist to determine if global cerebral hyperaemia or ischaemia is present.[43,44] Cerebral hyperaemia may then be treated with hyperventilation. Cerebral ischaemia may respond to elevation of CPP, mannitol and/or a reduction in the degree of hyperventilation.

Transcranial Doppler (TCD)

Transcranial Dopplers allow transcranial measurements of CBF velocity to be made on an intermittent or continuous basis.[41,43] In addition, a pulsatility index (PI) can be derived. Monitoring of CBFV and PI may assist in determining the optimum CPP for a particular patient.[43] By using a combination of CPP, TCD and Sjo_2 it is possible to determine states of cerebral ischaemia or hyperaemia and to assess the effects of changes in therapy on ICP.

Recordings of cerebral activity: multimodality evoked potentials (MEP) and the electroencephalogram (EEG)

These may be useful after the initial stabilization of the patient. They can aid in the monitoring of the patient's clinical course and possibly provide information on specific neurological function.[45]

Management

Once the immediate and surgically amenable intracranial problems (e.g. epidural and subdural haematomas, hydrocephalus and depressed skull fractures) have been dealt with, the aims of ICU management for severe head injuries become:

1 early detection of changes in neurological status through constant observation and monitoring;
2 prevention of secondary cerebral insults, especially those related to hyponatraemia, hypotension, hypoxaemia, hypercarbia and raised ICP;[12,46,47]
3 early diagnosis and treatment of medical and surgical problems, particularly intracranial mass lesions, cerebral oedema and epilepsy, which may be intercurrent or in the process of developing.

The main principles of management are as follows:

Constant observation

Nursing observation as per the GCS is extremely important, as head injuries are a dynamic rather than static process. If deterioration (a decrease of 2 points on the GCS or changes in pupillary or lateralizing signs) occurs, the cause must be sought.

Patient position

The patient should be nursed in the head-up position (approximately 30–45°) with the head in a neutral plane relative to the body, in order to facilitate ventilation and reduce ICP.

Respiratory care

Hypoxia, hypercarbia and respiratory obstruction must be prevented. The ventilatory parameters and inspired oxygen concentration should be adjusted to achieve a $Pao_2 > 80$ mmHg (10.6 kPa) and a $Paco_2$ of approximately 30 mmHg (4 kPa). Hyperventilation to a $Paco_2 < 25$ mmHg (3.4 kPa) has been shown to produce cerebral ischaemia and to affect outcome adversely.[48] Endotracheal suction and physiotherapy will increase ICP, and should be preceded by adequate sedation and analgesia.

Blood pressure control

Control of the blood pressure is aimed at keeping the systolic blood pressure within the normal limits of autoregulation. Varying degrees of autoregulatory dysfunction occur following head injuries. It is therefore important to prevent the blood pressure being in the ranges where CBF is pressure-dependent.[48] The critical CPP with reference to cerebral ischaemia is about 70 mmHg (9.2 kPa).[43] In the early phases of acute severe head injuries, the vascular factors probably account for a greater proportion of the increases in ICP than do cerebrospinal fluid (CSF) parameters.[50] Many of these ICP changes are due to cerebral ischaemia, as generally the CBF velocities are low in the first hours after a severe head injury,[40,41] hence the need for multimodality monitory.

Surgery

Early operative treatment is indicated for the recurrence of surgically amenable lesions such as intracranial collections and hydrocephalus.

Treatment of raised intracranial pressure (see Chapter 43)

Intracranial hypertension occurs in 54% of severe head injuries. Once intracranial mass lesions and hydrocephalus are excluded, then raised ICP in head injuries is due to cerebral vasodilatation, cerebral oedema or varying combinations of both.[51] In the acute stages, cerebral vasodilatation may be more important in the genesis of raised ICP, whereas in the later stages cerebral oedema secondary to ischaemia may be more important. Measurements of cerebral perfusion pressure, SjO_2 and CBF velocity can assist in optimizing therapy.[43] Therapy for raised ICP includes the following.

Controlled ventilation

Hyperventilation will produce a reduction in ICP. The arterial $Paco_2$ should be maintained at approximately 30 mmHg (4 kPa) and it is important to ensure that cardiac output and CPP are not reduced. Hyperventilation is useful for acute short-term control of ICP, particularly in the presence of cerebral hyperaemia.[41,43] Excessive hyperventilation to a $Paco_2 < 25$ mmHg (3.4 kPa) can aggravate cerebral ischaemia.[48] The efficacy of hyperventilation can be tracked by monitoring ICP, CPP, Sjo_2 and CBF. Duration of ventilation is generally 48–72 h in the first instance, followed by an attempt to wean the patient off the ventilator, provided the ICP is controlled. If the ICP rises during weaning, ventilation is continued for a further 24–48 h. Increases in ICP during controlled ventilation necessitate the checking of CPP and arterial blood gases, plus reassessment of ventilation and consideration of CT scanning.

Maintenance of CPP

When CPP is reduced in focal head injuries or vasospasm is present, then use of inotropes, particularly when autoregulation is intact, may improve SJo_2 and the ICP.[41,43]

Osmotic diuretics

If the blood–brain barrier is intact, osmotic diuretics such as mannitol and urea will lower ICP by drawing fluid across the blood–brain barrier (thus reducing the bulk of the normal brain). Mannitol is the agent generally used, as there is less rebound than with urea. If a patient is deteriorating rapidly in the acute stage of a head injury, mannitol 0.5–1.0 g/kg body weight IV is used. The subsequent dose of mannitol is 0.25–0.5 g/kg every 6 h. The osmotic diuresis should not be pursued at the expense of cardiovascular stability. If a diuresis does not occur, mannitol should not be continued. Serum osmolality can be used as a guide to mannitol therapy. It should not rise above 310 mosmol/kg as mannitol itself will enter the brain and interfere with the efficacy of the dehydration therapy.[52] If serum osmolality exceeds 350 mosmol/kg, serious cellular damage may occur.[53] Treatment with mannitol is continued for only 24–48 h, as eventually mannitol will cross into the brain and cause an increase in brain volume (rebound phenomenon). In one study, empirical mannitol therapy without ICP monitoring produced similar results to mannitol therapy given for ICP elevations > 25 mmHg (3.2 kPa).[59]

Steroids

The value of steroids to treat cerebral oedema associated with intracranial tumours is well-documented and accepted. However, the value of steroids in the treatment of cerebral oedema associated with head injuries remains unproven,[54] although there may be a subgroup of patients who are early responders to the overall treatment for head injury, whose outcome may be improved by steroids.[55] None the less, several prospective double-blind studies[56-58] have indicated that steroids do not significantly alter the morbidity, mortality or ICP in severely head-injured patients. Consequently, use of steroids in the management of head injuries has declined markedly (although steroids may be beneficial after spinal injury – see Chapter 69).

Diuretics

There is some evidence that the reduction in brain oedema with frusemide is due to more that the diuresis *per se*.[59] Frusemide is the diuretic of choice in patients with congestive heart failure plus cerebral oedema. It may produce less marked changes in serum electrolytes and osmolality than mannitol.[60] Animal experiments have suggested that frusemide can act synergistically with mannitol and thereby sustain the osmotic gradient established with mannitol,[61] and that oncodiuretic therapy (i.e. albumin plus frusemide) has similar cerebral effects to mannitol or frusemide.[62]

Cerebral metabolic depression

A number of drugs that reduce cerebral metabolic rate in tandem with a reduction in CBF have been used to control ICP, and with an expectation that they might contribute to preservation of neuronal function. The barbiturates,[10,63] propofol and lignocaine,[64] have been used for this purpose in patients with raised ICP unresponsive to conventional treatment modalities, and who do not have surgically correctable mass lesions on repeat CT scanning. High doses of these agents are often required; if used on a continuous basis, extensive ICP and cardiovascular monitoring and support are required.

Barbiturate therapy is generally commenced at an ICP > 20–25 mmHg (2.7–3.3 kPa) with a closed skull, and an ICP > 15 mmHg (2 kPa) with a craniectomy. Barbiturates have been shown to reduce ICP,[10] but prophylactic use of pentobarbitol failed to improve outcome from severe head injuries.[65] Eisenberg *et al.*[11] suggested that high-dose barbiturates are only indicated in a small subset of patients, and are an effective adjuvant to conventional therapy for ICP control. There was a marked difference in 1-month survival between responders and non-responders to therapy directed at ICP control (conventional ± pentobarbitol), but no other outcome details were reported.[11] Lee *et al.*[66] have suggested that barbiturate coma may be useful when other conventional therapies fail to control intracranial hypertension. Moderate hypothermia (32–33°C) may also reduce ICP and improve outcome.[67,68]

Fluid balance

Following initial resuscitation and stabilization, strict control of fluid balance will help to control cerebral oedema. It is important to prevent hyponatraemia and water overload. However, fluid restriction should not be pursued at the expense of cardiovascular stability or renal function.

Electrolytes

Electrolyte disturbances are frequently seen in patients with head injuries as a result of the head injury, stress response, use of osmotic diuretics, diabetes insipidus, fluid restriction, feeding regimens and medications. Regular monitoring of electrolytes, urea, creatinine, blood sugar and osmolalities are important in determining appropriate fluid and electrolyte therapy.

Physiotherapy

Physiotherapy has an important role to play in the removal of lung secretions and prevention of contractures plus rehabilitation. Adequate sedation and blood pressure control prior to chest physiotherapy are required in order to prevent ICP elevation.

Antibiotics

Despite lack of good data, many clinicians recommend prophylactic antibiotics for patients with CSF rhinorrhoea, compound wounds, and when operative fixation of fractures is performed. Antibiotics may also be used prophylactically following the insertion of an ICP monitoring device. Prophylactic antibiotics are not recommended for skull fractures (see Chapter 64), but penicillin or co-trimoxazole is used by some. Appropriate tetanus prophylaxis should be given.

Treatment of epileptic seizures

Epileptic seizures will markedly increase cerebral metabolic demands. Routine use of phenytoin has been recommended for postoperative neurosurgical patients, including those with head injuries.[69] However, the efficacy of prophylactic administration of phenytoin to prevent early posttraumatic seizures has yet to be firmly established.[70] Acute seizures should be treated with a barbiturate or a benzodiazepine, then phenytoin should be commenced for longer-term therapy.

Prophylaxis against gastric ulceration

Gastroduodenal lesions, particularly erosive gastritis, on endoscopy are very frequent in patients with severe head injuries, but significant haemorrhage only occurs in 10–14% of cases. Prophylaxis using anti-antacids ± H_2-receptor blockers should be considered for severe head injuries pending the introduction of enteral feeding.

Nutrition

Patients with severe head injuries, irrespective of whether they are receiving steroids, demonstrate markedly increased energy requirement, a negative nitrogen balance, weight loss and hypoalbuminaemia.[71,72] Early enteral/parenteral feeding is recommended.[73–75]

Other additional treatment

Other aspects of management which deserve comment are:

1 *Temperature control*: Fever increases the metabolic demands of the brain and may thus exacerbate neuronal injury. Hence it is important to determine the cause of the fever and to treat appropriately. Hypothermia has been shown experimentally to be protective to the brain in head injury and cerebral oedema, and moderate hypothermia (32–33°C) has been shown to reduce ICP with a suggestion of improved outcome.[67,68]

2 *Syndrome of inappropriate antidiuretic hormone*: This syndrome may be seen following a head injury and is managed as described in Chapter 51.

3 *Diabetes insipidus* may also follow a head injury (see Chapter 51).

4 *Coagulopathy*: Coagulopathies are not uncommon in patients with severe head injuries and must be looked for and treated promptly, in order to reduce the occurrence of intracranial haemorrhage.[76]

Prognosis of head injuries

A number of factors are important, including the age of the patient, time-lag between injury and treatment, type of injury, GCS score and severity of neurological deficit, plus complications, particularly hypoxaemia and hypotension. In general, poor motor function indicates a poor outcome, especially in the older age groups. Patients under 30 years of age have a better prognosis than those over 30 with the same degree of head injury. However, it is important to avoid making a rash prognostic decision too early, as many head-injured patients, particularly the very young, show a remarkable improvement with time.

Brain death, which is an indication for cessation of all active treatment, is described in Chapter 45.

References

1. Kalsbeek WD, McLaurin RL, Harris BSH and Hiller JD (1980) The national head and spinal cord injury survey: major findings. *J Neurosurg* **53**:S19–S31.

2. Kraus JF, Black MA, Hessel N *et al.* (1984) The incidence of acute brain injury and serious impairment in a defined population. *Am J Epidemiol* **119**:186–201.

3. Stening WA (1984) Understanding the epidemic of neurotrauma. *Med J Aust* **141**:5–6.

4. Jennett B and MacMillan R (1981) Epidemiology of head injury. *Br Med J* **282**:101–104.

5. Klauber MR, Marshall LF, Barrett-Connor E and Bowers SA (1981) Prospective study of patients hospitalized with head injury in San Diego County, 1978. *Neurosurgery* **9**:236–241.

6. Jennett B and Teasdale G (1977) Aspects of coma after severe head injury. *Lancet* **1**:878–881.

7. Miller JD, Butterworth JF, Gudeman SK *et al.* (1981) Further experience in the management of severe head injury. *J Neurosurg* **54**:289–299.

8. Becker DP, Miller JD, Ward JD, Greenberg RP, Young HF and Sakalas R (1977) The outcome from severe head injury with early diagnosis and intensive management. *J Neurosurg* **47**:491–502.

9. Moss E, Gibson JS, McDowall DG and Gibson RM (1983) Intensive management of severe head injuries. *Anaesthesia* **38**:214–225.

10. Marshall LF, Smith RW and Shapiro HM (1979) The outcome with aggressive treatment in severe head injuries. *J Neurosurg* **50**:20–30.

11. Eisenberg HM, Frankowski RF, Contant CF, Marshall LF, Walker MD and The Comprehensive Central Nervous System Trauma Centres (1988) High-dose barbiturate control of elevated intracranial pressure in patients with severe head injury. *J Neurosurg* **69**:15–23.

12. Miller JD, Sweet PC, Narayan R and Becker RD (1978) Early insults to the injured brain. *J Am Med Assoc* **240**:439–442.

13. Jones PA, Andrews PJD, Midgley S *et al.* (1994) Measuring the burden of secondary insults in head injured patients during intensive care. *J Neurol Anesth* **6**:4–14.

14. Teasdale G and Jennett B (1974) Assessment of coma and impaired consciousness. A practical scale. *Lancet* **ii**:81–84.

15. Langfitt TCS (1978) Measuring the outcome from head injuries. *J Neurosurg* **48**:673–678.

16. Jennett B, Teasdale G, Braakman R, Minderhoud J and Knill-Jones R (1976) Predicting outcome in individual patients after severe head injury. *Lancet* **i**:1031–1034.

17. Jennett B, Teasedale G, Braakman R, Minderhoud J, Heiden J and Kurze T (1979) Prognosis of patients with severe head injury. *Neurosurgery* **4**:283–289.

18. Young B, Rapp RP, Norton JA, Haack D, Tibbs PA and Bean JR (1981) Early prediction of outcome in head-injured patients. *J Neurosurg* **54**:300–303.

19. Narayan RK, Greenberg RP, Miller JD *et al.* (1981) Improved confidence of outcome prediction in severe head injury. *J Neurosurg* **54**:751–762.

20. Levati A, Farina ML, Vecchi G, Rossanda M and Marrubini MB (1982) Prognosis of severe head injuries. *J Neurosurg* **57**:779–783.

21. Choi SC, Ward JD and Becker DP (1983) Chart for outcome prediction in severe head injury. *J Neurosurg* **59**:294–297.

22. Selhorst JB, Gudeman SK, Butterworth JT, Harbison JW, Miller JD and Becker DP (1983) Papilloedema after acute head injury. *Neurosurgery* **16**:357–363.

23. Group of neurosurgeons (1984) Clinical topics. Guidelines for initial management after head injury in adults. *Br Med J* **288**:983–985.

24. Gennarelli TA, Spielman GM, Langfitt TW *et al.* (1982) Influence of the type of intracranial lesion on outcome from severe head injury. *J Neurosurg* **56**:26–32.

25. Hounsfield GN (1973) Computerised transverse axial scanning (tomography) part 1. Description of system. *Br J Radiol* **46**:1016–1022.

26. Narayan RK, Kishore PRS, Becker DP *et al.* (1982) Intracranial pressure: to monitor or not to monitor? A review of our experience with severe head injury. *J Neurosurg* **56**:650–659.

27. Van Dongen KJ, Braakman R and Gelpke GJ (1983) The prognostic value of computerized tomography in comatose head-injured patients. *J Neurosurg* **59**:951–957.

28. Uzzell BP, Dolinskas CA, Wiser RF and Langfitt TW (1987) Influence of lesions detected by computed tomography on outcome and neurophysiological recovery after severe head injury. *Neurosurgery* **20**:396–402.

29. Toutant SM, Klauber MR, Marshall LF *et al.* (1984) Absent or compressed basal cisterns on first CT scan: ominous predictions of outcome in severe head injury. *J Neurosurg* **61**:691–694.

30. Mendelow AD, Teasdale G, Jennett B, Bryden J, Hessett C and Murray G (1983) Risks of intracranial haematoma in head injured patients. *Br Med J* **287**:1173–1176.

31. Cooper PR and Ho V (1983) Role of emergency skull X-ray films in the evaluation of the head-injured patient: a retrospective study. *Neurosurgery* **13**:136–140.

32. Feuerman T, Wackym PA, Gade GI and Becker DP (1988) Value of skull radiography, head computed tomographic scanning, and admission for observation in cases of minor head injury. *Neurosurgery* **22**:449–453.

33. Snow RB, Zimmerman RD, Gandy SE and Deck MDF (1986) Comparison of magnetic resonance imaging and computed tomography in the evaluation of head injury. *Neurosurgery* **18**:45–52.

34. Barnett GH, Ropper AH and Johnson KA (1988) Physiological support and monitoring of critically ill patients during magnetic resonance imaging. *J Neurosurg* **68**:246–250.

35. Levin HS, Amparo E, Eisenberg HM *et al.* (1987) Magnetic resonance imaging and computerized tomography in relation to the neurobehavioural sequelae of mild and moderate head injuries. *J Neurosurg* **66**:706–713.

36. Turner JM and McDowall DG (1976) The measurement of intracranial pressure. *Br J Anaesth* **48**:735–740.

37. Saul TG and Ducker TB (1982) Effect of intracranial pressure monitoring and aggressive treatment on mortality in severe head injury. *J Neurosurg* **56**:498–503.

38. Galbraith S and Teasdale G (1981) Predicting the need for operation in the patient with an occult traumatic intracranial haematoma. *J Neurosurg* **55**:75–81.

39. Smith HP, Kelly DL, McWhorter JM *et al.* (1986) Comparison of mannitol regimens in patients with severe head injury undergoing intracranial monitoring. *J Neurosurg* **65**:820–824.

40. Stuart GG, Merry GS, Smith JA and Yelland JDN (1983) Severe head injury managed without intracranial pressure monitoring. *J Neurosurg* **59**:601–605.

41. Miller JD, Dearden NM, Piper IR and Chan KH (1992) Control of intracranial pressure in patients with severe head injury. *J Neurotrauma* **9**:S317–S326.

42. O'Sullivan MG, Statham PF, Jones PA *et al.* (1994) Role of intracranial pressure monitoring in severely head injured patients without signs of intracranial hypertension on critical computerized tomography. *J Neurosurg* **80**:46–50.

43. Chan KW, Miller JD, Dearden NM, Andrews PJD and Midgley S (1992) The effect of changes on cerebral perfusion pressure upon middle cerebral artery blood flow velocity and jugular bulb venous oxygen saturation after severe brain injury. *J Neurosurg* **77**:55–61.

44. Bourne GJ, Muizelaar JP, Choi SC, Newlon PG and Young HF (1991) Cerebral circulation and metabolism after severe traumatic brain injury: the elusive role of ischaemia. *J Neurosurg* **75**:685–693.

45. Greenberg RP, Newlon PG, Hyatt MS, Narayan RK and Becker DP (1981) Prognostic implications of early multi-modality evoked potentials in severely head-injured patients. *J Neurosurg* **55**:227–236.

46. Bowers SA and Marshall LF (1980) The outcome of 200 consecutive cases of severe head-injury treated in San Diego County. A prospective analysis. *Neurosurgery* **6**:237–242.

47. Baigelman W and O'Brien JC (1981) Pulmonary effects of head trauma. *Neurosurgery* **9**:729–740.

48. Muizelaar JP, Marmarou A, Ward JD *et al.* (1991) Adverse effects of prolonged hyperventilation in patients with severe head injury: a randomized clinical trial. *J Neurosurg* **75**:731–739.

49. Lewelt W, Jenkins LW and Miller JD (1980) Autoregulation of cerebral blood flow after experimental fluid percussion injury of the brain. *J Neurosurg* **53**:500–511.

50. Marmarou A, Maset AL, Ward JD *et al.* (1987) Contribution of CSF and vascular factors to elevation of ICP in severely head-injured patients. *J Neurosurg* **66**:883–890.

51. Miller JD and Corales RL (1981) Brain edema as a result of head injury: fact or fallacy? In: De Vlieger M, De Lange S and Beks JWF (eds) *Brain Edema*. New York: John Wiley.

52. Silber SJ and Thompson N (1972) Mannitol induced central nervous system toxicity. *Invest Urol* **9**:310–312.

53. Stuart FP, Torres E, Fletcher R, Crocker D and Moore FD (1970) Effects of single, repeated and massive mannitol infusion in the dog. Structural and functional changes in brain and kidney. *Ann Surg* **172**:190–204.

54. Molofsky WJ (1984) Steroids and head trauma. *Neurosurgery* **15**:424–426.

55. Saul TG, Ducker TB, Salcman M and Carro E (1981) Steroids in severe head injury. A prospective randomized clinical trial. *J Neurosurg* **54**:596–600.

56. Cooper PR, Moody S, Clark WK *et al.* (1979) Dexamethasone and severe head injury. *J Neurosurg* **51**:307–316.

57. Braakman R, Schouten HJA, Blaauw-Van Dishoeck M and Minderhoud JM (1983) Megadose steroids in severe head injury – results of prospective double-blind clinical trial. *J Neurosurg* **58**:326–330.

58. Dearden NM, Gibson JS, McDowall DG, Gibson RM and Cameron MM (1986) Effect of high-dose dexamethasone an outcome from severe head injury. *J Neurosurg* **64**:81–88.

59. Clasen RA, Pandolfi S and Casey D (1974) Furosemide and pentobarbital in cryogenic cerebral injury and edema. *Neurology* **24**:642–648.

60. Cottrell JE, Robustelli A, Post K and Turndorff H (1977) Furosemide and mannitol induced changes in intracranial pressure and serum osmolality and electrolytes. *Anesthesiology* **47**:28–30.

61. Pollay M, Fullenwider C, Roberts PA and Stevens FA (1983) Effect of mannitol and furosemide on blood–brain osmotic gradient and intracranial pressure. *J Neurosurg* **59**:945–950.

62. Albright AL, Latchaw RE and Robinson AG (1984) Intracranial and systemic effects of osmotic and oncotic therapy in experimental cerebral oedema. *J Neurosurg* **60**:481–489.

63. Shapiro HM, Galindo A, Wyte SR and Harris AB (1973) Rapid intra-operative reduction of intracranial hypertension with thiopentone. *Br J Anaesth* **45**:1057–1061.

64. Bedford RF, Persing JA, Pobereskin L and Butler A (1980) Lidocaine or thiopental for rapid control of intracranial hypertension. *Anesth Analg* **59**:435–437.

65. Ward JD, Becker DP, Miller JD *et al.* (1985) Failure of prophylactic barbiturate coma in the treatment of severe head injury. *J Neurosurg* **62**:383–388.

66. Lee MW, Deppe SA, Sipperley MC, Barrette RR and Thompson DR (1993) The efficacy of barbiturate coma in management of uncontrolled intracranial hypertension following neurosurgical trauma. *J Neurotrauma* **11**:325–331.

67. Marion DW, Obrist WD, Carlier PM, Penrod LC and Darby JM (1993) The use of moderate therapeutic hypothermia with severe head injuries: a preliminary report. *J Neurosurg* **79**:354–362.

68. Clifton GL (1995) Systemic hypothermia in treatment of severe brain injury. *J Neurol Anesth* **7**:152–156.

69. North JB, Penhall RK, Hanieh A, Frewin DB and Taylor WB (1983) Phenytoin and postoperative epilepsy. *J Neurosurg* **58**:672–677.

70. Young B, Rapp RP, Norton JA, Haack D, Tibbs PA and Bean JR (1983) Failure of prophylactically administered phenytoin to prevent early post-traumatic seizures. *J Neurosurg* **58**:231–235.

71. Young B, Ott L, Norton J *et al.* (1985) Metabolic and nutritional sequelae in the non-steroid treated head injury patient. *Neurosurgery* **17**:784–791.

72. Turner WW (1985) Nutritional considerations in the patient with disabling brain disease. *Neurosurgery* **16**:707–713.

73. Clifton GL, Robertson CS, Grossman RG, Hodge S, Foltz R and Garza C (1984) The metabolic response to severe head injury. *J Neurosurg* **60**:687–696.

74. Rapp RP, Young B, Twyman D *et al.* (1983) The favourable effect of early parenteral feeding on survival in head-injured patients. *J Neurosurg* **58**:906–912.

75. Young B, Ott L, Twyman D *et al.* (1987) The effect of nutritional support on outcome from severe head injury. *J Neurosurg* **67**:668–676.

76. Touho H, Hirakawa K, Hino A, Karasawa J and Ohno Y (1986) Relationship between abnormalities of coagulation and fibrinolysis and postoperative intracranial haemorrhage in head injury. *Neurosurgery* **19**:523–531.

GM Joynt and TE Oh

Severe faciomaxillary and upper airway injuries present with complex management problems.[1] Primary causes of death are occlusion of the airway by displaced bone and soft tissue, traumatic disruption of laryngeal structures and aspiration of blood and secretions.[2–4] Urgent airway management is required. Associated injuries to the cranium, cervical spine, oesophagus, thorax and skeleton are common, and further complicate management and worsen outcome.[1,5,6]

Faciomaxillary injury

Faciomaxillary trauma is due to blunt or sharp injuries. Blunt injuries cause facial skeleton fractures, haemorrhage and soft-tissue damage. Sharp injuries result in lacerations and penetrating injuries.

Blunt faciomaxillary injuries

Blunt facial injuries are commonly due to motor vehicle accidents, physical assaults, contact sports, falls and industrial accidents.[7–9] Faciomaxillary injuries from motor vehicle accidents are decreasing due to improved vehicle designs, but assault injuries are increasing.[8,9] The severity of facial injury is directly related to the degree and velocity of force applied.[10] Important injuries are facial fractures, haemorrhage, soft-tissue damage and oedema.[4] Over 50% of blunt faciomaxillary injuries have other associated injuries, e.g. thoracic (9%), abdominal (5%), limb fractures (30%) and, especially, head injury (55%).[7,11] There is no strong association with cervical spine injury unless vehicular trauma is the cause.[12,13]

Fractures

Evaluation of facial fractures begins with a history of the injury. Physical examination includes inspection for deformity, asymmetry, dental malocclusion, nasal septal deviation or haematoma, enophthalmos and abnormal eye movement. Tenderness, bony defects, crepitus and false motion should be sought in injured areas.[14] Useful radiographic studies include a posteroanterior, lateral oblique, stereo Water's view, stereo Caldwell's view and Panorex views. Two-dimensional and three-dimensional computed tomography (CT) provide additional information about patterns of fracture and soft-tissue disruption.[15] Attention should be paid to bony integrity and also to fluid-filled sinuses.[14] Common fractures of facial bones are nasal bones (32–45%), zygoma and zygomatic arch (13–15%), mandible (10–13%), orbital floor (3%), and maxilla (2–10%).[9]

Mandibular fractures

The mandible has a unique horseshoe shape that plays an important role in redistributing and dispersing forces.[3,16] It is a tubular bone and is weakest where the cortices are thinnest; most fractures thus occur at vulnerable points, regardless of the point of impact.[16] Common sites are the ramus (condylar neck and angle of mandible) and body at the level of the first or second molar. Multiple fractures are common (64%).[16,17] Body of mandible fractures are often accompanied by fractures of the opposite angle or neck, due to transmitted forces. Mandibular fragments are often distracted due to the action of lower jaw muscles. Respiratory obstruction may thus occur following bilateral mandibular angle or body fractures (i.e. Andy Gump fractures), due to posterior displacement of the tongue.[18] Mechanical temporomandibular joint impairment may result from condylar or zygomatic arch fractures, and can prevent jaw opening, even after administration of muscle relaxants.[3]

Midface fractures

LeFort described a classification of midface fractures in 1901[19] (Fig. 67.1). Isolated maxillary fractures are

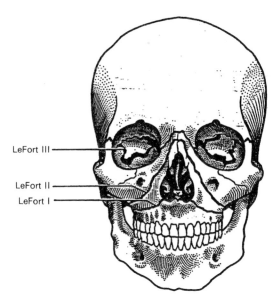

Fig. 67.1 LeFort classification of facial fractures. From Cantrill,[14] with permission.

rare, because the impact needed to cause fractures is usually sufficiently severe to break other facial bones. Fractures of nasal bones, zygoma, orbit and skull (particularly base of skull), and extensive soft-tissue injuries, including ocular injuries, are often associated with maxillary fractures.

LeFort I fracture (also known as Guerin's fracture)

This fracture involves only the maxilla at the level of the nasal fossa. It follows a horizontal plane above the floor of the nose. The fracture separates the palate from the remainder of the facial skeleton (i.e. palate facial dysjunction), and is usually caused by direct low-maxillary blows or by a lateral blow to the maxilla.

LeFort II fracture

This is the most common midface fracture[20] involving the maxilla, nasal bones and medial aspect of the orbit, resulting in a freely mobile pyramidal-shaped portion of the maxilla (i.e. pyramidal dysjunction). The fracture line extends from the lower nasal bridge through the medial wall of the orbit, and crosses the zygomaticomaxillary process. It is caused by direct blows to the mid alveolar area, or by lateral impacts and inferior blows to the mandible when the mouth is open.

LeFort III fracture

This is known as a craniofacial dysjunction because the fracture line runs parallel to the base of the skull, separating the mid facial skeleton from the base of the cranium. The fracture extends through the upper nasal

bridge and most of the orbit and across the zygomatic arch. It involves the ethmoid bone, and thus may transect the cribriform plate at the base of the skull.[20,21] LeFort III fractures usually result from superiorly directed blows to the nasal bones.[20]

Midface fractures rarely occur in a pure form and most are mixed (e.g. right hemi-LeFort I and left hemi-LeFort II).[3,14] Associated basal skull fractures occur frequently in LeFort III and occasionally in LeFort II fractures.[3,14] This may lead to cerebrospinal fluid (CSF) leakage (i.e. rhinorrhoea, common in LeFort II and III fractures), meningitis and pneumocranium.[3,22] Nasal intubation may cause the endotracheal or nasopharyngeal tube to pass through the cribriform plate and into the cranial cavity.[23,24] Airway obstruction often accompanies LeFort injuries. Posterior movement of the mobile maxilla causes the soft palate to collapse against the tongue and posterior pharynx.[4] Airway narrowing is worsened by haematoma or oedema in the pharyngeal wall. Secretions and teeth or bone debris may be present in the mouth and posterior pharynx. Nasal obstruction may result from septal dislocation, swelling, blood clots and foreign bodies.

Fractures of zygoma and orbit

Zygoma fractures are uncommon, but its attachments to the maxilla, frontal and temporal bones are vulnerable and may be disrupted. When the zygoma is displaced, disruption of the lateral wall and floor of the orbit may ensue. Eye function and integrity must be carefully examined when fractures involving the orbit are suspected. Orbital blow-out fractures occur when pressure is directly applied to the eye, and is hydraulically transmitted via the globe to the interior bony structures. The weaker inferior wall usually fractures, causing enophthalmos, diplopia, impaired eye movement and infraorbital hypoaesthesia.[11,14]

Nasal fractures

These are the most common fractures of the facial skeleton. Diagnosis is largely clinical, and major concerns are epistaxis and septal haematoma.[4] The more complicated nasoethmoid fracture caused by trauma to the nasal bridge may cause persistent epistaxis and CSF rhinorrhoea. CT scan and neurosurgical consultation are indicated.[14]

Soft-tissue injuries

These are characterized by abrasions, contusions, lacerations and avulsion injuries. Injuries to the cheek between the ear tragus and the vertical mid pupillary line must alert suspicion of injuries to the facial nerve, parotid salivary gland or the parotid duct.[11,14] Careful neurological assessment to exclude facial nerve injury is required in conscious patients.

Haemorrhage

The nose and tongue are the chief sites of haemorrhage. Severe bleeding usually involves a lingual artery, the internal maxillary artery or the anterior or posterior ethmoidal arteries.[4] Bleeding must be actively sought, as unnoticed epistaxis can lead to haemorrhagic shock and death.[25]

Management of blunt faciomaxillary injuries

Treatment priorities are to clear and secure the airway, treat hypovolaemia, control haemorrhage and evaluate possible associated life-threatening injuries. When these are satisfied, management is directed towards the specific facial injuries.

Airway management (see Chapter 25)

Immediate assessment of the airway must be made. Even an unobstructed airway should be carefully

monitored, as increasing oedema, swelling and haematoma may later compromise the airway. Signs of partial obstruction include restlessness, throat clutching and noisy respiration or stridor. Vigorous respiratory efforts with supraclavicular and rib retraction may be present. Complete obstruction may suddenly follow partial obstruction.

Management depends on the degree of obstruction (Fig. 67.2). Simple measures such as clearing the airway, positioning and inserting an oropharyngeal airway will suffice in many cases. Soft-tissue injuries and facial lacerations may mitigate against using an air-tight facemask for oxygen therapy or general anaesthesia. Obstruction from bimandibular fractures can be relieved by anterior traction on the jaw or tongue – a towel clip or suture is placed vertically through the tongue midline, and traction is applied.[3,4] Anterior traction on the mobile segment of maxilla in a LeFort fracture may clear posterior pharyngeal obstruction.[26] Failure of these measures to allow unobstructed ventila-

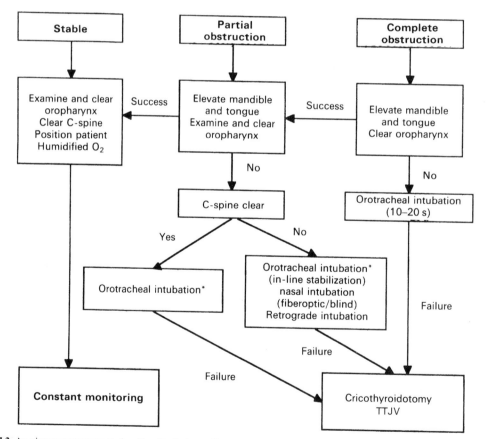

Fig. 67.2 An airway management algorithm for faciomaxillary trauma. C-spine = Cervical spine; TTJV = transtracheal jet ventilation.

*Mechanical immobility of the jaw may prevent orotracheal intubation (see text).

†Attempts at orotracheal intubation should not persist beyond 10–20 s in complete obstruction.

tion necessitates endotracheal intubation. Successful intubation can be achieved with different techniques depending on the type of injury, patient condition and available skills. If difficult visualization of the larynx is anticipated, the trachea must be intubated with the patient awake and breathing spontaneously.[3] Personnel and equipment to perform an urgent surgical airway (e.g. cricothyroidotomy) must be available before elective intubation is attempted.

Orotracheal intubation is the technique of choice in a base-of-skull fracture, and can be achieved in the awake patient with local analgesia. Analgesia is achieved with a combination of sprayed or nebulized lignocaine (4%) to the posterior pharynx and transcricoid injection of 2–3 ml of 2% lignocaine.[27,28] Blockade of the superior laryngeal and glossopharyngeal nerves will improve analgesia and facilitate intubation.[29,30] In the combative patient, or if urgent intubation is necessary, a rapid-sequence intubation can be used if airway difficulty is not anticipated.[3]

Nasotracheal intubation can be achieved in the awake, spontaneously breathing patient by blind technique or with fibreoptic guidance[31–33] Mechanical impairment of the temporomandibular joint is an indication. Analgesia is achieved as above with the addition of topical lignocaine (2–3%) and phenylephrine (0.25–0.5%) to the nasal mucosa.[34] Nasotracheal intubation is avoided in base-of-skull fractures.[2,14]

Alternative methods include retrograde intubation over a guide wire introduced through the cricothyroid membrane[35,36] and lighted stylet intubation.[37] In patients with fractures or suspected fractures of the cervical spine, orotracheal intubation with in-line stabilization, fibreoptic-guided intubation and retrograde techniques will produce minimal cervical spine movement[36,38] (see Chapter 69).

When anatomical disruption makes intubation difficult or impossible, a surgical airway may be life-saving. Techniques include cricothyroidotomy[39] transtracheal jet ventilation,[40] and, rarely, tracheostomy (see Chapter 25). Tracheostomy is best performed as a planned procedure in the operating room under local anaesthesia.

Control of haemorrhage

Haemorrhage may occasionally be massive and difficult to control.[25] Once the airway is secured, topical vasoconstrictors, anterior nasopharyngeal packs and a Foley balloon catheter inflated with air placed in the posterior nasopharynx should control or reduce blood loss.[4,25] Operative reduction of fractures and direct ligation of bleeding vessels are undertaken when simple measures fail. If all measures fail, ligation of the external carotid artery or intra-arterial embolization performed under angiographic control should be considered.

Definitive management

General measures

After the above considerations and other associated life-threatening injuries have been assessed and managed, definitive management of the facial injury can proceed. Patients without airway obstruction are nursed in 30° head-up position to drain blood, saliva and CSF away from the airway. When gross facial swelling is present, definitive surgery should be delayed while measures are instituted to reduce swelling. These include irrigation and debridement of open wounds, removal of foreign bodies, closure of facial lacerations (within 24 h), head-up position and ice packs.[4] There is a 'grace period' of 4–10 days for definitive surgery,[4,11,14] but in some cases, particularly orbital injuries with ocular function at risk, early surgery is preferred.[21] Despite lack of good data, many clinicians recommend prophylactic antibiotics for patients with CSF rhinorrhoea, compound wounds and when operative fixation of fractures is performed.[4,11] Prophylactic antibiotics are not recommended for skull fractures and any resulting cerebrospinal fluid leak[41] (see Chapter 64). Appropriate tetanus prophylaxis should be given.

Management of fractures

Unstable fractures (i.e. most mandibular and LeFort II and III fractures) are treated by internal wiring or plating and intermaxillary fixation. Isolated zygomatic arch fractures are often stable after operative reduction, and may require no other active management. Autogenous bone grafts and alloplastic materials may be required to reconstruct the orbital floor, if bone is lost or severely comminuted.[11] Closed reduction and external splinting may be required to manage nasal fractures, and must be performed within 10 days of injury.[42]

Management of soft-tissue injuries

The rich regional vascular supply protects against nutrient devitalization. Minimal debridement and delayed wound closure provide the best approach in managing a heavily contaminated wound.[42] Meticulous cleaning, removal of foreign bodies and debridement should be undertaken. Primary repair (within 24 h) should be undertaken if possible. Extensive skin debridement should be avoided. Extensive tissue loss may require myocutaneous or osteocutaneous grafts by microsurgery. Nerve lacerations lateral to the pupil should be repaired by a primary procedure before wound closure is performed.[42] Simple lacerations of the parotid capsule are repaired by closure with absorbable suture. The occasional formation of a sialocele is resolved by serial aspirations. Major duct injury requires microsurgical reconstruction.[4] Ophthalmological injuries usually require urgent specialist management.

Sharp faciomaxillary injuries

Sharp injuries result in lacerations or penetrating injuries. Causes include stab wounds, impaling injuries and gunshots. Lacerations are usually uncomplicated, and are treated by cleansing and primary closure. Damage to bone and important soft tissue is managed in the same way as blunt injury. An impaling object should be left *in situ* until skilled surgical management is available, if vital structures appear involved.

Gunshot injuries are the result of high- or low-velocity weapons. High-velocity missiles transmit high kinetic energy to tissues if bony structures are struck, and severe comminuted compound fractures, bleeding and massive soft-tissue disruption result.[1,4] Oedema develops rapidly, and an endotracheal airway should be secured *as soon as possible*.[26] Cricothyroidotomy may be required in severe cases.[4,26] In low-velocity wounds, airway control need not be as aggressive (Fig. 67.2). However, about 33% will still require intubation.[43] Bleeding is controlled by pressure packs until definitive surgery is undertaken. If the bullet trajectory is above the lower face, CT scan of the head and neck and angiography are indicated to detect cervical spine, intracerebral and major vessel (carotid or vertebral artery) damage.[4,43] Conservative debridement, closed fracture reduction and early repair of palate injuries is recommended. Open reductions are best delayed.[43] Tetanus and antibiotic prophylaxis are universally recommended.

Injuries to the larynx and cervical trachea (Table 67.1)

Although an uncommon injury, failure to recognize and treat laryngotracheal trauma promptly may have fatal consequences.[6,44,45] Common causes are blunt trauma from motor vehicle accidents and assaults, strangulation and penetrating trauma from stab wounds and gunshots.[6,44,46,47] The 'clothesline injury' occurs when a motorcyclist or bicyclist collides with a cable or wire, causing direct injury to the upper airway.[47]

Definitive investigation and management depend on the airway status and presence of associated injuries (Fig. 67.3). In upper airway trauma, blind nasal and orotracheal intubation can lead to complete airway obstruction and irreversible loss of the airway.[6,26,48] Similarly, cricoid pressure is contraindicated because of possible cricoid fracture or dislocation.[6] Tracheostomy is generally safe and also allows retrieval of the distal trachea from the mediastinum in the case of complete transection.[5] Common associated injuries include cervical spine fracture, head injury, oesophageal injury, pneumothorax, pneumomediastinum and multisystem trauma.[44,47,49,50] Panendoscopy or contrast radiog-

Table 67.1 Clinical features of acute laryngotracheal injury[6,44,45,47,51]

Likely mechanisms of injury
Motor vehicle accidents
'Clothesline' injury
Associated facial, neck or upper chest trauma
Strangulation

Symptoms
Respiratory distress
Hoarseness
Dysphonia
Cough
Noisy breathing and stridor
Dysphagia

Physical signs
Abnormal laryngeal contour
Subcutanous emphysema
Cervical ecchymosis
Haemoptysis

Findings on investigation
Radiography
   Air in soft tissues
   Pneumomediastinum
   Pneumothorax
   Cervical spine fracture
CT scan
   Cartilage and soft-tissue injury
   Altered airway patency
Laryngoscopy
   Vocal cord paralysis
   Mucosal or cartilage disruption
   Haematoma
   Laceration

CT = Computed tomography.

raphy (to exclude oesophageal injury) and chest X-rays are routinely indicated.[51]

Once the airway and associated life-threatening injuries have been stabilized, definitive investigation of the laryngeal injury is completed (Fig. 67.3), as early surgery (within 24 h) is important in preventing long-term morbidity.[47,51,52] Use of steroids to reduce swelling is unproven but recommended by some.[51] Prophylactic antibiotics are recommended.[47,51,53]

Penetrating wounds to the neck are easily recognized and more readily managed.[5] Gaping airway wounds can be intubated under direct vision, pending subsequent surgery.[6] Rapid-sequence induction and oral intubation are preferred unless direct laryngotracheal injury is suspected.[46] Clinical evidence of airway injury (Table 67.1) should lead to a more conservative approach (Fig. 67.3). In these cases, facilities for an emergency surgical airway should always be immediately available.[46] Patients with

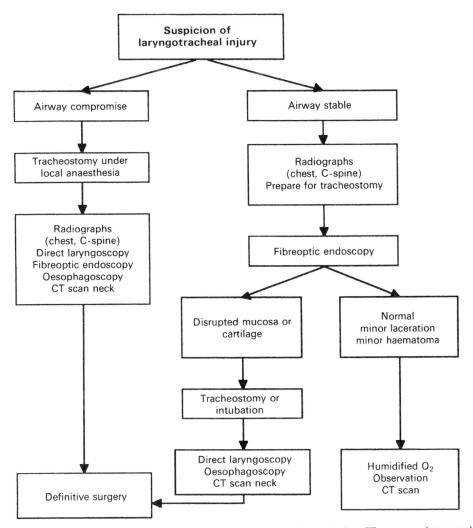

Fig. 67.3 A management algorithm for acute upper airway trauma. C-spine = Cervical spine; CT = computed tomography.

penetrating trauma (especially gunshot injuries) are likely to have concurrent vascular, oesophageal, nervous system (e.g. spinal cord, brachial plexus, cranial nerves or peripheral nerves) and thoracic injuries. Mortality is more closely related to vascular than airway injury,[6,45] and surgical exploration or urgent angiography and oesophagoscopy is recommended.[54,55]

Outcome

Priorities in the care of the traumatized patient are management of the airway and other life-threatening injuries. Mortality can be influenced by management in the acute phase.[6,45] Morbidity from facial injuries includes loss of sight, smell, hearing,

jaw function and facial form, which can be minimized by comprehensive surgical and supportive care. Proper treatment of laryngotracheal injuries will reduce the severe complications of laryngeal dysfunction (causing compromised phonation) and tracheal stenosis. Emphasis is placed on intensive investigation and early surgical management.[51,52]

References

1. Cantrill SV (1992) Massive facial trauma and direct neck trauma. In: Dailey RH, Simon B, Young GP and Stewart RD (eds) *The Airway: Emergency Management*. St Louis: Mosby Year Book, pp. 259–269.

2. Kline SN (1989) Maxillofacial trauma. In: Kreis DJ and Gomez GA (eds) *Trauma Management*. Boston: Little Brown, pp. 131–145.

3. Gotta AW (1993) Maxillofacial trauma. In: Grande CM (ed.) *Textbook of Trauma Anesthesia and Critical Care*. St Louis: Mosby, pp. 529–539.

4. Weiner SL and Barrett J (1986) *Trauma Management for Civilian and Military Physicians*. Philadelphia: WB Saunders.

5. Alfille PH and Hurford WE (1991) Upper airway injuries. *J Clin Anesth* 3:88–90.

6. Cicala RS, Kudsk KA, Butts A, Nguyen H and Fabian TC (1991) Initial evaluation and management of upper airway injuries in trauma patients. *J Clin Anesth* 3:91–98.

7. Davidoff G, Jakubowski M, Thomas D and Alpert M (1988) The spectrum of closed-head injury in facial trauma victims: incidence and impact. *Ann Emerg Med* 17:6–9.

8. Covington DS, Wainwright DJ, Teichgraeber JF and Parks DH (1994) Changing patterns in the epidemiology and treatment of zygoma fractures: 10 year review. *J Trauma* 37:243–248.

9. Hussain K, Wijetunge DB and Jackson IT (1994) A comprehensive analysis of craniofacial trauma. *J Trauma* 36:34–47.

10. Karlson TA (1982) The incidence of hospital-treated facial injuries from vehicles. *J Trauma* 22:303–310.

11. Schultz RC and Oldham RJ (1977) An overview of facial injuries. *Surg Clin North Am* 57:987–1010.

12. Davidson JSD and Birdsell BD (1989) Cervical spine injury in patients with facial skeletal trauma. *J Trauma* 29:1276–1278.

13. Hills MW and Deane SA (1993) Head injury and facial injury: is there an increased risk of cervical head injury? *J Trauma* 34:549–554.

14. Cantrill SV (1992) Facial trauma. In: Rosen P and Barkin RM (eds) *Emergency Medicine – Concepts and Clinical Practice*. St Louis: Mosby Year Book, pp. 355–370.

15. Mayer JS, Wainwright DJ, Yeakley JW, Lee KF, Harris JH and Kulkarni M (1988) The role of three-dimensional computed tomography in the management of maxillofacial trauma. *J Trauma* 28:1043–1053.

16. Halazonetis JA (1968) The 'weak' regions of the mandible. *Br J Oral Surg* 6:37–48.

17. Chu L, Gussack GS and Muller T (1994) A treatment protocol for mandible fractures. *J Trauma* 36:48–52.

18. Seshul MB, Sinn DP and Gerlock AJ (1978) The Andy Gump fracture of the mandible: a cause of respiratory obstruction or distress. *J Trauma* 18:611–612.

19. LeFort R (1901) Experimental study of fractures of the upper jaw. *Rev Chir Paris* 23:208–227,360–379 (Reprinted in *Plast Reconstr Surg* 1972;50:497–506.)

20. Manson PN, Hoopes JE and Su CT (1980) Structural pillars of the facial skeleton: an approach to the management of LeFort fractures. *Plast Reconstr Surg* 66:54–61.

21. Cruise CW, Blevins PK and Luce EA (1980) Naso-ethmoid-orbital fractures. *J Trauma* 20:551–556.

22. Kitahata LM and Collins WF (1970) Meningitis as a complication of anesthesia in a patient with a basal skull fracture. *Anesthesiology* 32:282–283.

23. Horellou M, Mathe D and Feiss P (1978) A hazard of nasotracheal intubation. *Anaesthesia* 33:73–74.

24. Muzzi DA, Losasso TJ and Cucchiara RF (1991) Complication from a nasopharyngeal airway in a patient with a basilar skull fracture. *Anesthesiology* 74:366–368.

25. Murakami WT, Davidson TM and Marshall LF (1983) Fatal epistaxis in craniofacial trauma. *J Trauma* 23:57–61.

26. Meislin HW, Iserson KV, Kaback KR, Kobernick M, Sanders AB and Seifert S (1983) Airway trauma. *Emerg Med Clin North Am* 1:295–312.

27. Bourke DL, Katz J and Tonneson A (1985) Nebulized anesthesia for awake endotracheal intubation. *Anesthesiology* 6:690–692.

28. Webb AR, Fernando SS, Dalton HR, Arrowsmith JE, Woodhead MA and Cummin AR (1990) Local anaesthesia for fiberoptic bronchoscopy: transcricoid injection or the spray as you go technique. *Thorax* 45:474–477.

29. Gotta AW and Sullivan CA (1984) Superior laryngeal nerve block: an aid to intubating the patient with fractured mandible. *J Trauma* 24:83–85.

30. Benumof JL (1991) Management of the difficult airway. *Anesthesiology* 75:1087–1110.

31. Mulder DS, Wallace DH and Woolhouse FM (1975) The use of the fiberoptic bronchoscope to facilitate endotracheal intubation following head and neck trauma. *J Trauma* 15:638–640.

32. Milnek EJ, Clinton JE, Plummer D and Ruiz E (1990) Fiberoptic intubation in the emergency department. *Ann Emerg Med* 19:359–362.

33. Delaney KA and Hessler R (1988) Emergency flexible fiberoptic nasotracheal intubation: a report of 60 cases. *Ann Emerg Med* 17:919–926.

34. Gross JB, Hartigan ML and Schaffer DW (1984) A suitable substitute for 4% cocaine before blind nasotracheal intubation: 3% lignocaine–0.25% phenylephrine nasal spray. *Anesth Analg* 63: 915–918.

35. King H, Huntington C and Wooten D (1994) Translaryngeal guided intubation in an uncooperative patient with maxillofacial injury: case report. *J Trauma* 36: 885–886.

36. Barriot P and Riou B (1988) Retrograde technique for tracheal intubation in trauma patients. *Crit Care Med* 16:712–713.

37. Verdile VP, Chiang JL, Bedger R *et al.* (1990) Nasotracheal intubation using a flexible lighted stylet. *Ann Emerg Med* 19:506–510.

38. Criswell JC and Parr MJA (1994) Emergency airway management in patients with cervical spine injury. *Anaesthesia* 49:900–903.

39. Salvino CK, Dries D, Gamelli R, Murphy-Macabobby M and Marshall W (1993) Emergency cricothyroidotomy in trauma victims. *J Trauma* 34:503–505.

40. Benumof JL and Scheller MS (1989) The importance of transtracheal jet ventilation in the management of the difficult airway. *Anesthesiology* 71:769–778.

41. Infection in Neurosurgery Working Party of the British Society for Antimicrobial Chemotherapy (1994) Antimicrobial prophylaxis in neurosurgery and after head injury. *Lancet* 344:1547–1551.

42. Walton RL, Bunkis J and Borah GL (1986) Maxillofacial trauma. In: Trunkey DD, Lewis FR (eds) *Current Therapy in Trauma*. Toronto: Decker, pp. 181–223.

43. Kihtir T, Ivatury RR, Simon RJ, Nassoura Z and Leban S (1993) Early management of civilian gunshot wounds to the face. *J Trauma* **35**:569–577.

44. Mathisen DJ and Grillo H (1987) Laryngotracheal trauma. *Ann Thorac Surg* **43**:254–263.

45. Kelly JP, Webb WR, Moulder PV, Everson C, Burch BH and Lindsey ES (1985) Management of airway trauma I: tracheobronchial injuries. *Ann Thorac Surg* **40**:551–555.

46. Shearer VE and Gieseke AH (1993) Airway management for patients with penetrating neck trauma. *Anesth Analg* **77**:1130–1134.

47. Angood PB, Attia EL, Brown RA and Mulder DS (1986) Extrinsic civilian trauma to the larynx and cervical trachea – important predictors of long term morbidity. *J Trauma* **26**:869–873.

48. Goodie D and Paton P (1991) Anaesthetic management of blunt airway trauma: three cases. *Anaesth Intens Care* **19**:271–274.

49. Chen FH and Fetzer JD (1993) Complete cricotracheal separation and third cervical spinal cord transection following blunt neck trauma: a case report of one survivor. *J Trauma* **35**:140–142.

50. Reddin A, Mirvis SE and Diaconis JN (1987) Rupture of the cervical oesophagus and trachea associated with cervical spine fracture. *J Trauma* **27**:564–566.

51. Myers EM and Iko BO (1987) The management of acute laryngeal trauma. *J Trauma* **27**:448–452.

52. Schaefer SD (1991) The treatment of acute external laryngeal injuries: state of the art. *Arch Otolaryngol Head Neck Surg* **117**:35–39.

53. Flynn AE, Thomas AN and Schecter WP (1989) Acute tracheobronchial injury. *J Trauma* **29**:1326–1330.

54. Scalfani SJA, Cavaliere G, Atweh N, Duncan AO and Scalea T (1991) The role of angiography in penetrating neck trauma. *J Trauma* **31**:557–563.

55. Campbell WH and Cantrill SV (1992) Neck trauma. In: Rosen P, Barkin RM (eds) *Emergency Medicine – Concepts and Clinical Practice*. St Louis: Mosby Year Book, pp. 371–412.

GM Clarke

The commonest form of chest trauma in Australia is closed chest injury secondary to road traffic accident. Serious associated extrathoracic injuries are often present. Initial management is directed towards the detection and correction of life-threatening disorders. Swift assessment and resuscitation are carried out simultaneously. A team approach is necessary, with the team leader having clear management priorities. In almost every case, respiratory and circulatory resuscitation take precedence.

A secondary assessment is made after the initial assessment. During this time, detailed radiological and other imaging investigations are undertaken. However, the chest X-ray is an integral part of initial assessment and should be obtained as soon as possible.

Immediate management

Obvious external bleeding is controlled and circulatory resuscitation initiated. Blood is sampled for cross-match, biochemistry and haematological tests. At the same time, respiratory and general measures (Table 68.1) are undertaken.

Table 68.1 Immediate management of chest trauma

Ensure patent airway, oxygenation and ventilation
Exclude or treat:
   Pneumothorax
   Haemothorax
   Cardiac tamponade
Assess for extrathoracic injuries
Decompress stomach
Provide pain relief
Reconsider endotracheal intubation, ventilation

Oxygenation

A clear airway must be ensured. Oxygen is administered by facemask, and ventilation assessed. Immediate endotracheal intubation and controlled ventilation are indicated in compromised airways, severe head injuries and gross hypoventilation and/or hypoxaemia unrelated to pneumothorax. Emergency cricothyroidotomy or tracheostomy is only rarely required when an upper respiratory tract obstruction cannot be bypassed by translaryngeal intubation (see Chapter 25).

Pneumothorax and haemothorax

Any pneumothorax and significant haemothorax is treated. Controlled ventilation in the presence of tension pneumothorax is potentially fatal. A 12 or 14 FG IV cannula may be inserted percutaneously to relieve tension pneumothorax in dire emergencies. Usually, however, there is time to insert a wide-bore intercostal catheter (ICC) under sterile conditions. An ICC directed superiorly through the second anterior intercostal space, 4 cm lateral to the sternal edge in adults, will usually adequately drain a non-loculated pneumothorax. Insertion through the mid axillary line at the level of the nipple or above is recommended if a more lateral position is required. This site is preferred if a haemothorax is to be drained, with the tube directed posteriorly. Pneumothoraces are expected to be situated anteriorly in the supine patient, and are hence more likely to be seen at the lung base. Radiological clues are basilar hyperlucency, distinct visualization of the diaphragm which may be depressed, distinct cardiac border and deepened costophrenic angle.

When inserting a chest tube, trocars are not recommended (to avoid penetration into lung or other organ). After sterile preparation and widespread infiltration with 1% lignocaine, the skin is incised and a pair of blunt forceps is used to dissect down to the

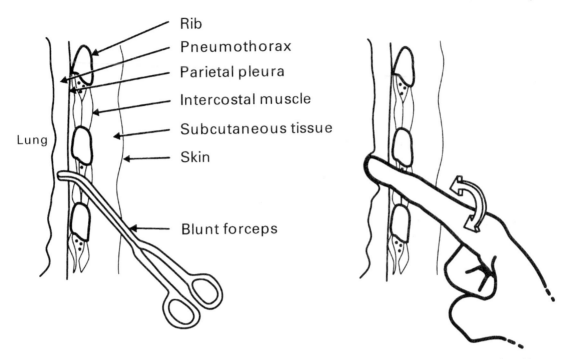

Rib
Pneumothorax
Parietal pleura
Intercostal muscle
Subcutaneous tissue
Skin

Lung

Blunt forceps

Fig. 68.1 Inserting an intercostal drain. Dissection is performed by blunt forceps. A gloved finger ascertains separation of lung from chest wall.

pleura, which is then gently ruptured (Fig. 68.1). A gloved finger through this tract ascertains that lung is not adhered to chest wall, and the ICC is inserted. The ICC is attached to an underwater seal drain, with applied suction if necessary. It is unusual to require more than 20 cm H_2O suction pressure, although the system should have the capacity for 40–60 cm H_2O suction, with an airflow volume of 15–20 l/min.[1,2]

Cardiac tamponade

Cardiac tamponade is suspected in any patient with thoracic trauma who has low blood pressure and raised venous pressure. Differential diagnoses include tension pneumothorax (most likely) and severe heart failure (usually due to gross myocardial contusion, or prolonged and inadequately treated shock). If readily available, transoesophageal echocardiography (TOE) can rapidly confirm or exclude tamponade. Computed tomography (CT) scan will also reveal pericardial effusion, but is unsuitable for the unstable patient. Hence in urgent situations, the clinical diagnosis should be acted upon.

Emergency treatment of cardiac tamponade is aspiration of the pericardial sac, preferably under continuous electrocardiogram (ECG) control. The patient is positioned supine 35° head-up. ECG limb leads are attached, and the chest lead is connected to the metal hub of a 16 FG aspirating needle by a sterile wire. The needle with its plastic cannula is advanced

towards the left shoulder at a 35° angle to the skin, from a point 2 cm below the apex of an angle formed between the xiphoid process and the left seventh costal cartilage (Fig. 68.2). Aspiration is made as the needle is slowly advanced. Remarkable improvement may follow the removal of as little as 30 ml of blood. Contact with the myocardium is denoted by ST elevation on the ECG, or ectopic beats. When a positive tap is obtained, the cannula is left *in situ* for continued drainage. Alternatively, a pigtail catheter (e.g. Pericardiocentesis set C-PCS-RPH-1, William A Cook, Australia) may be placed into the pericardial sac using a guide wire. Subsequent thoracotomy and full exploration will usually be necessary.

Many centres proceed to prompt thoracotomy with pericardial decompression, bypassing attempts at aspiration.[3,4] The surgical approach for penetrating chest wounds has been described.[5]

Extrathoracic injuries

Extrathoracic trauma, i.e. head, neck and abdominal injuries, and significant concealed blood loss must be excluded. This initial rapid assessment should be made before potent analgesics are administered.

Gastric decompression

Gastric distension with the attendant risks of regurgitation, vomiting and aspiration is extremely com-

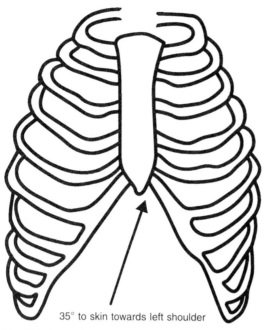

35° to skin towards left shoulder

Fig. 68.2 Approach to drain a pericardial effusion.

mon, especially in patients with associated head injury. The stomach should be decompressed by a nasogastric tube (or orogastric tube in suspected base-of-skull fractures). If urgent endotracheal intubation is necessary, a rapid-sequence crash intubation (with applied cricoid pressure) is recommended.

Pain relief

Pain relief is usually obtained at this early stage with IV opioids. This will frequently relieve respiratory distress in patients with fractures of the ribs and/or sternum.

Reconsideration of mechanical ventilatory support

After the initial management, mechanical ventilatory support should be reconsidered (Table 68.2). Ventilation should also be considered for patients with borderline respiratory distress associated with:

1 gross obesity;
2 significant pre-existing lung disease,
3 severe pulmonary contusion or aspiration,
4 severe abdominal injuries requiring surgery.

Specific thoracic injuries

Specific thoracic injuries should be systematically excluded.

Table 68.2 Major indications for endotracheal intubation and ventilation

Dangerous hypoxaemia and/or hypercarbia
Significant head injury
Gross flail segment and contusion and respiratory distress

Ruptured aorta

A widened mediastinum should always arouse suspicion of a ruptured aorta.[6] In one series, mediastinal width greater than 8 cm was present in all 10 patients with ruptured thoracic aorta.[7] Diagnosis is enhanced by one or more of the following radiological features:

1 left haemothorax;
2 depressed left main bronchus;
3 blurred outline of the arch or descending aorta;
4 fractured first rib or left apical haematoma;
5 displacement of the mid-oesophagus to the right (easily detectable with a nasogastric tube *in situ*).

Other suspicious radiological features include loss of the aorticopulmonary window, anterior or lateral deviation of the trachea, loss of the paraspinal 'stripe', and calcium layering in the aortic arch. Aortography remains the gold-standard investigation, although contrast-enhanced CT scan may be employed first, proceeding to angiography only if necessary.[8] TOE can provide excellent images of the distal aortic arch and descending aorta, especially the isthmus, where the majority of traumatic ruptures occur.[8-11] It may enable diagnosis in an unstable patient without transfer to an imaging department.[9] The isthmus is at the junction of the mobile arch and fixed descending aorta, immediately beyond the origin of the left subclavian artery. Rupture at this site is attributed to forward movement of the mobile arch against the tethered descending aorta in a deceleration situation (e.g. motor vehicle accident). In about 10% of cases, rupture is in the ascending aorta or near the origin of the other great vessels. These tears are usually due to direct trauma.

Treatment is prompt surgery and often necessitates cardiopulmonary or left atriofemoral bypass. These techniques do not necessarily protect against consequent paraplegia.[12] Many workers question the priority of aortography and immediate surgery over management of other life-threatening injuries, in patients who are not exsanguinating.[13-16] β-Blockers and antihypertensive agents have been used to enable elective delayed operation. However, only exceptional circumstances would justify an elective approach to aorta rupture.

Ruptured diaphragm and diaphragmatic paresis

The usual cause of a ruptured diaphragm is gross abdominal compression, and the incidence may have risen since seat belts were made compulsory.[17] Rupture of the left diaphragm is more common.[18] A haemopneumothorax is commonly misdiagnosed when the dilated stomach gives a horizontal air–fluid interface on erect chest X-ray. Misdiagnosis is less likely if a nasogastric tube is *in situ*, when the distal end is noted to be in an abnormal position. A ruptured diaphragm as an isolated injury is often surprisingly well-tolerated by the patient. Nevertheless, with a left diaphragmatic rupture, there is significant risk of gut strangulation, and surgical repair should follow basic resuscitation.

Rupture of the right diaphragm is more difficult to diagnose because of the liver. The radiographic appearance is similar to a paralysed right diaphragm. In the absence of right-sided rib fractures, a small haemothorax with a high right diaphragm is suggestive evidence. Magnetic resonance imaging (MRI) provides coronal and sagittal imaging, and direct visualization of the diaphragm. It has been recommended to diagnose ruptured diaphragm if CT is non-diagnostic.[19] Repair of ruptured diaphragm via an abdominal approach is recommended, as more than 75% of such cases have associated intra-abdominal injury.[20]

Unilateral and bilateral phrenic nerve palsy are occasionally seen after blunt chest trauma. The bilateral form results in classical paradoxical abdominal-to-chest wall movement, orthopnoea, reduced vital capacity and difficulty in weaning from ventilation.[21] Diaphragmatic dysfunction may also occur following upper abdominal surgery. This is possibly due to reflex inhibition of diaphragmatic activity.[22] Any respiratory dysfunction secondary to diaphragmatic paresis will be greatly magnified by the presence of other chest wall or lung injury.

Disruption of major airways

Although signs and symptoms may vary according to the level of the rupture, the clinical picture is frequently that of respiratory distress, subcutaneous emphysema and haemoptysis.[23] A pneumothorax, which may be under tension, is invariably present with ruptured bronchus. Mediastinal emphysema is commonly seen on chest X-ray. With tracheal injuries, immediate management involves endotracheal intubation (with the cuff positioned distal to the tear) to prevent aspiration and ablate air leak. Any pneumothorax must be drained. Suction to the intercostal catheter may be necessary.

When initial priorities are achieved, bronchoscopy and early primary repair are undertaken. A double-lumen tube may be necessary for operative repair and if air leak is significant. If a neck wound is large, an endotracheal tube can be passed via the neck and tracheal wound in emergency situations. Difficult intubation may be accomplished by a flexible bronchoscope. Once the airway is secured, general anaesthesia and other interventions may be undertaken.[24]

Massive haemothorax

Disruption of intercostal and/or internal mammary arteries is a common cause.[23] The condition is usually fatal if caused by massive bleeding from the aorta or major pulmonary arteries. Immediate management involves insertion of a wide-bore ICC and adequate resuscitation. Continued significant blood loss is an indication for early thoracotomy.[25] Inadequate drainage of a haemothorax may require a thoracotomy and decortication at a later date, but this is rarely necessary.[26]

Pulmonary contusion

The classical view of pulmonary contusion is that bruised lung is not confined within anatomical segments, and becomes more oedematous over the next 48 h. However, CT evaluation has revealed that such pulmonary infiltration and consolidation is, in fact, a pulmonary laceration surrounded by intra-alveolar haemorrhage ('blood pneumonia'), without significant interstitial injury.[27] Such lacerations have been classified into four types according to CT pattern, mechanism of injury, location of rib fracture and surgical findings.[28] When pulmonary contusion is associated with a severe flail segment and respiratory distress, assisted ventilation is required (which is usually short-term).[29]

Myocardial contusion

Myocardial contusion is common in blunt chest trauma, and may result in arrhythmias and cardiac failure. Both complications should be managed as in myocardial infarction. A standard 12-lead ECG may show a variety of abnormalities, ranging from non-specific T-wave changes to pathological Q waves. TOE may show cardiac wall motion abnormalities.[8] Abnormalities can also be demonstrated by myocardial nuclear scanning (not normally undertaken in the acutely injured patient). Serious damage to virtually every cardiac structure has been reported.[30] Cardiac injuries, e.g. rupture of the ventricular free wall, interventricular septum and valvular apparatus, and disruption of major coronary arteries are usually associated with penetrating injuries, but have also been reported in non-penetrating chest trauma.[31] Again, TOE may aid in diagnosis. Creatine kinase and CKMB enzymes should be measured in all cases of suspected myocardial contusion. Sternal fractures (more common in females, the elderly and in those wearing seat belts) are associated with a low incidence of cardiac contusion and arrhythmias.[32,33]

Systemic air embolism

This is more commonly seen in penetrating injuries and is immediately life-threatening. Although uncommon, it is probably underdiagnosed, as it is unlikely to be proven at conventional autopsy.[34] Air embolism is usually caused by a bronchopulmonary vein fistula. It is suspected in the chest-injured patient if:

1 focal neurological signs exist in the absence of head injury;
2 circulatory collapse immediately follows controlled ventilation in the absence of tension pneumothorax;
3 froth is obtained when arterial blood is sampled from a collapsed patient.

When suspected, the Fio_2 should be increased to 1.0, and ventilation pressures and volumes reduced to a minimum. Hyperbaric oxygen therapy, though indicated, is unlikely to be practical. Mattox[35] recommends urgent thoracotomy, to clamp the ascending aorta, remove air source (e.g. by clamping the pulmonary hilum) and aspirate free air from the left ventricle and ascending aorta.

Oesophageal perforation

Although usually due to penetrating injury, it can occur rarely with closed chest trauma. The patient may complain of retrosternal pain and difficulty in swallowing, and exhibit haematemesis and cervical emphysema. A chest X-ray may show mediastinal emphysema, widened mediastinum, pneumothorax, hydrothorax or hydropneumothorax. If suspected, a Gastrografin swallow and/or endoscopy is performed. Treatment is immediate surgical repair. A gastrostomy and feeding jejunostomy are usually performed at the same time.

Significance of a flail chest

A flail segment is no longer the dominant issue in chest injuries, but its significance should not be overlooked. The concept of pendulluft (to-and-fro movement of air between the flail and non-affected sides of the thorax) has been shown to be incorrect.[36] With flail chest, overall ventilation may be reduced, but is distributed to both lungs, because the mediastinal shift equalizes the pleural pressures. Nevertheless, there is poor expansion in contused, low compliant lung areas, impairment of coughing and seriously reduced ventilation in gross cases. Moreover, the greater the flail segment, the less the negative intrapleural pressure that can be generated for inspiration. Gross mediastinal shifts may impair systemic circulation.

Pain control

Adequate pain relief is extremely important. It is the major determinant of whether deep breathing and efficient coughing are possible, thereby avoiding endotracheal intubation in non-severe injuries. Choice of pain relief may vary during the course of management (see Chapter 79). Options include:

1 IV opioids by frequent, intermittent small doses, or by continuous infusion;
2 Entonox inhalation during physiotherapy;
3 intercostal nerve block:
   (a) multiple individual nerve blocks (repeated as necessary);
   (b) single large volume (e.g. 20 ml 0.5% bupivacaine) into one intercostal space (unilaterally or bilaterally), spreading to block nerves above and below the site injected;[37] or
   (c) intrapleural bupivacaine (0.25–0.5%) via unilateral or bilateral ICCs (epidural catheters have been used), using intermittent injections or continuous infusion;[38]
4 epidural analgesia;
5 epidural or spinal opioids;
6 non-steroidal anti-inflammatory agents (in fully resuscitated patients with normal renal function).

Respiratory support

While several basic approaches to managing the chest-injured patient have emerged (Table 68.3), the ultimate strategy is determined by the severity of chest injury, associated injuries and effectiveness of pain relief. All these factors influence respiratory dysfunction.

Table 68.3 Respiratory support of the chest-injured patient

Conservative
Non-invasive respiratory assistance (via facemask)
   Continuous positive airways pressure (CPAP)
   Pressure support ventilation (PSV)
   Bi-level positive airway pressure (BiPAP)
Invasive respiratory assistance (via a tracheal tube)
   CPAP
   PSV ± positive end-expiratory pressure (PEEP)
   Intermittent mandatory ventilation ± PEEP ± PSV
   Pressure control ventilation ± PEEP
   Volume control ventilation ± PEEP
   Independent lung ventilation ± PEEP
Surgical stabilization ± other measures

Conservative therapy

Conservative treatment involves oxygen by mask, adequate pain relief and physiotherapy. It is the treatment in mild injury (i.e. isolated thoracic injury with fractured ribs, but without significant flail or disturbed blood gases). Similarly, it may be employed in moderate chest injury (i.e. significant flail but with adequate blood gases and ability to cough). Prophylactic ventilation in these two groups is deemed inappropriate, with possible disadvantages of barotrauma, infection, tracheostomy complications and prolongation of hospitalization.[39,40]

Non-invasive respiratory assistance

Even with moderately severe, isolated chest injuries, endotracheal intubation can be avoided, provided adequate analgesia is assured, and the patient can tolerate a close-fitting facemask for non-invasive respiratory assistance. A preset airway pressure and the facemask lessen the risk of barotrauma. Patient tolerance for these non-invasive methods is variable. Non-invasive ventilation is promising, but controlled studies comparing this with conventional mechanical ventilation are lacking.[41]

Invasive respiratory assistance

This is necessary in severe chest injuries and if head injury is associated. Tracheal intubation is achieved by oral or nasal routes or a tracheostomy. Tracheostomy offers advantages over translaryngeal intubation in the conscious patient (e.g. decreased discomfort, need for sedation and resistance to breathing). Percutaneous tracheostomy may be undertaken in the ICU (see Chapter 23). Early use of intermittent mandatory ventilation is claimed to result in a shorter duration of assisted ventilation.[42] Currently, most centres use pressure control and pressure support ventilation in preference to volume control ventilation, to promote early weaning and reduce the incidence of barotrauma. Pressure ventilatory modes also provide some compensation for air leaks. Continuous positive airway pressure alone has not been fully evaluated, although it is used extensively during weaning. In patients with flail segments, inappropriate conservative therapy or poor ventilatory support may result in increased residual chest deformity. Independent lung ventilation may be used to treat a unilateral pulmonary contusion and/or flail.[43]

Surgical stabilization

There is revived interest in surgical stabilization of the chest wall. Advantages claimed are a shorter period of assisted ventilation or a shorter hospital stay.[44,45] Internal surgical stabilization undoubtedly reduces deformity, and a stable chest wall will help a patient cope with an underlying lung problem. However, except for a fractured sternum, rupture of the diaphragm, and in the course of an otherwise necessary thoracotomy, the case for surgical repair has yet to be established.[46]

Complications

Following resuscitation and initial management, complications may follow which usually require treatment.

Sputum retention

Sputum retention can precipitate or worsen respiratory distress and lead to pulmonary collapse. Infection is then more likely. Minimizing sputum retention in the spontaneously breathing patient includes adequate analgesia without marked respiratory depression. In the intubated/ventilated patient, efficient humidification and endobronchial toilet are essential. Frequent position changes are important. If clearing secretions remains difficult despite adequate pain relief, a minitracheostomy (e.g. 5.4 mm OD tube via a percutaneous cricothyroidotomy) may avoid conventional endotracheal intubation or tracheostomy.

Bronchospasm

Bronchospasm is managed conventionally. Its occurrence suggests the possibility of aspiration.

Barotrauma

Barotrauma is more common in the mechanically ventilated patient. It may also occur in the spontaneously breathing patient with chest injuries several days after admission, especially if respiratory distress is present. Surgical emphysema, mediastinal emphysema, pneumothorax, pulmonary interstitial emphysema and pneumoperitoneum can all occur.

In patients with surgical and/or mediastinal emphysema, some authorities recommend insertion of ICCs if anaesthesia or mechanical ventilation is planned, even though pneumothorax is not evident on chest X-ray. CT scan is very sensitive to confirm or exclude pneumothorax, and may be used to avoid ICC tube insertion.

Acute respiratory failure

Acute respiratory failure is common. When the acute lung injury (or acute respiratory distress syndrome (ARDS), see Chapter 29) occurs early after trauma, possible causes include pulmonary contusion, aspiration, prolonged shock or delayed resuscitation, and massive mediator release following multitrauma and fat embolism. When ARDS develops many days after injury, infection, which may originate from a site remote from the lungs, is a more likely cause.

Infection

Infection remains a major cause of death in chest injuries. The source of infection is invariably endogenous, mainly from bacteria colonizing the patient's oropharynx and alimentary tract. Some authorities recommend parenteral antibiotic prophylaxis (e.g. cefotaxime) active against community bacteria (e.g. *Streptococcus pneumoniae, Hoemophilus influenzae, Branhamella catarrhalis, Staphylococcus aureus* or *Escherichia coli*) from the time of admission for 4 days. At the same time, oral and intragastric non-absorbable combinations of polymyxin E, tobramycin and amphotericin B are administered, to prevent colonization and infection by *Enterobacter, Pseudomonas* and fungi such as *Candida*.[47] However, this strategy requires further rigorous study[48] (see Chapter 62).

The importance of hand-washing between attending patients and meticulous attention to sterile techniques in respiratory care and management of invasive catheters cannot be overemphasized. Early enteral feeding may decrease translocation of bacteria and toxins from the gut, and thus reduce the incidence of sepsis.[49]

Thromboembolism

Preventive measures include frequent movement, leg stockings, avoidance of pressure on limbs, and low-dose subcutaneous heparin (5000 units b.d. or t.d.s.), or low-molecular-weight sodium heparin (2500 units daily).

Inadequate nutrition

Gastric atony and stasis are common. In many cases, adequate enternal nutrition is possible by appropriate posturing (e.g. on right side during feeding). Metoclopramide or cisapride may be used to promote gastric emptying. Parenteral nutrition may be necessary.

Stress ulceration

Sucralfate 1 g q.i.d. nasogastrically is given as prophylaxis until enteral feeding is established. Alternatively H_2 blockers may be used. Early resuscitation is considered to be an important factor in reducing the incidence of this complication.

Coagulopathies

Prompt resuscitation, control of haemorrhage and possibly use of blood filters for massive blood transfusion help in this regard.

Prognosis

Reported mortality rates in chest-injured patients vary greatly, reflecting varied severity of the chest injury and associated extrathoracic injuries. In one Australian series,[50] of 1119 patients with chest and other injuries, the overall mortality was 5.3%. The three commonest causes of death were respiratory tract sepsis (35.6%), severe head injury (33.9%) and exsanguination (18.6%). Mortality was 37.5% for patients over 60 years who had respiratory failure, and 22.8% for all age groups requiring mechanical ventilation. Trunkey reported a 16% mortality in patients with isolated pulmonary contusion. When combined with a significant flail chest, mortality rose to 42%.[51]

References

1. Symbas PN (1989) Chest drainage tubes. *Surg Clin North Am* **69**:41–46.
2. Munnel ER and Thomas EK (1975) Current concepts in thoracic drainage systems. *Ann Thorac Surg* **19**:261–268.
3. Bodai BI, Smith JP and Blaisdell FW (1982) The role of emergency thoracotomy in blunt trauma. *J Trauma* **22**:487–490.
4. Baker CC, Thomas AN and Trunkey DD (1980) The role of emergency room thoracotomy in trauma. *J Trauma* **20**:848–855.
5. Mitchell ME, Muakkassa FF, Poole GV *et al.* (1993) Surgical approach of choice for penetrating cardiac wounds. *J Trauma* **34**:17–20.
6. Turney SZ, Attar S, Ayella R, Cowley R and McLaughlin J (1976) Traumatic rupture of the aorta. A five year experience. *J Thorac Cardiovasc Surg* **72**:727–732.
7. Kram HB, Wohlmuth DA, Appel PL and Shoemaker WC (1987) Clinical and radiological indications for aortography in blunt chest trauma. *J Vasc Surg* **6**:168–175.
8. Riou B, Goarin JP and Saada M (1993) Assessment of severe blunt chest trauma. In: Vincent J-L (ed.) *Yearbook of Intensive Care and Emergency Medicine*. Berlin: Springer-Verlag, pp. 611–618.
9. Brathwaite CE, Cilley JM, O'Connor WH, Ross SE and Weiss RL (1994) The pivotal role of transesophageal echocardiography in the management of traumatic thoracic aortic rupture with associated intra-abdominal haemorrhage. *Chest* **105**:1899–1901.
10. Books SW, Young JC, Cmolik B *et al.* (1992) The use of transesophageal echocardiography in the evaluation of chest trauma. *J Trauma* **32**:761–765.
11. Goarin JP, Le Bret F, Riou B, Jacquens Y and Viars P (1993) Early diagnosis of traumatic aortic rupture by transesophageal echocardiography. *Chest* **103**:618–619.
12. Mattox KL, Holzman M, Pickard LR *et al.* (1985) Clamp/repair: a safe technique for treatment of blunt injury to the descending thoracic aorta. *Ann Thorac Surg* **40**:456–463.
13. Pate JW (1994) Is traumatic rupture of the aorta misunderstood *Ann Thorac Surg* **57**:530–531.
14. Hilgenberg AD, Logan DL, Akins CW *et al.* (1992) Blunt injuries of the thoracic aorta. *Ann Thorac Surg* **53**:233–239.
15. Lee RB, Stahlman GC and Sharp KW (1992) Treatment priorities in patients with traumatic rupture of the thoracic aorta. *Am Surg* **58**:37–43.

16. Walker WA and Pate JW (1990) Medical management of acute traumatic rupture of the aorta. *Ann Thorac Surg* **50**:965–967.

17. Ryan P and Ragazzon R (1979) Abdominal injuries in survivors of road trauma before and since seat belt legislation in Victoria. *Aust NZ J Surg* **49**:200–202.

18. Aronoff RJ, Reynolds J and Thal ER (1982) Evaluation of diaphragmatic injuries. *Am J Surg* **144**:671–674.

19. Mirvis SE, Keramati B and Anderson JC (1988) MR imaging of traumatic diaphragmatic rupture. *J Comput Assist Tomogr* **12**:147–149.

20. Strug B, Noon GP and Beall AC Jr (1974) Traumatic diaphragmatic hernia. *Ann Thorac Surg* **17**:444–449.

21. Sandham JD, Shaw DT and Guenter CA (1977) Acute supine respiratory failure due to bilateral diaphragmatic paralysis. *Chest* **72**:96–98.

22. Ford GT, Whitelaw WA, Rosenal TW *et al.* (1983) Diaphragm function after upper abdominal surgery in humans. *Am Rev Respir Dis* **127**:431–436.

23. Lewis FR (1982) Thoracic trauma. *Surg Clin North Am* **62**:97–104.

24. Pate JW (1989) Tracheobronchial and oesophageal injuries. *Surg Clin North Am* **69**:111–123.

25. Kish G, Kozloff L, Joseph WL and Adkins PC (1976) Indications for early thoracotomy in the management of chest trauma. *Ann Thorac Surg* **22**:23–28.

26. Wilson JM, Boren CH Jr, Peterson SR and Thomas AN (1979) Traumatic hemothorax: is decortication necessary? *J Thorac Cardiovasc Surg* **77**:489–494.

27. Wagner RB and Jamieson PM (1989) Pulmonary contusion. *Surg Clin North Am* **69**:31–40.

28. Wagner RB, Crawford WO Jr and Schimpf PP (1988) Classification of parenchymal injuries of the lung. *Radiology* **167**:77–82.

29. Richardson JD, Adams L and Flint LM (1982) Selective management of flail chest and pulmonary contusion. *Ann Surg* **196**:481–486.

30. Bancewicz J and Yates D (1983) Blunt injury to the heart. *Br Med J* **286**:497.

31. Madoff IM and Desforges G (1972) Cardiac injuries due to non-penetrating thoracic trauma. *Ann Thorac Surg* **14**:504–511.

32. Hills MW, Delprado AM and Deane SA (1993) Sternal fractures: associated injuries and management. *J Trauma* **35**:55–60.

33. Brookes JG, Dunn RJ and Roger IR (1993) Sternal fractures: a retrospective analysis of 272 cases. *J Trauma* **35**:46–54.

34. Thomas AN and Stephen BG (1974) Air embolism: a cause of morbidity and death after penetrating chest trauma. *J Trauma* **14**:633–638.

35. Mattox K (1989) Indicators for thoracotomy: deciding to operate. *Surg Clin North Am* **69**:47–58.

36. Maloney JV, Schmutzer KJ and Raschke E (1961) Paradoxical respiration and 'Pendulluft'. *J Thorac Cardiovasc Surg* **41**:291–298.

37. O'Kelly E and Garry B (1981) Continuous pain relief for multiple fractured ribs. *Br J Anaesth* **53**:989–991.

38. Rocco A, Reiestad F, Gudman J and McKay W (1987) Intrapleural administration of local anesthetics for pain relief in patients with multiple rib fractures. *Reg Anesth* **12**:10–14.

39. Shackford SR, Smith DE, Zarins CK, Rice CL and Virgilio RW (1976) The management of flail chest. A comparison of ventilatory and non-ventilatory treatment. *Am J Surg* **132**:759–762.

40. Trinkle JK, Richardson JD, Franz JL, Grover FL, Arom KV and Holmstrom FMG (1975) Management of flail chest without mechanical ventilation. *Ann Thorac Surg* **19**:355–363.

41. Tobin MJ (1994) Mechanical ventilation. *N Engl J Med* **330**:1056–1061.

42. Cullen P, Modell JH, Kirby RR, Klein EF and Long W (1975) Treatment of flail chest. Use of intermittent mandatory ventilation and positive end expiratory pressure. *Arch Surg* **110**:1099–1103.

43. Hillman KM and Barber JD (1980) Asynchronous independent lung ventilation (AILV). *Crit Care Med* **8**:390–395.

44. Paris F, Tarazona V, Blasco E *et al.* (1975) Surgical stabilization of traumatic flail chest. *Thorax* **30**:521–527.

45. Moore BP (1975) Operative stabilisation of non-penetrating chest injuries. *J Thorac Cardiovasc Surg* **70**:619–630.

46. Editorial (1977) Management of the stove-in chest with paradoxical movement. *Br Med J* **1**: 1242.

47. Van Saene HKF, Stoutenbeek CHP, Miranda DR, Zandstra DF and Langrehr D (1986) Symposium paper: recent advances in the control of infection in patients with thoracic injury. *Injury* **17**:332–335.

48. Cook D (1993) Selective digestive decontamination: a critical appraisal. In: Vincent J-L (ed.) *Yearbook of Intensive Care and Emergency Medicine*. Berlin: Springer-Verlag, pp. 281–286.

49. Alexander JW (1992) Prevention of bacterial translocation with early enteral feeding – a feasible approach? In: Faist E, Meakins J and Schildberg FW (eds) *Host Defense Dysfunction in Trauma, Shock and Sepsis*. Berlin: Springer-Verlag, pp. 903–909.

50. James OF and Moore PG (1983) Causes of death after blunt chest injury. *Aust NZ J Surg* **53**: 37–42.

51. Trunkey DD (1987) Torso trauma. *Curr Probl Surg* **24**:209–265.

Spinal injuries

GM Joynt and KK Young

Trauma to the spine, especially when the spinal cord is damaged, may be life-threatening and may cause severe permanent disability. Hospital survival rates in large centres are now greater than 90% due to improved management.[1] None the less, long-term morbidity is high, and better vehicle design, passenger restraints, anti-drink driving programmes and safety education remain important.[2]

Aetiology

The incidence of spinal injuries in Australia is 20–25 per million population per year. In modern societies, traumatic spinal cord injuries are most commonly due to automobile accidents (45%), falls (20%), diving and other sporting accidents (15%) and physical violence (15%).[1,3,4] Automobile and diving accidents are strongly associated with alcohol ingestion.[3,5] Head-injury victims have a greater risk of spinal injury, but apparently not victims of facial injuries.[6] Ischaemic spinal cord injury may also occur after aortic trauma or surgical cross-clamping.[7]

Certain pre-existing spinal pathologies predispose to cord injury. These include degenerative disease, spinal canal stenosis, ankylosing spondylitis, Down's syndrome, Klippel–Feil syndrome, Chiari malformation, metastatic cancer, osteomyelitis, rheumatoid arthritis and unrecognized previous odontoid fracture.[8–10]

Pathophysiology

Mechanical trauma to the spinal cord results in immediate (primary) as well as delayed (secondary) injury processes.

Primary injury

Primary spinal cord injuries occur at the time of impact, and include both focal (i.e. avulsion, contusion, laceration and intraparenchymal haemorrhage) and diffuse lesions (i.e. concussive and diffuse axonal injury).[11,12] Further mechanical disruption of the cord can be caused by external compression or angulation. Ischaemic damage may occur due to occlusion of the vertebral arteries, or the branches of the thoracolumbar aorta which form the anterior spinal arteries.[13,14]

Secondary injury

Following primary injury, delayed spinal cord damage can result from cellular hypoxia, oligaemia and oedema.[12] Clinically, there are progressive sensory and motor disturbances.[3] Spinal cord blood flow decreases, and microscopy shows characteristic evolutionary changes that progress to necrosis.[13] Axonal degeneration occurs after approximately 8 h. This secondary spinal cord injury results from an injury-activated neurochemical cascade, which triggers changes including excessive neurotransmitter release, abnormal ion homeostasis and synthesis, and release or activation of various autodestructive factors (e.g. neural proteases, free radicals, eicosanoids and kinins).[11,12] The final result is impairment of blood flow, metabolic dysfunction, cellular ischaemia and death. Secondary spinal cord injury is exacerbated by systemic hypotension.[14]

Assessment of spinal injury
Radiographic evaluation

Plain X-rays remain the primary screening tool in suspected spinal injury (Fig. 69.1). Fractures, dislocation, subluxation and soft-tissue swelling can be detected (Table 69.1). However, *absence of a detectable lesion does not exclude injury*. The lesion may not be visualized because of the views used, poor-quality films or an inexperienced observer. Some cervical spine lesions may not easily be seen on plain X-rays (e.g. transverse process fractures).[15]

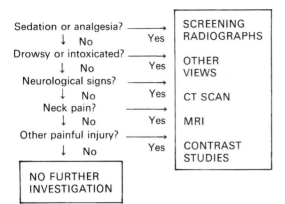

Fig. 69.1 Indications for screening radiographs. CT = Computed tomography; MRI = magnetic resonance imaging.

Once an injury is detected, stability should be assessed. Stability can mean either mechanical (orthopaedic) or neurological (i.e. spinal cord is at risk); the two are not necessarily concurrent. A mechanically stable fracture can be neurologically unstable, e.g. due to cord compression from extra-dural haematoma. X-rays can assess only mechanical stability.

Cervical spine

Nearly two-thirds of spinal injuries occur in the cervical spine – in adults mostly in the lower cervical spine (below C2), but in children mostly in the upper cevical spine. Multiple injuries are common, with each patient averaging 2.2 injuries.[16] It is important to note that 5–15% of cervical fractures are missed by portable screening films.[17] Although all acute abnormalities should be considered unstable, the assessment of stability is important to determine definitive management. The lesion is considered unstable if more than one column is disrupted.[16] Subluxation of more than 3 mm,[18] widening or narrowing of the disc space and increase of the interspinous distance strongly suggest instability.[16,19] The three-view trauma series is standard in most institutions.

Lateral view
Most significant injuries (75–90%) can be detected on this view. All seven vertebrae must be visualized. Features to evaluate are shown in Table 69.2 and Figures 69.2 and 69.3. Difficulties in visualizing C6, C7 and upper thoracic regions may require special techniques, such as traction on the arms or a 'swimmer's view'.[16]

Anteroposterior (AP) view
This view is useful for detecting unilateral facet injuries, lower spinous process fractures, anterior subluxations and pillar fractures.

Table 69.1 Basic examination of spinal radiographs

Check for:
Alignment
Vertebral bodies
Spinous processes

Bony changes
Bony density
Contour
Vertebral body height (anterior and posterior)
Spines and transverse processes

Spaces
Intervertebral spaces
Interspinous spaces

Damaged tissues
Retropharyngeal space
Posterior mediastinum
Retroperitoneum

Table 69.2 Cervical spine – lateral X-ray evaluation

C1–C2
Predental space or atlas–dens interval: i.e. distance between posterior aspect of anterior arch C1 and anterior aspect odontoid process normally: 2.0–2.5 mm in adults; 4.0–4.5 mm in children

Posterior cervical line: i.e. a straight line connecting the bases of C1 and C3 spinous processes should be within 2 mm of the base of C2 spinous process (the exception is pseudosubluxation of C2/C3 and C3/C4 in infants and children)

C3–C7
Anterior spinal, posterior spinal and spinolaminar lines: i.e. smooth lines connecting the anterior vertebral bodies, posterior vertebral bodies and bases of spinal processes

Prevertebral fat stripe: i.e. line overlying the soft tissue from C1 to C6 should parallel the anterior vertebrae

Retropharyngeal space: i.e. space between the posterior pharyngeal wall and:
    anterior body C2 normally < 7 mm in children and adults
    anterior body C3 and C4 normally < one-half of vertebral body width

Retrotracheal space: i.e. space between posterior tracheal wall and anterior inferior body C6 normally:
    ≤ 22 mm in adults; ≤ 14 mm in children less than 15 years

Disc spaces: anterior narrowing = flexion injury; anterior widening = extension injury

Facet joints should be parallel

Interspinous distance should decrease from C3 to C7

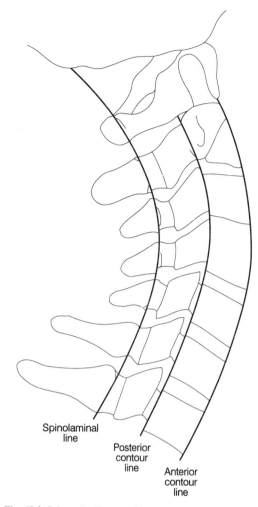

Fig. 69.2 Schematic diagram of lateral cervical spine. From Rosen,[63] with permission.

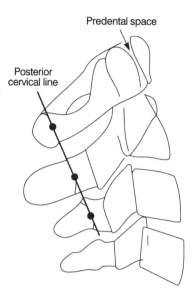

Fig. 69.3 Lateral view of upper cervical spine. From Rosen,[63] with permission.

Odontoid (open-mouth) view

This view is essential for evaluation of the odontoid process and the C1–C2 relationship.

The addition of *supine oblique views* results in a five-view trauma series, which is now recommended to improve diagnostic yield.[20,21]

Thoracolumbar spine

The above assessment principles apply equally to AP and lateral views of the thoracolumbar spine. The three-column model of Denis[22] is frequently used to classify thoracolumbar injuries. Disruption of two of the three vertebral columns implies mechanical instability.[16,22] Bulging of the mediastinal stripe or mediastinal widening may be evidence of an underlying fracture.[3] Most thoracic fractures are stable, but kyphosis of greater than 30° usually requires stabilization. Kyphosis of greater than 40° with some scoliosis indicates fracture-dislocation and potential instability.[17]

Computed tomography (CT) scanning

CT scanning is now the tomographic technique of choice. Indications for CT scanning include:

1 *inadequate plain radiography*: CT scanning is especially useful in the acute setting (often with CT scans for head injury) to visualize C1/C2 and C7/T1–T2 regions, where visualization with plain X-rays is difficult. Manipulation of the neck is also unnecessary;
2 *suspicious plain X-ray findings*;
3 *further investigation of fractures seen on plain X-rays*;
4 *high clinical suspicion of injury despite normal plain X-rays*. CT has a higher fracture detection rate.[23]

More sophisticated three-dimensional CT and CT myelography may be used to evaluate complex fractures and spinal canal contents.[24]

Magnetic resonance imaging (MRI)

MRI is difficult to use in the acute trauma setting. It is most useful in defining the extent of neural, vascular, ligamentous, disc and other soft-tissue injury (e.g. whiplash injury) and also the severity of cord injury.[25,26]

Clinical evaluation

General assessment

Talking to the patient establishes the level of consciousness. Clinical examination may reveal mechanisms of injury (e.g. abrasions and haematoma), overt signs of spinal injury (e.g. deformity) and associated injuries. Careful palpation of the entire spine and paraspinous musculature may reveal tenderness, muscle spasm or the classic 'step-off' deformity.

Neurological assessment

A careful, structured neurological examination is mandatory. Neurological deficits are present in 15–70% of patients with vertebral injuries.[3,27] However, vertebral injury need not be present for a spinal cord injury to exist. The 'spinal cord injury without radiographic abnormality' (SCIWORA) syndrome is not uncommon in adults,[28] is frequent in children, and occurs in both the cervical and thoracic spine.[29]

A full neurological examination covers motor function, tendon reflexes and sensory function, including assessment of pain, temperature, touch, vibration sense and proprioception. Breathing pattern may be abnormal with high spinal lesions. In the unconscious patient, clinical findings suggestive of cord injury are summarized in Table 69.3.[27] The examination should determine the level of a lesion, and whether it is complete or incomplete. Spinal shock may mimic a complete lesion, with total loss of motor power and sensation distal to the site of injury. In complete spinal cord lesion, this total loss of neurological function persists after the period of spinal shock. A complete lesion is excluded if there is any – even minimal – cord function, such as anal sphincter tone, perianal sensation or flexor toe movement.[3] Nearly all (99%) patients with a complete lesion over 24 h will not have a functional recovery.[30] Of patients with incomplete spinal injuries, 90% fall into one of four clinical syndromes: central cord syndrome, Brown–Séquard syndrome, anterior cord syndrome or cauda equina syndrome.[31]

Table 69.3 Signs of spinal cord injury in comatose patients

Relaxed anal sphincter
Flaccid areflexia
Response to pain above but not below suspected level of lesion
Unexplained hypotension and bradycardia
Priapism (characteristic but uncommon)
Ability to flex but not extend at the elbow suggests cervical injury

Central cord syndrome

Central grey matter is affected. There is greater loss of motor power in the upper limbs, usually with retention of urine and variable sensory loss below the lesion.

Brown–Séquard syndrome (cord hemisection)

Ipsilateral paralysis is present, with contralateral loss of pain and temperature sensation.

Anterior cord (anterior spinal artery) syndrome

Paralysis is present, with hypalgesia and hyaesthesia below the level of injury, but with preservation of posterior column functions (position and vibration senses).

Cauda equina syndrome

This is due to lumbar fracture, and produces a loss of bladder and bowel function, with paresis of the lower motor neurone type. Sensory loss may be patchy, and there may be radicular pain exacerbated by straight leg raising.

Management

Field management

Unless there are skilled personnel in the field, initial care must be limited to manoeuvres which can be easily and quickly performed. These include ensuring an adequate airway and ventilation and immobilization.

Ensuring an adequate airway and ventilation[32]

The upper airways are cleared of foreign matter. An obstructed airway must be supported by jaw thrust, rather than chin lift and neck extension.[33] A nasopharyngeal or oral airway is inserted if appropriate. Oxygen is administered by facemask. Hypotension is treated as necessary (e.g. with Trendelenburg position, fluids and drugs).[32]

Immobilization

Any suspected spinal injury must be immobilized. Soft neck collars are inadequate for cervical immobilization; rigid collars are more effective. The head and torso are best immobilized using a rigid backboard with strapping of the head (between sandbags), thorax, abdomen and lower limbs.[3,34] Cervical spine immobilization aims to maintain the neutral position, defined as that obtained when looking directly in front. Children less than 8 years may require back elevation with padding to achieve this position.[35] Immobilized patients are moved by 'log rolling'.

Hospital management

Initial assessment of a patient with known or suspected spinal injury should follow usual triage principles. Nearly two-thirds of trauma patients will have multiple injuries. The incidence of cervical spine injury in severe trauma is about 2.5%, rising to about 10% in severe head injuries.[16,27,32] Once a careful primary survey has been performed, appropriate resuscitation should be completed before definitive management of the spinal injury.

Airway control

A patent airway must be secured and maintained. Foreign matter is removed manually and by suction. A nasal or oral airway can be inserted with minimal cervical movement.[36] Jaw thrust, chin lift and ventilation with a bag and mask can cause displacement of unstable fractures, but the clinical significance of this is unknown.[27]

Controversy surrounds the safest method of tracheal intubation. Most methods can be performed safely in trained hands under appropriate circumstances.[37] Common techniques include awake nasotracheal intubation, orotracheal intubation under general anaesthesia and awake fibreoptic intubation. Choice of technique depends on the skill and preference of the operator, and may be modified by factors such as urgency and coexisting injuries (e.g. nasal and faciomaxillary fracture, basal skull fracture and laryngeal injury). The *Advanced Trauma Life Support* (ATLS) guidelines recommend nasotracheal intubation in the spontaneously breathing patient.[32] In the unconscious patient or during orotracheal intubation with general anaesthesia, manual axial traction of the neck aims to minimize fracture displacement during airway manoeuvres.[32] Excessive force should not be applied, as vertebral distraction occurs experimentally[38] and may cause further cord injury. Awake fibreoptic intubation is recommended if the necessary skills, equipment and time are available. If direct laryngoscopy and oral intubation are deemed appropriate, an assistant should hold the head to maintain in-line stabilization with minimal traction.[39] Cricoid pressure causes subluxation of the unstable cervical spine, but evidence that this is harmful is lacking.[38] If intubation fails, the airway is secured by emergency procedures such as cricothyroidotomy and tracheostomy. Such airways should normally be avoided, as their cervical site will compromise any future anterior decompression surgery. Other intubation alternatives claimed to maintain spinal immobility include retrograde tracheal intubation[40] and the use of a lighted stylette.[41] Unproven airway devices in spinal injuries include the laryngeal mask airway, and Combitube[27] (see Chapter 27).

Breathing[3]

Respiratory failure may occur. Possible causes are multiple, and include central nervous system causes (i.e. associated head injury or intoxication), loss of intercostal function (i.e. cord lesion above C8) and diaphragmatic function (i.e. cord lesion above C3), aspiration pneumonia, sputum retention and airway and pulmonary trauma. Management includes oxygen therapy, mechanical ventilatory support, pulmonary toilet and treating any reversible underlying cause.

Circulation

Although hypertension may occur immediately after spinal cord trauma, most patients are hypotensive on presentation to hospital.[42] This may be due to one or a combination of spinal shock, haemorrhagic shock and cardiogenic shock.

Spinal shock

Injuries above T1 cause sympathetic paralysis below the injury, resulting in vasodilatation and distributive shock. Venous return is reduced, due to paralysis of the muscles of the lower extremities and abdomen. Bradycardia may occur, as vagal tone is unopposed. Ensuing hypotension is treated by infusion of fluids, atropine and, if necessary, inotropes or vasopressors.[3,4] Central venous pressure monitoring is usually necessary.[43] Pulmonary artery catheter monitoring may be useful in unstable cases,[42] but is not universally recommended.[44] Spinal shock is a diagnosis of exclusion, after all other causes have been ruled out.

Haemorrhagic shock

Clinical examination to detect abdominal visceral injuries is unreliable in a patient with spinal cord injury, especially if unconscious. Examination of the abdomen may be undertaken with diagnostic peritoneal lavage, ultrasound, CT scan or laparotomy, depending on institutional preferences and haemodynamic stability.[45]

Cardiogenic shock

Cardiac function may be impaired by myocardial contusion, pericardial tamponade, ischaemia, tension pneumothorax, severe hypoxaemia and metabolic disturbances.

ICU management

Initial management aims to prevent extension of the primary injury and to reduce secondary injury. Subsequent management involves supportive care of resultant complications.

Primary injury

Spinal stabilization should be meticulously continued (e.g. by traction, brace and/or surgical stabilization) until definitive treatment is instituted. Timing of decompression and stabilization of vertebral fractures is a surgical decision, with no consensus on the best timing of both cervical and thoracolumbar surgery.[46,47]

Secondary injury

Attenuation of secondary cord injury is achieved by general and specific measures. General measures centre around the prevention of hypotension and hypoxia. Specific measures have included hypothermia, hyperbaric oxygen, and drugs such as glucocorticoids, 21-aminosteroids, superoxide dismutase and pentoxifylline.[11,12,48–50] Results of human studies on specific measures to prevent secondary injury have been disappointing, except the second national acute spinal cord injury study (NASCIS 2), which found that high-dose methylprednisolone given within 8 h of injury led to improved neurological function at 6 weeks, 6 months and 1 year.[51] The regimen consisted of 30 mg/kg IV over 15 min followed by an infusion of 5.4 mg/kg per h for 23 h from the second hour.[51] Those who received the regimen 8 h after injury had less recovery of motor function at 1 year than the placebo group.[52] The optimal dose and timing of administration are being investigated in a third NASCIS trial.[53]

Complications

Patients with lesions above C3 have total loss of respiratory function, and will require immediate intubation and ventilation. Expiratory muscles receive innervation from below C8, so all cervical spinal injuries result in limited expiratory function.[54] Lesions at C3, C4 or C5 demonstrate similar levels of inspiratory dysfunction, but the higher lesions have a greater respiratory complication rate.[55]

Respiratory complications are the leading cause of death following spinal cord injury. Most deaths are due to pneumonia.[56] Prevention of atelectasis and pneumonia relies on regular physiotherapy and bronchial hygiene. Suggested protocols include deep breathing exercises, incentive spirometry, chest percussion and assisted coughing. Aggressive management of lobar atelectasis includes bronchoscopy and saline lavage.[54] Ventilatory dysfunction should be monitored by serial lung function tests (e.g. vital capacity, negative inspiratory force or PI_{max}, FEV_1 and peak flow). Early intubation should be considered if reduced pulmonary mechanics persist.[54] Patients who develop respiratory failure invariably require mechanical ventilation. Suxamethonium (succinylcholine) is avoided between 3 days and 6 months postinjury as it may precipitate hyperkalaemia.[57]

Tracheostomy should be considered if ventilatory support for longer than 2 weeks is likely, and if surgery in the region is not contemplated.[42,54]

Pulmonary function can be expected to improve as muscle flaccidity changes to spasticity. Over a period of 3–4 months, an increase in vital capacity of 65–80% can be expected, and most patients can be weaned from the ventilator.[54] Inspiratory muscle training may improve respiratory muscle function.[58] Prophylactic antibiotics are not recommended.

Initial haemodynamic management is described above. Following the acute phase, low to normal blood pressure and pulse usually persist for weeks to months. However, about 50% of patients with lesions above T7 will demonstrate episodes of hypertension, bradycardia, muscular hypertonus and cutaneous changes (either pallor or vasodilatation with flushing and sweating).[59] Triggering factors of this mass autonomic reflex include cutaneous, proprioceptive or visceral irritation, which is often an overdistended bladder or rectum. This mass spinal sympathetic reflex is normally inhibited from above. The sudden increase in blood pressure stimulates a vagal response, which can produce bradycardia, heart block and vasodilatation above the injury level. Management is preventive (e.g. good bladder and bowel care) and supportive (e.g. α-adrenergic blockers). Bradycardia seen with tracheal suctioning is due to unimpeded vagal discharge, and can be abolished with IV atropine.[54]

During the acute phase, an indwelling urinary catheter is necessary, but after 2–3 weeks, intermittent bladder catheterization is favoured. Urinary infection is common, but should be distinguished from colonization before treatment is undertaken.[42] A nasogastric tube should be placed to decompress the stomach, as gastric stasis and ileus may occur. Enteral feeding is started when bowel function returns. Gentle rectal disimpaction may be necessary in the early stages.

Prevention of pressure sores is a high priority as they greatly increase morbidity and cost of hospitalization.[1] Poikilothermia occurs in patients with lesions above T1, and hypo- or hyperthermia should be detected and treated.[42] Spinal cord injury has a high risk of venous thromboembolism. Recommended prophylaxis is the use of graduated stockings or intermittent pneumatic calf compression, with low-dose heparin (5000 units/8 h) added for high-risk groups. Low-molecular-weight heparins and heparinoids may be more effective and have less risk of bleeding.[60,61] Eight weeks of prophylaxis seems adequate.[61] Hyponatraemia is common in the first week after spinal cord injury, and should be treated to prevent complications.[62]

Outcome

Improved care has led to greater than 90% hospital survival for spinal cord injuries. Rehabilitation allows over half of the survivors to achieve self-care independence. New drugs offer promise in reducing secondary spinal cord injury. To achieve optimal outcome, the above principles of resuscitation and intensive supportive care must be rigorously applied.

References

1. Ditunno JF and Formal CS (1994) Chronic spinal cord injury. *N Engl J Med* **330**:550–556.
2. Yeo JD (1993) Prevention of spinal cord injuries in an Australian study. *Paraplegia* **31**:759–763.
3. Hockberger RS, Kirshenbaum K and Doris PE (1992) Spinal trauma. In: Rosen P and Barkin RM (eds) *Emergency Medicine – Concepts and Clinical Practice*. St Louis: Mosby-Year Book, pp. 371–412.
4. Weesner CL, Hargarten SW, Aprahamian C and Nelson DR (1994) Fatal childhood injury patterns in an urban setting. *Ann Emerg Med* **23**:231–236.
5. Kluger Y, Jarosz D, Paul DB, Townsend RN and Doamond DL (1994) Diving injuries: a preventable catastrophe. *J Trauma* **36**:349–351.
6. Hills MW and Deane SA (1993) Head injury and facial injury: is there an increased risk of cervical head injury? *J Trauma* **34**:549–554.
7. Waters RL, Sie I, Yakura J and Adkins R (1993) Recovery following ischemic myelopathy. *J Trauma* **35**: 837–839.
8. Houser OW, Onofrio BM, Miller GM, Folger WN, Smith PL and Kallman DA (1993) Cervical neural foraminal canal stenosis: computerized tomographic myelography diagnosis. *J Neurosurg* **79**:84–88.
9. Murali R (1990) Special problems in patients with preexisting spine disease. In Cooper PR (ed.) *Management of Posttraumatic Spinal Instability*. Illinois: American Association of Neurological Surgeons, pp. 173–180.
10. Crockard HA, Heilman AE and Stevens JM (1993) Progressive myelopathy secondary to odontoid fractures: clinical, radiological, and surgical features. *J Neurosurg* **78**:579–586.
11. Anderson DK and Hall ED (1993) Pathophysiology of spinal cord trauma. *Ann Emerg Med* **22**:987–992.
12. Gentile NT and McIntosh TK (1993) Antagonists of excitatory amino acids and endogenous opioid peptides in the treatment of experimental central nervous system injury. *Ann Emerg Med* **22**:1028–1034.
13. Fairholm DJ and Turnbull IM (1971) Microangiographic study of experimental spinal cord injuries. *J Neurosurg* **35**:277–286.
14. Shackford SR, Mackersie RC, Davis JW *et al.* (1989) Epidemiology and pathology of traumatic deaths occurring at a level I trauma centre in a regionalized system: the importance of secondary brain injury. *J Trauma* **29**:1392–1397.
15. Woodring JH, Lee C and Duncan V (1993) Transverse process fractures of the cervical vertebrae: are they insignificant? *J Trauma* **34**:797–802.
16. Berquist TH (1990) Spinal trauma. In: McCort JJ (ed.) *Trauma Radiology*. New York: Churchill-Livingstone, pp. 31–74.
17. Trauma Committee – Royal Australasian College of Surgeons (1990) *Early Management of Severe Trauma (EMST)*. Melbourne: Royal Australasian College of Surgeons.
18. Scher AT (1979) Anterior cervical subluxation: a unstable proposition. *Am J Radiol* **133**:275–280.
19. Murphy MD, Baatnitzky S and Bramble JM (1989) Diagnostic imaging of spinal trauma. *Radiol Clin North Am* **27**:855–872.
20. Turetsky DB, Vines FS, Clayman DA and Northup HM (1993) Technique and use of supine oblique views in acute cervical spine trauma. *Ann Emerg Med* **22**:685–689.
21. Murphey MD (1993) Editorial: trauma oblique cervical spine radiographs. *Ann Emerg Med* **22**:728–730.
22. Denis F (1983) The three column spine and its significance in the classification of acute thoracolumbar spinal injuries. *Spine* **8**:817–831.
23. Acheson MB, Livingstone RR, Richardson ML and Stimac GK (1987) High-resolution CT scanning in the evaluation of cervical spine fractures: comparison with plain film examinations. *Am J Radiol* **148**: 1179–1185.
24. Cooper PR and Cohen W (1984) Evaluation of cervical spinal cord injuries with metrizamide myelography-CT scanning. *J Neurosurg* **61**:281–289.
25. Schaefer DM, Flanders A, Northrup DE, Doan HT and Osterholm JL (1989) Magnetic resonance imaging of acute cervical spine trauma. Correlation with severity of neurologic injury. *Spine* **14**:1090–1095.
26. Bondurant FJ, Cotler HB, Kulkarni MV, McArdle CB and Harris JH Jr. (1990) Acute spinal cord injury: a study using physical examination and magnetic resonance imaging. *Spine* **15**:161–168.
27. Abrams KJ and Grande CM (1994) Airway management of the trauma patient with cervical spine injury. *Curr Opin Anaesthiol* **7**:184–190.
28. Hardy AG (1977) Cervical spinal cord injury without bony injury. *Paraplegia* **14**:296–305.
29. Pang D and Wilberger JE (1982) Spinal cord injury without radiographic abnormalities in children. *J Neurosurg* **57**:114–129.
30. Young J and Dexter W (1978) Neurologic recovery distal to the zone of injury in 172 cases of closed traumatic spinal cord injury. *Paraplegia* **16**:39–49.
31. Bouzarth WF and Goldman HW (1986) Spinal injuries. In: Schwartz GR, Safar P, Stone JH, Storey PB and Wagner DK (eds) *Principles and Practice of Emergency Medicine*. Philadelphia: Saunders, pp. 1308–1138.
32. American College of Surgeons Committee on Trauma (1988) *Advanced Trauma Life Support for Physicians*. Chicago: American College of Surgeons.
33. Finucane BT and Santora AH (1988) *Principles of Airway Management*. Philadelphia: FA Davis.
34. Mazolewski P and Manix TH (1994) The effectiveness of strapping techniques in spinal immobilization. *Ann Emerg Med* **23**:1290–1295.
35. Nypaver M and Treloar D (1994) Neutral cervical spine positioning in children. *Ann Emerg Med* **23**: 208–211.
36. Aprahamian C, Thompson B, Finger W and Darin J (1984) Experimental cervical spine injury model: exam-

ination of airway management and splinting techniques. *Ann Emerg Med* **13**:584–587.

37. Crosby ET (1992) Tracheal intubation in the cervical spine-injured patient. *Can J Anaesth* **39**:105–106.

38. Crosby ET and Lui A (1990) The adult cervical spine: implications for airway management. *Can J Anaesth* **37**:77–93.

39. Criswell JC, Parr MJA and Nolan JP (1994) Emergency airway management in patients with cervical spine injuries. *Anaesthesia* **49**:900–903.

40. Barriot P and Riou B (1988) Retrograde technique for tracheal intubation in trauma patients. *Crit Care Med* **16**:712–713.

41. Verdile VP, Chiang JL, Bedger R *et al.* (1990) Nasotracheal intubation using a flexible lighted stylet. *Ann Emerg Med* **19**:506–510.

42. Luce JM (1985) Medical management of spinal cord injury. *Crit Care Med* **13**:126–131.

43. Mangiardi JR, Moser FG, Spitzer D and Bouzarth WF (1992) Spinal injuries. In: Schwartz GR (ed.) *Principles and Practice of Emergency Medicine*. Philadelphia: Lea & Febiger, pp. 955–993.

44. Levi L, Wolf A and Belzberg H (1993) Hemodynamic parameters in patients with acute cervical cord trauma: description, intervention, and prediction of outcome. *Neurosurgery* **33**:1007–1017.

45. Mirvis SE and Shanmuganathan (1994) Trauma radiology: part I computerized tomographic imaging of abdominal trauma. *J Intensive Care Med* **9**:151–163.

46. Levi L, Wolf A, Rigamonti D, Ragheb J, Mirvis S and Robinson WL (1991) Anterior decompression of cervical spine trauma: does the timing of surgery affect outcome? *Neurosurgery* **29**:216–222.

47. Errico TJ and Bauer RD (1990) Thoracolumbar spine injuries. In: Cooper PR (ed.) *Management of Posttraumatic Spinal Instability*. Illinois, American College of Neurological Surgeons, pp. 135–162.

48. Hall ED (1993) Lipid antioxidants in acute central nervous system injury. *Ann Emerg Med* **22**: 1022–1026.

49. Muizelaar JP, Marmarou A, Young HF, Choi SC, Wolf A, Schneider RL and Kontos HA (1993) Improving the outcome of severe head injury with the oxygen radical scavenger polyethylene glycol-conjugated superoxide dismutase: a phase II trial. *J Neurosurg* **78**:375–382.

50. Toung TJK, Kirsch JR, Maruki Y and Traystman RJ (1994) Effects of pentoxifylline on cerebral blood flow, metabolism, and evoked response after total cerebral ischaemia in dogs. *Crit Care Med* **22**: 273–281.

51. Bracken MB, Shepard MJ, Collins WF, Holford TR, Young W, Baskin DS *et al.* (1990) A randomized, controlled trial of methylprednisolone or naloxone in the treatment of acute spinal-cord injury. *N Engl J Med* **322**:1405–1411.

52. Bracken MB, Shepard MJ, Collins WF, Holford TR, Baskin DS, Eisenberg HM *et al.* (1992) Methylprednisolone or naloxone treatment after acute spinal cord injury: 1-year follow-up data. *J Neurosurg* **76**:23–31.

53. Bracken MB and Holford TR (1993) Effects of timing of methylprednisolone or naloxone administration on recovery of segmental and long-tract neurological function in NASCIS 2. *J Neurosurg* **79**: 500–507.

54. Mansel JK and Norman JR (1990) Respiratory complications and management of spinal cord injuries. *Chest* **97**: 1446–1452.

55. Jackson AB and Groomes TE (1994) Incidence of respiratory complications following spinal cord injury. *Arch Phys Med Rehab* **75**:270–275.

56. Carter RE (1987) Respiratory aspects of spinal cord injury management. *Paraplegia* **25**:262–266.

57. Gronert GA and Theye RA (1975) Pathophysiology of hyperkalemia induced by succinylcholine. *Anesthesiology* **43**:89–99.

58. Gross B, Ladd HW, Riley EJ, Macklem PT and Grossino A (1980) The effect of training on strength and endurance of the diaphragm in quadriplegia. *Am J Med* **68**: 27–35.

59. Roizen MF (1986) Anesthetic implication of concurrent diseases in anesthesia. In: Miller RD (ed.) *Anesthesia*. New York: Churchill-Livingstone, pp. 903–1014.

60. Hamilton MG, Hull RD and Pineo GF (1994) Venous thromboembolism in neurosurgery and neurology patients: a review. *Neurosurgery* **34**:280–296.

61. Green D, Chen D, Chmiel JS *et al.* (1994) Prevention of thromboembolism in spinal cord injury: role of low molecular weight heparin. *Arch Phys Rehabil* **75**:290–292.

62. Peruzzi WT, Shapiro BA, Meyer PR, Krumlovsky F and Seo BW (1994) Hyponatremia in acute spinal cord injury. *Crit Care Med* **22**:252–258.

63. Rosen P (ed.) (1992) *Emergency Medicine: Concepts and Clinical Practice*, 3rd edn, vol.1. St Louis: CV Mosby, p. 397.

70 Abdominal and pelvic injuries

CJ McArthur and JA Judson

Although important abdominal injuries are present in only 16–27% of hospital trauma admissions,[1,2] abdominal and pelvic injuries can represent up to 60% of missed diagnoses in preventable trauma deaths.[3] Most abdominal and pelvic injuries are caused by blunt trauma; penetrating aetiologies account for 6–21% of cases, depending on the society concerned.[1,4] Important considerations with abdominal and pelvic injuries are

1 potential for severe haemorrhage;
2 difficulties in diagnosing visceral injury;
3 severity of associated injuries (e.g. chest and head);
4 complications, especially sepsis.

Mechanisms of injury

Blunt injuries

Road crashes account for most abdominal and pelvic blunt injuries. Injuries may also result from falls, assaults and industrial accidents.[1,2] Associated injuries are frequent, involving the thorax (most common),[5] head and extremities. Seat belts reduce mortality in motor vehicle crashes (mainly by limiting brain injury),[6,7] but are associated with more gastrointestinal injuries (3.4% versus 1.8% of victims not wearing seat belts).[6] Abdominal and pelvic injuries are more likely with vehicular side-on collisions, and passengers at either side are equally at risk.[5] Crashes resulting in a deformed steering wheel, dashboard intrusion or irreparable vehicle also have more abdominal injuries.[7]

Penetrating injuries

Stab and gunshot wounds account for most penetrating injuries to the abdomen.[1,4]

Stab and laceration wound

Entry sites do not accurately predict the nature of deeper injury.[8] Penetration of the thoracic cavity should be suspected with upper abdominal wounds; conversely, lower chest wounds may involve abdominal structures. Intra-abdominal injury occurs in 44% of anterior abdominal wounds, 29% of flank wounds and 15% of back wounds.[8] Mandatory laparotomy has been superseded by algorithms involving repeated physical examination, wound exploration, peritoneal lavage and laparoscopy that predict intra-abdominal injury with 95% accuracy.[8] Posterior wounds may require additional investigations to diagnose retroperitoneal injury.[8,9]

Gunshot wound

Injuries depend on missile calibre, and its velocity and trajectory. Intra-abdominal, thoracic and multiple organ injuries and mortality are substantially greater than with stab wounds.[8,10] Laparotomy should be performed in all cases when peritoneal violation cannot be excluded, as 89% of such patients have intra-abdominal injury.[8]

Initial treatment and investigations

Resuscitation

Ensuring adequacy of airway, ventilation and oxygenation and restoration of blood volume are immediate priorities.[11] However, resuscitation should *not* delay surgery for uncontrolled haemorrhage. If rapid surgical haemostasis is provided in penetrating trauma, delaying or limiting fluid resuscitation before surgery may possibly improve outcome.[12,13]

The use of pneumatic antishock garments (PASG) is controversial. It does not improve overall mortality in penetrating trauma, and is associated with increased mortality in penetrating cardiothoracic vascular injuries.[14] Nevertheless, PASG can tamponade haemorrhage, and may be useful in blunt trauma when definitive therapy is delayed.

Clinical assessment

A full clinical examination (including the back) by experienced clinicians is most important. The mechanism of injury may direct attention to particular anatomical areas.[5-7] Contusions, external wounds and their relationship to underlying viscera are noted. Abdominal distension, tenderness and peritonism are sought. The rectum is examined for prostatic position, anal tone, blood or other evidence of injury. Gastric aspirate and urine are inspected for blood. Auscultation for bowel sounds is not useful.

Isolated penetrating injuries present few diagnostic problems, but the decision to explore the abdomen can be difficult.[8] Blunt abdominal trauma is often part of multiple injuries, and is more difficult to diagnose clinically, except when abdominal signs are obvious. Nevertheless, in conscious patients serial assessments can accurately identify those with significant intra-abdominal pathology. In the presence of impaired consciousness, intellectual disability or spinal, chest or pelvic injury, clinical assessment is unreliable.[11] Other more visually spectacular injuries may also divert attention from the abdomen.

Laparotomy is indicated on clinical grounds when there is shock with signs of intra-abdominal haemorrhage (e.g. peritonism or increasing distension). Also, in penetrating trauma, laparotomy is indicated for evisceration or peritonism without shock. In all other situations where clinical examination is inadequate, further investigations must be undertaken.[15]

Plain X-rays

A chest X-ray (preferably erect) is essential. It may demonstrate free intraperitoneal gas, herniation of abdominal contents through a ruptured diaphragm, or other abnormalities. Plain films of the abdomen are of no benefit. 'One-shot' IV urograms (IVU) have been advocated in the unstable patient prior to laparotomy, but are inaccurate in delineating renal injury,[16] and can delay definitive therapy. They are, however, useful to confirm kidney function. An anteroposterior pelvic X-ray is indicated for all victims of blunt trauma, except conscious patients with normal pelvis on examination.[17,18]

Peritoneal lavage

Diagnostic peritoneal lavage (DPL) with 1 litre (or 10 ml/kg) of isotonic saline is indicated in blunt trauma, when there is haemodynamic instability with uncertain clinical findings, and in penetrating trauma when peritoneal breach is suspected. DPL detects free blood in the abdominal cavity with over 97% accuracy,[19] and has replaced abdominal paracentesis and four-quad-

Table 70.1 Criteria for positive diagnostic peritoneal lavage

Clinical
Initial aspiration of >10 ml of frank blood
Egress of lavage fluid via chest tube or urinary catheter
Bile or vegetable material in lavage fluid

Laboratory

	Blunt injury	*Penetrating injury*
Red cells		
Definite	>100 000/mm^3	>20 000/mm^3
Indeterminate	50 000–100 000/mm^3	5000–20 000/mm^3
White cells	>500/mm^3	>500/mm^3
Amylase	>20 IU/l	>20 IU/l
Alkaline phosphatase	>10 IU/l	>10 IU/l

Laboratory criteria, especially for penetrating injury, remain debatable.

rant taps. Its safe use requires prior placement of a gastric tube and bladder catheter. Open and closed (percutaneous guide wire) methods are both satisfactory, and the choice is debatable.[20,21] DPL is unjustified when an indication for laparotomy already exists. It is relatively contraindicated in pregnancy, significant obesity and previous abdominal surgery. If required in these situations (or with pelvic fractures), the supraumbilical open method should be considered. Recent evidence suggests that *early* DPL remains reliable in the presence of pelvic fractures.[22]

The high sensitivity of DPL can result in a non-therapeutic laparotomy rate of up to 29%,[19] which can be reduced if DPL findings are integrated with clinical information.[23] Cell counts of lavage effluent are more accurate than qualitative methods.[24] Hollow viscus injury is difficult to detect; lavage amylase[25] and alkaline phosphatase[25,26] levels may be helpful, but the value of an isolated raised white cell count is controversial.[27] Serum amylase estimations are not useful in identifying pancreatic or bowel injury.[28] Generally accepted criteria for a positive DPL are shown in Table 70.1.

Computed tomography (CT)

CT requires a still patient, IV and enteral contrast, a high-resolution scanner and experienced interpretation to match the sensitivity of peritoneal lavage.[29] Cuts from the top of the diaphragm to the symphysis pubis are required. CT should only be undertaken in stable patients. It is particularly useful to assess the retroperitoneum and pelvic fractures, and delineate the nature of abdominal injury (thus guiding non-operative management of some solid organ injuries).[30] However, CT may not detect all hollow viscus trauma.[29,30] Magnetic resonance imaging offers no advantage over CT in evaluating acute abdominal trauma, and poses significant logistical problems.[31]

DPL versus CT

DPL is invasive, rapid and accurate in identifying intraperitoneal bleeding or contamination, but may miss diaphragmatic injuries and does not examine the retroperitoneum. Its primary role is in *unstable* patients with blunt trauma and stable patients with anterior stab wounds. CT is non-invasive, time-consuming, but also accurate, and has a primary role in defining the location and magnitude of intra-abdominal injuries in *stable* patients with blunt trauma or penetrating trauma to the flank or back.[29] The two modalities are complementary,[32] and should both be available. If CT is unavailable, DPL is indicated in the stable patient with blunt trauma.

Ultrasonography

Ultrasonography in the resuscitation room can be performed rapidly without compromising resuscitation. It is 91–100% sensitive and over 98% specific in detecting haemoperitoneum.[33–36] However, it is less sensitive in demonstrating the nature of organ injury, particularly in the liver, pancreas and bowel.[33,34,36] It is particularly useful in the evaluation of trauma in pregnancy, but requires experience to reach adequate levels of accuracy.[35,37] It is extensively used in Europe,[33–35] and is under evaluation in North America,[36,37] but its place in the diagnostic process depends on local circumstances.

Laparoscopy

Diagnostic laparoscopy may be useful in the haemodynamically stable patient. It is good at visualizing the diaphragm and identifying a need for laparotomy, but may miss specific organ injuries, particularly of the bowel.[38,39] Laparoscopy appears best suited for the evaluation of equivocal penetrating wounds.[40]

Angiography

Selective angiography and embolization are valuable in detecting and treating the source of major haemorrhage from pelvic fractures or retroperitoneal structures.[41]

Laparotomy

Laparotomy can be regarded as both therapeutic and diagnostic. Intra-abdominal injury may be detected by means discussed above, but often only laparotomy can accurately diagnose specific injuries. In severe and multiple trauma, the morbidity of a negative laparotomy is insignificant when compared with the dire consequences of not diagnosing and treating a serious injury.

Specific injuries
Spleen

The spleen is the organ most frequently injured by blunt trauma. Injuries vary from a small subcapsular haematoma to hilar devascularization or shattered spleen, but are rarely fatal with good medical care.[42] Diagnosis may be delayed in mild trauma.[43] When associated chest or neurological injuries are severe, minor splenic injury may not initially be detected unless further investigation is undertaken. Fractures of the lower left ribs are a common association. Minor trauma may cause splenic injury when the spleen is enlarged (e.g. from malaria, lymphomas and haemolytic anaemias).

Immediate splenectomy is indicated in patients with severe multiple injuries, splenic avulsion, fragmentation or rupture, extensive hilar injuries, failure of haemostasis, peritoneal contamination from gastrointestinal injury or rupture of diseased spleen.[42] However, overwhelming infection by encapsulated organisms, such as *Pneumococcus*, can occur early or late (even years) after splenectomy in 0–2% of individuals. It is a particular risk following splenectomy in children and young adults.[42] Polyvalent pneumococcal vaccine (Pneumovax) should be administered following splenectomy.

A conservative non-operative approach is possible in stable patients under 55 years, in whom associated abdominal injuries have been excluded.[42,44] Using these criteria, surgery is required in less than 10%.[44,45] Hospital observation is required for 10–14 days; strenuous activity is avoided for 6–8 weeks, and contact sports for 6 months.[42] CT grading systems do not identify patients in whom expectant management will fail.[45]

Other treatment alternatives include operative procedures to conserve splenic tissue (e.g. topical haemostatic agents, suture repair, absorbable mesh, partial splenectomy and splenic artery ligation).[42] Benefits of splenectomy with autotransplantation of splenic tissue are unproven.

Liver

The liver is the second most commonly injured organ after blunt abdominal trauma, and is the most frequently missed injury in deaths from trauma.[3] Diagnosis is made by laparotomy is unstable patients, or CT in stable patients. Injuries range from small subcapsular haematomas to major parenchymal disruption and laceration of hepatic veins or even hepatic avulsion.[46]

CT enables selected patients to be managed without operation. This is common in children; criteria for adults are still evolving.[46] Patients should be haemodynamically stable, have associated abdominal injuries excluded, and be assessed repeatedly.[46,47] Follow-up CT scans can show the resolution of injury, which typically takes 2–3 months.[46]

Operative treatment of more severe injuries can be difficult due to hypothermia, acidosis and coagulopathy.[48] If definitive haemostasis cannot be achieved, intraperitoneal packing with elective re-exploration and removal of packs 24–72 h later can be attempted.[49] Survival is better when the decision to terminate the initial procedure is made earlier.[50]

ICU management involves rewarming, blood transfusion, correction of coagulation defects and respiratory, cardiovascular and nutritional support. Dilutional coagulopathy and thrombocytopenia are common. Early complications of liver injury relate to complications of hypoperfusion or massive blood transfusion. Late complications are usually associated with sepsis.

Gastrointestinal tract (GIT)

Injury to the GIT is more common following penetrating trauma; the incidence in blunt trauma is under 5%.[51] The very high likelihood of bowel injury in abdominal gunshot wounds mandates laparotomy. DPL can be used to identify those with stab wounds for laparotomy, when peritoneal violation cannot be excluded.[8] Posterior stab wounds may damage retroperitoneal structures. CT examination with contrast enema may identify colonic injury better than clinical assessment or DPL.[8,9]

Blunt abdominal injuries to stomach, duodenum, small intestine, colon and their mesenteries are increasing with the use of seat belts,[6] and are difficult to evaluate. Physical signs may be absent initially. DPL may provide a general indication for laparotomy, but is less accurate in diagnosing isolated bowel trauma (especially of the duodenum) because of its retroperitoneal location.[51] CT is a sensitive indicator of free intraperitoneal air, but signs of duodenal perforation or haematoma are subtle, even with enteral contrast.[52] Consequently, duodenal injury is often missed. A high index of suspicion should be maintained in patients with persistent abdominal pain and tenderness.

Bleeding from mesenteric vessels is often self-limiting and may not require surgical control. However, vessel damage can cause ischaemia and infarction, and may require resection of affected bowel. Uncomplicated blunt bowel injury can often be managed by primary repair and anastomosis. In penetrating injuries, colostomy or, increasingly, primary repair in selected patients[53] are used. A faecal diversion procedure with delayed repair is indicated in significant peritoneal soiling. With massive multiorgan trauma, haemostasis and control of GIT soiling may be appropriate initially, to allow stabilization before later definitive operation.[48–50,54]

Pancreas

Blunt injuries to the pancreas are often associated with duodenal, liver and splenic trauma. CT is the most useful investigation. Acute hyperamylasaemia does not predict pancreatic or hollow viscus injury.[28] Severe injuries to the body of the pancreas are best managed by distal pancreatectomy. The majority of penetrating injuries can be managed with sump drainage alone. Pancreaticoduodenectomy may be indicated in fewer than 5% of cases.[55] Complications such as fistula, abscess and pseudocyst are common.

Kidney and urinary tract

Blunt injury to the urinary tract is more common than penetrating injury. Identification and treatment of other major injuries often take precedence. Gross haematuria should be investigated; contrast-enhanced CT is the examination of choice if the patient is haemodynamically stable. Unless there is unexplained shock, microscopic haematuria does not require further investigation.[56] Renovascular pedicle or ureteric injuries may not cause any haematuria. Most renal injuries resolve with expectant management. Lacerations involving the collecting system or injury to the renal pedicle usually require operative intervention, although restoration of renal function following long warm ischaemic times is unusual. If major renal injury is discovered at emergency laparotomy, intraoperative IVU is prudent to ensure contralateral function.[57]

Bladder rupture is commonly associated with pelvic fractures. Over 95% of patients have macroscopic haematuria. Retrograde cystography is the investigation of choice, as CT is neither sensitive nor specific enough.[58] Intraperitoneal bladder rupture requires operative repair and urinary drainage. Selected patients with sterile urine and extraperitoneal rupture can be managed with catheter drainage alone.

Urethral trauma is caused by direct blunt injury, or occurs in association with pelvic injury. It should be suspected if there is blood at the urinary meatus, perineal injury or abnormal position of the prostate on rectal examination in the male. In the absence of these findings, cautious urethral catheterization is appropriate. Treatment of urethral trauma is suprapubic drainage and subsequent definitive repair.

Diaphragm

Diaphragmatic injury occurs in fewer than 5% of cases of blunt injury, is left-sided in 80% of cases,[59] and is commonly associated with injuries to abdominal organs.[60] It should also be suspected in penetrating trauma below the fifth rib. Diagnosis can be difficult, especially in the presence of positive-pressure ventilation, and may become evident only after ventilatory support is discontinued. Chest X-rays are commonly abnormal but often with non-specific findings. DPL is insensitive for isolated diaphragmatic injuries. Ultrasound may be better than CT because of its variable angle of view. Laparoscopy provides good views of the diaphragm. Spontaneous healing does not occur, and all defects should be repaired. The risk of associated injuries in acute cases mandates an abdominal approach.

Bony pelvis and perineum

Pelvic fractures are primarily caused by vehicular trauma or falls. Associated injuries to the bladder, urethra and intra-abdominal organs are common.[61] Injuries may be life-threatening initially from major haemorrhage, or later from sepsis. Significant morbidity can result from damage to pelvic nerves, urethra or the structural integrity of the pelvis. Pelvic injury is suggested by pain on movement, structural instability, gross haematuria or peripelvic ecchymosis. Rectal examination is mandatory to identify rectal injury and prostatic position. Radiography can confirm bony injury, but CT is required to identify associated intra-abdominal injuries (in the haemodynamically stable) and can assist in planning operative stabilization.

Patients with haemodynamic instability and pelvic fractures must have intra-abdominal haemorrhage excluded. Early open supraumbilical DPL is the investigation of choice.[22,62] If grossly positive, laparotomy should precede external fixation or angiography. If DPL is positive by cell count alone, the risk of life-threatening intra-abdominal haemorrhage is low, and achieving haemostasis for pelvic bleeding becomes the priority; laparotomy should follow if the patient is still unstable.[61,62] PASG are useful in the pre-hospital and emergency setting. External fixation of the pelvis can control venous and small arteriolar bleeding near fracture sites, and will reduce the volume of an open pelvis, thus improving tamponade. Angiography and selective embolization are often successful in controlling arterial haemorrhage,[63] but the logistics can be formidable. Bleeding from large vessels such as the aorta, common and external iliac arteries, and common femoral artery requires surgical control.

Pelvic fractures range from simple fractures of individual bones requiring bed rest alone to complex fractures. Early operative stabilization of complex pelvic fractures is preferred in ICU, as it facilitates respiratory care, pain control and early mobilization. Compound pelvic fractures involving the perineum, rectum or vagina require aggressive surgery (including diversion of the faecal stream) to avoid high mortality.[64]

Retroperitoneal haematoma

Retroperitoneal haematoma is frequent following blunt trauma, and is commonly caused by injury to the lumbar spine, bony pelvis, bladder or kidney or, less commonly, to the pancreas, duodenum or major vascular structures. Diagnosis may be inferred by excluding other sites of major blood loss, or presumed by signs of underlying organ injury. CT with enteral contrast is the most useful investigation in the stable patient. A central haematoma should be explored with proximal vascular control, because of the risk of pancreatic, duodenal or major vascular injury. A lateral or pelvic haematoma should not be explored, unless there is evidence of major arterial injury, intraperitoneal bladder rupture or colonic injury. Treatment of major renal injury remains controversial.[65]

Trauma in pregnancy

Women injured during pregnancy pose problems of altered physiology, risk to the gravid uterus and fetus, and conflict of priorities between mother and fetus. High-flow oxygen must be given until maternal hypoxaemia, hypovolaemia and fetal distress have been excluded. Reduced respiratory reserve demands earlier intervention. Maternal compensation for blood loss is at the expense of uteroplacental blood flow. Mothers should be positioned to avoid aortocaval compression and intravenous access should be in the upper limbs. Abdominal (but not lower limb) PASG are contraindicated. Transfusions should be Rhesus-compatible. All Rhesus-negative mothers should receive immune globulin, because of the immunological risk of even minor fetomaternal haemorrhage.[66]

Only X-rays that may significantly alter therapy should be taken (with appropriate shielding), especially if under 20 weeks' gestation. DPL is safe if performed by the open method above the fundus. CT may miss injuries due to abdominal crowding. Ultrasound is safe and can accurately detect free intra-abdominal fluid, confirm gestation and fetal well-being, and identify placental abnormalities.[66]

Retroperitoneal haemorrhage is more common in pregnant patients. Placental abruption may conceal significant blood loss. Treatment may be expectant or by caesarean section, depending on the condition of the mother and fetus. Uterine rupture is unusual and will usually require hysterectomy. Rarely, perimortem caesarean section may be indicated in a dead or dying mother, to attempt to save the fetus.[66]

Placental abruption, fetal distress and fetal loss are rare following blunt injury, but premature uterine contractions are common.[67,68] Continuous cardiotocography is the most sensitive test to detect obstetric complications, but is required for only 6 h[67] unless abnormalities are noted. Kleihauer–Betke tests to identify fetomaternal haemorrhage are not predictive of fetal or maternal morbidity.[67,68]

Complications

Haemorrhage

Patients with haemorrhage from abdominal and pelvic injuries can suffer the same complications of shock and massive transfusion as any patient with severe haemorrhage (see Chapter 14).

Dilutional coagulopathy is common following resuscitation with fluids deficient in haemostatic factors. Patients resuscitated with crystalloids, colloids and red cells often require platelet and fresh frozen plasma transfusions. Disseminated intravascular coagulation (DIC) occurs infrequently in trauma, usually when shock has been prolonged.

Sepsis

Intra-abdominal sepsis remains an important preventable cause of death after trauma. Predisposing factors include peritoneal contamination from GIT injury, external wounds, invasive procedures, delayed diagnosis of hollow viscus injuries, splenectomy and devitalized tissue. Early diagnosis and effective lavage and drainage procedures may reduce the incidence of intra-abdominal sepsis. Prophylactic antibiotics for 24 h are satisfactory for penetrating injuries.[69] The development of unexplained fever and/or neutrophil leukocytosis, or multiple organ failure, points to intra-abdominal sepsis. Septic shock may represent a second shock insult to the trauma patient, leading to multiorgan dysfunction.

Gastrointestinal failure

GIT failure in various forms, ranging from stress ulceration and delayed gastric emptying to paralytic ileus, is a frequent occurrence. Stress ulceration is generally treated with sucralfate or H_2 antagonists. The value of prophylactic administration is debated[70] (see Chapter 35). Parenteral nutrition may be necessary in patients with bowel injuries or severe retroperitoneal haematoma. Enteral nutrition is preferred as it is associated with a lower incidence of sepsis following trauma.[71,72] Feeding through a jejunostomy tube placed during surgery or radiologically in the ICU is often feasible.

Raised intra-abdominal pressure

Abdominal distension with raised intra-abdominal pressure may be seen in the critically injured, as a consequence of haemorrhage, bowel oedema, ileus or surgical packs. This can have severe adverse effects on respiratory, cardiovascular and renal function.[73] Alleviation is by abdominal decompression using interposed synthetic mesh,[73] or by leaving the abdomen open, with or without visceral packing.[74] The abdomen is subsequently closed by staged repair as the distension resolves.

References

1. Cameron P, Dziukas L, Hadj A, Clark P and Hooper S (1995) Patterns of injury from major trauma in Victoria. *Aust NZ J Surg* **65**:848–852.
2. Streat SJ, Donaldson ML and Judson JA (1987) Trauma in Auckland: an overview. *NZ Med J* **100**:441–444.
3. Anderson ID, Woodford M, de Dombal FT and Irving M (1988) Retrospective study of 1000 deaths from trauma in England and Wales. *Br Med J* **296**:1305–1308.
4. Champion HR, Copes WS, Sacco WJ *et al.* (1990) The Major Trauma Outcome Study: establishing norms for trauma care. *J Trauma* **30**:1356–1365.
5. Pattimore D, Thomas P and Dave SH (1992) Torso injury patterns and mechanisms in car crashes: an additional diagnostic tool. *Injury* **23**:123–126.
6. Rutledge R, Thomason M, Oller D *et al.* (1991) The spectrum of abdominal injuries associated with the use of seat belts. *J Trauma* **31**:820–826.
7. Fox MA, Fabian TC, Croce MA, Mangiante EC, Carson JC and Kudsk KA (1991) Anatomy of the accident scene: a prospective study of injury and mortality. *Am Surg* **57**:394–397.
8. McCarthy MC, Lowdermilk GA, Canal DF and Broadie DA (1991) Prediction of injury caused by penetrating wounds to the abdomen, flank and back. *Arch Surg* **126**:962–966.
9. Himmelman RG, Martin M, Gilkey S and Barrett JA (1991) Triple-contrast CT scans in penetrating back and flank trauma. *J Trauma* **31**:852–855.
10. Feliciano DV, Burch JM, Spjut-Patrinely V, Mattox KL and Jordan GL (1988) Abdominal gunshot wounds. *Ann Surg* **208**:362–367.
11. American College of Surgeons Committee on Trauma (1993) *Advanced Trauma Life Support Program for Physicians: Instructor Manual.* Chicago: American College of Surgeons.
12. Civil IDS (1993) Resuscitation following injury: an end or a means? *Aust NZ J Surg* **63**:921–926.
13. Bickell WH, Wall MJ, Pepe PE *et al.* (1994) Immediate versus delayed resuscitation for hypotensive patients with penetrating torso injuries. *N Engl J Med* **331**:1105–1109.
14. Mattox KL, Bickell WH, Pepe PE, Burch J and Feliciano D (1989) Prospective MAST study in 911 patients. *J Trauma* **29**:1104–1112.
15. Prall JA, Nichols JS, Brennan R and Moore EE (1994) Early definitive abdominal evaluation in the triage of unconscious normotensive blunt trauma patients. *J Trauma* **37**:792–797.
16. Stevenson J and Battisella FD (1994) The 'one-shot' intravenous pyelogram: is it indicated in unstable trauma patients before celiotomy? *J Trauma* **36**:828–834.
17. Salvino CK, Esposito TJ, Smith D *et al.* (1992) Routine pelvic X-ray studies in awake blunt trauma patients: a sensible policy? *J Trauma* **33**:413–416.
18. Koury HI, Peschiera JL and Welling RE (1993) Selective use of pelvic roentgenograms in blunt trauma patients. *J Trauma* **34**:236–237.
19. Bilge A and Sahin M (1991) Diagnostic peritoneal lavage in blunt abdominal trauma. *Eur J Surg* **157**:449–451.

20. Cue JI, Miller FB, Cryer HM, Malangoni MA and Richardson JD (1990) A prospective, randomized comparison between open and closed peritoneal lavage techniques. *J Trauma* **30**:880–883.

21. Lopez-Viego MA, Mickel TJ and Weigelt JA (1990) Open versus closed diagnostic peritoneal lavage in the evaluation of abdominal trauma. *Am J Surg* **160**:594–596.

22. Mendez C, Gubler KD and Maier RV (1994) Diagnostic accuracy of peritoneal lavage in patients with pelvic fractures. *Arch Surg* **129**:477–482.

23. Day AC, Rankin N and Charlesworth P (1992) Diagnostic peritoneal lavage: integration with clinical information to improve diagnostic performance. *J Trauma* **32**:52–57.

24. Driscoll P, Hodgkinson D and Mackway-Jones K (1992) Diagnostic peritoneal lavage: it's red but is it positive. *Injury* **23**:267–269.

25. McAnena OJ, Marx JA and Moore EE (1991) Peritoneal lavage enzyme determinations following blunt and penetrating abdominal trauma. *J Trauma* **31**:1161–1164.

26. Jaffin JH, Ochsner MG, Cole FJ, Rozycki GS, Kass M and Champion HR (1993) Alkaline phosphatase levels in diagnostic peritoneal lavage fluid as a predictor of hollow visceral injury. *J Trauma* **34**:829–833.

27. Jacobs DG, Angus L, Rodriguez A and Militello PR (1990) Peritoneal lavage white count: a reassessment. *J Trauma* **30**:607–612.

28. Boulanger BR, Milzman DP, Rosati C and Rodriguez A (1993) The clinical significance of acute hyperamylasemia after blunt trauma. *Can J Surg* **36**:63–69.

29. Feliciano DV (1991) Diagnostic modalities in abdominal trauma. Peritoneal lavage, ultrasonography, computed tomography scanning, and arteriography. *Surg Clin North Am* **71**:241–256.

30. Wolfman NT, Bechtold RE, Scharling ES and Meredith JW (1992) Blunt upper abdominal trauma: evaluation by CT. *Am J Roentgenol* **158**:493–501.

31. McGehee M, Kier R, Cohn SM and McCarthy-SM (1993) Comparison of MRI with postcontrast CT for the evaluation of acute abdominal trauma. *J Comput Assist Tomogr* **17**:410–413.

32. Meredith JW, Ditesheim JA, Stonehouse S and Wolfman N (1992) Computed tomography and diagnostic peritoneal lavage. Complementary roles in blunt trauma. *Am Surg* **58**:44–48.

33. Goletti O, Ghiselli G, Lippolis PV *et al.* (1994) The role of ultrasonography in blunt abdominal trauma: results of 250 consecutive cases. *J Trauma* **36**:178–181.

34. Rothlin MA, Naf R, Amgwerd M, Candinas D, Frick T and Trentz O (1993) Ultrasound in blunt abdominal and thoracic trauma. *J Trauma* **34**:488–495.

35. Forster R, Pillasch J, Zielke A, Malewski U and Rothmund M (1993) Ultrasound in blunt abdominal trauma: influence on the investigators' experience. *J Trauma* **34**:264–269.

36. McKenney M, Lentz K, Nunez D *et al.* (1994) Can ultrasound replace diagnostic peritoneal lavage in the assessment of blunt trauma. *J Trauma* **37**:439–441.

37. Rozycki GS, Oschner MG, Jaffin JH and Champion HR (1993) Prospective evaluation of surgeons' use of ultrasound in the evaluation of trauma patients. *J Trauma* **34**:516–527.

38. Ivatury RR, Simon RJ and Stahl WM (1993) A critical evaluation of laparoscopy in penetrating abdominal trauma. *J Trauma* **34**:822–828.

39. Livingston DH, Tortella BJ, Blackwood J, Machiedo GW and Rush BF (1992) The role of laparoscopy in abdominal trauma. *J Trauma* **33**:471–475.

40. Fernando HC, Alle KM, Chen J, Davis I and Kein SR (1994) Triage by laparoscopy in patients with penetrating abdominal trauma. *Br J Surg* **81**:384–385.

41. Klein SR, Saroyan RM, Baumgartner F and Bongard FS (1992) Management strategy of vascular injuries associated with pelvic fractures. *J Cardiovasc Surg* **33**:348–357.

42. Wilson RH and Moorehead RJ (1992) Management of splenic trauma. *Injury* **23**:5–9.

43. Farhat GA, Abdu RA and Vanek VW (1992) Delayed splenic rupture: real or imaginary? *Am Surg* **58**: 340–345.

44. Smith JS, Wengrovitz MA and DeLong BS (1992) Prospective validation of criteria, including age for safe, non-surgical management of the ruptured spleen. *J Trauma* **33**:363–368.

45. Kohn JS, Clark DE, Isler RJ and Pope CF (1994) Is computed tomographic grading of splenic injury useful in the nonsurgical management of blunt trauma? *J Trauma* **36**:385–390.

46. Sherman HF, Savage BA, Jones LM, Berrette RR, Latenser BA and Varcelotti JR (1994) Nonoperative management of blunt hepatic injuries: safe at any grade? *J Trauma* **37**:616–621.

47. Hammond JC, Canal DF and Broadie TA (1992) Nonoperative management of adult blunt hepatic trauma in a municipal trauma center. *Am Surg* **58**:551–556.

48. Burch JM, Ortiz VB, Richardson RJ, Martin RR, Mattox KL and Jordan GL (1992) Abbreviated laparotomy and planned reoperation for critically injured patients. *Ann Surg* **215**:476–484.

49. Rotondo MF, Schwab CW, McGonigal MD *et al.* (1993) 'Damage control': an approach for improved survival in exsanguinating penetrating trauma. *J Trauma* **35**:375–383.

50. Hirshberg A, Wall MJ and Mattox KL (1994) Planned reoperation for trauma: a two year experience with 124 consecutive patients. *J Trauma* **37**:365–369.

51. Enderson BL and Maull KI (1991) Missed injuries: the trauma surgeon's nemesis. *Surg Clin North Am* **71**:399–418.

52. Kunin JR, Korobkin M, Ellis JH, Francis IR, Kane NM and Seigel SE (1993) Duodenal injuries from blunt trauma: value of CT in differentiating perforation from hematoma. *Am J Roentgenol* **160**:1221–1223.

53. Schultz SC, Magnant CM, Richman MF, Holt RW and Evans SR (1993) Identifying the low-risk patient with penetrating colonic injury for selective use of primary repair. *Surg Gynecol Obstet* **177**:237–242.

54. Carillo C, Fogler RJ and Shaftan GW (1993) Delayed gastrointestinal reconstruction following massive abdominal trauma. *J Trauma* **34**:233–235.

55. Jones RC (1985) Management of pancreatic trauma. *Am J Surg* **150**:698–704.

56. Knudson MM, McAninch JW, Gomez R, Lee P and Stubbs HA (1992) Hematuria as a predictor of abdominal injury after blunt trauma. *Am J Surg* **164**:482–486.

57. Schneider RE (1993) Genitourinary trauma. *Emerg Med Clin North Am* **11**:137–145.

58. Rehm CG, Mure AJ and O'Malley KF (1991) Blunt traumatic bladder rupture: the role of retrograde cystogram. *Ann Emerg Med* **20**:845–847.

59. Sukul DM, Kats E and Johannes EJ (1991) Sixty-three cases of traumatic injury of the diaphragm. *Injury* **22**:303–306.

60. Voeller GR, Reisser JR, Fabian TC, Kudsuk K and Mangiante EC (1990) Blunt diaphragm injuries. A five year experience. *Am Surg* **56**:28–31.

61. Jerrard DA (1993) Pelvic fractures. *Emerg Med Clin North Am* **11**:147–163.

62. Evers BM, Cryer HM and Miller FB (1989) Pelvic fracture hemorrhage. *Arch Surg* **124**:422–424.

63. Ben-Menachem Y, Coldwell DM, Young JW and Burgess AR (1991) Hemorrhage associated with pelvic fractures: causes, diagnosis and emergent management. *Am J Roentgenol* **157**:1005–1014.

64. Davidson BS, Simmons GT, Williamson PR and Buerk CA (1993) Pelvic fractures associated with open perineal wounds: a survivable injury. *J Trauma* **35**:36–39.

65. Feliciano DV (1990) Management of traumatic retroperitoneal haematoma. *Ann Surg* **211**:109–123.

66. Esposito TJ (1994) Trauma during pregnancy. *Emerg Med Clin North Am* **12**:167–199.

67. Towery R, English P and Wisner D (1993) Evaluation of pregnant women after blunt injury. *J Trauma* **35**: 731–736.

68. Dahmus MA and Sibai BM (1993) Blunt abdominal trauma: are there predictive factors for abruptio placentae or maternal–fetal distress? *Am J Obstet Gynecol* **169**:1054–1059.

69. Fabian TC, Croce MA, Payne LW, Minard G, Pritchard FE and Kudsk KA (1992) Duration of antibiotic therapy for penetrating trauma: a prospective trial. *Surgery* **112**:788–794.

70. Cook DJ, Witt LG, Cook RJ and Guyatt GH (1991) Stress ulcer prophylaxis in the critically ill: a meta-analysis. *Am J Med* **91**:519–527.

71. Kudsk KA, Croce MA, Fabian TC *et al.* (1992) Enteral versus parenteral feeding. Effects on septic morbidity after blunt and penetrating abdominal trauma. *Ann Surg* **215**:503–513.

72. Streat SJ and Hill GL (1987) Nutritional support in the management of critically ill patients in surgical intensive care. *World J Surg* **11**:194–201.

73. Torrie J, Hill AA and Streat S (1966) Staged abdominal repair in critical illness. *Anaesth Intens Care* **24**:368–374.

74. Bender JS, Bailey CE, Saxe JM, Ledgerwood AM and Lucas CE (1994) The technique of visceral packing: recommended management of difficult fascial closure in trauma patients. *J Trauma* **2**:182–185.

Part XI

Environmental injuries

71 | Near-drowning

TE Oh

Death by drowning claims over 700 lives each year in the UK,[1] 500 in Australia,[2] and 8000 in the USA.[3] Drowning and accidents are the leading causes of death in children and adolescents in many countries,[3-6] and drowning rates, especially in toddlers, appear unchanged.[7] Alcohol consumption is associated with the majority of adult drownings.[8,9] Others result from boating accidents, fishing mishaps,[10] suicides, epileptic attacks,[11,12] and surf and river misadventures. Childhood drownings involve swimming pools, bathtubs, buckets, ponds, creeks and the sea with older children.[3,6,9,13] Nearly all paediatric drownings are caused by inadequate adult supervision,[3,6] but epilepsy (especially in bathtub drownings) and child abuse are also factors.[9,14,15] Near-drowning may then be defined as 'survival, at least temporary, following asphyxia while immersed in a liquid medium'.[16] Useful figures of near-drowning cases are unknown, but are estimated to be three to five times more frequent than drownings.

Pathophysiology[3,17,18]

Upon submersion, there is an initial period of voluntary apnoea. The 'diving reflex'[19,20] (as induced by cold-water immersion of the face), consisting of apnoea, bradycardia and intense peripheral vasoconstriction with preferential blood shunting to the heart and brain, occurs in infants and toddlers, and to a lesser extent, in adults. Initial voluntary apnoea reaches a breakpoint (determined by hypercarbic and hypoxic drives) when involuntary inspiration is made. Water then enters the lungs, and gasping occurs. Laryngeal spasm may follow in some victims. Airway resistance is increased, reflex pulmonary vasoconstriction occurs, surfactant is diminished, and lung compliance is decreased. Water shifts from alveoli into the circulation. Swallowing, vomiting and aspiration of vomitus are likely. A phase of secondary apnoea follows within seconds of immersion, proceeded by further involuntary gasping and loss of consciousness. Respiratory arrest and cardiac arrhythmias occur several minutes later and precede death.

Hyperventilation before diving increases the risk of death by drowning. The resultant hypocarbia will suppress the central drive to breathe, even in the presence of severe hypoxaemia from the prolonged voluntary breath-holding. Consciousness is lost before spontaneous central respiratory efforts resume.

Aspirated fluid

In fresh-water drowning, water is quickly absorbed into the circulation and may cause haemolysis. Pulmonary surfactant characteristics are altered (denatured) producing widespread atelectasis. Electrolyte changes are usually insignificant and transient. Haemolysis may rarely produce haemoglobinuria and acute renal failure. Any chlorine and soap in fresh water does not appear to be of any adverse consequence to the lungs.

In sea-water drowning, the hypertonic salt water promotes rapid fluxes of water and plasma proteins into the alveoli (i.e. pulmonary oedema) and interstitium, dilutes or washes out surfactant, and may disrupt the alveolar–capillary membrane. However, alveolar epithelial function may be well-preserved after salt-water aspiration.[21] Both inhaled fresh and sea water may produce an inflammatory reaction in the alveolar–capillary membrane, leading to an outpouring of plasma-rich exudate into the alveoli. Inhaled gastric contents may contribute to this reaction.

Lung injury

Regardless of the immersion medium, the above changes lead to increased peripheral airway resistance, widespread atelectasis, pulmonary oedema, severe intrapulmonary shunting, gross ventilation: perfusion mismatch, increased pulmonary vasoconstriction, decreased compliance and marked hypoxaemia. Hypoxaemia and large increases in intrapulmonary shunting can occur with inhalation of as little as 2.5 ml/kg body weight.[22]

Denaturization of surfactant can continue despite successful resuscitation. The term secondary drowning has been used to describe pulmonary insufficiency which may develop any time up to 72 h after the event.[23] This occurs after a period of improvement following resuscitation and is seen in a small percentage of survivors. In fresh-water immersion, this sudden pulmonary deterioration may be pulmonary oedema due to altered capillary permeability.[3] Hyaline membrane formation in small airways and alveoli has been demonstrated at autopsy in patients who have survived from 12 to 72 h.[24] Infection and the acute respiratory distress syndrome (ARDS) may follow a near-drowning incident.

Cardiovascular effects

The cardiovascular system of most near-drowned victims shows remarkable stability. A wide variety of electrocardiogram (ECG) changes have been reported. Blood pressure changes are secondary to oxygenation, acid–base status, systemic vascular resistance and cardiac function. Blood volume changes secondary to fresh- or salt-water aspiration are rarely significant enough to be life-threatening. Consequently, changes in haemoglobin and haematocrit are usually not marked.

Superimposed hypothermia

Hypothermia may aid survival. Victims of prolonged submersion (e.g. over 1 h) in very cold water, especially children, have recovered completely, suggesting protective effects of induced cooling. However, the true mechanism of brain protection is unknown. Physiologically, body temperature cannot be cooled sufficiently within 10 min (before irreversible brain damage occurs) by surface cooling or ingestion and aspiration of large amounts of cold water.[20] Hypothermia may adversely complicate drowning. Cold water impairs motor activity and movement. Even strong swimmers with lifejackets drown within minutes if the water is very cold (e.g. 4°C).[25] Uncontrolled involuntary hyperventilation occurs in cold immersion,[26] and consciousness may be impaired, resulting in drowning. Hence submersion is not essential for drowning, and lifejackets will not always prevent drowning.

Mechanisms of death

Different mechanisms of death can occur in a drowning victim. The final outcome – brain death – can be caused by cerebral hypoxia, laryngeal spasm, lung reflexes and vagally mediated cardiac

arrest. The last three are immersion or submersion causes alone, rather than true drowning with water aspiration.[27] An estimated 10% of drownings are 'dry', i.e. little or no fluid is found in the lungs at autopsy. It has been suggested that initial entry of water into the larynx may produce a (vagal) reflex laryngospasm, which persists until asphyxial death supervenes.[3,17–19] The laryngospasm is immediately followed by an outpouring of thick mucus which, with bronchospasm, may prevent entry of water when the spasm relaxes shortly before death. 'Dry drowning' appears to be more common in adults, and facilitation of such pulmonary reflexes by raised blood alcohol levels has been suggested.[28]

Management[3,29]

The basic pathophysiological problems of fresh- and salt-water drownings are similar – hypoxaemia, pulmonary oedema, metabolic acidosis and circulatory dysfunction. Initial management of the critically ill survivor is thus similar, discounting whether fresh or salt water was the immersion medium. Therapy is directed towards restoring adequate oxygenation and circulation, correcting acid–base imbalance, and cerebral resuscitation and protection.

Immediate first-aid treatment

Immediate on-site resuscitation is the most important factor of good outcome.[30–33] Basic life support must be initiated without delay (see Chapter 7). In children, about 30% of survivors would have died if not for proper cardiopulmonary resuscitation.[9] Lung drainage procedures or the Heimlich manoeuvre are controversial.[34] There is a likelihood of inducing vomiting, since over half the immersion victims vomit during resuscitation.[25] Advanced life support is started when experienced personnel arrive. Oxygen is given and the victim kept warm while *en route* to hospital. The possibility of head and spinal injury, especially in diving or surfing accidents, must be remembered during resuscitation.

Hospital and ICU treatment

Significant benefits of intensive care after near-drowning are doubtful.[35,36] Resuscitation must continue on arrival at hospital. A nasogastric tube must be inserted to decompress the stomach and drain possible large volumes of water. Details of the time, place and medium of immersion and the water temperature should be obtained. Other helpful information includes resuscitation details (e.g. duration of apnoea or asystole and level of consciousness), whether head or neck injuries were sustained, and the past health of the victim (e.g. whether an epileptic, asthmatic or alcoholic).

Restoring ventilation and oxygenation

Oxygen is given by a semi-rigid mask if the patient is breathing spontaneously. Bronchospasm, if present, is relieved by aminophylline and β2-adrenergic agents. Continuous positive airway pressure (CPAP) with a mask will improve oxygenation if the patient is conscious and able to breathe adequately. Mechanical ventilation is instituted in patients with severe hypoxaemia and pulmonary oedema. Positive end-expiratory pressure (PEEP) improves pulmonary oedema as well as ventilation : perfusion mismatch. Treatment of ARDS is described in Chapter 29.

Restoring circulation

Low cardiac output is corrected by positive inotropic agents (e.g. adrenaline or dobutamine infusion) and fluid replacement. Isotonic fluids are usually all that is required, but plasma and blood may be needed if haemolysis is severe. Fluid replacement is guided by central venous pressure and pulmonary capillary wedge pressure measurements if indicated. Arrhythmias from acidosis, hypoxia, hypothermia and electrolyte abnormalities are treated conventionally.

Correcting acidosis

Sodium bicarbonate 50–100 mmol IV is given if the metabolic acidosis is significant (e.g. pH < 7.0).

Rewarming

Core temperatures should be rewarmed to above 28°C, as lower temperatures may give rise to spontaneous ventricular fibrillation and prolong coma. Induced hypothermia for brain protection (e.g. using surface ice packs) is controversial (see below). Normothermia should probably be maintained. Rewarming can be accomplished by warmed intravenous fluids, humidification of inspired gases and heated blankets. Hot baths are difficult to carry out in practice. More aggressive forms of treatment include warm peritoneal lavage and cardiopulmonary bypass[37,38] but are rarely indicated.

Cerebral protection

Attempts at brain resuscitation and protection are probably important (see Chapter 44). Treatment protocols include lowering *raised* body temperature, maintaining adequate oxygenation, blood pressure and circulation, correcting hyperglycaemia and controlling seizures. Monitoring and management of intracranial pressure (ICP) are controversial.[3] Proponents recommend maintaining ICP below 20 mmHg (2.7 kPa) and cerebral perfusion pressure above 50 mmHg (6.7 kPa)[39] while detractors contend that ICP monitoring does not influence outcome.[40,41] Induced hypothermia lacks beneficial evidence and may increase the risk of infection by altering white blood cell function.[3] There is no evidence to support the use of steroids and barbiturates for brain protection, and they should not be given.

Other treatment

Usual supportive care is given (e.g. correction of electrolye abnormalities, nutrition and physiotherapy. Prophylactic antibiotics are not useful.[3] A broad-spectrum antibiotic (e.g. second-generation cephalosporin) is indicated if there are signs of infection. The immersion site may influence on the type of inhaled organism and thus antibiotics. Hyperbaric oxygen therapy has been used in a few isolated reports,[42] but proper data are lacking.

Investigations and monitoring

Conventional ICU monitoring

This includes body temperature, ECG, arterial and central venous pressures, pulmonary artery pressures if indicated, arterial blood gases and saturation (by pulse oximetry). Lung shunting equations (e.g. alveolar–arterial oxygen gradient) will indicate progress and guide therapy.

Serum biochemistry

Theoretically, serum electrolyte levels are decreased in fresh-water drowning and increased in salt-water drowning. However, gross changes are rarely seen, because aspiration of large volumes of water is required to produce persistent changes in serum concentrations. Serum osmolality estimation on admission may be useful.

Haematological

Haemoconcentration may disguise the presence of anaemia. Tests for haemolysis are:

1 free haemoglobin in urine and plasma;
2 decreased serum haptoglobins. Free plasma haemoglobin combines with serum haptoglobins, and the resultant complex is taken up by the liver;
3 increased serum methaemalbumin. Free plasma haemoglobin divides into globin and haem.

The haem moiety is oxidized into methaem, which combines with serum albumin.

Radiology and imaging

A chest X-ray may show infiltrates and pulmonary oedema. Skull and cervical X-rays are required if spinal injury is suspected. Head CT scans are indicated for comatose patients. Single-photon emission CT can identify hypometabolic, but viable cortical brain areas.[42] Where there is suspicion of child abuse (e.g. bathtub immersion), consideration is given to a skeletal survey examination.

Neurological

Evoked brain potential tests and electroencephalograms may help to assess progress and outlook.[43] Psychometric assessments are recommended in survivors with suspected intellectual damage.

Drug assays

Estimations of blood alcohol and serum concentrations of anticonvulsant and sedative drugs may be indicated on admission.

Microbiological

Cultures of aspirated water, tracheal swabs and sputum may be indicated in severely polluted water immersion.

Complications

ICU complications of near-drowning include late pulmonary oedema (see above), fits, hyperpyrexia, pneumonia, septicaemia, gastrointestinal bleeding, ARDS and multiorgan failure.

Table 71.1 Predictors of death or severe neurological deficits after near-drowning

---

At the site of immersion
Immersion duration > 10 min and CPR duration > 25 min[33]

First respiratory effort after 30 min of CPR[44]

In the emergency department
Unreactive pupils and Glasgow coma score ≤ 5[36]

CPR still required on arrival[31]

Fixed dilated pupils and an arterial pH < 7.0[48]

CPR duration > 25 min[49]

In the ICU
No spontaneous, purposeful movements and abnormal brainstem function 24 h after immersion.[45]

Abnormal CT within 36 h of immersion. A normal CT on admission is a poor predictor[46]

Lower cerebral metabolic rate and lower cross-brain oxygen difference (systemic arterial oxygen content minus jugular venous bulb oxygen content)[47]

CPR = Cardiopulmonary resuscitation; CT = computed tomography.

Prognosis[3,31–33,36,42–49]

A short duration of immersion and immediate resuscitation undoubtedly favours better outcome[31–33] Children, cold-water immersion and low core temperatures appear to have a better prognosis. The best outcome predictors are obtained in the field. On arrival at hospital, sinus rhythm, reactive pupils and neurological responsiveness (especially an awake or rousable state) are good prognostic indicators,[33] but not arterial blood gases (even though hypoxaemia and metabolic acidosis frequently correlate with severity of pulmonary injury). Predictors of death or severe neurological impairment are listed in Table 71.1.

Of all child survivors in Queensland, about 70% recovered completely, 30% have selective deficits and 3% exist in a permanent vegetative state.[9] Debate currently exists on whether aggressive intensive care management should continue in initial survivors with poor outcome predictors. In general, field predictors are reasonably reliable, and intensive care may not significantly alter outcome. However, there are well-documented case reports of adult and child immersion victims with abysmal outcome predictors who have made complete or good recoveries.[20,50,51] Resuscitation and treatment should probably not be abandoned early, especially in young victims of cold-water immersion.

References

1. Golden F St C and Rivers JF (1975) The immersion accident. *Anesthesia* **30**:364–373.
2. Pearn J (1977) Drowning in Australia: a national appraisal with particular reference to children. *Med J Aust* **ii**:770–771.
3. Levin DL, Morriss FC, Toro LO, Brink LW and Turner GR (1993) Drowning and near-drowning. *Pediatr Clin North Am* **40**:321–336.
4. Pearn J, Nixon J and Wilkey I (1976) Freshwater drowning and near-drowning accidents involving children. *Med J Aust* **2**:942–946.
5. Mizuta R, Fujita H, Osamura T, Kidowaki T and Kiyosawa NT (1993) Childhood drownings and near-drownings in Japan. *Acta Paediatr Jpn* **35**:186–192.
6. Kemp A and Sibert JR (1992) Drowning and near drowning in children in the United Kingdom: lessons for prevention. *Br Med J* **304**:1143–1146.
7. Brenner RA, Smith GS and Overpeck MD (1994) Divergent trends in childhood drowning rates, 1971 through 1988. *J Am Med Assoc* **271**:1606–1608.
8. Mackie I (1979) Alcohol and aquatic disasters. *Practitioner* **222**:662–665.
9. Pearn J (1992) Medical aspects of drowning in children. *Ann Acad Med Singapore* **21**:433–435.
10. Rafnsson V and Gunnarsdottir H (1992) Fatal accidents among Icelandic seamen: 1966–86. *Br J Ind Med* **49**:694–699.

11. Saxena A and Ang LC (1993) Epilepsy and bathtub drowning. Important neuropathological observations. *Am J Forensic Med Pathol* **14**:125–129.

12. Lip GY and Brodie MJ (1992) Sudden death in epilepsy: an avoidable outcome? *J R Soc Med* **85**:609–611.

13. Jensen LR, Williams SD, Thurman DJ and Keller PA (1992) Submersion injuries in children younger than 5 years in urban Utah. *West J Med* **157**:641–644.

14. Diekema DS, Quan L and Holt VL (1993) Epilepsy as a risk factor for submersion injury in children. *Pediatrics* **91**:612–616.

15. Kemp AM and Sibert JR (1993) Epilepsy in children and the risk of drowning. *Arch Dis Child* **68**:684–685.

16. Modell JH (1981) Drown versus near-drowning: a discussion of definitions. *Crit Care Med* **9**:351–352.

17. Gonzalez-Rothi RJ (1987) Near drowning: consensus and controversies in pulmonary and cerebral resuscitation. *Heart Lung* **16**:474–482.

18. Pearn J (1985) Pathophysiology of drowning. *Med J Aust* **142**:586–588.

19. Gooden BA (1972) Drowning and the diving reflex in man. *Med J Aust* **2**:583–587.

20. Gooden BA (1992) Why some people do not drown. Hypothermia versus the diving response. *Med J Aust* **157**:629–632.

21. Cohen DS, Matthay MA, Cogan MG and Murray JF (1992) Pulmonary edema associated with salt water near-drowning: new insights. *Am Rev Respir Dis* **146**:794–796.

22. Modell JH, Calderwood HW, Ruiz BC, Downs JB and Chapman R Jr. (1974) Effects of ventilatory patterns on arterial oxygenation after near-drowning in sea water. *Anesthesiology* **40**:376–384.

23. Pearn JH (1980) Secondary drowning in children. *Br Med J* **281**:1103–1105.

24. Fuller RH (1963) Drowning and the post immersion syndrome. A clinicopathologic study. *Military Med* **128**:22–36.

25. Editorial (1978) Near-drowning. *Lancet* **2**:194–195.

26. Keatinge WR and Evans M (1961) The respiratory and cardio-vascular response to immersion in cold and warm water. *Q J Exp Physiol* **46**:83–94.

27. Editorial (1981) Immersion or drowning? *Br Med J* **282**:1340–1341.

28. Pearn J (1984) Drowning and alcohol. *Med J Aust* **141**:6–7.

29. Pearn J (1985) The management of near drowning. *Br Med J* **291**:1447–1452.

30. Olshaker JS (1992) Near drowning. *Emerg Med Clin North Am* **10**:339–350.

31. Fields AI (1992) Near-drowning in the pediatric population. *Crit Care Clin* **8**:113–129.

32. Kyriacou DN, Arcinue EL, Peek C and Kraus JF (1994) Effect of immediate resuscitation on children with submersion injury. *Pediatrics* **94**:137–142.

33. Quan L and Kinder D (1992) Pediatric submersions: prehospital predictors of outcome. *Pediatrics* **90**:909–913.

34. Quan L (1993) Drowning issues in resuscitation. *Ann Emerg Med* **22**:366–369.

35. Kallas HJ and O'Rourke PP (1993) Drowning and immersion injuries in children. *Curr Opin Pediatr* **5**:295–302.

36. Lavelle JM and Shaw KN (1993) Near drowning: is emergency department cardiopulmonary resuscitation or intensive care unit cerebral resuscitation indicated? *Crit Care Med* **21**:368–373.

37. Letsou GV, Kopf GS, Elefteriades JA, Carter JE, Baldwin JC and Hammond GL (1992) Is cardiopulmonary bypass effective for treatment of hypothermic arrest due to drowning or exposure? *Arch Surg* **127**:525–528.

38. Waters DJ, Belz M, Lawse D and Ulstad D (1994) Portable cardiopulmonary bypass: resuscitation from prolonged ice-water submersion and asystole. *Ann Thorac Surg* **57**:1018–1019.

39. Nussbaum E and Galant SP (1983) Intracranial pressure monitoring as a guide to prognosis in the early drowned, severe comatosed child. *J Pediatr* **102**:215–218.

40. Bohn DJ, Biggar WD, Smith CR *et al.* (1986) Influence of hypothermia, barbiturate therapy, and intracranial pressure monitoring on morbidity and mortality after near-drowning. *Crit Care Med* **14**:529–533.

41. Modell JH (1986) Treatment of near-drowning. Is there a role for the HYPER therapy? *Crit Care Med* **14**:593–594.

42. Neubauer RA, Gottlieb SF and Miale A Jr (1992) Identification of hypometabolic areas in the brain using brain imaging and hyperbaric oxygen. *Clin Nucl Med* **17**:477–481.

43. Fisher B, Peterson B and Hicks G (1992) Use of brainstem auditory-evoked response testing to assess neurologic outcome following near drowning in children. *Crit Care Med* **20**:578–585.

44. Pearn JH (1985) Drowning. In: Dickerman JD and Lucey JF (eds) *The Critically Ill Child. Diagnosis and Management*, 3rd edn. Philadelphia: W B Saunders, pp. 129–156.

45. Bratton SL, Jardine DS and Morray JP (1994) Serial neurologic examinations after near drowning and outcome. *Arch Pediatr Adolesc Med* **148**:167–170.

46. Romano C, Brown T and Frewen TC (1993) Assessment of pediatric near-drowning victims: is there a role for cranial CT? *Pediatr Radiol* **23**:261–263.

47. Connors R, Frewen TC, Kissoon N *et al.* (1992) Relationship of cross-brain oxygen content difference, cerebral blood flow, and metabolic rate to neurologic outcome after near-drowning. *J Pediatr* **121**:839–844.

48. Frates RC (1981) Analysis of predictive factors in the assessment of warm water near-drowning in children. *Am J Dis Child* **135**:1006–1008.

49. Waugh JH, O'Callaghan MJ and Pitt WR (1994) Prognostic factors and long term outcomes for children who have nearly drowned. *Med J Aust* **161**:594–599.

50. Mahoney PF, Williams L and Andrews JI (1993) Successful resuscitation from sea water drowning. *Arch Emerg Med* **10**:120–122.

51. Johnstone B and Bouman DE (1992) Anoxic encephalopathy: a case study of an eight-year-old male with no residual cognitive deficits. *Int J Neurosci* **62**:207–213.

72   Burns

RC Freebairn and TE Oh

Burns can result from temperature extremes (i.e. frostbite to severe heat) as well as from radiation or electrical injuries. Victims commonly tend to be young or elderly. Severe burns produce devastating physical and psychological effects. Therapy ranges from initial resuscitation to eventual surgery and rehabilitation. Burns patients are most effectively treated by specially trained staff in an isolated environment controlled in temperature and humidity.[1] This chapter will limit discussion to resuscitation and ICU management.

Pathophysiology[2,3]

Human skin can tolerate temperatures up to 40°C, but cellular destruction follows exposure to temperatures above 45°C.[2] Skin and deeper tissues are injured by direct cellular injury and delayed progressive ischaemia. Three zones of thermal injury can be delineated: a central zone of coagulation; a zone of stasis extending from the epicentre, in which viable tissue will undergo ischaemic necrosis if resuscitation is inadequate; and a distant zone of hyperaemia which will recover.[2]

Oedema formation follows burn injuries, with maximal effects within 24 h. This is due to fluid and protein shifts, as a result of vascular permeability, low oncotic capillary pressure and increased interstitial osmotic pressure.[3] Increased interstitial osmotic pressure is felt to be due to sodium binding to injured collagen. Vasoactive substances, e.g. leukotrienes, prostaglandins, oxygen radicals, serotonin and histamine are believed to be important factors of increased vascular permeability. Generalized oedema (i.e. also in non-burn tissue) occurs in burns above 20–30% of total body surface area (BSA). In these major burns, there is a decrease in cell transmembrane potential of non-burn tissue, leading to a shift of interstitial sodium and water into the cells.

Since the skin is a protective barrier and a thermoregulator, heat and water loss and invasion by microorganisms are major early pathophysiological changes following severe burns. The systemic inflammatory response syndrome is also precipitated by inflammatory mediators in major burn injuries.

Cardiovascular and circulatory effects

Significant cardiovascular changes are likely in the first 48 h in burns over 20% BSA. 'Burn shock' is a combination of hypovolaemic and cellular shock.[4] There is decreased circulating blood volume and extracellular fluid volume, coupled with an inadequate supply of substrates at the cellular level. Cardiac output is significantly decreased, due to the reduced plasma volume and myocardial depression (possibly the effect of circulating cytokines). Red cell loss from haemolysis and intravascular coagulation may reach 1% red cell mass per 1% of full-skin-thickness burn. Coagulopathy may occur in the resuscitation phase. Apart from dilutional effects, clotting factors are reduced and platelet aggregation occurs. Disseminated intravascular coagulation is common in extensive burns. A hypercoagulable state may develop 2 weeks after the burn injury.

Respiratory effects

Pulmonary dysfunction is a major cause of mortality or morbidity. Burns in a closed environment may cause inhalation injury plus intoxication from combustion products. Of these, carbon monoxide and cyanide are extremely important (Table 72.1). Toxic combustion products arise mainly from the burning of synthetic materials in clothes and furnishings. Burns impair respiratory function by causing injuries to the airway, lung and respiratory cells.

Airway injury

Direct heat injury caused by inhalation of heated air results in burns to the oropharynx and upper airways (i.e. above vocal cords). Inhalation of chemicals,

Table 72.1 Common causes of inhalational injury

Gas	Source	Effect
Carbon monoxide	Any organic matter	Tissue hypoxia, lipid peroxidation
Carbon dioxide	Any organic matter	Narcosis, tachycardia, hypertension, increased cardiac output
Nitrogen dioxide	Wallpaper, wood	Bronchial irritation, dizziness, pulmonary oedema
Hydrogen chloride (phosgene)	Plastics (polyvinyl chloride)	Severe mucosal irritation
Hydrogen cyanide	Wood, silk, nylons, polyurethane	Headache, respiratory failure, coma, persistent metabolic acidosis
Benzene	Petroleum, plastics	Mucosal irritation, coma
Ammonia	Nylon	Severe mucosal damage, extensive lung damage
Aldehyde	Wood, cotton, paper	Mucosal irritation

steam and gas vapour over 150°C, and direct flame injury affect upper and middle airways.[5] Most tracheobronchial damage is from products of incomplete combustion and noxious fumes. Mucosal injury is similar to that of the skin.[6] Inflammation from direct injury is exacerbated by oedema formation to compromise airway lumen. Maximal oedema formation is at around 24 h, but depends on various factors, including adequacy of resuscitation.[4] Inflammatory changes may externally compress the larynx, further distorting airway anatomy. Bronchospasm and bronchiolar oedema give rise to early symptoms of wheezing and bronchorrhoea, but *symptoms may be absent for the first 24 h.*

Lung injury

The pathophysiology of parenchymal lung damage is still uncertain. Possible causative factors include direct heat injury, chemical irritation, fluid overloading, secondary infection, aspiration and pulmonary embolism. Impairment of gas exchange is due to ventilation : perfusion mismatch consequent to airway injury rather than alveolar oedema. Lung complications can still result from major skin burns without inhalation injury. There is significant tissue oedema of unclear pathogenesis. The acute respiratory distress syndrome (ARDS) may arise (see Chapter 29).

Work of breathing increases significantly from increased airway resistance and reduced lung compliance. Arterial hypoxaemia with hypocarbia is a common finding on blood-gas analysis. Lung changes are most marked during the first 10–14 days. Bronchopneumonia is usually caused by air-borne organisms rather than by haematogenous spread from infected burn wounds, and increases mortality.[7]

Cellular injury

Inhalation of carbon monoxide (CO), cyanide and other noxious gases affects respiration at the cellular level. Cyanide inhibits cytochrome oxidase to prevent cellular respiration, and leads to cellular hypoxia; poisoning is difficult to detect. CO binds avidly to the haemoglobin, myoglobin, and mitochondrial and cellular enzymes (e.g. cytochrome P_{450}) to inhibit oxygen delivery, uptake and utilization. CO also causes direct lipid peroxidation, ultimately resulting in cellular hypoxia and destruction. The risk of inhaling noxious gases is greatly increased in enclosed-space fires, and CO appears to be synergistic with cyanide in toxicity.[8] (see Chapter 77).

Inflammatory response

Burn injury precipitates an inflammatory cascade.[9] The inflammatory response activates and releases mediators (e.g. cytokines and arachidonic acid metabolites) that direct and modulate wound healing, but may cause tissue destruction at other sites.[10] Circulating endotoxin from both the wound and the gut may be involved. Intervention with mediator inhibitors has potential, but is yet unproven for general use[11] (see Chapter 85).

Metabolic effects

Increased metabolic rate associated with nitrogen loss is greater with burn injury than any other form of trauma. There is a proportionate increase in oxygen consumption with hyperpyrexia, tachycardia, hyperventilation and hyperglycaemia. The mediators are humoral, including catecholamines and other anti-insulin hormones (see Chapter 82). Plasma insulin concentration initially decreases, but a prolonged insulin resistance phase usually follows. Hyper-metabolism increases with cooling, pain and sepsis. Hence efforts are directed to raise the environmental temperature, reduce evaporative loss by grafting the wound, and provide pain relief.

Immunological effects

Burn tissues are easily colonized by bacteria. Inflammatory and immune responses are elicited, but depression of both host defence systems in severe burns is common. A plasma inhibitor of immune function has been identified.[12] Despite advances in wound care and in topical and systemic antibiotics, infection still accounts for more than 50% of mortality in burns.[13]

Renal effects

Renal failure may occur as a complication of renal hypoperfusion, haemoglobinuria, myoglobinuria or septicaemia. It is associated with a high mortality, even after renal replacement therapy. There is progressive azotaemia, acidosis and hyperkalaemia. Renal creatinine clearance may be falsely elevated by fluid loss through open burn wounds.[14]

Gastrointestinal effects

Acute ulceration of the stomach or duodenum, known as Curling's ulcer, occurs in about 11% of burn victims. Major bleeding episodes from this ulceration may require surgical intervention.

Associated trauma effects

Burns victims may also have concomitant injuries, e.g. from motor vehicle accidents. The diagnosis and treatment of major internal injuries must not be forgotten because of an obvious and visible burn injury.

Psychological effects

Burn injuries bring pain, severe illness, disfigurement, loss of independence and long-term rehabilitation to survivors. It is hardly surprising that burns are associated with psychological problems.[15] Posttraumatic stress disorder has been described, and may contribute to agitation, sleep disturbance, low mood and diminished alertness.[16]

Management

Assessment of severity

Determinants of severity are BSA involved, depth of burn, anatomical site, age, airway involvement or noxious gas inhalation, and other morbidity-contributing factors, e.g. multiple trauma. Assessment includes a complete physical examination, with the patient fully exposed. A good history from rescuers and family is helpful.

Estimations of BSA burned use the age-adjusted BSA approximations of Lund and Browder[17] or the rule of nine for adult patients (Figs. 72.1 and 72.2). A palmar surface is 1% BSA. Electrical injury may involve extensive deep injury with little surface markings except entry, exit and arc points; estimation of severity is difficult.

The depth of a burn can be classified as:

1 *superficial dermal wound* (or first-degree burn) which involves only the epithelial layer. It is very painful but resolves within 2 weeks with no residual scarring;
2 *deep dermal wound* (or second-degree burn) which involves epithelium and a varying degree of dermis. Scarring varies according to the depth of the dermal injury. Healing is slow, over many weeks, in the absence of infection;
3 *full-thickness burn* (or third-degree burn) which loses eschar spontaneously at 2–3 weeks, and will lead to scarring and contracture. Wound closure by grafting or artificial dermis is required.[18]

Various techniques have been used to assess burn depth, including detection of dead cells, blood flow and degree of oedema, but none has emerged as a 'gold standard'. Clinical evaluation remains commonly used.

Fluid resuscitation

Intravenous fluid resuscitation is indicated in adults if the burn involves more than 20% BSA or 15% with inhalation injury. The objectives are to avoid organ ischaemia, preserve viable tissue by restoring tissue perfusion and minimize tissue oedema.[2] There is no universal consensus on the ideal fluid regimen.

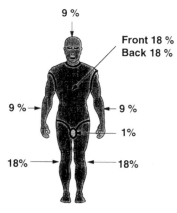

Fig. 72.1 Rule of nine to estimate body surface area burns in adults.

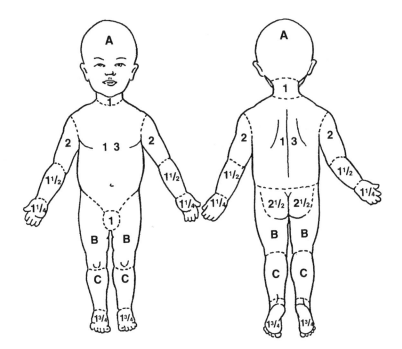

Fig. 72.2 Surface area percentages by age.

Age	<1 year	1 year	5 years	10 years	15 years	Adult
Area A = ½ of head (%)	9.5	8.5	6.5	5.5	4.5	3.5
Area B = ½ of one thigh (%)	2.75	3.25	4.0	4.25	4.5	4.75
Area C = ½ of one leg (%)	2.5	2.5	2.75	3.0	3.25	3.5

By permission of *Surgery, Gynecology & Obstetrics*, now known as the *Journal of the American College of Surgeons*.

Table 72.2 Various burns fluid resuscitation formulae[4]

	Electrolytes	ml/kg per % BSA per day	Colloids	ml/kg per % BSA per day	Volume in 8 h
Parkland	Ringer's lactate	4			50%
Modified Brooke	Ringer's lactate	2			50%
Brooke	Ringer's lactate	1.5	Albumin	0.5	50%
Evans	Normal saline	1.0	Albumin	1.0?	50%
Slater	Ringer's lactate	2 l/24 h	FFP	3.0	
Monafo	Hypertonic saline 250 mmol/l	Maintain 30 ml/h urine output			
Warden	(Modified hypertonic saline) Ringer's lactate plus 50 mmol HCO$_3^-$ (180 mmol Na/l) then Ringer's lactate	Maintain 30–50 ml/h urine output for 8 h			

BSA = Body surface area burned; FFP = fresh frozen plasma.

Recommended regimens (Table 72.2) should be titrated to individual requirements. Larger volumes are given in the first 8–12 h when fluid loss is greatest, with a gradual reduction over the next 16 h. Inhalation injuries may require more fluids (e.g. 6 ml/kg per % BSA).[19,20] The optimal composition of resuscitation fluids remains unknown.[4] Most regimens recommend giving salt solutions, about 0.5 mmol sodium/kg body weight per % BSA burned.[2] Hypertonic saline achieves the same resuscitation with less volume than isotonic saline, and weight gain is less.[21] Colloids may be extravasated to tissues, because of the increased vascular permeability, but withholding protein replacement may further decrease plasma oncotic pressure. Fluid administration is titrated to achieve a urine output of at least 1–2 ml/kg per min in children or 30–50 ml/h in adults.[4] Invasive haemodynamic monitoring may be necessary.[22] Inotropes should be given if shock persists despite adequate fluid replacement. Plasma exchange may be useful in refractory burns shock.[4]

Respiratory support

There may be no respiratory symptoms in the first 24 h. Upper airway patency requires careful assessment with a high index of suspicion. Cautious laryngoscopy is essential; airway obstruction may develop precipitously. Bronchoscopy may be necessary, usually after securing the airway. Chest X-rays and estimations of peak expiratory flow, arterial blood gases, co-oximetric Sao_2 and carboxyhaemoglobin are common investigations. Xenon 133 scanning is highly sensitive but fairly non-specific.[20,23]

In mild mucosal injury, management may be expectant, but endotracheal intubation should be undertaken if any doubt exists. Similarly, the presence of oedema, hypoxia, hypoventilation, stridor, dysphonia, respiratory distress, carbonaceous sputum and deep facial or neck burns obligates early tracheal intubation. Tracheostomy may occasionally be required on presentation, because of facial or upper airway burns. Suxamethonium must be avoided 2–60 days after injury, as it may give rise to severe hyperkalaemia.[24] Burn patients are relatively insensitive to non-depolarizing muscle relaxants, and large doses may be required. Ventilatory support is given if respiratory failure develops. Positive end-expiratory pressure (PEEP) may reduce airway hyperaemia.[25] The lungs are particularly sensitive to barotrauma, and high-frequency ventilation and permissive hypercapnia have been advocated to reduce complications and mortality.[26,27]

Oxygen, as 100%, is given for carbon monoxide (CO) poisoning. Pao_2 and Sao_2 measurements by pulse oximetry may be normal in CO poisoning. Low co-oximeter Sao_2 values with raised carboxyhaemoglobin concentrations are diagnostic.[28] However, carboxyhaemoglobin has a short half-life and absence of elevated concentrations does not exclude

significant exposure. Hyperbaric oxygen therapy may be beneficial for both CO poisoning and the burn wound, but proper evidence is lacking[29] (see Chapter 22). Transporting the burns patient and care in a hyperbaric chamber present significant risks. Treatment of cyanide poisoning is discussed in Chapter 77.

Correction of electrolyte disturbances

Electrolyte disturbances following resuscitation are common and require treatment.

1 Hypernatraemia due to salt loading and inadequate replacement of insensible water losses is treated by salt restriction and dextrose infusion.
2 Hyponatraemia and hypokalaemia from bathing wounds in water (instead of isotonic solutions) are managed by sodium and potassium replacement.
3 Hyperkalaemia may be severe in the acute phase due to tissue and red cell destruction. Dextrose and insulin may be required. Later renal losses of potassium may be high.
4 Hypocalcaemia is usually due to albumin depletion and should not be prematurely treated.
5 Hypophosphataemia is frequent and requires phosphate supplements.

Managing the burn wound

Early wound debridement and resurfacing reduce blood loss[30] and improve survival.[31] This is done after resuscitation, usually 24–36 h after the burn. However, mortality is high in patients at extremes of age and in those with more than 60% BSA burn. The best wound coverage is split-thickness autografts, but donor sites are limited and there is an associated morbidity (Table 72.3).[32] Allogeneic skin grafts have problems of availability and disease transmission. Auto- and allogeneic keratinocytes, cross-linked collagen and glycoaminoglycan dermal substitutes and collagen matrix with allogeneic fibroblasts are newer alternative skin substitutes.[32]

The burn wound is swabbed and biopsied to assess wound status and identify infective organisms.[1] Strict infection control procedures are mandatory. Topical chemotherapy is applied with wound excision and closure.[33] Those used are described below:

1 *Silver sulphadiazine*[34] inhibits growth of nearly all pathogenic bacteria. Hypersensitivity reactions, transient leukopenia and hyperpigmentation are possible complications.
2 *Mafenide acetate* 10% provides deep wound penetration, but can produce pain or metabolic acidosis by carbonic anhydrase inhibition.
3 *Silver nitrate* solution is effective and safe in concentrations of up to 0.5% but may occasionally cause hypotonic hyponatraemia and methaemoglobinaemia.

Table 72.3 Skin substitutes

Dressings	Allogeneic skin (cadaveric)
	Xenogeneic skin (porcine)
	Embryonic membranes
	Synthetic material ± growth factors
Epidermal substitutes	Cultured autologous keratinocytes
	Cultured allogeneic keratinocytes
Dermal substitutes	Acellular 'artificial skin'
Bilayer skin substitutes	Cultured autologous keratinocytes + allogeneic dermis
	Cellular artificial skin
	Cultured composite skin grafts

4 *Chlorhexidine gluconate* (0.2% solution or 1% cream) is effective against many bacteria, yeasts and viruses.

5 *Povidine-iodine*[35] has a wide range of bactericidal activity. It is associated with metabolic acidosis, renal insufficiency and thyroid function abnormalities, the validity of which has recently been questioned.

6 *Antibiotic solutions*: Numerous topical antibiotic solutions have been advocated, including neomycin, gentamicin, mupirocin and fusidic acid. Problems of resistance, hypersensitivity, skin irritation and limited efficacy reduce their usefulness.

Wound dressing changes can precipitate significant haemodynamic changes. Comprehensive monitoring and care by an experienced clinician are important.

Administration of antibiotics and tetanus toxoid

Systemic antibiotics are indicated when infection is present. There is little evidence to support the use of prophylactic antibiotics. These must be restricted to only a few situations, such as in the perioperative period of excision and grafting. First-generation cephalosporins or β-lactamase-resistant penicillins are commonly prescribed. Tetanus toxoid is given if indicated (see Chapter 47).

Nutrition

Early enteral feeding may reduce loss of gut mucosa, subsequent bacterial translocation and sepsis, and mortality.[36,37] However, intravenous supplementation of enteral feeds can be associated with increased mortality.[38] Parenteral nutrition should be reserved for patients unable to receive enteral feeding. Formulae to derive energy requirements are available (Table 72.4),[39] but requirements of burn patients are not significantly different from those of other trauma victims.[40] High caloric loads are not recommended. Pharmacological attempts to blunt the hypermetabolic response (e.g. β-adrenergic blockade) are

Table 72.4 Formulae for caloric requirements in burns[39]

Curreri	25 kcal/kg body weight + 40 kcal/BSA*
Molnar	Twice the BEE from the Harris–Benedict equation
Galveston	1800 kcal/m² + 2200 kcal/m² of burn

BEE = Basal energy expenditure.

* To a maximum of 50% body surface area (BSA) burned.

controversial. Optimal protein intake in burns is unknown, but additional protein may improve immune function and mortality.[39] Fat should complement carbohydrate to give calories. Formulations with high protein, low fat and linoleic acid, but enriched with vitamins A and C, zinc, histidine, cysteine, arginine and Ω_3 fatty acids are said to be superior to standard regimens.[41] The addition of glutamine enhances bacterial phagocytosis.[42] Insulin-like growth factor hormone (IGF-1) has been advocated as a primary anabolic mediator. IGF-F increases net tissue growth[43] and improves wound healing in children.[44]

Renal failure therapy

Prevention of renal failure is a primary objective of fluid resuscitation. Use of haptoglobin to reduce myoglobin toxicity to renal tubules has been advocated. Continuous renal replacement therapy should be implemented at an early stage of renal dysfunction. Infection in renal failure remains a major hazard.

Pain relief

Pain in the immediate post-burn period can aggravate shock. Immersion or showering with cool water reduces the extent of thermal damage and provides pain relief. The widely held belief that third-degree burns are painfree is not true; pain increases with larger BSA burns.[9] Low-dose opioid infusions are recommended in the initial phase. Patient-controlled analgesia can be introduced later. Bolus IV opioid supplements can be given with changes of dressings. Analgesic requirements increase over time. Ketamine is a useful anaesthetic and analgesic agent, but may cause unpleasant sensory disturbances. Small doses of benzodiazipines may reduce these disturbances.[33] Epidural and regional analgesia techniques may be appropriate if no contraindications exist. Non-steroidal anti-inflammatory agents may be used but have their unwanted side-effects. Hypnosis[45] and parental support can be useful.

Prognosis

Survival after a serious burn injury has improved significantly in the last 50 years. The association of 50% mortality in children was 49% BSA burn in the 1950s, but is 98% burn today.[23] Survival from a 100% burn has been recorded. Mortality is related to the extent and depth of burn, age, inhalational and other injuries, and to underlying disease states. Inhalational injuries increase mortality by 20%.[7]

References

1. Pruitt BA and McManus AT (1992) The epidemiology of infection in burn patients. *World J Surg* **16**:57–67.
2. Robson MC, Burns BF and Smith DJ (1992) Acute management of the burned patient. *Plast Reconstr Surg* **89**:1155–1168.
3. Lund T, Onarheim H and Reed R (1992) Pathogenesis of edema formation in burn injuries. *World J Surg* **16**:2–9.
4. Warden GD (1992) Burn shock resuscitation. *World J Surg* **16**:16–23.
5. Cahalane M and Demling RH (1984) Early respiratory abnormalities from smoke inhalation. *J Am Med Assoc* **251**:771–773.
6. Osguthorpe D (1991) Head and neck burns: evaluation and current management. *Arch Otolaryngol Head Neck Surg* **117**:969–974.
7. Shirani KZ, Pruitt BA and Mason A (1987) The influence of inhalational injury and pneumonia on burn mortality. *Ann Surg* **205**:82–87.
8. Gorman GF and Runciman WB (1991) Carbon dioxide poisoning. *Anaesth Intens Care* **19**:506–511.
9. Ward PA and Till GO (1990) Pathophysiologic events related to thermal injury of the skin. *J Trauma* **30**:S75–S79.
10. Smith DJ, Thomson PD, Garnier WL and Rodriguez JL (1994) Burn wounds: infections and healing. *Am J Surg* **167**:46S–48S.
11. Yeo-Kyu Y, Lalonde C and Demling R (1992) The role of mediators in the response to thermal injury. *World J Surg* **16**:30–36.
12. Ninneman JL and Ozkan AN (1985) Definition of a burn injury immunosuppressive serum component. *J Trauma* **24**:201–207.
13. Dasco CC, Luterman A and Curreri PW (1987) Systemic antibiotic treatment in burns patients. *Surg Clin North Am* **67**:57–68.
14. Sosa JL, Ward CG and Hammond JS (1992) The relationship of burn wound fluid to serum creatinine and creatinine clearance. *J Burn Care Rehab* **13**:437–442.
15. Königová R (1992) The psychological problems of burns patients. The Rudy Hermans Lecture 1991. *Burns* **18**:189–199.
16. Courtemanche DJ and Robinow O (1989) Post-traumatic stress disorders in the burn victim. *J Burn Care Rehab* **10**:247–250.
17. Lund CC and Browder NC (1944) The estimation of areas of burns. *Surg Gynecol Obstet* **79**:352–358.
18. Heimbach D, Engrav L, Grube B and Marvin J (1993) Burn depth: a review. *World J Surg* **16**:10–15.
19. Navar PD, Saffle JR and Warden GD (1985) Effect of inhalational injury on fluid resuscitation requirements after thermal injury. *Am J Surg* **150**:716–720.
20. Herndon DN, Barrow RE, Linares HA *et al.* (1988) Inhalational injury in burned patients: effects and treatment. *Burns* **14**:349–356.
21. Du G, Slater H and Goldfarb IW (1991) Influences of different resuscitation on acute early weight gain in extensively burned patients. *Burns* **17**:147–150.
22. Dries DJ and Waxman K (1991) Adequate resuscitation of burn may not be measured by urine output and vital signs. *Crit Care Med* **19**:327–329.
23. Clark WR, Bonaventura M and Myers W (1989) Smoke inhalation and airway management at a regional burn unit: 1975–1983. Part 1; Diagnosis and consequences of smoke inhalational injury. *J Burn Care Rehab* **10**:52–62.
24. Tolmie JD, Joyce TH and Mitchell GD (1967) Succinylcholine danger in the burned patient. *Anesthesiology* **28**:467–470.
25. Abdi S, Traber LD, Herndon DN, Redl G, Curry B and Traber DL (1990) Bronchial blood flow reduction with positive end-expiratory pressure after acute lung injury in sheep. *Crit Care Med* **18**:1152–1157.
26. Cioffi WG, Rue L, Graves TA, McManus WF, Mason AD and Pruitt BA (1991) Prophylactic use of high-frequency percussive ventilation in patients with inhalational injury. *Ann Surg* **213**:575–580.
27. Reynolds EM, Ryan DP and Doody DP (1993) Permissive hypercapnia and pressure-controlled ventilation as treatment of severe adult respiratory distress syndrome in a pediatric burn patient. *Crit Care Med* **21**:944–947.
28. Buckley RG, Aks SE, Eshom JL, Rydman R, Schaider J and Shayne P (1994) The pulse oximetry gap in carbon monoxide intoxication. *Ann Emerg Med* **24**:252–255.
29. Tibbles PM and Perrotta PL (1994) Treatment of carbon monoxide poisoning: a critical review of human outcome studies comparing normobaric with hyperbaric oxygen. *Ann Emerg Med* **24**:269–276.
30. Desai MH, Herndon DN, Broemling L *et al.* (1990) Early burn wound excision significantly reduces blood loss. *Ann Surg* **211**:753–759.
31. Herndon DN, Barrow RE, Rutan RL *et al.* (1989) A comparison of conservative versus early excision. Therapies in severely burned patients. *Ann Surg* **209**:547–552.
32. Nanchahal J and Ward CM (1992) New grafts for old? A review of alternatives to autologous skin. *Br J Plast Surg* **45**:354–363.

33. Andreassi L and Flori L (1992) Pharmacologic treatment of burns. *Clin Dermatol* **9**:453–458.

34. Dupuis LL, Shear NH and Zuker RM (1985) Hyperpigmentation due to topical application of silver sulphadiazine cream. *J Am Acad Dermatol* **12**:112–114.

35. Steen M (1993) Review of the use of povidone-iodine (PVP-1) in the treatment of burns. *Postgard Med J* **69**(suppl 3):s84–s92.

36. Alexander JW, Macmillan BG, Stinnet JD *et al.* (1980) Beneficial effects of protein feeding in severely burned children. *Ann Surg* **192**:505–557.

37. Ziegler TR, Smith RJ, O'Dwyer ST *et al.* (1988) Increased intestinal permeability associated with infections in burn patients. *Arch Surg* **123**:1313–1319.

38. Herndon DN, Barrow RE, Stein M *et al.* (1989) Increased mortality with intravenous supplemental feeding in severely burned patients. *J Burn Care Rehab* **10**:309–313.

39. Waymack JP and Herndon DN (1992) Nutritional support of the burned patient. *World J Surg* **16**:80–86.

40. ASPEN Board of Directors (1993) Guidelines for the use of parenteral and enteral nutrition in adult and pediatric patients. *JPEN* **17**:1SA–51SA.

41. Gotschlich MM, Jenkins M and Warden GD (1990) Differential effects of three enteral dietary regimens on selected outcome variables in burns patients. *JPEN* **14**:225–236.

42. Ogle CK, Ogle JD, Mao J-X *et al.* (1994) Effect of glutamine on phagocytosis and bacterial killing by normal and pediatric burn patient neutrophils. *JPEN* **18**:128–133.

43. Huang KF, Chung DH and Herndon DN (1993) Insulin like growth factor (IGF-1) reduces gut atophy and bacterial translocation after severe burn injury. *Arch Surg* **128**:47–54.

44. Herndon DN, Barrow RE, Kunkel KR *et al.* (1990) Effects of recombitant human growth hormone on donor site healing in severe burned children. *Ann Surg*, **211**:424–431.

45. Patterson DR, Everett J, Burns GL and Marvin JA (1992) Hypnosis for the treatment of burn pain. *J Consult Clin Psychol* **60**:713–717.

CST Aun

Thermal disorders occur as a result of impaired thermoregulation or overstress of the normal thermoregulatory system. Important ones encountered in the ICU are hypothermia, heat stroke, malignant hyperthermia and neuroleptic malignant syndrome.

Regulation of body temperature[1-3]

Temperature varies within the body. A 'core and shell' model is commonly used to describe the distribution of body heat. In health, core temperature is maintained within 36–37.5°C.[2] The balance between heat production and loss is regulated by complicated and sensitive feedback system based on three components: afferent input, central regulation and efferent responses.

Afferent input

Temperature is sensed by the cold and warm sensitive receptors found throughout the body. Signals from these sensors are conveyed up the $A\delta$ (cold signals) and unmyelinated C (warm signals) fibres, and the spinothalamic tracts in the anterior spinal cord to the central regulatory system, primarily the hypothalamus.

Central regulation[1]

Integrated thermal inputs from the skin and deep tissues are compared with the set threshold temperature in the hypothalamus. Normally, core temperature is set at 37°C with an interthreshold range of 0.2°C. Within this range, no thermoregulatory responses are triggered. However, appropriate responses (either warm or cold) are activated when the thermal input exceeds the interthreshold range. Many physiological factors affect the interthreshold range such as circadian rhythm, menstrual cycle and temperature adaptation.

Efferent responses

Efferent responses, either voluntary or autonomic, change metabolic heat production or alter heat loss. In general, energy-efficient effectors such as vasoconstriction are maximized before metabolically costly responses such as shivering are activated.

Temperature monitoring[1,4,5]

Electronic thermometers have supplanted the mercury-in-glass thermometer. They are faster in response, safer and are able to provide continuous readings. Thermistor and thermocouple are the two electronic thermometers most commonly used. In choosing the site for monitoring core temperature, the tympanic membrane, although closest to the brain, is potentially traumatic. Clinically, nasopharynx, distal oesophagus, pulmonary artery and rectum are commonly used alternative sites. Nasopharyngeal temperature may be affected by air leak around the endotracheal tube. Oesophageal probes should be positioned accurately in the lower one-quarter of the oesophagus. Rectal temperature is relatively inaccurate. It is influenced by local blood supply and rectal contents. Pulmonary artery temperature is useful during cardiac surgery.

Hypothermia[3,6-15]

Hypothermia is defined as a core temperature of 35°C or less.[6,8] It is frequently underdiagnosed and underreported. In the UK, 0.7% of all hospital admissions during winter (3% of elderly patients admitted) had hypothermia.[3] The true incidence in the USA is unknown.[9] Accidental hypothermia is a major public-health problem affecting the urban poor. In the USA, death rates from accidental hypothermia range from 2.2 to 4.3 per million population. In Ireland, it is estimated to be as high as 18.1 per million.[15]

Classifications

Clinically, hypothermia is arbitrary, classified according to the core body temperature.[8]

1 mild hypothermia: 32–35°C;
2 moderate hypothermia: 28–32°C;
3 severe hypothermia: below 28°C.

The four mechanisms of heat loss are radiation, conduction, convection and evaporation. Aetiologically, hypothermia can be divided into:

1 *Induced hypothermia*: The body temperature has deliberately been lowered as part of a therapeutic regimen.
2 *Accidental hypothermia*: Unintentional decrease in body temperature. This can be further differentiated into:[9]
   (a) Primary accidental hypothermia, in which the body possesses normal thermoregulation, but the cold stress is overwhelming (e.g. in immersion and cold exposure).
   (b) Secondary accidental hypothermia, in which mild to moderate cold exposure leads to hypothermia because of impaired thermoregulation.

Causes and pathogenesis (Table 73.1)

Hypothermia can occur in all ages, climates and ambient temperatures. The most frequent causes appear to be exposure, hypoglycaemia and use of depressant drugs, including alcohol. The elderly are more susceptible to accidental hypothermia from an impaired thermoregulatory system. In trauma patients, thermoregulation is altered, and the initial temperature has been found to have an inverse relationship with injury severity score (ISS) and mortality.[12]

Pathophysiology[3,7,8,10,12–14]

Cardiovascular effects

Sympathetic stimulation in mild hypothermia causes peripheral vasoconstriction, tachycardia and increased cardiac output. With increasing hypothermia, there is a progressive cardiovascular depression leading to a reduction in tissue perfusion. Electrocardiogram (ECG) changes include bradycardia and prolongation of P–R, QRS and Q–T intervals. The characteristic J or Osborn wave, an extra deflection at the QRS–ST junction, may be observed when core temperature is below 33°C. Below that, first-degree block and T-wave inversion are also common. At 20°C, third-degree block may be seen. Atrial fibrillation is common below 34°C and ventricular fibrillation (VF) below 28°C. Asystole is common when core temperature drops below

Table 73.1 Causes and predisposing conditions of hypothermia

Age	Extremes of age
Environmental	Exposure to cold
	Immersion
	Poor living conditions
Drugs	Anaesthetic agents
	Phenothiazines
	Barbiturates
	Alcohol
Central nervous system disorders	Cerebrovascular accidents
	Head injury
	Brain tumours
	Wernicke's encephalopathy
	Alzheimer's disease, Parkinson's disease
	Mental illness
	Spinal cord transection
Endocrine dysfunction	Hypoglycaemia
	Diabetic ketoacidosis
	Hyperosmolar coma
	Panhypopituitarism
	Hypoadrenalism
	Hypothyroidism
Trauma	Major trauma
Debility	Severe cardiac, renal, hepatic
	Malnutrition, sepsis
Skin disorders	Burns
	Exfoliative dermatitis

20°C.[3] Asystole and VF usually form the final pathway of hypothermic death. Fibrillation can occur earlier in the presence of diseased or ischaemic myocardium, or with stimuli such as insertion of a central venous line or endotracheal intubation.

Respiratory system

Initial reflex stimulation of respiration is followed by a progressive depression, both in respiratory rate and tidal volume. Respiration drive does not cease until 24°C. There are no clinically significant changes in respiratory mechanics in the 30–36°C temperature range.[14] Cold-induced bronchorrhoea may increase the difficulty of airway management.[8] Associated depression of cough reflex increases the hazard of aspiration pneumonia.

The solubility of respiratory gases, including anaesthetic agents in plasma, increases with hypothermia. The oxyhaemoglobin dissociation curve is shifted to the left, resulting in a decreased oxygen delivery to the tissues. This shift is balanced by the right shift from the underlying acidosis. Management to ensure adequate oxygenation requires a delicate balance between these competing forces.

Metabolic system

The metabolic changes in response to hypothermia occur in two phases: shivering and non-shivering. The shivering phase, observed in the 35°C to 30°C range, is characterized by intense energy production from the breakdown of stored body fuels. Compensatory mechanisms are activated to restore homeostasis. When temperature falls below 30°C, the non-shivering phase commences. Thermoregulation begins to fail, and metabolism slows dramatically, resulting in multiorgan decompensation, and eventually failure.[3] Metabolic processes slow by approximately 6% for each degree Celsius reduction in body temperature.[13] At 28°C, the basic metabolic rate falls by half.[13] Oxygen consumption is also reduced – about 75% of basal value at 30°C, 35–53% at 26°C and 25% by 20°C.[3] It is only at this stage that hypothermia affords significant protection against hypoxic organ damage.

The acidosis contains both a respiratory and a metabolic component. Inadequate ventilation causes CO_2 retention and reduces tissue perfusion, leading to accumulation of lactate and other acid metabolites from anaerobic metabolism. A reduction in tubular H^+ ion secretory capacity contributes to the acidosis in long-standing hypothermia.

Traditionally, arterial blood gases were corrected for temperature. However, more recent clinical,[16] physiochemical[17] and comparative physiological[18] data suggest that uncorrected values for pH and Pa_{CO_2} at the patient's actual temperature give a better reflection of the physiological state and indicator for appropriate therapy.[3,13,19] Pa_{O_2} values measured *in vitro* at 37°C may be substantially higher than the actual values in hypothermia. Hence significant hypoxaemia may be overlooked if uncorrected. The recommended formula is to decrease Pa_{O_2} (measured at 37°C) by 7.2% for each degree (°C) of the patient's temperature that is below 37°C.[3]

Liver function is depressed, affecting most enzymatic processes and detoxifying processes.

Central nervous system

There is a generalized cerebral depression. Confusion can cause illogical behaviour (e.g. paradoxical undressing and continued hiking or climbing instead of turning back). Loss of consciousness and pupillary dilatation supervene at 30°C. Cerebral blood flow reduces at a rate of 7% per degree (°C) drop in temperature.[14] There is a corresponding reduction in cerebral metabolic rate so that demand does not outstrip supply. The electroencephalogram (EEG) is usually flat at temperature below 20°C. Shivering is gradually replaced by muscular rigidity at 33°C and a rigor mortis-like appearance develops at 24°C.

Endocrine system

Hypothermia suppresses both exocrine and endocrine pancreatic functions. Below 30°C, insulin secretion decreases, and the peripheral tissue insulin resistance increases. Increase in blood sugar concentration is contributed by glycogenolysis and increased corticosteroids. Prolonged hypothermia may exhaust glycogen stores and ensure hypoglycaemia. Increased plasma cortisol concentration, despite a reduced adrenocorticotrophic hormone (ACTH) secretion, is probably due to reduced hepatic hormone clearance.[7]

Renal system

Initial peripheral vasoconstriction produces cold diuresis, as blood is shunted from the periphery to the central circulation. This relative central hypervolaemia suppresses antidiuretic hormone (ADH) secretion and hence promotes diuresis. The resultant decrease in total blood volume is partially responsible for the haemoconcentration that occurs in hypothermia. After the initial cold diuresis, there is a reduction in renal blood flow and glomerular filtration consequent to decreased cardiac output and increased vascular tone.[8] Changes in electrolyte levels are usually unpredictable.

Haematology

Increase in haematocrit values reflects the effects of haemoconcentration from dehydration and fluid shifts.[8] Splenic sequestration induced by hypothermia results in a decrease in white cell and platelet counts. Lowering temperature also interferes with the intrinsic clotting cascade.[3] Disseminated intravascular coagulation (DIC) may occur in severe cases, without any clear cause-and-effect relationship.

Gastrointestinal system

Intestinal motility decreases below 34°C, with ileus occurring frequently.

Immune function

There is an increased susceptibility to infection in hypothermic patients. The exact cause is not clear and is probably multifactorial.[3]

Diagnosis

The diagnosis of hypothermia requires a reliable, low-temperature recording device and a high index of suspicion. It may be difficult to differentiate from death, especially in the immersion victim. Death should not be assumed until resuscitation has failed in an adequately rewarmed patient (at least 35°C[15]; see Chapter 71).

Investigations for clarifying the underlying cause and to detect complications include full blood count, serum electrolytes, urea, creatinine, glucose and amylase, arterial blood gases, liver function studies, blood culture, drug and alcohol concentrations, toxin screen, chest X-ray, ECG and thyroid function tests.

Management[3,12,13,15,20]

The following areas should be focused in the management:

Prevention of further heat loss

The patient should be removed from the cold environment as soon as possible. Rough handling of the victim must be avoided to prevent induction of VF during transport. Transport in the upright position must be avoided because seizures may result from orthostatic hypotension.

Stabilization of cardiopulmonary status

Prehospital assessment of cardiac activity without monitors is difficult. Recommendations for basic and advanced life support for hypothermic patients are unresolved.[10] Cardiopulmonary resuscitation (CPR) should be withheld if obviously lethal injuries are present. Aggressive rewarming should be continued during resuscitation until the core temperature is at least 35°C. CPR during hypothermia may induce VF.[13] A resuscitation protocol based on core temperature and cardiac monitoring can be used:[20]

1 If core temperature is unknown or known to be above 28°C, CPR should be started for apparent arrest.
2 If the patient is known to be severely cold (<28°C) and ECG monitoring shows sinus rhythm, chest compression may precipitate VF and may be best avoided.

Patients in coma or in respiratory failure should be intubated and ventilated with warm oxygen.

Fluid resuscitation should be started preferably with central venous pressure (CVP) monitoring. Vascular cannulation may be difficult and drug delivery ineffective in the presence of intense peripheral vasoconstriction. Dextrose 5% in normal saline without potassium is a good choice. Lactated Ringer's should be avoided because the liver may not be able to metabolize lactate to bicarbonate. All IV fluids should be prewarmed if possible.

Relatively few drugs are useful during severe hypothermia because of diminished effectiveness, and prolonged half-lives may cause undesirable side-effects after rewarming. Among the inotropes, dopamine has been shown to be effective.[21] Vasopressors such as adrenaline, isoprenaline and metaraminol should be avoided because of their arrhythmoge-

nicity.[8] Atrial arrhythmia and heart block generally resolve spontaneously on rewarming. For persistent VF despite aggressive resuscitation and rewarming, IV bretylium 5–10 mg/kg may be considered. Electrical defibrillation may not be effective until the temperature is above 30°C. Sodium bicarbonate should be avoided, because of the slowness of transport across cell membranes, and severe alkalosis on rewarming may induce refractory VF and shift of the oxyhaemoglobin curve to the left (thereby reducing tissue oxygenation availability).

Treatment of the cause of hypothermia

The cause of hypothermia should be diagnosed and treated. Insulin administration in diabetics should be delayed until the temperature is above 30°C; it should be given in small IV doses, because degradation is slow and accumulation may occur with rebound hypoglycaemia as the patient is warmed.

Prevention of complications

Common complications can be prevented by careful monitoring and early intervention. Presence of infection should be evaluated and early antibiotics considered. Pneumonia can be prevented by protecting the airway. Intubation should be considered early in comatose patients.

Rewarming[3,8,9,15]

The mainstay of treatment is rewarming – to restore heat lost without precipitating fatal side-effects. Various methods of rewarming have been employed (Table 73.2). However, so far no randomized control trial exists to evaluate their efficacy, morbidity and mortality. Careful monitoring and supportive therapy during rewarming are mandatory.

Table 73.2 Rewarming methods

Passive
Warm environment
Insulating cover (warm blanket)

Active
External
  Warmed pads, blanket
  Hot air blower cover (e.g. Bair Hugger)
  Body-trunk hot-water immersion
  Radiant heat
Core
  Humidified warm inspired gases
  Gastrointestinal irrigation (intragastric, intracolonic)
  Pleural irrigation
  Dialysis (peritoneal, haemodialysis)
  Cardiopulmonary bypass

Passive external rewarming (PER)

The patient is allowed to rewarm spontaneously in a warm room, covered with a warm blanket. The patient must be stable and capable of generating heat. This can be used in mild hypothermia. Rewarming is gradual (about 0.5°C/h).

Active external rewarming (AER)

AER involves warming the skin with heating devices (Table 73.2) to raise the core temperature, and is recommended in mild to moderate hypothermia in alert and stable patients. It can also be used as an adjunct to active core warming in patients with severe hypothermia. Associated hazards are:

1 *Afterdrop of core temperature* – when peripheral vasodilatation causes increased flow of cold blood from the periphery to the central circulation. This may trigger fatal arrhythmias.
2 *Rewarming shock* – circulatory volume depletion is worsened by peripheral vasodilatation on warming the skin. This problem can be mitigated by leaving the limbs cooled while warming the trunk.

Active core rewarming (ACR)

ACR methods are fast but invasive. The inherent risks should be considered in the management.

1 *Airway rewarming*: Inspired gas is heated and humidified up to 40°C, and delivered through a facemask or an endotracheal tube. The rate of warming is about 1.5°C/h.
2 *Gastrointestinal rewarming*: Warm gastric lavage or oesophageal balloon can provide considerable heat transfer. However, VF during placement of gastric tube, aspiration and gut perforation are associated risks.
3 *Peritoneal lavage*: Dialysate is warmed up to around 40–42°C. Rewarming is rapid because of the high heat capacity of fluid. Electrolyte imbalance can be corrected by adjusting the dialysate fluid.
4 *Pleural lavage*: A closed method using thoracostomy tubes has been reported to be effective.
5 *Haemodialysis employing a blood warmer* may be useful in drug overdose cases.
6 *Cardiopulmonary bypass (CPB)* has theoretical advantages of controlling the rate of rewarming, oxygenation, composition of fluid and haemodynamic support. However, associated risks are heparinization, haemolysis and air embolism. Despite these problems, CPB is the method of choice for resuscitation in cases with profound hypothermia, especially those presenting with cardiac arrest.[20]

Outcome

While the search for the ideal rewarming technique continues, the outcome of hypothermia appears to be related to the severity of hypothermia, underlying conditions and the time lag prior to treatment. Many elderly patients may have a residual hypothalamic dysfunction, rendering them susceptible to recurrent hypothermia.

Heat stroke[22–26]

Heat stroke is defined as hyperthermia associated with neurological abnormality, resulting from exposure to a high ambient temperature or from vigorous physical activity.[22] It occurs in two distinct settings:

1 *Exertional heat stroke*, in which muscular exertion in hot, humid weather results in excessive storage of heat – often seen in military recruits or athletes.
2 *Classic heat stroke* is commonly seen in sedentary, elderly patients with underlying illnesses during heat waves. The urban poor are particularly at risk. In the USA, classic heat stroke is responsible for about 200 deaths in a typical summer; the toll may exceed 1200 with heat waves.[23]

Table 73.3 Predisposing factors to heat stroke

Age	Elderly
Environmental	High ambient temperature and humidity
	Heat waves
	Poor ventilation
Personal/behaviour	Lack of acclimatization
	Obesity
	Salt and water depletion
Underlying conditions	Infection/fever
	Fatigue
	Diabetes
	Malnutrition
	Alcoholism
	Hyperthyroidism
	Impaired sweat production
	Healed thermal burn
	Ectodermal dysplasia
	Prickly heat
	Sweat gland injury following
	Acute heat stroke
	Barbiturate poisoning
	Cardiovascular diseases
	Congestive heart failure
	Postassium deficiency
Drugs	Anticholinergics
	Antiparkinsonians
	Antihistamines
	Butyrophenones
	Phenothiazines
	Tricyclics
	Diuretics
	Sympathomimetic amines

Pathophysiology[22–29]

Hyperthermia is either due to an excessive heat production (as in exertional heat stroke) or an interference of thermoregulation from high ambient temperature and humidity, or both. Many risk factors predispose to heat stroke (Table 73.3). The critical temperature and duration of exposure that trigger heat stroke are not well-defined.

During heat stroke, there is a substantial fluid shift from the central compartment to the periphery which is reversible on cooling. Cardiac output is increased tremendously (3 l/min per °C increase in rectal temperature) due to redistribution of blood from splanchnic organs to the skin. This compensatory mechanism may fail earlier in patients with limited cardiac reserve. Obesity and anticholinergic drugs may also interfere with heat dissipation.

Major complications are seizures, acute respiratory distress syndrome (ARDS), cardiac failure from temperature-induced myocardial haemorrhage and necrosis, rhabdomyolysis, acute renal failure, liver failure and disseminated intravascular coagulation (DIC). Intractable DIC is the usual mode of demise in fatal cases. Mediators such as endotoxin and cytokines[27–29] are implicated in the pathogenesis of organ damage in heat stroke.

Clinical presentation[22–26]

The three cardinal signs are:

1 central nervous system dysfunction;
2 hyperpyrexia (core temperature above 40°C);
3 hot, dry skin which is pink or ashen depending on the circulatory state. However, clammy and sweaty skin may be seen.

Neurological system

Confusion, aggressive behaviour, delirium, convulsions and pupillary abnormalities may progress rapidly to coma. There may be decorticate posturing, faecal incontinence, flaccidity or hemiplegia. Cerebellar symptoms, including ataxia and dysarthria, may be permanent in a few patients. Lumbar puncture may show increased protein level, xanthochromia and a slight lymphocytic pleocytosis.

Cardiovascular system

Tachycardia, hypotension or normotension with a wide pulse pressure are seen. Haemodynamic profile is usually hyperdynamic (unless limited by pre-existing cardiac disease) with high cardiac output, low systemic vascular resistance, normal or low central venous and pulmonary wedge pressure.[30]

Respiratory system

There is extreme tachypnoea (respiratory rate up to 60 breaths/min) and hypoxaemia (Sa_{O_2} <90%). Rales and cyanosis are late signs of pulmonary oedema.

Other signs

Dehydration follows excessive sweating. Bleeding diathesis from DIC, thrombocytopenia and liver damage may be present.

Investigations

Urgent blood biochemistry profile is essential, because there is a significant difference between classic and exertional heat stroke (Table 73.4). In heat stroke, hepatic and pancreatic abnormalities are mild initially, but may develop into overt hepatic failure and pancreatitis later. Anaemia is frequent, platelet count may be low or normal, and leukocytosis is seen with mainly lymphocytosis.[31] Coagulation parameters are usually deranged when DIC sets in. A urinalysis screen is undertaken for signs of rhabdomyolysis and acute renal failure. Brain scan and cerebrospinal fluid analyses are indicated if intracranial bleeding or infection is suspected.

Table 73.4 Some biochemical differences between the two settings of heat stroke

	Classic heat stroke	Exertional heat stroke
Arterial blood gases	Mixed respiratory alkalosis	Severe metabolic acidosis
Serum electrolytes	Na^+, K^+, Ca^{2+}, Mg^+ are usually normal Hypophosphataemia in 20–80% of cases	Hyperkalaemia Hypocalcaemia Hyperphosphataemia
Blood glucose	Hyperglycaemia (90% of cases)	Hypoglycaemia may occur
Creatinine kinase	Moderately increased	Marked increase

Management[22–24,26]

Heat stroke is a medical emergency. Rapid and effective cooling and support of vital organ systems are the principal therapeutic objectives. Cooling methods include:

1 *Conduction*: by immersing the patient in ice water or packed ice. Internal cooling by cold gastric lavage can be used.
2 *Evaporation*: repeated wetting of the skin with water sprays, and fanning the patient at room temperature. This method is more effective than that by conduction.

Pharmacological treatment (including dantrolene) is ineffective.[23,32] Core and skin temperature should be monitored to avoid overshoot hypothermia and rebound hyperthermia. Skin temperature should be kept at 30–33°C. Cooling can be stopped when core temperature is about 39°C.

Fluid imbalance and electrolyte and acid–base disturbances must be corrected cautiously with crystalloids, guided by CVP, urine output, serum electrolyte values and haematocrit. A pulmonary artery catheter may be indicated in fragile patients.[30] Mannitol may be required to promote renal blood flow. Anuria, uraemia and hyperkalaemia are indications for early dialysis.

Oxygen therapy and controlled ventilation may be indicated. Anticonvulsants may be required. Prophylactic steroids or antibiotics are not recommended. Hypoglycaemia may be present, and must be treated. Evidence for underlying illness should be sought and treated accordingly.

Outcome

The mortality of heat stroke ranges from 5 to 50%, and the incidence of permanent neurological damage is between 7 and 14%.[22] Prognostic factors include age, severity, neurological deficits, plasma concentrations of liver and muscle enzymes, and the presence of lactic acidosis.

Malignant hyperthermia[33,34]

Malignant hyperthermia (MH) is a pharmacogenetic disorder (autosomal dominant) characterized by acute accelerated metabolism and rigidity in skeletal muscle, triggered by certain drugs (mainly anaesthetic drugs) and stresses.[33] Triggering anaesthetic drugs include any of the potent inhalational agents, and depolarizing muscle relaxants (i.e. suxamethonium and decamethonium). The evidence of local anaesthetics in triggering MH is weak.[34] The true incidence of MH is unknown, but estimates vary from 1 in 50 000[35] to 1 in 250 000,[36] possibly related to lack of uniform diagnostic criteria and the variety of anaesthetics used. The incidence is higher in childhood (1: 10 000).[35]

Aetiology and pathophysiology[34,37]

The exact pathophysiology of human MH is still unclear. The current theory is that MH is caused by an abnormality in calcium homeostasis within skeletal muscles. The excessive amount of myoplasmic calcium is primarily due to a defect in the calcium release channels (ryanodine receptors) of sarcoplasmic reticulum (SR). These channels, being hypersensitive to stimulators (such as halothane, suxamethonium), stay open and thus release an excessive amount of calcium into the myoplasm, which subsequently triggers a chain of events:

1 activation of muscle contractile elements, resulting in sustained contraction instead of the normal contraction–relaxation cycle. This accounts for the muscle rigidity;
2 enhanced glycolytic and aerobic metabolism causing hydrolysis of adenosine triphosphate, heat production, increased O_2 consumption, excessive CO_2 and lactate production, uncoupling of oxidative phosphorylation, and eventually cell breakdown and release of intracellular contents.

Clinical presentation[33,38]

The clinical presentation is very variable. MH typically occurs during induction of anaesthesia, but can be delayed for some hours. Early signs are:

1 rigidity of jaw muscles which may later become generalized (in 75% of human patients);
2 a rising end-tidal CO_2 tension ($ETCO_2$) during constant minute ventilation. The temperature of carbon dioxide absorption canisters may rise due to the accelerated chemical reaction within the soda-lime;
3 sweating, tachycardia and cardiac arrhythmias which include frequent ventricular extrasystoles, bigeminy and ventricular tachycardia. ECG may show tall peaked T waves characteristic of hyperkalaemia;
4 unstable blood pressure. Hypertension during the early stage and hypotension is a late sign as cardiac failure sets in;
5 cyanosis and mottling of the skin due to intense peripheral vasoconstriction.

Late signs are:

1 pyrexia, the hallmark of MH, is usually a late sign, and is influenced by the agents used. Suxamethonium in conjunction with halothane induces an earlier and more rapid rise. The rate of rise in core temperature is variable;[33]
2 acute pulmonary oedema, as a result of left ventricular failure, commonly occurs in the late stage;

3 generalized oedema: muscle swelling and pain including cerebral oedema resulting in coma and seizures;
4 bleeding diathesis from DIC;
5 renal failure, probably secondary to myoglobinuria;
6 hepatic failure and gastrointestinal bleed.

Investigations

1 *Arterial blood-gas analyses*: There is a rise in $Paco_2$, a decrease in Pao_2 and acidosis (mixed metabolic and respiratory). However, central venous CO_2 levels are more accurate in reflecting whole-body CO_2 stores. An increased central venous or femoral venous CO_2 to $Paco_2$ gradient may help confirm the diagnosis of MH.[39]
2 *Serum electrolyte concentrations*: These are variable. Serum potassium is usually elevated initially, followed by a decrease. Serum ionized calcium, sodium, phosphorus and magnesium concentrations vary with the duration and peak of hyperthermia, and severity of rhabdomyolysis.
3 *Serum enzyme concentrations*: Creatinine kinase concentration increases markedly during the crisis. This increase may be attenuated or absent if dantrolene is given early.
4 *Myoglobinaemia and myoglobinuria*: This is indicated by a cola-coloured urine.
5 *Coagulation screen*: This is carried out for signs of DIC.
6 *Blood glucose, lactate* and *urea nitrogen* estimation.

Diagnosis

The diagnosis of an acute MH reaction by clinical criteria can be difficult because of the non-specific clinical picture.[40] Diagnosis requires skeletal muscle biopsy. Currently caffeine halothane contracture test is the most common test used.[41] Standardization of protocols[42,43] has led to more uniform contracture testing. Studies are in progress to establish guidelines on diagnostic criteria with an acceptable specificity (frequency of negative results in true negatives) and sensitivity (frequency of positive results in true positives).[40,41]

Management[25,34,44]

MH is an emergency. A treatment protocol is:

1 Discontinue the triggering agents immediately.
2 Cancel/postpone the surgery if possible.
3 Hyperventilate with 100% oxygen (at least 10 l).
4 Give dantrolene while adequate muscle perfusion is present. The dose is 2–3 mg/kg in increments until symptoms resolve (up to a maximum of 10 mg/kg). Dantrolene acts by inhibiting SR calcium release without affecting uptake.[34] Dan-

trolene is repeated 1–2 mg/kg 6-hourly IV (biological half-life 5 h)[34] for at least 24–48 h, and then given orally 1 mg/kg when the patient is alert. Dantrolene is supplied in vials containing 20 mg of lyophilized dantrolene sodium together with 3.0 g mannitol and sodium hydroxide to raise the pH to 9.5. It must be dissolved in 60 ml water. The solution is irritant to veins and should be injected into a fast-running drip or large vein.
5 Correct acidosis with bicarbonate.
6 Simultaneously cool the patient (an active method is preferred). Core temperature is monitored and cooling is stopped at 38–39°C to avoid overshoot.
7 Arrhythmias usually respond to treatment of acidosis and hyperkalaemia. If arrhythmias persisted, standard antiarrhythmic agents (except calcium-channel blockers) may be used. Interaction of calcium antagonists with dantrolene may produce hyperkalaemia and profound myocardial depression.
8 Control serum potassium if necessary using glucose and insulin. Calcium may be needed in life-threatening hyperkalaemia.
9 Monitor $ETco_2$ oximetry, temperature, arterial and central venous blood gases and pressure, ECG, serum electrolytes, glucose, enzyme levels, clotting profile and urine output.
10 Maintain hydration and urine output over 2 ml/kg per h with IV fluid. Mannitol and frusemide help to reduce cerebral and muscle oedema, and prevent acute renal failure. Mannitol dose should be adjusted accordingly (dantrolene contains mannitol).
11 Movement and handling of the patient should be minimized as they may precipitate ventricular arrhythmias.

Outcome

The mortality rate from MH has declined from 70% in the 1960s to about 5% in the 1980s.[34] This is attributed to better understanding of MH, advanced monitoring leading to early diagnosis and vigorous treatment with early use of dantrolene.

Neuroleptic malignant syndrome[24,45–48]

The neuroleptic malignant syndrome (NMS) is a relatively rare but potentially fatal idiosyncratic response to neuroleptic drugs, characterized by mental status changes, muscular rigidity, hyperthermia and autonomic dysfunction. The estimated incidence varies from 0.07 to 2.2% in patients on neuroleptics.[47] All ages are affected; 80% of cases are under 40 years, and there is a male:female ratio of 2:1.[46,47]

Pathophysiology[45–48]

The pathophysiology of NMS remains unclear. Current theory proposes precipitation by blockade of the central dopamine receptors (D_1 and D_2) in the hypothalamus and basal ganglia, and of the peripheral dopamine receptors in the smooth-muscle and post-ganglionic sympathetic neurones. Interference with hypothalamic central dopamine action may lead to disturbances in thermoregulation and hence hyperthermia. Interference in the basal ganglia, specifically in the nigrostriatal dopaminergic pathways, causes skeletal muscle hypertonicity and prolonged muscle contractions, leading to further heat production and muscle breakdown.

Neuroleptic agents (e.g. butyrophenones, phenothiazines, thioxanthenes and dibenoxazepines) are the primary agents that trigger the syndrome. However, other non-neuroleptic agents have been reported to cause NMS (e.g. monoamine oxidase inhibitors, tricyclic antidepressants and lithium). It may also occur on withdrawal of parkinsonian medication.

Predisposing factors are inconsistent. Patients with organic brain disease, psychosis, previous NMS episodes, dose changes of neuroleptics, dehydration and exhaustion, are prone to develop NMS.

Clinical presentation[45–48]

The syndrome may occur at any time during treatment with neuroleptic medication. Classically, NMS is characterized by:

1 pyrexia (around 40°C);
2 muscle rigidity (usually 'lead-pipe');
3 altered sensorium;
4 autonomic dysfunction (e.g. tachycardia, labile blood pressure, tachypnoea, sweating, urinary incontinence, pallor and cardiac arrest).

The symptoms of NMS usually progress rapidly over 1–3 days,[46] with hyperthermia (around 40°C), muscle rigidity, akinesia, mutism, coarse tremor and myoclonus. Autonomic signs of hypermetabolism (i.e. tachycardia, labile blood pressure and sweating) usually suggest onset of hyperthermia. Mental status varies from confusion to coma. Other associated neurological signs include disorders of speech and swallowing. Predisposing factors include functional psychoses and organic brain diseases.

Complications[46]

These include acute renal failure from rhabdomyolysis,[49] respiratory failure from rigidity of chest wall muscle, aspiration pneumonia from muscle dysfunction, pulmonary embolism, myocardial infarction with pulmonary oedema, DIC and sepsis. Irreversible cerebellar or other brain damage may result from extreme temperatures.[50]

Investigations[47,48]

Laboratory findings are non-specific: increased creatinine phosphokinase concentration,[51] leukocytosis, increased platelet count, abnormal liver function tests, acidosis, hypoxia, hypercarbia and elevated plasma and urinary catecholamine concentrations.[52] Examination of cerebrospinal fluid is unremarkable. Computed tomography scan of the brain is usually negative.

Management[45,47,53]

1 The offending agent or agents should be withdrawn immediately.
2 Supportive therapy:
  (a) cooling procedures as in MH;
  (b) treatment of cardiovascular instability;
  (c) mechanical ventilatory support if necessary;
  (d) treatment of dehydration with fluid therapy to maintain renal function;
  (e) correction of acidosis;
  (f) dialysis may be required.
3 Exclude other differential diagnosis of hyperthermia (e.g. infection, hyperthyroidism and MH), or neurological structural abnormalities.[47,48]
4 Specific pharmacotherapy has been used with varying degrees of success:
  (a) bromocriptine, a D_2 agonist (acting at the postsynaptic site) given as 2.5 mg b.d. to 10 mg t.i.d. orally until creatinine phosphokinase concentrations return to normal. It may worsen psychosis,[54] and is contraindicated in patients receiving monoamine oxidase inhibitors before the syndrome.
  (b) amantadine, an *N*-methyl-D-aspartate (NMDA) antagonist, is given 100 mg t.i.d. orally.[55] It restores the balance between glutamatergic and dopaminergic systems.
  (c) dantrolene, given as 0.8–1.5 mg/kg IV 6-hourly, has few side-effects, but hepatotoxicity is a risk of long-term therapy.
  (d) L-dopa and carbidopa for patients caused by withdrawal of parkinsonian drugs.
  (e) azumolene, a new drug structurally related to dantrolene but easier to administer, is currently under investigation.[56]
5 Non-specific therapy includes the following:
  (a) benzodiazepines may control agitation or reverse catatonia.
  (b) non-depolarizing neuromuscular blockers can reduce the temperature by muscle relaxation.
  (c) calcium-channel blockers have been used in refractory cases. The mechanism is uncertain.[57]
  (d) the use of anticholinergic agents to relieve rigidity is controversial.[53]
  (e) electroconvulsive therapy (ECT) has been found useful in some cases.

The duration of treatment must be adjusted according to the metabolism of the inciting agent.

Haemodialysis is not helpful in removing the offending drug, since neuroleptic drugs are protein-bound and too large to dialyse.[58] A 2-week interval after resolution of symptoms has been suggested before neuroleptics are reinstituted.[59]

Outcome

A mortality rate of 20% before 1980 has been reduced to below 12% after 1986.[45] This is related to early diagnosis, therapy and advances in critical care management. Renal failure increases the mortality to nearly 60% and therefore must be prevented. The recovery may be slow and the stay in the ICU may be prolonged owing to the high frequency of complications. Prognosis is good in survivors.

References

1. Sessler DI (1994) Temperature regulation. In: Gregory GA (ed.) *Pediatric Anesthesia*, 3rd edn. New York: Churchill Livingstone, pp. 47–81.
2. Guyton AC (1991) Body temperature, temperature regulation and fever. In: *Textbook of Medical Physiology*, 8th edn. Philadelphia: WB Saunders, pp. 797–808.
3. Curley FJ and Irwin RS (1991) Disorders of temperature control. Part 1. Hypothermia. In: Rippe JM, Irwin RS, Alpert JS and Fink MP (eds) *Intensive Care Medicine*, 2nd edn. Boston: Little, Brown, pp. 658–674.
4. Ilsley AH, Rutten AJ and Runciman WB (1983) An evaluation of body temperature measurement. *Anaesth Intens Care* **11**:31–39.
5. Cork RC, Vaughan RW and Humphrey LS (1983) Precision and accuracy of intraoperative temperature monitoring. *Anesth Analg* **62**:211–214.
6. Sheehy TW and Navari RM (1985) Hypothermia. *Intens Crit Care Diges* **4**:12–18.
7. Lonning PE, Skulberg A and Abyholm F (1986) Accidental hypothermia. Review of the literature. *Acta Anaesthesiol Scand* **30**:601–613.
8. Jolly BT and Ghezzi KT (1992) Accidental hypothermia. *Emerg Med Clin North Am* **10**:311–327.
9. Bracker MD (1992) Environmental and thermal injury. *Clin Sports Med* **11**:419–436.
10. Danzl DF, Pozos RS, Auerbach PS *et al.* (1987) Multicenter hypothermia survey. *Ann Emerg Med* **16**:1042–1055.
11. Kurtz KJ (1982) Hypothermia in the elderly. The cold facts. *Geriatrics* **37**:85–93.
12. Pavlin EG (1993) Hypothermia in traumatized patients. In: Grande CM (ed.) *Textbook of Trauma Anesthesia and Critical Care*. St Louis: Mosby-Year Book, pp. 1131–1139.
13. Corneli HM (1992) Accidental hypothermia. *J Pediatr* **120**:671–679.
14. Morley-Forster PK (1986) Unintentional hypothermia in the operating room. *Can Anaesth Soc J* **33**:516–527.
15. Larach MG (1995) Accidental hypothermia. *Lancet* **345**:493–498.
16. Reuler JB (1978) Hypothermia: pathophysiology, clinical settings, and management. *Ann Intern Med* **89**:519–527.
17. Swain JA (1988) Hypothermia and blood pH: a review. *Arch Intern Med* **148**:1643–1646.
18. White FN (1981) A comparative physiological approach to hypothermia. *J Thorac Cardiovasc Surg* **82**:821–831.
19. Ream AK, Reitz BA and Silverberg G (1982) Temperature correction of P_{CO_2} and pH in estimating acid–base status: an example of the emperor's new clothes? *Anesthesiology* **56**:41–44.
20. Zell SC and Kurtz KJ (1985) Severe exposure hypothermia: a resuscitation protocol. *Ann Emerg Med* **4**:339–345.
21. Nicodemus HF, Chaney RD and Herold R (1981) Hemodynamic effects of inotropes during hypothermia and rapid rewarming. *Crit Care Med* **9**:325–328.
22. Bouchama A and Hammami MM (1994) Heatstroke: diagnosis, pathophysiology and treatment. *Intensive Care* Summer 44–47.
23. Simon HB (1993) Hyperthermia. *N Engl J Med* **329**:483–487.
24. Curley FJ and Irwin RS. Disorders of temperature control. Part 2. Hyperthermia. In: Rippe JM, Irwin RS, Alpert JS and Fink MP (eds) *Intensive Care Medicine*, 2nd edn. Boston; Little, Brown, pp. 674–688.
25. Knochel JP (1989) Heat stroke and related heat stress disorders. *Dis Month* **35**:301–378.
26. Tek D and Olshaker JS (1992) Heat illness. *Emerg Med Clin North Am* **10**:299–310.
27. Editorial (1989) Endotoxins in heatstroke. *Lancet* **ii**:1137–1138.
28. Bouchama A, Parhar RS, El-Yazigi A, Sheth K and Al-Sedairy S (1991) Endotoxemia and release of tumor necrosis factor and interleukin-1a in acute heatstroke. *J Appl Physiol* **70**:2640–2644.
29. Bouchama A, Al-Sedairy S, Siddiqui S, Shail E and Rezeig M (1993) Elevated pyrogenic cytokines in heatstroke. *Chest* **104**:1498–1502.
30. Dahmash NS, Al-Harthi SS and Akhtar J (1993) Invasive evaluation of patients with heat stroke. *Chest* **103**:1210–1214.
31. Bouchama A, AI Hussein K, Adra C, Rezeig M, Al Shail E and Al-Sedairy S (1992) Distribution of peripheral blood leukocytes in acute heat stroke. *J Appl Physiol* **73**:405–409.
32. Bouchama A, Cafege A, Devol EB, Labdi O, El-Assil K and Seraj M (1991) Ineffectiveness of dantrolene sodium in the treatment of heatstroke. *Crit Care Med* **19**:176–180.
33. Britt BA (1985) Malignant hyperthermia. *Can Anaesth Soc* **32**:666–677.
34. Gronert GA and Antognini JF (1994) Malignant hyperthermia. In: Miller RD (ed.) *Anesthesia*. New York; Churchill Livingstone, pp. 1075–1093.
35. Ball SP and Johnson KJ (1993) The genetics of malignant hyperthermia. *J Med Genet* **30**:89–93.
36. Ording H (1985) Incidence of malignant hyperthermia in Denmark. *Anesth Analg* **64**:700–704.
37. MacLennan DH and Phillips MS (1992) Malignant hyperthermia. *Science* **256**:789–794.

38. Rosenberg H (1988) Clinical presentation of malignant hyperthermia. *Br J Anaesth* **60**:268–273.

39. Karan SM, Crowl F and Muldoon SM (1994) Malignant hyperthermia masked by capnographic monitoring. *Anesth Analg* **78**:590–592.

40. Larach MG, Localio AR, Allen GC *et al.* (1994) A clinical grading scale to predict malignant hyperthermia susceptibility. *Anesthesiology* **80**:771–779.

41. Larach MG, Landis JR, Bunn JS and Diaz M (1992) The North American Malignant Hyperthermia registry. Prediction of malignant hyperthermia susceptibility in low-risk subjects. An epidemiologic investigation of caffeine halothane contracture responses. *Anesthesiology* **76**:16–27.

42. Ellis ER, Halsall PJ, Ording H *et al.* (1984) The European Malignant Hyperpyrexia Group: a protocol for the investigation of malignant hyperpyrexia (MH) susceptibility. *Br J Anaesth* **56**:1267–1269.

43. Larach MG for The North American Malignant Hyperthermia Group (1989) Standardization of the caffeine halothane muscle contracture test. *Anesth Analg* **69**:511–515.

44. MHAUS (1993) *Emergency Therapy for Malignant Hyperthermia, Acute Phase Treatment.* Westport: Malignant Hyperthermia Association of the United States.

45. Prager LM, Millham FH and Stern TA (1994) Neuroleptic malignant syndrome: a review for intensivists. *J Intens Care Med* **9**:227–234.

46. Lev R and Clark RF (1994) Neuroleptic malignant syndrome presenting without fever: case report and review of the literature. *J Emerg Med* **12**:49–55.

47. Caroff SN and Mann SC (1993) Neuroleptic malignant syndrome. *Med Clin North Am* **77**:185–202.

48. Heiman-Patterson TD (1993) Neuroleptic malignant syndrome and malignant hyperthermia. Important issues for the medical consultant. *Med Clin North Am* **77**:477–492.

49. Becker BN and Ismail N (1994) The neuroleptic malignant syndrome and acute renal failure. *J Am Soc Nephrol* **4**:1406–1412.

50. Lee S, Merriam A, Kim T-S, Liebling M, Dickson DW and Moore GRW (1989) Cerebellar degeneration in neuroleptic malignant syndrome: neuropathologic findings and review of the literature concerning heat-related nervous system injury. *J Neurol Neurosurg Psychiat* **52**:387–391.

51. Gurrera RJ and Romero JA (1993) Enzyme elevations in the neuroleptic malignant syndrome. *Biol Psychiat* **34**:634–640.

52. Gurrera RJ and Romero JA (1992) Sympathoadrenomedullary activity in the neuroleptic malignant syndrome. *Biol Psychiat* **32**:334–343.

53. Gratz SS, Levinson DF and Simpson GM (1992) The treatment and management of neuroleptic malignant syndrome. *Prog Neuro-Psychopharmacol Biol Psychiat* **16**:425–443.

54. Rosebush PI, Stewart T and Mazurek MF (1991) The treatment of neuroleptic malignant syndrome. Are dantrolene and bromocriptine useful adjuncts to supportive care? *Br J Psychiat* **159**:709–712.

55. Kornhuber J, Weller M and Riederer P (1993) Glutamate receptor antagonists for neuroleptic malignant syndrome and akinetic hyperthermic parkinsonian crisis. *J Neural Transm* **6**:63–72.

56. Shader RI and Greenblatt DJ (1992) A possible new approach to the treatment of neuroleptic malignant syndrome. *J Clin Psychopharmacol* **12**:155.

57. Talley BJ and Taylor SE (1994) Nifedipine use in neuroleptic malignant syndrome. *Psychosomatics* **35**:168–170.

58. Byrd C (1993) Neuroleptic malignant syndrome: a dangerous complication of neuroleptic therapy. *J Neurosci Nurs* **25**:62–65.

59. Rosebush PI, Stewart TD and Gelenberg AJ (1989) Twenty neuroleptic rechallenges after neuroleptic malignant syndrome in 15 patients. *J Clin Psych* **50**:295–298.

| 74 | **Electrical safety and injuries** |

LAH Critchley and TE Oh

Patients suffering from the consequences of electrocution and associated burns occasionally require ICU management. Patients and staff in the ICU are at risk of electrocution from faulty electrical equipment. The necessity of direct patient contact with electrical equipment increases this risk, and when therapy involves an invasive contact close to the heart, microshock is an additional hazard. Faulty electrical equipment can also result in power failures, fires and explosions.

Physical concepts

Electricity is produced by the movement of negatively charged electrons. A potential difference or voltage, measured in volts (V), exists between two points if the number or density of electrons is greater at one point. When these points are connected by a conductor, the potential difference will cause electrons or an electric current (I), measured in amperes (A), to flow. Resistance (R), measured in ohms (Ω), opposes this flow of electrons. Resistance is low in a conductor, because electrons can move freely from atom to atom. However, resistance is high in an insulator as electrons are unable to move. Voltage, current and resistance are related by Ohm's law:

$$V = I \times R$$

When an electric current flows through a resistance, it dissipates energy as heat. The heating effect per second, or power, is measured in joules per second or watts:

$$\text{Power} = V \times I = I^2 \times R$$

When a current flows in one direction, such as produced by a battery, it is called a direct current. Electricity to homes, hospitals and factories is supplied as an alternating current which flows back and forth at a frequency, i.e. cycles per second or hertz (Hz). Two configurations are commonly used. Australasia and the UK use 240 V at 50 Hz, and North America uses 120 V at 60 Hz.

A current flowing in a circuit produces electric and magnetic fields which induce currents to flow in neighbouring circuits. When this results in a current flowing between the two circuits, it is called capacitive and inductive coupling respectively. With capacitive coupling, high-frequency currents are most easily passed, and the size of the current is greatest when the circuits are close. Inductive coupling can result from the strong magnetic fields produced by heavy-duty electrical equipment, such as transformers, electric motors and magnetic resonance imaging machines. The most common problem associated with coupling is electrical interference or 'noise'. Monitoring equipment is designed to filter out this noise. However, in certain circumstances, such as the use of high-frequency surgical diathermy and magnetic resonance, sufficient amperage can be induced to cause microshock and burns.[1,2]

Static electricity has no free flow of electrons. Insulated objects can become highly charged, usually by repeated rubbing. The charge is dissipated by electrons jumping on to another neighbouring object of a different potential. 'Jumping' electrons ionize and heat the air through which they pass, causing a spark which may ignite an inflammable liquid or gas. Lightning is a type of static electrical discharge. Currents of 12 000–200 000 A and voltages in the millions are involved, which flow for only a fraction of a second.[3]

Physiological considerations

For a current to flow through the body, the body must complete a circuit. Usually this involves the current flowing from its source to ground through the body. The pathophysiological effects depend on the size of the current, and this depends on the voltage and electrical resistance of the body, most of which occurs

Table 74.1 Origin and pathophysiological effects of different levels of electrical injury

Current	Source	Effects on victim
10–100 µA	Earth leakage	Microshock (ventricular fibrillation)
300–400 µA	Faulty equipment	Tingling (harmless)
>1 mA	Faulty equipment	Pain (withdraw)
>10 mA	Faulty equipment	Tetany (cannot let go)
>100 mA	Faulty equipment	Macroshock (ventricular fibrillation)
>1 A	Faulty equipment	Burns and tissue damage
>1000 A	High-tension injury	Severe burns and loss of limbs
>12 000 A	Lightning	Coma, severe burns and loss of limbs

in the skin. Dry skin has a resistance in excess of $100\,000\,\Omega$.[4] However, skin resistance is markedly reduced (to approximately $1000\,\Omega$)[5] if the skin is wet, or if a conductive jelly has been applied. Hence, from Ohm's law, dry skin in contact with 240 V mains supply will result in a 0.24 mA current flowing through the body, whereas moist or wet skin will result in a 240 mA current.

Electrocution

Most cases of electrocution occur in the workplace (about 60%) or at home (about 30%).[5] Pathophysiological processes involved in true electrical injuries are poorly understood. The extent of injury depends on first, the amount of current that passes through the body; second, the duration of the current; and third, the tissues traversed by the current (Table 74.1).

The extent of injury is most directly related to amperage. However, usually only the voltage involved is known. In general, lower voltages causes less injury, although voltages as low as 50 V have caused fatalities. An electric current passing through the body produces these main effects.

Tissue heat injury

Currents in excess of 1 A generate sufficient heat energy to cause burns to the skin and internal tissues and organs. Blood vessels and nervous tissue appear to be particularly susceptible.[5]

Depolarization of muscle cells

An alternating current of 30–200 mA will cause ventricular fibrillation.[6] Currents in excess of 5 A cause sustained cardiac asystole. (This is the principle used in a defibrillator.) Apart from ventricular fibrillation, other arrhythmias may occur. Myocardial damage may result in ST and T-wave changes, and global left ventricular dysfunction may occur hours or days later, despite initial minimal electrocardiogram (ECG) changes.[7,8] Myocardial infarction has been reported, and the diagnosis is often difficult, because

of the elevated creatine phosphokinase concentrations (even MB isoenzymes) from the extensive muscle injury.[9,10]

Tetanic contractions of skeletal muscle occur with currents in excess of 15–20 mA. The threshold is particularly low with alternating currents at the household frequency of 50–60 Hz. Tetanic contraction will prevent voluntary release of the source of electrocution, and violent muscle contractions may cause fractures of long bones and spinal vertebrae.[5]

Vascular injuries

Blood vessels may become thrombosed and occluded as a result of the thermal injury, causing tissue ischaemia and necrosis. Affected limbs may even require amputation.[11]

Neurological injuries

Neurological injuries may be central or peripheral, and immediate or late in onset. Spinal cord damage resulting in para- or quadriplegia can result from a current traversing both arms.[5,12] Monoparesis may occur in affected limbs, and the median nerve is particularly vulnerable.[5,12] Electrocution to the head may result in unconsciousness, paralysis of the respiratory centre and late complications such as epilepsy, encephalopathy and parkinsonism.[5,12] Autonomic dysfunction may also occur, causing acute vasospasm or a late sympathetic dystrophy.[5]

Renal failure

Acute renal failure may result from the myoglobinuria secondary to extensive muscle necrosis.[12]

Other injuries

Electrocution can cause the victim to fall or be thrown, and clothing to catch fire, resulting in associated injuries. Intrauterine fetal death has been known. High-voltage injuries can rupture the eardrum. Cataracts may develop later.[11]

Microshock

The above domestic/industrial electrocution is known as macroshock, when current flowing through the intact skin and body passes through the heart. In the ICU, potential microshock electrocution exists. Microshock occurs when there is a direct current path to the heart muscle. The pathway may be provided by a saline-filled monitoring catheter, pulmonary artery catheter or transvenous pacemaker wires. The current required to produce ventricular fibrillation in micro-shock is extremely small, in the order of 60 μA.[13] Currents of 1–2 mA are barely perceptible and produce tingling of the skin (Table 74.1). Hence a lethal microshock may be transmitted to a patient via a staff member who is unaware of the conducted current. Microshock can result from direct contact with faulty electrical equipment, or stray currents from capacitive coupling or earth leakage. Such small currents are potentially lethal because a high current density is produced at the heart (Fig. 74.1).

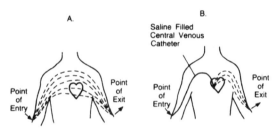

Fig. 74.1 Microshock. (A) Low current density at the heart; (B) high current density at the heart if there is a conducting pathway such as a saline-filled catheter.

High-tension and lightning injuries

High-tension electricity involves voltage much greater than domestic supply – usually many thousands of volts. Tissue damage is mainly due to the generation of heat, as high-amperage currents are involved. Witnesses have described tissues actually exploding.[14]

Lightning injury is a type of high-tension injury. It is rare and its incidence depends upon geographical location. Victims can be thrown a few metres as a result of violent muscular contractions. Electrical arcing of the air causes intense heat, resulting in superficial burns and clothes igniting. Characteristic entrance and exit site burns are seen, which have a spider-like appearance with redness and blistering.

Victims are usually unconscious in the initial phase. However, many victims survive,[3] and good recovery has been reported despite initial hopeless neurological responsiveness (e.g. fixed dilated pupils).[15] Immediate death usually results from cardiorespiratory arrest; asystole is more common than ventricular fibrillation.[3]

Management of electrical injuries

Treatment of electrical injuries is mainly supportive. They include the following.

First aid and resuscitation

It is imperative to make the immediate environment safe for rescuers. Power sources should be switched off and wet areas avoided where possible. Instinctive attempts to grab the electrocuted victim must be avoided until it is safe to do so. Cardiopulmonary resuscitation is carried out when indicated, and continued even if the prognosis seems hopeless.

Investigations

Investigations are indicated to detect damaged organs. They include ECG, echocardiography, computed tomography (CT) of the head, electroencephalogram (EEG), X-rays of the spine and long bones, haemoglobin, serum electrolytes, creatine kinase and urine myoglobin to assess muscle damage, and nerve conduction studies. Arteriograms may help in decision-making to amputate limbs.[11]

Hospital and ICU management

Management is directed towards the treatment of burns, ischaemic and necrotic tissue and injured organs. The principle of treating electrical burns is complete excision. Fasciotomies and amputations may be necessary. Tetanus toxoid and antibiotics, especially penicillin, are given if indicated.

Electrical hazards in ICU

The ICU has the potential to inflict both macroshock and microshock injuries to staff and patients. Potential sources of these electrical hazards are described below.

Major electrical faults

The casing and insulated wiring of electrical equipment protect against electric shock. Faulty wiring or components, and deterioration of internal insulation, can result in the casing becoming live. Contact with live casing or wires can result in an electric current flowing through the victim to ground. The outcome largely depends on the resistance offered by the body to the current. If it is low, such as in a wet environment, sufficient current can flow to cause death.

Microshock currents

Earth leakage currents

Within all pieces of electrical equipment, stray low-amperage electrical currents exist that usually flow to earth, called earth leakage currents. They originate from current leaks across imperfect insulation of wires, capacitive and inductive coupling within the equipment, and coupling from electric and magnetic fields that exist in the working environment, such as the 50–60 Hz mains supply. Normally these currents are small and harmless, but they have the potential to cause microshock.

Pacing wires and central venous lines

In certain circumstances, sufficient current to cause microshock can be passed by capacitive and inductive coupling to intracardiac pacing wires and central venous lines. Ventricular fibrillation has resulted from capacitive coupling with thermistor wires in a pulmonary artery catheter.[1]

Different earth potentials

Inadequate or faulty earthing can result in separate earthing points being at different resting potentials. If contact is made between the two earthing points, sufficient current can flow to cause microshock.

Staff–patient contact

Small currents capable of causing microshock can be transmitted unknowingly to a patient by a staff member who simultaneously touches faulty electrical equipment and the patient. If this current returns to earth via an intracardiac connection, a high current density will pass through the heart, resulting in microshock.

Inductive currents

Inductive coupling from the strong magnetic fields produced by magnetic resonance imaging can cause overheating of wires and equipment. Severe burns have resulted from the use of pulse oximetry during magnetic resonance imaging, and specially designed wiring and probes are recommended.[2] Similar problems can exist with any intravascular device containing wires, such as a pulmonary artery catheter.

Other related hazards

Electrical equipment have the potential to cause other hazards such as thermal injury, fires and power failures. Preliminary critical incident reports suggest that power failures are the most commonly encountered incidents involving electricity in the ICU.

Power failures can be disastrous, as many patients' lives depend on electrically driven life support equipment. As the intensivist frequently works outside the ICU, he or she should also be aware of potential electrical hazards outside ICU.

Electrical safety standards

Most western countries have standards of electrical safety that apply to the use of medical equipment. For example, Australian Standards (AS 3003 and AS 3200) set minimum requirements for Australian hospitals. AS 2500 covers the safe use of electricity in patient care areas.[6] The UK and Europe follow the International Electrotechnical Commission code[17] and the USA follows the National Electric Code 1993.[18] Hospitals should establish their own committees to ensure that adequate standards are applied. However, patient care areas differ in their safety requirements and commonly used classifications are listed below. The ICU should conform to 1b and preferably 1c.

1 (a) unprotected areas – where only routine electrical safety standards are applied;
   (b) body-protected areas – where the level of electrical safety is sufficient to minimize the risk of macroshock when the patient is in direct contact with electrical equipment and the skin impedance is reduced or bypassed;
   (c) cardiac-protected areas – where the level of electrical safety is sufficient to minimize the risk of direct microshock to the heart;
2 wet locations – where spillage of water and physiological solutions, such as saline and blood, frequently occurs;
3 until recently, standards existed for the safe use of inflammable anaesthetic agents.

Measures to protect staff and patients[19,20]

Earthing, fuses and circuit breakers

Earthing reduces the risk of macroshock. The casing in most electrical equipment is connected to ground by a very-low-resistance wire. If a fault arises, the earth wire offers a low-resistance path to ground. The high-amperage current that results will blow the main fuse or circuit breaker, thus warning that a fault is present. Additional protection can be achieved by connecting all the earthing points in a patient care area together by a very-low-resistance wire. This reduces the risk of microshock occurring from earthing points at different potentials, and is commonly used in cardiac-protected areas.

Power supply isolation

Mains isolation

The power supply is isolated from earth using a mains isolation transformer. If contact is made with live faulty circuitry, the risk of electric shock is reduced because stray currents no longer preferentially flow through a patient or staff member to earth. The presence of stray earth leakage currents can be detected by using a line isolation monitor. This type of system is particularly useful in wet locations where the body may offer a very low resistance to earth.

Internal isolation

The mains power supply is isolated from the patient connection by using transformers and photoelectric diodes. The casing is still earthed to protect against faulty circuitry. This method of protection is commonly used in ICU equipment.

Earth leakage circuit breakers

These are devices that switch off the electrical supply if small currents are detected flowing to earth. They can be used to protect against microshock. A major disadvantage is that the power supply to essential life-supporting equipment is switched off.

Equipment checks

The purchase of new equipment should be strictly controlled, and circuit diagrams should be provided. All new equipment should be checked for function and current leaks before use in the ICU. Preventive maintenance of equipment should be done regularly. Dated stickers should be used to show when the equipment was last checked. All faulty equipment must be removed from service, labelled appropriately and recommissioned only after thorough checking.

Reserve power supplies and alarms

All essential equipment should have a reserve power supply (usually a battery) and alarms that warn of power failure. All hospitals should provide an emergency back-up power supply in case of power cuts.

Personnel education

Staff should be taught correct ways to handle electrical equipment. Equipment with frayed wires should never be used, plugs should never be tugged, trolleys should never be wheeled over power cords, and two pieces of equipment should never be handled simultaneously. Staff should also respond appropriately to alarms.

References

1. McNulty SE, Cooper M and Staudt S (1994) Transmitted radiofrequency current through a flow directed pulmonary artery catheter. *Anesth Analg* **78**:587–589.
2. Peden CJ, Menon DK, Hall AS, Sargentoni J and Whitwam JG (1992) Magnetic resonance for the anaesthetist. *Anaesthesia* **47**:508–517.
3. Apfelberg DB, Masters FW and Robinson DW (1974) Pathophysiology and treatment of lightning injuries. *J Trauma* **14**:453–460.
4. Bruner JMR (1976) Hazards of electrical apparatus. *Anesthesiology* **28**:396–424.
5. Fontneau NM and Mitchell A (1991) Miscellaneous neurologic problems in the intensive care unit. In: Rippe JM, Irwin RS, Alpert JS and Fink MP (eds) *Intensive Care Medicine*, 2nd edn. Boston: Little, Brown, pp. 1602–1603.
6. Loughman J and Watson AB (1971) Electrical safety in hospitals and proposed standards. *Med J Aust* **2**:349–355.
7. Lewin RF, Arditti A and Sclarovsky S (1983) Non-invasive evaluation of cardiac injury. *Br Heart J* **49**:190–192.
8. Jensen PJ, Thomsem PEB, Bagger JP, Norgaard A and Baandrup U (1987) Electrical injury causing ventricular arrhythmias. *Br Heart J* **57**:279–283.
9. Walton AS, Harper RW and Coggins GL (1988) Myocardial infarction after electrocution. *Med J Aust* **148**:365–367.
10. McBride JW, Labrosse KR and McCoy HG (1986) Is serum creatine kinase-MB in electrical injured patients predictive of myocardial injury? *J Am Med Assoc* **255**:764–768.
11. Hunt JL, McManus WF, Haney WP and Pruitt BA (1974) Vascular lesions in acute electric injuries. *J Trauma* **14**:461–473.
12. Solem L, Fischer RP and Strate RG (1977) The natural history of electrical injury. *J Trauma* **17**:487–492.
13. Watson AB, Wright JS and Loughman J (1973) Electrical thresholds for ventricular fibrillation in man. *Med J Aust* **1**:1179–1182.
14. Burke JF, Quinby WC, Bondoc C, McLaughlin E and Trelstad RL (1977) Patterns of high tension electric injury in children and adolescents and their management. *Am J Surg* **133**:492–494.
15. Hanson GC and Mcllwaith GR (1973) Lightning injury: two case histories and a review of management. *Br Med J* **4**:271–274.
16. Australian Standard 2500 (1988) *Guide to the Safe Use of Electricity in Patient Care*. Sydney: Standards Association of Australia.
17. CEI-IEC 601–1&2 (1988) *Medical Electrical Equipment*, Geneva: International Electrotechnical Commission.
18. Early MW, Murray RH and Caloggero JM (1993) *National Electrical Code Handbook*, 6th edn. Quincy: National Fire Protection Association.
19. Litt L (1994) Electrical safety in the operating room. In: Miller RD (ed.) *Anesthesia*, 4th edn. New York: Churchill Livingstone, pp. 2625–2634.
20. Ehrenwerth J (1994) *Electrical Safety in and around the Operating Room. ASA Refresher Course in Anesthesia*. Philadelphia: JB Lippincott, p. 123.

75 | Envenomation

MM Fisher

Australia's unique geography and climate provide a home for over 25 000 animal species, of which at least 200 have venom glands. The more highly venomous of these species far outrank any overseas species in their ability to kill.[1] Despite this, deaths due to envenomation are infrequent (less than 10 per annum).

General principles of management of envenomation

First aid

First-aid manoeuvres are used to delay systemic absorption of venom until definitive treatment is available. The first-aid method used in Australia for all rapid-acting venoms is the bandage-and-splint method, first described by Sutherland *et al.*[2] The technique is based on earlier demonstrations that venom moves in superficial lymphatics and capillaries, and relies on emptying these vessels. A firm bandage is applied over the bitten area and up the limb, which is then splinted. The patient should be carried to a transport facility and not permitted to move, as muscle activity may allow systemic absorption. When bites occur on the trunk, pressure should be applied over the bitten area and a firm bandage applied. The bandage-and-splint technique has been validated experimentally and in clinical practice. Apart from being effective, the technique has advantages over arterial tourniquets; it is less damaging and painful, and upon removal, does not produce reactive hyperaemia in the limb, which may lead to catastrophic envenomation. There is definitely no role for arterial tourniquets in envenomation. Localization of venom by bandage may lead to its local detoxification.

For venoms which produce late life-threatening effects, such as in stonefish and red back spider envenomation, bandage-and-splint techniques are not indicated, as such measures may increase pain.[1]

Pain from stonefish, fortescue and bull rout envenomation responds to warm water. The pain of bluebottle stings may be relieved by a number of methods, and ice is the most effective. Liberal application of vinegar is recommended in box jellyfish envenomation as it paralyses the stinging apparatus

Emergency room treatment

The treatment in the emergency room is based on the type of first aid which has been used (Table 75.1). Virtually all serious envenomations produce symptoms within 4 h. Children should be observed for 24 h after a history of envenomation. A history of headache, abdominal pain, nausea and vomiting, or abnormal coagulation, accurately predict envenomation in children who have a presumptive diagnosis of envenomation.[3]

Anaphylactic shock

In snake handlers, zoo keepers and people who have been previously been bitten, anaphylaxis to the venom may occur, and confuse and complicate the presenting features and treatment. Bluebottles, bees, wasps and jumper ants are more likely to kill through allergic than toxic mechanisms. Severe hypotension in snake bite due to Australian snakes should lead to a consideration of anaphylaxis. Use of mast cell tryptase assays may confirm the diagnosis of anaphylaxis in reactions to the venoms of snakes and Hymenoptera (see Chapter 58).

Venepuncture

Many Australian snake venoms contain potent prothrombin activators, and many produce very prolonged bleeding times. Although complications from bleeding vascular malformations and gastric ulcers have been described, it is unusual for severe bleeding to occur in the absence of multiple puncture sites.

Table 75.1 Emergency room treatment of envenomation

Presenting first aid	No symptoms	Minor symptoms	Significant envenomation
None	Observe 6 h*	Observe 6 h*	Bandage Definitive treatment Remove bandage
Bandage and splint	Remove bandage Observe 6 h*	Remove bandage Observe 6 h*	Definitive treatment Remove bandage
Arterial tourniquet	Remove tourniquet Observe 6 h*	Prepare for definitive treatment Remove tourniquet Observe or treat	Definitive management Remove tourniquet

* Observe 24 h in children.

Nevertheless, it is good practice to keep injections to a minimum, insert an IV cannula, and to draw blood and administer therapy. The two exceptions to this are adrenaline pretreatment and tetanus toxoid when indicated.

Snake handlers

Zoo keepers and snake collectors present particular difficulties in the management of snake bite.[4] If they are bitten by exotic snakes, antivenoms are available from Taronga Zoo, Gosford Wildlife Park and Royal Melbourne Hospital. In addition, handlers usually have a history of previous bites, and are at increased risk from anaphylaxis to antivenom and venom. They will invariably require pretreatment. However, they are often resistant to receiving antivenom, wishing only to have it in life-threatening circumstances because of the perceived risk of anaphylaxis. It is useful if possible to have one member of staff whom they know and trust involved in their treatment early.

Tetanus toxoid

All envenomated patients should have tetanus immunoglobulin status checked and appropriate prophylaxis administered.

Use of antivenom

Indications for antivenom

Antivenom is indicated if there is evidence of significant envenomation. It is not necessary to wait for life-threatening symptoms prior to its use, and nor is it necessary for minor symptoms.

Pretreatment

There are no controlled trials of pretreatment to prevent allergic reactions to antivenoms in Australia. However, pretreatment appears significantly to reduce the incidence of adverse reactions to antivenoms.[5,6] The current Commonwealth Serum Laboratory's recommendations are parenteral antihistamine and IM adrenaline prior to antivenom administration, with the addition of steroids in known allergic patients.[6] Use of adrenaline is controversial, particularly with respect to its possible role in cerebral haemorrhage. However, an equal number of patients suffer cerebral haemorrhage whether or not adrenaline is used; cerebral haemorrhage is usually associated with IV use, and subcutaneous adrenaline 0.5 mg is unlikely to cause hypertension.[5]

Method of administration

The major principles in antivenom administration are as follows:

1 Dosage is related to the amount of venom injected, and not the size of the patient. Dosage is not reduced in children.
2 Antivenom should be administered via a drip after dilution in at least 500 ml of saline. Careful monitoring and observation should be employed during infusion.

Assessing effects of antivenom

The usual consequence of administering antivenom is prompt improvement. If the patient continues to deteriorate or does not improve, the possibilities are that a further dose is necessary or that the wrong antivenom was given.

Prevention of serum sickness

Sutherland[6] also recommends a 5-day course of steroids after polyvalent or large doses of antivenom, and possibly after any exposure. The incidence of delayed reactions to Australian antivenoms is about 5% of cases. There are no controlled trials of such therapy.

Management of envenomation of specific Australian species

Snakes[1,7]

The known toxic effects of snake venoms in Australia and their management are as follows:

1 *Muscular paralysis*: treatment is by artificial ventilation and antivenom.
2 *Coagulopathy and disseminated intravascular coagulopathy*: treatment is with fresh frozen plasma and antivenom.
3 *Rhabdomyolysis*: treatment is by maintaining high urine output and mannitol infusion and with antivenom. Careful and frequent measurement of potassium levels is indicated and use of calcium salts, glucose and insulin, sodium bicarbonate, resonium and, occasionally, dialysis may be necessary. The brown snake also has a nephrotoxin, and renal failure in the absence of rhabdomyolysis has been described.
4 *Hypotension* should be treated with colloid infusion and antivenom.
5 *Local tissue damage* is treated with symptomatic relief. Necrotic tissue should be debrided, but tissue necrosis is less common with Australian snakes than foreign species such as rattlesnakes and cobras.
6 *Sudden collapse and death* may occur in brown snake bite.[8]

Spiders

Funnel web spiders[9]

Venomous species are largely confined to the east coast of Australia. The commonest offender is the Sydney funnel web (*Atrax robustus*), although envenomation has been described from *Hadronychae formidabilis*, *H. infensus*, *H. versutus* and *H. ex bermagui*. Bites from spiders of this genus are often associated with envenomation. Envenomation produces a dramatic syndrome due to the release of endogenous transmitters which produce an 'autonomic storm' leading to salivation, hypertension, tachycardia, gastric dilatation, massive membrane pulmonary oedema, muscle spasms, metabolic and respiratory acidosis,[10] and possibly raised intracranial pressure. Symptomatic treatment consists of muscle paralysis, artificial ventilation, vasodilators, high levels of positive end-expiratory pressure to control pulmonary oedema, and volume replacement with colloid. The use of antivenom rapidly reverses all symptoms, and appears to be effective in all species.[11]

Red back spider (Latrodectus hasselti macens)[1]

This spider's bites are usually administered on the trunk rather than the limbs. The female spider is poisonous. Symptoms are related to release of acetylcholine and catecholamines from autonomic terminals, which produces severe local pain within minutes. The pain then spreads across the body. Localized sweating occurs, which also spreads. Other features may include lymphadenopathy, shivering, headache, nausea and vomiting, and pyrexia. Hypertension, tachycardia and paralysis are the life-threatening features. Icepacks may produce symptomatic relief. Antivenom is administered IM in a dose of 500 units. Pretreatment is indicated in patients allergic to horse serum. There is a higher incidence of serum sickness than with other Australian antivenoms. Antivenom is repeated in 2 h if no improvement occurs, and may be given IV after pretreatment in severe cases. Diazepam may help muscle spasms. It is effective up to 2 weeks after envenomation. Rhabdomyolysis has been described in one case.[12]

Other spiders produce a range of symptoms, from minor to severe. Funnel web antivenom produced improvement in a child bitten by a wolf spider. Of increasing concern is the syndrome of necrotizing arachnidism, which ranges from ulcers to a systemic inflammatory response with skin and muscle necrosis. Ulcers may persist and recur for some years. The profusion of recommended treatments (e.g. dapsone, heparin and hyperbaric oxygen) is distinguished by lack of proven efficacy. The white-tailed spider, black widow spider and common house spider have all been implicated, but all may produce harmless bites. It has been suggested that the syndrome may be due to *Mycobacterium ulcerans*.[13]

Ticks

Ticks are found in scrub and bush country on the east-coast regions of Australia. The tick buries the byostome into the host tissues, and produces symptoms via acquired allergy to the secretions, introduced microorganisms, or a potent neurotoxin in the saliva. The symptoms produced are ataxia and progressive weakness leading to paralysis, and the condition may be mistaken for Guillain–Barré syndrome or poliomyelitis. The presenting complaint may be difficulty in reading. Toxic myocarditis and rhabdomyolysis have been described. Lymphadenopathy is a common clinical presentation.

A careful search for ticks should be carried out in all cases presenting with muscle weakness. The ticks should be removed by dousing with kerosene and prising the tick free with curved forceps. Antitoxin should be administered for significant paralysis, the dosage being two ampoules in serious cases.

Jellyfish[1]

The commonly found jellyfish *Pelagia noctiluca* (the little mauve stinger) and *Physalia physalis* (the bluebottle or Portuguese man of war) are found in all coastal waters of Australia. They produce marked local pain and redness (which is relieved by the application of cold compresses) and may produce anaphylaxis.

In the northern coastal waters *Carukia barnsei*, the Irukandji, produces pain, nausea, vomiting, profuse sweating and backache. Vinegar is used for first aid, and treatment is with analgesia. *Cliropsolins quadrigatis* produce similar but less severe effects than the box jellyfish. Box jellyfish antivenom neutralizes the effects of the venom in mice but has not been used in humans. The box jellyfish, *Chironex fleckeri southcott*, is the most dangerous jellyfish in the world, and has caused more than 70 deaths in Australian waters. Box jellyfish envenomation causes severe pain and skin whealing, which leads to necrosis. This is followed rapidly by hypotension and paralysis. Treatment is by dousing with vinegar and applying a bandage-and-splint over envenomated areas. Ventilatory support is necessary until antivenom can be administered. Plasma expanders and analgesia may be required.

Blue-ringed octopus

This small (less than 100 g) octopus is found in all Australian waters, and is normally brown in colour, with bright blue rings appearing when disturbed. The bite may be totally painless. Mild cases may produce cerebellar signs, but the usual outcome is paralysis from tetradotoxin. The treatment involves bandage-and-splint first aid and mechanical ventilation. There is no antivenom. The role of anticholinesterases in accelerating return of muscle power is not established but worthy of trial.

Stonefish

Stonefish are found in northern waters of Australia and characteristically envenomate through dorsal spines when trodden on. The stings are extremely painful, and may be associated with muscle paralysis, weakness, cardiovascular collapse and skin necrosis. First aid consists of applying warm to hot water, or injection of local anaesthesia if available. Regional block should be considered in multiple stings. The puncture wound should be debrided and antivenom given, unless minor discomfort is the sole feature. Dosage of antivenom is based on one ampoule for every two punctures, up to three ampoules.

Bees and ants[14,15]

Reaction to the venom of the universal European honey been (*Apis ellifera*) is common, but fatalities are rare.[14] Direct toxic effects with pain and swelling may occur as a result of bee and ant stings, but the most life-threatening feature is anaphylaxis. In those who have had severe reactions, desensitization should be considered. They should otherwise learn to administer adrenaline by themselves, if and when the need arises.

References

1. Sutherland SK (1983) *Australian Animal Toxins*. Melbourne: Oxford University Press.
2. Sutherland SK, Coulter AR and Harris RD (1979) Rationalisation of first aid measures for elapid snakebite. *Lancet* **i**:183–186.
3. Tibballs J (1992) Diagnosis and treatment of confirmed and suspected snake bite. Implications from an analysis of 46 paediatric cases. *Med J Aust* **156**:270–272.
4. Fisher MM and Bowey CJ (1989) Urban envenomation. *Med J Aust* **150**:695–697.
5. Tibballs J (1994) Premedication for snake antivenom. *Med J Aust* **160**:4–7.
6. Sutherland SK (1992) Antivenom use in Australia. Premedication, adverse reactions and the use of venom detection kits. *Med J Aust* **157**:734–739.
7. Sutherland SK and King K (1991) *Management of Snakebite Injuries*. Monograph series number 1. Sydney: The Royal Flying Doctor Service of Australia.
8. Sutherland SK (1992) Deaths from snake bite in Australia, 1981–1991. *Med J Aust* **157**:740–746.
9. Gray MR (1984) A guide to funnel-web spider identification. *Med J Aust* **141**:837–840.
10. Fisher MM, Carr GA, McGuinness R and Warden JC (1980) *Atrax robustus* envenomation. *Anaesth Intens Care* **8**:410–420.
11. Dieckmann J, Prebble J, McDonogh A *et al.* (1989) Efficacy of funnel-web spider antivenom in human envenomation by *Hydronyche* species. *Med J Aust* **151**:706–707.
12. Gala S and Katalaris CH (1992) Rhabdomyolysis due to redback spider envenomation. *Med J Aust* **157**:66.
13. Harvey MS and Raven RJ (1991) Necrotising arachnidism in Australia: a simple case of misidentification. *Med J Aust* **154**:856.
14. Harvey P, Sperber S, Kette F *et al.* (1988) Bee sting mortality in Australia. *Med J Aust* **1**:209–211.
15. Southcott RV (1988) Some harmful Australian insects. *Med J Aust* **149**:656–661.

Part XII

Pharmacological considerations

Pharmacokinetics, pharmacodynamics and drug monitoring in acute illness

TG Short and T Gin

Critically ill patients usually receive multiple drug therapy for specific treatment of their illness (e.g. antibiotics), managing pathophysiological consequences of their condition (e.g. inotropes) and for sedation (e.g. benzodiazepines and opioids). These drugs are nearly always given IV and often have a narrow therapeutic index. Critically ill patients may have altered pharmacokinetics, and multiple drug therapy may lead to unexpected interactions between drugs, and interventions such as haemodialysis and plasmapheresis may profoundly affect drug disposition. The individual response to drugs can also change quickly. A detailed knowledge of pharmacological changes in the critically ill is required to administer drugs safely. However, information about changes in drug handling and drug response has been derived mostly from normal patients and those with stable, chronic single-organ failure, and may be less relevant to critically ill patients with multiple organ dysfunction. It is thus essential to monitor the effects of all drug treatment regularly. Individualizing drug therapy has been shown to improve the survival of critically ill patients.

Pharmacokinetics

Pharmacokinetics is the study of the absorption, distribution, metabolism and elimination of drugs. Several mathematical models can be used to describe drug disposition, but common pharmacokinetic concepts include volume of distribution (V), clearance (Cl) and half-time ($t_{1/2}$), which can be used to design rational dosing regimens.[1]

Volume of distribution

The *apparent* volume of distribution (V) of a drug is the volume into which an amount (A) of drug appears to be dispersed, given the concentration (C) measured in the blood according to the formula $V = A/C$. Drug dispersion is not instantaneous, and hence more than one apparent volume of distribution can be calculated. The apparent *initial* volume of distribution (V_1) is the volume into which drug appears to be dispersed immediately after IV injection. The apparent volume of distribution at *steady state* (V_{ss}) is the larger volume calculated after distribution of drug throughout the body has occurred or when the rate of drug administration equals the rate of elimination. The V_1 is useful for calculating the initial IV loading dose (D_L) to achieve a target concentration (C), i.e. $D_L = V_1 \times C$, if high initial concentrations may cause unwanted effects (e.g. theophylline). The V_{ss} similarly allows calculation of the loading dose, when the therapeutic index is high and it is desirable to achieve and maintain therapeutic concentrations quickly (e.g. penicillin). Volumes of distribution depend upon physicochemical characteristics of drugs and can be altered by pathophysiological changes.

Clearance

Clearance (Cl) is defined as the volume of blood completely cleared of drug per unit time, and can be calculated for specific organs or the total body. The liver is the main organ for drug metabolism, and it has a different intrinsic clearance (metabolizing capacity) for different drugs. Depending on the drug, metabolism may be altered by enzyme inhibition, enzyme induction or changes in hepatic blood flow and protein binding. The rate of elimination of drugs is usually proportional to the amount of drug – a first-order process. However, when the concentration of some drugs (e.g. ethyl alcohol, phenytoin or high-dose barbiturates) is relatively large, the metabolic pathway becomes saturated, and drug is slowly eliminated at a fixed rate – a zero-order process. A corollary is that small doses of drug will cause marked sustained increases in plasma concentration during zero-order kinetics, compared with administration during first-order kinetics. Total body clearance (Cl_{TB}) can be used to calculate the infusion rate (k_{01}) of a drug to maintain a given blood concentration, when steady-state conditions have been reached (C_{ss}) by the formula k_{01} = $C_{ss} \times Cl_{TB}$. Clearance is the most useful indicator of drug elimination, and clearance and volume of distribution determine the elimination half-time.

Half-time

Half-time is the time taken for the drug concentration in the blood to decrease by 50%. After a bolus dose of drug or after stopping an infusion, blood concentrations decrease because of redistribution and metabolism. The initial distribution half-life of a drug ($t_{\frac{1}{2}\alpha}$) describes the initial rapid decrease in concentration mainly caused by drug redistribution to tissue. The elimination half-time ($t_{\frac{1}{2}\beta}$) describes the slower decrease in blood concentration caused mainly by drug elimination. If the concentration–time curve is best fitted by a triexponential curve, a terminal elimination half-time ($t_{\frac{1}{2}\gamma}$) can be calculated to describe drug elimination when there is a slow return of drug from peripheral reservoirs. The relevance of these elimination half-times depends on the drug concentration required to have an effect relative to the concentration in the patient. Elimination half-time is of limited use if termination of drug effect is caused by redistribution (e.g. IV anaesthetic agents). The half-time after stopping a short infusion will thus be less than the terminal elimination half-time. However, as the infusion is prolonged to achieve steady state, the half-time upon stopping the infusion will increase until the terminal elimination half-time is reached.[2] Half-time, none the less, determines the time required for an exponential process to approach an equilibrium or steady state. For a given dose rate, whether given by boluses or infusion, four half-times are required for 94% completion of steady-state and five half-times required for 97% completion.

Protein binding

In general, only the unbound drug can be distributed across membranes, exert a pharmacological effect and be metabolized or eliminated. Changes in protein binding are thus important for drugs which are highly protein-bound (>80%) because small changes in protein binding will result in large changes in the free concentration (e.g. warfarin displacement by phenytoin) with changes in the volume of distribution, clearance of drug and drug effect. Most acidic drugs, including all antibiotics, bind to albumin, with binding being proportional to the log of the concentration of albumin. When albumin concentrations are below 20 g/l, increases in free concentration are likely to be significant. Basic drugs, such as lignocaine, pethidine, phenytoin and propranolol, bind mainly to α_1 acid glycoprotein. During acute illness, α_1 acid glycoprotein concentrations increase with increased binding.[3]

Practical applications

A knowledge of pharmacokinetics enables use of appropriate dosing regimens. If a drug has limited toxicity in overdose, a large loading dose can be given to achieve and maintain a therapeutic concentration quickly (e.g. penicillins). With a drug of narrow therapeutic index, a small loading dose (calculated with initial volume of distribution) is better; maintenance doses are then based on clearance and closely monitored response (e.g. aminophylline).

The immediate effect of changing the rate of drug infusion will depend on the half-time of the drug. For drugs with long half-times (e.g. midazolam and morphine), an increase in dose requirements should

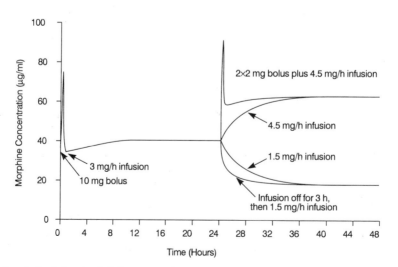

Fig. 76.1 Effect of methods of changing infusion rate on plasma concentration of morphine in a healthy patient

be met by titrating small boluses to achieve the new state, and then increasing the infusion rate by an appropriate amount. Decreases in requirements should be met by switching off the infusion, and then restarting at a lower rate after the new desired state has been reached. Simply decreasing or increasing the infusion rate is only appropriate for very-short-acting drugs such as adrenaline. To change the infusion rate for morphine (which has an elimination half-time of at least 3 h in healthy individuals) will require 15 h for the drug concentration to reach the new steady state (Fig. 76.1).

Pharmacodynamics

Pharmacodynamics is the study of the effects of drug on the body. The relationship between drug dosage or concentration and drug effect is complex. Drug effects are caused by the presence of active drug at its sites of action. The logarithmic dose–response curve is sigmoid in shape (see below) and this may be modified by complicating factors such as drug interactions and patient tolerance.

Biophase

Drugs do not usually work in the blood, but rather at sites in various organs (e.g. muscle relaxants at receptors in the neuromuscular junction, and antibiotics in bronchial secretions in a patient with pneumonia). This site of action is known as the biophase. There is a delay between achieving an adequate concentration of drug in the blood and a therapeutic concentration at the biophase. This delay is the result of two factors – the amount of blood flow to the organ and the time for the drug to pass from the blood to the biophase. Intravenous drug therapy differs from enteral routes of administration in that very high drug concentrations are achieved in the blood and highly perfused organs, compared with organs that are poorly perfused (Table 76.1). Thus, rapid administration of drugs with a narrow therapeutic index may cause transient toxicity at the main or secondary sites of action (e.g. rapid IV administration of vancomycin can cause severe hypotension secondary to histamine release).

Dose–response curve

Drug effect is usually proportional to the logarithm of the free concentration of drug, and is described by a sigmoid shaped dose–response curve (Fig. 76.2). This relationship means that the dose of drug required to significantly increase or decrease its effect at a certain concentration is highly variable. In the middle part of the curve, small changes in dose (and thus concentration) will have large clinical effects; at the high or low ends of the curve, large changes in dose are required to obtain a change in clinical effect. The sigmoid shape of the curve results from the fact that for any drug there is a maximal observable therapeutic effect. Dose–response curves can be drawn for any aspect of drug pharmacology, and the ratio between the median toxic dose and the median effective dose is termed the therapeutic index. When this ratio is low, it is essential to titrate drug effect carefully, and observe or measure response carefully (e.g. aminoglycosides and aminophylline). Drug effects also depend upon interactions with other drugs and concurrent disease. The effects of drugs with similar effects are not necessarily additive – sedative effects of an opioid plus a benzodiazepine or propofol are up to 50% more than expected if the effects were simply additive.[4,5]

Table 76.1 Distribution of cardiac output in healthy and critically ill patients

Organ	% Body weight	% Cardiac output	Change in % cardiac output in critical illness
Lungs	2	100	Nil
Heart	0.5	5	+++
Brain	2	14	+++
Kidneys	0.5	23	− − −
Liver/splanchnic	10	28	− − −
Endocrine/bone marrow	2	6	− −
Skin	6	9	− −
Muscle	50	16	− −
Fat	15	5	− −
Other	12	5	− −

After intravenous injection in a healthy patient, initial organ concentrations depend on their blood flow and mass. In the critically ill, cardiac output may vary widely depending on therapy, and distribution will depend on the amount of peripheral vasoconstriction (e.g. from hypovolaemic shock) or vasodilatation (e.g. systemic inflammatory response syndrome).

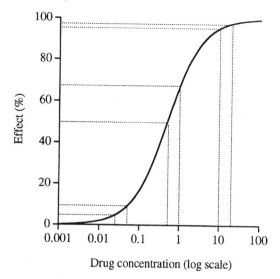

Fig. 76.2 A typical dose–response curve. In the middle part of the curve, a small change in drug concentration causes a large change in effect. At the extremes of the curve, large changes in concentration are required to observe much change in effect.

Changes in critical illness

Route of administration

The enteral route is usually best avoided because of alterations in gut motility, blood flow, pH, function and first-pass metabolism. Anticholinergics, antacids, phenothiazines and opioids all delay gastric emptying. Subcutaneous and IM injection suffer from similar problems with systemic transfer of drug being dependent on blood flow at the site of injection, which in turn depends on posture, activity, site of injection and degree of vasoconstriction or vasodilatation at that site.

The IV route is used because of speed of onset, convenience, reliability and lack of enteral formulations of some drugs. Intravenous apparatus including glass, plastics and rubber may absorb drugs, decreasing the dose delivered (e.g. insulin, heparin and isosorbide). When several drugs are delivered through the same IV line, chemical incompatibility may also occur. This may be a result of pH effects altering solubility, solvent effects (e.g. precipitation of the propylene glycol used to dissolve some preparations of diazepam when diluted excessively) and cation–anion interactions causing precipitation or formation of less active yet soluble complexes (e.g. thiopentone or calcium in combination with most other drugs). Although precipitation can be detected by visual inspection, lack of visual changes does not preclude loss of potency (e.g. heparin and dopamine, insulin and total parenteral nutrition).[6,7]

When infusing drugs IV, the method of administration can alter the amount delivered dramatically.

Simple infusions using a drip chamber to regulate flow are not adequate when infusing inotropes, and mechanical drop counters and peristaltic pumps are also erratic. Syringe pumps are the most accurate, but are erratic at low rates (e.g. 1–2 ml/h) so dilution may be needed to allow an increase in flow rate to more reliable speeds. Siphoning from or flushing of IV lines can also result in drug overdose.

Pharmacokinetic and pharmacodynamic changes

Critically ill patients often have multiple organ dysfunction, causing alterations in drug handling and effect in the body at all levels. The net effect of these multiple changes is difficult to predict. Frequently, the main effect is to increase interpatient variability in response, even if the average response is little altered. Intrapatient variability also occurs over very brief periods in response to changes in the patient's condition. Midazolam may fail to be metabolized in septic shock, and cardiogenic shock can cause rapid increases in lignocaine concentrations, even after the infusion has been ceased.[8,9]

Circulatory failure

Circulatory failure causes a greater percentage of cardiac output to go to essential organs (e.g. heart and brain) and decreased blood flow to peripheral tissues (Table 76.1). The net effect is increased blood concentrations in the heart and brain, and decreased blood concentrations in the periphery. There is decreased renal blood flow and shunting of blood from cortical to juxtamedullary nephrons. Glomerular filtration rate and tubular excretion are decreased, decreasing extraction of drugs and metabolites. Liver blood flow is decreased and hepatocellular function impaired, thus decreasing clearance of both highly extracted drugs (because of failure of delivery) and poorly extracted drugs (because of failure of cellular metabolism).[10] Mechanical ventilation may cause further decreases in liver blood flow by increasing intrathoracic, and therefore, venous pressure.

The initial effect of circulatory failure is a large decrease in V_1, and a decrease in VD_{ss} and clearance of drugs. The effects are more profound on normally rapidly distributed drugs (e.g. sedatives or lignocaine, where standard doses may cause central nervous system toxicity) than slowly distributed drugs such as digoxin. Fluid and inotropic therapy may alter these effects over brief periods of time. With volume overload, there may be an increase in V_1 but with a more prolonged distribution half-time. Acidaemia may exacerbate these changes by increasing the free concentration of highly bound drugs, but decrease the pharmacological response to some drugs by altering receptor affinity (e.g. catecholamines). Hypovolaemic shock causes increased sensitivity to central nervous system depressants, even after restoration of circulating volume, and this is probably secondary to (as yet unidentified) circulating factors.[11]

Hepatic failure

Hepatic failure may increase or decrease volume of distribution and total body clearance, and increases elimination half-time of hepatically metabolized drugs. Loading doses are often not greatly affected. Extrahepatic metabolism is considerable in anhepatic animal models. In the severely ill, there is usually a decrease in liver blood flow, and therefore, the rate at which drugs are delivered to the liver for metabolism. Flow-dependent drugs include lignocaine, morphine and midazolam. Vasopressors do not usually decrease liver blood flow because increases in cardiac output compensate for potential vasoconstriction. Phase 1 reactions, which involve cytochrome P_{450}, are usually more affected than phase 2 reactions. There is a poor correlation between derangement of conventional tests of liver function and the degree of impairment of drug metabolism; the impairment may also vary widely over short periods of time. In the severely ill, metabolism of some drugs will almost cease, as indicated by a lack of formation of metabolites and very high plasma concentrations (e.g. midazolam).[8]

Hepatic failure tends to decrease the amount of drug bound because of accumulation of metabolites which compete for binding sites on protein. For instance, elevated concentrations of bilirubin decrease in protein binding of sulphonamides, tetracyclines, penicillins and cephalosporins. A decrease in protein binding will offset increases in volume of distribution when the drug is highly protein-bound, such as most penicillins and erythromycin. For drugs with low protein binding such as aminoglycosides, a decrease in protein binding will have little effect on free plasma concentrations.

Renal failure

Total body clearance is reduced by renal failure, and volumes will increase if there is significant fluid retention. Renal failure tends to decrease renal clearances and increase half-times of drugs cleared by the kidneys. Drug doses may be decreased to as little as 10% of normal. In the case of drugs which are metabolized by the liver with metabolites excreted by the kidneys, there may be accumulation of active metabolites in renal failure (e.g. morphine-6-glucuronide). Renal failure usually affects glomerular function more than tubular function, so excretion of aminoglycosides, which depend more on glomerular filtration, are affected more than excretion of penicillins, which are dependent on tubular function.

Creatinine clearance is usually a poor guide in the critically ill because there may be alterations in the rate of formation of creatinine as well as its excretion by the kidneys. Some assays of creatinine are also inaccurate in jaundiced patients. The effects of disease may also be paradoxical. For instance, propranolol elimination is thought to be via metabolism in the liver, but elimination is impaired in renal failure by an unknown mechanism. Phenytoin excretion is increased in uraemia. Accumulation of metabolic products causes decreases in protein binding of drugs (e.g. uraemia decreases binding of penicillins, sulphonamides and cephalosporins).

Renal replacement (dialytic) therapy drastically alters volumes and clearances of drugs. Effects vary with the mode of dialysis, the type of membrane in use and the drugs in question. For most modern membranes little information is available, but several reviews of what is known are available.[12,13]

Systemic inflammatory response syndrome

In acute severe illness such as sepsis, and multiple organ failure, there is an increase in capillary permeability and total body water secondary to the leaky capillaries. This usually increases volume of distribution of drugs, so that increased loading doses may be required to attain a satisfactory therapeutic concentration. Similar changes occur in patients with major burns and may be a result of circulating leukotrienes. The volume of distribution may also change over short periods of time. When patients start to recover, serum concentrations may increase because of the decreasing volume of distribution of the drug (e.g. vancomycin)[14] or decrease because of resumption of normal metabolism and clearance (e.g. midazolam).[8] Circulatory, hepatic and renal failure will also add the characteristic changes already described, of decreased metabolism and accumulation of active metabolites.

Changes in receptors in acute illness

Many drugs act at receptors, and some receptors may change in the critically ill, affecting drug response. One cause of tolerance (i.e. decreased drug effect for a given dose or plasma concentration) is altered receptor function. Catecholamines show an increase in receptor numbers in response to a lack of agonist (*up-regulation*) and a decrease in receptor numbers in response to increased concentrations of agonist (*down-regulation*). Proliferation of extrajunctional acetylcholine receptors on muscle after acute injuries such as burns and denervation can lead to hyperkalaemia following the use of suxamethonium. Drug affinity for receptors is also pH-dependent. Acidosis decreases the affinity of catecholamines for their receptors, and is a significant problem when the pH < 7.1. Hypothermia also decreases drug affinity for receptors.

Drug monitoring

When a drug has a narrow therapeutic index, it is essential to monitor response to the drug. This can be either via clinical observation (e.g. sedatives or inotropes) or measuring drug concentrations (e.g. aminoglycosides and theophyllines). When measuring drug concentrations, toxicity may either be associated with peak concentrations (e.g. theophylline-induced arrhythmias) or mean concentrations (e.g. gentamicin-induced ototoxicity; hence trough concentrations are measured).

For some drugs, there are accepted therapeutic and toxic ranges. Acute illness may alter the relationship between drug concentration and effect, so that plasma concentration data should be interpreted with caution, and the clinical signs of efficacy and toxicity actively searched for. Systemic drug concentrations may be a poor indication of the drug concentration at its site of action. Drug concentrations may also increase dramatically after cessation of infusions, as a result of physiological changes such as a decrease in cardiac output or changes in regional organ perfusion.

Gastrointestinal, respiratory and central nervous system side-effects or toxic effects of drugs may be difficult to detect in the critically ill. Most commercial drug assays measure total concentration of drug in plasma, and do not assess the effects of changes in protein binding. Because of the poor correlation between drug concentration and effect for many commonly monitored drugs, the value of therapeutic monitoring has recently been questioned. Some examples of changes in commonly used drugs are given in Table 76.2. Detailed information on specific drugs is available in standard pharmacology textbooks.[15]

Sedatives

Most ICUs use midazolam and/or opioids for sedation. Propofol may be appropriate in certain cases (see Chapter 78). Pharmacokinetic differences contribute to the more predictable adjustment and monitoring of sedation with propofol compared with midazolam. However, recovery from sedation will also depend upon concurrent elimination of any opioid component. For midazolam, elimination half-time is increased in the critically ill, and the metabolism of midazolam may change in parallel with patient condition.[8] In renal failure, decreased protein binding is compensated by increased clearance of the free drug, although there may be increased effect, because midazolam is normally 96% bound.[16]

For propofol, pharmacokinetics have been studied during 2–4-day infusions only in patients without hepatic impairment[17–19] Both fixed and variable infusion rates adjusted to degree of sedation were used, with most infusion rates falling in the range 1–3 mg/kg per h. After stopping the infusion, propofol concentrations decreased by half within 10 min, and then declined more slowly. Given the lower blood concentration required for sedation compared with anaesthesia, the rapid decrease in propofol concentration usually led to rapid awakening, although concomitant drugs and disease could delay full recovery. The rapid decrease in blood concentration is a result of the high clearance of propofol. The long terminal elimination half-time (12–50 h) in these studies described blood concentrations that were too small to have clinical effect. Propofol is 98% bound, to albumin and erythrocytes, and severe hypoalbuminaemia and anaemia cause increases in the free fraction.

Table 76.2 Therapeutic drug monitoring in the critically ill

Drug	Therapeutic levels	Toxic effects and guidelines to dosage
Antiarrhythmics		
Digoxin	0.8–2.5 μg/ml	> 5 μg/ml. Monitor ECG for conduction defects and arrhythmias
Lignocaine	3–6 mg/ml	Increased toxicity in congestive heart failure
Antibiotics		
Gentamicin	Peak 5–10 μg/ml, trough < 2	Renal and ototoxicity: increase dose. Give once a day and monitor level pre-dose
Amikacin	Peak 8–16 μg/ml, trough < 4	As above
Vancomycin	Peak 20–40 μg/ml, trough < 10	
Anticonvulsants		
Phenytoin	10–20 mg/ml	Arrhythmias, monitor free concentration in uraemia and hypoalbuminaemia
Bronchodilators		
Theophylline	10–20 mg/l	> 25 mg/l

ECG = Electrocardiogram.

Opioids

Opioid requirements may vary over 10-fold between patients, and tolerance develops quickly so that the dose must be titrated and monitored. Opioids given primarily for analgesia are best controlled by patients themselves with a patient-controlled analgesia (PCA) device, while analgesia and side-effects are regularly monitored with a variety of visual analogue or ordinal scales. The most commonly used opioids are morphine and fentanyl. Pethidine is seldom used because accumulation of the toxic metabolite norpethidine readily occurs. Morphine is metabolized mainly by the liver but hepatic failure seldom affects morphine metabolism,[20] while renal failure causes accumulation of both morphine and the active metabolite morphine-6-glucuronide, with half-times of up to 38 h for the latter. Fentanyl is perceived to be a shorter-acting drug than morphine, but this is a result of rapid distribution after small doses are given. When stopping infusions of fentanyl, one can expect the half-time to be dependent on the duration of infusion.[2] The terminal elimination half-time of fentanyl is 6 h but there are no active metabolites. Fentanyl is 84% protein-bound and metabolized in the liver, but hepatic and renal failure appear to have little effect apart from reductions in protein binding.[21]

Muscle relaxants

Neuromuscular blocking agents should be relatively easy to administer because simple, inexpensive and real-time monitoring of neuromuscular block is available. Variable neuromuscular block may be caused by changes in elimination, drug interactions, electrolyte disturbances and altered patient responses, especially with neuromuscular disease.[22] Apart from atracurium, the elimination (and thus the effect) of common neuromuscular blocking agents is prolonged in hepatic and renal failure. Regular monitoring during infusion may reveal changes in organ function before standard laboratory tests. Decreased plasma cholinesterase may prolong the action of suxamethonium, but this is not clinically a problem compared with the potential for potassium release in patients with denervation.

Antiarrhythmic drugs

Lignocaine clearance and VD_{ss} are decreased in cardiac and hepatic failure. Active metabolites accumulate in renal failure. α_1-Acid glycoprotein binding is significant in severe illness, and this may increase total lignocaine concentrations without apparent toxicity, probably because free concentrations may be little changed. When possible, early signs of toxicity such as drowsiness, confusion and numbness should be actively searched for, and therapeutic concentrations measured daily.[23]

Digoxin maintenance doses are reduced when there is renal function impairment and concurrent use of amiodarone, calcium-channel blockers, erythromycin, quinidine, tetracycline or verapamil therapy. Toxicity is enhanced by hypokalaemia, hypocalcaemia and hypomagnesaemia, and may present as almost any arrhythmia or cardiac conduction block. Digoxin monitoring is routine in the critically ill and should be carried out regularly. Toxicity is rare if concentrations are <2.5 μmol/l and common if > 5 μmol/l. In renal or hepatic failure, the assay may be unreliable due to the endogenous production of a digoxin-like immunoreactive factor.[24]

Antibiotics

Aminoglycosides and vancomycin have a narrow therapeutic index, causing nephrotoxicity and ototoxicity. There is an association between adequate peak concentrations and clinical response. However, it is not necessary to maintain the peak level, due to a post-antibiotic effect, which is the inability of organisms to grow subsequent to exposure to a high concentration of aminoglycoside. Clinical outcome is improved and toxicity decreased by adequate single daily doses of aminoglycosides. Standard normograms fail to achieve adequate plasma concentrations in most critically ill patients due to increases in volume of distribution.[25–29] Doses of gentamicin and tobramicin need to be increased by 80% on average to achieve adequate concentrations. Dose requirements are also highly variable between patients. For example, the VD_{ss} of vancomycin is 0.2–1.5 l/kg, and serum creatinine concentrations do not predict drug elimination rates.[30] Vancomycin nephrotoxicity is associated with trough concentrations of 20–30 μg/ml and ototoxicity associated with concentrations of 22–100 μg/ml. Vancomycin nephrotoxicity is enhanced when it is used with an aminoglycoside. Gentamicin volume of distribution varies by up to six-fold between patients and within patients over time. Its excretion half-life varies from 1.1 to 69.0 h and its VD_{ss} by 20–30% between sequential readings in patients. It is essential that these drugs are monitored.

β-Lactam antibiotics show bacteriocidal activity which is slow and dependent on maintaining concentrations in tissue above a threshold of 4–5 times minimum inhibitory concentration (MIC). Higher concentrations do not increase efficacy. Studies in ventilated patients have shown variability of 10 times in plasma concentrations using standard dosing regimens, and serum concentrations frequently decrease by 8 h to below MIC. Animal data and case reports indicate that therapeutic efficacy may be improved by giving these drugs as infusions.[25,31]

In burns patients, volumes are increased and clearances decreased for most antibiotics. The exception is imipenem, whose clearance is little different after thermal injury. Aminoglycosides and vancomycin follow the changes already mentioned.[32]

Anticonvulsants

The hepatic metabolism of phenytoin is saturable so that concentration monitoring is essential to determine the effects of a change in dose at higher concentrations.[33] The target range is 10–20 mg/ml (40–80 μmol/l) to minimize toxicity, but control of seizures may be achieved well outside this range. Decreased protein binding will increase the free concentration of phenytoin and low total concentrations may be misleading. Total and unbound concentrations of phenytoin are low during and after barbiturate therapy,[34] suggesting that enzyme induction can further complicate phenytoin dosage and reaffirming the importance of concentration monitoring.

Bronchodilators

Aminophylline has a long half-time and a narrow therapeutic index because of cardiotoxicity. Effects cannot be directly assessed by measuring change in airways resistance, because mucosal swelling and mucosal plugging contribute to airways resistance. A loading dose followed by infusion may be unreliable because of changes in plasma concentrations due to gender, smoking, cimetidine, erythromycin, acute viral illness, pulmonary oedema and hepatic cirrhosis. Theophylline excretion is dependent on liver metabolism rather than liver blood flow because it has a low extraction ratio. Clearance is decreased in sepsis to 10–66% of values obtained in healthy volunteers.[35] Clearance and protein binding may both be decreased in the presence of hypoxia.[36] Large variations between patients combined with low therapeutic index mean concentrations should be monitored daily, and concentrations kept between 50 and 110 μmol/l. A subtherapeutic concentration is corrected by an appropriate 'top-up' bolus infusion, and excessive concentrations should be managed by stopping the infusion and restarting later at a lower rate.

Salbutamol can be given by IV or aerosol for status asthmaticus, and side-effects can be monitored by continuous haemodynamic and electrocardiographic monitoring. Adrenaline is useful and has the advantage that it wears off quickly, whereas adverse effects of salbutamol may last up to 4 h.

References

1 Hull CJ (1991) *Pharmacokinetics for Anaesthesia*. Oxford: Butterworth-Heinemann.

2 Hughes MA, Glass PSA and Jacobs JR (1992) Context-sensitive half-time in multicompartment pharmacokinetic models for intravenous anesthetic drugs. *Anesthesiology* **76**:334–341.

3 Craig WA and Welling PG (1977) Protein binding of antimicrobials: clinical pharmacokinetic and therapeutic implications. *Clin Pharmacokinet* **2**:252–268.

4 Short TG, Plummer JL and Chui PT (1992) Interactions between propofol, alfentanil and midazolam. *Br J Anaesth* **69**:162–167.

5 Smith C, McEwan AI, Jhaveri R *et al.* (1994) The interaction of fentanyl on the Cp50 of propofol for loss of conciousness and skin incision. *Anesthesiology* **81**:820–828.

6 Rudy AC and Brater DC (1994) Drug interactions. In: Chernow B (ed.) *The Pharmacologic Approach to the Critically Ill Patient*, 3rd edn. Philadelphia: Williams & Wilkins, pp. 18–40.

7 Florence AT and Attwood D (1988) *Physicochemical Principles of Pharmacy*, 2nd edn. London: Macmillan.

8 Shelly MP, Mendel L and Park GR (1987) Failure of critically ill patients to metabolise midazolam. *Anaesthesia* **42**:619–626.

9 Runciman WB, Myburgh JA and Upton RN (1990) Pharmacokinetics and pharmacodynamics in the critically ill. In: Dobb GJ (ed.) *Clinical Anaesthesiology*. London: Baillière Tindall, pp. 271–303.

10 Wagner BKJ, Angaran DM and Fuhs DW (1994) Therapeutic drug monitoring. In: Chernow B (ed.) *The Pharmacologic Approach to the Critically Ill Patient*, 3rd edn. Philadelphia: Williams & Wilkins, pp. 182–201.

11 Klockowski PM and Levy G (1988) Kinetics of drug action in disease states. XXV. Effect of experimental hypovolaemia on the pharmacodynamics and pharmacokinetics of desmethyldiazepam. *J Pharmacol Exp Ther* **245**:508–512.

12 Reetze-Bonorden P, Böhler J and Keller E (1993) Drug dosage in patients during continuous renal replacement therapy: pharmacokinetic and therapeutic considerations. *Clin Pharmacokinet* **24**:362–379.

13 Freebairn RC and Lipman J (1993) Renal replacement therapy in the critically ill – precarious progress: Part II. Technical aspects and clinical application. *S Afr J Surg* **31**:147–151.

14 Gous AGS, Dance M, Luyt D *et al.* (1994) Vancomycin pharmacokinetics in critically ill septic infants. *Crit Care Med* **22**:A181.

15 Chernow B (ed.) (1994) *The Pharmacologic Approach to the Critically Ill Patient*, 3rd edn. Philadelphia: Williams & Wilkins.

16 Vinik HR, Reves JG, Greenblat DJ *et al.* (1983) The pharmacokinetics of midazolam in chronic renal failure patients. *Anesthesiology* **59**:390–394.

17 Albanese J, Martin C, Lacarelle B, Saux P, Durand A and Gouin F (1990) Pharmacokinetics of long term propofol infusion used for sedation in ICU patients. *Anesthesiology* **73**:214–217.

18 Bailie GR, Cockshott ID, Douglas EJ and Bowles BJM (1992) Pharmacokinetics of propofol during and after long term continuous infusion for maintenance of sedation in ICU patients. *Br J Anaesth* **68**:486–491.

19 Beller JP, Pottecher T, Lugnier A, Mangin P and Otteni JC (1988) Prolonged sedation with propofol in ICU patients: recovery and blood concentration changes during periodic interruptions in infusion. *Br J Anaesth* **61**:583–588.

20 Shelley MP, Cory EP and Park GR (1986) Pharmacokinetics of morphine in two children before and after liver transplantation. *Br J Anaesth* **58**:1218–1223.

21 Haberer JP, Schoeffler P, Couderc E and Duvaldstin P (1982) Fentanyl pharmacokinetics in anaesthetized patients with cirrhosis. *Br J Anaesth* **54**:1267–1270.

22 Hanson CW III (1994) Pharmacology of neuromuscular blocking agents in the intensive care unit. *Crit Care Clin* **10**:779–797.

23 Park GR (1993) Pharmacokinetics and pharmacodynamics in the critically ill patient. *Xenobiotica* **23**:1195–1230.

24 Howarth DM, Sampson DC, Hawker FH and Young A (1990) Digoxin like immunoreactive substances in the plasma of intensive care unit patients: relationship to organ dysfunction. *Anaesth Intens Care* **18**:45–52.

25 van Dalen R and Vree TB (1990) Pharmacokinetics of antibiotics in critically ill patients. *Intensive Care Med* **16**:S235–S238.

26 Reed RL, Wu AH, Miller-Crotchett P, Crotchett J and Fischer RP (1989) Pharmacokinetic monitoring of nephrotoxic antibiotics in surgical intensive care patients. *J Trauma* **29**:1462–1470.

27 Moore RD, Lietman PS and Smith CR (1987) Clinical response to aminoglycoside therapy: importance of the ratio of peak concentration to minimal inhibitory concentration. *J Infect Dis* **155**:93–99.

28 Marik PE, Havlik I, Monteagudo FSE and Lipman J (1991) The pharmacokinetics of amikacin in critically ill adult and paediatric patients: comparison of once-versus twice-daily dosing regimens. *J Antimicrob Chemother* **27C**:81–89.

29 Marik PE, Lipman J, Kobiliski S and Scribante J (1991) A prospective randomised study comparing once-versus twice-daily amikacin dosing in critically ill adult and paediatric patients. *J Antimicrob Chemother* **28** 753–764.

30 Dasta JF and Armstrong DK (1988) Variability in aminoglycoside pharmacokinetics in critically ill surgical patients. *Crit Care Med* **16**:327–330.

31 Daenan S and de Vries-Hospers H (1988) Cure of *Pseudomonas aeruginosa* infection in neutropenic patients by continuous infusion of ceftazidime. *Lancet* **1**:937.

32 Boucher BA, Kuhl DA and Hickerson WL (1992) Pharmacokinetics of systemically administered antibiotics in patients with thermal injury. *Clin Infect Dis* **14**:458–463.

33 Brodie MJ and Feely J (1988) Practical clinical pharmacology. Therapeutic drug monitoring and clinical trials. *Br Med J* **296**:1110–1114.

34 Yoshida N, Oda Y, Nishi S *et al.* (1993) Effect of barbiturate therapy on phenytoin pharmacokinetics. *Crit Care Med* **21**:1514–1522.

35 Toft P, Hansen M and Klitgaard NA (1991) Theophylline and ethylenediamine pharmacokinetics following administration of aminophylline to septic patients with multiorgan failure. *Intensive Care Med* **17**:465–468.

36 Richer M and Lam YWF (1993) Hypoxia, arterial pH and theophylline disposition. *Clin Pharmacokinet* **25** 283–299.

JWN Weekes

Poisoning or drug intoxication is frequently intentional. It may be accidental or iatrogenic, or may result from manipulative or criminal intent. Specific antidotes are available for only a very small number of poisons and drugs. Despite the vast array of toxins available, the majority of patients will recover with basic supportive care. This chapter describes the general management of poisons and drug intoxication. Common or important agents are selected for discussion. Readers should refer to major tomes for detailed information.

ICU admission guidelines for adults (Table 77.1)

Guidelines are helpful in selecting patients who will truly benefit from ICU admission.[1] Clinical judgement must be exercised whenever doubt exists. Guidelines are most useful in centres having the capacity to observe patients for some hours in the emergency room.

Table 77.1 ICU admission guidelines for adult patients with drug overdose and poisoning

Unresponsive to verbal stimuli
Requires airway protection
Seizures
$Pa\text{CO}_2$ >45 mmHg (6 kPa) and/or
$Pa\text{O}_2$ <60 mmHg (7 kPa) on room air
Cardiac rhythm other than sinus
Sinus tachycardia >110 beats/min with tricyclics
Second- or third-degree atrioventricular block
QRS >0.12 s (>0.1 s with tricyclics)
Systolic blood pressure <90 mmHg (11 kPa)
(despite simple volume expansion)

Priority poisons

Paracetamol, carbon monoxide, methanol, ethylene glycol, cyanide and paraquat are dangerous poisons requiring priority treatment. Limiting the period from ingestion to supportive treatment is always important. It is also essential to introduce specific treatment (Table 77.2)[2–7] with minimal delay to prevent or reduce possible damage.

General principles

The general principles of management are diagnosis, assessment and resuscitation, drug manipulation and continued supportive care. Attending staff need to observe universal precautions, and must be protected from contamination (e.g. from organophosphate or expired cyanide).

Diagnosis

Drug overdose should always be considered in the unconscious patient. Relatives, friends, general practitioners or pharmacists can frequently provide valuable information. The administration of thiamine and/or glucose should be considered at this stage.

Assessment and resuscitation

These should proceed simultaneously.

Airway and ventilation

Dentures are removed. The oropharynx is cleared of food and vomitus. Tolerance of an oropharyngeal airway usually indicates the need for endotracheal intubation for airway protection. With the exception of paraquat, oxygen 8–10 l/min is given by facemask, and intravenous access is established. Inadequate spontaneous respiration, clinically or on arterial blood gas (ABG) analysis, requires ventilatory support.

Table 77.2 Special treatment regimens

Poison	Additive treatment
Paracetamol[2]	*N*-acetylcysteine 150 mg/kg in 200 ml 5% dextrose infuse over 15 min, followed by 50 mg/kg in 500 ml 5% dextrose over 4 h. Then 100 mg/kg in 100 ml 5% dextrose over 16 h
Methanol[3]	Oral or IV ethanol 0.6 g/kg loading dose. Then 109 mg/kg per h adjusted to maintain blood concentration at 1 g/l (IV use 5–10% solution; orally use 20% solution)
Ethylene glycol[3]	As for methanol
Cyanide[4]	1 Sodium thiosulphate 150 mg/kg IV followed by 30–60 mg/kg per h 2 Cobalt EDTA 600 mg IV over 1 min, with further 300 mg IV if no response (cobalt EDTA (Kelocyanor) one 20 ml 1.5% ampoule contains 300 mg)
Carbon monoxide[5,6]	Hyperbaric oxygen 3 atm absolute for 60 min, repeated at 24 h
Paraquat[7]	1 l 15% aqueous suspension of fuller's earth orally, followed by 200 ml 20% mannitol. Repeat 2-hourly until fuller's earth is seen in stools

IV = Intravenous; EDTA = ethylenediaminetetraacetic acid.

Expired air resuscitation is contraindicated in cyanide poisoning.

Haemodynamic status

Blood pressure, pulse rate, peripheral perfusion and urine output are assessed and recorded. Hypovolaemia is corrected. The use of invasive monitoring, inotropic agents and supportive therapy is discussed elsewhere.

Conscious level and neurological signs

Thorough examination cannot be over-stressed. Descriptive documentation is preferable to various classifications which have been used.

Body temperature

Disturbance of central thermoregulatory mechanisms, vasodilatation and prolonged exposure may result in profound hypothermia with its associated problems. Salicylates and drugs with anticholinergic properties may produce hyperthermia.

Body surface

Signs of head or body injury should be sought. Skin blisters may be seen. A specific search must be made for venepuncture marks in suspected addicts. Surface contamination by drugs (e.g. organophosphates) should not be overlooked. Indurated muscle groups due to prolonged pressure may herald rhabdomyolysis and acute renal failure.

Investigations

1 urinalysis;
2 chest X-ray – aspiration is common;
3 electrolytes and creatinine – many drugs are dependent on renal elimination. Significant renal insufficiency may alter management;
4 osmolality – differences between measured and calculated osmolalities may indicate ethanol, methanol or ethylene glycol poisoning;
5 ABG analysis – metabolic acidosis occurs with salicylate, methanol, ethylene glycol, paraldehyde, phenformin, iron and isoniazid.

Drug assays[8,9]

Specific drug assay may have diagnostic, therapeutic and prognostic importance, e.g. timed serum concentrations of paracetamol and paraquat. However, routine screening should be limited to salicylates and paracetamol. Urine, blood and gastric contents can be taken and analysed if required.

Drug manipulation (Table 77.3)
Decrease absorption

Emesis
Efficacy is disputed.[10–12] Ipecacuanha (Ipecac syrup, Australian Pharmaceutical Formulary 6% containing 0.12% alkaloids) is a useful emetic in children in doses of 10–30 ml. It is less effective in adults. Administration–emetic interval in children averages 14 min.[11] Airway protection may be lost during this interval, resulting in aspiration. Excessive Ipecac is itself a poison.

Table 77.3 Drug manipulation

Decrease absorption	Emesis, lavage, charcoal
Increase excretion	Diuresis, pH manipulation
	Dialysis
	Haemoperfusion
	Plasmapheresis
	Faecuresis
Alter drug metabolism	
Antidotes	

Table 77.4 Activated charcoal – effectiveness

Repeat doses increase non-renal elimination of:

Phenobarbitone	Digoxin
Salicylate	Meprobamate
Dapsone	Theophylline
Diazepam	Carbamazepine
Digitoxin	

Table 77.5 Activated charcoal – not effective

Elemental metals – iron, lithium, boron
Pesticides – malathion, DDT, carbamate
Strong acids and alkalis
Cyanide

Gastric lavage

Unless performed within 1 h of drug ingestion, its efficacy is disputed.[10,12] Safe technique demands airway protection. Prior intubation is essential when laryngeal competence is absent or doubtful. In the majority of overdoses, aspiration is more lethal than the ingested drug. The patient is positioned head-down on the left side, with the pylorus pointing upwards. A large-bore tube (30 FG) with large side holes is passed into the stomach. The tube is aspirated before lavage is started. Water at body temperature is instilled, and recovered completely before continuing. Volumes greater than 1 ml/kg may promote drug passage through the pylorus. Lavage is continued until return is clear. Sodium, water and heat balance are of major importance in children. Stomach massage or gastroscopy may assist removal of coalesced drug masses. Lavage is contraindicated in ingestions of corrosives, caustics and acids; oesophageal or gastric perforation may occur. Inhalation of petroleum derivatives causes intense pneumonitis.

Charcoal

Activated charcoal has now replaced Ipecac as first-line treatment for most acute poisonings – 50 g is given after lavage and repeated 4-hourly. Preparations vary in their adsorptive capacity,[13] and an appropriate preparation should be chosen. Numerous reports confirm the efficacy of repeated charcoal administration in the elimination of various drugs.[14–16] This effect is not limited to drugs with significant enterohepatic circulation. Charcoal adsorption is also thought to maintain a drug concentration gradient between mucosal blood and gut lumen, with continued elimination of drug down this gradient. Cyclic charcoal administration is effective for drugs shown in Table 77.4 and ineffective for drugs listed in Table 77.5. However, charcoal prevents the actions of Ipecac and oral *N*-acetylcysteine, and charcoal aspiration followed by death has been reported.[17]

Faecuresis

Benefits are doubtful. Controversy surrounds the use of charcoal cathartics.[18] If a cathartic is to be used, sorbitol is the most effective in reducing transit time.[19] Commercial preparations of 70% sorbitol and charcoal are available.

Increase excretion

Forced diuresis

The technique is hazardous and has dubious value. It depends on bulk flow to reduce the time available for drug reabsorption. Intravenous fluids are combined with diuretics to produce a urine output of 2–5 ml/kg per h. Osmotic diuretics (e.g. mannitol) act at the proximal tubule where most reabsorption occurs. Hence they are preferable to loop diuretics. Volume status and electrolyte balance must be meticulously monitored. Forced diuresis is contraindicated in the presence of cardiac failure or impaired renal function.

Alkalinization

This technique uses hyperventilation[20] and/or sodium bicarbonate[21] 1 mmol/kg per h with monitoring of ABGs to maintain urine pH 7–8 and blood pH >7.45. It has been combined with forced diuresis.

Acidification

Acidification of the urine may increase the elimination of phencyclidine and amphetamines. This is achieved by infusing ammonium chloride 4 g every 24 h or as a 1–2% solution in normal saline. ABG and urine pH are monitored to maintain urine pH 5.5–6.5. Although frequently recommended for quinine poisoning, the evidence is contradictory.[22]

Extracorporeal techniques[23–27]

Haemodialysis effectively removes compounds of low molecular weight and those with low protein binding, small volume of distribution and low spontaneous clearance.

Table 77.6 Dialytic therapy of choice

Haemodialysis	*Haemoperfusion*
Methanol	Theophylline
Ethylene glycol	Phenobarbitone
Salicylates	
Lithium	

Haemoperfusion using charcoal or resin columns is effective in removing lipid-soluble drugs.

Plasmapheresis[28] is of unproven benefit, and at present must be regarded as an experimental procedure.

Table 77.6 indicates the preferred technique according to the poison ingested. The exact role of these specialized, expensive techniques has yet to be defined. Decisions to institute dialytic treatment should be based on the poison and dose ingested, the patient and the response to conservative treatment (see Chapter 39).

Altered drug metabolism

Ethanol may be used to saturate the pathways responsible for metabolizing methanol and ethylene glycol into their toxic metabolites. *N*-acetylcysteine is used in paracetamol poisoning as a source of sulphydryl groups which provide attachment sites for the toxic metabolite.

Antidotes

Antidotes are available in some cases of poisoning (Table 77.2 and Table 77.7).

Continued supportive therapy

The following protocols should be applied:

1 Care of the unconscious patient is instituted.
2 Vital functions are monitored and recorded. Organ function is supported where indicated.
3 The patient is rewarmed using humidified gases, space blankets and warmed infusion fluids.
4 Antibiotics are started if aspiration has occurred.
5 Intermittent IV diazepam to treat convulsions may be required.
6 Cardiac arrhythmias and/or cardiac failure are treated when indicated.
7 Fluid, electrolytes and nutritional support are maintained.

Specific therapy of some common or difficult overdoses

This section emphasizes only those features which may aid clinical diagnosis or prognosis. Treatment suggestions are always intended to support those measures described under general principles. Controversial therapies are mentioned.

Anticholinergics

Features

Pupils are dilated and accommodation is paralysed. Parasympathetic block is characterized by dry mouth, ileus and urinary retention. Agitation, delirium, disorientation and hallucinations are common. Convulsions, arrhythmias and hyperpyrexia may occur.

Table 77.7 Selected antidotes and pharmacological or physiological antagonists

Poison	*Antidote/antagonist*
Digoxin	Fab fragments of digoxin-specific antibodies. Fab required (mg) = digoxin nmol/l $\times$ 0.278 $\times$ body weight (kg) or digoxin ng/ml $\times$ 0.358 $\times$ body weight (kg)
β-Blockers	Glucagon 5–10 mg IV. An infusion of 2–10 mg/h may be required. Isoprenaline, adrenaline and pacing as required
Organophosphates	1 Atropine 0.3–5.0 mg IV stat to reverse bradycardia and/or reduce excessive secretions. An infusion of 0.5 mg/min or greater may be necessary 2 Pralidoxime 1 g IV bolus followed by 0.5 g/h
Calcium-channel blockers	Calcium chloride 1 g over 5 min with ECG monitoring. Repeated doses with continuous ECG monitoring and measurement of calcium concentrations may be required Isoprenaline, adrenaline and pacing as indicated

IV = Intravenous; ECG = electrocardiogram.

Treatment
Treatment is supportive.

Controversial
The use of physostigmine is controversial (see section on tricyclics, below).

Antidepressants

Tricyclics

Points of interest
A QRS duration ≥ 0.1 s in the limb leads of an electrocardiogram (ECG) is the best predictor of arrhythmia and/or seizures.[29] Amoxapine is the exception to the rule.[30] Status epilepticus occurs in the setting of normal QRS duration.

Features
Anticholinergic effects are described above. All forms of rhythm and conduction disturbances have been described. The volume of distribution is large. Rapid hepatic metabolism usually results in improvement within 24 h.

Treatment
Increasing arterial pH to ≥ 7.45 significantly reduces the available free drug.[29] This may be achieved by hyperventilation[20] and/or sodium bicarbonate[21] in 25–50 mmol aliquots. The duration of ECG monitoring remains arbitrary. Monitoring for 12 h after the normalization of the ECG is suggested.

Controversial
Physostigmine has been used to treat all the toxic manifestations with variable success. Asystole and convulsions have followed its use.[31] It is not recommended.[32]

Monoamine oxidase inhibitors (MAOI)

Features
Hypertensive crisis with tyramine-containing foods (e.g. cheese) and sympathomimetic agents can be dramatic.

Treatment
1 diazoxide 150–300 mg IV;
2 phentolamine 5 mg IV;
3 sodium nitroprusside infusion (see Chapter 16).

Antihistamines

Features
Anticholinergic symptoms and signs are features.

Treatment
Treatment is supportive.

Barbiturates

Features
The central nervous system (CNS), cardiovascular and respiratory systems are depressed. Cardiovascular depression is due to vasomotor centre depression and a toxic effect on myocardium and peripheral vessels. Hypotension and relative hypovolaemia may be extreme.

Treatment
Treatment is supportive. Urine alkalinization will hasten elimination of phenobarbitone.

Benzodiazepines

Features
Overdose is common, but features are not usually severe unless complicated by other drugs, pre-existing disease and the extremes of age.

Treatment
Treatment is supportive. Flumazenil is a specific antagonist. However, its brief duration of action limits its use to diagnostic purposes.

Cardiac glycosides

Features
Any cardiac arrhythmia may occur. Severe poisoning may produce hyperkalaemia which is resistant to usual therapies.

Treatment
Hypokalaemia is corrected. Phenytoin 250–500 mg IV at 50 mg/min may be useful for tachyarrhythmias. Transvenous pacing may be necessary to control symptomatic bradyarrhythmias. DC shock, if essential, should be initiated at low energy levels, e.g. 20–50 J. Fab fragments of digoxin-specific antibodies (Table 77.7) are indicated in severe cases.[33,34]

Carbon monoxide (CO)

Points of interest
Symptoms of CO toxicity were first described by Haldane[35] in 1919. The mechanisms of toxicity remain unclear.[36] Smokers may have up to 10% of their haemoglobin bound to CO (i.e. carboxyhaemoglobin, COHb) without deleterious effects.[37] During CO poisoning, oxygen delivery to the heart and brain is increased.[37] There is no marker which reliably detects CO poisoning. Whilst coma and/or COHb levels >40% always indicate serious poisoning, delayed deterioration can occur in their absence. Only one randomized, prospective study on the use of oxygen at normal atmospheric pressure and hyperbaric oxygen (HBO) has been published.[38] Affinity of CO for haemoglobin is approximately 240 times that of oxygen.

Features

Neurological signs vary from mild confusion through to fitting or coma. A history of loss of consciousness should always be sought and may be the only indicator of significant poisoning. ST segment changes may be present on ECG. In the absence of respiratory depression or aspiration, Pa_{O_2} will be normal. It is essential that Sa_{O_2} is measured directly by co-oximeter, and not calculated. Cherry-pink skin and mucosa are rarely seen. Cyanosis is far more common.

Treatment

There is universal agreement to use HBO. The pressure, duration, timing and frequency of treatment remain controversial. A review of 13 published series of 2441 patients[5] and a longitudinal study of 100 patients[6] suggest HBO at 3 atm absolute for 1–2 h on admission, and repeated at 24 h for all patients with signs or symptoms of CO poisoning, regardless of severity. Hospitals without HBO facilities should refer patients with severe poisoning or those who fail to respond to conventional oxygen therapy (see Chapter 22).

Chloral hydrate

Features

CNS depression is common. Cardiac arrhythmias may occur. Chloral hydrate is metabolized to trichlorethanol which may sensitize the heart to endogenous catecholamine.

Treatment

β-Adrenergic blockers may be used to control tachyarrhythmias.

Chloroquine[39]

Features

Hypotension and sudden cardiac arrest result from severe poisoning.

Treatment

Adrenaline 0.25 μg/kg per min IV, cautiously increasing the infusion dose until hypotension is reversed, together with diazepam 2 mg/kg over 30 min, followed by 1–2 mg/kg per day.

Cyanide[4]

Features

Onset of cell toxicity is very rapid. The ability to detect the odour of bitter almonds is genetically determined and is therefore unreliable. Attendant staff must not undertake expired air resuscitation.

Treatment

Oxygen 100% is given together with:

1 sodium thiosulphate 150 mg/kg IV followed by infusion of 30–60 mg/kg per h to convert cyanide to thiocyanate;
2 cobalt ethylenediaminetetraacetic acid (EDTA; Kelocyanor, one 20 ml 1.5% ampoule contains 300 mg) 600 mg IV over 1 min, with a further 300 mg if there is no response. Kelocyanor chelates cyanide. Dextrose 50% 25 ml IV is recommended by the manufacturers;
3 hydroxocobalamin IV. The dose is not established; 100 μg/kg is suggested.

Ethylene glycol[3]

Features

Odourless inebriation, increased measured osmolality and severe metabolic acidosis are due to oxalic acid. Oxalate crystalluria leads to rapidly progressive renal failure.

Treatment

Treatment is as for methanol (Table 77.2).

Heavy metals

Features

Renal, hepatic and gastrointestinal damage are common.

Treatment

Treatment is dimercaprol (BAL) 4 mg/kg by deep IM injection every 4 h for 2 days, then 2–4 mg/kg daily for about 1 week.

Iron

Features

The corrosive action on gastric mucosa results in vomiting, pain, haematemesis and melaena and gastric perforation. Severe poisoning is reflected by plasma concentrations more than 90 μmol/l in children and 145 μmol/l in adults within 4 h of ingestion.

Treatment

Desferrioxamine mesylate (an iron chelator) 5 g is left in the stomach after lavage. Simultaneously, 2 g is injected IM and an infusion of 15 mg/kg per h (maximum 80 mg/kg in 24 h) is commenced. Treatment is continued until serum concentrations and clinical status are satisfactory.

Lead

Features

Abdominal pain, vomiting and diarrhoea precede coma and convulsions. Liver and renal failure and haemolysis may occur.

Treatment

BAL (see heavy metals, above) plus calcium disodium edetate (EDTA) are infused in a daily dose of 50 mg/kg for 5 days.

Lithium[40]

Features

Serum lithium levels >1.5 mmol/l are toxic. Neurological signs and symptoms are varied and many. Severe poisoning may result in permanent damage. Renal toxicity includes nephrogenic diabetes insipidus adding to the problems of fluid management.

Treatment

Serum concentrations >3.5–4.0 mmol/l generally require haemodialysis. Patients with lower concentrations, but with signs of severe toxicity may also require dialysis. The majority of patients respond to general supportive measures.

Methanol

Features

Methanol itself is non-toxic. Acidosis and blindness are thought to be due to the metabolism of methanol to formaldehyde and then to formic acid. A latent period of 12–18 h may occur. Measured osmolality is elevated and the anion gap increased.

Treatment (Table 77.2)

1 Ethanol (competitively inhibits metabolism) is given 0.6 g/kg orally or IV followed by 109 mg/kg per h to maintain plasma ethanol concentrations at 1 g/l.
2 Haemodialysis[41] should be considered if the blood methanol concentration is more than 500 mg/l, or the minimal lethal dose (30 ml) has been taken, or where acidosis, visual and mental disturbances are present.

Opioids

Features

Overdose patients may be infected with hepatitis B or HIV. Staff must take appropriate precautions.

Treatment

Treatment is supportive. Naloxone 0.1–0.4 mg IV (half-life 30–45 min) is given hourly.

Organophosphates[42]

Features

Signs are salivation, bronchorrhoea, bronchospasm, sweating, colicky abdominal pain, diarrhoea, miosis, fasciculation progressing to muscle paralysis, and bradycardia, leading to asystole.

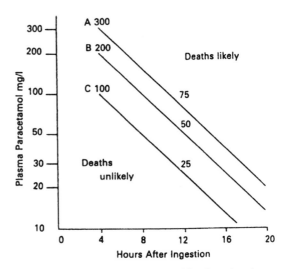

Fig. 77.1 Assessment using paracetamol levels against time. Death is likely with levels above line A, and unlikely with levels below line C. Treatment is recommended with levels at line B.

Treatment (Table 77.7)

Contaminated clothing or gastric aspirate must not be handled. Thorough washing is essential where surface contamination is present.

1 atropine starting at 0.6 mg hourly IM or IV to control parasympathetic overactivity. In massive overdose, atropine doses may have to be equally massive;
2 pralidoxime (PAM) 1 g IV over 5–10 min and 0.5 g hourly;
3 plasma cholinesterase levels are monitored until recovery is apparent.
Note: Do not use PAM for carbamate poisoning.

Paracetamol[43–48]

Points of interest

In normal adults, doses >10 g may exceed the ability of hepatic glutathione to conjugate the toxic metabolite. Plasma concentrations >250 mg/l at 4 h or ≥ 50 mg/l at 12 h (Fig. 77.1) are usually associated with hepatic damage. The treatment nomogram (Fig. 77.1) must be interpreted with caution in the presence of prolonged alcohol consumption. While intravenous acetylcysteine administered more than 16 h after ingestion may not prevent severe liver damage,[46] outcome in paracetamol-induced fulminant hepatic failure is improved.[47] Severe hepatic injury has a 10% mortality.[46] The majority of patients recover within 1–2 weeks.

Features

Nausea and vomiting may be the only features present in the first 24 h.

Treatment

1 Gastric lavage, administration of activated charcoal, and assaying drug concentrations are performed as described in general principles.

2 *N*-acetylcysteine 150 mg/kg in 200 ml 5% dextrose is infused over 15 min, followed by 50 mg/kg in 500 ml 5% dextrose over 4 h, and 100 mg/kg in 1 l 5% dextrose over 16 h (total dose 300 mg/kg in 20 h). Maximum protective effect is time-dependent. An ingestion–treatment interval of less than 10 h gives the best result.

3 In fulminant hepatic failure, the last dose (100 mg/kg in 1 l 5% dextrose over 16 h) is repeated until the patient recovers from the encephalopathy.[45]

4 A pH <7.3 regardless of the stage of encephalopathy, or international normalized ratio >6.5 and creatinine >300 μmol/l and grade 3 or 4 encephalopathy are suggested as criteria for liver transplantation.[47]

Paraquat[48]

Points of interest

In adult humans the LD_{50} is 3–5 g (i.e. 15–25 ml of 20% w/v liquid concentrate). The mortality rate in patients ingesting the liquid concentrate is 25–75%. The lung is the primary target organ. Injury is enhanced by oxygen. Peak concentrations are achieved between 0.5 and 2.0 h.

Features

Corrosive effects on mouth, pharynx and oesophagus are seen. Dyspnoea and pulmonary oedema follow within 24 h, progressing to irreversible fibrosis and death. Cardiac, renal and hepatic dysfunction are common.

Treatment

After establishing the diagnosis, the lowest inspired oxygen concentration to produce a safe Pao_2 is given. Following gastric lavage, 1 l 15% aqueous suspension of fuller's earth is instilled down the gastric tube, followed by 200 ml 20% mannitol. This is repeated until stools contain fuller's earth.

Prognosis

This can be determined from the nomogram (Fig. 77.2).[49]

Controversial

Extracorporeal techniques are of unproven benefit. This is expected, given the very brief time to reach peak plasma concentrations and the large volume of distribution.

Phenothiazines

Features

Anticholinergic and cardiac effects are similar to tricyclic overdose.

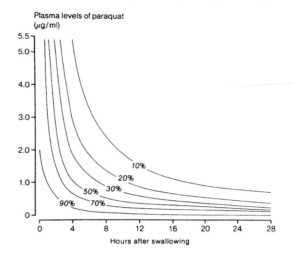

Fig. 77.2 Relationship between plasma paraquat concentration and survival. Percentages denote the probability of survival. From Hart *et al.*,[49] with permission. Copyright The Lancet Ltd, 1984.

Treatment

Treatment is supportive.

Quinine

Features

Cinchonism, visual defects and cardiac effects are signs.

Treatment

Treatment is supportive.

Controversial

Stellate ganglion block and forced acid diuresis have no proven benefit.[22,50]

Salicylates

Points of interest

Moderate toxicity occurs with serum concentrations 500–750 mg/l (3600–5500 μmol/l), and severe toxicity with concentrations >750 mg/l.[51] Serum concentrations alone do not determine prognosis.[52] The elimination half-life increases significantly with increasing concentrations. Small reductions in pH produce large increases in non-ionized salicylate which then penetrates tissues.[51]

Features

Tinnitus, deafness, diaphoresis, pyrexia, hypoglycaemia, haematemesis, hypokalaemia and increased prothrombin time may occur. Acid–base status is variable. Delayed presentation, coma, hyperpyrexia, pulmonary oedema and acidaemia are reported as more common in fatal cases.[52]

Treatment

Multiple doses of activated charcoal significantly reduce the elimination half-life.[53] Vitamin K and glucose are used to correct hypoprothrombinaemia and hypoglycaemia. Elevating the arterial pH to ≥ 7.4 with hyperventilation and/or aliquots of sodium bicarbonate will decrease the amount of non-ionized drug available to enter tissues. Forced diuresis is hazardous and is not recommended. Haemodialysis is very effective in removing salicylate and correcting acid–base disturbance. Indications for its use are yet to be defined, but should be considered for severe cases.

Theophylline

Points of interest

Toxic levels result from intentional overdose in 10–30% of cases.[54] Serum concentrations >30 mg/l (167 μmol/l) produce toxic symptoms in over 90% of patients. Peak concentrations in acute overdose correlate with severity and hypokalaemia. In chronic medication, toxic symptoms occur at lower concentrations. Sustained-release preparations may result in delayed peaks and prolonged toxicity.

Features

Concentrations <30 mg/l (167 μmol/l) are frequently associated with agitation, tremor, nausea, vomiting and sinus tachycardia. Concentrations >100 mg/l (555 μmol/l) in acute poisoning or >40 mg/l (222 μmol/l) in chronic medication frequently result in seizures, malignant ventricular arrhythmias, severe hypotension and death.

Treatment

Multiple doses of activated charcoal will decrease the elimination half-life from approximately 10 ± 2.1 to 4.6 ± 1.27 h.[51] Theophylline concentrations must be monitored 1–2-hourly until they no longer increase. Hypokalaemia requires potassium replacement. Rebound hyperkalaemia has been reported.[55] Ondansetron may prove useful to combat vomiting.[56]

Controversial

Charcoal haemoperfusion is controversial – proposed indications include concentrations >100 mg/l (555 μmol/l), seizures, malignant arrhythmias and the presence of pre-existing liver disease or congestive heart failure.

References

1. Brett AS, Rothschild N, Gray R and Perry M (1987) Predicting the clinical course in intentional drug overdose. *Arch Intern Med* **147**:133–137.
2. Prescott LF (1981) Treatment of severe acetaminophen poisoning with intravenous acetylcysteine. *Arch Intern Med* **141**:386–389.
3. Peterson CD, Collins AJ, Himes MJ, Bullock ML and Keane WF (1981) Ethylene glycol poisoning. *N Engl J Med* **304**:21–23.
4. Vogel SN and Sultan TR (1981) Cyanide poisoning. *Clin Toxicol* **18**:367–383.
5. Gorman DF and Runciman WB (1991) Carbon monoxide poisoning. *Anaesth Intens Care* **19**:506–511.
6. Gorman DF, Clayton D, Gilligan JE and Webb RK (1992) A longitudinal study of 100 consecutive admissions for carbon monoxide poisoning to the Royal Adelaide Hospital. *Anaesth Intens Care* **20**:311–316.
7. ICI Australia Operations (1985). *The Treatment of Paraquat Poisoning* Melbourne: ICI.
8. Snyder JW and Vlasses PH (1988) Role of the laboratory in treatment of the poisoned patient. *Arch Intern Med* **148**:279–280.
9. Brett AS (1988) Implications of discordance between clinical impression and toxicology analysis in drug overdose. *Arch Intern Med* **148**:437–441.
10. Kulig K, Bar-Or D, Cantrill SV, Rosen P and Rumack BH (1985) Management of acutely poisoned patients without gastric emptying. *Ann Emerg Med* **14**:562–567.
11. MacLean WC Jr (1973) A comparison of ipecac syrup and apomorphine in the immediate treatment of ingestion of poisons. *J Pediatr* **82**:121–124.
12. Prescott LF (1983) New approaches in managing drug overdose and poisoning. *Br Med J* **287**:274–276.
13. Greensher J, Mofenson HC, Pichioni AL and Fallon P (1979) Activated charcoal updated. *JACEP* **8**:261–263.
14. Editorial (1987) Repeated oral activated charcoal. *Lancet* **i**:1013–1015.
15. Editorial (1985) Activated charcoal reborn. Progress in poison management. *Arch Intern Med* **145**:43–44.
16. McLuckie A, Forbes AM and Ilett KF (1990) Role of repeated doses of activated charcoal in the treatment of acute intoxications. *Anaesth Intens Care* **18**:375–384.
17. Harsch HH (1986) Aspiration of activated charcoal. *N Engl J Med* **314**:318.
18. McNamara RM, Aaron CK, Gemboryo M and Davidheiser S (1988) Sorbitol catharsis does not enhance efficacy of charcoal in a simulated acetaminophen overdose. *Ann Emerg Med* **17**:243–246.
19. Krenzeolk EP, Keller R and Steard RD (1985) Gastrointestinal transit times of cathartics combined with charcoal. *Ann Emerg Med* **14**:1152–1155.
20. Kingston M (1979) Hyperventilation in tricyclic antidepressant poisoning. *Crit Care Med* **7**:550–551.
21. Brown TCK, Barker GA, Dunlop ME *et al.* (1973) The use of sodium bicarbonate in the treatment of tricyclic antidepressant arrhythmias. *Anaesth Intens Care* **1**:203–210.
22. Bateman DN, Blain PG, Woodhouse KW *et al.* (1985) Pharmo-kinetics and clinical toxicity of quinine overdosage: lack of efficacy of techniques intended to enhance elimination. *Q J Med New Series* **214**:125–131.
23. Winchester JF, Gleford MC, Kepshield JH and Schreiner GP (1987) Dialysis and hemoperfusion of poisons and drugs – update. *Trans Am Soc Artif Intern Organs* **XXIII**:762–773.
24. Knepshield JH and Winchester JF (1982) Hemodialysis and hemoperfusion for drugs and poisons. *Trans Am Soc Artif Intern Organs* **XXVIII**:666–669.

25. Garella S (1982) Conservative approach to treatment of acute drug intoxication. *Trans Am Soc Artif Intern Organs* **XXVII**:671–676.

26. Uldall PR (1982) Controlled trial of resin hemoperfusion for the treatment of drug overdose at Toronto Western Hospital. *Trans Am Soc Artif Intern Organs* **XXVIII**:676–677.

27. Pond SM (1991) Extracorporeal techniques in the treatment of poisoned patients. *Med J Aust* **154**:617–622.

28. Jones JS and Dougherty J (1986) Current status of plasmapheresis in toxicology. *Ann Emerg Med* **15**:474–482.

29. Boehnert MT and Fovejoy FH (1985) Value of the QRS duration versus the serum drug level in predicting seizures and ventricular arrhythmias after an acute overdose of tricyclic antidepressants. *N Engl J Med* **313**:474–479.

30. Frommer DA, Kulig KW, Marx JA and Rumack B (1987) Tricyclic antidepressant overdose. A review. *J Am Med Assoc* **257**:521–526.

31. Pertil P and Peterson CD (1980) Asystole complicating physostigmine treatment of tricyclic antidepressant overdose. *Ann Emerg Med* **9**:588–590.

32. Dziukas LJ and Vohra J (1991) Tricyclic antidepressant poisoning. *Med J Aust* **154**:344–350.

33. Smith TW, Butler VP, Haber E *et al.* (1982) Treatment of life-threatening digitalis intoxication with digoxin-specific Fab antibody fragments. *N Engl J Med* **307**:1357–1362.

34. Antman EM, Wenger TL, Butler VP, Haber E and Smith TW (1990) Treatment of 150 cases of life-threatening digitalis intoxication with digoxin-specific Fab antibody fragments. *Circulation* **81**:1744–1752.

35. Haldare JS (1919) Symptoms, causes and prevention of anoxaemia and the value of oxygen in its treatment. *Br Med J* **2**:65.

36. Runciman WW and Gorman DF (1993) Carbon monoxide poisoning; from old dogma to new uncertainties. *Med J Aust* **158**:439–440.

37. Mark P (1992) Carbon monoxide poisoning: a review. *South Pacific Underwater Med Soc J* **22**: 127–135.

38. Raphael JC, Jaro-Guincestse MC, Chastang C *et al.* (1989) Trial of normobaric and hyperbaric oxygen for acute carbon monoxide intoxication. *Lancet* **ii**:414–419.

39. Riou B, Barriot P, Rimailho A and Baud FJ (1988) Treatment of severe chloroquine poisoning. *N Engl J Med* **318**:1–6.

40. Simard M and Gumbiner B (1989) Lithium carbonate intoxication. *Arch Intern Med* **149**:36–46.

41. Gonda A, Gault H, Churchill D and Hollomby D (1978) Hemodialysis for methanol intoxication. *Am J Med* **64**:749–757.

42. Bardin PG, van Eeden SF, Moolman JA, Foden AP and Joubert JR (1994) Organophosphate and carbamate poisoning. *Arch Intern Med* **154**:1433–1441.

43. Cheung L, Potts RG and Meyer KC (1994) Acetaminophen treatment nomogram. *N Engl J Med* **330**:1907–1908.

44. Prescott LF, Illingworth RN, Critchley JAJH, Stewart MJ, Adam RD and Proudfoot AT (1979) Intravenous *n*-acetylcysteine: the treatment of choice for paracetamol poisoning. *Br Med J* **2**:1097–1100.

45. Keays P, Harrison PM, Windon JA *et al.* Intravenous acetylcysteine in paracetamol induced fulminant hepatic failure: a prospective controlled trial. *Br Med J* **303**:1026–1029.

46. Prescott LF (1983) New approaches in managing drug overdosage and poisoning. *Br Med J* **287**:274–276.

47. Riegler JL and Lake JR (1993) Fulminant hepatic failure. *Med Clin North Am* **77**:1057–1083.

48. Pond SM (1990) Manifestations and management of paraquat poisoning. *Med J Aust* **152**:256–259.

49. Hart TB, Nevitt A and Whitehead A (1984) A new statistical approach to the prognostic significance of plasma paraquat concentrations. *Lancet* **ii**:1222–1223.

50. Boland ME, Brennan Roper SM and Henry JA (1985) Complications of quinine poisoning. *Lancet* **i**:384–385.

51. Worthley LIG (1994) *Synopsis of Intensive Care Medicine*. Edinburgh: Churchill Livingstone, pp. 845–869.

52. Chapman BJ and Proudfoot AT (1989) Adult salicylate poisoning: deaths and outcome in patients with high plasma salicylate concentrations. *Q J Med* **72**:699–707.

53. Hillman RJ and Prescott LF (1985) Treatment of salicylate poisoning with repeated oral charcoal. *Br Med J* **291**:1472.

54. Sessler CN (1990) Theophylline toxicity: clinical features of 116 consecutive cases. *Am J Med* **88**:567–576.

55. Henderson A, Wright DM and Pond SM (1992) Management of theophylline overdose patients in the intensive care unit. *Anaesth Intens Care* **20**:56–62.

56. Brown SGA and Prentice DA (1992) Ondansetron in the treatment of theophylline overdose. *Med J Aust* **156**: 512.

78 | Sedation in intensive care

JF Bion and TE Oh

Although sleep deprivation has adverse physiological and psychological effects, there is no formal consensus on how sedation should contribute to the comfort of critically ill patients (e.g. which drugs to use or how their effects should be monitored). Sedation in intensive care has shifted from deep sedation, often using muscle relaxants,[1] to light sedation.[2] This has been due to widespread use of assisted mechanical ventilatory modes, easier delivery of sedative drugs by syringe infusion and knowledge of adrenocortical inhibition from long-term infusion of some sedatives[3] (e.g. etomidate which was attributed to cause increased mortality in trauma patients).[4]

Definition and patient perceptions

Sedation in intensive care means caring for the physical and psychological comfort of critically ill patients receiving organ-system support. Competence, compassion and communication are basic elements; drugs only provide part of the care.[5] Aims of sedation can be determined to some extent by interviewing patients following discharge.[6] Although memory and awareness are not the same, and survivors represent a selected population, survivors of critical illness none the less recall anxiety, pain, thirst and lack of rest as particular problems. Recollection of therapeutic paralysis is rare, but particularly distressing when it occurs. Anxiety is commonly related to concern about the welfare of relatives in the event of death, which is unlikely to be abolished by anxiolytic sedatives. Thirst may be related to cerebral angiotensin levels as much as mouth care. Pain should not be a common experience with skilled ICU care. Other potential sources of distress are the endotracheal tube impeding communication, loss of control over one's physical state and environment and depersonalization. The presence of relatives is uniformly reassuring to patients, and relatives should be involved in comfort care.

Aims of sedation

In general terms, critically ill patients should receive a sedative regimen which allows them to sleep when undisturbed, minimizes discomfort, abolishes pain, alleviates anxiety and facilitates organ-system support and nursing care. Sedation should aim for a level at which communication (i.e. coherent intellectual contact) with the patient remains possible. This will aid patient assessments and, if mechanical ventilation is instituted, expedite weaning. This level of sedation will not be appropriate for all ICU patients. For example, patients with raised intracranial pressure (ICP), low pulmonary compliance or severe intra-pulmonary shunting will need close physiological control, for which deeper sedation with neuromuscular paralysis will be required. Thus, clear sedation protocols are important for different patient groups.

Methods of assessing sedation

Methods of assessment of sedation include measures of level of consciousness, pain or discomfort, comprehension, tolerance of organ-system support and severity of illness. The precise variables and methods selected will depend upon case mix and research considerations.

1 *Level of consciousness* (i.e. depth of sedation) should be recorded. A graded scale describing responses to speech or stimuli can be used. Ramsay's ordinal scaling system[7] is acceptable, and there are several variants. However, this scale is not a scoring system, and it does not provide information about quality of sedation.
2 *Linear analogue scales* are more useful for research purposes. Recording by trained observers allows the various components of sedation to be measured independently, to derive an index of quality. Linear analogue scales are descriptively flexible, and can be analysed either numerically or graphically.[6]

3 *Electroencephalography (EEG)* can help to distinguish metabolic and hypoxic encephalopathies, but is less reliable for distinguishing drug effects from those of disease (see below).

Sedation in multiple organ dysfunction

The presence of multiple organ dysfunction (MOD) has implications for sedation practice:

1 *Cerebral dysfunction* is common in critically ill patients with MOD and sepsis.[8] The encephalopathy of MOD is complex, and may be due to drugs, intracranial haemorrhage or infarction, hypoxaemia, hypoperfusion or systemic metabolic disturbances. Cerebral dysfunction in sepsis has been called septic encephalopathy,[9] and is characterized on EEG by a featureless amplitude trace and a shift to the slower frequencies (θ and δ bands). Septic encephalopathy has some clinical features of hepatic encephalopathy (and hepatic impairment is common in MOD). Pathogenetic mechanisms seem to be cerebral oedema and toxins. Cerebral oedema may follow hyponatraemia, accumulation of progesterone and oestrogen, antidiuretic hormone, angiotensin, hypoalbuminaemia and increased vascular permeability. Potential toxins include so-called middle molecules (possibly breakdown products of cytokines of catabolic hormones), ammonia, glutamine excess, aromatic and sulphated amino acids and immunoinflammatory mediators.

Distinguishing disease from drug effects can be difficult. Cautious use of naloxone or flumazenil may be necessary to exclude opioid or benzodiazepine accumulation respectively. Physostigmine may have a role in increasing intracerebral acetylcholine concentrations and reversing anticholinergic agents.

2 *Hepatic dysfunction* has a variable effect on drug clearance which depends upon the lipid-solubility of the drug, hepatic blood flow and hepatocellular function. Clearance of lipid-soluble drugs (e.g. benzodiazepines) is affected primarily by liver blood flow (i.e. flow-limited). Other relatively lipid-insoluble drugs (e.g. alfentanil) depend more on liver enzymes for metabolism (i.e. rate-limited).

3 *Renal dysfunction* results in reduced clearance of water-soluble drug metabolities, e.g. morphine-6-glucuronide. Renal blood flow autoregulation for changes in perfusion pressure is also impaired. The renal medulla is critically dependent on vasa recta blood flow for oxygenation, and tubular function and renal repair mechanisms are at risk if renal perfusion pressure is impaired by careless sedation. Cyclo-oxygenase inhibitors (non-steroidal anti-inflammatory analgesics) should be avoided in renal impairment, because they block the production of intrarenal prostaglandins (mainly PGE_2) which preserve vasa recta blood flow.[10] Renal replacement therapy has a variable effect on drug clearance (see Chapter 39).

Agents used for therapeutic sedation

No available drug offers all the properties of an ideal sedative drug or regimen (Table 78.1). Drugs used for ICU sedation can be considered as analgesics and hypnotics.

Table 78.1 Properties of the ideal sedative drug or sedative regimen

Analgesia
Hypnosis
Water-soluble and stable in solution at room temperature
Short onset and offset of action
No effect on cardiovascular or respiratory function
Metabolic pathways independent of hepatic or renal function
Non-cumulative
Inactive metabolites
Modest cost

Analgesia – opioids and alternatives

Opioids are the most important component of any sedative regimen. They are probably not truly sedative in their own right, but certainly permit sleep by relieving pain and discomfort. Respiratory depression is usually not a problem in a monitored environment, but can interfere with the rapid processing of short-stay patients such as following cardiac surgery. In these circumstances, a compromise may be necessary between patient comfort and weaning from mechanical ventilation. Reduced gastrointestinal motility is commonly blamed on opioids, but severity of illness is probably a more important cause.[11] Nausea and vomiting are a feature of short-term administration.

Morphine

Morphine is the standard opioid analgesic, being both effective and cheap. It is relatively slow in onset, and inadequate pain relief requires supplementary bolus doses. It should be used cautiously in patients with renal failure, as the glucuronide will accumulate.[12] Morphine-6-glucuronide has approximately 20 times the potency of the parent compound.[13] In high doses, morphine has been shown to impair immune responses in animals,[14] and its safety in critically ill patients should not be assumed. Tolerance to and dependence on opioids can occur, but is rare and usually follows prolonged and excessively high doses in the absence of pain. Morphine clearance is substantially slower in neonates,[15] and is also impaired in sepsis as a result of hepatic hypoperfusion.

Alfentanil

Alfentanil is a fentanyl derivative with one-quarter of the potency. It is 92% protein-bound, is less lipophilic than fentanyl, and hence has a smaller volume of distribution. Its effect reaches a peak about 90 s after IV injection, and rapidly declines, due to metabolism by the liver to inactive metabolites. The elimination half-life in healthy subjects is 90 min.[16] A single case has been reported of prolonged elimination following infusion, but the cause was not determined.[17] In acute hepatic failure, alfentanil infusion is highly effective at obtunding deleterious stress responses, without clinical evidence of accumulation. It is the most appropriate opioid for patients with impaired renal function. Alfentanil has been used in combination with midazolam to provide effective sedation of ventilated patients.[18] The combination of alfentanil with propofol has attractions in that both agents have high plasma clearances and short half-lives.

Fentanyl

Fentanyl is much more lipid-soluble and has a larger volume of distribution than alfentanil. Large doses may take a long time to clear. It is less suitable for long-term administration, particularly in patients with impaired hepatic function.

Non-steroidal anti-inflammatory analgesics

Non-steroidal anti-inflammatory analgesics are useful alternatives to opioids provided that splanchnic oxygenation can be assured. They are best reserved for postoperative analgesia in physiologically stable patients without an oxygen debt, and who have no pre-existing renal dysfunction or gastrointestinal ulceration. They are contraindicated if there is any possibility of intestinal or renal dysoxia,[10] whether from haemodynamic instability, systemic oxygen debt or sepsis. They should be prescribed with great caution in ICU.

Regional blockade

Regional blockade with local anaesthetic agents has limited application in critically ill patients who often have multiple sources of pain or discomfort. Epidural bupivacaine with diamorphine or fentanyl can provide excellent analgesia, and thereby facilitate earlier extubation following upper gastrointestinal surgery or abdominal vascular surgery.

Hypnotic agents

Benzodiazepines

Benzodiazepines bind to specific receptors in the brain and spinal cord, thereby facilitating the inhibitory actions of γ-aminobutyric acid (GABA). This results in hypnotic, anxiolytic, muscle-relaxation and anticonvulsant activity.[19] As with any sedative, rapid IV injection in an unstable patient may produce airway compromise and cardiovascular depression. Benzodiazepines, like other flow-limited drugs, may accumulate in patients with impaired hepatic blood flow. Overdose or accumulation can be corrected by flumazenil, which has a shorter half-life than agonist benzodiazepines and may need to be given by continuous infusion for effective reversal.

Midazolam

Midazolam is a water-soluble hypnotic imidazo-benzodiazepine extensively bound to plasma proteins. Metabolism involves hydroxylation by hepatic microsomal enzymes[20] and subsequent conjugation with glucuronic acid before renal excretion. The hydroxy-metabolites have limited sedative activity.[21] Its elimination half-life ranges from 1 to 4 h in healthy subjects, but may be increased unpredictably in the critically ill patients,[22] particularly septic patients with impaired hepatic blood flow. Midazolam can be administered as a continuous infusion for sedation at a dose range of 0.02–0.20 mg/kg per h. It is cardiovascularly stable in fit people, and it is a satisfactory hypnotic in patients who are not critically ill and who are also receiving analgesia. It is also a suitable choice for paediatric sedation.[23] In patients with MOD however, the unpredictable half-life may cause concern. Moreover, it may impair verbal contact and cooperation, particularly during weaning from ventilation, because of its potent amnesic properties. Attempts to control agitated patients with larger doses result in over-sedation.[24]

Diazepam and lorazepam

Diazepam and lorazepam may be used in intermittent bolus, and not by infusion. Unlike diazepam, lorazepam has no active metabolites. Both drugs have a long half-life (over 90 h for desmethyldiazepam, the active metabolite of diazepam), and accumulation is a significant risk. Their only advantage is that they are cheap. IV administration of a few milligrams of diazepam at night may be all that is needed to facilitate sleep in long-term ventilator-dependent patients who have become tolerant of shorter-acting benzodiazepines such as temazepam.

Propofol

Propofol (2,6-di-isopropylphenol) is a short-acting IV anaesthetic agent. The drug is 97% bound to plasma proteins, is highly lipophilic, and following a single induction dose (2.5 mg/kg) undergoes rapid and extensive distribution from blood into brain and other tissues. The volume of distribution at steady state is 329 l/kg and the clearance 1.81 l/min.[25] Propofol is rapidly metabolized by the liver primarily to its inactive glucuronide and sulphate conjugates. Metabolites are excreted in the urine, and extrahepatic mechanisms may contribute to the metabolism.[10] Given as an infusion at 1–3 mg/kg per h, propofol can produce a controllable level of sedation with rapid recovery.[26] When compared with midazolam for intensive care sedation, propofol has shorter arousal times, but no difference in quality of sedation.[27] A similar study following cardiac surgery failed to demonstrate a difference in duration of ventilation or ICU stay.[28] Infusions of propofol for up to 96 h do not appear to lead to tachyphylaxis, and adequate recovery can be obtained in most patients by 10 min.[29] However, more information is needed on the pharmacokinetics in patients with MOD.

Propofol has several disadvantages. It causes hypotension from a reduction in cardiac output and arterial and venous tone.[30] Prolonged infusions will lead to increased serum triglycerides and cholesterol concentrations.[31] In patients on fluid restriction, the large volumes of infusion pose problems (although these will be resolved by the introduction of a 2% formulation). There is a reported association of propofol infusions and sudden death in children with severe viral infections.[32] Hence it should not be used by infusion in paediatric patients without further investigation. It is also expensive.

Isoflurane

Isoflurane delivered into the ventilator circuit in concentrations of around 0.25–0.50% has been used to provide satisfactory sedation of patients for limited periods without adverse effects or evidence of fluoride accumulation.[24,33] Main problems are the need for scavenging of expired vapours and vasodilatation.

Ketamine

Ketamine is a phencyclidine derivative which produces potent analgesia and dissociative anaesthesia. It increases heart rate and blood pressure indirectly by vasomotor stimulation through the sympathetic nervous system. It has myocardial depressant properties, and should be avoided in patients with high cervical spinal cord lesions. Its bronchodilator properties may be useful for sedating asthmatics requiring mechanical ventilation, including children.[34] In low doses (0.5 mg/kg) it is a useful analgesic for facilitating brief, but painful surface procedures (e.g. changing adherent burns dressings).

Chlormethiazole

Chlormethiazole is a sedative anticonvulsant presented as a 0.8% solution in 5% dextrose for IV infusion. A rate of 4–10 ml/min is given initially until the desired effect is achieved, after which it is reduced to 1–2 ml/h. The ease of administration probably accounts for its popularity in ordinary wards for managing patients with clinical problems ranging from acute confusional states to status epilepticus and eclampsia. Bioavailability is increased in alcoholics,[35] and careless use has caused deaths. Nasal irritation, thrombophlebitis, haemolysis, large low-sodium fluid volumes, and accumulation after 48 h with delayed recovery limit the usefulness of this drug.

Chloral hydrate

Chloral hydrate is used in paediatric practice as an adjunct to IV sedation, particularly during weaning from ventilation. It is metabolized by the liver to the active substance trichlorethenol. This is in turn metabolized to the acetate and glucuronide, both of which will accumulate in renal dysfunction.[36]

Butyrophenones and phenothiazines

Butyrophenones and phenothiazines have no real sedation role in the ICU. Haloperidol may occasionally be useful in agitated and confused elderly patients. Droperidol, and particularly chlorpromazine, have significant α-adrenergic blocking activity, which in critically ill patients may cause marked hypotension.

Barbiturates

Barbiturates are unsuitable for therapeutic sedation. Thiopentone may be useful as an agent of last resort for the management of status epilepticus or critically raised ICP if other drugs have failed. It is cardiovascularly depressant and cumulative; recovery after prolonged infusions will take many days. The dose should be adjusted according to continuous EEG monitoring and plasma concentrations.

Muscle relaxants

Muscle relaxants may form part of a sedation regimen, although they have no sedative properties of their own. ICUs should establish clear policies for the use of relaxants,[37] including preconditions (Table 78.2), indications (Table 78.3) and standards of monitoring. No patient should be paralysed without first being sedated to the point of unrousability, and the adequacy of sedation should be checked at least daily.

Table 78.2 Preconditions for the use of muscle relaxants

Patients must be receiving mechanical ventilatory support

The ICU must have full-time dedicated cover by experienced medical staff

The ICU nursing staff should be appropriately trained in the use of muscle relaxants

Patients must be free from pain, and not consciously aware

Neuromuscular monitoring equipment should be available

Table 78.3 Indications for muscle relaxants in ICU

To facilitate short procedures under general anaesthesia in ICU

To facilitate mechanical ventilation when adequate sedation alone is unable to:

Increase chest wall compliance

Prevent incoordinate respiratory movements

Reduce peak airway pressures

Reduce the risk of barotrauma

Allow optimal gas exchange

Facilitate permissive hypercapnia

To reduce respiratory muscle Vo_2 in patients with critically impaired systemic Do_2

To ensure physiological control in patients with critically raised intracranial pressure

To control muscle spasms in tetanus or the malignant neuroleptic syndrome

Choice of muscle relaxants and monitoring

Dependence on hepatic and renal function for clearance and concerns about myopathy limit the safe use of steroidal relaxants. They are best reserved for intermittent bolus administration in patients with normal hepatic and renal function. The metabolism of the benzylisoquinolinium atracurium is independent of hepatic and renal function. Rapid clearance allows predictable recovery even from very prolonged infusions. Its major metabolite laudanosine, which has convulsant activity in animals, accumulates in patients with profound hepatic failure,[38] but there is no evidence that this is clinically important in humans. The new stereoisomer of atracurium, cisatracurium, is more potent, and the lower doses needed result in generation of less laudanosine.

Monitoring neuromuscular blockade in intensive care is required to avoid overdosage. The degree of neuromuscular blockade can be assessed either clinically by stopping the infusion or withholding further doses, or by regular measurement of neuromuscular transmission using a peripheral nerve stimulator and accelerometer. The accelerograph has a small probe containing a piezoelectric crystal, attached to the thumb. This produces a voltage proportional to the rate of acceleration when the thumb moves in response to ulnar nerve stimulation. As the mass of the thumb is constant, acceleration is directly proportional to the strength of muscle contraction. The most suitable stimulation modes are train-or-four (TOF) count, posttetanic count (PTC) and double-burst stimulation (DBS). Measurements made at the adductor pollicis may not reflect the degree of paralysis of the diaphragm.

Problems with muscle relaxants

1 *Accumulation* of the parent compound or the active metabolites will occur with the steroidal muscle relaxants, particularly pancuronium, in patients with hepatic or renal impairment. Saturation of peripheral storage sites may also account for delayed recovery.

2 *Histamine release* producing vasodilatation or bronchospasm may occur following bolus administration of atracurium, but this is not seen when administered by infusion.

3 *Protective reflexes* are abolished, and care must be taken to prevent corneal abrasions, conjunctivitis, pressure sores, ventilator disconnections, peripheral nerve injuries and deep venous thrombosis.

4 *Neurological assessment* is unreliable, and exclusion of residual neuromuscular block using a nerve stimulator is mandatory if the patient is unconscious.

5 *Drugs and disease* may potentiate neuromuscular blockade; aminoglycosides, hypo- and hyperkalaemia and hypophosphataemia are the most common.

6 *Prolonged weakness* in association with a myopathy lasting weeks or months has been reported in association primarily with the steroidal relaxants. Common associated factors have included high doses, impaired renal function and concurrent corticosteroids or aminoglycoside antibiotics.

Clinical considerations and sedative regimens

Patients admitted following elective surgery, or those with isolated respiratory failure, rarely present with sedation problems. If renal and hepatic function are unimpaired, then morphine by continuous infusion is the first choice for relief of pain or discomfort. A hypnotic agent may only be required at night; a benzodiazepine, propofol, or an inhalational agent (isoflurane) can all be used equally satisfactorily. Propofol is convenient and has a predictable duration of action, but costs much more.

Patients with MOD are more complicated to manage. Cerebral dysfunction makes neurological assessment difficult, and it is preferable not to use drugs with active and accumulating metabolites. Morphine, diamorphine and pethidine should not be

Table 78.4 Acute confusional states

Hypoxaemia
Systemic infection
Cerebral hypoxia–ischaemia
Other central nervous system lesions
Postictal
Drug dependence and withdrawal
Metabolic encephalopathies

used in the presence of renal impairment (particularly oliguric renal failure), as their active metabolites will accumulate. Midazolam and diazepam will accumulate in hepatic failure or when hepatic blood flow is impaired, and their water-soluble active metabolites are partly dependent on renal function for clearance. Alfentanil is the most appropriate opioid, with propofol, for hypnosis. Midazolam is an acceptable alternative if sedation is needed long-term. Neuromuscular blockade with atracurium may be considered if sedative drugs alone do not adequately facilitate organ-system support without unacceptable cardiovascular depression. Encephalopathic patients with raised ICP must not be rendered hypotensive with sedative drugs; the most appropriate regimen is alfentanil with a muscle relaxant.

Acute confusional states in non-intubated patients are also difficult to manage. Common or important causes are listed in Table 78.4. Confusion also delays weaning from ventilation and extubation. Sedative drugs must never be used as an alternative to identifying and treating the cause of confusion or distress, particularly in the elderly.[39] Skilled nursing care and the presence of relatives are more important than drugs if the patient can communicate. Any pain must be relieved. Hypoxaemia must be identified and corrected. Bacteraemias may not be accompanied by pyrexia, and blood cultures should be taken if infection is a possibility. Hypoxic–ischaemic cerebral damage is common in cardiovascularly unstable patients with vascular disease, and recovery from confusion is usually good, given time. Clonidine has been used successfully to manage delirium tremens following alcohol withdrawal.[40] If sedation is required, small doses are given with continuous monitoring of effect.

References

1. Bion JF and Ledingham IMcA (1986) Sedation in intensive care – a postal survey. *Intensive Care Med* **13**:215–216.
2. Merriman H (1981) The techniques used to sedate ventilated patients. A survey of methods used in 34 ICUs in Great Britain. *Intensive Care Med* **7**:217–224.
3. Lambert A, Mitchell R, Frost J *et al.* (1983) Direct *in vitro* inhibition of adrenal steroidogenesis by etomidate. *Lancet* **ii**:1085–1086.
4. Watt I and Ledingham IMcA (1984) Mortality amongst multiple trauma patients admitted to an intensive therapy unit. *Anaesthesia* **39**:973–981.
5. Lassen HCA (1953) A preliminary report on the 1952 epidemic of poliomyelitis in Copenhagen, with special reference to the treatment of acute respiratory insufficiency. *Lancet* **i**:37–41.
6. Wallace PGM, Bion JF and Ledingham IMcA (1988) The changing face of sedative practice. In: Ledingham IMcA (ed.) *Recent Advances in Critical Care Medicine 3*. Edinburgh: Churchill Livingstone.
7. Ramsay MAE, Savage TH, Simpson BRG and Goodwin R (1974) Controlled sedation with alphaxalone and alphadolone. *Br Med J* **2**:656–659.
8. Sprung CL, Peduzzi PN, Shatney CH *et al.* (1990) Impact of encephalopathy on mortality in the sepsis syndrome. *Crit Care Med* **18**:801–805.
9. Hasselgren P-O and Fischer JE (1986) Septic encephalopathy. *Intensive Care Med* **12**:13–16.
10. Osborne RJ, Joel SP and Slevin MI (1986) Morphine intoxication in renal failure: the role of morphine-6-glucuronide. *Br Med J* **292**:1548–1549.
11. Shimomura K, Kamata O and Ueki S (1971) Analgesic effects of morphine glucuronides. *Tohuku J Exp Med* **105**:45–52.
12. Tubaro E, Borelli G, Groce C *et al.* (1983) Effect of morphine on resistance to infection. *J Infect Dis* **148**:656–666.
13. Lynn AM and Slattery JT (1987) Morphine pharmacokinetics in early infancy. *Anesthesiology* **66**:136–139.
14. Macnab MSP, Macrae DJ, Grant IS and Feely J (1986) Profound reduction in morphine clearance and liver blood flow in shock. *Intensive Care Med* **12**:366–369.
15. Bower S and Hull CJ (1982) Comparative phamacokinetics of fentanyl and alfentanil. *Br J Anaesth* **54**:871.
16. Yate PM, Thomas D, Short SM *et al.* (1986) Comparison of infusions of alfentanil or pethidine for sedation of ventilated patients on the ITU. *Br J Anaesth* **58**:1091–1099.
17. Cohen AT and Kelly DR (1987) Assessment of alfentanil by intravenous infusion as long-term sedation in intensive care. *Anaesthesia* **42**:545–548.
18. Saidman LJ (1985) Midazolam: pharmacology and uses. *Anesthesiology* **62**:310–324.
19. Wandel C, Bocker R, Bohrer H *et al.* (1994) Midazolam is metabolized by at least three different cytochrome P450 enzymes. *Br J Anaesth* **73**:658–661.
20. Ziegler WH, Schalch E, Leishman B and Eckert M (1983) Comparison of the effects of intravenously administered midazolam, triazolam and their hydroxy metabolites. *Br J Clin Pharmacol* **16**:63S–69S.
21. Dirksen MSC, Vree TB and Driessen JJ (1987) Clinical pharmacokinetics of long-term infusion of midazolam in critically ill patients – preliminary results. *Anaesth Intens Care* **15**:440–444.
22. Hartwig S, Roth B and Theisohn M (1991) Clinical experience with continuous intravenous sedation using midazolam and fentayl in paediatric intensive care. *Eur J Pediatr* **150**:784–788.

23. Kong KL, Willatts SM and Prys-Roberts C (1989) Isoflurane compared with midazolam for sedation in the intensive care unit. *Br Med J* **298**:1277–1280.

24. Kay NH, Sear JW, Uppington J *et al.* (1986) Disposition of propofol in patients undergoing surgery. A comparison in men and women. *Br J Anaesth* **58**:1075–1079.

25. Servin F, Haberer JP, Cockshott ID, Farinotti R and Desmonts JM (1986) Propofol pharmacokinetics of patients with cirrhosis. *Anesthesiology* **65**:A554.

26. Newman LH, McDonald JC, Wallace PGM and Ledingham IM (1987) Propofol infusion for sedation in intensive care. *Anaesthesia* **42**:929–937.

27. Aitkenhead AR, Pepperman ML, Willatts SM *et al.* (1989) Comparison of propofol and midazolam for sedation in critically ill patients. *Lancet* **2**:704–709.

28. Higgins TL, Yared J-P, Estafanous FG *et al.* (1994) Propofol versus midazolam for intensive care unit sedation after coronary artery bypass grafting. *Crit Care Med* **22**:1415–1423.

29. Beller JP, Pottecher T and Lugnier A (1988) Prolonged sedation with propofol in ICU patients: recovery and blood concentration changes during periodic interruption in infusion. *Br J Anaesth* **61**:583–588.

30. Boer F, Ros P, Borill JG, Van Brummelen P and Van Der Krogt J (1990) Effects of propofol on peripheral vascular resistance during cardiopulmonary bypass. *Br J Anaesth* **65**:184–189.

31. Gottardis M, Khunl-Brady KS and Koller W (1989) Effect of prolonged sedation with propofol on serum triglyceride and cholesterol concentrations. *Br J Anaesth* **62**:393–396.

32. Park GR, Stevens JE and Rice AS (1992) Metabolic acidosis and fatal myocardial failure after propofol infusion in children. *Br Med J* **305**:613–616.

33. Spencer EM and Willatts SM (1992) Isoflurane for prolonged sedation in the intensive care unit; efficacy and safety. *Intensive Care Med* **18**:415–421.

34. Tobias JD, Martin LD and Wetzel RC (1990) Ketamine by continuous infusion for sedation in the pediatric intensive care unit. *Crit Care Med* **18**:819–821.

35. Editorial (1987) Chlormethiazole and alcohol: a lethal cocktail. *Br Med J* **294**:592.

36. Reimche LD, Sankaran K, Hindmarsh KW *et al.* (1989) Chloral hydrate sedation for neonates and infants: clinical and pharmacological considerations. *Dev Pharmacol Ther* **121**:57–64.

37. Elliot M and Bion JF (1995) Neuromuscular blocking drugs in intensive care. *Acta Anaesthesiol Scand* **106**:70–82.

38. Bion JF, Bowden MI, Chow L, Honisberger L and Weatherley BC (1993) Atracurium infusions in patients with fulminant hepatic failure awaiting liver transplantation. *Intensive Care Med* **19**:S94–S98.

39. O'Keeffe ST and Ni Chonchubhair A (1994) Postoperative delirium in the elderly. *Br J Anaesth* **73**:673–687.

40. Ip Yam PC, Forbes A and Kox WJ (1992) Clonidine in the treatment of alcohol withdrawal in the intensive care unit. *Br J Anaesth* **68**:106–108.

GD Phillips

Many patients in the ICU experience pain. The pain may be related to surgical operations, traumatic injuries or organ disease (e.g. myocardial ischaemia). Pain has a number of adverse effects. It produces anxiety and lack of sleep and contributes to delirium.[1] It exaggerates the hormonal response to injury, resulting in sodium and water retention and hyperglycaemia. Increased sympathetic output due to pain increases heart rate, blood pressure and peripheral resistance, with consequent increased cardiac work and myocardial oxygen consumption leading to ischaemia.[2] Pain from chest and abdominal wounds or injury results in muscle splinting, decreased tidal volume, vital capacity, functional residual capacity and alveolar ventilation. Poor coughing leads to sputum retention, atelectasis, pulmonary infection, hypoxia and hypercarbia. Other effects of pain include venous stasis due to immobility, with subsequent deep venous thrombosis and decreased intestinal motility. Apart from humanitarian grounds, pain relief is important, as it will reduce physical morbidity due to the above effects.

Some pain characteristics

Pain is 'an unpleasant sensory and emotional experience, associated with actual or potential tissue damage, or described in terms of such damage.[3] Perception of pain depends not only on the degree of tissue injury, but also on modification of the message by other simultaneously occurring sensory input. Personality traits influence pain perception, and it seems likely that differences in pain perception between individuals will be found to be of greater significance than the types and locations of the surgery or trauma.[4] Pain perception is influenced by cultural background, previous pain experience, fear, uncertainty, misinterpretation of events and helplessness[5] – assessment is complex.[6]

Age can influence analgesic requirements. The elderly and the very young may require less analge-

sics, but there is not much difference between the sexes. Recent evidence suggests that children experience as much pain as adults, which they often fail to communicate to nurses, and their pain management is often poor.[7]

Chronic disease may influence analgesic response. Patients on long-term medications may develop a tolerance to analgesics, and thus require larger doses. Pain is exacerbated by many factors which contribute to a vicious cycle of pain, anxiety and sleeplessness. These include discomfort from tubes, drains, incisions, catheters, plasters, traction, light, noise, dressings, as well as inability to communicate (see Chapter 78).

Pain following surgery is self-limiting, being most severe on the first day, and becoming minimal by the third day. The severity of the pain depends on the site of the operation, being most marked following operation in the thorax and upper abdomen, with less severity in lower abdominal operations and operations on the head, neck and limbs.

Two different types of pain may be present: a dull, steady, background pain at rest, and a severe, acute stabbing pain associated with movement, coughing and physiotherapy. The pain itself may be referred from another site (e.g. shoulder-tip pain of diaphragmatic origin). Assessment of pain based on response to coughing and physiotherapy has been found useful in determining the response to various analgesic measures.

Management of pain

Supportive measures will minimize overall pain and anxiety. Constant communication and reassurance are important, and noise levels should be reduced as much as possible. Troublesome symptoms such as flatulence, urinary retention, nausea and vomiting should be treated. Fractures should be immobilized. Adequate sleep may be achieved with hypnotics, by reducing the frequency of recording vital signs, and by minimizing disturbance from lights. Anxiolytics (e.g. diazepam) may be useful in the over-anxious patient. Many patients, however, are prepared to offset pain against side-effects of therapy, and are satisfied if their pain is made bearable.

Guidelines for pain management in different circumstances are now readily available. The US Department of Health and Human Services *Clinical Practice Guidelines*[8] is one such example, itself referencing others.[3,9] This booklet makes some important points in successful pain management:

1 *Prevention* is better than treatment. Pain relief should be effective on awakening from surgery, or as soon as possible in non-surgical conditions. Spinal cord pathways 'remember' painful stimuli.
2 *Assessment and reassessment* of the patient's pain are essential, and must lead to modifications to the pain management plan.
3 *Drugs and techniques* used to control pain should be governed by policies and procedures that define levels of monitoring and the roles for health care providers involved.
4 *Patient satisfaction* is the ultimate indication of the quality of pain relief.

Kehlet[10] suggested that management of pain should be considered as use of four treatment modalities:

1 *pre-emptive analgesia* to reduce post-injury neuroplasticity which leads to pain hypersensitivity;
2 *multimodal pain therapy* or balanced analgesia;
3 *search for new drugs* such as tachykinin and bradykinin antagonists;
4 *search for new techniques* which concentrate on peripheral treatment of pain at the site of injury.

Parenteral drugs

Opioid analgesics

Morphine

Morphine remains the mainstay of opioid therapy despite the introduction of newer drugs. There is a direct relationship between blood concentration of opioid and pain relief, and it is possible to predict blood concentrations. Irregular absorption following IM injection results in fluctuating blood concentrations, with periods of pain until the next dose takes effect. If IM opioids are used, the dose which relieves pain (usually morphine 0.15 mg/kg) should be available to the patient *as often as required*, rather than on a rigid p.r.n. basis. If the circulatory status is unstable, opioid analgesics are best given IV, carefully titrated in small increments on an individual basis. Pain relief is better managed by shortening the time between injections rather than by increasing individual dosage.

IV opioid infusions produce better, more consistent analgesia.[11] A loading dose of 10 mg morphine over 30 min, followed by a constant infusion of morphine 2.5 mg/h, is often effective in a 70 kg adult. Both loading dose and constant infusion may have to be varied depending on age, haemodynamic status and clinical effect. Opioid analgesia may also be self-administered by the patient. Increments of morphine (0.025 mg/kg) can be delivered IV on demand, by a patient-controlled apparatus (i.e. patient-controlled analgesia, PCA), with a maximum dose limit.[12–14]

Pethidine

Pethidine remains a useful alternative to morphine, but has the disadvantage of norpethidine toxicity in patients requiring large doses, resulting in muscle twitching, rigidity and convulsions.[15] It has the greatest atropine-like activity.

Fentanyl

Fentanyl is a potent, lipid-soluble synthetic opioid, which is rapidly and widely distributed to tissues. It has fewer adverse effects on the cardiovascular system, and can be used in patients with haemodynamic instability in whom morphine may cause severe hypotension. (Morphine is clearly much cheaper for maintenance, once the patient becomes stable.) Its duration of action is short, making it useful for painful procedures. Prolonged administration results in a prolonged elimination half-life. New derivatives of fentanyl include the more potent and longer-acting sufentanil and lofentanil, and the less potent ultrashort-acting alfentanil.[16]

Methadone

Methadone is an alternative for long-duration postoperative pain relief, as a single dose, which may produce up to 24 h analgesia.[17] The low systemic clearance of methadone enables analgesic blood concentrations to be sustained for long periods. There is considerable individual variability both in the terminal half-life of methadone and in pain relief. Thus, there is potential for accumulation if doses are given at inappropriate intervals. Titration of supplementary methadone doses is suggested.

Side-effects

All opioids have similar side-effects if given in equianalgesic doses (Table 79.1). The side-effects are dose-related, and include cardiorespiratory depression, dysphoria, nausea and vomiting. Opioid agents depress the ventilatory response to hypercarbia, but not to hypoxia. Hence, uncontrolled administration of oxygen to some patients may lead to a respiratory arrest. Routine prescribing of an antiemetic with every dose of opioid is probably not justified, because

Table 79.1 Opioid analgesics

Drug	Rapid half-life (min)	Slow half-life (h)	Equipotent dose (mg)	Duration of pain relief (h)
Pethidine	4–11	3–7	100	3–4
Morphine	25	2–4	10	3–4
Methadone	10	20–50	10–20	18–24
Fentanyl	2–3	2–5	0.1	0.5–1

Repetitive dosing at high dose levels results in low clearance with a potential for accumulation.
Modified from Cousins and Phillips.[50]

of the potential of unwanted phenothiazine and additive central nervous system depressant effects.

Naloxone

Naloxone is the antagonist of choice. Unfortunately it reverses analgesia as well as cardiorespiratory depression, and the patient may become restless and agitated. The dose is 0.1–0.4 mg IV, repeated hourly if necessary. Detailed descriptions of other opioid agents are reviewed elsewhere. Spinal administration of opioids is discussed below.

Agonist–antagonists[18,19]

Agonist–antagonists such as pentazocine, butorphanol, buprenorphine and nalbuphine have not made much headway in pain management, especially in the intensive care setting, and the availability of naloxone removes the original reason for their development.

Oral analgesics[20]

Oral analgesics are useful for minor pain, or for postoperative pain after the second or third day. Some minor analgesics are listed in Table 79.2. Again, use of these drugs should form part of the multimodel armamentarium. They also have side-effects, including altered platelet function (aspirin), and worsening

Table 79.2 Some mild (oral) analgesics

Drug	Oral dose (mg)	Half-life (h)
Aspirin	600–900	0.25
Paracetamol (acetaminophen)	600–900	4
Codeine	30–60	4
Ibuprofen	200–400	2.1
Indomethacin	25–50	4.6
Naproxen	250–500	14

of renal failure, fluid retention and peptic ulceration in some patients (non-steroidal anti-inflammatory drugs).

Transdermal opioids[21]

Recent studies have confirmed that fentanyl can be delivered to the circulation via the skin, using a skin patch which contains a drug reservoir and a rate-controlling membrane. After a lag of about 6–12 h, reasonably stable plateau blood concentrations are achieved. When the patches are removed, the skin acts as a sink so that blood concentration of fentanyl remains elevated for 12–24 h. These limitations can probably be overcome by supplementary IV doses at the start of treatment, and careful observation for 12–24 h after treatment. This option of opioid use may be valuable in children and situations where other routes are not available or appropriate.

Regional analgesia

Many local analgesia techniques may be used for pain relief. Epidural block has the widest scope in the ICU. However, all regional techniques are time-consuming, and require trained personnel. Complications, although uncommon, may be serious.

Epidural (extradural) blocks

Epidural blocks are most advantageous following upper abdominal and chest surgery, where coughing, deep breathing and mobility are facilitated.

Epidural local anaesthetic agents

Bupivacaine has a longer duration of action than lignocaine. The most consistently reported advantage of epidural block is improved FEV_1 and ability to cough.[22] For lower limb, lower abdominal and pelvic pain relief, the catheter is inserted in the lumbar region at L1–2 or L2–3. A loading dose of 10–15 ml 0.5% bupivacaine is followed by an infusion of 5–20 ml/h 0.125% bupivacaine.

Upper abdominal and thoracic pain is best treated with a mid thoracic catheter inserted at an accessible interspace between T7 and T10 levels. An initial dose of 4–6 ml 0.5% bupivacaine is followed by an infusion of 6–10 ml/h 0.125% bupivacaine. If analgesia becomes inadequate with the dilute 0.125% infusion, it is necessary to top up with an appropriate dose (4–8 ml) of the 0.5% solution.

The complications of epidural blockade in inexpert hands are serious, and include:

1 subarachnoid injection causing coma, hypotension, bradycardia and respiratory arrest;
2 sympathetic blockade, with hypotension and bradycardia;
3 respiratory muscle paralysis due to a high block;
4 epidural haematoma or abscess;
5 side-effects of the local anaesthetic agent itself.[23,24]

Full resuscitation facilities must be available. The patient's pulse, blood pressure, respiratory rate and sensory level of blockade must be monitored closely with each injection.[25] Continuous epidural infusions of local anaesthetic may produce fewer and less acute episodes of hypotension than incremental injections.

Epidural opioids

The use of epidural opioid injections offers pain relief without postural hypotension.[26,27] Morphine 5 mg, pethidine 50 mg and fentanyl 50 μg reach the cerebrospinal fluid (CSF) rapidly in high concentrations, and produce analgesia by direct action on opiate receptors in the posterior horn cells of the spinal cord. Analgesia with morphine may last 12–24 h. Experimental work has defined the principles of action of spinal opiate analgesia.[28] There are fundamental differences between local anaesthetic and opioid epidural blockade.[29] Epidural opioids do not provide the dense analgesia of local anaesthetics, but produce effective analgesia which lasts for up to 24 h, without the troublesome hypotension of local anaesthetics (Table 79.3). However, epidural opioids may produce some hypotension, itching, nausea, vomiting, urinary retention and delayed respiratory depression (Table 79.4). Side-effects are antagonized by naloxone without altering analgesic effect.[80]

There is clear evidence that epidural local anaesthetic and opioid drugs act synergistically. Thus careful selection of doses of these two different drugs will decrease the risk of toxicity from each component, while increasing the analgesic efficacy. There is also good documentation of minimizing or eliminating tachyphylaxis to epidural local anaesthetics, when local anaesthetic is combined with opioid. Several well-controlled studies have reported clear superiority of a combined infusion of bupivacaine (0.1% at 3–4 ml/h) and morphine (0.3–0.4 mg/h) compared to either treatment alone.[31] Fentanyl has also been reported to be additive to bupivacaine epidural infusion. Usually, the dose (rate) of 0.125% bupivacaine can be halved by adding 25–50 μg/h of fentanyl. However, the dose of opioid and local anaesthetic must be titrated carefully to suit the needs of individual patients.[32]

The potential advantage of superior analgesia with epidural opioid or local anaesthetic has to be justified

Table 79.3 Comparison of actions and efficacy of spinally applied opioids and local anaesthetic block

	Opioids	*Local anaesthetics*
Actions		
Site of action	Substantia gelatinosa of dorsal horn spinal cord and other opioid receptors	Nerve roots (and long tracts in spinal cord)
Type of blockade	Presynaptic and (postsynaptic) inhibition of *neurone cell* excitation	Blockade of nerve impulse conduction in *axonal* membrane
Modalities blocked	Selective block of pain conduction	Blockade of sympathetic and pain fibres; often also loss of sensation and motor function
Efficacy		
Type of pain and efficacy of blockade:		
Surgical or traumatic pain	Partial relief	Complete relief possible
Postoperative pain – early		
First 24 h	Fair relief (high dose)	Complete relief
Over 24 h	Good relief (low dose)	Complete relief

Adapted from Cousins *et al.*[29]

Table 79.4 Effects and side-effects of spinally applied opioids and local anaesthetic block

Side-effects	Spinal opioids	Spinal local anaesthetics

Cardiovascular	Minor heart rate changes	Low block (below T10)
		  Sympathetic blockade
		  Postural hypotension

	Usually no postural hypotension	High block (above T4)
		  Sympathetic blockade
		  Postural hypotension

	Vasoconstrictor response intact	Cardioaccelerator block $\downarrow$ Heart rate, $\downarrow$ inotropic drive
Respiratory	Early depression*† (1–2 h) – systemically absorbed drug Late depression *† (6–24 h) – opioid in cerebrospinal fluid migrating to brain	Usually unimpaired unless C5 level reached
Central nervous system		
Sedation	May be marked*	Mild or absent, depending on agent
Convulsions	Usually not seen	Expected toxicity from high dose
Other neurological abnormalities	Confusion, amnesia, catalepsy, hallucinations (reported with high doses intrathecally)	Not usually seen
Nausea	Yes*	Yes – low incidence
Vomiting	Yes*	Yes – low incidence
Urinary retention	Yes*†	Yes
Skin itching	Yes*	No
Meiosis	Yes	No

* Antagonized by naloxone but repeated doses may be required.
† Prevented by naloxone infusion.
Adapted from Cousins *et al.*[29]

in individual cases against the price of greater invasiveness and complications of these techniques. In an ICU, epidural opioids offer a useful alternative to continuous infusion of local anaesthetics when control of severe pain is required.[33]

Intercostal nerve blocks[34]

Intercostal nerve blocks are useful to provide analgesia to appropriate dermatomes. The technique allows coughing without pain. Bilateral blocks are necessary for midline wounds. Unfortunately, visceral nerves are not blocked, multiple injections are required, and there is the added risk of pneumothorax. The action of bupivacaine can be prolonged with the use of adrenaline, and 3–5 ml of 0.5% is usually effective. When more than three or four ribs are fractured, or there are bilateral fractures, epidural blockade may be preferable.

Intrapleural catheter[35,36]

Use of local anaesthetics injected into the pleural space to produce analgesia may be of value in specific situations.

Inhalation agents

The use of inhalation agents requires additional apparatus. Moreover, the problem of atmospheric pollution with possible adverse effects on staff is a definite disadvantage. Nevertheless, inhalation analgesic agents are useful in time-limited procedures such as change of dressings and physiotherapy.

Nitrous oxide

The use of 50% nitrous oxide : 50% oxygen (Entonox) provides good analgesia.[37] Ten to 12 breaths are necessary to produce an adequate brain concentration. Entonox can be given by a demand apparatus, by positive-pressure ventilation and by semi-rigid plastic oxygen masks (e.g. MC, Edinburgh, or Hudson masks). The last technique allows 10–25% nitrous oxide and 25–35% oxygen to be inspired with satisfactory analgesia.[38] Use of Entonox should be confined to 36 h, as marrow depression can occur with prolonged usage.[39]

Other methods of pain relief

Transcutaneous electrical nerve stimulation[40]

This technique involves electrical stimulation of large-diameter afferent nerve fibres, thus selectively inhibiting pain (the gate control theory of pain). Electrical stimulation has been used postoperatively and for pain from rib fractures. The technique is often not effective on its own, but may achieve a reduction in analgesic requirements.

Acupuncture and hypnosis

Stimulation of designated body sites by manual rotation of a needle to produce a unique sensation and pain relief, and manipulation of attention, together with strong suggestion, are of little value in the ICU. Both hypnosis and acupuncture are too time-consuming to be widely applicable. Some degree of patient cooperation is usually necessary.

Pain relief in different circumstances[41]

Conscious non-intubated patient

The choice of analgesia is usually between staff-controlled IV infusion of an opioid, PCA or an epidural block with bupivacaine and/or opioid. In the former situation, for peak pain during physiotherapy, a small bolus of opioid or inhalation of nitrous oxide and oxygen will usually be effective. The aim is effective deep breathing and coughing, with minimal cardiovascular compromise. Most studies of postoperative analgesia have studied rest pain, not pain during effort, which is a vital concern.[10]

Ventilated patient

Continuous IV infusion of morphine is usually satisfactory. Large doses may be given if necessary, or smaller doses supplemented by administration of diazepam or midazolam.[42] A mixture of morphine 50 mg and midazolam 45 mg in 50 ml normal saline may be infused at 1–5 ml/h. Fentanyl is an expensive alternative, while high-dose pethidine may result in norpethidine toxicity.

Opioid-tolerant patient

Patients already receiving opioids before an acute illness may require large doses to produce analgesia.

Clinical approach

Morphine is still the most widely used analgesic agent for severe pain. The discovery of several different populations of opiate and non-opiate receptors and endogenous morphine-like compounds would appear to offer potential advances.[43,44] Regional analgesia is useful and should, perhaps, be employed more often. The use of opioids by epidural injection represents a real advance in selected patients. Research into newer methods of pain prevention and management continues.[45] Effective analgesia depends on a variety of approaches, including pre-emptive analgesia,[46] and multimodal therapy,[47] and more attention to peripheral mechanisms of producing analgesia.[48,49]

References

1. Phillips GD and Cousins MJ (1986) Neurological mechanisms of pain and the relationship of pain, anxiety, and sleep. In: Cousins MJ and Phillips GD (eds) *Acute Pain Management. Clinics in Critical Care Medicine.* New York: Churchill Livingstone, pp. 21–48.
2. Kehlet H (1982) The modifying effect of general and regional anesthesia on the endocrine–metabolic response to surgery. *Reg Anaesth* (suppl 7):538–548.
3. National Health and Medical Research Council (1988) *Management of Severe Pain.* Canberra: Australian Government Publishing Service.
4. Boyle P and Parbrook GD (1977) The interrelation of personality and postoperative factors. *Br J Anaesth* **49**:259–264.
5. Peck C (1986) Psychological factors in acute pain management. In: Cousins MJ and Phillips GD (eds) *Acute Pain Management. Clinics in Critical Care Medicine.* New York: Churchill Livingstone, pp. 251–274.
6. Scott LE, Clum GA and Peoples JB (1983) Preoperative predictors of postoperative pain. *Pain* **15**:283–393.
7. Mather LE and Mackie J (1983) The incidence of postoperative pain in children. *Pain* **15**:271–282.
8. Department of Health and Human Services (1992) *Clinical Practice Guidelines Acute Pain Management: Operative or Medical Procedures and Trauma.* AHCPR publication no. 92–0032. Rockville, MD: Department of Health and Human Services.
9. American Pain Society (1989) *Principles of Analgesic Use in the Treatment of Acute Pain and Chronic Cancer Pain. A Concise Guide to Medical Practice*, 2nd edn. Skokie, IL: American Pain Society.
10. Kehlet H (1994) Postoperative pain relief – what is the issue? *Br J Anaesth* **72**:375–378.
11. Stapleton JV, Austin KL and Mather LE (1979) A pharmacokinetic approach to postoperative pain: continuous infusion of pethidine. *Anaesth Intens Care* **7**:25–32.
12. Check WA (1982) Results are better when patients control their own analgesia. *J Am Med Assoc* **247**:945–947.
13. Hull CJ and Sibbald A (1981) Control of postoperative pain by interactive demand analgesia. *Br J Anaesth* **53**:385–391.
14. Rowbotham DJ (1992) The development and safe use of patient-controlled analgesia. *Br J Anaesth* **68**:331–332.

15. Kaiko RF, Foley KM, Grabinski PY *et al.* (1983) Central nervous system excitatory effects of meperidine in cancer patients. *Ann Neurol* **13**:180–185.

16. Mather LE and Phillips GD (1986) Opioids and adjuvants: principles of use. In: Cousins MJ and Phillips GD (eds) *Acute Pain Management. Clinics in Critical Care Medicine.* New York: Churchill Livingstone, pp. 77–104.

17. Gourlay GK, Willis RJ and Wilson PR (1984) Post-operative pain control with methadone: influence of supplementary methadone dose and blood concentration – response relationship. *Anesthesiology* **61**:19–26.

18. Galloway FM, Hrdlicka J, Losada M, Noveck RJ and Caruso FS (1977) Comparison of analgesia by intravenous butorphanol and meperidine in patients with postoperative pain. *Can Anaesth Soc* **34**:90–102.

19. Dobkin AB, Esposito B and Philbin C (1977) Double-blind evaluation of buprenorphine hydrochoride for postoperative pain. *Can Anaesth Soc J* **24**:195–202.

20. Kehlet H, Mather LE (eds) The value of non-steroidal anti-inflammatory drugs in postoperative pain. *Drugs* **44** (suppl 5):1–63.

21. Duthie DJR, Rowbotham DJ, Wyld R, Henderson PD and Nimmo WS (1988) Plasma fentanyl concentrations during transdermal delivery of fentanyl to surgical patients. *Br J Anaesth* **60**:614–618.

22. Sundberg A, Wattwil M and Arvill A (1986) Respiratory effects of high thoracic epidural anaesthesia. *Acta Anaesthesiol Scand* **30**:215–217.

23. Reiz S and Nath S (1986) Cardiotoxicity of local anaesthetic agents. *Br J Anaesth* **58**:736–746.

24. Hasselstrom LJ and Mogensen T (1984) Toxic reaction of bupivacaine at low plasma concentration. *Anesthesiology* **61**:99–100.

25. Cousins MJ and Bromage PR (1988) Epidural neural blockade. In: Cousins MJ and Bridenbaugh PO (eds) *Neural Blockade in Clinical Anaesthesia and Management of Pain*, 2nd edn. Philadelphia: Lippincott, pp. 253–360.

26. Bromage PR, Camporesi E and Chestnut D (1980) Epidural narcotics for postoperative analgesia. *Anesth Analg* **59**:473–480.

27. Behar M, Magora F, Olshwang D and Davidson JT (1979) Epidural morphine in treatment of pain. *Lancet* **1**:527–528.

28. Yaksh TL and Nouethead R (1985) The physiology and pharmacology of spinal opiates. *Ann Rev Pharmacol Toxicol* **25**:433–462.

29. Cousins MJ, Mather LE and Wilson PR (1984) Intrathecal and epidural administration of opioid analgesics. *Anesthesiology* **61**:276–310.

30. Rawal N, Schott U, Dahlstrom B *et al.* (1986) Influence of naloxone on analgesia and respiratory depression following epidural morphine. *Anesthesiology* **64**:194–201.

31. Torda TA and Pybus DA (1984) Extradural administration of morphine and bupivacaine: a controlled comparison. *Br J Anaesth* **56**:141–146.

32. Cullen ML, Staren ED, El-Ganzouri A *et al.* (1985) Continuous epidural infusion for analgesia after major abdominal operations. A randomized, prospective double blind study. *Surgery* **98**:718–728.

33. Cousins MJ, Gourlay GK and Cherry DA (1988) Acute and chronic pain: use of spinal opioids. In: Cousins MJ and Bridenbaugh PO (eds) *Neural Blockade in Clinical Anaesthesia and Management of Pain*, 2nd edn. Philadelphia: Lippincott, pp. 955–1030.

34. Cronin KD and Davies MJ (1976) Intercostal block for postoperative pain relief. *Anaesth Intens Care* **4**:259–261.

35. Reistad F and Stromskag KE (1986) Intrapleural catheter in the management of postoperative pain – a preliminary report. *Reg Anaesth* **11**:89–91.

36. Blake DW, Bjorksten A, Dawson P and Hiscock R (1994) Pharmacokinetics of bupivacaine enantiomers during intra-pleural infusion. *Anaesth Intens Care* **22**:522–528.

37. Stewart RD (1988) Nitrous oxide. In: Paris PM and Stewart RD (eds) *Pain Management in Emergency Medicine.* Connecticut: Appleton and Lange, pp. 221–238.

38. Parbrook GD (1972) Entonox for postoperative analgesia. *Proc R Soc Med* **63**:8–9.

39. Editorial (1978) Nitrous oxide and the bone-marrow. *Lancet* **2**:613–614.

40. Burton C (1976) Transcutaneous electrical nerve stimulation to relieve pain. *Postgrad Med* **59**:105–108.

41. Phillips GD and Cousins MJ (1986) Practical decision making. In: Cousins MJ and Phillips GD (eds) *Acute Pain Management. Clinics in Critical Care Medicine.* New York: Churchill Livingstone, pp. 275–290.

42. Dundee JW, Holliday NJ, Harper KW *et al.* (1984) Midazolam: a review of its pharmacological properties and therapeutic use. *Drugs* **28**:519–543.

43. Snyder SH (1977) Opiate receptors and internal opiates. *Sci Am* **236**:44–58.

44. Bullingham RED (ed) (1983) *Opiate Analgesia. Clinics in Anesthesiology.* London: W.B. Saunders.

45. Wall PD (1988) The prevention of postoperative pain. *Pain* **33**:289–290.

46. Woolf CJ and Chong M-S (1993) Preemptive analgesia-treating postoperative pain by preventing the establishment of central sensitisation. *Anesth Analg* **77**:362–379.

47. Kehlet H and Dahl JB (1993) The value of 'multimodal' or 'balanced analgesia' in postoperative pain treatment. *Anesth Analg* **77**:1048–1056.

48. Dahl JB, Møiniche S and Kehlet H (1994) Wound infiltration with local anaesthetics for postoperative pain relief – a review. *Acta Anaesthesiol Scand* **38**:7–14.

49. Stein C (1993) Peripheral mechanisms of opioid analgesia. *Anesth Analg* **76**:182–191.

50. Cousins MJ and Phillips GD (1986) *Acute Pain Management. Clinics in Critical Care Medicine.* New York: Churchill Livingstone.

Part XIII

Metabolic homeostasis

LIG Worthley

By affecting the charge on reactive groups of enzymes, the alteration in concentration of hydrogen ions can profoundly influence the rate of metabolic reactions.[1] Despite the abundance of hydrogen in body fluids, the concentration or chemical activity of the hydrogen ion (or hydronium ion, H_3O) is remarkably small and constant. This is largely due to buffer systems which allow for a rapid turnover of protons with minimal alteration in hydrogen ion activity. In humans, the acid–base balance is maintained and regulated by the renal and respiratory systems, which modify the extracellular fluid (ECF) pH by changing the bicarbonate pair ($[HCO_3^-]$ and P_{CO_2}); all other body buffer systems adjust to the alterations in this pair.

Definitions[2]

pH

The negative logarithm of the hydrogen ion activity (Ha^+) is equal to the hydrogen ion concentration when the activity coefficient is unity. It is measured using a glass membrane electrode, porous only to H^+ ions, which develops a transmembrane potential proportional to the log of the H^+ ion activity (Ha^+). This potential is compared to the potential which is recorded using a standard solution of selected pH value. As the hydrogen ion activity coefficient is unity, and as the measurement of H^+ provides a practical scale of acidity and alkalinity, the linear consideration of the H^+ concentration has merit when compared to its logarithmic counterpart pH.[3] For example, it allows use of the Henderson equation to assess clearly the acid–base consequences of alteration in the P_{CO_2} and bicarbonate values:[4]

$$[H^+] = K \times \frac{CO_2}{[HCO_3^-]} \qquad \text{(equation 1)}$$

The plasma concentration of the H^+ ion at a pH of 7.4 is 40 nmol/l. Doubling or halving the H^+ concentration reduces or increases the pH by log 10 respectively (i.e. by approximately 0.3):

pH	H^+ (nmol/l)
6.8	160
7.1	80
7.4	40
7.7	20

Definitions of terms

Acid:	a proton donor or hydrogen ion donor.
Base:	a proton acceptor or hydrogen ion acceptor.
Acidaemia:	arterial blood pH less than 7.36 (H^+ greater than 44 nmol/l).
Alkalaemia:	arterial blood pH greater than 7.44 (H^+ less than 36 nmol/l).
Acidosis:	an abnormal condition which tends to decrease arterial pH if there are no secondary changes in response to the primary disease process.
Alkalosis:	an abnormal condition which tends to increase arterial pH if there are no secondary changes in response to the primary disease process.
Mixed disorder:	two or more primary acid–base abnormalities coexisting.
Compensation:	Normal body process tending to return the arterial pH to normal (respiratory or renal).
Acid–base balance:	Difference in quantity between input and output of acids and bases (Table 80.1).
Buffer:	a solution containing substances which have the ability to minimize changes in pH when an acid or base is added to it.

Table 80.1 Daily H⁺ balance

	Input (mmol/day)		Output (mmol/day)
Volatile			
CO_2	13 000	Lungs	13 000
Lactate	1500	Liver, kidney	1500
Non-volatile			
Protein SO_4	45	Titratable acid	30
Phospholipid PO_4	13		
Other	12	NH_4^+	40

pKa: the negative logarithm of the dissociation constant. If it describes a buffer system, then it is numerically equal to the pH of the system when the acid and its anion are present in equal concentrations.

Regulation of pH [H⁺] in body fluids

Despite wide variations in dietary acid and base, there seems to be no specific centre for H⁺ ion regulation. The body's respiratory and renal systems coordinate to regulate H⁺ homeostasis by regulating HCO_3^- and P_{CO_2}. The initial body defence against a change in pH is carried out by the body's buffer systems.[5]

Body buffering

Dilution

A comparison of the effect of adding the daily non-volatile H⁺ load (70 mmol H⁺) to a 70 kg man and to an equal volume of non-buffered water, at the same temperature and pH shows:

	Water volume (l)	pH (H⁺nmol/l) Before	After
70 kg man	42	7.4 (40)	7.39 (41)
Non-buffered water	42	7.4 (40)	2.78 (1 666 666)

It is clear that dilution is a poor defence against pH changes.

Buffer systems

These are present in the ECF and intracellular fluid (ICF). Their effectiveness or capacity is proportional to the amount of buffer, the pKa of the buffer, the pH of the carrying solutions and whether the buffer operates as an open or closed system.

Mechanisms of buffers

Any chemical reaction reaching an equilibrium can be expressed by the law of mass action. In the case of a weak acid:

$$HA \rightleftharpoons [H^+] + [A^-] \qquad \text{(equation 2)}$$

At equilibrium, the product of the concentrations of H⁺ and A⁻ is a constant fraction of the concentration of HA, or:

$$K = \frac{[H^+] [A^-]}{[HA]} \qquad \text{(equation 3)}$$

The value of K at equilibrium is always the same and independent of the concentrations of the reactants present initially. With the addition of another acid (H⁺ donor) to the system, the ionization of the weak acid HA is reduced (to keep K constant). If a base is added, the reduction in the H⁺ ion concentration produces further ionization of the acid, HA. Both reduce the change in H⁺ ion concentration (pH). However, the ionization of a weak acid is small. Thus, only a small addition of H⁺ can be tolerated before the pH falls. Supplementing the ion A⁻ by adding a salt of a strong base (e.g. NaA) provides a reservoir for combining with the added H⁺. A buffer system, therefore, can be produced by mixing a weak acid with the salt of that acid and a strong base.

Equation 3 can be rearranged as:

$$[H^+] = K \times \frac{[HA]}{[A^-]} \qquad \text{(equation 4; Henderson equation)}$$

The negative log of equation 4 is:

$$pH = pKa + \log \frac{[A^-]}{[HA]} \qquad \text{(equation 5; Henderson-Hasselbalch equation)}$$

Most (80%) of the buffering occurs within ± 1 pH unit of the pKa value of the buffer system (Fig. 80.1). Considering equation 5, this occurs when:

$$\log \frac{[A^-]}{[HA]} \text{ is } \pm 1 \text{ i.e. } \frac{\text{Base}}{\text{Acid}}$$

$$= \frac{10}{1} \text{ or } \frac{1}{10} \qquad \text{(equation 6)}$$

Buffer systems

The major body buffer systems involve bicarbonate, protein, haemoglobin and phosphate.

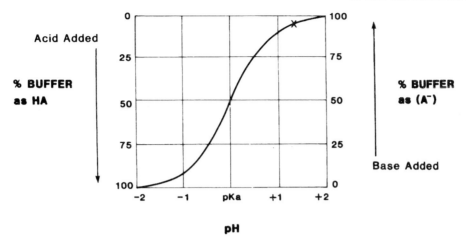

Fig. 80.1 Reaction curve for the buffer HA:(A⁻) where pH = pKa ± 2.

Bicarbonate–carbonic acid buffer pair

The arterial H⁺ ion activity can be represented by the Henderson equation:

$$[H^+] = 24 \times \frac{Paco_2}{[HCO_3^-]} \qquad \text{(equation 7)}$$

or the Henderson–Hasselbalch equation:

$$pH = 6.1 + \log \frac{[HCO_3^-]}{Paco_2 \times 0.03} \qquad \text{(equation 8)}$$

where 24 = the numerical value of the product of the solubility coefficient of CO_2 and the dissociation constant of carbonic acid; $Paco_2$ = arterial blood CO_2 partial pressure in mmHg; $[HCO_3^-]$ = arterial blood bicarbonate concentration in mmol/l; $[H^+]$ = arterial blood hydrogen ion concentration in nmol/l; 0.03 = solubility coefficient of carbon dioxide; 6.1 = negative logarithm of the dissociation constant of carbonic acid.

This system is quantitatively the most important ECF buffer, and functions better as a physiological (or open-system) buffer than chemical (or closed-system) buffer. Its pKa is 6.1, therefore its chemical buffering capacity at a pH of 7.4 (see position X in Fig. 80.1) is poor.

The benefit of an open compared to a closed buffer system can be demonstrated if one considers both systems subjected to a pH change of 0.3 units by the addition of acid. The normal equation:

$$7.4 = 6.1 + \log \frac{20}{1} \qquad \text{(equation 9)}$$

is changed by the acid addition to:

Closed system	Open system
$7.1 = 6.1 + \log \dfrac{19}{1.9}$	$7.1 = 6.1 + \log \dfrac{10}{1}$
	(equation 10)

In the open system, the denominator, in this case $Paco_2$, is kept constant. The buffer anion in the closed system falls from 20 to 19, whereas in the open system it falls from 20 to 10, thereby buffering more H⁺.

The bicarbonate – carbonic acid system also has the added advantage of further CO_2 change with respiratory compensation, reducing even further the pH defect. These responses are shown, in stages, in Figure 80.2.

The utility of this buffer system can be fully appreciated when it is realized that it is open-ended for both the numerator and the denominator. The $Paco_2$ can be modified by change in ventilation, and the HCO_3^- concentration can be regulated by renal mechanisms. All other body buffer systems adjust accordingly to alterations in this pair – an interrelationship which is known as the isohydric principle.

Haemoglobin, protein and phosphate buffers

Proteins have a series of titratable groups within their molecular structure, with the ability to buffer pH changes. The buffering characteristic of haemoglobin is almost entirely dependent upon the imidazole group of histidine, which dissociates less when haemoglobin is in the oxygenated compared to the

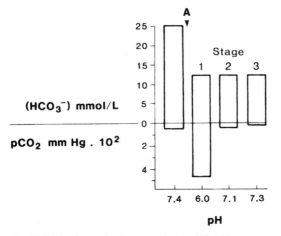

Fig. 80.2 Bicarbonate buffer system in blood if acid were added at A to reduce plasma HCO_3^- to 50%. The histograms show buffering at different stages 1–3.

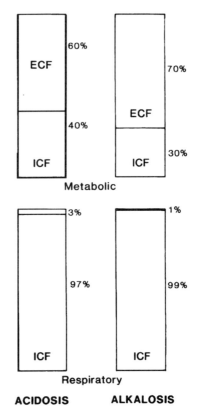

Fig. 80.3 Buffering contributions of the intracellular fluid (ICF) and extracellular fluid (ECF) with primary respiratory or metabolic acid–base changes.[16]

deoxygenated form. Thus, deoxygenated blood is a better buffer than oxygenated blood; the haemoglobin molecule accommodates 0.7 mmol of H^+ for each mmol of O_2 released, without change in pH. As the respiratory quotient is normally 0.8, a slight reduction in pH usually occurs when blood travels from the arterial to the venous system.

The haemoglobin buffer is an important one, since it is involved in handling the largest daily acid load of the body, i.e. carbonic acid. Gram for gram, plasma proteins have one-third the buffering capacity of haemoglobin. However, as haemoglobin has twice the concentration of plasma protein, it has six times the capacity to buffer H^+.

The phosphate buffer system has a pKa of 6.8 and so is a better chemical (or closed) buffer system than the bicarbonate buffer system. However, in plasma it has 1/20 the concentration, and also operates only as a closed system, so its capacity is far less than that of the bicarbonate–carbonic acid buffer. In the ICF and in urine, the phosphate buffer system assumes greater importance.

Total body buffering

The contributions of ICF and ECF buffers vary depending upon the nature of the acid or base disturbance. In dogs in which respiratory or metabolic acid–base defects were produced, the respiratory pH changes were buffered mainly by ICF buffers, whereas metabolic pH changes had a greater ECF buffering component[6-8] (Fig. 80.3). Preferential utilization of extracellular buffers occurs in the initial phase of a metabolic acidosis, with the contribution of ICF buffers becoming greater as the acidosis increases in severity.[9]

Experiments using rat diaphragm and human leukocytes reveal that conditions simulating respiratory acidosis or alkalosis produce a greater ICF pH change than do conditions simulating metabolic acidosis or alkalosis.[10-12] Furthermore, when metabolic acidosis or alkalosis is simulated and appropriate respiratory compensatory (CO_2) changes are also included, the ICF pH remains remarkably constant, suggesting a greater *in vivo* tolerance to metabolic pH change than there is to respiratory pH change[10,13,14]

Respiratory response

It is clear, when considering the Henderson equation (equation 2), that variations in $Paco_2$ alter the pH. The effect is rapid and influences both the ICF and ECF. Arterial $Paco_2$ varies inversely with alveolar ventilation, and directly with CO_2 production. Normal CO_2 production is 13 000 mmol/day; and if pulmonary ventilation ceased for 20 min, $Paco_2$ would rise to 110 mmHg (13.3 kPa) and pH would fall to 7.03. If renal function ceased for a similar period, no change in arterial pH would occur.

Regulation of ventilation involves a complex interplay between mechanical and chemical stimuli. Any change in arterial HCO_3^-, Pco_2, pH, Po_2 or stimuli from pulmonary mechanoreceptors alters ventilation and thus Pa_{CO_2} and pH. The respiratory response to a metabolic pH change follows peripheral chemoreceptor stimulation, and provides the compensatory response to metabolic pH change.

Renal response

This determines the final outcome to the acid or base load, by altering the denominator of the Henderson equation (i.e. $[HCO_3^-]$). The response is slow and the maximum excretory capacity of 300 mmol H^+ per day can only be reached after 7–10 days.[15]

Unlike all other ions, HCO_3^- has no permanence. It may be generated from CO_2 or lost with CO_2 excretion. The accompanying H^+ generated or lost is dealt with by the body's buffers. The kidney uses the bicarbonate ion for alkali reserve, and as an anion for sodium reabsorption or excretion when maintaining the ECF volume. The lungs use the bicarbonate ion for CO_2 transport and excretion.

Renal regulation of H^+ balance is due to reabsorption or excretion of filtered HCO_3^-, excretion of titratable acidity (TA), and excretion of ammonia. Tubular H^+ secretion usually involves Na^+ reabsorption, maintaining electrical neutrality.

Reabsorption of filtered HCO_3^-

About 85–90% of the filtered HCO_3^- is reclaimed by the proximal tubule. Further reabsorption occurs in the distal nephron, with the luminal fluid being free of HCO_3^- at a luminal pH of 6.2.[16] The amount of HCO_3^- reaching the distal nephron is influenced by the filtered load of HCO_3^- (thus, with a metabolic acidosis, the total proximal H^+ secretion is less than normal) and the functional ECF volume.[17] The mechanism of proximal tubular HCO_3^- reabsorption relies upon H^+ secretion. Cellular carbonic anhydrase (CA) supplies H^+ for the hydrogen pump, and the brush border CA facilitates the combination of HCO_3^- with H^+.

Formation of titratable acidity

The majority of the urinary TA is formed with the conversion of monohydrogen phosphate to dihydrogen phosphate, which occurs throughout the nephron.[16] The pKa of this system is 6.8, and at maximum urinary acidity (i.e. pH 4.5), almost all of the filtered phosphate is in the dihydrogen form. At this urinary pH, two-thirds of the filtered creatinine (pKa 4.97) and 95% of the uric acid (pKa 5.8) are in the acidic mode, and may account for 25% of the urinary TA at maximum urinary acidity. Normally, 20–30 mmol of H^+/day is excreted as TA, and this is proportional to the amount of buffer excreted, pKa of the buffer and pH of the urine. In diabetic ketoacidosis, the rate of excretion of betahydroxybutyrate (pKa

4.8) is large, and this compound forms the major component (up to 250 mmol H^+/day) of urinary TA. Normally, urinary excretion of phosphate is determined by the need to maintain phosphate balance rather than acid–base homeostasis. Thus TA appears to play a supportive, rather than an active, role in H^+ balance.

Formation of ammonia

Ammonia (NH_3) is formed in tubular epithelia throughout the nephron.[18] Deamidation and deamination of glutamine accounts for 60% of the urinary NH_3; 30–35% comes from free arterial NH_3. The NH_3 diffuses into the renal tubular lumen, where it binds a hydrogen ion to form a non-diffusible ammonium ion (NH_4^+) which is then excreted.[19] This process permits Na^+/H^+ exchange to occur without further change in urinary pH, although an acidic urine allows a greater sink into which free NH_3 can diffuse, and is thus one of the determinants of urinary NH_4^+ excretion. Renal tubular synthesis of NH_3 is coupled to renal gluconeogenesis, which in turn is attuned to the body's acid–base requirements. Systemic acidosis, hypokalaemia and mineralocorticoids increase ammonia production.[18] Normally, 30–50 mmol of H^+/day are excreted as NH_4^+, which may increase to 300 mmol/day in severe acidosis.

Mechanisms of proximal and distal H^+ secretions

Proximal H^+ secretions

This is a low gradient (minimal luminal pH achievable is 7.0), high capacity (its H^+ secretion is responsible for reabsorbing most of the filtered HCO_3^-, ie 4000–5000 mmol/day) system. The proximal H^+ secretion is increased with hypokalaemia, hypercarbia, increased luminal HCO_3^-, increased tubular Na^+ reabsorption, presence of non-reabsorbable anions, and increase in CA activity.

Distal H^+ secretion

This is a high-gradient (minimal luminal pH achievable is 4.5), low-capacity (H^+ secretion ranges from 0 to 300 mmol/day) system. Unlike the proximal tubule, the distal nephron is influenced by mineralocorticoid activity. In hyperaldosteronism, distal Na^+ reabsorption and excretion of H^+ and K^+ are enhanced. In the presence of hypokalaemia, H^+ loss is augmented due to electroneutrality requirements for some of the distal Na^+ reabsorbed. In secondary hyperaldosteronism, the K^+ and H^+ loss may be less than in primary hyperaldosterone states, due to a reduction in distal luminal flow induced by avid proximal Na^+ reabsorption. Thus an increase in distal H^+ or K^+ urinary secretion may only become evident when distal Na^+ delivery is increased, e.g. with the use of diuretics.

Clinical approach to acid-base disorders

Classification of an acid–base defect

The primary defect is usually defined by its initiating process, e.g. lactic, keto- or renal tubular acidosis. A broader classification, however, divides them into metabolic and respiratory, the latter relating to changes in carbonic acid (CO_2) only. Compensatory responses may be qualified as partial.[2] Thus, one speaks of:

1 chronic respiratory acidosis with partial renal compensation;
2 lactic acidosis with respiratory compensation;
3 metabolic alkalosis without respiratory compensation.

Biochemical description of an acid–base defect

Three values are necessary to describe an acid–base defect:

1 pH or [H^+] nmol/l (a measure of acidity or alkalinity);
2 Pa_{CO_2} mmHg or kPa (a measure of the respiratory component);
3 HCO_3^- mmol/l (a measure of the metabolic component).

While pH and Pa_{CO_2} may be measured directly, there is no direct method to measure HCO_3^- concentration. Also, HCO_3^- concentrations may vary with changes of P_{CO_2}. To separate the respiratory from the non-respiratory HCO_3^- components, derived indices of standard bicarbonate, base excess and buffer base have been proposed, although these *in vitro* values have the disadvantage of not accurately reflecting the *in vivo* situation.[20] For clinical purposes, however, in addition to the history and physical examination, the HCO_3^- concentration calculated from the Henderson equation, with the Pa_{CO_2} and pH, are all that is required to interpret the acid–base disorder fully.[20,21]

Diagnosis of an acid–base defect

Here one seeks to define the primary attack upon the H^+ homeostasis, and to assess the body's compensatory response. Biochemical data, including arterial blood-gas analysis, anion gap and renal and hepatic serum profiles, should all be taken into account. In mixed pH disorders, an acid–base diagram may be used as an aid to the diagnostic process. The diagram (Fig. 80.4) has the advantage of demonstrating the *in vivo* relationship between H^+ concentration and Pa_{CO_2} in primary acid–base disorders. The appropriate compensatory Pa_{CO_2} for the primary metabolic acid–base disorder, and the (H^+) or pH change associated with variation in primary acid–base dis-

orders, are represented by confidence bands for each disorder.[22]

In the absence of a diagram, various rules of thumb have been proposed to facilitate the bedside diagnosis.[5] For example:

1 A *primary metabolic acidosis* is associated with a respiratory compensatory decrease in Pa_{CO_2}, the numerical value (in mmHg) of which is usually within ± 5 mmHg (0.67 kPa) of the number denoted by the two digits after the decimal point of the pH value, down to a pH of 7.15–7.10. A *primary metabolic alkalosis* is associated with a similar Pa_{CO_2} change, increasing until the pH value reaches 7.55–7.60.
2 In a *primary respiratory acidosis* the calculated HCO_3^- value rises 1 mmol/l for each 10 mmHg (1.3 kPa) rise in Pa_{CO_2} up to a HCO_3^- value of 30 mmol/l.
3 In a *primary respiratory alkalosis* the calculated HCO_3^- decreases 2.5 mmol/l for each 10 mmHg (1.3 kPa) reduction in Pa_{CO_2} down to a HCO_3^- value of 18 mmol/l.
4 In *chronic respiratory acidosis*, renal compensation elevates the calculated HCO_3^- 4 mmol/l for each 10 mmHg (1.3 kPa) rise in Pa_{CO_2} up to a HCO_3^- value of 36 mmol/l.

Clinical acid–base disorders

Metabolic (non-respiratory) acidosis

This arises from an abnormal process generating excess non-carbonic acid, or abnormal loss of HCO_3^- (Table 80.2). Characteristically, arterial blood gas analysis reveals pH < 7.36 (H^+ > 44 nmol/l), Pa_{CO_2} < 35 mmHg (4.7 kPa), and calculated HCO_3^- < 18 mmol/l. An increased anion gap may also exist, reflecting the accumulation of unmeasured acid anions, the anion in question approximating the increased gap.[23]

Treatment of metabolic acidosis

Therapy in all acid–base disorders should initially focus upon treatment of the underlying disorder, e.g. insulin for diabetic ketoacidosis or measures to improve the cellular redox state in lactic acidosis. These measures terminate the production of (H^+) and allow metabolism of the organic acid present to return the pH towards normal. To maintain homeostasis of the intracellular pH while treatment takes effect, appropriate compensatory P_{CO_2} for the metabolic acidosis should be maintained. While bicarbonate replacement is commonly used for renal tubular acidosis and gastrointestinal bicarbonate loss, sodium bicarbonate administration is now no longer recommended as a routine for the metabolic acidosis associated with diabetes[24] or cardiac arrest,[25] as there is no evidence that it reduces mortality. Furthermore,

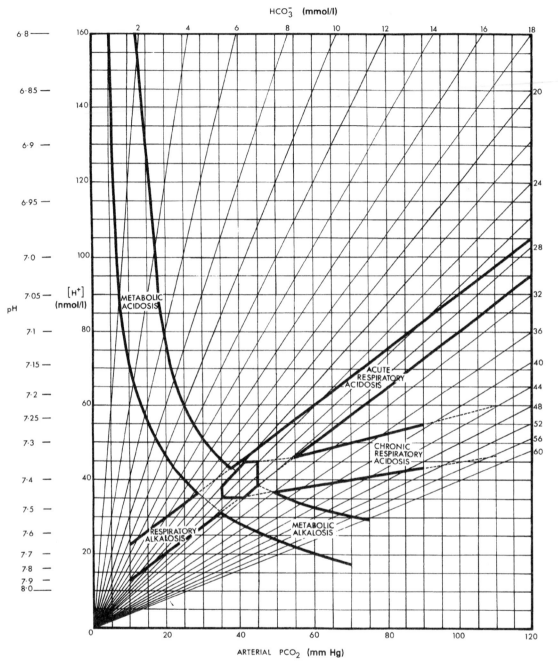

Fig. 80.4 Acid–base diagram.

excess generation of CO_2, hyperosmolality, hypocalcaemia and rebound alkalosis are possible hazards with its use. Small doses of 50–100 mmol $NaHCO_3$ IV are only used if hyperkalaemia is present. Other agents such as THAM or carbicarb (an equimolar mixture of Na_2CO_3 and $NaHCO_3$, which, during buffering, generates two-thirds of the amount of CO_2

in comparison to $NaHCO_3$) have not improved mortality in metabolic acidosis.[26,27]

Diabetic ketoacidosis

With fluid and electrolyte therapy to correct the fluid and electrolyte losses, and insulin therapy to correct

Table 80.2 Aetiology of metabolic acidosis

Disorder	Acid
Accumulation of acid (anion gap > 18 mmol/l)	
Ketoacidosis	β-Hydroxybutyrate, acetoacetate
Lactic acidosis	Lactate
Methanol	Formate, lactate
Renal failure	Sulphate, phosphate
Salicylic acid	Salicilate, lactate, ketoacids
Paraldehyde	Lactate, acetate, formate, pyruvate
Ethylene glycol	Oxalate
Intravenous fructose	Lactate
Sorbitol	Lactate
Ethanol	Lactate
Xylitol	Lactate
Accumulation of HCl (anion gap < 18 mmol/l)	
Releasing HCl with metabolism	
Arginine hydrochloride, lysine hydrochloride	
NH$_4$Cl	
Synthetic amino acid solutions	
Direct administration of HCl	
Intravenous HCl	
Loss of HCO$_3^-$ (anion gap < 18 mmol/l)	
Gastrointestinal loss	
Small bowel, biliary or pancreatic fistula	
Diarrhoea	
Ureteroenterostomy	
Cholestyramine	
Renal loss	
Renal tubular acidosis	
Carbonic anhydrase inhibition	

Table 80.3 Classification of lactic acidosis

Type A
Severe exercise
Cardiac arrest
Shock
Hypoxia < 35 mmHg (4.7 kPa)
Anaemia

Type B
Thiamine deficiency
Diabetes
Hepatic failure
Renal failure
Infection
Leukaemia, lymphoma
Pancreatitis
Short bowel syndrome (D-lactate)

Drug-induced
Phenformin, metformin, ethanol, methanol, salicylates
Intravenous fructose, xylitol or sorbitol

Hereditary
Glucose-6-phosphatase deficiency
Fructose-1,6-diphosphatase deficiency

the metabolic defect, specific therapy for the metabolic acidosis is not required.

Lactic acidosis

This is a metabolic acidosis due to excess production or reduced metabolism of lactic acid. It may be classified as either type A, where an inadequate delivery of oxygen for tissue requirements generates lactate faster than it can be removed, or type B, where overt tissue hypoxia does not appear to play a major role (Table 80.3). Nevertheless, both types share mechanisms of overproduction and underutilization. While arterial blood lactate levels are often used to assess the presence or absence of lactic acidosis, assessment of the cellular redox state by measuring blood lactate:pyruvate (L:P) ratios is of questionable value, since it assumes that the cytoplasmic redox state (measured by the L:P ratio) reflects the mitochondrial redox potential, which may not be so.[28] Moreover, the cytosolic and mitochondrial redox states may be reversed.[29]

Many forms of therapy for lactic acidosis have been tried, indicating a general dissatisfaction with any one form of treatment. NaHCO$_3$,[30] sodium acetate,[31] THAM,[30] insulin and glucose,[32] dichloroacetate,[33] haemo-and peritoneal dialysis, methylene blue, thiamine, pantothenic acid, biotin and nitroprusside[34] have all been tried. Animal studies suggest that in all disorders where lactic acidosis is present, cardiac dysfunction is commonly the fundamental problem. Thus, treatment should be aimed at correcting tissue perfusion. Oxygen delivery must be optimized, which often requires the use of a Swan–Ganz catheter to monitor cardiac output, left and right heart pressures and mixed venous oxygen tension. Anaemia and metabolic deficiencies of thiamine, pantothenic acid, biotin or magnesium should be corrected, and optimal hepatic and renal perfusion ensured, since the latter are the major sites of lactate metabolism. The traditional therapy of massive alkalinization is now no longer recommended.[35,36]

Renal tubular acidosis (RTA)

RTA is a disorder characterized by excess urinary loss of HCO$_3^-$, normal anion gap and an elevated serum level of Cl$^-$. It is classified into proximal or distal types[8] depending on the renal tubular site of the defect.

Distal RTA (classic RTA or type 1)
This arises from an inability of the distal nephron to generate and maintain a steep lumen-to-peritubular

H^+ gradient. With a standard acid load of 0.1 g NH_4Cl/kg body weight, the urine pH does not fall below 5.4. There is usually evidence of nephrocalcinosis, nephrolithiasis, hypokalaemia and osteomalacia, and therapy with alkaline solutions of potassium and sodium citrate is often required.

Proximal RTA (type 2)

This arises from a reduced proximal tubular capacity to secrete H^+ (required to reabsorb filtered HCO_3^-). Therefore, a reduced serum concentration of HCO_3^- is reached, at which normal urinary acidification occurs, reflecting normal distal acidification mechanisms. Usually, other proximal tubular defects also exist, i.e. amino aciduria, glycosuria and phosphaturia. Therapy with alkaline solutions is often not undertaken unless the acidosis is severe (i.e. HCO_3^- < 16 mmol/l).

Hyperkalaemic RTA (type 4)

Failure of the kidneys to liberate renin, failure of the adrenals to synthesize or excrete aldosterone, or failure of the distal nephron to respond to aldosterone can cause hyperkalaemic hyperchloraemic metabolic acidosis, due to failure of the distal Na^+/H^+ or Na^+/K^+ exchange mechanism. If there is a reduced distal delivery of sodium, distal H^+ excretion is likewise reduced. Therefore, to diagnose a distal Na^+/K^+ or Na^+/H^+ exchange defect, urinary sodium should be greater than 40 mmol/l.[37] Type 4 RTA may be caused by Addison's disease, urinary tract obstruction, diabetes, interstitial nephritis, spironolactone, triamterene, amiloride, non-steroidal anti-inflammatory drugs and cyclosporin.

Metabolic (non-respiratory) alkalosis

This condition arises from an abnormal process generating excess HCO_3^-, or an abnormal loss of non-carbonic acid. Characteristically, arterial blood-gas measurements reveal pH > 7.44 (H^+ < 36 mmol/l), $Paco_2$ > 45 mmHg (6.0 kPa), and HCO_3^- > 32 mmol/l. Normally, the kidney has a large capacity to excrete HCO_3^-; thus, once metabolic alkalosis is generated, maintenance of this state requires an abnormal retention of HCO_3^- (Table 80.4). The process of generating a metabolic alkalosis can be terminated if therapy is directed at the underlying disease. However, correction of the pH defect only occurs with renal excretion of the excess HCO_3^-, which often requires therapy to be directed at the abnormal renal HCO_3^- retention mechanisms. Renal maintenance of the metabolic alkalosis is usually effected by a proximal or a distal mechanism.[17]

Proximal mechanism

In the proximal tubule, there is an obligatory uptake of Na^+ controlled by the ECF volume. Normally, some of the Na^+ uptake occurs with H^+ secretion.

Table 80.4 Generation of metabolic alkalosis

Generation
Loss of H^+
  Renal
    Secondary hyperaldosteronism with K^+ depletion
    Conn's syndrome
    Cushing's syndrome
    Bartter's syndrome
    ACTH-secreting tumours
    Drugs – corticosteroids, carbenoxolone, diuretics, liquorice
    Post-hypercarbic alkalosis
  Gastrointestinal
    Nasogastric suction, vomiting
    Villous adenoma
    Congenital alkalosis with diarrhoea
Gain of HCO_3^-
    $NaHCO_3$ administration
    Metabolic conversion of organic acid anions, citrate, acetate, lactate

Maintenance
Diminished functional ECF volume
Mineralocorticoid excess with K^+ depletion
Severe K^+ depletion > 450 mmol/l
Chronic renal failure

ACTH = Adrenocorticotrophic hormone; ECF = extracellular fluid.

With diminished ECF volume, this Na^+/H^+ exchange mechanism is exaggerated, and hence, if a metabolic alkalosis exists, it will be maintained. Reversal of the pH defect, even in the presence of a mild hypokalaemia, can be achieved with saline infusions, but not with Na^+ solutions of a non-reabsorbable anion. Correction of the alkalosis can also occur with the administration of saline-free albumin solutions, suggesting that nephron recognition of a diminished ECF volume is the major determinant in the maintenance of the alkalosis (and not just a chloride deficiency). Although correction of a metabolic alkalosis may be achieved without the use of saline or potassium chloride solutions, it should not be interpreted as being desirable if saline or potassium chloride deficiencies exist. Moreover, correction of an existing hypokalaemia enhances the ability of saline solutions to correct metabolic alkalosis.[5]

Distal mechanism

Under the influence of mineralocorticoids, distal Na^+ reabsorption promotes K^+ and H^+ excretion. In the presence of hypokalaemia, H^+ excretion is augmented. In primary hyperaldosteronism, mechanisms to generate and maintain the metabolic alkalosis exist, although, to generate the alkalosis, hypokalaemia is also required. In secondary hyperaldosteronism, the

Table 80.5 Treatment of metabolic alkalosis

Indirect
Inhibition of renal mechanisms maintaining alkalosis
  Proximal
    Increased functional ECF–
      Saline infusions
      Blood, plasma or albumin infusions
      Inotropic agents
    Carbonic anhydrase inhibition –
      Acetazolamide
  Distal
    KCl
    Aldosterone inhibition (spironolactone)
    Triamterene, amiloride
Following metabolism to urea and HCl
  Arginine or lysine hydrochloride
  NH_4Cl

Direct
Intravenous HCl

ECF = Extracellular fluid.

excess proximal Na^+ reabsorption reduces distal nephron flow, and thus reduces K^+ and H^+ loss. Hence, while the metabolic alkalosis may be maintained, it is not generated unless there is concomitant use of diuretics, which increases the distal delivery of Na^+.

Treatment of metabolic alkalosis

Therapy should be directed at correcting both proximal and distal mechanisms (Table 80.5). In the presence of renal insufficiency, these manoeuvres may be insufficient, and treatment with NH_4Cl, arginine hydrochloride or lysine hydrochloride is often recommended. However, in the presence of hepatic failure, these agents are unable to be metabolized to HCl, and may produce hyperammonaemia. In such situations, administration of IV HCl (200 mmol in 1 l of 5% dextrose) through a central venous line at a maximum rate of 300–350 mmol/day may be used.[38]

Respiratory acidosis

This arises from an acute or chronic excess CO_2 and depends on the rate of production as well as excretion of CO_2. Therapy is aimed at improving ventilation. In chronic respiratory acidosis, there often coexists an iatrogenic metabolic alkalosis caused by corticosteroid or diuretic administration.

Respiratory alkalosis

This is caused by a reduction in CO_2 which often accompanies the increased ventilation associated with hypoxia, hysteria, hepatic failure, shock or sepsis. Therapy is directed at correcting the underlying abnormality causing the hyperventilation.

References

1. Relman AS (1972) Metabolic consequences of acid–base disorders. *Kidney* 1:347–359.
2. Anderson OS, Astrup P, Bates RG *et al.* (1966) Report of *ad hoc* committee on acid–base terminology. *Ann NY Acad Sci* 133:251–253.
3. Campbell EJM (1962) RlpH. *Lancet* i:681–683.
4. Henderson LJ (1908) The theory of neutrality regulation in the animal organism. *Am J Physiol* 21: 427–448.
5. Worthley LIG (1977) Hydrogen ion metabolism. *Anaesth Intens Care* 5:347–360.
6. Giebisch G, Berger L and Pitts RF (1955) The extrarenal response to acute acid base disturbances of respiratory origin. *J Clin Invest* 34:231–245.
7. Swan RC and Pitts RF (1955) Neutralization of infused acid by nephrectomized dogs. *J Clin Invest* 34:205–212.
8. Swan RC, Axelrod DR, Seip M and Pitts RF (1955) Distribution of sodium bicarbonate infused into nephrectomized dogs. *J Clin Invest* 34:1795–1801.
9. Schwartz WB, Orning KJ and Porter R (1957) The internal distribution of hydrogen ions with varying degrees of metabolic acidosis. *J Clin Invest* 36:373–382.
10. Adler S, Roy A and Relman AS (1965) Intracellular acid–base regulation. II: The interaction between CO_2 tension and the extracellular bicarbonate in the determination of muscle cell pH. *J Clin Invest* 44:21–29.
11. Relman AS (1966) The participation of cells in disturbances of acid–base balance. *Ann NY Acad Sci* 133:160–171.
12. Levin GE, Collinson P and Baron DN (1976) The intracellular pH of human leucocytes in response to acid–base changes *in vitro*. *Clin Sci* 50:293–299.
13. Schwartz WB, Brackett NC Jr and Cohen JJ (1965) The response of extracellular hydrogen ion concentration to graded degrees of chronic hypercapnia: the physiological limits of the defense of pH. *J Clin Invest* 44:291–302.
14. Adler S, Roy A and Relman AS (1965) Intracellular acid–base regulation, I The response of muscle cells to changes in CO_2 tension or extracellular bicarbonate concentration. *J Clin Invest* 44:8–20.
15. Sartorius OW, Roemmelt JC and Pitts RF (1949) The renal regulation of acid–base balance in man. The nature of renal compensations in ammonium chloride acidosis. *J Clin Invest* 28:423–439.
16. Pitts RF (1968) *Physiology of the Kidney and Body Fluids*, 2nd edn. Chicago: Year Book Medical Publishers.
17. Seldin DW and Rector FC (1972) The generation and maintenance of metabolic alkalosis. *Kidney Int* 1:306–321.
18. Toto RD (1986) Metabolic acid–base disorders. In: Kokko JP and Tannen RL (eds) *Fluids and Electrolytes*. Philadelphia: WB Saunders, pp. 229–304.

19. Pitts RF (1971) The role of ammonia production and excretion in regulation of acid base balance. *N Engl J Med* **284**:32–38.

20. Schwartz WB and Relman AS (1963) A critique of parameters used in the evaluation of acid–base disorders. *N Engl J Med* **268**:1382–1388.

21. Editorial (1974) Acids, bases and nomograms. *Lancet* **ii**:814–816.

22. Worthley LIG (1976) A diagram to facilitate the understanding and therapy of mixed acid base disorders. *Anaesth Intens Care* **4**:245–253.

23. Editorial (1977) The anion gap. *Lancet* **i**:785–786.

24. Morris LR, Murphy MB and Kitabchi AE (1986) Bicarbonate therapy in severe diabetic ketoacidosis. *Ann Intern Med* **105**:836–840.

25. Standards and Guidelines for Cardiopulmonary Resuscitation (CPR) and Emergency Medical Care (EMC) (1992) *J Am Med Assoc* **268**:2172–2288.

26. Blecic S, deBacker D, Deleuze M, Vachiery J-L and Vincent J-L (1988) Correction of metabolic acidosis in CPR: bicarbonate vs carbicarb. *Intens Care Med* **14** (suppl 1):269.

27. Bleich HL and Schwartz WB (1966) Tris buffer (THAM). *N Engl J Med* **274**:782–787.

28. Cohen RD and Simpson R (1975) Lactate metabolism. *Anesthesiology* **43**:661–673.

29. Williamson DH, Lund P and Krebs HA (1967) The redox state of free nicotinamide-adenine-dinucleotide in the cytoplasm and mitochondria of the liver. *Biochem J* **103**:514–527.

30. Woods HF (1971) Some aspects of lactic acidosis. *Br J Hosp Med* **6**:668–676.

31. Wain RA, Wiernik PH and Thompson WL (1973) Metabolic and therapeutic studies of a patient with acute leukemia and severe lactic acidosis of prolonged duration. *Am J Med* **55**:255–260.

32. Hems RA, Ross BP, Berry MN and Krebs HA (1966) Gluconeogenesis in the perfused rat liver. *Biochem J* **101**:284–292.

33. Alberti KGMM and Natrass M (1977) Lactic acidosis. *Lancet* **ii**:25–29.

34. Taradash MR and Jacobson LB (1975) Vasodilator therapy of idiopathic lactic acidosis. *N Engl J Med* **293**:468–471.

35. Graf H and Arieff AI (1986) The use of sodium bicarbonate in the therapy of organic acidosis. *Intensive Care Med* **12**:285–288.

36. Cooper DJ and Worthley LIG (1987) Adverse haemodynamic effects of sodium bicarbonate in metabolic acidosis. *Intensive Care Med* **13**:425–427.

37. Battle DC, von Riotte A and Schlueter W (1987) Urinary sodium in the evaluation of hyperchloremic metabolic acidosis. *N Engl J Med* **316**:140–144.

38. Worthley LIG (1977) The rational use of intravenous hydrochloric acid in the therapy of metabolic alkalosis. *Br J Anaesth* **49**:811–817.

Fluid and electrolyte therapy

LIG Worthley

Management of patients with fluid and electrolyte disorders requires an understanding of body fluid compartments and of water and electrolyte metabolism. These principles will be considered along with commonly encountered fluid and electrolyte disturbances.

Fluid compartments (Table 81.1, Fig. 81.1)

Total body water (TBW)

Water contributes to approximately 60% of body weight, with organs varying in water content (Table 81.2). Men normally have less body fat than women, and thus have a higher percentage of body weight as water. The average water content as a percentage of total body weight is 60% for males and 50% for females. TBW as a percentage of total body weight decreases with age, due to a progressive loss of muscle mass, causing bone and connective tissue to assume a greater percentage of total body weight[1-3] (Table 81.3).

TBW can be measured by techniques involving dilution of substances which are distributed throughout the TBW space. Antipyrine is one such substance which is easily measured and slowly metabolized and excreted. Alternatively, isotopes of water may be used. Deuterium oxide (D_2O) is non-radioactive and thus difficult to measure, whereas tritium (THO) is a weak β-emitter and can be easily measured. Equilibrium of a small dose takes 4–6 h and the results are predictable to within ± 2%.[3,4]

TBW is commonly divided into two volumes, the extracellular fluid (ECF) volume and the intracellular fluid (ICF) volume.[2] Sodium balance regulates ECF volume, whereas water balance regulates the ICF volume. Sodium excretion is normally regulated by various hormonal and physical ECF volume sensors, whereas water balance is normally regulated by hypothalamic osmolar sensors.[5]

Table 81.1 Body fluid compartments

Fluid compartment	Volume (ml/kg)	% Total body weight
Plasma volume	45	4.5
Blood volume	75	7.5
Interstitial volume	200	20
Extracellular fluid volume	250	25
Intracellular fluid volume	350	35
Total body fluid volume	600	60

Table 81.2 Water content of various tissues

Tissue	% Water content
Brain	84
Kidney	83
Skeletal muscle	76
Skin	72
Liver	68
Bone	22
Adipose tissue	10

Table 81.3 Water content as a percentage of total body weight

Age (years)	Males (%)	Females (%)
10–15	60	57
15–40	60	50
40–60	55	47
>60	50	45

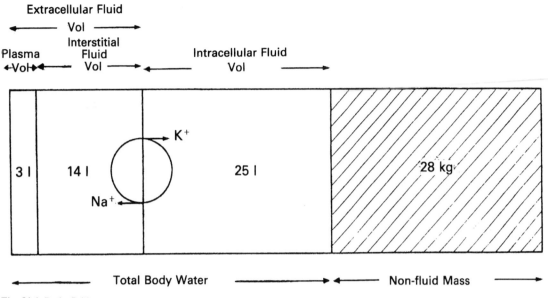

Fig. 81.1 Body fluid compartments.

Extracellular fluid

ECF is defined as all body water external to the cell, and is commonly subdivided into plasma and interstitial fluid volumes. The ECF is normally 40% of TBW and 25% of total body weight. With acute or chronic illness, ICF volume is reduced, and ECF volume is increased, and may even exceed the ICF volume. Measurement of ECF is performed using substances which diffuse throughout the ECF space without penetrating the cell.

Plasma volume

This may be measured using Evans blue, or radio-iodine-labelled albumin (^{131}I). However, as 7–10% of ^{131}I albumin escapes from the vascular compartment per hour, plasma volume may be overestimated using this method. To counter this effect, multiple readings may be taken and extrapolation to zero time can be performed.[6]

Red blood cell volume

This is part of the ICF volume, and can be calculated from plasma volume and haematocrit values. However, total blood haematocrit is about 85–92% of venous haematocrit, therefore estimations of red blood cell mass may be overestimated by about 5–7% using this method. Red blood cells tagged with chromium (^{51}Cr) will give a more accurate recording.[6]

Extracellular fluid volume

Depending upon the tracer used, values ranging from 15 to 27% of total body weight are described. The tracers used are either ionic (e.g. isotopes of bromide, chloride or sulphate) or non-ionic (e.g. insulin, mannitol and sucrose) substances. Non-ionic substances are large molecules, and often fail to distribute throughout the ECF in a reasonable time, whereas ionic substances distribute throughout the ECF compartment and also partly through the ICF compartment. Thus, ionic substances give larger measurements of ECF volume than non-ionic substances.

Bromide equilibrates in about 20–24 h, during which time 3–5% is lost in the urine. The latter can be measured and allowed for in the calculations, to give results with a variability of 2%. When reporting ECF volumes, the tracer used should be stated as well as the time taken to equilibrate, e.g. a '20-h bromide space'. Most ECF tracers show two decay curves. The first is a rapidly equilibrating pool of 20 min, delineating an ECF space which is in dynamic equilibrium with the plasma. This is about 20% of TBW or about 8–10 l in volume. The second is a slowly equilibrating ECF space (24 h), and includes the ECF of dense connective tissue and bone.

Electrical conductivity methods can be applied simply at the bedside, and have been used to measure the ratio of TBW and ECF volumes. If TBW is also measured, then the ECF volume can be derived. However, the accuracy of these methods, compared to conventional methods, particularly in patients with liver disease, has not been confirmed.[7]

Overall ECF volume, as a percentage of total body weight, shows little change with age. Therefore, most of the change in TBW due to age is from a decrease in ICF volume.

Interstitial space

This cannot be measured directly and is often calculated from the difference between the ECF volume and plasma volume.

Intracellular fluid

ICF is defined as all the body water within cells and, unlike the ECF compartment, is an inhomogeneous, multicompartmental entity, with different pH and ionic composition depending upon the organ or tissue being considered. The ICF volume is often determined by inference, from the difference in measurements of the TBW and ECF spaces. This estimation suffers from the inaccuracies inherent in both ECF and TBW measurements. In general, the ICF is considered to be 60% of TBW and 35% of total body weight.

Transcellular fluid

Fluids in this compartment have a common characteristic of being formed by transport activity of cells. The fluid is extracellular in nature and will be considered as part of the interstitial volume. It may vary from 1 to 10 l, the larger volumes occurring in diseased states (e.g. bowel obstruction or cirrhosis with ascites), and is formed at the expense of the remaining interstitial and plasma volumes.

Water metabolism

Water balance is maintained by altering the intake and excretion of water. Intake is controlled by thirst, whereas excretion is controlled by the renal action of antidiuretic hormone (ADH). In health, plasma osmolalities of about 280 mosmol/kg suppress plasma ADH to levels low enough to permit maximal urinary dilution.[8] Above this value, an increase in ECF tonicity of about 1–2% or a decrease in TBW of 1–2 l causes the posterior pituitary to release ADH, which acts upon the distal nephron to increase water reabsorption. Maximum plasma ADH levels are reached at an osmolality of 295 mosmol/kg.[8] The osmotic stimulation also changes thirst sensation, and in the conscious ambulant human, initiates water repletion (drinking), which is more important in preventing dehydration than ADH secretion and action. Thus, in health, the upper limit of the body osmolality (and therefore serum sodium) is determined by the osmotic threshold for thirst, whereas the lower limit is determined by the osmotic threshold for ADH release.[9]

Table 81.4 Drugs affecting antidiuretic hormone secretion

Stimulate	Inhibit
Nicotine	Ethanol
Narcotics	Narcotic antagonists
Vincristine	Dilantin
Barbiturates	
Cyclophosphamide	
Chlorpropamide	
Clofibrate	
Carbamazepine	
Amitryptylline	

Increase in osmolality caused by permeant solutes (e.g. urea) does not stimulate ADH release. ADH may also be released in response to hypovolaemia and hypotension, via stimulation of low- and high-pressure baroreceptors. The ADH release is extremely marked when more than 30% of intravascular volume is lost. ADH release may also be stimulated by pain and nausea, which are thought to act through the baroreceptor pathways.[5] ADH release may also be stimulated by a variety of pharmacological agents (Table 81.4). Renal response to ADH depends upon an intact, distal nephron and collecting duct and a hypertonic medullary interstitium. The capacity to conserve or excrete water also depends upon the osmolar load presented to the distal nephron.[5]

Water requirements

Water is needed to eliminate the daily solute load, and to replace daily insensible fluid loss (Table 81.5). With a normal daily excretion of 600 mosmol solute, maximal and minimal secretions of ADH will cause urine osmolality to vary from 1200 to 30 mosmol/kg respectively, and urine output to vary from 500 ml to 20 l/day respectively. Skin and lung water losses vary, and may range from 500 ml to 8 l/day, depending on physical activity, ambient temperature and humidity.

Table 81.5 Daily fluid balance (for a 70 kg man at rest in a temperate climate)

	Input (ml)			Output (ml)	
	Seen	Unseen		Seen	Unseen
Drink	1000		Urine	1000	
Food		650	Skin		500
Water of oxidation		350	Lungs		400
			Faeces		100
Total	1000	1000	Total	1000	1000

Disorders of osmolality

Tonicity

Osmolality is a measure of the number of osmoles per kilogram water. The osmolality of the ECF is due largely to sodium salts. Clinical effects of hyperosmolality, due to excess solute, depend upon whether the solute distributes evenly throughout the TBW (e.g. permeant solutes of alcohol or urea) or distributes in the ECF only (e.g. impermeant solutes of mannitol or glucose). With impermeant solutes, hyperosmolality is associated with a shift of fluid from the ICF to the ECF compartment.[10] Hyperosmolality due to increased impermeant solutes is known as hypertonicity. This condition may also be associated with a reduction in the serum sodium concentration (see below).

Water excess

In a 70 kg man, for every 1 l excess water, ECF increases by 400 ml and ICF increases by 600 ml, on average. The osmolality also decreases by 6–7 mosmol/kg, and the serum sodium falls by 3.0–3.5 mmol/l.

Water deficiency

In a 70 kg man, for every 1 l water loss, 600 ml is lost from the ICF and 400 from the ECF. The osmolality also increases by 7–8 mosmol/kg, and the serum sodium rises by 3.5–4.0 mmol/l.

Electrolytes

Chemical compounds in solution may either:

1 remain intact (i.e. undissociated), in which case they are called non-electrolytes (e.g. glucose or urea); or

2 dissociate to form ions, in which case they are called electrolytes. Ions carry an electrical charge, e.g. Na^+, Cl^-. Ions with a positive charge are attracted to a negative electrode or cathode, and hence are called cations. Conversely, ions with a negative charge travel towards a positive electrode or anode and are called anions. Each body water compartment contains electrolytes with different composition and concentration (Table 81.6).

Sodium

Sodium is the principal cation of the ECF and accounts for 86% of ECF osmolality. In a 70 kg man, total body sodium content is 4000 mmol (58 mmol/kg), 70% of which is exchangeable (i.e. exchanges with isotopic tracer sodium within 24 h). The majority of the exchangeable sodium (85%) resides in the ECF compartment; the remainder resides in the ICF compartment and the exchangeable bone compartment[11] (Table 81.7). Non-exchangeable sodium resides in bone[12] (Table 81.7). ECF concentration of sodium varies between 134 and 146 mmol/l. The intracellular sodium concentration varies between different tissues, and ranges from 3 to 20 mmol/l.

Table 81.7 Sodium compartments (in a 70 kg man)

	Total (mmol)	mmol/kg
Total body sodium	4000	58
Non-exchangeable bone sodium	1200	17
Exchangeable sodium	2800	40
Intracellular sodium	250	3
Extracellular sodium	2400	35
Exchangeable bone sodium	150	2

The standard western society dietary sodium intake is about 150 mmol/day, but the daily intake varies widely, with urinary losses ranging from <1 to >240 mmol/day.[13] Sodium balance is influenced by renal hormonal and ECF physical characteristics. The complete renal adjustment to an altered sodium load usually requires 3–4 days before balance is restored.

Hyponatraemia

Hyponatraemia is defined as a serum sodium less than 135 mmol/l and may be classified as isotonic, hypertonic or hypotonic, depending upon the measured serum osmolality (Table 81.8).

Table 81.6 Electrolyte composition of body fluid compartments

Electrolyte	ICF (mmol/l)	ECF (mmol/l)	
		Plasma	Interstitial
Sodium	10	140	145
Potassium	155	3.7	3.8
Chloride	3	102	115
Bicarbonate	10	28	30
Calcium (ionized)	< 0.01	1.2	1.2
Magnesium	10	0.8	0.8
Phosphate	105	1.1	1.0

Table 81.8 Common causes of hyponatraemia

Misleading result
Isotonic
  Hyperlipidaemia
  Hyperprotinaemia
Hypertonic
  Hyperglycaemia
  Mannitol, glycerol, glycine or sorbitol excess

Water retention
Renal failure
Hepatic failure
Cardiac failure
Syndrome of inappropriate antidiuretic hormone secretion
Drugs
Psychogenic polydipsia

Water retention and salt depletion
Postoperative, post trauma or excess fluid losses
  inappropriately replaced
Adrenocortical failure
Diuretic excess

Isotonic hyponatraemia

Plasma normally contains 93% water and 7% solids (5.5% proteins, 1% salts and 0.5% lipids). If the solid phase is increased significantly (e.g. in hyperlipidaemia or hyperprotinaemia), any device which dilutes a specific amount of plasma for analysis will give falsely lower values for all measured compounds. This effect produces factitious hyponatraemia and is associated with a normal measured serum osmolality.[14] Measurement of plasma sodium by an ion-selective electrode is not affected by the volume of plasma solids, and therefore pseudohyponatraemia will not occur with this method.[14]

Hypertonic hyponatraemia

In patients who have hypertonicity due to increased amounts of impermeant solutes (e.g. glucose, mannitol, glycerol or sorbitol), a shift of water from the ICF to the ECF occurs to provide osmotic equilibration, thus diluting the ECF sodium. Such resultant hyponatraemia is often associated with an increased measured osmolality. For example, in the presence of hyperglycaemia, for every 3 mmol/l rise in glucose, the serum sodium decreases by 1 mmol/l.[15]

Hypotonic hyponatraemia

Hyponatraemia is almost always caused by an excess of TBW, due to excessive hypotonic or water-generating IV fluids (e.g. 1.5% glycine, 0.45% saline or 5% dextrose) or excessive ingestion of water, particularly in the presence of high circulating ADH levels. It may rarely be caused by loss of exchangeable sodium or potassium.[16] In the latter circumstances, a loss of approximately 40 mmol sodium or potassium, without a change in TBW content, is required to lower the serum sodium by 1 mmol/l. As hyponatraemia may be associated with an alteration in both TBW and total body sodium, the ECF may be increased (hypervolaemia), decreased (hypovolaemia) or exhibit no change (isovolaemia).[8]

In health, a fluid intake up to 15–20 l may be tolerated before water is retained and hyponatraemia occurs. In psychogenic polydipsia, if water intake exceeds the renal capacity to form dilute urine, water retention and hyponatraemia will occur. With this disorder, plasma osmolality exceeds urine osmolality. In circumstances where ADH is increased (e.g. hypovolaemia, hypotension, pain or nausea), or where renal response to ADH is altered (i.e. in renal, hepatic, pituitary, adrenal or thyroid failure), water retention occurs with lower intakes of fluid.

Syndrome of inappropriate ADH secretion (SIADH)

This syndrome is a form of hyponatraemia in which there is an increased level of ADH inappropriate to any osmotic or volume stimuli that normally affect ADH secretion.[17,18] Diagnostic criteria and possible causes are listed in Table 81.9 and Table 81.10 respectively.

Clinical features

While cerebral manifestations are usually absent when the sodium concentration exceeds 125 mmol/l, progressive symptomatology of headache, nausea, confusion, disorientation, coma and seizures is often observed when plasma sodium falls below 120 mmol/l.[19]

Table 81.9 Criteria to diagnose syndrome of inappropriate antidiuretic hormone (SIADH)

Hypotonic hyponatraemia
Urine osmolality greater than plasma osmolality
Urine sodium excretion greater than 20 mmol/l
Normal renal, hepatic, cardiac, pituitary, adrenal and thyroid
  function
Absence of hypotension, hypovolaemia, oedema and drugs
  affecting antidiuretic hormone secretion
Correction by water restriction

Table 81.10 Aetiologies of syndrome of inappropriate antidiuretic hormone (SIADH)

Ectopic ADH production by tumours
Small-cell bronchogenic carcinoma
Adenocarcinoma of the pancreas or duodenum
Leukaemia
Lymphoma
Thymoma

Central nervous system disorders
Cerebral trauma
Brain tumour (primary or secondary)
Meningitis or encephalitis
Brain abscess
Subarachnoid haemorrhage
Acute intermittent porphyria
Guillain–Barré syndrome
Systemic lupus erythematosus

Pulmonary diseases
Viral, fungal and bacterial pneumonias
Tuberculosis
Lung abscess

Table 81.11 Causes of hypernatraemia

WATER DEPLETION
Extrarenal loss
Exposure
Gastrointestinal tract losses (often with excess saline replacement)

Renal loss
Osmotic diuresis – urea, mannitol, glycosuria
Diabetes insipidus
  Neurogenic
    Posttraumatic, fat embolism
    Metastatic tumours, craniopharyngioma, pinealoma, cysts
    Meningitis, encephalitis
    Granulomas (tuberculosis, sarcoid)
    Guillain–Barré syndrome
    Idiopathic
  Nephrogenic
    Congenital
    Hypercalcaemia, hypokalaemia
    Lithium
    Pyelonephritis
    Medullary sponge kidney
    Polycystic kidney
    Postobstructive uropathy
    Multiple myeloma, amyloid, sarcoid

SALT GAIN
Hypertonic, saline or sodium bicarbonate

Treatment

Treatment depends on clinical manifestations, which may also relate to the speed of onset of hyponatraemia. If the patient is asymptomatic and hyponatraemia has been present for many weeks, simple fluid restriction and reversal of any precipitating factor may be all that is required. In hyponatraemia of rapid onset, particularly if associated with cerebral symptoms, treatment consists of IV hypertonic saline (50–70 mmol/h) to increase the serum sodium by 2 mmol/l per h, until a concentration of 130 mmol/l is attained.[20] If seizures are present, rapid treatment of cerebral oedema is required. While mannitol 500 ml of 20% IV may be used, 250 mmol of sodium chloride IV over 10 min provides the same osmotic effect, and has the advantage of simultaneously increasing the serum sodium (usually by about 7 mmol/l).[21] Normally, with symptomatic hyponatraemia (serum sodium less than 120 mmol/l), the patient has both water excess (approximately 6–8 l) and sodium deficiency (200–400 mmol).

Complications reported with hypertonic saline therapy include congestive cardiac failure and central pontine and extrapontine myelinolysis (osmotic demyelination syndrome).[22] Monitoring of central venous pressure or pulmonary capillary wedge pressure throughout saline administration is required. If a spontaneous diuresis has not occurred with the administration of saline, a diuretic may be required. There is still no uniform agreement that osmotic demyelination is produced by a rapid correction of hyponatraemia.[23,24] Nevertheless, serum sodium should be increased up to only 130 mmol/l, and maintained at this level for the next 24–48 h.

Hypernatraemia

Hypernatraemia is defined as a serum sodium greater than 145 mmol/L (Table 81.11). It is always associated with hyperosmolality and may be caused by:

1 excessive administration of sodium salts (bicarbonate or chloride);
2 water depletion;
3 excess sodium and loss of water.

Excessive administration of sodium salts is rare, and usually results from a therapeutic misadventure. Pure water depletion is uncommon, unless water restriction is applied to a patient who is unconscious or unable to ingest water, as the thirst response normally corrects water depletion. The serum sodium level rises, and is associated with a loss of volume in both ECF and ICF.

Clinical features

Hypernatraemia usually produces symptoms if the serum sodium exceeds 155–160 mmol/l (i.e. osmolality >330 mosmol/kg). Clinical features include pyrexia, restlessness, irritability, drowsiness, lethargy, confusion and coma.[25] Convulsions are uncommon. The diminished ECF volume may reduce cardiac output, thereby reducing renal perfusion and leads to prerenal failure.

Treatment

Treatment of pure water depletion consists of water administration. If IV fluid is required, 5% dextrose or hypotonic saline solutions (0.45% saline) are often used, as sterile water infusion causes haemolysis. In rare cases, IV sterile water may be used, by administering through a central venous catheter.[26] Since rapid rehydration may give rise to cerebral oedema, the change in serum sodium should be no greater than 2 mmol/l per h.[20]

Potassium

Potassium is the principal intracellular cation and accordingly (along with its anion) fulfils the role of the ICF osmotic provider. It also plays a major role in the functioning of excitable tissues (e.g. muscle and nerve). As the cell membrane is 20 times more permeable to potassium than sodium ions, potassium is largely responsible for the resting membrane potential. Potassium also influences carbohydrate metabolism and glycogen and protein synthesis.

Total body potassium is 45–50 mmol/kg in the male (3500 mmol/70 kg) and 35–40 mmol/kg (2500 mmol/65 kg) in the female; 95% of the total body potassium is exchangeable. The ECF potassium ranges from 3.1 to 4.2 mmol/l, thus the total ECF potassium ranges from 55 to 70 mmol. About 90% of the total body potassium is intracellular; 8% resides in bone, 2% in ECF water and 70% in skeletal muscle.[27,28] With increasing age (and decreasing muscle mass), total body potassium decreases.

The daily intake of potassium in a standard western society diet varies from 40 to 150 mmol, and the urinary loss varies from 30 to 150 mmol/l.[13,28,29] In certain cultures, potassium ingestion may be as low as 25 mmol, or as high as 500 mmol/day.

Factors affecting potassium metabolism

The potassium content of cells is regulated by a cell-wall pump-leak mechanism. Cellular uptake is by the Na^+/K^+ pump which is driven by Na^+/K^+-ATPase. Movement of potassium out of the cell is governed by passive forces (i.e. cell membrane permeability and chemical and electrical gradients to the potassium ion).

Acidosis promotes a shift of potassium from the ICF to the ECF, whereas alkalosis promotes the reverse shift. Hyperkalaemia stimulates insulin release, which promotes a shift of potassium from the ECF to the ICF, an effect independent of the movement of glucose.[28] β_2-Adrenergic agonists promote cellular uptake of potassium by a cyclic adenosine monophosphate-dependent activation of the Na^+/K^+ pump, whereas α-adrenergic agonists cause a shift of potassium from the ICF to the ECF.[30] Aldosterone increases renal excretion of potassium, but whether it also causes a general transcellular shift of potassium is not clear. Glucocorticoids are also kaluretic – an effect which may be independent of the mineralocorticoid receptor.

Normally, mechanisms to reduce the ECF potassium concentration (by increasing renal excretion and shifting potassium from the ECF to the ICF) are very effective. However, mechanisms to retain potassium in the presence of potassium depletion are less efficient, particularly when compared to those of sodium conservation. Even with severe potassium depletion, urinary loss of potassium continues at a rate of 10–20 mmol/day. Metabolic alkalosis also enhances renal potassium loss, by encouraging distal nephron Na^+/K^+, rather than Na^+/H^+ exchange.

Hypokalaemia

Hypokalaemia is defined as a serum potassium of less than 3.5 mmol/l (or plasma potassium less than 3.0 mmol/l). It may be due to decreased oral intake, increased renal or gastrointestinal loss, or movement of potassium from the ECF to the ICF (Table 81.12).

Clinical features

Clinical features include weakness, hypotonicity, depression, constipation, ileus, ventilatory failure, ventricular tachycardias (characteristically torsade de pointes), atrial tachycardias, and even coma.[31] With prolonged and severe potassium deficiency, rhabdomyolysis and thirst and polyuria (due to the development of renal diabetes insipidus) may occur. The ECG changes are relatively non-specific, and include prolongation of the PR interval, T-wave inversion and prominent U waves.

Treatment

Treatment with IV or oral potassium chloride will correct hypokalaemia, particularly if it is associated with metabolic alkalosis. If the patient has renal tubular acidosis and hypokalaemia, potassium acetate or citrate is required. Intravenous administration of potassium should normally not exceed 40 mmol/h, and plasma potassium should be monitored at 1–4-hourly intervals.[27,28] In patients with acute

Table 81.12 Causes of hypokalaemia

Inadequate dietary intake (urine K^+ < 20 mmol/l)

Abnormal body losses

Gastrointestinal (urine K^+ < 20 mmol/l)
    Vomiting, nasogastric aspiration
    Diarrhoea, fistula loss
    Villous adenoma of the colon
    Laxative abuse

Renal (urine K^+ < 20 mmol/l)
    Conn's syndrome
    Cushing's syndrome
    Bartter's syndrome
    Ectopic ACTH syndrome
      Small cell carcinoma of the lung
      Pancreatic carcinoma
      Carcinoma of the thymus
    Drugs
      Diuretics
      Corticosteroids
      Carbenicillin, amphotericin B, gentamicin
      Cisplatin
    Renal tubular acidosis
    Magnesium deficiency

Compartmental shift

Alkalosis
Insulin
Na^+/K^+-ATPase stimulation
    Sympathomimetic agents with β_2 effect
    Methylxanthines
Barium poisoning
Hypothermia
Toluene intoxication
Hypokalaemic periodic paralysis

ACTH = Adrenocorticotrophic hormone.

Table 81.13 Causes of hyperkalaemia

Collection abnormalities

Delay in separating red blood cells
Specimen haemolysis
Thrombocythaemia

Excessive intake

Exogenous (i.e. intravenous or oral potassium chloride
    massive blood transfusion)
Endogenous (i.e. tissue damage)
    Burns, trauma
    Rhabdomyolysis
    Tumour lysis

Decrease in renal excretion

Drugs
    Spironolactone, triamterine, amiloride
    Indomethacin
    Captopril, enalapril
Renal failure
Addison's disease
Hyporeninaemic hypoaldosteronism

Compartmental shift

Acidosis
Insulin deficiency
Digoxin overdosage
Succinylcholine
Arginine hydrochloride
Hyperkalaemic periodic paralysis
Fluoride poisoning

myocardial infarction and hypokalaemia, IV potassium is recommended at a rate of 10 mmol/30 min (in 50–100 ml 5% dextrose), and repeated as necessary until serum potassium is 4.0–4.5 mmol/l (or plasma potassium is 3.5–4.0 mmol/l).[32] The potassium concentration should be measured hourly during potassium replacement.

Hyperkalaemia

Hyperkalaemia is defined as a serum potassium greater than 5.0 mmol/l or plasma potassium greater than 4.5 mmol/l. It may be artifactual (from sampling errors), or may be due to excessive intake, severe tissue damage, decreased excretion or body fluid compartment shift (Table 81.13).

Clinical features

Clinical features include tingling, paraesthesia, weakness, flaccid paralysis, hypotension and bradycardia.

The characteristic ECG effects include peaking of the T waves, flattening of the P wave, prolongation of the PR interval (until sinus arrest with nodal rhythm occurs), widening of the QRS complex and the development of a deep S wave. Finally, a sine-wave ECG pattern develops which deteriorates to asystole, which may occur at serum potassium levels of 7 mmol/l or greater.

Treatment

Treatment is directed at the underlying cause, and may include dialysis. Rapid management of life-threatening hyperkalaemia may be achieved by:

1. IV dextrose, 50 g with 20 U of soluble insulin;
2. IV sodium bicarbonate, 50–100 mmol;
3. IV calcium chloride 5–10 ml of 10% (3.4–6.8 mmol, which is used to reduce the cardiac effects of hyperkalaemia);
4. Oral and rectal Resonium A 50 g.

Calcium

Almost all (99%) of the body calcium (30 mol or 1100 g or 1.5% body weight) is present in the bone. A small but significant quantity of ionized calcium exists in the ECF, and is important for many cellular activities, including secretion, neuromuscular impulse formation, contractile functions and clotting. Normal daily intake of calcium is 15–20 mmol, although only 40% is absorbed. The average daily urinary loss is 2.5–7.5 mmol. The total ECF calcium of 40 mmol (2.20–2.55 mmol/l) exists in three forms. Forty per cent (1.0 mmol/l) is bound to protein (largely albumin), 47% is ionized (1.15 mmol/l), and 13% is complexed (0.3 mmol/l) with citrate, sulphate and phosphate. The ionized form is the physiologically important form, and may be acutely reduced in alkalosis by causing a greater amount of the serum calcium to be bound to protein.[33,34] While the serum ionized calcium can be measured, total serum calcium is usually measured, which can vary with the serum albumin levels. A correction factor can be used to offset the effect of serum albumin on serum calcium. This is 0.02 mmol/l for every 1 g/l increase in serum albumin (up to a value of 40 g/l), added to the measured calcium level. For example, if measured serum calcium is 1.82 mmol/l, and serum albumin 25 g/l, corrected serum calcium = 1.82 + [(40–25) × 0.02] mmol/l = 2.12 mmol/l.

Clinical features of a reduced serum ionized calcium include tetany, cramps, mental changes and decrease in cardiac output. The clinical features of hypercalcaemia, on the other hand, include nausea, vomiting, pancreatitis, polyuria, polydipsia, muscular weakness, mental disturbance and ectopic calcification (see Chapter 54).

Magnesium

Magnesium is primarily an intracellular ion which acts as a metallocoenzyme in numerous phosphate transfer reactions. It thus has a critical role in the transfer, storage and utilization of energy.

In humans, the total body magnesium content is 1000 mmol, and the plasma concentrations range from 0.70 to 0.95 mmol/l. The daily oral intake is 8–20 mmol (40% of which is absorbed) and the urinary loss, which is the major source of excretion of magnesium, varies from 2.5 to 8 mmol/day.[33,35]

Hypomagnesaemia

Hypomagnesaemia is caused by decreased intake or increased loss (Table 81.14). Clinical features include neurological signs of confusion, irritability, delirium tremors, convulsions and tachyarrhythmias. Hypomagnesaemia is often associated with resistant hypokalaemia and hypocalcaemia. Treatment consists of IV magnesium sulphate as a bolus of 10 mmol,

Table 81.14 Causes of magnesium deficiency

Gastrointestinal disorders
Malabsorption syndromes
Gastrointestinal tract fistulas
Short-bowel syndrome
Prolonged nasogastric suction
Diarrhoea
Pancreatitis
Parenteral nutrition

Alcoholism

Endocrine disorders
Hyperparathyroidism
Hyperthyroidism
Conn's syndrome
Diabetes mellitus
Hyperaldosteronism

Renal diseases
Renal tubular acidosis
Diuretic phase of acute tubular necrosis

Drugs
Aminoglycosides
Carbenicillin, ticarcillin
Amphotericin B
Diuretic therapy
Cis-platinum
Cyclosporin

administered over 5 min, followed by 20–60 mmol/day.

Hypermagnesaemia

Hypermagnesaemia is often caused by excessive administration of magnesium salts or conventional doses of magnesium in the presence of renal failure. Clinical features include drowsiness, hyporeflexia and coma. Cardiovascular effects of vasodilatation and hypotension and conduction defects of sinoatrial and atrioventricular nodal block and asystole may occur. Treatment is directed towards increasing excretion of the ion, which may require dialysis. Intravenous calcium chloride may be used for rapidly treating the cardiac conduction defects.[35]

Phosphate

While most of the body phosphate exists in bone, 15% is found in the soft tissues as adenosine triphosphate, red blood cell 2,3-diphosphoglycerate and other cellular structural proteins, including phospholipids, nucleic acids and phosphoproteins. Phosphate also acts as a cellular and urinary buffer.[33,36]

Table 81.15 Causes of hypophosphataemia

Hyperparathyroidism
Vitamin D deficiency
Vitamin D-resistant rickets
Renal tubular acidosis
Alkalosis
Parenteral nutrition
Alcoholism

Table 81.16 Causes of hyperphosphataemia

Rhabdomyolysis
Renal failure (acute or chronic)
Vitamin D toxicity
Acidosis
Tumour lysis
Hypoparathyroidism
Pseudohypoparathyroidism
Diphosphonate therapy
Excess intravenous administration

Table 81.17 Daily volume and electrolyte composition of gastrointestinal tract secretions

	Volume (l)	*Electrolytes* (mmol/l)				
		H+	*Na+*	*K+*	*Cl−*	*HCO₃*
Saliva	0.5–1.0	0	30	20	10–35	0–15
Stomach	1.0–2.5	0–120	60	10	100–120	0
Bile	0.5	0	140	5–10	100	40–70
Pancreatic	0.75	0	140	5–10	70	40–70
Small and large gut	2.0–4.0	0	110	5–10	100	25

Hypophosphataemia

Hypophosphataemia may be caused by a decreased intake, increased excretion or intracellular redistribution (Table 81.15). While hypophosphataemia may be symptom-free, clinical features have been described, which include paraesthesiae, muscle weakness, seizures, coma, rhabdomyolysis and cardiac failure. Treatment consists of oral or IV sodium or potassium phosphate, 50–100 mmol/24 h.

Hyperphosphataemia

Hyperphosphataemia is usually caused by an increased intake or decreased excretion (Table 81.16). Clinical features include ectopic calcification of nephrocalcinosis, nephrolithiasis and band keratopathy. Treatment may require haemodialysis; otherwise oral aluminium hydroxide and even hypertonic dextrose solutions to shift ECF phosphate into the ICF can be used.

Replacement therapy

Gastrointestinal losses

The daily volumes and composition of gastrointestinal secretions in mmol/l are shown in Table 81.17. Clinical effects of fluid loss from the gastrointestinal tract are largely determined by the volume and composition of the fluid, and therapy is usually directed at replacing the losses. Gastric fluid loss (e.g. from vomiting and nasogastric suction) results in water, sodium, hydrogen ion, potassium and chloride depletion. Hence, metabolic alkalosis, hypokalaemia, hypotension and dehydration develop if the saline and potassium chloride losses are not correctly replaced.

Pancreatic and biliary fluid losses

Pancreatic and biliary fluid losses (e.g. pancreatic or biliary fistula) may result in hyperchloraemic acidosis with hypokalaemia, hypotension and dehydration if the losses of bicarbonate, potassium and saline are not correctly replaced.

Intestinal losses

Intestinal losses (e.g. fistula or ileostomy losses, diarrhoea and ileus) result in hypokalaemia, hypotension and dehydration if the saline and potassium losses are not replaced.

References

1. Edelman I and Leibman J (1959) Anatomy of body water and electrolytes. *Am J Med* **27**:256–277.
2. Gamble J (1954) *Chemical Anatomy, Physiology and Pathology of Extracellular Fluid*. Cambridge, MA: Harvard University Press.

3. Moore FD, Olesen KH, McMurrey JD, Parker HV, Ball MR and Boyden CM (1963) *Body Composition in Health and Disease*. Philadelphia: WB Saunders.

4. Streat SJ, Beddoe AH and Hill GL (1985) Measurement of total body water in intensive care patients with fliud overload. *Metabolism* **34**:688–694.

5. Bie P (1980) Osmoreceptors, vasopressin and control of renal water excretion. *Physiol Rev* **60**:961–1048.

6. Pain RW (1977) Body fluid compartments. *Intensive Care Med* **5**:284–294.

7. Holt TL, Cui C, Thomas BJ *et al.* (1994) Clinical applicability of bioelectric impedance to measure body composition in health and disease. *Nutrition* **10**:221–224.

8. Humes HD (1986) Disorders of water metabolism. In: Kokko JP and Tannen RL (eds) *Fluid and Electrolytes*. Philadelphia: WB Saunders Co, pp. 118–149.

9. Phillips PJ (1977) Water metabolism. *Anaesth Intens Care* **5**:295–304.

10. Gennari FJ (1984) Serum osmolality. Uses and limitations. *N Engl J Med* **310**:102–105.

11. McKeown JW (1986) Disorders of total body sodium. In: Kokko JP and Tannen RL (eds) *Fluid and Electrolytes*. Philadelphia: WB Saunders, pp. 63–117.

12. Cohn SH, Abesamis C, Zanzi J, Aloia JF, Yasumura S and Ellis KJ (1977) Body elemental composition: comparison between black and white adults. *Am J Physiol* **232**:419–422.

13. Intersalt Cooperative Research Group (1988) Intersalt: an international study of electrolyte excretion and blood pressure. Results for 24 hour urinary sodium and potassium excretion. *Br Med J* **297**:319–328.

14. Weisberg LS (1989) Pseudohyponatremia: a reappraisal. *Am J Med* **86**:315–318.

15. Katz MA (1973) Hyperglycemia-induced hyponatremia – calculation of expected serum sodium depression. *N Engl J Med* **289**:843–844.

16. Fuisz RE (1963) Hyponatremia. *Medicine* **42**:149–168.

17. Robinson AG (1985) Disorders of antidiuretic hormone secretion. *Clin Endocrinol Metab* **14**:55–88.

18. Bartter FC and Schwartz WB (1967) The syndrome of inappropriate secretion of antidiuretic hormone. *Am J Med* **42**:790–806.

19. Arieff AI (1984) Central nervous system manifestations of disordered sodium metabolism. *Clin Endocrinol Metab* **13**:269–294.

20. Arieff AI and Guisado R (1976) Effects of the central nervous system of hypernatremic and hyponatremic states. *Kidney Int* **10**:104–116.

21. Worthley LIG and Thomas PD (1986) Treatment of hyponatraemic seizures with intravenous 29.2% saline. *Br Med J* **292**:168–170.

22. Sterns RH, Riggs JE and Schochet SS Jr (1986) Osmotic demyelination syndrome following correction of hyponatraemia. *N Engl J Med* **314**:1535–1542.

23. Ayus JC, Krothapalli RK and Arieff AI (1985) Changing concepts in treatment of severe symptomatic hyponatremia. Rapid correction and possible relation to central pontine myelinolysis. *Am J Med* **78**:897–902.

24. Tien R, Arieff AI, Kucharczyk W, Wasik A and Kucharczyk J (1992) Hyponatremic encephalopathy: is central pontine myelinolysis a component? *Am J Med* **92**:513–522.

25. Ross EJ and Christie SBM (1969) Hypernatremia. *Medicine* **48**:441–472.

26. Worthley LIG (1986) Hyperosmolar coma treated with intravenous sterile water. A study of three cases. *Arch Intern Med* **146**:945–947.

27. Stockigt JR (1977) Potassium metabolism. *Anaesth Intens Care* **5**:317–325.

28. Tannen RL (1986) Potassium disorders. In: Kokko JP and Tannen RL (eds) *Fluid and Electrolytes*. Philadelphia: WB Saunders, pp. 150–228.

29. Kliger AS and Hayslett JP (1978) Disorders of potassium balance. In: Brenner BM and Stein JH (eds) *Acid–base and Potassium Homeostasis in Contemporary Issues in Nephrology*, vol. 2. New York: Churchill Livingstone, pp. 168–204.

30. Sterns RH, Cox M, Felig PU *et al.* (1981) Internal potassium balance and the control of the plasma potassium concentration. *Medicine* **60**:339–354.

31. Phelan DM and Worthley LIG (1985) Hypokalaemic coma. *Intens Care Med* **11**:257–258.

32. Standards and guidelines for cardiopulmonary resuscitation (CPR) and emergency cardiac care (ECC). *J Am Med Assoc* **268**:2172–2188.

33. Thomas DW (1977) Calcium, phosphorus and magnesium turnover. *Anaesth Intens Care* **5**:361–371.

34. Pak CYC (1986) Calcium disorders: hypercalcemia and hypocalcemia. In: Kokko JP and Tannen RL (eds) *Fluid and Electrolytes*. Philadelphia: WB Saunders, pp. 472–501.

35. Cronin RE (1986) Magnesium disorders. In: Kokko JP and Tannen RL (eds) *Fluid and Electrolytes*. Philadelphia: WB Saunders, pp. 502–512.

36. Lau K (1986) Phosphate disorders. In: Kokko JP and Tannen RL (eds) *Fluid and Electrolytes*. Philadelphia: WB Saunders, pp. 398–471.

82 Metabolic response to illness, injury and infection

IKS Tan

Illness, injury and infection evoke a constellation of metabolic changes in the host. A transitory ebb or shock phase is followed by a hypermetabolic flow phase (Fig. 82.1). The magnitude of the response is proportional to the extent of injury. Additional components of illness, such as ischaemia/reperfusion, starvation/nutrition, surgical procedures, drugs/anaesthetic techniques and concurrent diseases have an impact on the response. The usefulness of some components of the metabolic response is unclear in the critically ill, and its modulation may be beneficial in improving survival.

Mediators of the metabolic response

Cytokines

Cytokines are soluble non-antibody regulatory proteins responsible primarily for the inflammatory response. Injury and infection result in the release of cytokines from a variety of cells, primarily macrophages and monocytes. Complex interactions occur between various cytokines, and between the cytokine network and the immune, endocrine and nervous systems. Cytokines generally exert their effects in a paracrine fashion, but in severe injury and infection they enter the circulation and act as hormones.[1] The following are the major cytokines involved in the response to stress:

1 *Tumour necrosis factor (TNF, cachectin)* is a key proximal mediator.[2] After endotoxin challenge, TNF concentrations increase and peak before other mediators. The administration of monoclonal antibodies against TNF attenuates the increase in other mediators. TNF administration reproduces all features of septic shock,[3] including hypermetabolism, fever, anorexia, hyperglycaemia, decreased lipogenesis, marked protein catabolism and lactic acidosis. TNF activates the hypothalamic–pituitary–adrenal axis.

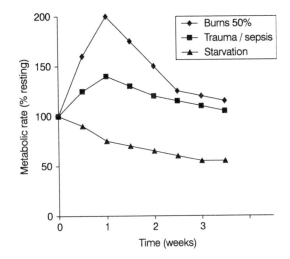

Fig. 82.1 Time course of metabolic response.

2 *Interleukins (IL):* IL-1 (endogenous pyrogen) produces much the same metabolic effects as TNF, and the combined effect of the two cytokines is greater than the effect of either alone. TNF and IL-1 induce each other's production. IL-1 is a potent inducer of the hypothalamic–pituitary–adrenal axis as well as central and peripheral noradrenergic neurones.[4] IL-6 is the main mediator of the acute-phase response.[5] Like TNF and IL-1, IL-6 levels correlate with severity of illness and outcome, but in mild injury, only serum IL-6 levels increase.[6] IL-8 induces neutrophil adhesion, chemotaxis and enzyme release.[7] IL-2 generation is decreased.

3 *Colony-stimulating* factors stimulate the proliferation of hemopoietic cells. They also stimulate superoxide and cytokine production by neutrophils and macrophages.

4 *Interferon-γ* up-regulates TNF receptors and induces TNF synthesis.[8]

Neuroendocrine mediators

Afferent neuronal impulses and cytokine release from the site of injury or infection activate the sympathetic nervous system and hypothalamic–pituitary hormone secretion (Fig. 82.2). Administration of adrenaline, cortisol and glucagon combinations reproduces only partially the metabolic response to stress. Protein catabolism is not of the magnitude observed after injury, and there is no fever or induction of the acute-phase response.[9] The following hormones are involved in the response to stress:

1 *Catecholamine* levels are increased with stress. There is tachycardia and calorigenesis with increased oxygen consumption. Blood flow redistribution occurs depending on tissue receptor balance. Glycogenolysis, gluconeogenesis and lipolysis are stimulated.

2 *Hypothalamic–pituitary–adrenal axis* activation results in gluconeogenesis, proteolysis and lipolysis. Anti-inflammatory and cell-protective effects[10] attenuate damage from excessive activation of the metabolic response.[11]

3 *Insulin and glucagon* levels are increased but the insulin levels are inappropriately low for the level of hyperglycaemia.[12] The increased glucagon : insulin ratio augments gluconeogenesis.

4 *Growth hormone* levels increase transiently but somatomedin (insulin-like growth factor, IGF-1) activity is depressed. Antidiuretic hormone, renin, angiotensin and aldosterone levels increase. Thyroid hormone (thyroxine; T_4) levels are usually low-normal. Low triiodothyromine (T_3), high reverse T_3 and normal thyroid-stimulating hormone levels are typical of the sick euthyroid syndrome.

The metabolic response

The metabolic response to injury and infection begins with the activation of receptors throughout the body by the above mediators. Many metabolic responses involve gene induction and regulation. In addition, catecholamines can initiate rapid functional changes via protein phosphorylation, which does not require gene induction. Behavioural effects such as anorexia also have an impact on the metabolic response. The metabolic effects may be described at three levels: cellular metabolic events, intermediary metabolism and systemic protein system responses.

Cellular metabolic events

Heat shock proteins (HSPs)

Heat shock proteins are synthesized in response to a variety of stress. Many HSPs are also expressed constitutively. HSPs act as chaperones, assisting in the assembly, dissasembly, stabilization and internal transport of other intracellular proteins.[13] They facilitate translocation of the glucocorticoid–receptor complex from the cytosol to the nucleus.[14] HSPs have cellular protective roles in sepsis[15] and ischaemia–reperfusion.[16]

Mitochondrial abnormalities

Mitochondrial abnormalities may limit cell metabolism.[17] The ketone body ratio (acetoacetate: β-hydroxybutyrate ratio) reflects liver mitochondrial redox potential, and correlates inversely with the magnitude of stress and catabolic response.[18]

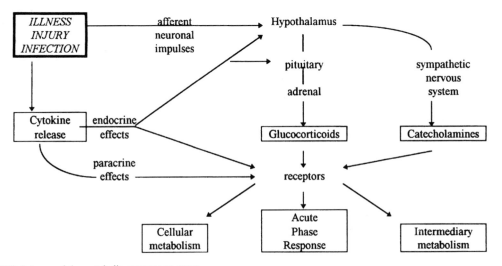

Fig. 82.2 Schema of the metabolic response to stress.

Leukocyte activation

Leukocyte activation occurs systemically. Following directed adhesion to endothelium and migration into tissue, leukocytes undergo an oxidative burst, producing oxygen-derived free radicals, proteases and arachidonic acid metabolites (i.e. leukotrienes, thromboxanes and prostaglandins).

Intermediary metabolism

Protein metabolism

Interleukin-1, TNF, related cytokines and hormonal changes trigger extreme protein catabolism, termed autocannibalism.[19] Glutamine, alanine and other amino acids are mobilized from skeletal muscle and taken up by hepatocytes and gut mucosa.[20] Excess glutamine utilization may lead to glutamine depletion. Increased ureagenesis occurs, leading to nitrogen loss. Levels of branch-chained amino acids (i.e. leucine, isoleucine, valine) fall with peripheral oxidation. The fraction of energy expenditure derived from glucose is reduced, while that derived from amino acid oxidation in the Krebs cycle is increased.[21]

Carbohydrate metabolism

Hyperglycaemia results from glycogenolysis, accelerated gluconeogenesis and peripheral insulin resistance. Lactate production increases from peripheral tissue, areas of injury and the white cell mass, and serves as substrate for gluconeogenesis in hepatocytes.[21] In the terminal phase of severe illness, hypoglycaemia may occur.

Fat metabolism

Lipolysis is increased with increased turnover of triglycerides and fatty acids. TNF, IL-1 and IL-6 decrease lipoprotein lipase activity,[1] contributing to hypertriglyceridaemia. Ketosis is suppressed, indicating that fat is not a major calorie source.

Electrolyte and micronutrient metabolism

Salt and water retention occurs, with hyponatraemia. Protein loss is accompanied by potassium, magnesium and phosphate loss. Zinc redistributes to liver and bone marrow. Zinc deficiency is associated with impaired IL-2 production and wound healing.[22] Iron levels decrease.

Systemic protein system responses

The acute-phase response

This is a systemic response to injury characterized by redirection of hepatic protein synthesis and haematological alterations. Production of proteins involved in defence is increased (e.g. protease inhibitors, fibrinogen, C-reactive protein, haptoglobin, complement C3), while synthesis of serum transport and binding molecules is reduced (i.e. albumin, transferrin).[23] Serum levels of acute-phase reactants like C-reactive protein can be used for diagnostic, monitoring and prognostic purposes.

Complement cascade

Complement cascade triggering produces chemoattractants (C3a, C5a), vasoactive anaphylatoxins (C3a, C4a, C5a), opsonins (C3b), stimulation of neutrophil and monocyte oxidative burst (C3b) and neutrophil adherence to endothelium (C5a).

Value of the metabolic response

The value of the metabolic response to stress has generated debate.[24] Cytokines and neuroendocrine mediators reprioritize metabolic processes to provide an increased supply of substrates to active tissues involved in defence against the results of injury. Cardiovascular changes divert blood flow to inflamed areas and vital organs. Inflammation localizes the area of injury. Sympathectomized and adrenalectomized animals fare poorly when stressed.

Disadvantages of the metabolic response include increased oxygen consumption and myocardial work. This may be detrimental to patients with marginal cardiovascular reserves.[25] The redistribution of blood flow away from the non-vital gut organ may result in translocation of bacteria and endotoxin into the circulation.[26] High catecholamine levels are arrythmogenic to the compromised heart.

In adrenalectomized animals, replacement with supraphysiologic stress doses of glucocorticoids did not confer a haemodynamic or survival advantage after injury as compared to replacement with physiological doses only.[27] This implies that hypercortisolaemia due to stress may be an epiphenomenon. Protein catabolism leading to loss of muscle has functional consequences such as respiratory muscle weakness.[28] A 25% body weight loss in the presence of injury may be fatal.[29] Wound healing and multiple facets of host defence are impaired, increasing the risk of nosocomial infection.[30]

A systemic stress response with prolonged production of cytokines is believed to contribute to shock and the multiple organ dysfunction syndrome[19] (see Chapter 85). Much research effort has been directed towards selectively blocking undesirable effects of the metabolic response to illness.

Factors affecting the metabolic response

Energy balance and oxygen delivery

Hypermetabolism increases oxygen demand and consumption. Inadequate oxygen delivery can lead to anaerobic metabolism and inadequate production of adenosine triphosphate and other high-energy phosphates. However, the existence of a *systemic* pathological supply-dependency of oxygen consumption on oxygen delivery in critically ill patients, and the implied widespread cellular hypoxia, is doubtful. Direct monitoring of intracellular pH and high-energy phosphate concentration during sepsis in a number of organs do not show a fall indicative of hypoxia.[31] Every study in which oxygen delivery and consumption were determined independently has not shown dependence of oxygen consumption on oxygen delivery[32] (see Chapter 22). Inadequate oxygen delivery may however be present in the gut.[26] Multiple causes contribute to raised lactate levels. *Aerobic* glycolysis rather than anaerobic glycolysis is characteristic of the metabolic response to stress.[21]

Surgical procedures and anaesthetic techniques

Total afferent neuronal blockade (somatic and autonomic block), for example, by epidural anesthesia, attenuates the metabolic changes of surgical injury. Analgesia *per se* has only a limited effect.[24] Minimally invasive procedures are associated with reduced cytokine release. This has translated to reduced morbidity and hospital stays.[33] The concept of stress-free anaesthesia and surgery may be important in reducing various aspects of postoperative morbidity.

Starvation and nutrition

Starvation alone produces adaptive hypometabolism with the use of fat as the primary fuel, sparing protein. In contrast, injury and infection result in hypermetabolism with prominent protein catabolism. Starvation in combination with the metabolic changes of stress produces a hypoalbuminaemic malnourished state, not unlike kwashiorkor. Malnutrition clearly contributes to morbidity and mortality. However, current forms of nutrition do not adequately reduce protein catabolism or promote protein synthesis, but result in fat and fluid gain instead.[34] It is likely that the quality of nutrients, the timing and the route of nutritional support can favourably influence the metabolic response to stress[35] (see Chapter 83 and 84). Early enteral nutrition with added glutamine and short-chain fatty acids is ideal. Vitamin E, zinc, Ω_3 fatty acids, arginine and nucleic acid supplementation of nutrition are all under active investigation.[36]

Drugs and disease

Adverse effects of steroids include increased infection rates and myopathy (particularly in conjunction with the use of neuromuscular blocking drugs).[37] The treatment of bacterial meningitis illustrates the use of steroids as a modulator of an excessive inflammatory response,[38] but its use in sepsis is dangerous.[39] To improve the efficacy of nutritional support, administration of growth hormone, IGF-1 and other anabolic adjuncts are under investigation.[40] Diseases like diabetes will clearly have an impact on the metabolic response to stress.

Secondary insults

Secondary insults like catheter-related sepsis, unnecessary interventions, fear, pain and hypothermia will increase the severity of the metabolic response and lead to unnecessary increases in catabolism, energy and oxygen need. Perhaps patients in the ICU today do not need the 'fright, fight, flight' response, but whether attenuation of the metabolic response will accelerate recovery, reduce convalescence, and improve morbidity and mortality remains to be proven.

References

1. Souba WW (1994) Cytokine control of nutrition and metabolism during critical illness. *Curr Probl Surg* **31**:577–652.
2. Deitch EA (1994) Cytokines yes, cytokines no, cytokines maybe? *Crit Care Med* **24**:817–819.
3. Michie HR, Spriggs DR, Manogue KR *et al.* (1988) Tumor necrosis factor and endotoxin induce similar metabolic responses in human beings. *Surgery* **104**:280–286.
4. Dunn AJ (1993) Infection as a stressor: a cytokine-mediated activation of the hypothalamo–pituitary–adrenal axis? *Ciba Found Symp* **172**:226–242.
5. Castell JV, Gomez–Lechon MJ, David M, Fabra R, Trullenque R and Heinrich PC (1990) Acute-phase response of human hepatocytes: regulation of acute-phase protein synthesis by interleukin-6. *Hepatology* **12**:1179–1186.
6. Pullicino EA, Carli F, Poole S, Rafferty B, Malik ST and Elia M (1990) The relationship between the circulating concentrations of interleukin 6 (IL-6), tumor necrosis factor (TNF) and the acute phase response to elective surgery and accidental injury. *Lymphokine Res* **9**:231–233.
7. Feuerstein G and Rabinovici R (1994) Importance of interleukin-8 and chemokines in organ injury and shock. *Crit Care Med* **22**:550–551.
8. Koerner TJ, Adams DO and Hamilton TA (1987) Regulation of tumor necrosis factor (TNF) expression: interferon-gamma enhances the accumulation of mRNA for TNF induced by lipopolysaccharide in murine peritoneal macrophages. *Cell Immunol* **109**:437–443.
9. Gelfand RA, Matthews DE, Bier DM and Sherwin RS (1984) Role of counterregulatory hormones in the catabolic response to stress. *J Clin Invest* **74**:2238–2248.
10. Pagliacci MC, Migliorati G, Smacchia M, Grignani F, Riccardi C and Nicoletti I (1993) Cellular stress and glucocorticoid hormones protect L929 mouse fibroblasts from tumor necrosis factor alpha cytotoxicity. *J Endocrinol Invest* **16**:591–599.

11. Munck A and Naray-Fejes-Toth A (1992) The ups and downs of glucocorticoid physiology. Permissive and suppressive effects revisited. *Mol Cell Endocrinol* **90**:C1–C4.

12. Weissman C (1990) The metabolic response to stress: an overview and update. *Anesthesiology* **73**:308–327.

13. Becker J and Craig EA (1994) Heat-shock proteins as molecular chaperones. *Eur J Biochem* **219**:11–23.

14. Pratt WB (1993) The role of heat shock proteins in regulating the function, folding, and trafficking of the glucocorticoid receptor. *J Biol Chem* **268**:21455.

15. Villar J, Ribeiro SP, Mullen JBM *et al.* (1994) Induction of the heat shock response reduces mortality rate and organ damage in a sepsis-induced acute lung injury model. *Crit Care Med* **22**:914–921.

16. Mestril R, Chi SH, Sayen MR, O'Reilly K and Dillmann WH (1994) Expression of inducible stress protein 70 in rat heart myogenic cells confers protection against simulated ischemia-induced injury. *J Clin Invest* **93**:759–767.

17. Dong Y, Sheng C, Herndon D and Waymack JP (1992) Metabolic abnormalities of mitochondrial redox potential in post burn multiple system organ failure. *Burns* **18**:283–286.

18. Kiuchi T, Shimahara Y, Wakashiro S *et al.* (1990) Reduced arterial ketone body ratio during laparotomy: an evaluation of operative stress through the changes in hepatic mitochondrial redox potential. *J Lab Clin Med* **115**:433–440.

19. Beal AL and Cerra FB (1994) Multiple organ failure syndrome in the 1990s; systemic inflammatory response and organ dysfunction. *J Am Med Assoc* **271**:226–233.

20. Austgen TR, Chen MK, Flynn TC and Souba WW (1991) The effects of endotoxin on the splanchnic metabolism of glutamine and related substrates. *J Trauma* **31**:742–751.

21. Cerra FB (1989) Metabolic manifestations of multiple systems organ failure. *Crit Care Clin* **5**:119–131.

22. Okada A, Takagi Y, Nezu R and Lee S (1990) Zinc in clinical surgery – a research review. *Jpn J Surg* **20**:635–644.

23. Fey GH and Gauldie J (1990) The acute phase response of the liver in inflammation. *Prog Liver Dis* **9**:89–116.

24. Kehlet H (1991) The surgical stress response: should it be prevented? *Can J Surg* **34**:565–567.

25. Breslow MJ (1992) The role of stress hormones in perioperative myocardial ischemia. *Int Anesthesiol Clin* **30**:81–100.

26. Mythen MG and Webb AR (1994) The role of gut mucosal hypoperfusion in the pathogenesis of post-operative organ dysfunction. *Intensive Care Med* **20**:203–209.

27. Udelsman R, Ramp J, Gallucci WT *et al.* (1986) Adaptation during surgical stress. A reevaluation of the role of glucocorticoids. *J Clin Invest* **77**:1377–1381.

28. Arora NS and Rochester DF (1982) Respiratory muscle strength and voluntary ventilation in undernourished patients. *Am Rev Respir Dis* **126**:5–8.

29. Apovian CM, McMahon MM and Bistrian BR (1990) Guidelines for refeeding the marasmic patient. *Crit Care Med* **18**:1030–1033.

30. Salo M (1992) Effects of anaesthesia and surgery on the immune response. *Acta Anaaesthesiol Scand* **36**:201–220.

31. Hotchkiss RS and Karl IE (1992) Reevaluation of the role of cellular hypoxia and bioenergetic failure in sepsis. *J Am Med Assoc* **267**:1503–1510.

32. Russell JA and Phang PT (1994) The oxygen delivery/consumption controversy. Approaches to management of the critically ill. *Am J Respir Crit Care Med* **149**:533–537.

33. Joris J, Cigarini I, Legrand M *et al.* (1992) Metabolic and respiratory changes after cholecystectomy performed via laparotomy or laparoscopy. *Br J Anaesth* **69**:341–345.

34. Streat SJ, Beddoe AH and Hill GL (1987) Aggressive nutritional support does not prevent protein loss despite fat gain in septic intensive care patients. *J Trauma* **27**:262–266.

35. Round table conference on metabolic support of the critically ill patients. *Intensive Care Med* **20**:298–299.

36. Bower RH, Cerra FB, Bershadsky B *et al.* (1995) Early enteral administration of a formula (Impact®) supplemented with arginine, nucleotides, and fish oil in intensive care unit patients: results of a multicenter, prospective, randomized, clinical trial. *Crit Care Med* **23**:436–449.

37. Zochodne DW, Ramsay DA, Saly V, Shelley S and Moffatt S (1994) Acute necrotizing myopathy of intensive care: electrophysiological studies. *Muscle-Nerve* **17**:285–292.

38. Nathavitharana KA and Tarlow MJ (1993) Current trends in the management of bacterial meningitis. *Br J Hosp Med* **50**:403–407.

39. Bone RC, Fischer CJ Jr, Clemmer TP *et al.* (1987) Effect of high-dose glucocorticoid therapy on mortality in patients with clinical signs of systemic sepsis. *N Engl J Med* **317**:659–665.

40. Ziegler TR, Gatzen C and Wilmore DW (1994) Strategies for attenuating protein-catabolic responses in the critically ill. *Annu Rev Med* **45**:459–480.

83 | Enteral nutrition

GJ Dobb

It is common for patients requiring intensive care to need nutritional support. For some, the episode of critical illness comes after a period of ill health with poor nutrition and weight loss. In nearly all patients, the critical illness is accompanied by anorexia or inability to eat because of impaired consciousness, sedation or intubation through the upper airway. The aims of nutritional support for critically ill patients proposed by the American Society for Parenteral and Enteral Nutrition[1] include:

1 detection and correction of pre-existing malnutrition;
2 prevention of progressive protein-energy malnutrition;
3 optimizing the patient's metabolic state;
4 reduction of morbidity and time to convalescence.

Enteral versus parenteral nutrition

The enteral route should always be used if feasible. Studies[2] have shown better nitrogen retention and weight gain, reduced frequency of hepatic steatosis and reduced incidence of epigastric and intestinal bleeding when patients are fed by the enteral when compared to the parenteral route. The lesser cost of enteral nutrition is a further significant advantage. To these must be added the now clear physiological benefits of enteral nutrition in helping maintain gut mucosal barrier integrity,[3] mucosal structure and function and release of gut trophic hormones. A meta-analysis of eight randomized clinical trials[4] comparing early enteral nutrition with parenteral nutrition in high-risk surgical patients shows nearly half the frequency of septic complication in patients given enteral nutrition (18% versus 35%). In patients needing intensive care, survival has been significantly better in patients enterally fed than those needing parenteral nutrition[5] despite similar illness severity scores.

Specific nutrients can be given enterally, but not parenterally, and their delivery to the luminal surface of the gut mucosa may be responsible for improved outcomes with enteral as compared with parenteral nutrition. These specific nutrients include glutamine, arginine, nucleotides, fibre (and the short-chain fatty acids resulting from its degradation in the gut), Ω_3 fatty acids and perhaps absorption of protein in the form of peptides rather than individual amino acids (see below).

Assessing nutritional status

A simple dietary history and clinical examination indicate when nutrition is inadequate in patients needing intensive care. Investigations showing hypoalbuminaemia and lymphocytopenia have limited usefulness in these patients. Changes in the body mass of intensive care patients are largely caused by changes in total body water rather than protein or fat, and skinfold measurements do not provide accurate estimates of body fat.[6] Other techniques for measuring body composition, including neutron activation analysis, dual-energy X-ray absorptiometry, magnetic resonance imaging and bioimpedance methods, have been used in research but not routine clinical practice.

Assessing nutritional requirements

Nitrogen balance studies and indirect calorimetry provide intellectual respectability to the prescription for enteral nutrition, but both have limitations in the critically ill. Estimation of urinary nitrogen excretion from urinary urea and protein measurements (Table 83.1) gives retrospective information of dubious value in unstable critically ill patients.[7] More accurate estimates of nitrogen losses are provided by pyro-chemiluminescence which measures total nitrogen in urine or other body fluids. However, the value of such

Table 83.1 Calculation of daily nitrogen loss for nitrogen balance

---

Loss in urine (24-h collection)

Urine urea (mmol) $\times$ 0.0336	= A
Urine protein loss (g) $\times$ 0.16	= B

Blood urea correction

Change in plasma urea (mmol/l) $\times$ body weight (kg) $\times$ 0.0168	= C
Daily nitrogen loss = A + B + C (g) + extrarenal losses*	

---

*Gastric aspirate, intestinal fistulae, etc. – usually ignored unless losses are large.

Table 83.2 Common constraints limiting ability to meet estimated nutritional requirements in critically ill patients

---

Restricted total fluid intake
Glucose intolerance
Impaired renal function
Delayed gastric emptying/reduced feed absorption
Diarrhoea
Fasting for procedures

---

measurements remains doubtful, when even the most aggressive nutritional support may fail to achieve nitrogen balance in critically ill patients.

Portable bedside calorimetry has been available for many years but has not been widely used. Technical problems caused by gas leaks between ventilator and the patient's lungs, high inspired oxygen concentrations and gases saturated with water vapour together with difficulty in achieving steady-state conditions have limited its usefulness. Studies in ventilated patients needing intensive care have given variable results, perhaps because of the technical problems.[8] It has been suggested that extrapolated estimates of 24 h energy expenditure in these patients from short periods of measurement can be fairly accurate. However, in other studies, estimates based on the Harris–Benedict equation have been as useful as more complex alternatives, and even estimates from indirect calorimetry vary considerably from day to day.[9] Newer devices for indirect calorimetry[10] may overcome previous difficulties and become more widely used, facilitating estimation of energy requirements. In the absence of such measurements, estimated energy expenditure can be derived from formulae which take into account the patient's height, weight, age and sex. Such estimates need to be modified by fever, sedation, neuromuscular paralysis or losses during dialysis.[11]

In practice, an energy intake of 125–145 kJ (30–35 kcal)/kg body weight and protein intake of 1.5–2.0 g/kg per day provides a suitable target nutritional intake for many critically ill patients. This gives 470–630 kJ (112–148 kcal) to each gram of protein nitrogen – within the range of most commercially available feeds which provide 420–765 kJ (100–180 kcal) per gram of nitrogen. A feed developed specifically for highly stressed patients (Traumacal, Mead Johnson) provides just 378 kJ (90 kcal) per gram of nitrogen.

Giving excessive amounts of energy, particularly as carbohydrate, increases fat synthesis with fat deposition in the liver, and increases carbon dioxide production. Increased carbon dioxide production can cause difficulty in weaning patients with impaired inspiratory function from mechanical ventilation. Further constraints on nutritional intake by critically ill patients are listed in Table 83.2. Some of these can be overcome by using diuretics and haemofiltration to prevent fluid overload, and early dialysis to avoid azotaemia. Even so, it seems patients generally receive only about three-quarters of estimated needs.[12]

There are considerable variations in electrolyte content between different commercially available feeds. This can affect the choice of feed, e.g. when sodium or potassium restriction is important. Commercial complete feeds generally contain the recommended daily amounts of vitamins for healthy adults in a feed volume corresponding to approximately 8400 kJ (2000 kcal). The vitamin requirements of critically ill patients may be greater, particularly for folic acid and vitamin C, or when losses of water-soluble vitamins are increased by dialysis or continuous haemodiafiltration.

Nasogastric/nasoenteric tube feeding[13]

Nasal tubes are preferred to oral because of better patient tolerance. The nasal route is relatively contraindicated in patients with a fractured base of skull, because of the risk of intracranial penetration. Complications include trauma and bleeding during insertion, erosion of the nares and sinusitis.[14] A double-lumen tube (Moss Tubes, West Sand Lake, New York, USA) which allows both gastric aspiration and jejunal feeding has been advocated for ICU patients, but performance has been disappointing in practice.[15]

Percutaneous jejunostomy or gastrostomy are alternatives to oral or nasal incubation. A feeding jejunostomy is usually created as an additional procedure during a laparotomy for other indications. There is a relatively high frequency of complications including leaks, wound infection and peritonitis.[16] Gastrostomy, now commonly performed as a percutaneous endoscopic procedure, is usually reserved for patients needing long-term enteral feeding. Complications occur in a quarter of all patients[17] and are similar to those associated with jejunostomy.

Unless there are specific contraindications, nasogastric feeding should be attempted as soon as possible in all ICU patients unable to eat, unless they are expected to be able to resume eating within a day or so.[18] Ventilated patients can have normal gastric emptying in the absence of bowel sounds,[19] but impaired gastric emptying is common in patients with increased intracranial pressure.[20] Early nasogastric feeding may reduce the frequency of gastric ileus. Nasogastric feeding is started through a 12–14 FG tube. Tubes of this size allow aspiration of gastric contents to check the absorption of feeds and administration of crushed tablets or viscous elixirs, and are less likely to become blocked than smaller tubes.

The place of starter regimens of increasing feed volume is unproven. However, it is common practice to start with 30–40 ml/h of feed, increasing to the full estimated requirement over 12–48 h, depending on tolerance. When enteral feeding is started after prolonged starvation or parenteral nutrition, feeds should be started at low volumes, increasing more slowly and with closer than usual clinical and biochemical monitoring, because of the risk of refeeding syndrome.[21] Tolerance is usually judged by gastric residual volume. While it has been found that residual volumes of up to 400 ml in critically ill patients do not necessarily indicate intolerance,[22] there is concern that large residual volumes may increase the risk of regurgitation. Factors further increasing the chance of regurgitation include a large- (as opposed to small) bore nasogastric tube, positioning patients supine[23] and increasing age.[24] When 4-hourly gastric aspirates are consistently greater then 200–300 ml, cisapride 10 mg 6-hourly often improves gastric emptying.[25] When aspirates remain large or feeds are not absorbed, insertion of a fine-bore nasoenteral feeding tube should be considered. Similar tubes can replace large-bore nasogastric tubes once nasogastric feeding is established and gastric residual volumes no longer need to be checked.

Many different fine-bore (<12 FG) nasogastric or nasoenteral feeding tubes are available. A stylet or guide wire is usually inserted through the tube during placement, and a weighted tip is common although there is little evidence that this assists duodenal or jejunal intubation. A number of techniques are described to assist nasogastric insertion of fine-bore tubes and for further passage beyond the pylorus.[26] Only 15–50% of fine-bore tubes pass spontaneously through the pylorus within 24 h of insertion, with the proportion in ICU patients probably being at the lower end of the range.[27] Drugs used to encourage passage through the pylorus include cisapride 10 mg 6-hourly, metoclopramide 10–20 mg IV 6-hourly/or erythromycin 100–200 mg IV over 15 min,[28] or erythromycin elixir 400 mg 8-hourly for three doses

Table 83.3 Potential complications during fine-bore feeding tube insertion

Pharyngeal
Trauma and bleeding
Perforation of retropharyngeal space
Abscess

Chest
Oesophageal perforation
Pneumomediastinum
Pneumothorax
Pulmonary haemorrhage
Clinical pneumonitis
Pleural effusion
Empyema

Abdominal
Gastric perforation
Bowel perforation

through the feeding tube.[29] A fine-bore feeding tube incorporating a pH sensor[30] has been suggested as a means of assisting transpyloric enteral access, but may have a limited place in severe critical illness because of achlorhydria or use of H_2-receptor antagonists. Insertion under fluoroscopic guidance or using gastroscopic assistance increases the certainty of placement and has a 95% success rate.

Once in place, the tube must be securely fixed and its position confirmed by an X-ray before feeding starts. With care, the complications of fine-bore tube insertion can be minimized (Table 83.3). Misplacement complicates 0.3–4.0% of insertions.

Feed composition

Many prepared feeds in liquid or powder form are commercially available. These vary in their protein, carbohydrate and fat sources, electrolyte, mineral and vitamin content, osmolality and the content of specific nutrients including fibre, branched-chain amino acids (BCAA), essential amino acids, glutamine, arginine, nucleotides and other nutrients. A lactose-free, isotonic liquid feed providing approximately two-thirds of the non-protein energy as carbohydrate meets the needs of most patients. When necessary, such a feed can be modified by the addition of individual carbohydrate, protein or fat sources to meet specific needs.

Specific feeds

Specific feeds are available for trauma and certain diseases (e.g. Traumacal, Pulmocare, Ross Products Division, Abbott Laboratories). In general, any clinical or nutritional benefit to justify the greater cost using these feeds has still to be shown. The exception are feeds with a reduced carbohydrate content (e.g. Glucerna, Pulmocare, Ross Products Division, Abbott Laboratories). Feeds providing approximately one-third of the non-protein energy as carbohydrate and two-thirds as fat reduce problems of glucose intolerance in diabetic patients, and can assist weaning from mechanical ventilation in patients with marginal respiratory function.[31]

Elemental feeds

Elemental feeds provide protein in the form of free amino acids or peptides. Overall, there is no advantage from using elemental feeds,[32] and they cost more than standard formulae. There may be a place for such feeds in patients after prolonged fasting (because of mucosal atrophy) and patients with the short-bowel syndrome, radiation enteritis, pancreatitis or pancreatic insufficiency. Elemental feeds cause less stimulation of pancreatic exocrine secretion than complex feeds, especially when given into the jejunum, but they do not promote intestinal growth factors[33] and may therefore perpetuate gut mucosal atrophy.

Branched-chain amino acids

The effect of feeds with a high proportion of amino acids as valine, leucine and isoleucine has been extensively investigated in post surgical and septic patients. It is unlikely there is any overall benefit.[34] Experimental studies show that BCAA can provide a source of glutamine.[35] Feeds enriched with BCAA have been advocated for patients with hepatic encephalopathy. BCAA do not significantly affect the outcome of patients with acute hepatic encephalopathy, but protein given in this form may allow a greater total protein intake in chronic hepatic encephalopathy without causing deterioration.[36]

Glutamine

Glutamine is the most abundant amino acid in plasma and intracellular fluid. It is the principal interorgan carrier of nitrogen, particularly between the organs of synthesis (i.e. muscle and liver) and the sites of utilization (i.e. gut, lymphocytes and lung). Glutamine has a key role in skeletal muscle synthesis and breakdown, ammoniagenesis in the kidney, gluconeogenesis and nucleotide biosynthesis. It is a major metabolic fuel for the enterocytes of the gut mucosa and lymphocytes.[37] Although not regarded as an essential amino acid, it becomes conditionally essential in catabolic states.[38] Plasma concentrations are decreased by surgery, trauma or sepsis. Adverse effects on the function of glutamine utilizing tissues may be reduced by feeds supplemented with glutamine.[39]

Inclusion of large amounts of glutamine in enteral feeds has been limited by its instability to heat sterilization with formation of ammonia and pyroglutamic acid.[40] Enteral feeds supplemented with glutamine are now available (e.g. Alitraq, Ross Products Division, Abbott Laboratories). Some, but not all, experimental studies show that glutamine-supplemented feeds reduce bacterial translocation. The place of glutamine-supplemented feeds for critically ill patients has still to be fully defined.

Arginine

Arginine-supplemented feeds can stimulate release of growth hormone, prolactin, insulin, glucagon and insulin-like growth factor. Arginine is the precursor of nitric oxide and enhances mitogen-stimulated T-cell proliferation after injury.[41]

Nucleotides

Nucleotides have an important role in maintaining normal immune function. Lack of dietary nucleotides suppresses helper T cells and production of IL-2.[42] Nucleotides are the precursors of deoxyribonucleic acid (DNA) and ribonucleic acid (RNA), which are essential to cell division and protein synthesis. Optimal growth and function of lymphocytes, macrophages and intestinal cells appears dependent on a dietary source of nucleotides.[43] There is a biochemical link between glutamine and nucleotides (Fig. 83.1).

Medium-chain triglycerides

Medium-chain triglycerides have attracted interest because absorption from the small intestine is relatively independent of pancreatic lipase. Providing up to 50% of total lipid as medium-chain triglyceride enhances gut mucosal protein synthesis,[44] but the optimal formulation for enteral nutrition is still uncertain.

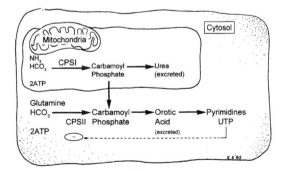

Fig. 83.1 Nucleotide synthesis in enterocytes from glutamine. CPS = Carbamoyl phosphate synthetase: ATP = adenosine triphosphate; UTP = uridine triphosphate.

Fish oils

Fish oils, and particularly the Ω_3 fatty acids, experimentally moderate the inflammatory response to injury or sepsis.[45] This may be through changes in arachidonic acid metabolism.[46]

Fibre

Fibre is a usual component of food. The short-chain fatty acids acetate, propionate and butyrate, derived from the bacterial breakdown of fibre, are important substrates for colonic mucosal nutrition. Fibre binds bile salts which would otherwise be irritant to the colonic mucosa, and fibre-containing diets promote absorption of water from the lumen of the colon. Fibre also slows glucose absorption and supports growth of the normal intestinal flora. Despite these potential benefits, a review of clinical trials[47] concluded that there was no firm basis for the routine use of fibre-supplemented enteral nutrition solutions. However, there are differences in the effect of different fibre sources, and possibly a mixture of fibre sources would provide more natural nutrition. The fibre-containing enteral feeding solutions available usually contain only one source of dietary fibre, often soy-polysaccharide. No adverse clinical effects have been reported.

Enhanced feeds

Enhanced feeds containing a mixture of the specific nutrients described as supplements to the basic formula are now available. They cost more than standard feeds. A feed supplemented with arginine, RNA and Ω_3 fatty acids (Impact, Sandoz Nutrition) improved nitrogen balance and markers of immune function, while reducing infective complications and mean length of hospital stay in patients having surgery for upper gastrointestinal cancer.[48] Mortality was low, but the only deaths occurred in those given supplemented feeds. A trial of the same feed in ICU patients found no difference in nitrogen balance compared to the use of Osmolite HN (Ross Laboratories).[49] The frequency of infection and length of stay in patients given the supplemented feed were again reduced, but without a significant effect on mortality. It is likely that the ideal feed for critically ill patients has still to be developed from the results of incremental research.

Growth factors

Growth factors are now manufactured using recombinant techniques. Their use as an adjunct to nutritional support has been investigated in studies using recombinant human growth hormone, insulin-like growth factor and epidermal growth factor. Growth hormone[50] consistently improves nitrogen balance and the rate of protein synthesis in critically ill patients, and enhances the healing of burns. An adequate source of glutamine appears important for growth hormone to be effective. A commonly used dose is 10 mg/day subcutaneously or 0.1–0.17 mg/kg per day. Its effects may be mediated by stimulation of insulin-like growth factor. Side-effects include glucose intolerance and hypercalcaemia.

Insulin-like growth factor has pronounced metabolic effects,[51] and has improved nitrogen balance in clinical studies of critically ill patients. Infusion of insulin-like growth factor can cause hypoglycaemia. Use of growth factors as adjuncts to enteral feeding appears promising, but they are expensive and effects on clinically important outcomes, such as duration of hospital stay or mortality, have still to be shown.

Administration of feeds

It has been common practice to give feeding continuously. Many units routinely use pump-assisted infusions, especially through fine-bore tubes. There is limited evidence that bolus feeds to the same total quantity given 4-hourly may be more physiological and improve nitrogen balance. An intermittent regimen also allows acidification of gastric contents, and so minimizes the risk of bacterial overgrowth. Theoretical benefits have still to be shown to affect outcome in ICU patients, and thus the continuous method continues to be preferred for its convenience.

The system used for administration of enteral feeds must be sterile, simple to use, safe and cheap with connectors that are incompatible with intravascular infusions sets. Distinctive colouring of enteral feeds reduces the risk of intravascular infusion – a catastrophic complication when it occurs.[52] Using a single reservoir to contain a whole day's feed, and changing this 24-hourly has the merit of simplicity, and seems more likely to result in the patient receiving the amount of feed prescribed. The disadvantage is an increased risk of bacterial contamination. Factors affecting the frequency of bacterial contamination are the time at room temperature, number of manipulations during feed preparation and feed composition. A feed 'hanging' time at room temperature of no more than 12 h is generally recommended.

Complications

Complications of enteral feeding are more frequent in patients needing intensive care than the less severely ill.[53] Complications associated with enteral feeding are listed in Table 83.4.

A high frequency of intolerance of early enteral feeding is seen in patients with inadequately resuscitated shock, and those with a pelvic fracture or retroperitoneal haematoma after repair of a leaking

Table 83.4 Complications associated with enteral feeding

Complications related to feeding tubes
Complications of tube insertion (see Table 83.3)
Failed insertion
Patient discomfort
Erosion of nares
Sinusitis
Tube displacement (infusion to inappropriate site)
Tube obstruction
Surgical complications of gastrostomy and jejunostomy
Aerophagy

Complications related to enteral feeding
Nosocomial infection from bacterial contamination of feed
Nausea, abdominal distension and discomfort
Regurgitation or vomiting
Pulmonary aspiration of feed
Diarrhoea
Intestinal pseudo-obstruction
Interactions with enteral medications

Complications related to feed content
Hyperglycaemia
Azotaemia
Hypercarbia
Electrolyte abnormalities
Specific deficiency disorders with long-term use

abdominal aortic aneurysm. In a study of mechanically ventilated blunt trauma patients, 36% could not tolerate enteral feeds, even after endoscopic transpyloric tube placement.[54] Conversely, two-thirds of the patients did tolerate enteral feeding. Intolerance of enteral feeding was associated with a high mortality.

Attention to tube placement, its care, the choice of feed, cleanliness and careful patient monitoring should minimize the risk of complications. Obstruction of fine-bore feeding tubes (<12 FG) can be minimized by not aspirating through them.[55] When obstruction does occur, instilling Coca-cola or a similar beverage sometimes dissolves the blockage.

Diarrhoea is one of the most troublesome complications associated with enteral feeding[56] in the ICU. The reported frequency has been 32–68%, but definitions of diarrhoea[57] vary considerably. It causes distress to the patients and staff, places heavy demands on nursing time and linen services, contaminates patient's skin and the surrounding area with potentially pathogenic organisms, causes problems with skin care and results in losses of fluid, electrolytes and nutrients that are difficult to quantify. Factors associated with diarrhoea in ICU patients include antibiotic use and administration of medications in the form of high-osmolality elixirs. Fibre does not reduce the frequency of diarrhoea during enteral feeding. When diarrhoea occurs, spurious diarrhoea caused by faecal impaction must be excluded by rectal examination, and a stool sample should be tested for *Clostridium difficile* and its toxin – the cause of pseudomembranous colitis. Diarrhoea is a common side-effect of many medications. Diarrhoea during enteral feeding usually resolves with time in the absence of an infective cause or continuation of the precipitating factor. Once an infective cause has been excluded, loperamide 4 mg initially, then 2 mg after each liquid stool, to a maximum of 16 mg in 24 h can be used for symptomatic relief.

Team approach

A team approach to enteral nutrition is widely advocated. Close liaison with a dietitian assists in the provision of a high-quality service, sensitive to individual patient's needs in the ICU, but the roles of team members must be clearly defined.[58]

References

1. American Society for Parenteral and Enteral Nutrition Board of Directors (1993) Guidelines for the use of parenteral and enteral nutrition in adult and pediatric patients. *JPEN* **14**:15A–25A.
2. Dobb GJ (1992) Enteral nutrition for the critically ill. In: Vincent J-L (ed.) *Yearbook of Intensive Care and Emergency Medicine 1992*. Berlin: Springer–Verlag, pp. 609–619.
3. Deitch EA (1994) Bacterial translocation: the influence of dietary variables. *Gut* **35**(suppl 1):S23–S27.
4. Moore FA, Feliciano DV, Andrassy RJ *et al.* (1992) Early enteral feeding, compared with parenteral, reduces postoperative septic complications: the results of a meta-analysis. *Ann Surg* **216**: 172–183.
5. Chang RWS, Jacobs S and Lee B (1987) Gastrointestinal dysfunction among intensive care unit patients. *Crit Care Med* **15**:909–914.
6. Plank LD and Hill GL (1995) Modern techniques for measuring body composition in patients who are critically ill. In: Bion J, Burchardi H, Dellinger RP and Dobb GJ (eds) *Current Topics in Intensive Care*. London: WB Saunders, pp. 125–143.
7. Konstantinides FN, Konstantinides NN, Li JC, Myaga ME and Cerra FB (1991) Urinary urea nitrogen: too insensitive for calculating nitrogen balance studies in surgical clinical nutrition. *JPEN* **15**: 189–193.
8. McClave SA, Snider HL, Greene L *et al.* (1992) Effective utilisation of indirect calorimetry during critical care. *Intensive Care World* **9**:194–200.
9. Vermeij CG, Feenstra BWA and Lanschot JBV (1989) Day to day variability of energy expenditure in critically ill surgical patients. *Crit Care Med* **17**:623–626.
10. Weissman C, Sardar A and Kemper M (1994) An *in vitro* evaluation of an instrument designed to measure oxygen consumption and carbon dioxide production during mechanical ventilation. *Crit Care Med* **22**:1995–2000.

11. Elwyn DH, Kinney JM and Askanazi J (1981) Energy expenditure in surgical patients. *Surg Clin North Am* **61**:545–556.

12. Evans NJ, Sorouri BK and Feurer ID (1991) Construction of nutrient supply in the intensive care unit. *JPEN* **15**:34S.

13. Payne-James JJ (1992) Enteral nutrition: accessing patients. *Nutrition* **11**:337–344.

14. Rouby JJ, Laurent P, Gosnach M *et al.* (1994) Risk factors and clinical relevance of nosocomial maxillary sinusitis in the critically ill. *Am J Respir Crit Care Med* **150**:776–783.

15. Gentello LM, Cortes V, Castro M *et al.* (1993) Enteral nutrition with simultaneous gastric decompression in critically ill patients. *Crit Care Med* **21**:392–395.

16. Adams MB, Seabrook GR, Quebbeman EAA and Condon RE (1986) Jejunostomy. A rarely indicated procedure. *Ann Surg* **121**:236–238.

17. George J, Crawford D, Lewis T, Shepherd R and Ward M (1990) Percutaneous endoscopic gastrostomy: a two year experience. *Med J Aust* **152**:17–19.

18. Minard G and Kudsk KA (1994) Is early feeding beneficial? How early is early? *New Horizons* **2**: 156–163.

19. Shelly MP and Church JJ (1987) Bowel sounds during intermittent positive pressure ventilation. *Anaesthesia* **42**:207–209.

20. Norton JA, Ott LG, McClain C *et al.* (1988) Intolerance to enteral feeding in the brain injured patient. *J Neurosurg* **68**:62–66.

21. Solomon SM and Kirby DF (1990) The refeeding syndrome: a review. *JPEN* **14**:90–97.

22. McClave SA, Snider HL, Lowen CC *et al.* (1992) Use of residual volume as a marker for enteral feeding intolerance: prospective blinded comparison with physical examination and radiographic findings. *JPEN* **16**:419–422.

23. Ibanez J, Penafiel A, Raurich JM, Marse P, Jorda R and Mata F (1992) Gastroesophageal reflux (GER) in intubated patients receiving enteral inutrition: effect of supine and semirecumbent positions. *JPEN* **16**:419–422.

24. Mullan H, Roubenoff RA and Roubenoff R (1992) Risk of pulmonary aspiration among patients receiving enteral nutrition support. *JPEN* **16**:160–164.

25. Spapen HD, Duinslaeger L, Diltoer M, Gillet R, Bossuyt A and Huyghens LP (1995) Gastric emptying in critically ill patients is accelerated by adding cisapride to a standard enteral feeding protocol: results of a prospective, randomized controlled trial. *Crit Care Med* **23**:481–485.

26. Zaloga GP (1991) Bedside method for placing small bowel feeding tubes in critically ill patients. A prospective study. *Chest* **100**:1643–1646.

27. Marian M, Rappaport W, Cunningham D *et al.* (1993) The failure of conventional methods to promote spontaneous transpyloric feeding tube passage and the safety of intragastric feeding in the critically ill ventilated patient. *Surg Gynecol Obstet* **176**:475–479.

28. Annese V, Janssens J, Vantrappen G *et al.* (1992) Erythromycin accelerates gastric emptying by inducing antral contractions and improved gastroduodenal co-ordination. *Gastroenterology* **102**:823–828.

29. Stern MA and Wolf DC (1994) Erythromycin as a prokinetic agent: a prospective randomized, controlled study of efficacy in nasoenteric tube placement. *Am J Gastroenterol* **89**:2011–2013.

30. Berry S, Schoettker P and Orr M (1994) pH measurements as guide for establishing short term postpyloric enteral access. *Nutrition* **10**:419–423.

31. Al-Saady NM, Blackmore CM and Bennett ED (1989) High fat, low carbohydrate enteral feeding lowers $P_{a}CO_2$ and reduces the period of ventilation in artificially ventilated patients. *Intensive Care Med* **15**:290–295.

32. Mowatt-Larssen CA, Brown RO, Wojtysiak SI and Kudsk KA (1992) Comparison of tolerance and nutritional outcome between a peptide and a standard enteral formula in critically ill hypoalbuminemic patients. *JPEN* **16**:20–24.

33. Playford RJ, Woodman AC, Clark P *et al.* (1993) Effect of luminal growth factor preservation on intestinal growth. *Lancet* **341**:866–867.

34. Jimenez FJJ, Leyba CO, Mendez SM, Barros Perez M and Munoz Garcia J (1991) Prospective study on the efficacy of branched chain amino acids in septic patients. *JPEN* **15**:252–261.

35. Platell C, McCauley R, McCulloch R and Hall J (1993) The influence of parenteral glutamine and branched chain amino acids on total parenteral nutrition-induced atrophy of the gut. *JPEN* **17**:348–354.

36. Lerebours E (1993) Nutritional support in liver disease. In: Wilmore DW and Carpentier YA (eds) *Metabolic Support of the Critically Ill Patient. Update in Intensive Care and Emergency Medicine 17.* Berlin: Springer-Verlag, pp. 377–389.

37. Smith RJ (1990) Glutamine metabolism and its physiologic importance. *JPEN* **14**:40–44.

38. Wilmore DW (1994) Glutamine and the gut. *Gastroenterology* **107**:1885–1886.

39. Ziegler TR, Smith RJ, Byrne TA and Wilmore DW (1993) Potential role of glutamine supplementation in nutrition support. *Clin Nutr* **12**(suppl 1):S82–S90.

40. Grimble G (1993) Glutamine, glutamate and pyroglutamate: facts and fantasies. *Clin Nutr* **12**:66–69.

41. Barbul A (1990) Arginine and immune function. *Nutrition* **6**:53–64.

42. Rudolph FB, Kulkarni AD, Fanslow WC, Pizzini RP, Kumar S and van Buren CT (1990) Role of RNA as a dietary source of pyrimidines and purines in immune fucntion. *Nutrition* **6**:45–52.

43. Grimble GK (1994) Dietary nucleotides and gut mucosal defence. *Gut* **35**(suppl):S46–S51.

44. Schwartz S, Farriol M, Garcia-Arumi E, Andrea AL, Lopez HJ and Arbos MA (1994) Effect of medium chain triglycerides (MCT) on jejunal mucosa mass and protein synthesis. *Gut* **35**(suppl 1): S39–S41.

45. Teo TC, Selleck KM, Wan JM *et al.* (1991) Long term feeding with structured lipid composed of medium chain and N-3 fatty acids ameliorates endotoxic shock in guinea pigs. *Metabolism* **40**: 1152–1159.

46. Kinsella JE and Lakesh B (1990) Dietary lipids, eicosanoids, and the immune system. *Crit Care Med* **18**:S92–S113.

47. Scheppach W, Burghardt W, Bartram P and Kasper H (1990) Addition of dietary fiber to liquid formula diets: the pros and cons. *JPEN* **14**:204–209.

48. Daly JM, Lieberman MD, Goldfine J *et al.* (1992) Enteral nutrition with supplemental arginine, RNA, and omega-3 fatty acids in patients after operation: immunologic, metabolic and clinical outcome. *Surgery* **112**:56–67.

49. Bower RH, Cerra FB, Bershadsky B *et al.* (1995) Early enteral administration of a formula (Impact) supplemented with arginine, nucleotides and fish oil in intensive care unit patients: results of a multicenter, prospective, randomized clinical trial. *Crit Care Med* **23**:436–449.

50. Ziegler TR (1994) Growth hormone administration during nutritional support: what is to be gained? *New Horizons* **2**:244–256.

51. Clemmens DR and Underwood LE (1991) Nutritional regulation of IGF-1 and IGF binding proteins. *Ann Rev Nutr* **11**:393–412.

52. Ulicny KS and Korelitz JL (1989) Multiorgan failure from the inadvertent intravenous administration of enteral feeding. *JPEN* **13**:658–660.

53. Dobb GJ (1990) Enteral nutrition. *Clin Anaesthesiol* **4**:531–557.

54. Dunham CM, Frankenfield D, Belzberg H, Wiles C, Cushing B and Grant Z (1994) Gut failure – predictor of or contributor to mortality in mechanically ventilated blunt trauma patients? *J Trauma* **37**:30–34.

55. Powell K, Marcuard SP, Farrior ES and Gallagher ML (1993) Aspirating gastric residuals causes occlusion of small bore feeding tubes. *JPEN* **17**:243–246.

56. Dobb GJ (1986) Diarrhoea in the critically ill. *Intensive Care Med* **12**:113–115.

57. Bliss DZ, Guenter PA and Settle RG (1992) Defining and reporting diarrhoea in tube fed patients: what a mess. *Am J Clin Nutr* **55**:753–759.

58. Adam SK and Webb AR (1990) Attitudes to the delivery of enteral nutrition support to patients in British intensive care units. *Clin Intensive Care* **1**:150–156.

84 | Parenteral nutrition

GD Phillips

An adequate daily supply of nutrients is necessary for the ICU patient to maintain health and offer resistance against illness. If oral or enteral feeding is inadequate or not possible, then nutrients must be given intravenously. IV feeding may thus be supplementary or complete (i.e. total parenteral nutrition, TPN). Hyperalimentation describes the IV administration of generous amounts of hypertonic glucose with amino acids, but no lipid.[1] Parenteral nutrition in children is discussed in Chapter 104.

The principles of balanced parenteral nutrition have been almost unchanged for the past 25 years. Benefits of special solutions for renal, liver and respiratory failure, stress, trauma and sepsis, and attempts to calculate individual patient requirements more accurately, have not yet been realized. Early proposals on vitamin and trace element requirements have been supported by time. Some new proposals require further evaluation before inclusion in routine practice.

Indications[2–4]

TPN may be indicated in any patient who cannot be fed via the gastrointestinal tract for more than a few days. Indications may be absolute (e.g. a patient with peritonitis, prolonged ileus or total small-bowel resection) or relative (e.g. in preoperative preparation of the cachectic patient or in inflammatory bowel disease, where nutrition may be achieved enterally; Table 84.1). Recommended guidelines[4] provide a useful basis for commencing parenteral nutrition. These guidelines include brief statements and rationale for such issues as nutrition support in critical care, organ failure, intestinal failure, malnutrition, etc. Enteral nutrition (EN) is preferred to parenteral nutrition whenever possible.

There are no absolute contraindications (except for a functioning gut), but renal and hepatic insufficiencies require careful attention in the use of amino acids and lipid. Severe disturbances of lipid metabo-

Table 84.1 Indications for parenteral nutrition[2–4]

Alimentary tract obstruction (e.g. adhesions, carcinoma of oesophagus)
Prolonged ileus (e.g. peritonitis, pancreatitis, post-surgery)
Enterocutaneous fistulae
Malabsorption and short-bowel syndromes
Inflammatory intestinal disease (e.g. Crohn's disease, ulcerative colitis)
Cachexia (e.g. starvation states, carcinoma)
Burns, severe trauma
As an adjunct to chemotherapy
Acute renal failure, hepatic failure
Other hypercatabolic states

lism preclude the use of IV lipid. The decision to progress from TPN to EN should be reviewed daily, since TPN is more expensive and is associated with more complications.

Requirements (Table 84.2)[5]

Water

The normal adult daily water requirement is 30–35 ml/kg. Extra water is required to replace losses such as those from vomiting, diarrhoea, sweating and fever (where approximately 150 ml is added for each 1°C rise). Water gain from metabolism must also be considered in the fluid balance (about 400 ml/day). Water requirements will be influenced by the presence of cardiac, respiratory, renal and hepatic diseases.

Energy and nitrogen[6–15]

Patients with malnutrition but who are physically active may tolerate up to 240 kJ (57 kcal)/kg per 24 h, with an energy (kcal) to nitrogen (g) ratio of 200:1.

Table 84.2 Daily allowances of nutrients and minerals in an adult. Adult allowances/kg body weight per 24 h. Basal allowances cover resting metabolism and some physical activity

Water	30 ml
Energy	125 kJ (30 kcal)
Nitrogen	0.1–0.2 g
Glucose	3 g
Lipid	2 g
Sodium	1.0–2.0 mmol
Potassium	0.7–1 mmol
Calcium	0.1 mmol
Magnesium	0.1 mmol
Phosphorus	0.4 mmol

Modified from Wretlind.[5]

It was common practice to provide such input to stressed, catabolic patients, but many studies now show that the metabolic changes under such conditions result in poor utilization of administered nutrients. Total energy input in the catabolic patient can be as low as 125 kJ (30 kcal)/kg per 24 h, with a calorie : nitrogen ratio of 150:1. Beyond a glucose infusion rate of 6–7 mg/kg per min, there is increased oxygen consumption (Vo_2), CO_2 production, and energy consumption associated with lipogenesis.[16,17]

Lipid should be used to provide 30–40% of non-protein energy input whenever possible. The energy value of lipid is 39 kJ (9.3 kcal)/g compared with 17 kJ (4.1 kcal)/g for carbohydrate. Nitrogen requirements are around 0.2 g/kg per 24 h, equivalent to 1.25 g/kg per 24 h of protein, or 1.5 g/kg per 24 h of amino acids. This may need to be reduced in renal or hepatic failure.

Sources of energy

The two principal sources of energy are carbohydrate and lipid.

Carbohydrate

Glucose is the carbohydrate of choice. It is a physiological substrate required by the brain and metabolized by all body tissues, besides being a prerequisite of protein anabolism. Concentrated solutions of glucose must be given to satisfy the caloric requirements. Most patients increase their endogenous insulin secretion to allow the blood glucose to remain within physiological limits. Diabetics will require added insulin. When insulin production is reduced, as in the early posttraumatic and septic state, infusion of excessive glucose results in lipogenesis with a marked increase in CO_2 production.[16] If

hyperglycaemia occurs, consideration should be given to reducing the glucose infusion rate, rather than adding insulin.

Fructose (laevulose) has been said to offer the advantages of being insulin-independent, less irritant to veins, more rapidly metabolized by the liver and having a better nitrogen-sparing effect. However, only the first few steps of hepatic metabolism are insulin-independent, and the conversion of substrates to glucose requires insulin. In susceptible patients, especially in children, and at high infusion rates, fructose can induce severe lactic acidosis. Parenteral solutions of fructose are no longer available in Australia and some other countries.

Sugar alcohols (e.g. sorbitol and xylitol) have no advantages over glucose. The risks of lactic acidosis, raised serum uric acid and osmotic diuresis have led to xylitol and sorbitol being banned in Australia. Ethanol is likewise unavailable.

Lipid[7–9,17–19]

Lipid provides more energy per unit volume than carbohydrate, and also avoids the complications of excess glucose administration. Lipid is necessary for cell wall integrity, prostaglandin synthesis and function of lipid-soluble vitamins. Manifestations of essential fatty acid (EFA) deficiency such as dermatitis, alopecia, fatty liver and defective immune response can be seen in long-term lipid-free parenteral nutrition. IV lipids are available as emulsions with egg yolk or phospholipids (lecithin) as the emulsifiers, and a sugar or sugar alcohol added. Soybean oil emulsion is better than cotton seed oil emulsion in avoiding adverse effects, although the reasons are unclear. The emulsions are similar in particle size to chylomicrons and are cleared as such by the body. The infusion rate should be limited to 0.5 g/kg per h so as not to exceed a maximum rate of lipid uptake. There is interest currently in the value of infusing fat emulsions containing medium-chain triglycerides in critically ill patients to improve lipid utilization.[18,19] The addition of heparin to facilitate lipid clearance is unnecessary, and may be contraindicated.

Allergic reaction or overloading syndrome[20] described previously with early cottonseed emulsions is rare with soybean oil emulsions. Similarly, previously described complications of long-term use such as anaemia, coagulopathy, impaired liver function and fat pigmentation are not recognized complications of soybean oil emulsions.

The ideal energy contribution from lipid is not known. Lipid given as a sole substrate has no protein-sparing effect. Efficient metabolism of lipid requires adequate carbohydrate intake, but the optimum combination of carbohydrate and lipid as non-protein energy substrates remains to be clarified. In general, it is usual to give 30–40% of the total caloric intake as lipid.

The emulsions are isotonic and can be given via a peripheral vein, or mixed with other ingredients, provided strict guidelines are followed (see below). Bedside determination of lipid clearance can be made by spinning down a blood sample, and visually assessing whether the serum is milky or hyperlipaemic. In patients likely to be lipid-intolerant, serum lipids should be monitored. If lipid cannot be given as a daily calorie source, it should be given twice weekly, to avoid development of EFA deficiency.

Sources of nitrogen

Blood, plasma and albumin are poor nitrogen sources for tissue synthesis because they must first be catabolized to their constituent amino acids, and they do not contain all the essential amino acids (EAA). Nevertheless, plasma proteins need to be given when deficient. Albumin in particular, may be required repeatedly in chronic illness when hypoalbuminaemia is common.

Amino acids occur in two isomeric forms, laevo (L) and dextro (D). With the exception of small amounts of D-methionine and D-phenylalanine, the body can utilize only L-amino acids for protein synthesis. In this way, correctly supplied amino acids will enter the body amino acid pool. Protein hydrolysates and D-racemic amino acid solutions were used before the preferred L-amino acid solutions became widely available.

L-amino acids

Synthetic crystalline amino acid solutions containing the L-form have replaced other solutions. Composition of the solution varies. While the need for EAA is beyond dispute, the optimal amounts of essential and non-essential amino acids still remain unknown. It is widely agreed that the most effective mixture of amino acids is one of high biological value, containing all the essential and most of the non-essential amino acids. A high content of a single non-essential amino acid, especially glycine, must be avoided. Cysteine and histidine are considered necessary in paediatric use. Branched-chain amino acids (BCAA, i.e. isoleucine, leucine and valine) should be present in amounts relatively greater than the other EAA, usually some 25%.[21] However, formulas enriched with BCAA, although slightly improving nitrogen balance in postoperative and trauma patients, do not improve the clinical outcome.[4,22] Table 84.3 lists the composition of two available L-amino acid solutions, but there are many others. For optimal utilization, amino acids should be infused simultaneously with energy sources and potassium.

Table 84.3 Comparison of two amino acid (AA) solutions

	Vamin 14 (Baxter)	Synthamin 17 (Baxter)
Essential AA (g/l)		
Isoleucine	4.2	6.0
Leucine	5.9	7.3
Lysine	6.8	5.8
Methionine	4.2	4.0
Phenylalanine	5.9	5.6
Threonine	4.2	4.2
Tryptophan	1.4	1.8
Valine	5.5	5.8
Semi-essential AA (g/l)		
Cysteine/cystine	0.42	
Histidine	5.1	4.8
Tyrosine	0.17	0.4
Non-essential AA (g/l)		
Arginine	8.4	11.5
Alanine	12	20.7
Proline	5.1	6.8
Aspartic acid	2.5	
Glutamic acid	4.2	
Serine	3.4	5.0
Glycine	5.9	10.3
Electrolytes (mmol)		
Sodium	100	71.5
Potassium	50	60.0
Magnesium	8	5.0
Calcium	5	
Chloride	100	70.0
Phosphorus	0	30.0
Acetate	135	150.0
Total AA (g/l)	83.3	100.0
Total nitrogen (g/l)	13.5	16.5
Osmolality (mosmol/kg)	1145	1260.0
pH (approximate)	5.6	6.0

Vamin 14 and Vamin 18 are available electrolyte-free. Synthamin 9, 13 and 17 are available with and without electrolytes.

Electrolytes

The electrolyte content of amino acid solutions are dissimilar (Table 84.3). The basic recommended daily allowances are shown in Table 84.2, but requirements may vary with the clinical situation. Additional electrolytes are thus frequently necessary. Analysis of urine and gastrointestinal fluid electrolyte content may aid in determining requirements.

Sodium

Excess sodium is to be avoided after injury, since sodium retention may occur. Sodium intake from other sources such as normal (0.9%) saline must be accounted for. An average adult requirement is 1–2 mmol/kg per 24 h.

Potassium

Potassium is essential for protein synthesis, with about 6 mmol/g nitrogen required for optimal amino acid utilization. The requirement for potassium is usually greatest during the first few days of TPN, presumably because of initial deposition in the liver and movement into cells. The basal daily requirement in an adult is 0.7–1.0 mmol/kg per 24 h. Gradual increase in glucose input, with daily monitoring of serum potassium, will minimize the risk of hypokalaemia.

Calcium

Calcium supplements are required in long-term TPN because of continuing endogenous losses from immobilization. Calcium may be required also in certain other conditions such as pancreatitis. An average 24-h supply of 0.1 mmol/kg is sufficient in the adult.

Phosphate

Phosphorus is necessary for bone metabolism, tissue synthesis and phosphorylation of energy bonds (adenosine triphosphate; ATP). Hypophosphataemia occurs early in phosphorus-free TPN. The principal dangers are the decrease in erythrocyte 2,3-diphosphoglycerate, which will result in a decreased oxygen supply to the tissues, and muscle weakness, which may interfere with respiration. Adults may require up to 0.7 mmol/kg per 24 h.

Magnesium

Magnesium is important in anabolism and in enzyme systems, especially those involving the metabolic activity of brain and liver. A normal adult requirement is 0.1 mmol/kg per 24 h, but this is increased in diarrhoea, polyuria, pancreatitis and hypercatabolic states. The main source of magnesium loss is in gastrointestinal fluid.

Chloride and acetate

Some of the crystalline L-amino acid solutions contain large amounts of acetate. When additional sodium or potassium is given, the chloride:acetate ratio of the salts must be balanced; otherwise metabolic acid–base problems may be produced, especially in patients with excessive gastrointestinal fluid loss.

Vitamins and trace elements

In order to supplement available amino acid solutions, additional electrolytes are frequently necessary as well as the following.

Vitamins[23–25]

Vitamins are necessary for the utilization of nutrient components. Deficiencies of water-soluble vitamins can occur rapidly. Vitamin deficiencies may result in development of classic syndromes such as beriberi and scurvy, pellagra and rickets, but the most common reported deficiencies in TPN from a few weeks to 3 months have been folic acid deficiency with pancytopenia, thiamine deficiency with encephalopathy and vitamin K deficiency with hypoprothrombinaemia. IV vitamin requirements are greater than by the oral route, presumably because of greater renal excretion. Vitamin recommendations vary from study to study.

An excess of most water-soluble vitamins can be taken without apparent toxic effects. However, excessive vitamin A and D intake can cause exfoliative dermatitis and hypercalcaemia respectively, and toxicity due to massive doses of some water-soluble vitamins has been reported. Two common parenteral vitamin preparations are listed (Table 84.4). MVI-12 (Rorer) contains both water- and lipid-soluble vitamins, but contains no vitamin K, which must be supplemented in those patients not receiving warfarin therapy.

Table 84.4 Two parenteral vitamin preparations and recommendations

Vitamin	AMA/1975[24] per 24 h	MVI-12 × 10 ml (Rorer)	B Group + C × 4 ml (Nicholas)
Vitamin A mg (IU)	1 (3300)	1 (3300)	0
Vitamin D μg (IU)	5 (200)	5 (200)	0
Vitamin E μg (IU)	10 (10)	10 (10)	0
Vitamin C (mg)	100	100	100
Folic acid (μg)	400	400	0
Nicotinamide (mg)	40	40	100
Riboflavin (mg)	3.6	3.6	10
Thiamine (mg)	3	3	20
Pyridoxine (mg)	4	4	5
Cyanocobalamin (μg)	5	5	0
Pantothenic acid (mg)	15	15	9
Biotin (μg)	60	60	0
Vitamin K (mg)	Not stated	0	0

Trace elements[23,26,27]

Zinc is an essential constituent of many enzymes (e.g. carbonic anhydrase). Deficiencies in zinc, with dermatitis and poor wound healing, are well-recognized, and may develop within a few weeks. *Iron* is essential for haemoglobin synthesis and body reserves are small. *Copper* is important for erythrocyte maturation and lipid metabolism. *Manganese* is important in calcium/phosphorus metabolism, and reproduction and growth. *Cobalt* is an essential constituent of vitamin B_{12}. *Iodine* is required for thyroxine synthesis. *Chromium* is necessary for normal glucose utilization, *molybdenum* is a component of oxidases, and *selenium* of glutathione peroxidase.

The exact requirements of trace elements in TPN still need to be clarified. Two recommendations are given in Table 84.5. For TPN of even a few weeks' duration, it is essential that zinc be given, since losses in the critically ill patient are high. Administration of plasma weekly will not provide adequate amounts of trace elements. The L-amino acid solutions do not contain trace elements, as did the old hydrolysate solutions.

Other additives

Insulin[28]

Insulin may be required when hypertonic glucose is infused, due to inadequate endogenous insulin, or insulin resistance. Attempts to force glucose utilization in the stressed patient may do more harm in promoting lipogenesis with increased CO_2 production. Significant amounts of exogenous insulin can be lost by adsorption to the infusion system. However, administration of insulin in the TPN fluid is safer than giving it separately, in which case hypoglycaemia may occur if the TPN infusion stops.

Heparin[29]

Heparin addition has been recommended to decrease the risk of venous thrombosis, but its value is controversial.

Planning a regimen

Regimens are best planned over a 24-h period. The patient's requirements are estimated, and the available nutrient solutions are then considered in order to choose the most appropriate solutions in the right proportions. Tabulating all the constituents will aid in the planning (Table 84.6). Modifications for use in renal failure and hepatic disease, and the use of amino acids as the sole substrate, are discussed below.

Table 84.5 Trace element recommendations (μg/24 h)

Trace element	AMA 1979[26]	Shenkin[23]
Iron	Not stated	1100
Zinc	2500–6000	6400
Copper	500–1500	1300
Iodine	Not stated	130–910
Manganese	150–800	270
Fluoride	Not stated	950
Chromium	10–15	10
Selenium	Not stated	200
Molybdenum	Not stated	20

Table 84.6 A regimen for total parenteral nutrition via a central vein

Infuse at 83 ml/h	H_2O (ml)	Energy (kJ)	CHO (g)	Protein (g)	Fat (g)	Na^+ (mmol)	K^+ (mmol)	Ca^{2+} (mmol)	Mg^{2+} (mmol)	P^- (mmol)
Solution 1										
500 ml Synthamin 17 and	500	–	–	50	–	35	30	–	2.5	15
500 ml Dextrose 30%	500	4300	250	–	–	–	–	–	–	–
with additives:										
Na^+						25				
Ca^{2+}								2.0		
Solution 1: Repeated	1000	4300	250	50	–	60	30	2.0	2.5	15
Solution 2: 500 ml Intralipid 20%	500	4200	–	–	100 + 22.5 g glycerol	–	–	–	–	+
24-h Total	2500	12 800	500	100	100	120	60	4.0	5	30

Vitamins and trace elements may be added to solution 1 in recommended amounts (see Tables 84.4 and 84.5).

Acute renal failure[4,30,31]

Parenteral nutrition is helpful in acute renal failure, a state of hypercatabolism. In order to be effective, certain criteria must be met:

1 adequate calories in a low volume load;
2 minimal rise in blood urea nitrogen;
3 low potassium content;
4 stringent sepsis control.

There is a disturbance of both glucose and lipid metabolism in acute renal failure. Concentrated glucose and lipid can be used if carefully monitored. Dialysis and improvements in blood biochemistry will improve the utilization of nutrients. Lipid may interfere with haemodialysis.

Amino acids should be limited to 0.5 g/kg per 24 h initially. All EAA need to be supplied. Endogenous urea can be utilized, although inefficiently, for non-essential amino acids. The synthetic L-amino acid solutions may be used. The electrolyte-free preparations are particularly useful. Loss of amino acids will occur if administered during dialysis.

Hepatic failure[4,30,32]

Lipid can be metabolized in jaundiced patients, but should be used cautiously in hepatic failure. The bulk of the caloric intake should be supplied as hypertonic glucose. Protein intake should be limited to 0.5 g/kg per 24 h, or eliminated in hepatic coma.

Respiratory failure[4,30,33]

Patients with respiratory muscle weakness, debilitation and/or pre-existing chronic respiratory disease are at risk of respiratory failure in acute illness. The infusion of excess glucose results in lipogenesis and a marked increase in CO_2 production. This effect is minimized if up to 50% of non-protein calories are provided from lipid.

Central venous infusion

Catheter and infusion set[34,35]

Central venous catheters are most commonly inserted percutaneously into the subclavian vein. Strict aseptic techniques of catheter insertion and care must be observed. Catheter dressing should be performed at least every alternate day with application of povidone-iodine at the wound site. Gauze dressings, if used, should be changed immediately they become wet. The use of a clear sterile dressing over the catheter site is recommended. The catheter is changed for specific reasons (e.g. wound infection or septicaemia). Catheters of different materials and varied placement techniques are continually being evaluated. Presently, the most commonly used catheter is

the polyurethane catheter inserted over a guide wire.

The infusion set is changed with the dressing, or after use of blood and blood products. The whole infusion system should be used only for TPN and no other purpose (e.g. blood sampling). Unnecessary manipulation of infusion lines and use of three-way stopcocks are to be discouraged. The efficacy of in-line bacterial filters is debatable, and their use is not possible when lipid-containing solutions are used. Use of a pump to regulate administration rate may be indicated.

Solutions

Parenteral nutrition solutions are best prepared under sterile conditions in the hospital pharmacy.[36,37] Such pre-mixed single unit solutions can be tailor-made daily to meet individual patient requirements, and are now being produced commercially. If such facilities are unavailable, glucose and amino acids can be administered simultaneously using Y-connections, twin giving sets and closed mixing chambers. Lipid emulsions may be mixed with other nutrient solutions, provided strict guidelines are followed, to avoid disturbing the stability of the emulsion. For central venous administration, it is thus possible to administer a high-calorie, balanced-energy, nitrogen-loaded single solution, with all necessary minerals, trace elements and vitamins added.

Peripheral intravenous infusion[38,39]

Peripheral infusion of isotonic amino acids without additional energy has been advocated to minimize nitrogen loss under conditions of negative energy balance. Energy requirement is provided by mobilization of body lipid and the ketone bodies produced by lipid catabolism. The weight loss which then occurs is derived from lipid and not muscle mass. This method may be helpful in postoperative patients in the short term (although true benefits are controversial), but has no place in complete parenteral nutrition. An alternative approach is to add lipid and a low concentration of glucose to the amino acids, so that the osmolality remains < 800 mosmol/kg.

Monitoring[40–42]

Assessment of progress and avoidance of metabolic complications are best achieved by a regular monitoring protocol (Table 84.7). Lipid in the serum can interfere with biochemical and haematological estimations. Blood sampling is best avoided following a recent lipid infusion, or during the infusion. Daily nitrogen balance can be estimated from the nitrogen loss as calculated by the sum of the urinary urea excretion, proteinuria and rise in blood urea, although

Table 84.7 Parenteral nutrition – relevant monitoring

Regular clinical
Nursing observations
   Temperature
   Blood pressure
   Pulse rate
   Respiratory rate
   Fluid balance

Regular ward testing
Medical assessment
   Urinalysis
   Dextrostix
   Reflectance meter
   Blood glucose

Daily (at least)
Fluid balance review
Nutrient input review
Biochemistry
   Serum electrolytes
   Serum urea/creatinine
   Blood glucose

Weekly (at least)
Complete blood count
Coagulation screen
Weight
Liver function tests
Serum calcium/magnesium/phosphate

As indicated
Serum lipids
Urine zinc
Serum uric acid
Blood gases
24-h urinary urea, electrolytes, osmolality

Special circumstances
Nitrogen balance
Body composition
Body protein turnover
Gas exchange measurements
Trace element balance
Vitamin assays

using this as a basis for calculating amino acid requirements is debatable.

Complications[34,43–47]

Parenteral nutrition is not a technique for the inexperienced or occasional therapist. Complications can be severe if not lethal, and can only be minimized if parenteral nutrition is carried out by experienced clinicians as a team effort. Important complications of TPN are described below.

Catheter complications[34,46]

Complications relating to central venous catheters include pneumothorax, vessel perforation, thrombosis and air or catheter embolism. Infection remains the biggest problem. The need for careful aseptic techniques and regulations is emphasized.[48]

Fluid overload

Circulatory overload may result from excessive fluid infusion, especially in the elderly and those with heart failure and renal insufficiency.

Hyperosmolar dehydration syndrome

This is attributable to allowing hyperglycaemia to occur. Consistent urine glucose levels greater than 2% and sudden increases in urine volume are warnings of osmotic diuresis. Blood glucose levels should normally not exceed 11 mmol/l. Serum osmolality estimations are necessary in difficult cases.

Electrolyte imbalances

Electrolyte imbalances may occur, especially hypokalaemia in the first 24–48 h, and hypomagnesaemia in the patient with gastrointestinal fluid loss.

Hypophosphataemia

Hypophosphataemia may occur, especially in the first 24–48 h.

Metabolic acidosis

Metabolic acidosis from amino acid solutions may be due to a large amount of hydrochlorides, a high titratable acidity or an excess of cationic amino acids which produce excess H^+ ions when metabolized. Clinically, metabolic acidosis does not present a problem and can be reduced with the use of bicarbonate or acetate salts.

Hyperammonaemia

Hyperammonaemia in parenteral nutrition has been described, particularly in infants and patients with liver failure. Hyperammonaemia has occurred with crystalline amino acid solutions containing excessive glycine or inadequate arginine concentrations

Essential fatty acid deficiency syndrome

See above.

Rebound hypoglycaemia[45]

Parenteral nutrition infusions should not be stopped suddenly, as hypoglycaemia may occur due to the high level of endogenous insulin, although this is probably rare. Patients should be gradually weaned off TPN over a period of 12 h using 10% glucose. A blocked catheter should be replaced immediately, or a peripheral infusion of 10% glucose commenced.

Vitamin and trace elements deficiencies[49]

See above.

Liver dysfunction

Liver dysfunction may occur for a number of reasons. Some abnormality of liver function tests is common during TPN.[47]

Pharmaceutical considerations[36,37]

Involvement of a pharmacist can minimize complications associated with interactions and incompatibilities in the mixtures, fluid contamination during preparation and mistakes in TPN orders. Classic examples are calcium phosphate precipitation, cracking of lipid emulsion, instability of vitamins[25,50] and precipitation or loss of activity of antibiotics.

Other clinical considerations

The aim of parenteral nutrition is to provide adequate nutrition until it can be replaced by adequate oral nutrition.[51-54] Transition from IV to oral feeding should be gradual, otherwise diarrhoea may result. Early mobilization of the patient is important. Apart from the other well-known advantages, it aids anabolism.

References

1. Dudrick SJ, Wilmore DW, Vars HM and Rhoads JE (1968) Long-term total parenteral nutrition with growth, development, and positive nitrogen balance. *Surgery* **64**:134–142.
2. Phillips GD (1985) Total parenteral nutrition in acute illness. *Anaesth Intens Care* **13**:288–299.
3. Shaw JHF (1986) Recent advances in the nutritional and metabolic management of critically ill surgical patients. *NZ Med J* **99**:655–667.
4. ASPEN Board of Directors (1993) Guidelines for the use of parenteral and enteral nutrition in adults and pediatric patients. *J Parent Enteral Nutr* **17**(suppl):1SA–51SA
5. Wretlind A (1978) Parenteral nutrition. *Surg Clin North Am* **58**:1055–1070.
6. Hill GL and Church J (1984) Energy and protein requirements of general surgical patients requiring intravenous nutrition. *Br J Surg* **71**:1–9.
7. Long CL (1987) Fuel preferences in the septic patient: glucose or lipid? *J Parent Ent Nutr* **11**:333–335.
8. Nordenstrom J, Askanazi J, Elwyn DH *et al.* (1983) Nitrogen balance during total parenteral nutrition. Glucose vs fat. *Ann Surg* **197**:27–33.
9. Nanni G, Siebel JH, Coleman D, Fader P and Castiglione R (1984) Increased lipid fuel dependence in the critically ill septic patient. *J Trauma* **24**:14–29.
10. Long CL, Kinney JM and Gieger JW (1976) Non-suppressibility of gluconeogenesis by glucose in septic patients. *Metabolism* **25**:193–200.
11. Quebbeman EJ, Ausman RK and Schweider TC (1982) An evaluation of energy expenditure during parenteral nutrition. *Ann Surg* **195**:282–286.
12. Pellett PL (1990) Food and energy requirements in humans. *Am J Clin Nutr* **51**:711–722.
13. Tracy KJ, Legaspi A, Albert JD *et al.* (1988) Protein and substrate metabolism during starvation and parenteral refeeding. *Clin Sci* **74**:123–132.
14. Konstantinides FN, Konstantinides NN, Li JC, Myaya ME and Cerra FB (1991) Urinary urea nitrogen. Too insensitive for calculating nitrogen balance studies in surgical clinical nutrition. *J Parent Enteral Nutr* **15**:189–193.
15. Frankenfield DC, Omert LA, Badellino MM *et al.* (1994) Correlation between measured energy expenditure and clinically obtained variables in trauma and sepsis patients. *J Parent Enteral Nutr* **18**:398–403.
16. Wolfe RR, O'Donnell TF, Stone MD, Richmond DA and Burke JF (1980) Investigation of factors determining the optimal glucose infusion rate in total parenteral nutrition. *Metabolism* **29**:892–900.
17. Askanazi J, Nordenstrom J, Rosenbaum SH *et al.* (1981) Nutrition for the patient with respiratory failure: glucose vs fat. *Anesthesiology* **54**:373–377.
18. Radermacher P, Santak B, Strobach H, Schrör K and Tarnow J (1992) Fat emulsions containing medium chain triglycerides in patients with sepsis syndrome: effect on pulmonary hemodynamics and gas exchange. *Intens Care Med* **18**:231–234.
19. Ball MJ (1993) Parenteral nutrition in the critically ill: use of a medium chain triglyceride emulsion. *Intens Care Med* **19**:89–95.
20. Solomons SM and Kirby DF (1990) The refeeding syndrome. A review. *J Parent Enteral Nutr* **14**:90–97.
21. Brennan MF, Cerra F, Daly JM *et al.* (1986) Report of a research workshop: branched-chain amino acids in stress and injury. *J Parent Ent Nutr* **10**:446–452.
22. Vente JP, Soeters PB, von Meyenfeldt MF, Rouflart MMJ, Van der Linden CJ and Guoma DJ (1991) Prospective randomised double-blind trial of branched chain amino acid enriched versus standard parenteral nutrition solutions in traumatized and septic patients. *World J Surg* **15**:128–133.
23. Shenkin A (1986) Vitamin and essential trace element recommendations during intravenous nutrition: theory and practice. *Proc Nutr Soc* **45**:383–390.
24. Nutritional Advisory Group, Department of Food and Nutrition, American Medical Association (1975) Statement on multivitamin preparations for parenteral use. Chicago: AMA. Cited in: Multivitamin preparations for practical use. *J Parent Ent Nutr* **3**:258–262.
25. Nordfjeld K, Pedersen JL, Rasmussen M and Jensen UG (1984) Storage of mixtures for total parenteral nutrition. III: Stability of vitamins in TPN mixtures. *J Clin Hosp Pharm* **9**:293–301.

26. Expert Panel, AMA Department of Foods and Nutrition (1979) Guidelines for essential trace element preparations for parenteral use. *J Am Med Assoc* **241**:2051–2054.

27. Wolman SJ, Anderson GH, Marliss EB and Jejeebhoy KN (1979) Zinc in total parenteral nutrition: requirements and metabolic effects. *Gastroenterology* **76**:458–467.

28. Marcuard SP, Dunham B, Hobbs A and Caro JF (1990) Availability of insulin from total parenteral nutrition solutions. *J Parent Enteral Nutr* **14**:262–264.

29. D'Angio R, Quercia R, Orlando R, Nightingale C and Drezner D (1987) The effect of heparin on the clearance of intravenous lipid emulsion in critically ill surgical patients. *J Parent Enteral Nutr* **11**(suppl):19S.

30. Panel Report (1981) Nutritional support of patients with liver, renal and cardiopulmonary diseases. *Am J Clin Nutr* **34**:1235–1245.

31. Mirtallo JM, Schneider PJ, Mauko K, Ruberg RL and Fabri PJ (1982) A comparison of essential and general amino acid infusions in the nutritional support of patients with compromised renal function. *J Parent Enteral Nutr* **6**:109–113.

32. Kanematsu T, Koyanagi N, Matsumata T, Kitano S, Takenaka K and Sugimachi K (1988) Lack of preventive effect of branched-chain amino acid solutions on post-operative hepatic encephalopathy in patients with cirrhosis: a randomized prospective trial. *Surgery* **104**:482–488.

33. Van den Berg B, Bogaard JM and Hop WCJ (1994) High fat, low carbohydrate enteral feeding in patients weaning from the ventilator. *Intensive Care Med* **20**:470–475.

34. Ryan JA, Abel RM, Abbott WM *et al.* (1974) Catheter complications in total parenteral nutrition: a prospective study of 200 consecutive patients. *N Engl J Med* **290**:757–761.

35. Murphy LM and Lipman TO (1987) Central venous catheter care: a review. *J Parent Ent Nutr* **11**:190–201.

36. Niemiec PW and Vanderveen TW (1984) Compatibility considerations in parenteral nutrient solutions. *Am J Hosp Pharm* **41**:893–911.

37. Lawrence RT, Flukes WK and Braithwaite PA (1981) Total parenteral nutrition using a combined nutrient. *Aust J Hosp Pharm* **11**:40–42.

38. Payne-James JJ and Khawaja HT (1993) First choice for total parenteral nutrition: the peripheral route. *J Parent Enteral Nutr* **17**:468–478.

39. Stokes MA and Hill GL (1993) Peripheral parenteral nutrition: a preliminary report on its efficacy and safety. *J Parent Enteral Nutr* **17**:145–147.

40. Marshall WJ and Mitchell PEG (1987) Total parenteral nutrition and the clinical chemistry laboratory. *Ann Clin Biochem* **24**:327–336.

41. Westonskow DR, Cutler CA and Wallace WD (1984) Instrumentation for monitoring gas exchange and metabolism in critically ill patients. *Crit Care Med* **12**:183–187.

42. Silberman H and Silberman AW (1986) Parenteral nutrition, biochemistry and respiratory gas exchange. *J Parent Enteral Nutr* **10**:151–154.

43. Wolfe BM, Ryder MA, Nishikawa RA, Halsted CH and Schmidt BF (1986) Complications of parenteral nutrition. *Am J Surg* **152**:93–99.

44. Freund HR (1991) Abnormalities of liver function with total parenteral nutrition. *Nutrition* **7**:1–5.

45. Wagman LD, Miller KB, Thomas RB, Newsome HH and Weir GC (1986) The effect of acute discontinuation of total parenteral nutrition. *Ann Surg* **204**:524–529.

46. Inove Y, Nezu R, Matsuda H *et al.* (1992) Prevention of catheter-related sepsis during parenteral nutrition: effect of a new connection device. *J Parent Enteral Nutr* **16**:581–585.

47. Buchmiller CE, Kleiman-Wexler RL, Epherave KS, Booth B and Hensley CE II (1993) Liver dysfunction and energy source: results of a standardized clinical trial. *J Parent Enteral Nutr* **17**:301–306.

48. McGee WT, Ackerman BL, Rouben LR, Prasad VM, Bandi V and Mallory DL (1993) Accurate placement of central venous catheters: a prospective, randomized, multi-center trial. *Crit Care Med* **21**:1118–1123.

49. Wasa M, Satani M, Tanano H, Nezu R, Takagi Y and Okada A (1994) Copper deficiency with pancytopenia during total parenteral nutrition. *J Parent Enteral Nutr* **18**:190–192.

50. Smith JL, Canham JE and Wells PA (1988) Effect of phototherapy light, sodium bisulfite, and pH on vitamin stability in total parenteral nutrition solutions. *J Parent Enteral Nutr* **12**:394–402.

51. Phillips GD and Odgers CL (1986) *Parenteral and Enteral Nutrition: A Practical Guide*, 3rd edn. Edinburgh: Churchill Livingstone.

52. ASPEN (1986) Guidelines for use of total parenteral nutrition in the hospitalised adult patient. *J Parent Enteral Nutr* **10**:441–445.

53. Christman JW and McCain W (1993) A sensible approach to the nutritional support of mechanically ventilated critically ill patients. *Intensive Care Med* **19**:129–136.

54. Heyland DK, Cook DJ and Guyatt GH (1993) Enteral nutrition in the critically ill patient: a critical review of the evidence. *Intensive Care Med* **19**:435–442.

Multiple organ dysfunction

IKS Tan and TE Oh

Successful resuscitation and support of the critically ill patient have allowed the emergence of a syndrome characterized by progressive dysfunction of several independent organ systems. The term *multiple organ dysfunction syndrome* (MODS) best describes the spectrum of derangement that may occur.[1] Various parameters can more accurately quantify the degree of dysfunction, but the use of these as criteria to define *organ failure* is arbitrary and varied. Also, failure of organ systems such as the gut are difficult to define. The older term multiple organ failure is thus unsatisfactory.

MODS typifies the *raison d'être* of an ICU. It is the leading cause of death in non-coronary ICUs, with mortality rates well over 50%.[2] MODS results in prolonged ICU stays and great emotional and financial costs. There is no specific treatment and prevention of MODS is thus crucial.

Pathogenesis

Systemic inflammation

MODS is thought to result from an uncontrolled systemic inflammatory and stress response gen-erated by an initial insult[3] (Fig. 85.1). The initial insult can be any severe illness, such as infection, trauma, burns, pancreatitis and prolonged shock. This initial insult may occasionally directly cause a primary multiple organ dysfunction from tissue ischaemia, ischaemia–reperfusion injury or direct cell damage.

The host response to stress includes inflammation (local and systemic), release of stress hormones, cardiovascular and pulmonary changes and activation of contact, complement, coagulation and fibrinolytic systems. An uncontrolled, persistent host stress response, even without a primary multiple organ dysfunction, results in a secondary MODS. The systemic inflammatory response is the major component of the host stress response that leads to MODS.[4] In MODS, the erstwhile beneficial inflammatory response becomes autodestructive.

Tumour necrosis factor (TNF) is a central cytokine in the genesis of the systemic inflammatory response and organ injury.[5] After endotoxin challenge, TNF concentrations increase and peak before other mediators. The administration of monoclonal antibodies against TNF may improve survival and attenuates the increase in other mediators (see

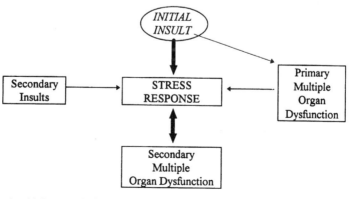

Fig. 85.1 Pathogenesis of multiple organ dysfunction syndrome.

below). TNF injection reproduces the features of the septic response, such as hypermetabolism and shock.

Many other products, including interleukin (IL) IL-1, IL-6, IL-8, interferon-γ, colony-stimulating factors and platelet-activating factor, participate in the inflammatory response with multiple effects and complex interactions. Some appear to mitigate rather than augment inflammation, such as C1 esterase inhibitor, IL-1 receptor antagonist and heat shock proteins.

Cytokines and other products of the inflammatory response activate integrins on leukocytes, leading to strong adhesion to the endothelium. Following migration into tissue, leukocytes produce oxygen-derived free radicals, proteases and arachidonic acid metabolites (i.e. leukotrienes, thromboxanes and protaglandins). These terminal effectors damage endothelium, cell membranes and intracellular organelles throughout the body, and add to the inflammatory process in addition to causing organ dysfunction.

Continuing ischaemia

Ongoing tissue ischaemia from blood flow maldistribution, disseminated intravascular coagulation (DIC), intravascular volume loss and tissue oedema cause further organ dysfunction. Gut ischaemia may result in bacterial translocation and endotoxin release into the circulation, augmenting systemic inflammation. The gut has been termed the motor of multiorgan failure.[6] Inadequate oxygen delivery can lead to anaerobic metabolism and inadequate production of adenosine triphosphate (ATP) and other high-energy phosphates, contributing to organ dysfunction. However, the existence of a *systemic* pathological supply-dependency of oxygen consumption on oxygen delivery, and the implied widespread cellular hypoxia, is doubtful.[7,8] Direct monitoring of intracellular pH and high-energy phosphate concentration during sepsis in a number of organs do not show a fall indicative of hypoxia.[7] Every study in which oxygen delivery and consumption were determined independently has not shown dependence of oxygen consumption on oxygen delivery[8] (see Chapter 22).

Altered metabolism

Altered metabolism contributes to organ dysfunction (see Chapter 82). Interleukin-1, TNF, related cytokines and hormonal changes trigger extreme protein catabolism, termed autocannibalism.[2] Loss of muscle has functional consequences. A 25% body weight loss in the setting of injury may be fatal. Wound healing and multiple facets of host defence are impaired, increasing the risk of nosocomial infection. Mitochondrial abnormalities may limit cell energy production.[9] The ketone body ratio (acetoacetate β-hydroxybutyrate ratio) reflects liver mitochondrial redox

potential, and a ratio of less than 0.4 is typical of multiorgan failure.

Clinical features

There are fever, tachycardia, tachypnoea and leukocytosis with systemic inflammation. Some patients may respond with lowered temperature or white cell count. If the initial insult causes shock from volume loss or cytokine-induced vasodilatation, there is early evidence of acute respiratory and renal failure, ischaemic hepatitis and DIC. A common pattern is one in which resuscitation is apparently adequate, but signs of acute lung injury develop in 24–72 h. Deterioration of other organ systems follows.

Acute lung injury is the commonest manifestation of MODS. Inflammatory injury of the alveolar epithelium and endothelium results in pulmonary oedema. There are hypoxaemia and respiratory distress and the chest X-ray shows consolidation (see Chapter 29).

Cytokines increase nitric oxide production through the induced form of nitric oxide synthase, leading to hypotension.[10] Increased endothelial permeability with loss of circulating volume and the effects of kinins and other vasodilators also contribute to hypotension. With resuscitation, increase in cardiac index and oxygen delivery occur.[11] The left ventricle dilates and myocardial contractility is depressed.[12] Maldistribution of blood flow occurs at the regional as well as the microcirculatory level. Splanchnic ischaemia may manifest as stress ulcer bleeding, ileus, hepatitis, acalculous cholecystitis and pancreatitis.[13] DIC will contribute to tissue ischaemia as well as bleeding.

Encephalopathy is very common and correlates with mortality in sepsis.[14] Heterogeneous neuropathies and myopathies may occur in the setting of multiorgan failure, with a reported incidence of 22 out of 23 patients studied.[15]

Marked protein catabolism with rapid reduction in muscle mass occurs. This is obscured by the generalized oedema that accompanies systemic inflammation and fluid resuscitation. Hyperglycaemia results from increased gluconeogenesis and impaired glucose clearance. Lipolysis increases plasma glycerol and free fatty acids. Ketone levels are low. With progression of MODS, hypertriglyceridaemia occurs from reduced triglyceride clearance, and preterminally gluconeogenesis fails, causing hypoglycaemia.[16]

Oliguric renal failure and liver failure herald impending death. Deleterious organ interactions may occur with renal and liver failure, Kupffer cell dysfunction and impaired drug and intermediary metabolism. Further bacterial translocation and endotoxaemia result and a vicious cycle develops.[3,17]

Normally, the hypermetabolism peaks on the third to fifth day post-insult, and abates by days 7–10.

During recovery, temperature and the hyperdynamic circulation return to normal values. A spontaneous diuresis ensues and azotaemia resolves. Long-term pulmonary fibrosis can complicate acute lung injury.

Management

The goals of management are resuscitation, source control and organ system and metabolic support. These goals are discussed separately but must be undertaken concurrently. Prompt resuscitation and definitive control of precipitating factors (see below) are vital in the prevention of organ dysfunction. With progression, the prospect of reversal decreases, and management is non-specific and supportive only. Treatable causes of organ dysfunction must be excluded.

Resuscitation

End-points of resuscitation

Normal values of physiological parameters in response to a severe insult appear inadequate in ensuring optimal survival. Survival from severe trauma[18] as well as septic shock[11] is associated with supranormal values of cardiac index, oxygen delivery and oxygen consumption. However, global indices of oxygen delivery may not reflect regional variations in perfusion and oxygen delivery,[19] and use of supra-normal values as end-point indices are controversial (see Chapter 22). Gastric intramucosal pH may be a more reliable index of outcome than systemic indices of oxygen delivery.[20-22] Therapy aimed at maintaining gastric intramucosal pH more than 7.35 may improve survival in critically ill patients.[23]

Methods of resuscitation

Rapid normalization of clinical signs and achievement of the end-points of resuscitation are associated with improved survival. Taking longer than 24 h attain supranormal circulatory values will increase mortality in traumatized patients.[18] Aggressive volume loading of more than 40 ml/kg within the first hour can improve survival in paediatric patients with septic shock.[24] Achieving and maintaining a hyper-dynamic state minimize the possibility of an oxygen debt or perfusion deficit. Since colloids restore circulating volume faster than crystalloids, an argument may be made for its early use. The use of hypertonic solutions[25] requires more experience. Use of red cell transfusion to improve oxygen delivery does not improve oxygen consumption significantly.[26] Vasoactive agents have differing effects on various tissue beds. The effect of a given inotrope on splanchnic perfusion is unpredictable, and close monitoring is required. Dopexamine appears to have

a favourable effect on the splanchnic circulation.[27] With severe hypotension, vasopressors such as adrenaline or noradrenaline may be used.

Control of precipitating factors

The initial insult and the factors that perpetuate MODS must be controlled. Suspicion of infection requires an aggressive search for the source leading to urgent treatment. Appropriate antibiotics at the earliest possible time are crucial in improving survival.[28] In the setting of trauma, bleeding needs prompt control. Aggressive resuscitation before definitive control of bleeding may worsen survival,[29] emphasizing the importance of prompt surgery. Early fracture fixation[30] and early burn excision[31] can reduce the incidence of sepsis and MODS, and may improve survival.

Organ system and metabolic support

Treatment is largely supportive in established MODS, since measures directed against components of the inflammatory response remain experimental. Nosocomial infections and iatrogenic complications must be guarded against. Invasive monitoring devices and interventions should be minimized.

Cardiovascular failure

Other causes of hypotension must be excluded. Covert as well as overt shock should be guarded against with continuous monitoring.

Respiratory failure

Acute lung injury has an extensive differential diagnosis. The possibilities of nosocomial pneumonia or fluid overload must be evaluated. Mechanical ventilatory support, by reducing the work of breathing, can beneficially divert oxygen delivery to other tissue beds in need. This is balanced against the overall reduction in cardiac output with positive-pressure ventilation and the risk of ventilator-associated lung injury.

Haematological support

Haematological support is required in DIC (see Chapter 89).

Renal failure

Azotaemia may be due to prerenal, renal or postrenal causes. Renal perfusion and urine output should be maintained with fluid therapy. Inotropic support is needed if the patient is hypotensive. Renal-dose dopamine may be detrimental.[32] Renal replacement therapy should be started early. Continuous renal replacement therapies allow gentle and progressive correction of fluid, electrolyte and acid–base imbalance, provision of space for nutrition, as well as blood purification. Filtration of pathogenic mediators is also achieved[33] (see Chapter 38).

Metabolic support and nutrition (see Chapters 83 and 84)

The goal of metabolic support is to obtain nitrogen equilibrium rather than isocaloric equilibrium.[2] Overfeeding can increase mortality,[34] as can malnutrition. Enteral nutrition is preferred over parenteral nutrition as blood flow to the gut mucosa is stimulated, maintaining gut barrier function and reducing infectious complications.[35] Early enteral nutrition has also been shown to decrease liver dysfunction, hospital length of stay and cost. Enteral formulae are complete and better balanced than parenteral formulations. Vitamin E, zinc, Ω_3 fatty acids, glutamine, arginine and nucleic acid supplementation of nutrition are all under active investigation.[36] It is likely that the quality of nutrients can favourably influence the metabolic response to stress.[37] Administration of growth hormone can improve nitrogen balance[38] and reduce body protein, potassium and phosphorus losses. The effect of growth hormone administration on muscle function, e.g. weaning from ventilatory support and rehabiliation, is presently unclear.

Reduce stress response

Measures should be undertaken to reduce detrimental host stress responses and unnecessary requirements for oxygen consumption. This includes appropriate sedation, analgesia, prevention of hypothermia, removal of residual foci of inflammation and avoidance of secondary insults such as catheter-related sepsis.

Experimental therapies

If systemic inflammation is the major factor in the pathogenesis of secondary MODS, it follows that organ dysfunction is unlikely to be reversed simply by better resuscitation. Anti-inflammatory and anti-cytokine therapy has generated considerable research effort. The brief duration, paracrine nature and often beneficial effects of cytokines work against the success of this approach.

The use of monoclonal anti-TNF in patients with septic shock has a non-significant 17% reduction in 28-day mortality.[39] No significant reduction in 28-day mortality was also reported with the use of IL-1 receptor antagonist in septic patients.[40] Ibuprofen has not been useful[41] and corticosteroids are dangerous.[42] Antagonists to platelet-activating factor and phospholipase A_2 are under investigation. Inhibitors of neutrophil adherence to endothelium may be harmful.[43] Conversely, augmenting neutrophil function with granulocyte colony-stimulating factor may be beneficial.[44] The use of antioxidants, *N*-acetyl cysteine, ATP-MgCl$_2$ and inhibitors of nitric oxide synthase require more research.

Prognosis

Better results may be achieved if patients at high risk for MODS can be identified so that MODS can be prevented by timely resuscitation and control of precipitating factors. Risk factors vary depending on the initial insult. Indices of the severity of the initial insult such as the injury severity score and the need for blood transfusions are predictive of MODS in the setting of trauma.[45] Failure of an organ system is also determined by the functional reserve of the organ, so that associated variables such as age may be predictive.

Mortality associated with each individual organ failure is quite high, and rises cumulatively with the number of failing organs. Failure of three or more organs persisting after 3 days has a 98% mortality.[46] Clearly, there are patients who will not benefit from intensive care. Justice in the fair distribution of finite health resources should also determine the decision to limit or withdraw therapy, as should patient autonomy. It remains for each society, the ICU and the individual patient–doctor relationship to resolve these issues.

References

1. Bone RC, Balk RA, Cerra F *et al.* (1992) Definitions for sepsis and organ failure and guidelines for the use of innovative therapies in sepsis. *Chest* **101**:1644–1655.
2. Beal AL and Cerra FB (1994) Multiple organ failure syndrome in the 1990s; systemic inflammatory response and organ dysfunction. *J Am Med Assoc* **271**:226–233.
3. Demling R, LaLonde C, Saldinger P and Knox J (1993) Multiple-organ dysfunction in the surgical patient: pathophysiology, prevention, and treatment. *Curr Probl Surg* **30**:345–424.
4. Border JR (1988) Hypothesis: sepsis, multiple organ failure, and the macrophage. *Arch Surg* **123**:285–286.
5. Deitch EA (1994) Cytokines yes, cytokines no, cytokines maybe? *Crit Care Med* **24**:817–819.
6. Marshall JC, Christou NV and Meakins JL (1993) The gastrointestinal tract: the 'undrained' abscess of multiple organ failure. *Ann Surg* **218**:111–119.
7. Hotchkiss RS and Karl IE (1992) Reevaluation of the role of cellular hypoxia and bioenergetic failure in sepsis. *J Am Med Assoc* **267**:1503–1510.
8. Russell JA and Phang PT (1994) The oxygen delivery/consumption controversy. Approaches to management of the critically ill. *Am J Respir Crit Care Med* **149**:533–537.

9. Dong Y, Sheng C, Herndon D and Waymack JP (1992) Metabolic abnormalities of mitochondrial redox potential in post burn multiple system organ failure. *Burns* **18**:283–286.

10. Lorente JA, Landin L, dePablo R, Renes E and Liste D (1993) L-arginine pathway in the sepsis syndrome. *Crit Care Med* **21**:1287–1295.

11. Shoemaker WC, Appel PL, Kram HB, Bishop MH and Abraham E (1993) Sequence of physiological patterns in surgical septic shock. *Crit Care Med* **21**:1876–1889.

12. Parillo JE, Parker MM, Natanson C *et al.* (1990) Septic shock in humans. Advances in the understanding of pathogenesis, cardiovascular dysfunction, and therapy. *Ann Intern Med* **113**:227–242.

13. Bersten A and Sibbald WJ (1989) Circulatory disturbances in multiple systems organ failure. *Crit Care Clin* **5**:233–254.

14. Bolton CF, Young GB and Zochodne DW (1993) The neurological complications of sepsis. *Ann Neurol* **33**:94–100.

15. Coakley JH, Nagendran K, Honavar M and Hinds CJ (1993) Preliminary observations on the neuromuscular abnormalities in patients with organ failure and sepsis. *Intensive Care Med* **19**:323–328.

16. Cerra FB (1989) Metabolic manifestations of multiple systems organ failure. *Crit Care Clin* **5**:119–125.

17. Hawker F (1991) Liver dysfunction in critical illness. *Anaesth Intens Care* **19**:165–181.

18. Bishop MH, Shoemaker WC, Appel PL *et al.* (1993) Relationship between supranormal circulatory values, time delays, and outcome in severely traumatized patients. *Crit Care Med* **21**:56–63.

19. Ruokonen E, Takala J, Kari A, Saxen H, Mertsola J and Hansen EJ (1993) Regional blood flow and oxygen transport in septic shock. *Crit Care Med* **21**:1296–1303.

20. Maynard N, Bihari D, Beale R *et al.* (1993) Assessment of splanchnic oxygenation by gastric tonometry in patients with acute circulatory failure. *J Am Med Assoc* **270**:1203–1210.

21. Marik PE (1993) Gastric intramucosal pH. A better predictor of multiorgan dysfunction syndrome and death than oxygen derived variables in patients with sepsis. *Chest* **104**:225–229.

22. Gutierrez G, Bismar H, Dantzker D and Silva N (1992) Comparison of gastric intramucosal pH with measures of oxygen transport and consumption in critically ill patients. *Crit Care Med* **20**:451–457.

23. Gutierrez G, Palizas F, Doglio G *et al.* (1992) Gastric intramucosal pH as a therapeutic index of tissue oxygenation in critically ill patients. *Lancet* **339**: 195–199.

24. Carcillo JA, Davis AL and Zaritsky A (1991) Role of early fluid resuscitation in pediatric septic shock. *J Am Med Assoc* **266**:1242–125.

25. Mattox KL, Maningan PA, Moore EE *et al.* (1991) Prehospital hypertonic saline/dextran infusion for post-traumatic hypotension. The USA multicenter trial. *Ann Surg* **213**:482–491.

26. Ronco JJ, Phang PT, Walley KR, Wiggs B, Fenwick JC and Russell JA (1991) Oxygen consumption is independent of changes in oxygen delivery in severe adult respiratory distress syndrome. *Am Rev Respir Dis* **143**:1267–1273.

27. Smithies M, Yee TH, Jackson L, Beale R and Bihari D (1994) Protecting the gut and the liver in the critically ill: effects of dopexamine. *Crit Care Med* **22**: 789–795.

28. Strang JR and Pugh EJ (1992) Menigococcal infections: reducing the case fatality rate by giving penicillin before admission to hospital. *Br Med J* **305**:141–143.

29. Stern SA, Dronen SC, Birrer P and Ewang X (1993) Effect of blood pressure on hemorrhage volume and survival in a near-fatal hemorrhage model incorporating a vascular injury. *Ann Emerg Med* **22**:155–163.

30. Border JR and Bone LB (1988) Multiple trauma: major extremity wounds; their immediate management and its consequences. *Adv Surg* **22**:261–291.

31. Herndon DN, Barrow RE, Rutan RL, Rutan TC, Desai MH and Abston S (1989) A comparison of conservative versus early excision therapies in severely burned patients. *Ann Surg* **209**:547–552.

32. Thompson BT and Cockrill BA (1994) Renal does dopamine: a siren song? *Lancet* **344**:7–8.

33. Bellomo R, Tipping P and Boyce N (1993) Continuous veno-venous hemofiltration with dialysis removes cytokines from the circulation of septic patients. *Crit Care Med* **21**:522–526.

34. Alexander JW, Gonce SJ, Miskell PN *et al.* (1989) A new model for studying nutrition in peritonitis: the adverse effects of overfeeding. *Ann Surg* **209**:334–340.

35. Gianotti L, Alexander JW, Nelson JL, Fukushima R, Pyles T and Chalk CL (1994) Role of early enteral feeding and acute starvation on postburn bacterial translocation and host defence: prospective randomized trials. *Crit Care Med* **22**:265–272.

36. McClave SA, Lowen CC and Snider HL (1992) Immunonutrition and enteral hyperalimentation of critically ill patients. *Dig Dis Sci* **37**:1153–1161.

37. Bower RH, Cerra FB, Bershadsky B *et al.* (1995) Early enteral administration of a formula (Impact®) supplemented with arginine, nucleotides, and fish oil in intensive care unit patients: results of a multicenter, prospective, randomized, clinical trial. *Crit Care Med* **23**: 436–449.

38. Voerman BJ, deBoer H and Thijs LG (1994) Recombinant growth hormone in critically ill patients. *Curr Opin Anaesthesiol* **7**:161–165.

39. Wherry J, Wenzel R, Abraham E *et al.* (1993) A controlled randomized double-blind trial of monoclonal antibody to human tumor necrosis factor (TNF Mab) in patients with sepsis syndrome. *Chest* **104**:35(abstract).

40. Fisher CJ Jr, Dhainaut JFA, Opal SM *et al.* (1994) Recombinant human Interleukin-1 receptor antagonist in the treatment of patients with sepsis syndrome. *J Am Med Assoc* **271**:1836–1843.

41. Haupt MT, Jastremski MS, Clemmer TP, Metz CA and Goris GB (1991) Effect of ibuprofen in patients with severe sepsis: a randomized double-blind multi-centre study. *Crit Care Med* **19**:1339–1347.

42. Bone RC, Fischer CJ Jr, Clemmer TP *et al.* (1987) Effect of high-dose glucocorticoid therapy on mortality in patients with clinical signs of systemic sepsis. *N Engl J Med* **317**:659–665.

43. Eichacker PQ, Hoffman WD, Farese A *et al.* (1993) Leucocyte CD18 monoclonal antibody worsens endotoxemia and cardiovascular injury in canines with septic shock. *J Appl Physiol* **74**:1885–1892.

44. Eichacker PQ, Waisman Y, Natanson C *et al.* (1993) Recombinant granulocyte colony-stimulating factor reduces endotoxemia and improves cardiovascular function and survival during bacterial sepsis in non-neutropenic canines.

Clin Res **41**:240.

45. Sauaia A, Moore FA, Moore EE, Haenel JB, Read RA and Lezotte DO (1994) Early predictors of post-injury multiple organ failure. *Arch Surg* **129**:39–45.

46. Knaus WA, Draper EA, Wagner DP and Zimmerman JE (1985) Prognosis in acute organ system failure. *Ann Surg* **202**:685–693.

Part XIV

Haematological management

86 | Blood transfusion

JP Isbister

When using blood transfusion therapy, the clinical problem and patient's needs must be identified and clearly understood.[1-4] Blood component therapy should only be regarded as supportive therapy and rarely, if ever, definitive therapy. In most circumstances, therapy is required for haematological deficiencies until the basic disease process can be corrected (e.g. surgical control for acute haemorrhage, or support for bone marrow suppression until the marrow recovers). Therapy may be given to control the effects of a deficiency or to prevent problems. In some circumstances, the therapeutic indication is passive immunotherapy rather than a haematological deficiency (e.g. Rh prophylaxis).

Homologous transfusion should not be the first line of therapy for haematopoietic defects. For many patients, it is possible to correct or manage the effects of haematopoietic deficiencies without transfusing homologous blood components, thus avoiding potential hazards. Decisions on blood component therapy can be difficult, and much debate continues on the indications for various homologous blood components.

In considering the use of homologous blood transfusion, these questions need to addressed:

1 What is the timeframe of the decision-making process?
2 Is it an elective decision?
3 What is the haematological defect?
4 What is the most appropriate therapy for the patient?
5 Can the risk of adverse effects be avoided or minimized?
6 Is there a role for autologous transfusion?
7 What component is indicated and where should it be obtained?
8 How should the component be administered and monitored?
9 What are the risks of the blood component therapy?

10 Will therapy jeopardize the safety of any future transfusions?
11 What is the cost of the haemotherapy?
12 Is the patient fully informed of the medical decisions?

Safe transfusion requires attention to the following details (Fig. 86.1):

1 clear indications and benefits of blood component therapy;
2 accurate patient identification for compatibility testing;
3 identification and careful management of high-risk patients;
4 communication of benefits and risks to the patient/relatives;
5 appropriate handling, administration and monitoring;
6 awareness of possible transfusion-related complications;
7 early diagnosis of adverse effects of transfusion and prompt action instituted;
8 accurate documentation;
9 input into quality assurance programmes.

Blood storage

Whole blood is collected into closed plastic packs mixed with an anticoagulant and stabilizer, to a final volume of approximately 500 ml (70 ml preservative and 430 ml whole blood). Acid citrate dextrose (ACD) has been used since the 1940s, but in recent years, solutions with added phosphate and adenine (CPD-A) are used to increase post-transfusion viability and red cell function (e.g. 2,3-diphosphoglycerate (DPG) levels). Blood is stored at 4°C in carefully designed and monitored refrigerators. Storage shelf-life is up to 35 days with CPD-A, but use of fresher blood (<2 weeks old) is advisable in critically ill patients, especially when rapid transfusion of large

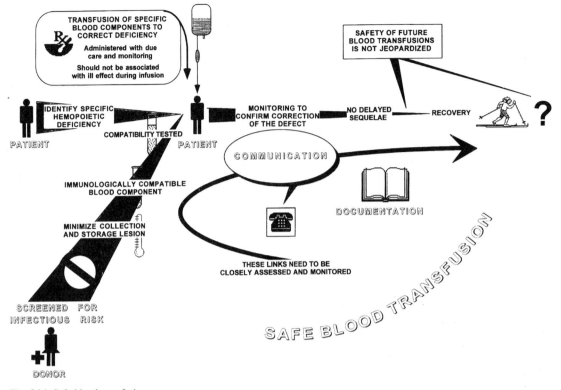

Fig. 86.1 Safe blood transfusion.

volumes is required or if coagulopathy is present. It is better to collect and store blood under appropriate conditions for each specific component. Red cells stored as whole blood are subjected to greater damage due to the presence of neutrophils and plasma proteolytic systems. Ongoing research increasingly recognizes that leukocytes (especially neutrophils) create an adverse storage environment for most blood components, and are responsible for a number of the adverse effects of blood component therapy.

Potential effects of storage on blood[5,6]

As with any biological fluid, blood degenerates with time during storage. Changes occur in both the cellular and plasma components (Fig. 86.2).

Metabolic effects

Adenosine triphosphate (ATP) is progressively depleted with storage and the pH falls; oxidant damage to the membrane occurs with rigid sphero-cyte formation, swelling and finally, potassium leak-age. Parallel to these changes, haemoglobin (Hb) function may be altered due to falling levels of both ATP and more significantly, 2,3-DPG, resulting in increasing oxygen affinity. These changes occur

earlier, and to a greater extent in whole blood than in red cell concentrates. Storage of blood as whole blood is associated with the greatest storage lesions, and in general, the only time for using whole blood is when it is relatively fresh. The implications for the storage of autologous whole blood are still being evaluated.

Removal of the buffy coat prior to storage should be standard practice, but the cost is prohibitive. Platelets and granulocytes in the buffy coat are foundations for microaggregate formation, with release of various cell-damaging enzymes into the storage medium. Thus, transfusion of large volumes of stored blood, although increasing intravascular volume, will not necessarily provide immediately available oxygen to the tissues to the degree antici-pated from the increased Hb.

Microaggregates

The plastic mesh filter used in conventional blood-giving sets only removes particulate material larger than 170 μm in size. Microaggregates of platelet/leukocyte/fibrin thrombi progressively form in blood during storage, ranging in size from 20 μm to over 170 μm. The adverse effects of microaggregates are still debated (Table 86.1). Nevertheless, it is generally agreed that an additional microfilter should be used

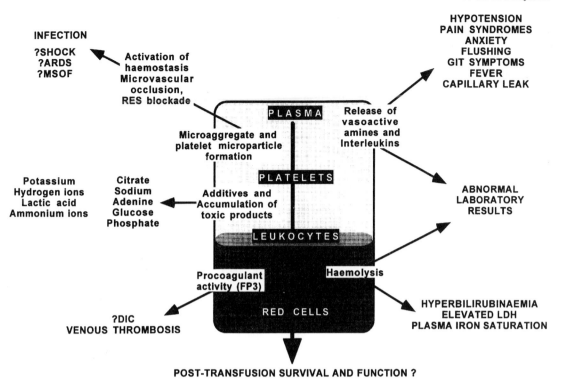

Fig. 86.2 Storage lesions. ARDS = Acute respiratory distress syndrome; MSOF = multisystem organ failure; RES = reticuloendothelial system; DIC = disseminated intravascular coagulation; GIT = gastrointestinal tract; LDH = lactate dehydrogenase.

when large volumes of stored blood (e.g. > 1 l) are transfused over short periods of time. Hence the quality of stored whole blood or blood components cannot be guaranteed, and the use of fresh blood products or the development of better blood preservative solutions is of paramount importance.

Table 86.1 Potential problems from infusion of microaggregates

Impaired pulmonary gas exchange, acute respiratory distress syndrome (ARDS)

General microcirculatory impairment

Depression of reticuloendothelial system (RES) function

Depression of fibronectin levels

Febrile reactions

Activation of the haemostatic system

Activation of the complement system

Unnecessary antigenic stimulation

Release of vasoactive substances

Transfusion management of acute haemorrhage[3,4,7]

Homologous blood is required in acute haemorrhage to restore blood volume and oxygen-carrying capacity. If blood loss has been massive, or there are defects in the haemostatic system, specific component therapy may be indicated. Volume is always the highest priority; whole blood or red cell concentrate transfusions are not usually indicated if less than 15–20% of the blood volume has been lost. A normal human may survive 30% deficit in blood volume without fluid replacement, in contrast to 80% loss of red cell mass if normovolaemia is maintained. Presently, minimization of homologous blood transfusion is an imperative, and haemodilution to low haematocrits is accepted practice if further haemorrhage is unlikely, and other aspects of oxygen transport are intact (e.g. cardiorespiratory function).

Haemotherapy is the mainstay of management for the resuscitation of haemorrhagic shock, and requires a coordinated priority-oriented clinical and laboratory approach. Rapid infusions of large volumes of stored blood have potential problems, largely related to storage lesions. It is not possible, nor necessary, for fresh blood to be immediately available for all acutely haemorrhaging patients. Whenever possible, blood less than a week from collection is desirable in the patient continuing to bleed. Whole blood is rarely indicated for a bleeding patient, and is usually used for logistic reasons or in situations of massive blood loss (i.e. > a blood volume) when fresh whole blood may need to be considered. If massive blood transfusion is anticipated, the hospital transfusion service and blood bank must be informed.

A protocol approach to blood component therapy is generally not recommended, as each patient should be treated individually. In an elective situation, when defects can be identified in advance and appropriate blood components prescribed, a protocol approach may be justified. This should be done in close consultation with the haematologist and hospital transfusion service.

Specific hazards of massive blood transfusion (Table 86.2)[8]

Adverse reactions of massive blood transfusion (usually defined as replacement of the circulating volume in 24 h) may manifest in many ways, and

Table 86.2 Potential hazards of massive and rapid blood transfusion

---

Impaired oxygen transport
Microaggregates*
Fluid overload
Defective red cell function*
Impaired haemoglobin function*
Disseminated intravascular coagulation (DIC)*
Acute respiratory distress syndrome (ARDS)*
Multiorgan dysfunction syndrome (MODS)?

Haemostatic failure
Dilution
Depletion
Decreased production
Disseminated intravascular coagulation*
Electrolyte and metabolic disturbances
Hyperkalaemia* or delayed hypokalaemia*
Sodium overload*
Acid–base disturbances*
Citrate toxicity*
Hypothermia*

Vasoactive reactions
Kinin activation*
Damaged platelets and granulocytes*

Serological incompatibility
Impaired reticuloendothelial function*

---

*Complications related to the method and time of storage.

each may be misinterpreted as being due to other mechanisms. Any patient receiving massive blood transfusion is likely to be seriously ill and have multiple problems. The complications caused or aggravated by massive blood transfusion are not always possible to define. Many effects must be considered in conjunction with the injuries and multiorgan dysfunction.

Citrate toxicity

The patient responds to citrate infusion by removing citrate and mobilizing ionized calcium. Citrate is metabolized by the Krebs cycle in all nucleated body cells, especially the liver. Marked elevation in citrate is seen with transfusion exceeding 500 ml in 5 min, with the concentration falling rapidly when the infusion is slowed. Citrate metabolism is impaired by hypotension, hypovolaemia, hypothermia and liver disease. Toxicity may also be potentiated by alkalosis, hyperkalaemia, hypothermia and cardiac disease. The clinical significance of minor depression of ionized calcium remains ill-defined, and it is accepted that a warm, well-perfused adult patient with normal liver function can tolerate a unit of blood each 5 min without requiring calcium supplements. The rate of transfusion is more significant than the total volume transfused. Common practice today is to administer 10% calcium gluconate 1.0 g IV, following each 5 units of blood or fresh frozen plasma. This is still controversial, as there is increasing concern regarding calcium homeostasis and cell function in acutely ill patients.

Acid–base and electrolyte disturbances
Acid–base

Stored bank blood contains an appreciable acid load, and is often used in a situation of pre-existing or continuing metabolic acidosis. The acidity of stored blood is mainly due to citric acid of the anticoagulant and the lactic acid generated during storage. Their intermediary metabolites are rapidly metabolized with adequate tissue perfusion, resulting in a metabolic alkalosis. Hence, routine use of sodium bicarbonate is usually unnecessary and is generally contraindicated. Alkali further shifts the oxygen dissociation curve to the left, provides a large additional sodium load, and depresses the return of ionized calcium to normal following citrate infusion. Acid–base estimations should be performed and corrected in the context of the clinical situation. With continuing hypoperfusion, however, metabolism of citrate and lactate will be depressed, lactic acid production will continue, and there may be an indication for IV bicarbonate and calcium to correct acidosis and low ionized calcium.

Serum potassium

Although controversial, it is unlikely that the high serum potassium concentrations in stored blood have pathological effects, except in acute renal failure. However, hypokalaemia may be a problem 24 h after transfusion, as the transfused cells correct their electrolyte composition, and potassium returns into the cells. Thus, although initial acidosis and hyperkalaemia may be an immediate problem with massive blood transfusion, the net result of successful resuscitation is likely to be delayed hypokalaemia and alkalosis. With CPD blood, the acid load and red cell storage lesion are less. Constant monitoring of the acid–base and electrolyte status is essential in such fluctuating clinical situations.

Serum sodium

The sodium content of whole blood and fresh frozen plasma is higher than the normal blood concentration due to the sodium citrate. This should be remembered when large volumes of plasma are being infused into patients who have disordered salt and water handling (e.g. renal, liver or cardiac disease).

Hypothermia[5]

Blood warmed from 4°C to 37°C requires 1255 kJ (300 kcal), the equivalent heat produced by 1 h of muscular work, with oxygen requirement of 62 1 oxygen. Hypothermia impairs the metabolism of citrate and lactate, shifts the oxygen dissociation curve to the left, increases intracellular potassium release, impairs red cell deformability, delays drug metabolism, masks clinical signs, increases the incidence of arrhythmias, reduces cardiac output and impairs haemostatic function. Thus, a thermostatically controlled blood-warming device should be routinely used when any transfusion episode requires rapid infusion of more than 2 units of blood.

Jaundice

Jaundice is common following massive blood transfusion. A significant amount of transfused stored blood (up to 30% of aged blood) may not survive, and the resulting bilirubin load will result in varying degrees of hyperbilirubinaemia. During hypovolaemia and shock, liver function may be impaired, particularly in sepsis or multiorgan failure. An important rate-limiting step in bilirubin transport is the energy-requiring process of transporting conjugated bilirubin from the hepatocyte to the biliary canaliculus. Thus, although an increased load of bilirubin from destroyed transfused red cells may be conjugated, there may be delayed excretion, leading to a conjugated hyperbilirubinaemia. This paradoxical conjugated hyperbilirubinaemia may be misinterpreted as biliary obstruction or cholangitis, leading to unnecessary investigations. The effect of resorbing haematoma and the possibility of an occult haemolytic transfusion reaction should also be considered.

Potential adverse effects of homologous transfusion[1]

The potential mechanisms of transfusion reactions include:

1 immunological differences between the donor and recipient, which result in varying degrees of blood component incompatibility. In order for a reaction to occur in these circumstances, the recipient needs to have been previously immunized to a cellular or plasma antigen;
2 alterations in blood products due to preservation and storage, i.e. quantitative and/or qualitative deficiencies in the blood components which will reduce efficacy of transfusion;
3 transmission of infectious disease.

The clinical presentations of transfusion reactions can be legion. Figure 86.3 gives an algorithm approach to analysing the possibility of a transfusion reaction.

Pyrexia

Mild febrile reactions are not usually a matter of concern, but rigors and temperatures above 38°C should not be ignored. The majority of febrile reactions are now considered due to an immunological reaction against transfused cellular or plasma components, usually leukocytes.

Transfusion-related infections[9] (Table 86.3)
Hepatitis

Post-transfusion hepatitis is a potential complication of homologous transfusion; identifying infectious donors became possible since the 1970s. Hepatitis B and C are almost totally preventable transfusion-transmitted diseases. Hepatitis C virus (HCV, first reported in 1989 and makes up the majority of what was formerly called non A, non B hepatitis) is a major cause of acute and chronic hepatitis. Virtually all persons with acute HCV infection seem to become chronically infected.

Human immunodeficiency virus (HIV) and acquired immunodeficiency syndrome (AIDS)

Understanding of the natural history of transfusion-associated HIV infection is still evolving. Fortunately, the antibody screening of blood donors has

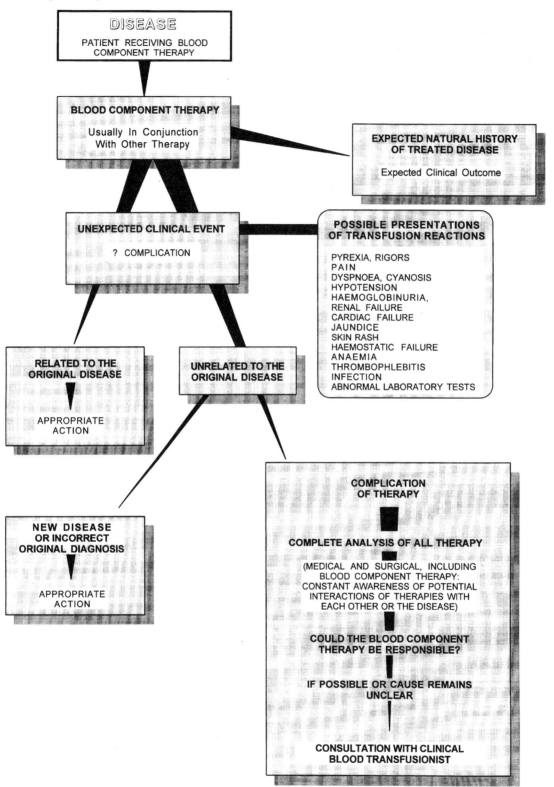

Fig. 86.3 An approach to a possible transfusion reaction.

Table 86.3 Transfusion-related infusions

Infection	Donor selection by questionnaire	Donor selection by laboratory screening
Hepatitis A	+	–
Hepatitis B	+	+
Hepatitis non-A non-B (commonest)	+/–	+
Cytomegalovirus infection	–	Antibody-positive blood should be avoided in neonates and immunosuppressed patients
HIV-associated viral infection	+	+
HTLV-I	+	+
Epstein–Barr infection	–	–
Other unidentified viral agents	–	–
Toxoplasmosis	–	–
Syphilis	+	+
Parasitic disease	+	+/–
Bacterial contamination	+/–	–

HIV = Human immunodeficiency virus;
HTLV-I = human T-lymphotrophic virus I.

almost eliminated transfusion-associated HIV transmission, but as the antibody test is an indirect measure of infectivity, it is not 100% certain of detecting all potentially infective donors, and donors may be in the 'window' period. Immunosuppressed patients and neonates appear to be more likely to sustain full-blown AIDS (see Chapter 60).

Mononucleosis syndromes

The development of a swinging pyrexia with varying degrees of peripheral blood atypical mononucleosis, 7–10 days following transfusion, can be a diagnostic confusion. The temperature may fluctuate markedly with associated rigors and drenching sweats, but the patient may feel reasonably well between febrile attacks. Abnormalities in liver function are common. Cytomegalovirus (CMV) infection is the commonest cause of this syndrome.

Endotoxaemia

Bacterial contamination of stored blood has always been recognized as a potential cause of fulminant endotoxic shock, but recent reports of transfusion-transmitted *Yersinia enterocolitica* have aroused concern. The clinical features of transfusion-related endotoxic shock in the non-anaesthetized patient include violent chills, fever, tachycardia and vascular collapse,[1,4,9] with prominent nausea, vomiting and diarrhoea. Anaesthetized patients may have delayed onset of symptoms (e.g. fever, tachycardia, hypotension and cyanosis), followed by disseminated intravascular coagulation (DIC), renal failure and sometimes acute respiratory distress syndrome (ARDS).

Haemolytic transfusion reactions[3]

Most severe acute haemolytic transfusion reactions have a clearly identifiable and avoidable cause and may occur under several circumstances (Table 86.4). Most delayed haemolytic reactions are immune in nature and usually cannot be prevented.

Initial symptoms and signs

Acute intravascular haemolysis, which is more typical of ABO incompatibility, may manifest in several ways. Classical symptoms and signs include apprehension, flushing, pain (e.g. at infusion site, headache, chest, lumbosacral and abdominal), nausea, vomiting, rigors, hypotension and circulatory collapse.

Haemostatic failure

Haemorrhagic diathesis due to DIC may be a feature, resulting in severe generalized haemostatic failure, with haemorrhage and oozing from multiple sites. As the responsible transfusion is likely to have been administered for haemorrhage, increasing severity of local bleeding may be the first clue to an incompatible transfusion, especially if the patient is anaesthetized in the operating room.

Table 86.4 Mechanisms by which blood may be haemolysed before or following transfusion

Immune destruction
Donor red-cell serological incompatibility
    Acute incompatible blood transfusion
    Delayed transfusion reaction
High-titre haemolysin in donor plasma
Interdonor incompatibility
?Destruction of donor cells without detectable antibodies
Non-immune destruction
Transfusion of incorrectly stored or outdated blood
Inadvertently frozen blood
Overheated blood
Infected blood
Mechanical destruction, e.g. infusion under pressure

Oliguria and renal impairment

Renal impairment may complicate a haemolytic transfusion reaction, and prevention or appropriate management of established renal failure is important. If circulating volume and urinary output are rapidly restored, established renal failure is unlikely to occur.

Anaemia and jaundice

A severe haemolytic transfusion reaction may be suspected from the development of jaundice or anaemia.

Allergic and anaphylactoid reactions[10]

Non-cellular blood components (plasma and plasma derivatives) are not usually considered as major causes of adverse reactions to transfusion therapy. However, the complexity and antigenic heterogeneity of plasma and its various components, presence of antibodies and changes effected by the preparation processes present a broader spectrum of potential adverse effects than is frequently recognized. Many of the adverse effects are ill-understood and probably remain undetected or undiagnosed clinically.

The classification of allergic reactions to blood transfusion has been debated. Clinical severity may range from minor urticarial reactions or flushing to fulminant cardiorespiratory collapse and death. Many reactions are probably true anaphylaxis, but in others, mechanisms are less clear, and the term anaphylactoid has been used. Currently, to avoid implying the mechanism of the reaction, the term immediate generalized reaction (IGR) is preferred. Clinical syndromes of IGR have been classified as follows:

1 Grade I: skin manifestations;
2 Grade II: mild to moderate hypotension, gastrointestinal disturbances (nausea) and respiratory distress;
3 Grade III: severe hypotension, shock and bronchospasm;
4 Grade IV: cardiac and/or respiratory arrest.

Plasma and plasma components may cause adverse effects by several pathophysiological mechanisms:

1 Immunological reactions to normal components of plasma may occur in two ways:
   (a) Plasma proteins being antigenic to the recipient; they may contain epitopes on their molecules different from those on the recipient's functionally identical plasma proteins (e.g. anti-immunoglobulin A (IgA) antibodies).
   (b) Antibodies in the donor plasma which react with cellular components of the recipient's blood cells or plasma proteins.

2 Physicochemical characteristics and contaminants of donor plasma, such as temperature, chemical additives, medications and micro-organisms may be responsible for immunological or non-immunological recipient reactions.
3 The preparation techniques and storage conditions of blood and blood products may potentially cause adverse reactions through:
   (a) accumulation of metabolites or cellular release products;
   (b) plasma activation, i.e. activation of some of the proteolytic systems, importantly, the complement and kinin/kininogen systems, with generation of vasoactive substances and anaphylotoxins. Some apparently allergic reactions to blood products may be due to vasoactive substances in the infusion, subjective sensations that may be missed in an unconscious patient. For example, hypotension occurring during rapid infusion of a hypovolaemic patient is likely to be interpreted as further volume loss (particularly with some plasma protein fractions reported to produce a transient fall in blood pressure).
   (c) Histamine generation, i.e. histamine concentrations increase in stored blood components and may be correlated with non-febrile, non-haemolytic transfusion reactions. Histamine release may be stimulated in the patient by plasma components, synthetic colloids and various medications.
   (d) Generation of cytokines, particularly interleukin-8, in high concentrations have been demonstrated in the supernates of stored platelet concentrates.

Postoperative infections[11,12]

Homologous transfusion has been shown to be an independent risk factor for postoperative infection. Indeed, it may be the single most important predisposing cause of postoperative bacterial infection. Most infections are distant from the wound site itself, suggesting a systemic reduction in host resistance to infection.

Transfusion-associated graft-versus-host disease

Graft-versus-host disease, classically observed in relationship to allogeneic bone marrow transplantation, may occur following blood transfusion due to infused immunocompetent lymphocytes precipitating an immunological reaction against the host tissues of the recipient. It is most commonly observed in immunocompromised patients, but may also be seen in recipients of directed blood donation from first-degree relatives, and occasionally, when donor and recipient are not related, due to homozygosity for human leukocyte antigen (HLA) haplotypes, for which the recipient is heterozygous. The syndrome usually occurs 3–30 days after homologous transfusion, with fever, liver function test abnormalities, profuse watery diarrhoea, erythematous skin rash and progressive pancytopenia.

Transfusion-related acute lung injury (TRALI)[13]

TRALI is potentially fulminant complication of blood transfusion, characterized by acute respiratory distress. Symptoms usually arise within hours of a recent blood transfusion. In contrast to ARDS, most patients improve clinically within 48 h if well-resuscitated, and will usually make a full recovery. TRALI is due to the presence of leuko-agglutinating or HLA-specific antibodies in the implicated components of donor plasma. When complement is activated, C5a promotes neutrophil aggregation and sequestration in the lung microvasculature, causing endothelial damage and leading to interstitial oedema. A broader spectrum of TRALI than just that related to leuko-agglutinins is likely. The term TRALI is now being expanded to include cases of posttransfusion ARDS in which other mechanisms may be responsible (e.g. anaphylactic reactions, platelet reactions, granulocyte transfusions, DIC and poorly stored blood).

Autologous transfusion[14,15]

Transfusion of autologous blood will eliminate the immunological and most infective risks associated with donor homologous blood, and are increasingly used. There are three main approaches (Fig. 86.4).

Preoperative banked autologous blood collection

Blood is collected from the patient at intervals in the weeks before elective surgery and stored as whole blood. Alternatively, but less economically, blood may be collected in the months before surgery and frozen. The latter approach is only used for patients with rare blood groups for whom compatible homologous blood is difficult to find. The storage lesion associated with the storage of autologous blood as whole blood for up to 5 weeks is of concern and in some centres the blood is fractionated. There is an increasing move more to intraoperative techniques to minimize homologous transfusion, e.g. perioperative haemodilution and intraoperative salvage.

Perioperative haemodilution[16]

Up to 4 units of blood is collected immediately prior to surgery, with simultaneous infusion of colloid (e.g. albumin or dextran 70) in order to lower the haematocrit to about 0.25. Retransfusion of autologous blood is started when intraoperative loss exceeds 300 ml. Blood losses up to 2 l can be replenished in this way, and additional homologous blood is seldom needed. The preparation of platelet-rich plasma, fresh plasma and platelet gel may all be used in conjunction with perioperative haemodilution.

Intraoperative autologous blood salvage[17–19]

Rapid, massive blood losses can occur in vascular surgery, liver surgery and ectopic pregnancies. Intraoperative salvaging of autologous shed blood may be useful in these situations, and the appropriate technology and expertise are available. The safest technique uses a red cell saver which washes the red cells prior to reinfusion, thus avoiding the risks of coagulopathy and air embolism. However, filtration systems have improved and have an economical advantage. Collection of chest drainage blood post-bypass is popular, as this blood is defibrinated so clotting is not a problem, but the use of large volume, especially in hypovolaemic patients, should be avoided.

Platelet transfusion therapy[20,21]

Platelet transfusion therapy may benefit most patients with platelet deficiency or dysfunction, but is unlikely to be of benefit to those whose problem is related to increased platelet consumption. In some disorders, such as immune thrombocytopenia or alloimmunized patients, platelet transfusions are usually ineffective and may be deleterious. The standard adult dose is 6 units, and general guidelines for administration are as follows:

1 prophylaxis: platelet count $< 15 \times 10^9/l$;
2 pre-surgery: platelet count $< 70 \times 10^9/l$;
3 active bleeding: platelet count $< 100 \times 10^9/l$.

Normal human immunoglobulin

Normal human immunoglobulin is available in IM and IV forms for the treatment or prevention of infection in patients with proven hypogammaglobulinaemia. IV immunoglobulin therapy is also finding a role in some autoimmune disorders, such as idiopathic thrombocytopenic purpura, autoimmune polyneuropathy and others (see Chapter 88).

Basic immunohaematology[3]

Red-cell serology has become a highly specialized area of knowledge, and clinicians cannot be expected to know the topic in depth. The following is a summary of core knowledge.

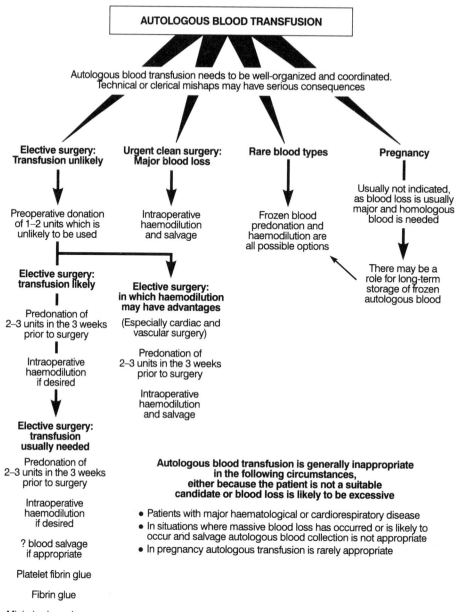

Fig. 86.4 Autologous blood transfusion.

Saline agglutination

Safe transfusion has revolved around this traditional serological technique. A saline suspension of red cells is mixed with serum and observed for agglutination. Saline agglutination is used for ABO blood grouping and is one of the techniques for compatibility testing of donor blood.

Direct and indirect antiglobulin test (AGT; Coombs test)

In red-cell serology, the antiglobulin test is used to detect IgG immunoglobulins or complement components. The direct antiglobulin test (DAGT) detects immunoglobulin or complement components present on the surface of the red cells circulating in the patient. The result is positive in autoimmune haemolytic anaemia and haemolytic disease of the newborn, and during a haemolytic transfusion reaction. The indirect antiglobulin test (IAGT) detects the presence of non-agglutinating antibodies in the patient's plasma, usually IgG type. Antibody screening for atypical antibodies and pretransfusion compatibility testing are the main applications of the IAGT.

Regular and irregular (atypical) antibodies

The regular alloantibodies (isoagglutinins) of the ABO system are naturally occurring agglutinins present in all ABO types except AB. Group O people have anti-A and anti-B isoagglutinins, group A have anti-B and group B have anti-A. Group A cells are the cause of the commonest and most dangerous ABO-incompatible haemolytic reactions. Atypical antibodies are not normally present in the plasma, but may be found in some people as naturally occurring antibodies or as immune antibodies. Immune antibodies result from previous antigenic exposure due to blood transfusion or pregnancy. Naturally occurring antibodies more frequently react by saline agglutination and, although they may be stimulated by transfusion, are usually of minimal clinical significance. In contrast, many of the immune atypical antibodies are of major

clinical significance, being the reason for pretransfusion compatibility testing and antenatal antibody screening. Most of the clinically significant immune atypical antibodies are detected by the IAGT. Blood group antigens vary widely in their frequency and immunogenicity. The D antigen of the Rhesus blood group system is common and highly immunogenic. Thus, when a Rh-negative (i.e. D-negative) patient is exposed to D-positive blood, formation of an anti-D antibody is highly likely. For this reason, the D antigen is considered when providing blood for transfusion, in contrast to the numerous other red-cell antigens which are less common or less immunogenic. Besides the Rh (D), and sometimes the Kell (K) blood group antigens, it is not practical nor necessary to take notice of other blood group antigens, unless an atypical antibody is detected during antibody screening procedures.

Antibody screen

On receipt of a blood sample, the transfusion service type red cells (ABO and Rh D) and screen the serum for atypical antibodies. This screen tests the patient's serum with group O screening cells. The screening panel consists of red cells obtained usually from two group O donors, which contain all common red-cell antigens occurring with a frequency of greater than

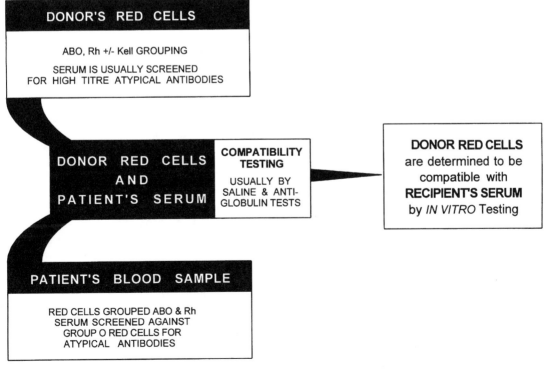

Fig. 86.5 Compatibility test (cross-match).

approximately 2% in the community. If an atypical antibody is detected on the antibody screen, further serological investigations are carried out to identify the specificity of the antibody.

Cross-match (compatibility test)

The major cross-match, i.e. donor–recipient compatibility, is the final compatibility test between the donor cells and the patient's serum (Fig. 86.5). The cross-match test tends to be overemphasized to the detriment of the antibody screen. With developments in red-cell serology and laboratory methods, emphasis is now concentrated on the steps prior to the final compatibility cross-match.

Type and screen system

Precompatibility testing has assumed a major role in the selection of blood for transfusion. Thus, when elective surgery requiring blood transfusion is planned, the blood transfusion service must receive a clotted blood sample well before the time of surgery. Precompatibility testing should be performed during routine working hours, when facilities and staff are geared for large workloads and all possible contingencies.

Provision of blood in emergencies

The decision to give uncross-matched or partially cross-matched blood, or to wait for cross-match-compatible blood is difficult. Clinicians should be aware of basic serological considerations and problems faced by the serologist. Depending upon the degree of urgency and prior knowledge of the patient's red-cell serology, blood can be provided with varying degrees of safety. However, when a patient is exsanguinating and likely to die, giving ABO-compatible uncross-matched blood, especially if the antibody screen is negative, is safe and appropriate therapy.

Universal donor group O blood

Group O blood under normal circumstances will be ABO-compatible with all recipients. The transfusions should be given only in extreme emergencies, as red-cell concentrates or as whole blood from donations which have been screened for high-titre A or B haemolysins. If the recipient is of child-bearing age, every attempt should be made to give Rh D-negative blood if her blood group is unknown.

ABO group-specific blood

Transfusion of blood of the correct ABO type circumvents all isoagglutinin problems above. Its safety is dependent on meticulous attention to

grouping. Previous blood group information (e.g. as denoted on the identification bracelet or by handwriting in the records) may be incorrect, and the clinician assumes a considerable risk if blood is administered on this information.

Saline-compatible blood

The administration of saline-compatible blood is, for practical purposes, the administration of ABO group-specific blood.

References

1. Harrison CR and Polesky HF (1994) Current transfusion medicine practices and issue. *Arch Pathol Lab Med* **118**:333–470.
2. Isbister JP (1994) The clinicians' approach to risk management. *Transf Sci* **3**:37–48.
3. Mollison PL, Engelfriet CP and Contreras M (1993) *Blood Transfusion in Clinical Medicine*, 9th edn. London: Blackwell Scientific Publications.
4. Rossi EC, Simon TL and Moss GS (1991) *Principles of Transfusion Medicine*. Baltimore, MD: Williams & Wilkins.
5. Isbister JP (1992) *Current Issues in Anaesthesiology: Blood Transfusion and Blood Component Therapy*. London: Current Science.
6. Moroff G and Holme S (1991) Concepts about current conditions for the preparation and storage of platelets. *Trans Med Rev* **5**:48–59.
7. Sawyer PR and Harrison CR (1990) Massive transfusion in adults. Diagnoses, survival and blood bank support. *Vox Sang* **58**:199–203.
8. Gillon J and Greenburg AG (1993) Transfusions: immunologic, volume-related, and storage-related complications. *Infect Urol* **6**:83–87.
9. Gillon J and Greenburg AG (1992) Transfusions: infectious complications. *Complications Surg* **11**: 19–28.
10. Isbister JP (1993) Adverse reactions to plasma and plasma components. *Anaesth Intens Care* **21**: 31–38.
11. Agarwal N, Murphy JG, Cayten CG and Stahl WM (1993) Blood transfusion increases the risk of infection after trauma. *Arch Surg* **128**:171–177.
12. Duke BJ, Modin GW, Schecter WP and Horn JK (1993) Transfusion significantly increases the risk for infection after splenic injury. *Arch Surg* **128**:1125–1132.
13. Popovsky MA, Chaplin Jr HC and Moore SB (1992) Transfusion related acute lung injury: a neglected serious complication of hemotherapy. *Transfusion* **32**:589–592.
14. Isbister JP (1985) Strategies for avoiding or minimizing homologous blood transfusion: a sequel to the AIDS scare. *Med J Aust* **142**:596–599.
15. Tulloh BR, Brakespear CP, Bates SC *et al.* (1993) Autologous predonation, haemodilution and intraoperative blood salvage in elective abdominal aortic aneurysm repair. *Br J Surg* **80**: 313–315.
16. Messner K (1975) Hemodilution. *Surg Clin North Am* **55**:659–668.

17. Chernow B (1993) Blood conservation in critical care – the evidence accumulates. *Crit Care Med* **21**:481–482.

18. Ouriel K, Shortell CK, Green RM and DeWeese JA (1993) Intraoperative autotransfusion in aortic surgery. *J Vasc Surg* **18**:16–22.

19. Dzik WH and Sherburne B (1990) Intraoperative blood salvage: medical controversies. *Transf Med Rev* **4**:208–235.

20. National Institute of Health Bethesda, MD (1987) Platelet transfusion therapy. *Transf Med Rev* **1**:195–200.

21. Rao GHR, Escolar G and White JG (1993) Biochemistry, physiology, and function of platelets stored as concentrates. *Transfusion* **33**:766–778.

AM Forbes

Colloids are plasma expanders used to restore blood volume in shocked patients. They include albumin, gelatin, dextran and starch. The blood volume is expanded by the volume infused and, with hyperosmotic solutions, by the passage of water from the extravascular space. Blood products[1,2] include fresh frozen plasma, which contains all the coagulation factors, and plasma derivatives such as coagulation factors and immunoglobulins, which are used to correct specific deficiencies. The available range of plasma-derived products is steadily increasing. All blood products except albumin carry a risk of virus transmission[3,4] including human immunodeficiency virus (HIV), hepatitis B and C, cytomegalovirus (CMV) and Epstein–Barr virus (infectious mononucleosis). Recent developments have tried to overcome these risks, and include careful screening of donors and use of pasteurization and fractionation techniques. Recombinant human plasma proteins are under investigation for their potential in providing coagulation factors for clinical use.[5]

Principle

Plasma expanders or colloids have molecular weights (MW) greater than 35 kDa, and infusion results in maintenance or initial increase in blood osmotic pressure (Table 87.1). The ideal properties of a plasma expander[6] are:

Table 87.1 Composition of blood and plasma expanders

	Molecular weight (kDa)	Albumin (g/l)	Globulin (g/l)	Polysaccharide (g/l)	Na^+ (mmol/l)	K^+ (mmol/l)	Ca^{2+} (mmol/l)	Cl^- (mmol/l)	pH	Osmolarity (mosmol/kg)
Whole blood		35–45	20–30		140–150	3–40	2.0–2.5	100–106	6.5–7.0	285–295
Serum albumin 5%	60–70	50	2		140	0.12	2	125	6.7–7.3	260
Fresh frozen plasma		35–45	20–30		168	3.2	8.2	76	7.1	310–330
Serum albumin 20%	50	200			50				7.0	80
Haemaccel	35	35 (degraded peptide)			145	5.1	6.25	145	7.3	293
Dextran 40* in 0.9% saline	40			100	150			150		346–368
Dextran 70* in 5% dextrose	70			60						335–337

* Available in either saline or 5% dextrose solution.

1 The solution is stable and easily stored for long periods.
2 The colloid is free of pyrogens, antigens and toxic substances.
3 There should be no risk of transmitted viral infection.
4 An adequate colloid osmotic pressure (COP) is achieved with a half-life of several hours. COP should be kept above 20 mmHg (2.7 kPa), produced by total serum protein of 50 g/l. This is 70% of the normal average COP of 28 mmHg (3.7 kPa).
5 Metabolism and excretion of the colloid do not adversely affect the recipient.
6 Infusion does not cause coagulopathy, haemolysis, red cell agglutination or problems with cross-matching.

Specific colloids

Normal serum albumin (NSA)

NSA possesses most of the properties of an ideal colloid, but because of its limited availability, synthetic and cheaper plasma expanders should be used whenever possible. Solutions (5% and 20%) are prepared from human plasma, and heat treatment is applied to ensure that neither HIV nor hepatitis can be transmitted. The plasma protein is mainly albumin (96%), and has a shelf-life of 5 years at 2–8°C and 1 year at 25°C.

NSA 5% is indicated in hypovolaemia due to haemorrhage or plasma loss (e.g. burns, crush injuries and peritonitis), and is particularly valuable when there is associated hypoalbuminaemia. About 80% of NSA remains in the intravascular compartment, and this volume expansion lasts for about 24 h. The intravascular half-life is 16 h, and this is similar for endogenous albumin. NSA is also used as a replacement fluid during plasma exchange. Concentrated salt-poor 20% albumin may be used in the presence of overloading of salt and water, and of hypoalbuminaemia.

The problem of hypotension during rapid transfusion[6,7] has been overcome by ensuring low levels of prekallikrein activator and sodium acetate in the final product. Side-effects of flushing, urticaria, fever and hypotension are rare.

Haemaccel

Haemaccel (Behringwerke) is a 3.5% solution of gelatin (35 kDa) cross-linked by urea bridges (Table 87.1). It is prepared by hydrolysis of animal collagen. Other gelatin preparations, modified fluid gelatin and oxypolygelatin, are not available in Australia.

Haemaccel is cheap and stable, with a shelf-life of 8 years at 25°C. It is iso-osmotic with plasma, increases plasma volume only by the volume infused, and has a short intravascular half-life of 2–3 h. It is

eliminated completely by hepatic metabolism and renal excretion. An advantage of Haemaccel over other plasma substitutes is the lower tendency to produce haemorrhagic complications. Incidence of reactions to gelatin solutions is low (0.04%), and range from skin rashes and pyrexia to life-threatening anaphylaxis. The reactions appear related to histamine release, which is probably the result of a direct effect of gelatin on mast cells.[6,8,9]

Apart from its use in hypovolaemic shock, Haemaccel is a useful carrier agent for insulin in the therapy of uncontrolled diabetes, because less insulin is lost to the glass or plastic container. Haemaccel contains sodium and a large amount of calcium ions (Table 87.1), and should not be infused in the same administration set as blood.

Dextran

Dextrans are polysaccharides which are produced by fermentation of sucrose with bacterium *Leuconostoc mesenteroides*, and then hydrolysed and fractionated into different molecular sizes. Dextran for clinical use includes dextran 70 (70 kDa) and dextran 40 (40 kDa), mixed with either saline or dextrose. Dextran preparations are stable at room temperature, non-pyrogenic and non-toxic.

Dextran 70 (Macrodex, Pharmacia)

Dextran 70 (6%) is used in hypovolaemic shock[10–12] and in the prophylaxis of thromboembolism. It exerts a colloid osmotic pressure greater than plasma (Table 87.1), and additional electrolyte solutions are required to replenish the extravascular space. Use of dextran to replace large volumes of plasma or blood should be limited to 1 l, because of the risk of abnormal bleeding. Volumes over 1 l may interfere with haemostasis, although evidence for this is conflicting.[10,12] Platelet dysfunction and decreased fibrinogen and factor VIII are suggested reasons for increased bleeding. Dextran is contraindicated in disseminated intravascular coagulation (DIC). Rouleaux formation and interference with blood cross-matching may be a problem with high MW dextran, but not with dextran 70 and 40.

Dextran 70 can also be infused perioperatively to lessen the risk of deep venous thrombosis and pulmonary embolism, because of its antithrombotic effect. Dextran has an intravascular half-life of about 6 h, and is eliminated by hepatic metabolism and renal excretion. Dextran 70 molecules are rapidly excreted by the kidney.

Dextran 40 (Rheomacrodex, Pharmacia)

Compared with dextran 70, 10% dextran 40 produces a greater expansion of blood volume (Table 87.1), but the effect is shorter-lasting (half-life of 2 h). Dextran 40 should not be used in hypovolaemic shock, since it may obstruct renal tubules and precipitate acute renal failure.

Dextran 40 may have anti-sludging properties (such as disaggregation of cells and decreased platelet adhesiveness) and be able to improve flow in small vessels. Clinical results in the treatment of peripheral perfusion disturbances are conflicting, but it may be used to prevent thromboembolism in stroke patients, to improve blood flow following vascular and neurosurgery, and in acute pancreatitis.

Other plasma expanders and blood substitutes

Crystalloids

Infusion of isotonic electrolyte solutions or 5% dextrose results in a brief expansion of plasma volume. After 30 min, only about one-fifth of the infused volume remains within the circulation.[6] These solutions are an important part of resuscitation,[13,14] but the relative merits of crystalloids and colloids remain controversial. Hypertonic saline (3.0–7.5%) can be used as a plasma expander, but is associated with increased plasma sodium levels and osmolarity.[6]

Hydroxyethyl starch

Hydroxyethyl starch is a 6% starch solution prepared by the hydrolysis of corn, with hydroxyethyl units attached to 70% of the glucose units. It has therapeutic effectiveness similar to dextran 70.[6] Like dextran, it may cause haemostatic disturbances when used in large volumes.

Stroma-free haemoglobin

Haemoglobin (Hb) preparations are being developed in an attempt to provide a colloid plasma substitute which carries oxygen and which is of low viscosity. Stroma-free Hb is a solution prepared by filtration of outdated lysed red cells. There is no coagulant activity and the Hb is rapidly cleared from the circulation. The risk of hepatitis B virus transmission is eliminated. The wide use of stroma-free Hb as a blood substitute awaits further evaluation.[15–18]

Perfluorochemicals

Liquid perfluorochemicals (perfluorocarbons) transport oxygen in solution, and have the potential to carry the same amount of oxygen as an equal volume of packed red cells.[19–21] Clinical studies of fluosol-DA 20% (Green Cross, Osaka, Japan) have been carried out in patients with surgical bleeding and anaemia.[22–25] This product also has potential uses for priming extracorporeal circuits, emergency resuscitation and in the management of cerebral and myocardial ischaemia. Circulatory half-life is 30–48 h.

Adverse effects have been minor, with 10% of patients showing a transient decrease in circulating white cells and platelets.[23] Perfluorochemicals are taken up by the reticuloendothelial cells and the macrophages, but methods of elimination from the cells and the body, presumably from the lung, are not known.[20] There is continuing investigation of optimal emulsification, particle size, stability at ambient temperature, compatibility with other products such as dextran and adverse effects on platelets.

Plasma derivatives[26,27]

Fresh frozen plasma (FFP)

FFP is prepared from a single unit of blood and contains all the coagulation factors.[1,28] One unit of 200 ml contains factor VIII 200 units, factor IX 200 units and fibrinogen 400 mg. It is kept at a temperature of –50°C in order to preserve coagulant levels. FFP is useful when a patient requires correction of a coagulation defect and also as volume replacement. Indications[29,30] include DIC, emergency reversal of warfarin and treatment of thrombotic thrombocytopenic purpura.

Fibrinogen (factor I)

Fibrinogen is available in FFP (400 mg/unit) and cryoprecipitate (250 mg/unit). Pooled fibrinogen concentrate has been withdrawn, because of the high risk of transmitting hepatitis. Fibrinogen is indicated when hypofibrinogenaemia is a problem, and particularly when the fibrinogen level is less than 100 mg/dl. This may occur after massive transfusion or during DIC, especially in obstetric haemorrhage.

Cryoprecipitate

Cryoprecipitate comprises 15 ml frozen plasma, is prepared from a single unit of blood, and contains about 50% of the coagulant factor activity of the original unit. It contains fibrinogen 250 mg, factor VIII 100 units, factor XIII, von Willebrand's factor and fibronectin. Cryoprecipitate is stored at –30°C and remains stable for 6 months. It is indicated in the treatment of coagulation defects, including massive haemorrhage, DIC, deficiency of fibrinogen, von Willebrand's disease and haemophilia A (factor VIII deficiency). In haemophilia, the aim is to raise the level of factor VIII to over 30% of normal.

Factor VIII

Traditional factor VIII concentrate is prepared from pools of FFP, and one freeze-dried vial contains factor VIII 300 units. It is stable for 2 years when stored at 4°C. Further purification of the concentrate by chromatography results in high-purity factor VIII, and the relative merits of high- and intermediate-purity products are being investigated. For haemophilia A, factor VIII 10–15 units/kg may be given IV, depending on the severity of the bleeding. It may be repeated 12-hourly, because of its 12-h half-life.

Factor IX

Factor IX concentrate (Prothrombinex) contains factor II, VII, IX and X in varying amounts, and is prepared from pools of plasma. It is available as a freeze-dried preparation, and is reconstituted with water immediately before use. Traditional factor IX concentrate of intermediate purity is used to treat haemophilia B, and to correct bleeding disorders due to deficiency of vitamin K-dependent factors II, VII, IX and X (e.g. to reverse coumarin anticoagulants and in liver disease). Purified factor IX concentrates are now available, and are 100 times purer than the traditional concentrate, with 75% of total protein being factor IX.

Other plasma concentrates

Von Willebrand's disease may be treated with desmopressin infusion, cryoprecipitate and the recently introduced intermediate and high-purity von Willebrand factor concentrates. Factor VII concentrate can be used in patients with inhibitors to factor VIII or IX, as it bypasses the requirement for factors VIII and IX. Antithrombin III concentrate is available for treating antithrombin III-deficient patients at times of risk, such as surgery.

Immunoglobulins (γ-globulins)

Immunoglobulins are plasma proteins with antibody activity, and are prepared from plasma pools obtained from normal blood donors. Immunoglobulin is given IV for prophylaxis against hepatitis A in travellers to areas where the disease is prevalent. It also contains useful levels of measles and poliomyelitis antibodies, but active immunization makes this application unnecessary. Immunoglobulins are indicated in the prevention or treatment of patients with hypogammaglobulinaemia, and may have a role in the treatment of autoimmune diseases such as thrombocytopenic purpura and myasthenia gravis. Recent reports of viral transmission[4] necessitate careful consideration of their use.

Specific immunoglobulins are available for tetanus and hepatitis B prophylaxis and treatment in patients who have not been actively immunized. Other specific immunoglobulins include Rh D immunoglobulin, which prevents sensitization of Rh-negative mothers, and zoster[31] and CMV immunoglobulin, for transplant recipients who are CMV antibody-negative.

Cellular components

Packed cells are red-cell concentrates half the volume of whole blood, with a haematocrit of 0.6–0.7. Apart from the smaller volume load, there is also less sodium, potassium, albumin and citrate. Packed cells also contain some white cells and platelets, and small amounts of plasma and additive solution. Washed red blood cells are produced after removing almost all of the leukocytes and plasma, and are sometimes necessary for patients with a history of transfusion reactions. The storage life of packed cells is 21–35 days, depending upon the anticoagulant in the original whole blood, but washed red cells must be given within 12 h of preparation.

Packed cells should be used in treating anaemia, particularly if there is associated cardiac failure, hepatic or renal disease. They can also be used for volume replacement, together with normal saline or other plasma expanders.

Granulocytes (white-cell concentrates or leukocytes)

Granulocyte transfusion may be indicated in the management of bacterial infections in the neutropenic patient,[32] particularly following chemotherapy for malignancies. Patients most likely to benefit[33] are those with a peripheral granulocyte count of under 0.5 $\times 10^9$/l, failure to improve after 24–48 h antibiotic therapy, prolonged aplasia and Gram-negative septicaemia. Histocompatible granulocytes, as identified by the human leukocyte antigen (HLA) system, should be given to avoid formation of alloimmune leukocyte and platelet antibodies.

Platelets

Platelet transfusion is indicated when a haemostatic defect is due to thrombocytopenia or abnormal platelet function (Table 87.2). Examples include acute leukaemia with the induction of remission, and aplastic anaemia. Other indications are platelet destruction during cardiopulmonary bypass and DIC. Platelets are of less value in idiopathic thrombocytopenic purpura, when antibodies significantly decrease platelet viability. In general, a platelet count of 20–50 $\times 10^9$/l carries a slight risk of spontaneous bleeding, between 10 and 20 $\times 10^9$/l moderate risk, and below 10 $\times 10^9$/l serious risk.

One unit of concentrates contains approximately 7 $\times 10^{10}$/l platelets, and is recovered from 1 unit of blood. The platelets are stored at room temperature (22°C), and should be given as soon as possible after collection, since they are viable for only 5 days. Refrigeration decreases platelet viability. Six units of concentrate raise the platelet count by about 30 $\times 10^9$/l, and can be repeated if necessary. Ideally, ABO and Rhesus-specific platelets should be used, and infused rapidly through a short infusion set without a

Table 87.2 Indications for platelet transfusion

Thrombocytopenia with decreased platelet production
Acute leukaemia
Aplastic anaemia
Myelodysplasia

Thrombocytopenia with platelet loss, sequestration or destruction
Cardiac bypass surgery
Massive transfusion
Disseminated intravascular coagulation
Splenomegaly
Idiopathic thrombocytopenic purpura

Abnormal platelet function
Congenital
Drug-induced

---

filter, which would otherwise trap platelets. The normal life span of platelets in the circulation is 10 days. HLA-matched platelets are given to alloimmunized patients with thrombocytopenia that is resistant to transfusion of platelet concentrates.

References

1. Mollison PL, Engelfriet CP and Contreras M (eds) (1993) *Blood Transfusion in Clinical Medicine*, 9th edn. Oxford: Blackwell Scientific Publications, pp. 638–676.

2. Williams WJ, Beutler E, Ersler AJ and Lichtman MA (eds) (1990) *Hematology*, 4th edn. New York: McGraw-Hill, pp. 1628–1673.

3. Bentop F (1994) Impact of replacement therapy on the evolution of HIV infection in hemophiliacs. *Thromb Haemost* **71**:678–683.

4. Schiff RI (1994) Transmission of viral infection through intravenous immune globulin. *N Engl J Med* **331**:1649–1650.

5. Storch H (1993) Rekombinante plasmaproteine zum therapeutischen einsatz – stand und entwick lungstendenzen. *Beitr Infusionther* **31**:31–37.

6. Griffel MI and Kaufman BS (1992) Pharmacology of colloids and crystalloids. *Crit Care Clin* **8**:235–253.

7. Isbister JP (1993) Adverse reactions to plasma and plasma components. *Anaesth Intens Care* **21**:31–38.

8. Lorenz W, Doenicke A, Messmer K *et al.* (1976) Histamine release in human subjects by modified gelatin (Haemaccel) and dextran: an explanation for anaphylactoid reactions observed under clinical conditions. *Br J Anaesth* **48**:151–164.

9. Messmer KFW (1983) Traumatic shock in polytrauma: circulatory parameters, biochemistry, and resuscitation. *World J Surg* **7**:26–30.

10. Schott U, Sjostrand UT and Berseus O (1985) Three percent dextran 60 as a plasma substitute in blood component therapy. An alternative in surgical blood loss replacement. *Acta Anaesthesiol Scand* **29**:767–774.

11. Schott U, Thoren T, Sjostrand U, Berseus O and Soderholm B (1985) Three per cent dextran 60 as a plasma substitute in blood component therapy. Comparative studies on pre- and postoperative blood volume. *Acta Anaesthesiol Scand* **29**:775–781.

12. Hedstrand O, Hogman C, Zaren B and Lundkvist B (1987) Postoperative complications after blood replacement with or without plasma. A trial in elective surgery. *Acta Chir Scand* **153**:501–505.

13. Haljamae H (1993) Volume substitution in shock. *Acta Anaesthesiol Scand* **98**(suppl):25–28.

14. Imm A and Carlson RW (1993) Fluid resuscitation in circulatory shock. *Crit Care Med* **9**:313–333.

15. Harringer W, Hodakowski GT, Svizzero T, Jacobs EE and Vlahakes GJ (1992) Acute effects of massive transfusion of a bovine hemoglobin blood substitute in a canine model of hemorrhagic shock. *Eur Cardiothorac Surg* **6**:649–654.

16. Crowley JP, Metzger J, Gray A, Pivacek LE, Cassidy G and Valeri CR (1993) Infusion of stroma-free linked hemoglobin during acute Gram negative bacteremia. *Circ Shock* **41**:144–149.

17. Roth RI, Levin J, Chapman KW, Schmeiz CM and Rickles FR (1993) Production of modified cross linked cell free hemoglobin for human use. *Transfusion* **33**:919–924.

18. Millis RM, Barber JD, Anderson WA, Dehkord O, Toussaint RM and Ertugrul L (1994) Acute beneficial effect of Fluosol DA on urinary excretion of stroma-free hemoglobin in the isolated rat kidney. *Ren Fail* **16**:325–335.

19. Colman RW, Chang LK, Mukherji B and Sloviter HA (1980) Effects of a perfluoro erythrocyte substitute on platelets *in vitro* and *in vivo*. *J Lab Clin Med* **75**:553–562.

20. Geyer GP (1985) *Artificial Blood Substitutes. Supportive Therapy in Haematology*. Boston: Martinus Nijhoff, pp. 388–396.

21. Kashimoto S, Nakamura T, Nomaka A, Kume M, Oguchi T and Kumazawa T (1994) Effects of artificial blood (FC-43 emulsion) on myocardial energy metabolism in the rat heart–lung preparation. *Br J Anaesth* **73**:380–383.

22. Mitsuno T, Ohyanagi H and Naito R (1982) Clinical studies of a perfluorochemical whole blood substitute (Fluosol-DA). *Ann Surg* **195**:60–69.

23. Tremper KK, Friedman AE, Levine EM, Lapin R and Camarillo D (1982) The preoperative treatment of severely anemic patients with a perfluorochemical oxygen-transport fluid, Fluosol-DA. *N Engl J Med* **307**:277–283.

24. Tremper KK and Cullen BF (1984) US clinical studies of the treatment of anemia with Fluosol-DA 20%. *Artif Organs* **8**:19–24.

25. Gould SA, Rosen AL and Sehgal LR (1986) Fluosol-DA as a red cell substitute in acute anaemia. *N Engl J Med* **314**:1653–1656.

26. Task Force of the College of American Pathologists (1994) Practice parameter for the use of fresh frozen plasma, cryoprecipitate and platelets. *J Am Med Assoc* **271**:777–819.

27. Soutar RL (1994) Recent advances in the development and use of plasma concentrates. *Br J Hosp Med* **51**:119–122.

28. Menitove JE (1990) Preparation and clinical use of plasma and plasma fractions. In: Williams WJ, Beutler E, Ersler AJ and Lichtman MA (eds) *Hematology*, 4th edn. New York; McGraw-Hill, pp. 1659–1673.

29. Thomson A, Napier JAF and Wood JK (1992) Use and abuse of fresh frozen plasma. *Br J Anaesth* **68**:237–238.

30. Donaldson MDJ, Seaman MJ and Park GR (1992) Massive blood transfusion. *Br J Anaesth* **69**:621–630.

31. Rice P, Simmons K, Carr R and Banatvala J (1994) Near fatal chickenpox during prednisolone treatment. *Br Med J* **309**:1069–1070.

32. Nushacher J (1990) Preservation and clinical use of leukocytes. In: Williams WJ, Beutler E, Ersler AJ and Lichtman MA (eds) *Hematology*, 4th edn. New York: McGraw-Hill, pp. 1647–1653.

33. Robinson AE (1986) White cell concentrate therapy. In: Cash JD (ed). *Progress in Transfusion Medicine*, vol. 1. Edinburgh: Churchill Livingstone, p. 54.

JP Isbister

Blood-letting to remove 'evil humours' has a long history over 2000 years. This principle of removing pathological components from blood continues as a mode of therapy today.[1] Exchange transfusions revolutionized the treatment of haemolytic disease in the newborn, and paved the way for plasmapharesis or plasma exchange – the removal of plasma, with replacement by albumin–electrolyte solutions or plasma proteins. Plasma exchange was initially used to manage hyperviscosity associated with malignant paraproteinaemia, but is now used to treat a wide range of autoimmune and other diseases (now > 100; Table 88.1). Nevertheless, it is expensive and not risk-free, and debate continues on its therapeutic role in some diseases.

Rationale for plasma exchange[1]

Theoretically, plasma exchange should be effective to treat any disorder in which there is a pathogenic circulating factor. However, this premise is probably too simplistic, and other mechanisms may contribute to its beneficial effects (Table 88.2). None the less, it is a non-specific and relatively crude procedure, which brings about numerous potentially undesirable alterations in the plasma's *milieu intérieur*.

Pathophysiology of autoimmune disease

Autoimmune disease originates from the break-down of immunoregulation (i.e. immune tolerance), allowing the immune system to become autoaggressive. Those having underlying humoral mechanisms result from either a circulating autoantibody against a self-antigen (alone or in combination with an environmental antigen), or circulating immune complexes (which may be deposited in the microcirculation of various organs, resulting in end-organ damage). Cellular and tissue damage are

Table 88.1 Acute diseases in which plasma exchange may be beneficial*

Immunoproliferative diseases with monoclonal immunoglobulins

Hyperviscosity syndrome
Cryoglobulinaemia
Renal failure in multiple myeloma

Autoimmune diseases due to autoantibodies or immune complexes

Goodpasture's syndrome
Myasthenia gravis
Guillain–Barré syndrome
Systemic lupus erythematosus
Thrombotic thrombocytopenic purpura
Rapidly progressive glomerulonephritits
Coagulation inhibitors
Autoimmune haemolytic anaemia
Pemphigus

Conditions in which replacement of plasma may be beneficial

Disseminated intravascular coagulation
Overwhelming sepsis syndromes (e.g. meningococcaemia)
Administration of large volume of specific plasma (e.g. humoral immune deficiency states)

Conditions in which the mechanisms are unknown

Reye's syndrome

Removal of protein-bound or large-molecular-weight toxins

Paraquat poisoning
Envenomation?

Rapid removal of plasma and replacement with red cells

Severely anaemic patients in gross congestive cardiac failure

*This is an incomplete list and only includes disorders which are relatively common or in which plasma exchange has a definitive role to play.

Table 88.2 Rationale for plasma exchange

Removal of circulating toxic factor antibodies
   Monoclonal antibodies
   Autoantibodies
   Alloantibodies, immune complexes, chemicals, drugs
Depletion of the mediators of inflammation
Replacement of deficient plasma factor(s)
Potentiation of drug action
Enhanced reticuloendothelial function
Altered immunoregulation
Potentiating effects of plasma exchange on other modes of therapy

effected by the autoantibody or immune complexes activating the cellular and humoral components of the inflammatory response. The circulating proteolytic systems involved include the complement, coagulation, fibrinolytic and kinin systems. On the cellular side, neutrophils and macrophages are involved, but eosinophils and basophils may also play a part.

The varied clinical manifestations of autoimmune disorders relate more to the cell, tissue or organ involved, rather than the pathophysiological process. However, basic pathophysiological mechanisms of autoimmune diseases need to be understood in order to standardize treatment. Although some cells of the host defence system, particularly macrophages and lymphocytes, may have special differentiation appropriate to individual organs, their basic functional processes are not much dissimilar between different organs.

In general, autoimmune disease can be an acute, self-limiting ('one-hit'), intermittent disorder or a chronic perpetuating one. Acute autoimmune disease may have an identifiable trigger, such as an infection. This is followed 10 days to 3 weeks later by the appearance of pathogenic humoral or cellular factors in circulating blood. At this point, end-organ damage commences, and clinical features of the disease appear. The course of the disease will be determined by:

1 biological function and importance of the system involved;
2 extent of damage;
3 replaceability or otherwise of the cells under attack;
4 time course of the damaging insult.

The extent of damage will depend on:

1 characteristics of the antibodies or lymphocytes involved (e.g. antibody affinity, complement-fixing capabilities and titre);

2 function of other components of the host defence system (e.g. neutrophils, platelets, proteolytic systems and reticuloendothelial system);
3 presence of other aggravating factors (e.g. infection, hormonal responses and circulatory responses).

The kinetics of the end-cell involved in the immunological damage are relevant in determining final outcome. Ultimate recovery of organ function after 'burn-out' of a self-limiting autoimmune disease or control of a chronic autoimmune disease is determined by the ability of the cell to replace and restore function to normal. Cells are broadly divided into three kinetic characteristics (Fig. 88.1):

1 *Continuous replicators*: These cells are continuously replaced in the normal state. They are readily replaced when damaged, and if the immunological insult is removed or controlled, full replacement of the end-cells occurs. This is typically seen with the haemopoietic system, the cells lining the gut and skin cells.
2 *Discontinuous or intermittent replicators*: These cells are not being constantly replaced in the normal state, but when damaged, they initiate cell division and replacement. This is seen with hepatocytes, renal tubular cells and the neuronal Schwann cell.
3 *Non-replicating cells*: These cells when damaged are irreplaceably destroyed, with permanent loss of function. This is seen with neuronal cells, muscle cells and glomeruli.

Thus, the clinical features and final outcome of any autoimmune disease are determined by many factors, including the ability of the end-organ to repair itself following removal/control of the immunological insult. In many self-limiting autoimmune disorders, if the end-cell is a continuous or intermittent replicator, full recovery can be expected, as long as appropriate support to end-organ function is given during the acute phase. However, in disorders with non-replicating cells such as acute glomerulonephritis, therapy must aim to remove the immunological insult or dampen its damaging affects, so as to minimize irreparable damage to end-cells. Immunological mediators may also produce disease without direct destruction of end-cells. This occurs when autoantibodies develop against cell receptors, with blocking or destruction of the receptor, as is typically seen in myasthenia gravis and thyrotoxicosis.

Thus, therapy in acute and chronic autoimmune disease aims to minimize irreparable end-organ damage and support patients during the acute illness. This can include:

1 non-specific therapy to suppress the effector mechanisms, e.g. corticosteroids, antiplatelet therapy,

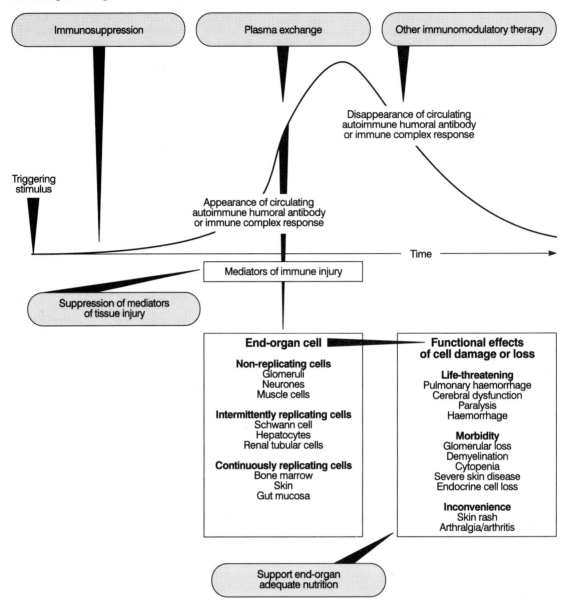

Fig. 88.1 Therapy of 'one-hit' autoimmune disease.

non-steroidal anti-inflammatory drugs, anticoagulation and depletion of humoral effector mechanisms by plasma exchange or defibrination;

2 therapy to reduce circulating levels of humoral factor by plasma exchange or immunoabsorption techniques;

3 specific or broad-spectrum immunosuppressive agents to suppress or block the immune response, e.g. corticosteroids, cytotoxic agents, antilymphocyte globulin and, possibly, high-dose γ-globulin therapy;

4 therapy directed at altering reticuloendothelial function, which may then affect autoantibody and immune complex clearance, or clearance of circulating damaged cells.

As most disorders are multifactorial, it is unlikely that a single form of therapy will be successful. A multipronged approach to therapy needs to be planned following an analysis of the basic underlying pathophysiology. The stage of the disease is also important (Fig. 88.1). Clearly, plasma exchange will have a different response when autoantibody production is rising rapidly, compared to a stage when autoantibody has ceased production. Also, immunoregulation is a complex process, and therapies may interfere at points in the immune system. In general, plasma exchange is a temporizing procedure, and concomitant immunosuppressive therapy is usually required to maintain control. Plasma exchange for autoimmune disease should be regarded as a first step in immunosuppression, and restricted to acute or fulminant situations with potential life-threatening or end-organ-damaging complications. In some situations, the humoral factor may be only transient ('one antigen hit' disorders), and no follow-up immunosuppression is required (e.g. acute postinfectious polyneuritis).

Technical considerations

Cell separators for plasma exchange therapy are broadly divided into two groups:

1 Machines which use centrifugation for the separation are also suitable for specific separation and removal of blood components (e.g. thrombopheresis and leukapheresis).
2 Machines which separate by membrane fitration can only be used for plasma separation.

Either of these can be combined with immunoabsorption techniques, in which immunoglobulins are specifically or non-specifically removed.

As plasma is removed, it is replaced volume for volume with a solution of adequate colloid (oncotic) activity (e.g. 5% albumin) and appropriate electrolyte composition. Although the levels of other plasma proteins are reduced by plasma exchange, clinically significant effects are rare in most patients. However, if extremely large volumes are exchanged, or exchanges are done frequently, it may be necessary to replace some plasma proteins. In patients with coagulation factor deficiencies or immunodeficiency, fresh frozen plasma (FFP) is usually required. Thrombocytopenic patients may require platelet transfusions at the conclusion of the procedure. The use of large volumes of fresh blood products results in substantial infusion of sodium citrate and a significant risk of posttransfusion hepatitis.

Indications (Table 88.1)

Plasma exchange is most beneficial for immunoproliferative and autoimmune diseases. In some conditions with unclear pathophysiology, beneficial effects of plasma exchange may be due to infusion of a deficient component rather than removal of a circulating factor.

Malignant monoclonal antibodies[2]

Monoclonal immunoglobulins are a classical feature of multiple myeloma and Waldenström's macroglobulinaemia, but may also be associated with other immunoproliferative and lymphoproliferative disorders. These monoclonal proteins are associated with numerous clinical effects, many of which may be reversed by plasma exchange.

1 *Hyperviscosity syndrome*: Characteristic clinical features of hyperviscosity in association with monoclonal proteins include visual disturbance, neurological dysfunction and hypervolaemia, all of which can be rapidly relieved by plasma exchange.
2 *Haemostatic disturbances*: Monoclonal proteins may impair haemostasis by affecting platelet function or inhibiting coagulation factors. Plasma exchange is usually effective in controlling haemorrhage and may also be helpful in preparing patients for surgery.
3 *Renal failure*:[3] The development of renal failure in the course of multiple myeloma is generally regarded as a sign of poor prognosis. In most cases, the renal failure is multifactorial in origin, but some of these factors may be reversible by plasma exchange. Patients presenting acutely with hyperviscosity, dehydration and hypercalcaemia may show recovery of renal function following adequate hydration, alkaline diuresis and plasma exchange.

Immunological diseases[4–10]

Diseases mediated by specific autoantibodies

Goodpasture's syndrome
Most cases are due to circulating antiglomerular basement membrane antibodies. The disease classically has a fulminant presentation with rapidly progressive renal failure and life-threatening pulmonary haemorrhage. Early diagnosis and intensive plasma exchange may be necessary to preserve renal function and control pulmonary haemorrhage. Patients already in anuric renal failure rarely show improvement in renal function.

Myasthenia gravis
Removal of the acetylcholine receptor autoantibody (anti-AChR) is associated with clinical improvement in the majority of patients with this disorder. The beneficial effects of plasma exchange are usually transient, and the procedure should usually be used with other forms of therapy (see Chapter 49). Although the indications for plasma exchange in myasthenia gravis are still debated, its major role is usually in myasthenic crisis, in patients whose condition is resistant to other forms of therapy, and prior to surgery. Therapy should be monitored by

anti-AChR assays and respiratory function tests. Patients undergoing plasma exchange may transiently deteriorate during the procedure, due to a combination of the physical exertion and removal of medication from the circulation; adequate ventilatory support should be available.

Autoimmune haematological disorders

Occasionally, plasma exchange may be indicated in severe autoimmune haemolytic anaemia and idiopathic thrombocytopenic purpura, when conventional forms of therapy have failed. Autoantibodies may also be directed against coagulation factors, presenting a major management problem. Antibodies directed against factor VIII are the commonest, occurring spontaneously or in association with replacement therapy in haemophiliacs.

Immune complex disease

Rapidly progressive glomerulonephritis

Immune complex-induced rapidly progressive glomerulonephritis may occur by itself or with several systemic disorders (e.g. systemic lupus erythematosus, polyarteritis nodosa and Wegener's granulomatosis). The therapeutic role of plasma exchange in this disorder is difficult to assess, but plasma exchange may improve renal function, even in fulminant, rapidly deteriorating cases. The decomplementing and defibrinating effects of plasma exchange when FFP is not used as replacement fluid may be partly responsible for clinical improvement. However, the ultimate prognosis of the disease depends on adequate immunosuppression to inhibit immune complex formation, or spontaneous disappearance of the inciting antigen.

Systemic lupus erythematosus

Plasma exchange has a role in acute life-threatening or organ-damaging relapses of systemic lupus erythematosus. Rapid deterioration in renal function, cerebritis and acute fulminant lupus pneumonitis are clinical situations in which plasma exchange should be considered.

Cryoglobulinaemia

The various forms of cryoglobulinaemia may be associated with vasculitis or hyperviscosity. In some cases, there may be an acute fulminant presentation with cutaneous vasculitis, renal failure and neurological impairment. In this situation, plasma exchange should be considered an urgent definitive form of therapy.

Miscellaneous acute disorders with unclear immune mechanisms

Renal transplant rejection

Humoral mechanisms appear to play a part in hyperacute renal allograft rejection. Plasma exchange may be useful in tiding patients over episodes of acute graft rejection, but results of clinical trials are conflicting. General opinion is that plasma exchange helps in a limited number of patients who cannot be preselected by clinical or laboratory criteria.

Thrombotic thrombocytopenic purpura

This rare disorder, with thrombocytopenia, microangiopathic haemolytic anaemia, fever, neurological dysfunction and renal impairment, is ill-understood. In some cases, damage to the microvascular endothelium secondary to deposition of immune complexes has been shown, while reports of remissions after infusion of fresh blood and frozen plasma in other cases suggest a deficient plasma component. The prognosis of this disorder has improved dramatically over the last decade. The exact role of each aspect of therapy remains unclear, but plasma infusion, plasma exchange and antiplatelet therapy all have a role.

Haemolytic–uraemic syndrome

In this condition, renal failure is associated with a microangiopathic haemolytic anaemia. The pathophysiology is probably similar to thrombotic thrombocytopenic purpura, with overlap syndromes being seen. Plasma exchange may have a role in therapy.

Guillain–Barré syndrome

This acute self-limiting disease of an acute demyelinating neuropathy (usually following a viral infection) commonly results in admission to the ICU (see Chapter 48). There is convincing evidence that the demyelination is due to postinfectious autoimmunity, with both cellular and humoral arms of the immune system attacking myelin. Controlled trials have now substantiated the benefits of plasma exchange in shortening the illness, reducing complications and cost savings. In general, all bed-ridden patients with severe disease or evidence of rapid progression should be exchanged. Indications for plasma exchange of patients with a lesser severity of disease are less clear. Plasma exchange should be instituted early and frequently. Some patients show rapid improvement after plasma exchange, suggesting the presence of neuronal blocking factors. The onset of recovery after plasma exchange may be delayed, probably due to time for remyelination to occur. Guillain–Barré syndrome also responds to high-dose IV immunoglobulin. However, availability and cost mitigate against this as first-line therapy.

Complications[11]

Plasma exchange is a relatively safe procedure, but close supervision by experienced staff is essential. A sound understanding of the haemodynamic, biochemical, haematological and immunological effects of plasma exchange is of paramount importance.

Potential complications include fluid imbalance, reactions to replacement fluids, vasovagal reactions, pyrogenic reactions, hypothermia, embolism (air or microaggregates), hypocalcaemia, anaemia, thrombocytopenia, haemostatic disturbances, hepatitis, hypogammaglobulinaemia and altered pharmacokinetics of drugs. Prevention and treatment of most of these complications are obvious. However, certain complications and ill-understood effects of plasma exchange should be emphasized.

Circulatory effects

Any extracorporeal procedure is likely to result in problems of circulatory instability. Intravascular volume changes, vasovagal reactions, medications and infusion fluids may all alone, or in combination, be responsible for circulatory problems. The patient will usually be able to compensate if there are no associated oxygen transport defects. However, if there are pre-existing defects (e.g. altered blood volume, vascular disease or renal failure), close monitoring is essential. A strict and accurate fluid and electrolyte balance is mandatory.

Plasma oncotic pressure

Most patients compensate for minor fluctuations in plasma oncotic pressure. Patients who have oedema or local factors which predispose to interstitial fluid accumulation (e.g. raised intracranial pressure, interstitial pulmonary oedema, deep venous thrombosis and renal impairment) need their plasma oncotic pressure monitored by estimations of total protein level.

Infection

Many patients presenting for plasma exchange are already immunosuppressed, either due to disease or secondary to drug therapy. In patients requiring recurrent and frequent plasma exchange, attempts should be made to maintain serum immunoglobulin levels. When FFP is not used as replacement fluid, the bactericidal and opsonic activities of blood are probably impaired, and it is probably advantageous to infuse at least 2 units of FFP at the conclusion of the procedure. The risk of post transfusion hepatitis must always be borne in mind.

Haemostasis

Plasma exchange causes major perturbations in the haemostatic system which may result in either bleeding or thrombosis. The significance of these alterations will largely depend on the volume and frequency of exchange, pre-existing defects in the system, anticoagulation, other risk factors for thrombosis, replacement fluids and invasive procedures.

Reactions to replacement fluids

The rapid infusion of any blood component may be associated with allergic or vasomotor reactions. Plasma exchange is a rather unique situation in which blood or blood products and plasma substitutes are being infused at resuscitation rates into normovolaemic, normotensive patients.

Effects of intravascular proteins

If plasma protein fractions or albumin are being used for replacement fluids, not only will coagulation and complement components be depleted, but various transport and binding proteins in the circulation are significantly reduced. These may have significant, as yet ill-understood, effects on drug activity and elimination. In particular, the reduction of antithrombin III levels may affect heparin activity, and there is an increased risk of venous thrombosis after plasma exchange. The effects of corticosteroids may be potentiated after plasma exchange owing to a reduction in binding proteins.

References

1. Isbister JP (1979) Plasma exchange: a selective form of blood-letting. *Med J Aust* **2**:167–169.
2. Reinhart WH, Lutolf O, Nydegger U, Mahler F and Werner Straub P (1992) Plasmapheresis for hyperviscosity syndrome in macroglobulinemia Waldenström and multiple myeloma: influence on blood rheology and the microcirculation. *J Lab Clin Med* **119**:69–76.
3. Isbister JP, Harris DCH and Ibels LS (1984) The management of renal failure in multiple myeloma. *Clin Exp Haemorrheol* **5**:373–384.
4. Douzinas EE, Markakis K, Karabinis A, Mandalaki T, Bilalis D and Fessas P (1992) Early plasmapheresis in patients with thrombotic thrombocytopenic purpura. *Crit Care Med* **20**:57–61.
5. Hayward CPM, Sutton DMC, Carter WH Jr *et al.* (1994) Treatment outcomes in patients with adult thrombotic thrombocytopenic purpura–hemolytic uremic syndrome. *Arch Intern Med* **154**:982–987.
6. Novitzky N, Jacobs P and Rosenstrauch W (1994) The treatment of thrombotic thrombocytopenic purpura: plasma infusion or exchange? *Br J Haematol* **87**:317–320.
7. Prick MJJ and Verhagen WIM (1991) Chronic inflammatory demyelinating polyneuropathy: immunoglobulins or plasmapheresis. *Arch Neurol* **48**:1118–1119.
8. Pusey CD, Rees AJ, Evans DJ, Peters DK and Lockwood CM (1991) Plasma exchange in focal necrotizing glomerulonephritis without anti-GBM antibodies. *Kidney Int* **40**:757–763.

9. Thornton CA and Griggs RC (1994) Plasma exchange and intravenous immunoglobulin treatment of neuromuscular disease. *Ann Neurol* **35**:260–268.

10. Van der Meché FGA, Schmitz PIM and Dutch Guillain-Barré Study Group (1992) A randomized trial comparing intravenous immune globulin and plasma exchange in Guillain–Barré syndrome. *N Engl J Med* **326**:1123–1129.

11. Mokrzycki MH and Kaplan AA (1994) Therapeutic plasma exchange: complications and management. *Am J Kidney Dis* **23**:817–827.

Haemostatic failure

JP Isbister

Failure of haemostasis is common in critically ill patients, and tends to be complex and multifactorial. As it complicates a wide range of disorders, definitive diagnosis and specific therapy may thus affect outcome. Frequently, complex tests are required for definitive diagnosis, but due to clinical urgency, therapy may be initiated on clinical evidence without waiting for full laboratory results. Consultation with a clinical haematologist is considered mandatory.

Normal haemostasis[1]

Haemostasis is achieved by highly integrated and regulated vascular, cellular and humoral responses. The triad of vascular constriction, platelet plugging and fibrin clot formation forms haemostatic plugs, and provides the framework for haemostasis (Fig. 89.1) and healing. Following injury, vascular constriction occurs to reduce bleeding and initiate haemostasis. This constriction is further accentuated by vasoconstrictors released in association with platelet plug formation. Vascular endothelial cells synthesize substances which act at the membrane surface and/or interact with platelets and the coagulation system (e.g. prostacyclin, antithrombin III, plasminogen activator, von Willebrand's factor, thrombomodulin, heparin cofactor II and nitric oxide). Thus difficulties will be encountered if different components of the haemostatic system are analysed in isolation. Following the initial vascular reactions, successful haemostasis depends on adequate numbers of functioning platelets, coagulation cascade function and poorly understood contributions from red cells and leukocytes.

Soluble plasma coagulation proteins are activated following the primary phase of haemostasis (formation of the platelet plug). These complex plasma proteins are responsible for forming the fibrin clot. Fibrin is the end-product of a proteolytic activity cascade, where precursor coagulation proteins are activated to potent proteolytic enzymes, which (with cofactors) activate precursors further down the coagulation amplifier.

The *intrinsic* coagulation system is initiated by activation of the contact phase, i.e. factors XII and XI. Other plasma proteolytic, fibrinolytic, kinin and complement systems may also be activated in concert with coagulation. After contact, initial activation factors IX, VIII, calcium and platelet phospholipid interact to activate factor X, which enters the common pathway of coagulation Xa, prothrombin (II), V, calcium and platelet phospholipid to generate thrombin. Thus thrombin is the potent final proteolytic enzyme of the coagulation sequence that converts fibrinogen to fibrin monomers, which subsequently polymerize to form the fibrin clot. This clot is further acted on by factor XIII to form stable fibrin.

Direct rapid activation of the common pathway can also occur via the *extrinsic* pathway, by which damaged tissues release a tissue thromboplastin, which activates factor VII, a potent converter of factor X (and thus common pathway activation). Rapid clotting of blood in a syringe during a difficult venepuncture is due to activation of this extrinsic system. The extrinsic system also has a role early in haemostasis, by generating small amounts of thrombin to facilitate platelet aggregation. Activated factor VII (VIIa) is also important in factor IX activation (of the intrinsic pathway). The contact phase of the intrinsic pathway is probably less important than was originally thought.

Parallel to and within the coagulation system are complex feedback mechanisms to ensure fine-tuning and protection against inappropriate and excessive activation (e.g. disseminated intravascular coagulation (DIC) or venous thromboembolism). There are several inhibitory proteins, including antithrombin III, α_2-macroglobulin, and protein C and S, as well as the fibrinolytic system, which are important in controlling the degree and site of fibrin formation. Massive activation, as may be seen in trauma and severe infections, can precipitate disseminated activation, but in general, the

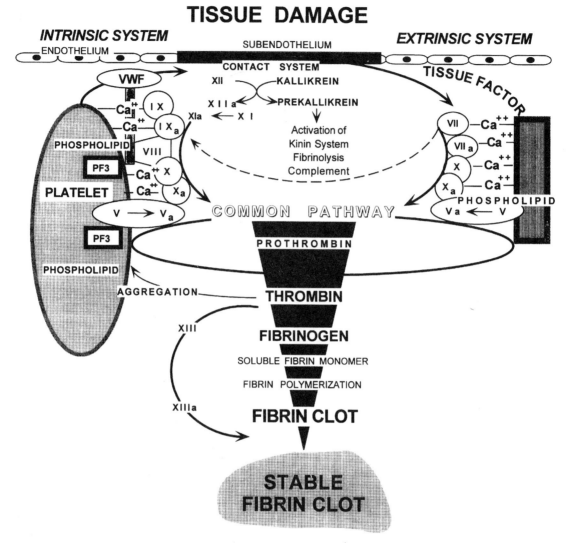

Fig. 89.1 The haemostatic system. VWF = von Willebrand factor; PF3 = platelet factor 3.

system is well-controlled and activity is localized to the area of stimulus. Perturbations in this complex defence system can produce a wide range of clinical disorders, from excessive arterial or venous thrombosis, microvascular obstruction and atheroma, to haemostatic failure.

Investigation for a systemic haemostatic defect[1–3] (Fig. 89.2)

Several clinical features suggest local or generalized failure of the haemostatic system (Fig. 89.2). History is important and is frequently underrated, especially with respect to drug ingestion. Laboratory investigations

(see below) will depend on the degree of urgency. It may be necessary to administer blood component therapy without a definitive haemostatic defect being proven. In more elective settings, the defect can be accurately identified, and specific blood component therapy given. Crude tests of whole blood clotting time (WBCT) and clot observation may have a role in emergency settings, especially while waiting for laboratory results. For this, blood must be collected in a *glass* tube – collected blood will not clot immediately in a plastic syringe – and kept at 37°C (e.g. under the axilla) and timed for clot formation. Clot size, retraction and possible lysis can all be crudely observed. Based on clinical evidence, laboratory results when available, and consultation with a

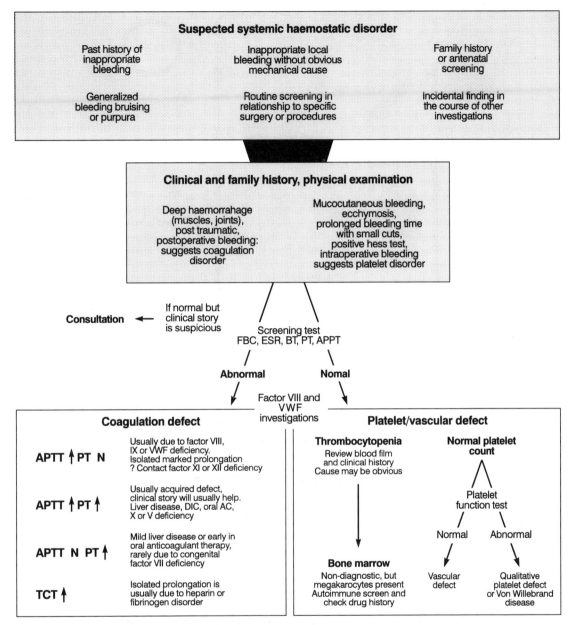

Fig. 89.2 Investigation for haemostatic defect. FBC = Full blood count; ESR = erythrocyte sedimentation rate; BT = bleeding time; PT = prothrombin time; VWF = Von Willebrand factor; APTT = activated partial thromboplastin time; TCT = thrombin clotting time; DIC = disseminated intravascular coagulation; AC = anticoagulants.

haematologist, further specific tests may be indicated (e.g. factor assays and platelet function tests).

Tests of the haemostatic system (Fig. 89.3)

Proper collection of blood samples, including good venepuncture technique, is crucial. Contam- ination with tissue factor due to traumatic venepuncture will activate the sample and inval- idate results. It is best to avoid arterial lines for sampling, as heparin contamination is possible, even if the first sample withdrawn is discarded. Collection from any vascular access line may result in a diluted sample. Most samples are col-

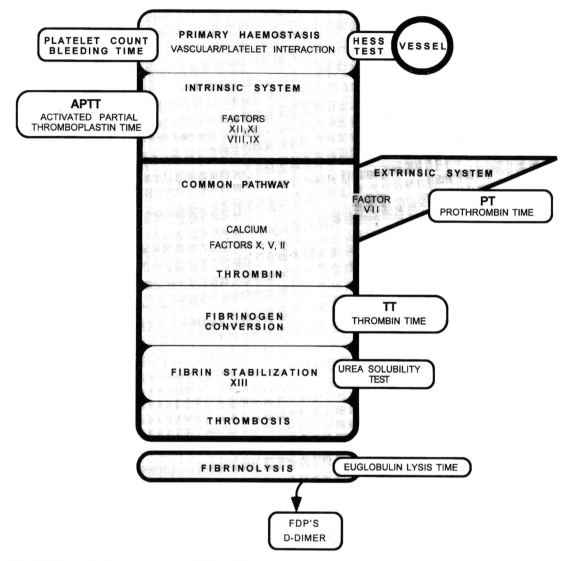

Fig. 89.3 Tests of the haemostatic system. FDPs = Fibrinogen degradation products.

lected into citrated tubes with an amount of anti-coagulant related to the filling volume. The correct amount of blood must be added to the tube (up the marked line) and mixed gently. Rapid transfer of the sample to the laboratory is important.

Laboratory tests to investigate haemostatic defects are presented below. In broad terms, prothrombin time (PT) tests integrity of the extrinsic system, activated partial thromboplastin time (APTT) the intrinsic system, and thrombin clotting time (TCT) fibrinogen conversion. D-Dimer measures the breakdown products of lysis of fibrin.

Bleeding time (BT; normal range: 3–9 min)

This is the most basic test to assess primary haemostasis (i.e. the vascular phase and platelet plug formation *in vivo*). It is usually performed by the Ivy method (tourniquet applied to 40 mmHg (5.3 kPa)) using a commercial disposable template to make a standard incision. The incision is made on the flexor surface of the forearm, and the accumulating blood is absorbed with blotting paper from the side. BT is progressively prolonged when the platelet count falls below $75–100 \times 10^9/l$ (with normal platelet function). BT is also prolonged when platelet function is defective, or in capillary/

vascular disease or certain coagulation defects. BT is not a good screening test for a haemostatic disorder in unselected patients.

Platelet count (normal range: 150–400 × 10⁹/l)

Counting of platelets is usually performed as part of the full blood count by automated cell counters. In emergencies, examination of the blood film by an experienced observer will usually give a good approximation. Accurate platelet counts are not possible on 'fingerprick' blood.

Thrombin clotting time (normal range <2 s longer than control 10–15 s)

TCT tests the final conversion of fibrinogen to fibrin, and bypasses the intrinsic and extrinsic systems, as thrombin is added to the test system. Prolonged TCT is due to hypofibrinogenaemia, dysfibrinogenaemia, heparin and fibrin degradation products (FDPs).

Prothrombin time (normal range <3 s of control) and international normalized ratio (INR)

PT is a test of the extrinsic pathway, where citrated plasma is recalcified at the same time as tissue factor (thromboplastin) is added and the clotting time recorded. Prolongation may be caused by factor VII deficiency, liver disease, vitamin K deficiency or oral anticoagulant therapy. INR is the ratio of sample PT to a control international standard PT. Anticoagulant therapy aims for an INR ratio of 2.0–2.5.

Activated partial thromboplastin time (normal range varies between laboratories: >6 s longer than control is probably abnormal)

APTT is a test of the intrinsic coagulation system. The contact phase of the coagulation cascade is activated before the sample is recalcified in the presence of a platelet substitute. Prolongation is due to contact-phase defect. A mild to moderate prolongation of APTT in the presence of a normal PT usually means that a haemophilic factor (i.e. factors VIII and IX) is deficient or inhibited. Prolonged PT and APTT indicate factor X, V and II deficiency. APTT is also prolonged in the presence of inhibition, e.g. by heparin, warfarin, FDPs or lupus anticoagulant, which is usually associated with the antiphospholipid syndrome.

Specific coagulation factor assays

All factors can be assayed, but factor VII components and fibrinogen are the ones most commonly performed.

D-dimer

When fibrin is lysed by the proteolytic activity of plasmin, various cleavage fragments are released. These are usually measured immunologically on a serum sample. Minor elevations of D-Dimer, as may be seen in the postoperative state, trauma, renal impairment, sepsis and venous thrombosis, do not indicate excessive fibrinolysis. High D-Dimer concentrations suggest excessive fibrinolysis (e.g. in DIC).

Euglobulin lysis time (ELT; normal range >90 min)

This test mainly reflects the presence of plasminogen activators. A shortened time is indicative of system fibrinolytic activation.

Congenital haemostatic defects[1-3]

Congenital bleeding disorders are relatively uncommon, and are usually confined to a single defect. It is important to identify the defect so that specific replacement therapy can be given. Commonly seen disorders are described below.

Haemophilia A (classical haemophilia)

This is a sex-linked disorder due to a deficiency of factor VIII. The mainstay of treatment is coagulation factor replacement. Factor VIII concentrates are given to prevent bleeding (e.g. for tooth extractions and invasive procedures, including arterial blood-gas sampling) and to control existing haemorrhage. The dose is calculated on the basis that 1 unit of factor is that amount present in 1 ml of pooled normal plasma. A normal individual with a plasma volume of 3000 ml would have 3000 U of factor VIII in the circulation. An equivalent haemophiliac with <1% factor VIII in the plasma would require a dose of 3000 U to raise the plasma concentration to 100% normal.

Experience has demonstrated that 15–20 U/kg body weight will control most haemarthroses, but doses of up to 30 U/kg are required for muscle haematomas or prevention of dental bleeding. Raising factor VIII concentrations to 100% normal is indicated for severe bleeding (e.g. intracranial or intra-abdominal haemorrhage), but patient response varies considerably, and empirical doses may be necessary. Measurement of factor VIII concentrations following replacement therapy is helpful. A factor VIII concentration of 25% (usually achieved with a dose of 15 U/kg) controls joint bleeding, whereas a concentration of 50% (generally obtained with a dose of 30 U/kg) prevents bleeding following tooth extraction.

The half-life of factor VIII in the circulation is approximately 12 h. Hence doses are repeated

12-hourly if a specific plasma concentration is targeted. The concentrate may also be given by continuous infusion. Recently developed recombinant factor VIII will alleviate the shortage of factor VIII concentrates, but at a prohibitive cost.

Haemophilia B or Christmas disease

This disorder is due to factor IX deficiency, and is less common than classical haemophilia. The general principles of management are similar, with factor IX concentrates being used.

Von Willebrand's disease

This is the commonest hereditary haemostatic disorder, being autosomal dominant, with marked phenotypic variation characterized by deficient or defective von Willebrand factors. This factor is the bridging molecule between the primary phase of haemostasis and coagulation. The coagulation part of factor VIII combines with von Willebrand factor to make up the whole factor VIII molecule. In general, management is not dictated by the variant, with cryoprecipitate or fresh frozen plasma (FFP) being used. However, desmopressin (DDAVP) infusion has reduced the need for blood products, especially in the elective setting. DDAVP induces a haemostatic state via release of factor VIII and von Willebrand factor; 0.3 µg/kg is infused slowly over 30 min, immediately prior to surgery.

Congenital platelet disorders

These are relatively rare, the commonest severe variety being Glanzmann's thrombasthenia. Platelet transfusions may be required for acute bleeds or elective surgery. DDAVP with or without antifibrinolytic therapy to boost haemostasis may obviate platelet transfusions, which risk alloimmunization and future refractoriness.

Acquired haemostatic disorders[1-3]

Acquired disorders of coagulation are usually more complex and multifactorial. A unified approach is essential for the successful management of these potentially life-threatening situations, and transfusion therapy cannot be isolated from other treatment.

Massive blood transfusion[4]

The nature and management of haemostatic defects secondary to massive blood loss and transfusion remain poorly understood. Some degree of haemostatic failure will inevitably result if blood more than a week old is used for resuscitation. The labile factors V and VIII are not well-preserved beyond 3–4 days; platelets are aggregated and non-functional even

Table 89.1 Possible factors contributing to haemostatic failure following massive blood transfusion

Pre-existing haemostatic defect

Loss of coagulation factors, platelets and inhibitors

Dilution of coagulation factors, platelets and inhibitors

Impaired synthesis due to effects of shock on liver and bone marrow function

Effects of trauma: disseminated intravascular coagulation (DIC) and fibrinolysis

Effects of storage lesion: depletion of coagulation factors and platelets, aggravation or precipitation of DIC

Depletion of modulators of haemostasis (e.g. antithrombin III, fibronectin and protein C)

Incompatible transfusion reaction: DIC

Hypothermia

? Citrate toxicity

before then; some coagulation factors may be activated; and microaggregates and degenerate cells may aggravate or initiate DIC. The relative importance of the different potential mechanisms of haemostatic failure (Table 89.1) is difficult to determine, but the identification of correctable defects will avoid or minimize complications.

Bleeding correlates poorly with the volume of transfusion or components administered, but nature of the insult, degree of hypovolaemic shock and time to resuscitation correlate with haemostatic failure. Trauma patients with major coagulopathy and microvascular haemorrhage usually have abnormal laboratory parameters prior to massive blood transfusion. Except for severe abnormalities, haemostatic laboratory parameters correlate poorly with clinical evidence of haemostatic failure. Thrombocytopenia and impaired platelet function are the most consistent significant haematological abnormalities; correction of these disorders may be associated with control of microvascular bleeding. Coagulation deficiency from massive blood loss is usually confined to factors V and VIII. Preventive protocol blood component replacement has not proved successful. DIC is usually related to the underlying pathology (see below), but may be compounded by massive blood transfusion.

Coagulation screening tests (APTT, PT and TCT) should be performed, but the usual urgent situation does not allow for specific factor assays. FFP is indicated if the test results are abnormal. Indeed, a case can be made for prophylactic FFP infusions in patients with massive blood loss which has been replaced with red-cell concentrates and plasma substitutes containing no coagulation factors. Fresh

Table 89.2 Potential problems with stored blood components

Failure to correct deficiency

Inadequate correction of deficiency

Blockade of reticuloendothelial system (microaggregates, coagulation)

Microvascular pathophysiology (acute respiratory distress syndrome, multiorgan dysfunction syndrome)

Accentuation of free radical pathology (leukocytes, iron)

Activation and consumption of the haemostatic system

Hyperkalaemia, hypocalcaemia, hypothermia

Vasoactive effects (hypotension)

Hyperbilirubinaemia

---

platelet concentrates are indicated in patients with continuing microvascular oozing, especially after receiving over 10 units of stored blood. Prophylactic platelet concentrates are, however, not indicated.

Potential problems associated with large volume blood component replacement are summarized in Table 89.2.

The role of fresh blood in bleeding associated with massive blood loss and transfusion has not been resolved. Fresh blood can provide immediately functioning oxygen-carrying capacity, volume and haemostatic factors. The benefit in controlling haemorrhage probably relates to the presence of immediately functioning platelets. Although using fresh blood reduces the number of homologous donors, the risk of transfusion-related viral infections is possibly higher than fully tested stored blood. In general, fresh blood should be given if bleeding is ongoing, when fresh platelet concentrates are not readily available.

Haemostatic failure associated with liver disease[1]

The liver is the production site of nearly all the factors involved in the formation and control of coagulation (Table 89.3). Bleeding associated with liver disease can be very difficult to manage. The diagnosis of any specific defect is difficult, and there may also be a combination of excessive consumption and/or impaired synthesis of coagulation factors, coagulation inhibitor proteins and activators of fibrinolysis. Moreover, effects of massive blood loss, shock and transfusion must also be considered.

Haemostatic defects due to deficient vitamin K-dependent coagulation factors (II, VII, IX and X) in patients with predominantly cholestatic liver disease may be rapidly reversed with vitamin K therapy, and blood transfusion may not be required. If vitamin K fails to reverse the abnormality, hepatocellular damage

Table 89.3 Haemostatic disturbances in liver disease

Deficiency of vitamin K-dependent clotting factors

Deficiency of fibrinogen and factor V

Dysfibrinogenaemia

Disseminated intravascular coagulation

Excessive fibrinolytic activity

Circulating anticoagulants

Platelet abnormalities

---

is likely. Vitamin K-dependent factors are stable during storage at 4°C; there is no need to use fresh blood or FFP for their replacement. When an elective procedure is planned on a patient with liver disease, prophylactic replacement of vitamin K-dependent factors, and possibly factor V, is usually all that is necessary. FFP, supernatant plasma or factor concentrates may be used. Unfortunately, the transfused factors, particularly factor VII, disappear rapidly from the circulation, so transfusions must be repeated if there is continuing bleeding or risk of bleeding.

Low fibrinogen levels in liver disease usually indicate advanced disease with a poor prognosis, or the presence of DIC. Fibrinogen concentrates have fallen into disrepute due to the high incidence of hepatitis B and possible aggravation of intravascular clotting. Cryoprecipitate is probably a safer method of administering fibrinogen in a small volume. The diagnosis of DIC in liver disease can be extremely difficult.

Disseminated intravascular coagulation[1,5–7]

DIC is a pathophysiological process and not a disease in itself. The disorder is an inappropriate, excessive and uncontrolled activation of the haemostatic process. This may initially occur with adequate compensation, when defects may only be demonstrated in laboratory tests. If the initiating disorder is severe enough, the clinical syndrome of acute uncontrolled DIC results, with systemic bleeding, possibly in conjunction with end-organ failure.

Pathophysiology

DIC is characterized by the consumption of clotting factors and platelets within the circulation, resulting in varying degrees of microvascular obstruction due to fibrin deposition (Fig. 89.4). Mechanisms which may inappropriately activate the haemostatic system include:

1 activation of the coagulation sequence by release of tissue thromboplastins into the systemic circulation (e.g. extensive tissue trauma, surgery, malignancy and acute intravascular haemolysis);

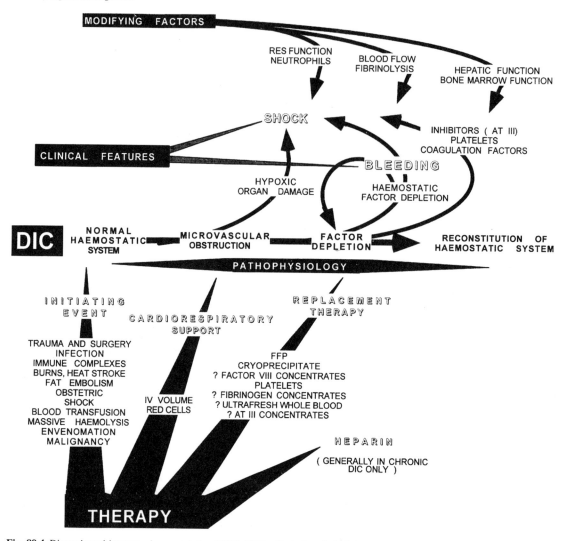

Fig. 89.4 Disseminated intravascular coagulation (DIC). RES = Reticuloendothelial system; AT III = antithrombin III; FFP = fresh frozen plasma.

2 vessel wall endothelial injury causing platelet activation, followed by activation of the haemostatic system, predominantly via the intrinsic pathway (e.g. Gram-negative sepsis from endotoxin release, viral infections, extensive burns and prolonged hypotension, hypoxia or acidosis);

3 induction of platelet activation (e.g. sepsis, viraemia, antigen–antibody complexes and platelet activation).

When platelet and coagulation factor consumption becomes significant, bleeding becomes a major feature. A compensatory secondary fibrinolysis occurs, which in some cases may accentuate the bleeding. Perpetuation of the process may be due to continuation of the stimulus or consumption of the natural inhibitors of haemostasis.

Clinical features

The clinical presentation of DIC varies, with patients showing thrombotic, haemorrhagic or mixed manifestations in various organ systems. The major problem and presenting feature of acute DIC is bleeding. This may manifest as generalized bruising, and bleeding at sites of therapeutic or traumatic invasion (e.g. venepuncture sites and surgical wounds). DIC may occur in association with a wide range of clinical disorders (Table 89.4). When DIC occurs in acutely ill patients with multiorgan dysfunction, the

Table 89.4 Conditions associated with disseminated intravascular coagulation

Infections
Malignancy
Shock
Liver disease
Transplantation
Extracorporeal circulations
Severe blood transfusion reaction
Snake bite
Vascular malformations
Extensive intravascular haemolysis
Septicaemia
Viraemia
Protozoal (malaria)
Carcinomas and leukaemia, especially acute promyelocytic leukaemia
Pregnancy
  Septic abortion
  Abruptio placentae
  Eclampsia
  Amniotic fluid embolism
  Placenta praevia
Extensive surgical trauma
Burns
Heat stroke
Acute hepatic necrosis

prognosis is poor. DIC may be an agonal event in some patients, when it should not be treated.

Acquired failure of haemostasis in pregnancy is usually a manifestation of DIC. The clinical picture is similar to other cases of DIC, except that onset may be more sudden and unexpected, with greater depletion of coagulation factors, especially fibrinogen. The trigger for this systemic activation of the coagulation system varies in different clinical situations. Procoagulation material in the systemic circulation may come from damaged placenta and decidua (abruptio placentae), amniotic fluid (amniotic fluid embolism) or dead products of conception (retained dead fetus). None the less, the end-result and management are similar. Massive blood loss may lead to further coagulation factor and platelet depletion, thus aggravating the situation. In many obstetric complications, there may be microcirculatory impairment secondary to prolonged shock or toxaemia, which will result in impaired liver synthesis of coagulation factors. Thus attempts to categorize the defects after obstetric complications are difficult.

Laboratory findings

The complexities of haemostasis are awesome. Results of tests may be variable and difficult to interpret. Significant DIC can be present despite normal standard coagulation tests (i.e. PT, APTT and TCT) and, conversely, some patients may have laboratory features of DIC without any clinical sequelae. Key diagnostic tests are those demonstrating excessive conversion of fibrinogen to fibrin within the circulation, and its subsequent lysis. There may be morphological evidence with fibrin deposition in the microcirculation, but this evidence is difficult to obtain during life. Platelet fibrin clots create a mesh in which passing red cells may be traumatized, resulting in red-cell fragmentation and haemolysis. The blood film may demonstrate fragmentation of the red cells (microangiopathic haemolytic anaemia), but this is more commonly seen in chronic DIC, especially that associated with malignancy.

The diagnosis is usually based on the clinical picture with a supportive pattern of laboratory tests (Table 89.5). Hypofibrinogenaemia, with prolongation of the APTT and TCT, in conjunction with an increase of FDPs (D-Dimer test), is excellent supportive evidence for the diagnosis. There is increasing agreement that the most reliable tests to diagnose DIC and follow the response to therapy are D-dimer measurement, presence of circulating fibrin monomer, increased fibrinopeptide A, and reduced concentrations of platelets and antithrombin III (AT III). The D-Dimer test is specific for fibrin breakdown and is more specific for DIC versus primary fibrinogenolysis.

Laboratory findings in chronic DIC are significantly different from acute DIC. Many of the usual tests of haemostasis, including platelet count and coagulation factors, are normal or near normal. However, this is a compensated state in which

Table 89.5 Tests to establish the diagnosis of disseminated intravascular coagulation

Prolongation of thrombin clotting time

Prolongation of activated partial thromboplastin time

Prolongation of prothrombin time

Hypofibrinogenaemia, thrombocytopenia, low factor VIII concentration

Elevated fibrin degradation products, elevated D-Dimer assay, shortened euglobulin lysis time, if fibrinolysis has become systemically activated

Elevated fibrinopeptide A, platelet factor IV and β-thromboglobulin

Reduced coagulation inhibitor levels, including antithrombin III, protein C and protein S

Microangiopathic haemolytic anaemia may be seen in subacute or chronic cases there is increased turnover of each of the haemo-static components. A microangiopathic red-cell picture on the peripheral blood film is usually present.

Management

Management of DIC remains controversial. Removal or treatment of the initiating cause is extremely important, in conjunction with resuscitation. Early recognition of DIC and initiation of treatment may allow the patient to survive hours or days, granting time for definitive diagnosis and treatment of the inciting disorder.

Blood component therapy should be given, but heparin should only be considered in selected cases.

1 *FFP* contains all the coagulation factors and the main inhibitors AT III and protein C in near normal quantities, and should be used.
2 *Cryoprecipitate*, which contains all components of the factor VIII complex as well as fibrinogen, factor XIII and fibronectin in concentrated form, may be especially useful if fibrinogen is depleted. Five to 10 units should be infused with FFP.
3 *Platelet* transfusion may be indicated in the presence of severe thrombocytopenia. However, this is controversial; patients tend to be resistant if the initiating cause of DIC has not been controlled.
4 *AT III concentrates* and possibly other inhibitors of haemostasis are likely to find a greater therapeutic role. Successful treatment of the bleeding phase of DIC probably depends to a variable degree on the patient being able to 'switch off' the coagulation system, irrespective of whether the initiating agent has been removed. Correcting low coagulation inhibitor levels, reticuloendothelial blockade and impaired or excessive fibrinolysis is probably important.
5 *Heparin* should only be used after initial adequate replacement therapy has failed to control bleeding. The decision to use heparin should not be undertaken lightly nor without due consultation. Small doses should be used initially (e.g. 50–100 units/kg followed by 10–15 units/kg per h), adjusted according to the clinical and laboratory response. Heparin is especially valuable in certain clinical situations, including acute promyelocytic leukaemia, early stages of amniotic fluid embolism, and immediately following severe incompatible blood transfusion.

Management of sudden massive obstetric haemorrhage due to DIC is similar. Fresh blood is probably warranted in many cases. Management includes attempts to empty and contract the uterus. Once the uterus is emptied and adequately contracted, the haemostatic failure quickly resolves.

Outcome

Factors which may affect the outcome of DIC include:

1 nature of the initiating event;
2 host factors, e.g. state of the reticuloendothelial system, concentrations of inhibitors of coagulation and fibrinolytic activity, and liver (synthesis) function;
3 the extent of end-organ damage sustained during the thrombotic phase and from shock during the haemorrhagic phase.

Anticoagulants and antiplatelet therapy[1]

Increasing use of these modes of therapy ultimately means more iatrogenic bleeding, and intensivists must be aware of the methods for rapid reversal of therapy. Bleeding problems in patients on well-controlled anticoagulation are usually due to surgery, trauma or a local lesion (e.g. peptic ulceration). Otherwise, bleeding is due to over-anticoagulation, sometimes as a result of drug interactions. Elective surgery in these patients requires careful planning to avoid haemorrhagic or thrombotic complications.

Oral anticoagulant agents

Oral anticoagulant agents induce a controlled deficiency of the vitamin K-dependent clotting factors (II, VII, IX and X), as measured by prolongation of PT. This is simply reversed with stored blood, supernatant plasma or FFP. The reversal is short-lived unless vitamin K is also given, as the infused coagulation factors have a short half-life, particularly factor VII (7 h). β-Lactam antibiotics may also inhibit vitamin K metabolism and induce a coagulopathy.

Heparin

Heparin acts on several sites of the clotting pathway by potentiating the action of AT III, a natural coagulation inhibitor. The anticoagulant effect of heparin is commonly measured by the APTT and TCT. Immediate reversal of heparin activity can be achieved with protamine sulphate. Formulas have been quoted (e.g. 1 mg protamine sulphate will neutralize 100 units of heparin), but it is better to titrate the dose using APTT, after an initial empirical dose of 50 mg. Protamine sulphate should be injected slowly IV; it may itself impair coagulation and be associated with anaphylactoid reactions.

Antiplatelet agents

Antiplatelet agents are being used increasingly for prophylaxis and therapy of arterial disease, and many of the non-steroidal anti-inflammatory agents are also platelet-inhibitory drugs. Aspirin has an irreversible effect on platelet function, and platelet function tests may show abnormalities for up to 10 days after medication. Most of the other antiplatelet agents have a reversible effect lasting a matter of hours or occasionally days (e.g. Naprosyn). Aspirin is now one of the commonest causes of postoperative bleeding. The bleeding is usually mild and of nuisance value, but may occasionally be serious, depending on the surgery (e.g. neurosurgery or cardiac surgery) and platelet transfusion may be necessary. Aspirin may also have a synergistic effect on an existing mild haemostatic defect (e.g. von Willebrand's disease), resulting in major haemostatic failure.

Acquired inhibitors of coagulation[1]

Devastating haemostatic failure may be seen with rare inhibitors of various coagulation factors. Immunoglobulin autoantibodies against factors VIII (commonest), IX, X, V, and von Willebrand factor have been reported. These patients are relatively resistant to factor replacement therapy. Removal of the offending autoantibody by plasma exchange should be attempted, with administration of FFP with or without factor concentrates.

Primary fibrinolysis

This rare acquired disorder is really primary fibrinogenolysis, because circulating plasmin is responsible for an uncontrolled proteolytic attack on the coagulation system (particularly factor VIII and fibrinogen). It may occur in malignancy or during certain types of surgery (e.g. neurosurgery, lung, pancreas, uterus and prostate) due to release of tissue plasminogen activators. The clinical picture of widespread bleeding is similar to DIC. Blood component therapy, especially FFP, is indicated. This is possibly a rare indication to use fibrinogen concentrates. Fibrinolytic inhibitors (e.g. ϵ-aminocaproic acid or tranaxemic acid) should be considered.

Extracorporeal circulation[8,9]

A range of haemostatic disturbances may arise from extracorporeal circulation, most commonly cardiopulmonary bypass. Abnormalities are generally related to the time on bypass, and are more likely with multiple valve replacements or reoperations. Inadequate reversal of heparin, increased fibrinolytic activity or platelet functional defects may contribute to bleeding. Appropriate laboratory investigations should be performed swiftly to allow logical therapy.

Thrombocytopenia and qualitative platelet defects[1,10]

Idiopathic thrombocytopenic purpura (ITP)

ITP is an autoimmune disorder where autoantibodies (immunoglobulin G; IgG) are directed against the platelets, which are subsequently destroyed by the reticuloendothelial system (predominantly in the spleen). The acute form, usually seen in children, commonly follows a viral infection, and recovery over weeks to months is usual. Chronic ITP, characteristically seen in adult women, has a variable course; spontaneous recovery may uncommonly occur.

Therapy remains controversial. Acute ITP is usually self-limiting in children and seldom needs active treatment. In adults, initial treatment is with prednisolone 50–75 mg daily, until remission occurs, when the dose is gradually reduced. Corticosteroids should be regarded as short-term therapy. There is little evidence that corticosteroids will raise the platelet count in the acute phase. However, their short-term role in reducing the incidence of bleeding, which is highest in the first weeks, may be important. High-dose IV gammaglobulin is effective in most patients, but limited availability restricts use to specific circumstances (e.g. fulminant acute disease, preoperatively, and in pregnancy).

Drug-induced thrombocytopenia

The clinical presentation of drug-induced thrombocytopenia is variable. Some may present with fulminant haemostatic failure. Possible causative drugs include quinine (also in bitter drinks), quinidine, antituberculous drugs, heparin, sedormid, thiazide diuretics, penicillins, sulphonamides, rifampicin and anticonvulsants. *Heparin-induced thrombosis thrombocytopenia syndrome* (HITTS) is an important and potentially life-threatening complication of heparin therapy. An immune reaction to heparin occurs after 7–10 days of therapy, when the patient's platelets aggregate and thrombocytopenia develops. This reactivity can be demonstrated by a variety of laboratory tests. In contrast to other causes of drug-induced thrombocytopenia, there may be arterial, microvascular or venous thrombosis associated with the platelet aggregation. The incidence of HITTS is unknown, but may be increasing with wider use of subcutaneous prophylactic heparin. The risk is considerably less with use of low-molecular-weight heparins or if heparin therapy is kept short.

Sepsis

Platelets play an important role in the inflammatory response and a reactive thrombocytosis is usually seen in infection. However, if there is overwhelming sepsis, associated DIC or marrow-suppressive influences, thrombocytopenia may be seen. Sepsis, shock, DIC, alcoholism and nutritional deficiency are common factors contributing to thrombocytopenia in critically ill patients.

Qualitative platelet defects

The effects of aspirin and other antiplatelet agents are discussed above. Haemostatic failure is a common manifestation of renal failure. The mechanism is unclear, but the defect can be substantially corrected by dialysis. Prolongation of BT, defects in aggregation responses, diminished adhesion and reduced platelet factor 3 availability have all been demonstrated. A relationship between the degree of anaemia and prolongation of bleeding is usually demonstrable – increasing the haemoglobin level reduces the bleeding time.

Patients with the myelodysplastic syndrome may also have a qualitative platelet function defect with the thrombocytopenia. β-Lactam antibiotics may also be responsible for a platelet function defect.

Thrombotic thrombocytopenic purpura (TTP)

This rare potentially fulminant and life-threatening disorder, characterized by platelet microthrombi in small vessels, results in tissue dysfunction and a microangiopathy. Activation of coagulation is not a prominent feature. The clinical syndrome is manifest by the pentad of thrombocytopenia, microangiopathic haemolytic anaemia, fever, renal dysfunction and neurological abnormalities. Abdominal symptoms, hepatic dysfunction and pulmonary abnormalities may also occur. Coagulation tests are usually normal or mildly abnormal. The diagnosis is made on the clinical features and a microangiopathic blood film with thrombocytopenia.

The aetiology of TPP is unknown. TPP has been associated with bacterial cytotoxins (of *Shigella dysenteriae* and certain *Escherichia coli* serotypes), cytotoxic agents, and bacterial and viral infections (i.e. cytomegalovirus, human immunodeficiency virus and herpesviruses). Pathologically, there appears to be an abnormal interaction between the vascular endothelium and platelets, but the primary event remains uncertain. Circulating platelet aggregating factors and a high-molecular-weight von Willebrand factor have been identified in some cases. An underlying autoimmune mechanism has been suggested.

TTP used to be fatal in 90% of patients, but outcome has dramatically improved over the past two decades with the development of effective therapy. Plasma infusion or exchange has become the cornerstones of treatment. Cryoprecipitate-poor plasma (depleted in von Willebrand factor) may offer advantages over whole FFP. Presently, remissions are possible in the majority of patients, and cures are common, but unfortunately, up to 50% relapse. The relapse is usually milder than the initial presentation, and may need less aggressive therapy. Patients resistant to this approach may respond to alternative therapies, including high-dose immunoglobulin, dextran, platelet-inhibitory drugs, corticosteroids, vincristine, or splenectomy.

Haemolytic–uraemic syndrome

This syndrome has many similarities to TTP, but renal involvement is the hallmark, in association with microangiopathic haemolytic anaemia and thrombocytopenia. Unlike TTP, neurological manifestations are uncommon. It usually occurs in children (related to bacterial or viral infections), but may rarely be seen in adults (commonly drug-related, and as a more chronic and serious course). Haemolytic–uraemic syndrome associated with quinine and Mitomycin C have been recently described. The prognosis and approach to management of haemolytic–uraemic syndrome are similar to TTP.

References

1. Loscalzo J and Schafer AI (1994) *Thrombosis and Hemorrhage*, 1st edn. Boston: Blackwell Scientific Publications.
2. Hoffman R, Benz EJ, Shattil SJ, Furie B and Cohen H (1991) *Hematology: Basic Principles and Practice*. New York: Churchill Livingstone.
3. Williams JW, Beutler E, Erslev AJ and Lichtman MA (1994) *Hematology*, 5th edn. New York: McGraw-Hill.
4. Sawyer PR and Harrison CR (1990) Massive transfusion in adults. Diagnoses, survival and blood bank support. *Vox Sang* **58**:199–203.
5. Bick RL (1992) Disseminated intravascular coagulation. *Hematol Oncol Clin North Am* **6**:1259–1285.
6. Bredbacka S, Blombäck M, Wiman B and Pelzer H (1993) Laboratory methods for detecting disseminated intravascular coagulation (DIC): new aspects. *Acta Anaesthesiol Scand* **37**:125–130.
7. Garcia GI and Lawrence WD (1992) Disseminated intravascular coagulation in infection. *Complications Surg* **11**:8–12.
8. Woodman RC and Harker LA (1990) Bleeding complications associated with cardiopulmonary bypass. *Blood* **76**:1680–1697.
9. Khuri SF, Wolfe JA, Josa M *et al.* (1992) Hematologic changes during and after cardiopulmonary bypass and their relationship to the bleeding time and nonsurgical blood loss. *J Thorac Cardiovasc Surg* **104**:94–107.
10. Boshkov LK, Warkentin TE, Hayward CPM, Andrew M and Kelton JG (1993) Heparin-induced thrombocytopenia and thrombosis: clinical and laboratory studies. *Br J Haematol* **84**:322–328.

Host defence failure

JP Isbister

There are coordinated haematological and immuno-logical responses to injury involving both cellular and humoral components. The ultimate prognosis of a life-threatening injury or infection may be determined by the body's ability to eliminate invading organisms and initiate repair. From this aspect, the haematological and immunological systems, with the liver, assume a vital role in the critically ill patient. Bone marrow and lymphoid cells are responsible for producing the necessary cellular components, and the liver for most of the circulating humoral factors.

Host defence system[1–11]

The non-specific (i.e. inflammatory response) and specific (i.e. adaptive immunity) host defence systems are closely integrated, and an inseparable relationship exists between the haemostatic system, the inflammatory response, the immune response and oxygen transport. However, there are conceptual advantages in dividing the systems into individual components to help understand and determine specific therapy. There are also specific clinical syndromes associated with individual defects in the system. In this chapter, the acute-phase response will be discussed from the cellular and humoral point of view. The haemostatic system is addressed in Chapter 89, and the immune system in Chapter 59.

Cellular components from the bone marrow and the humoral factors from the liver are, first, a non-specific defence system, and second, function as final attack mediators for the immune system. The immune system is a specific antigen-directed system and not the body's initial front-line defence against invasion, unless previously preprogrammed (i.e. immunized). Body defence systems (Fig. 90.1) can be divided into local and systemic. Each system has its own specialized protective mechanisms, including local activation of the various cellular and humoral factors, which may have specific purposes (e.g. secretory immunoglobulin A (IgA), organ-specific macrophages and lymphoid cells; Table 90.1).

Any defence system requires meticulous control at a systemic and local level to avoid inappropriate and excessive activation which may damage the host. A certain degree of host damage is inevitable during the response to injury and the subsequent healing process. Provided this is maintained locally, the overall host defence system is beneficial to the individual. However, if there is systemic activation, inappropriate host damage may occur. Conversely, under-activity of the host defence system has equally devastating consequences if an invading insult cannot

Table 90.1 Components of the host defence system

Defence factor	Source
Granulocytes	Bone marrow
Monocytes and macrophages (+ cytokines)	Bone marrow
Eosinophils	Bone marrow
Basophils	Bone marrow
Platelets and related proteins	Bone marrow
Lymphocytes and lymphoid organs (+ cytokines)	Bone marrow
Antibodies	Plasma cells
Complement system	Predominantly liver
Coagulation and fibrinolysis	Predominantly liver
Kinin system	Predominantly liver
Adhesion molecules	Endothelial cells
Histamine	Basophils, mast cells
Prostaglandins	Various sites
Inhibitory 'control' proteins (e.g. antithrombins, α_1-antitrypsin antiplasmins, α_2-macroglobulin C1 esterase inhibitor, histaminases, kininases)	Liver

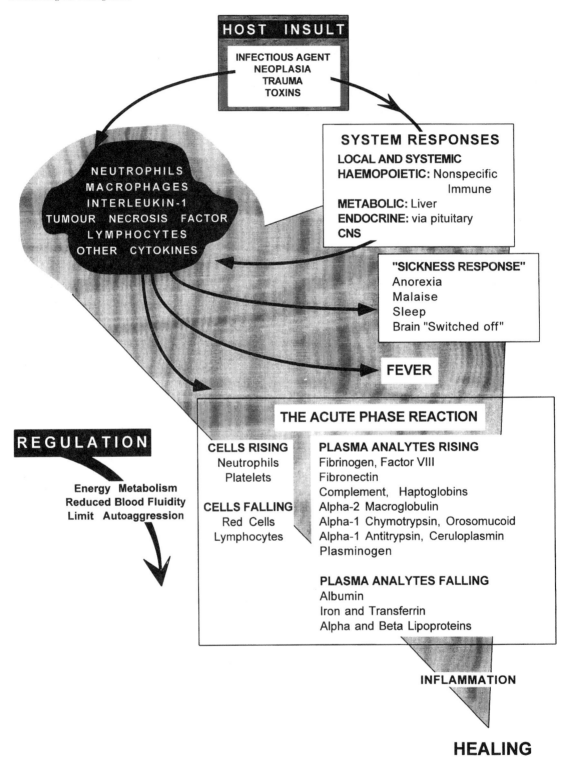

Fig. 90.1 Body defence systems. CNS = Central nervous system.

be neutralized. Thus, there is a wide range of disorders within this spectrum of activities of the host defence system.

With overactivity, disseminated intravascular coagulation (DIC) and thrombosis, excessive activation of inflammatory response, and acute anaphylactic/anaphylactoid reactions may occur. Apart from host damage during the activation phase, the patient host may not be able to reproduce depleted factors. The resultant consumption syndromes may be life-threatening or, at least, adversely affect the repair process. Imbalance in the immune system may 'tip' the patient towards allergy and autoimmune disease as well as the possibility of malignancy. With underactivity of the host defence system, haemorrhage, poor wound healing and infection may result. In some patients, there may be a delicate balance between underactivity and overactivity of the host defence system.

Adequate functioning of the circulatory system, especially the microcirculation, is vital for host defence function. Although bone marrow and liver can tolerate significant degrees of hypoxia, function will ultimately be impaired if adequate oxygenation is

not maintained. Second, the host defence system mediates most of its actions at a microcirculatory level, where the interface between the delivery of host defence factors and the site of tissue damage or invasion exists. These are probably important in the pathogenesis of the multiorgan dysfunction syndrome (MODS), and much research on this centres on the host defence system.

Acute-phase reaction[12-14]

The acute-phase reaction (Fig. 90.2) is the coordinated reaction of the haemopoietic and hepatic systems, which involve some 20 plasma proteins and all the cellular components of the blood (Table 90.2). The reaction occurs within hours or days of acute physical or chemical trauma, infection, tissue infarction, immunological reactions and pregnancy. Certain cells and plasma proteins are seen to rise and others to fall. The functions of many of these acute-phase proteins remains unclear, but teleologically, they should be assumed to be beneficial to the patient, and

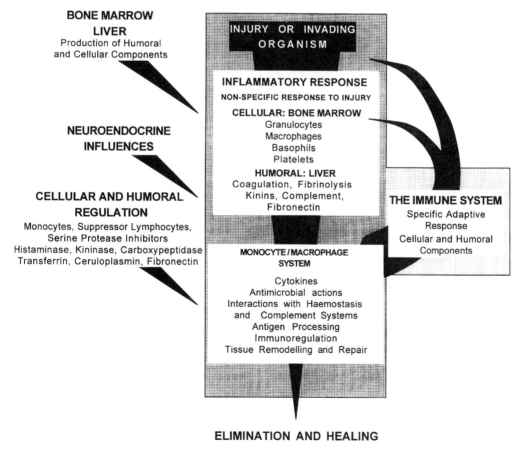

Fig. 90.2 Acute-phase response to injury.

Table 90.2 The acute-phase response

Rise	Fall
Cells	
Neutrophils	Haemoglobin
Platelets	Lymphocytes
Plasma proteins	
Fibrinogen and factor VIII	Albumin
Complement	Serum iron and total
	iron-binding capacity
Haptoglobins	
C-reactive protein	
α_2-Macroglobulin	
α_1-Antitrypsin	
Caeruloplasmin	
Plasminogen	

Table 90.3 Compromised hosts

Congenital
Rare haemopoietic or immunological deficiencies
   Qualitative granulocyte defects
   Hypogammaglobulinaemia
   Combined immunodeficiency

Acquired
Bone marrow failure
Liver disease
Acquired immune deficiency
   Haematological malignancies
   HIV/AIDS
   Immunosuppressive therapy
   Plasma exchange
Malnutrition
Alcoholism
Uraemia
Drug addicts
Elderly
Malignancy
Post-splenectomy
Diabetes
Corticosteroids and other immunosuppressive agents

HIV = Human immunodeficiency virus; AIDS = acquired immunodeficiency syndrome.

should not be tampered with unless there is good reason. The falls in haemoglobin, serum iron and albumin are all normal in the acute-phase reaction. Most of the proteins altered are inflammatory mediators, inhibitors or transport proteins.

Fibrinogen, the bulk protein of the coagulation system, is one of the plasma proteins to show the greatest rise in the acute-phase reaction, and is responsible for the elevation in the erythrocyte sedimentation rate. The rise in haptoglobins would suggest an important role which remains unclear. They may be important in having a bacteriostatic action by binding haemoglobin in the tissues which would otherwise promote bacterial growth. The complement proteins are important mediators in the inflammatory response. When such a potent system as the acute-phase response is activated, a well-tuned parallel response in the control proteins is necessary to avoid overactivity. The fall in albumin is due to redistribution and decreased synthesis; it is a normal response, possibly to compensate for the rise in other plasma proteins. No attempt should be made to correct the serum albumin unless a specific adverse clinical feature directly attributable to the hypoalbuminaemia can be established (e.g. severe oedema in protein-losing states). Cosmetic albumin infusions may not only be detrimental to the patient, but are a waste of a valuable blood product.

Host defence failure[15–18]

The host defence system may fail as a result of the current disease, or a pre-existing congenital or acquired defect (Table 90.3). Pre-existing defects may also interact with the current problem. A patient may have enough reserve in host defences to prevent spontaneous infections or haemostatic failure, but if stressed by an unexpected insult, rapid consumption of limited resources leaves the host defence system exhausted, with limited or no ability to replace the expended components, thus accentuating the overall defects (Table 90.4)

Table 90.4 Factors in host defence failure secondary to illness

Circulatory shock
Overwhelming defence system activation and consumption
   Disseminated intravascular coagulation
   Granulocyte aggregation
   Consumption opsinopathy (fibronectin)
   Reticuloendothelial system blockade
Plasma dilution from IV fluids
Homologous blood transfusion
   Reticuloendothelial system blockade with massive stored blood transfusion
   Immunosuppression with any homologous transfusion
Specific organ failure (e.g. liver and bone marrow)
Multiorgan dysfunction syndrome
Malnutrition
Continuing sepsis
Drugs, e.g. antibiotics and anaesthetic agents
Invasive procedures

Table 90.5 Causes of acute marrow failure in the critically ill

Acute megaloblastosis
  Acute folate deficiency
  Nitrous oxide effects on B_{12}
Overwhelming sepsis
  Alcoholics, in particular
Marrow infarction
Drug-induced aplasia
Multiorgan dysfunction syndrome

Acute bone marrow failure

Failure of cellular production by the bone marrow is uncommon in critically ill patients, and is usually the cause, rather than the result of acute illness. Patients with severe aplastic anaemia or marrow suppression secondary to haematological malignancy (including the effects of cytotoxic therapy) are susceptible to life-threatening infections. In general, such patients are usually cared for in special isolation wards rather than the ICU. However, with the use of increasingly aggressive cytotoxic drug regimens in the management of malignant disease, more patients are likely to be admitted to the ICU for organ-supportive therapy.

The management of pancytopenia due to acute marrow failure includes bone marrow examination to establish a diagnosis, and rapid correction of reversible factors. Acute marrow failure should be suspected in any patient with a sudden fall in the platelet and granulocyte count (Table 90.5). As red cells have a longer life-span, development of anaemia is more delayed following an acute marrow insult. Unless there are clearly identifiable contributory factors, development of pancytopenia due to consumption and decreased production carries a poor prognosis, and is commonly a manifestation of the MODS. Replacement therapy (e.g. platelet and plasma transfusions) may have a temporizing role, but unless the underlying insult can be controlled, recovery is unlikely.

Neutropenia

Neutropenia is one of the most common and important leukocyte abnormalities seen in clinical practice. With severe agranulocytosis, the patient is at risk from overwhelming bacterial sepsis. If associated thrombocytopenia is present, the combination of sepsis and haemorrhage is poorly tolerated. The neutrophil count needs to fall below 1×10^9/l before there is an increased incidence of spontaneous infection. However, the risk rises exponentially when the count drops below 0.2×10^9/l.

Consumption opsinopathy

This term describes the clinical situation where many of the mediators and opsonic components of the host defence system have been consumed, and production is unable to keep up with demand. Traumatic or septic shock are common clinical associations which may be responsible for increasing demand and reducing supply.

Fibronectin is an important glycoprotein in assisting intravascular clearance of debris, maintaining microcirculatory function and cell interactions. Depletion of this opsonic factor may impair host defences and contribute to MODS. Fibronectin is present in cryoprecipitate fraction of plasma, and replacement may have a role in treating overwhelming sepsis with multiorgan dysfunction, although results have been conflicting.

The alcoholic as a compromised host

The alcoholic's host defence system may be impaired in a number of ways (Table 90.6). Alcoholics are prone to a range of disorders which may result in ICU admission (e.g. trauma, metabolic derangements, pneumonia, liver failure and gastrointestinal haemorrhage). Thus, recognition of a poor host response is important.

Assessment of host defence function[19,20] (Fig. 90.3)

Constant awareness of cellular and humoral components in the host defences is essential for critically ill patients. Ensuring an adequately functioning oxygen transport chain, with rapid and efficient resuscitation, will greatly help maintain host defences. Each patient should be assessed for pre-existing risk factors (Fig. 90.3) and monitored for the development of defects during the course of the illness.

Important haematological factors are considered when assessing a patient for elective surgery (Table 90.7). The central contribution of adequate haemotherapy, haemostasis and prevention of postoper-

Table 90.6 Host defence defects in alcoholics

Bone marrow suppression
Malnutrition
Nutritional anaemia (especially folic acid)
Sideroblastic anaemia
Liver disease
Thrombocytopenia
Poor neutrophil response
Poor acute-phase response
Qualitative platelet and neutrophil defects

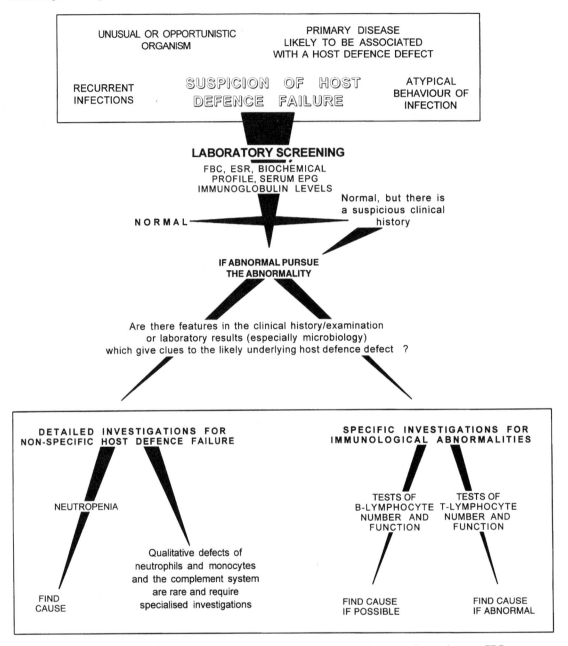

Fig. 90.3 Assessment of host defence function. FBC = Full blood count; ESR = erythrocyte sedimentation rate; EPG = electrophoretogram.

ative infection and venous thrombosis to the outcome of major elective surgery highlights the importance of the host defence system. Suspicion of haematological deficiency is usually apparent from the clinical history and examination, and only minimal laboratory investigations, if any, are required in an otherwise healthy patient. However, if the clinical history and findings suggest any predisposition to infection, bleeding, poor wound healing or thrombotic tendency, further clinical laboratory investigation may be necessary to delineate the defect in more detail. In some cases, specific blood component therapy may be available to correct the defect temporarily (e.g. immunoglobulins, plasma, coagulation factors and platelet or granulocyte transfusions).

Table 90.7 Preoperative haematological and host defence assessment

Oxygen transport	Red-cell indices
Haemostasis	Platelets and coagulation
Venous thromboembolism	Risk factor assessment
Host defences	Granulocytes, monocytes, immune function

References

1. Craddock CG (1980) Defences of the body: the initiators of defence, the ready reserves, and the scavengers. In: Maxwell I (ed.) *Blood Pure and Eloquent*. New York: McGraw-Hill, pp. 417–444.
2. Roitt I, Brostoff J and Male D (1993) *Immunology*, 3rd edn. St Louis: Mosby.
3. Abbas AK, Lichtman AH and Pober JS (1991) *Cellular and Molecular Immunology*. Philadelphia: WB Saunders.
4. Marino JA and Spagnuolo PJ (1988) Fibronectin and phagocytic clearance mechanisms. *J Lab Clin Med* **111**:493–494.
5. Molloy RG, Mannick JA and Rodrick ML (1993) Cytokines, sepsis and immunomodulation. *Br J Surg* **80**:289–297.
6. Tracey KJ and Cerami A (1994) Tumor necrosis factor: a pleiotropic cytokine and therapeutic target. *Annu Rev Med* **45**:491–503.
7. Patarroyo M (1991) Leukocyte adhesion in host defense and tissue injury. *Clin Immunol Immunopathol* **60**:333–348.
8. Kinashi T and Springer TA (1994) Adhesion molecules in hematopoietic cells. *Blood Cells* **20**:25–44.
9. Abbassi O, Kishimoto TK, McIntire LV and Smith CW (1993) Neutrophil adhesion to endothelial cells. *Blood Cells* **19**:245–260.
10. Smith CW (1993) Leukocyte–endothelial cell interactions. *Semin Hematol* **30**(suppl 4):45–55.
11. Ochs HD, Nonoyama S, Farrington ML, Fischer SH and Aruffo A (1993) The role of adhesion molecules in the regulation of antibody responses. *Semin Hematol* **30**(suppl 4):72–81.
12. Dowton SB and Colten HR (1988) Acute phase reactants in inflammation and infection. *Semin Hematol* **25**:84–90.
13. Baumann H and Gauldie J (1994) The acute phase response. *Immunol Today* **15**:74–80.
14. Steel DM and Whitehead AS (1994) The major acute phase reactants: C-reactive protein, serum amyloid P component and serum amyloid A protein. *Immunol Today* **15**:81–88.
15. Polk HC Jr (1993) Factors influencing the risk of infection after trauma. *Am J Surg* **165**(suppl):2S–7S.
16. Tichelli A (1993) Hematological and immunological aspects of spleen loss. *Chir Gastroenterol* **9**:103–107.
17. Waymack JP, Fernandes G, Cappelli PJ *et al.* (1991) Alterations in host defense associated with anesthesia and blood transfusions: II. Effect on response to endotoxin. *Arch Surg* **126**:59–62.
18. Girard DE, Kumar KL and McAfee JH (1987) Hematologic effects of acute and chronic alcohol abuse. *Hematol/Oncol Clin North Am* **1**:301–334.
19. Isbister JP (1986) *Clinical Haematology: A Problem Oriented Approach*. Sydney: Williams & Wilkins.
20. Tellado-Rodriguez J and Christou NV (1988) Clinical assessment of host defense. *Surg Clin North Am* **68**:41–55.

91 | Haematological malignancies

JP Isbister

Treatment of haematological malignancy is successfully evolving. In recent years, the prognosis for patients with acute leukaemia has changed from death within 1–3 months without effective therapy to long-term survival and cure in many cases. In some diseases, including Hodgkin's disease, childhood acute lymphoblastic leukaemia, some high-grade lymphomas and some adult leukaemias, the potential for cure has been realized. These advances have predominantly resulted from a wide range of new cytotoxic chemotherapeutic regimens which obliterate the disease in conjunction with comprehensive supportive therapy. In some cases, supralethal therapy is necessary with the use of bone marrow transplantation (autologous or allogeneic).

It is thus important that clinicians unfamiliar with the care of these patients do not take a nihilistic approach. If patients can be adequately supported, and complications treated during the severe neutropenic stage of chemotherapy, clinical improvement rapidly occurs following marrow recovery. However, patients requiring prolonged ventilatory support and/or dialysis have a poor prognosis; intensive therapy can only be justified if marrow recovery is imminent, and anticipated life expectancy is reasonable once they survive the crisis.

Classification and pathophysiology[1-3]

The heterogeneous nature and individual kinetic characteristics of the haemopoietic and lymphoid cells, and the disseminated nature of haemopoietic and lymphoid tissue, demonstrate the complexity of haematological malignancy. The numerous classification systems are confusing for the non-expert. In broad terms, haematological malignancies originating from the marrow are classified as *leukaemias* or multiple myeloma, and those arising in the peripheral lymphoid organs are classified as *lymphomas* – (nodal and extranodal) Hodgkin's and non-Hodgkin's lymphomas.

The leukaemias are divided into acute and chronic, generally according to the time span of their clinical course (Table 91.1). In general, acute leukaemias (which are blastic in appearance) have a rapid, fatal clinical course without effective treatment. In contrast, chronic leukaemias have more differentiated cells and have a more prolonged natural history. All leukaemias are classified on the basis of their cell of origin. The broad division is into those of myeloid origin (i.e. of haemopoietic marrow origin) and those of lymphoid origin (arising from the cells of the immune system; Table 91.1). Leukaemias can be further subdivided using the FAB (French–American–British) system.

Most patients with acute myeloid leukaemia present with features of bone-marrow failure. Acute promyelocytic leukaemia (M3) is a unique subtype of acute myeloid leukaemia, which may typically present with disseminated intravascular coagulation (DIC) requiring expert haematological management. Acute lymphoblastic leukaemia is the commonest type encountered in children. The lymphomas are a complex and heterogeneous group of malignancies ranging from highly malignant disorders through to low-grade indolent disease not requiring therapy. An adequate discussion is not within the scope of this chapter.

Table 91.1 Broad classification of leukaemias

Type of leukaemia	Abbreviation
Acute lymphoblastic leukaemia	ALL
Acute myelogenous leukaemia	AML
Chronic lymphatic leukaemia	CLL
Chronic myeloid leukaemia	CML

Complications of haematological malignancies[3]

Metabolic disturbances

Haematological malignancy may be initially associated with a range of metabolic derangements. Hyperuricaemia and hypercalcaemia are well-recognized complications, which may be associated with renal failure. The tumour lysis syndrome is a rarer complication which may occur spontaneously or shortly after initiation of therapy. There is sudden liberation of intracellular contents in quantities which overwhelm the excretory capacity of the kidneys, resulting in hyperkalaemia, hyperphosphataemia, hypocalcaemia and, occasionally, lactic acidosis. Pre-empting the development of the syndrome usually allows control of the metabolic effects. This includes maintaining a high IV fluid intake, alkalinizing the urine and administration of allopurinol. Multiple myeloma is most commonly associated with metabolic disturbances, e.g. renal insufficiency, hypercalcaemia, hyperviscosity and hyperuricaemia. Most of these can be managed conventionally. However, when large amounts of monoclonal protein are present in the plasma, fluid management can be difficult due to the hypervolaemia with or without hyperviscosity, and plasma exchange may be indicated (see Chapter 88).

Coagulopathies

A range of haemostatic disturbances may occur with haematological malignancy and its therapy. These disturbances are considered in Chapter 89.

Acute respiratory distress syndrome

Acute (or adult) respiratory distress syndrome (ARDS) remains a potentially lethal complication of autodestructive inflammation. As most of the mediators (e.g. cytokines, neutrophils and endothelial adherence molecules) initiating the disease process are haemopoietic in origin, it is not surprising that ARDS may occur in haemopoietic malignancies. However, ARDS is relatively uncommon in the neutropenic septic patient, perhaps because of the fact that the neutrophil is one of the central mediators of this syndrome. ARDS and interstitial pneumonitis may be problems in hyperleukocytosis, transfusion-associated lung injury, cytomegalovirus (CMV) infection, DIC, colony-stimulating factor therapy, post marrow transplantation (see below), and sometimes in relation to chemotherapy and radiotherapy. The use of *all-trans* retinoic acid (ATRA) may be associated with the development of a potentially lethal ARDS/pulmonary leukostasis syndrome (retinoic acid syndrome), usually accompanied by a rising leukocyte count. Early recognition of the symptom complex of fever and dyspnoea with or without pulmonary infiltrates is important, and therapy with high-dose corticosteroids decreases morbidity and mortality.[4]

Side-effects of chemotherapy

The wide range of cytotoxic chemotherapeutic agents used in haematological malignancies may be responsible for a plethora of toxicities other than bone-marrow suppression.[3] Haematologists will be aware of these, and should communicate the necessary information to the ICU staff.

Bone-marrow failure

Most of the acute leukaemias present with clinical and laboratory features of marrow failure, with anaemia, bleeding or infection. If it is not a problem at presentation, marrow failure is almost universal during remission induction and subsequent chemotherapy.

Neutropenia

Neutropenia should be considered in the following terms; absolute neutrophil count, rate of fall, nadir and duration. Duration of the neutropenia is a critical factor determining management and outcome. Patients with profound prolonged neutropenia of $<0.1 \times 10^9/l$ granulocytes for >10 days require special attention and may require different initial therapy. For practical purposes, neutropenia has been divided into the following groups:-

1. neutropenia $< 0.5 \times 10^9/l$;
2. neutropenia between 0.5 and $1.0 \times 10^9/l$ and potentially decreasing;
2. neutropenia $0.5–1.0 \times 10^9/l$ and counts remain stable or are increasing;
4. profound prolonged neutropenia.

Figure 91.1 illustrates the numerous interacting factors to be considered when managing neutropenic patients with haematological malignancy. Table 91.2 lists the organisms which may be associated with various defects in the host defence system.

Principles of management of haematological malignancies

ICU admission

Patients with haematological malignancy may be critically ill from their disease or therapy. At times during their therapy, they may require intensive supportive therapy and can develop a range of life-threatening complications. None the less, it is rarely necessary to admit critically ill patients with haematological disorders to the ICU. Admission of

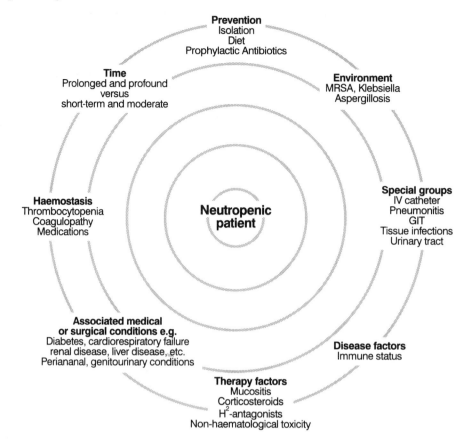

Fig. 91.1 Interacting factors in the management of neutropenic patients with haematological malignancy. MRSA = Methicillin-resistant *Staphylococcus aureus*; GIT = gastrointestinal tract.

such patients is best avoided, as they have severely impaired host defences and poor tolerance for invasive procedures. However, severe respiratory infections or pneumonitis requiring mechanical ventilation are indications for ICU admission. Such patients present specific problems for the ICU staff, e.g. severe marrow failure requiring intensive transfusion support and nutritional difficulties.

There must be good communication between the ICU staff and the haematologists, and clear policies on admission and treatment. The purpose of the admission to ICU and the ultimate treatment goals must be well-understood. If the patient's ultimate prognosis is poor, extraordinary invasive measures cannot be justified. A palliative approach will be instituted if the patient does not respond to treatment within a specific period of time. However, if the haematological malignancy has a high likelihood of cure or long-term good-quality survival, more strenuous and extended intensive care is given.

Infection prevention

Prevention of infection is extremely important. Infection may be endogenously or exogenously acquired. Most patients when admitted to hospital become colonized with the hospital flora (see Chapter 62). The major sources of infecting organisms, however, are the patients themselves, e.g. from the oropharynx, gastrointestinal tract, IV line sites, lung and local lesions.

All ICUs must demand strict adherence to infection control guidelines. The most effective procedure is hand-washing by all health care workers involved with the immunocompromised patient. Other preventive measures include sterile techniques for invasive procedures, maintaining a clean environment, cooked patient meals and limited use of prophylactic antibiotics. Many would argue that the efficacy of empirical therapy in the neutropenic patient makes prophylactic antibiotics unnecessary. Reverse barrier nursing is instituted to minimize exposure to exogenous

Table 91.2 Organisms associated with immune deficiency states

NEUTROPENIA
Bacteria
Gram-negative bacilli
 Escherichia coli
 Pseudomonas aeruginosa
 Klebsiella pneumoniae
Gram-positive cocci
 Staphylococcus epidermidis
 Staphylococcus aureus
 Streptococcus viridans
Fungal
 Candida
 Aspergillus
 Mucormycosis

CELLULAR IMMUNE DYSFUNCTION
Bacteria
 Listeria monocytogenes
 Salmonella
 Mycobacterium
 Nocardia asteroides
 Legionella
Fungi
 Cryptococcus neoformans
 Histoplasma capsulatum
 Coccidioides immitis
Viruses
 Varicella-zoster
 Cytomegalovirus
 Herpes simplex
Protozoa
 Pneumocystis carinii
 Toxoplasma gondii
 Cryptosporidium

HUMORAL IMMUNE DYSFUNCTION
Bacteria
 Streptococcus pneumoniae
 Haemophilus influenzae

infection. This can be difficult in an ICU setting and will not prevent infections of endogenous origin.

Invasive procedures

Invasive procedures should be kept to a minimum, and appropriate steps taken to minimize bleeding and the risk of infection. Endotracheal intubation should be avoided or minimized. Tissue biopsies, arterial access, physiotherapy and other invasive procedures, if indicated, should be planned and discussed beforehand with the haematologists.

Blood component therapy[5]

During the period of marrow suppression, red-cell concentrates need to be administered regularly to maintain the level around 10 g/dl. If a higher oxygen delivery is desired (i.e. in acute respiratory failure), the haemoglobin level should be higher (> 12 g/dl). Blood viscosity is not clinically significant until the haemoglobin level exceeds 16 g/dl.

Haemostasis is usually secured with regular transfusions of platelet concentrates to maintain the platelet count above $15 \times 10^9/l$. In the presence of sepsis, platelets are consumed rapidly and transfusions may be necessary on a daily basis; otherwise every other day is usually adequate. The patient should be examined daily for signs of haemostatic failure (e.g. purpura, ecchymoses and fundal haemorrhages). Granulocyte transfusions rarely have a role in supportive therapy, especially since haemopoietic growth factors were introduced. However, they may be required when bacterial sepsis is unresponsive in a patient with absent neutrophils, particularly if the problem is local infection.

Antimicrobial therapy

The febrile neutropenic patient

After resistance of the malignant cell to therapy, infection is the commonest cause of death in patients with haematological malignancy. Patients usually tolerate neutropenia without developing infection until the count is $< 1.0 \times 10^9/l$. It is not until the neutrophil count drops below $0.2 \times 10^9/l$ that sepsis becomes a major problem. These patients must be watched closely for infection, and treated early if necessary. When the neutrophil count is less than 0.5 $\times 10^9/l$, any temperature above 38°C should be regarded as representing serious sepsis until proven otherwise. High-risk patients include those with pneumonitis, severe mucositis, infected IV catheter and evidence of local sepsis. Patients with haematological malignancy may have pre-existing immunodeficiency.

Early empirical antibiotic therapy (see below) may be life-saving. With most patients, the fever resolves, especially if marrow function returns in the short term. Ultimate proof of infection is frequently not established. Patients with agranulocytosis will not show the typical features of inflammation. For example, lung consolidation may not be seen, cellulitis or sputum may not be clinically obvious and urinary tract symptoms may be minimal. The role of steroids in suppressing temperature and clinical features of inflammation must be considered. Non-infectious causes of fever (e.g. malignancy or drug-related) must also be considered. Pulmonary investigations such as computed tomography (CT) scan, bronchial alveolar lavage and transbronchial biopsy may be required in patients with features suggesting pneumonitis.

Presence of rigors, hypotension and shock may suggest Gram-negative sepsis. Gram-negative sepsis is potentially rapidly fatal in the neutropenic patient, but is less common than in the past. Less virulent Gram-positive organisms now predominate. This may be related to increased use of permanent indwelling vascular devices, mucositis (particularly associated with high-dose cytosine arabinoside, viral mucositis, H_2 antagonists, and quinolones as antibiotic prophylaxis. However, streptococcal and staphylococcal sepsis can be severe and empirical use of vancomycin in high-risk patients is justified. *Staphylococcus epidermidis* is an indolent form of sepsis; time is usually available for optimal therapy, with most patients recovering.

Choice of empirical antibiotic therapy

Antibiotic therapy should be empirical, aggressive and cover against Gram-negative sepsis. Agents effective against anaerobic organisms may need to be included when there are gastrointestinal problems, and against viral and fungi infections when necessary. The following factors must be considered:

1 probable nature and site of infection;
2 the host defence defect;
3 time course of neutropenia;
4 local microbiological ecology;
5 prior antibiotic usage;
6 haemostasis;
7 presence of indwelling lines (including endotracheal tube and urinary catheter);
8 type of chemotherapy;
9 nature of disease;
10 patient factors (e.g. hepatic, renal and respiratory function).

Antibiotic regimens

Initial empirical therapy should cover against *Pseudomonas aeruginosa*, *Escherichia coli*, *Klebsiella* spp., *Streptococcus viridans*, and *Staphylococcus*, depending on the clinical circumstances, described above. Cover against *Staphylococcus epidermidis* is not necessary until bacteraemia is demonstrated.

Single-drug therapy
Single-drug therapy with a third-generation cephalosporin (e.g. cefotaxime, ceftriaxone or cefatzidime) or imipenem may be adequate in low-risk patients (i.e. those with > 0.5×10^9/l neutrophils and expected to stay above that count, or neutropenia expected to last less than 7 days).

Two-drug therapy
Two-drug therapy with an added aminoglycoside (e.g. gentamicin, tobramycin, amikacin or netilmicin) is recommended in patients with prolonged and profound neutropenia, but no additional risk factors.

Three-drug therapy
Three-drug therapy with a glycopeptide (e.g. vancomycin or teicoplanin) added to the aminoglycoside and cephalosporin is indicated for patients particularly likely to be infected with coagulase-negative staphylococci, methicillin-resistant *Staphylococcus aureus*, *Corynebacterium* species and penicillin-resistant *Streptococcus viridans* (e.g. those with an infected indwelling catheter, pneumonitis, rash and severe mucositis).

Daily clinical assessment and review of microbiological results are essential. Antibiotic therapy is modified according to microbiological results. If no helpful microbiological information is available in single- or two-drug therapy, the regimen should be re-evaluated at 48 h, and a glycopeptide added if there is no response. If the fever resolves and microbiological cultures are negative, the aminoglycoside may be ceased. With three-drug therapy, reassessment at 72 h is appropriate. If there is no response, further investigations (e.g. computed tomography (CT) chest scan and bronchoalveolar lavage) may be indicated. Introduction of antifungal therapy, haemopoietic growth factors or granulocyte transfusions needs to be considered.

Haemopoietic growth factors and immunotherapy[6]

Genetically engineered haemopoietic growth factors are now widely used to minimize the degree and time of neutropenia. Granulocyte and granulocyte–macrophage colony-stimulating factors are glycoproteins which stimulate the proliferation and maturation of bone marrow progenitor cells, and increase the number and function of these committed cell populations. Treatment reduces the duration and severity of neutropenia in patients receiving chemotherapy, and after haemopoietic stem cell transplantation. Growth factors do not prevent neutropenia, but shorten its duration. Their use, although expensive, is well-tolerated and has been associated with fewer infectious febrile episodes. Use of such agents may be beneficial and can be justified in patients with prolonged neutropenia. This is not necessarily the case with short-duration neutropenia under a week, where the risk of infection is low.

Certain patient subgroups

Patients with indwelling IV catheters

Indwelling IV Silastic catheters present with infectious and non-infectious complications. The incidence of catheter-associated infections varies. Indwelling IV catheters present an increased risk of bacteraemia for both neutropenic patients and those with normal neutrophil counts. Coagulase-negative *Staphylococcus* is the most common cause of catheter-associated bacteraemia, but *Staphylococcus aur-*

eus, *Bacillus* spp., *Corynebacterium*, Gram-negative organisms (especially *Acinetobacter* and *Pseudomonas* spp.) and *Candida* can also cause catheter infections. Infections at the exit site and along the catheter subcutaneous tunnel can be caused by aerobic bacteria, mycobacteria and fungi.

If bacteraemia is thought to be catheter-related, it may be possible to avoid removal of the catheter, particularly if the organism is coagulase-negative *Staphylococcus*. Even patients with Gram-negative infections can often be successfully treated with antibiotics infused through the catheter. In patients with multiple-lumen catheters, the administration of antibiotics should be rotated through all the lumens, as infection may be restricted to only one. However, removal of the catheter is usually necessary in the following circumstances:

1 bacteria (e.g. species of *Bacillus*) which are not eradicated, despite being sensitive to the antibiotics used;
2 candidaemia, due to the high incidence of disseminated infection;
3 patients with tunnel infections.

Lung infiltrates in febrile patients with neutropenia[7]

Lung infiltrates in febrile patients with neutropenia represent a high risk of treatment failure. Prolonged neutropenia has a significantly adverse effect on the outcome of infection. Incorporation of systemic antifungal agents into first-line therapy, particularly in selected high-risk subgroups, may improve outcome. Involvement of a respiratory physician with experience in managing immunocompromised patients is important. Further investigations (e.g. fine-cut chest CT, bronchoscopy, bronchoalveolar lavage with or without transbronchial biopsy) may be necessary. Pulmonary haemorrhage can be a sudden and life-threatening cause of pulmonary infiltration and respiratory insufficiency. This usually occurs in severe thrombocytopenia associated with infection, and in patients who have become resistant to platelet transfusions.

Bone marrow (haemopoietic stem-cell) transplantation[3,8,9]

Haemopoietic stem-cell transplantation is increasingly used in the treatment of a number of malignant and non-malignant disorders. Allogeneic bone marrow transplantation has been used as an adjunct in the treatment of acute leukaemia, with an impressive success rate, translated into long-term survival and cure. It is now being extended to the management of a wider range of haematological malignancies, and more recently, some solid tumours.

Haemopoietic stem cells can be obtained from either marrow aspiration, or from the peripheral blood by apheresis, using a blood-cell separator following stimulation of the marrow with cytotoxic therapy and haemopoietic growth factors. Allogeneic transplantation unfortunately has a number of potentially serious or even fatal complications related to graft-versus-host disease (GvHD). It does however have the advantage of using normal marrow, which need not be stored. A limited degree of GvHD may have a beneficial antitumour effect. Autologous stem-cell transplantation is of particular advantage when relatively normal bone marrow can be obtained, in which case GvHD is not a problem. The principles for using bone marrow transplantation in the management of malignancy include the following:

1 The tumour must be responsive to chemotherapy and/or radiotherapy.
2 The dose limitation of chemotherapeutic agents used must relate to marrow toxicity, and not other end-organs.
3 There should be a source of uncontaminated haemopoietic stem cells.
4 Appropriate haemopoietic supportive therapy must be available during the marrow aplastic period.
5 High-quality clinical and laboratory facilities must be available for the collection and preservation of haemopoietic stem cells.
6 An integrated team of medical, nursing and scientific staff is essential.

A well-prepared clinical protocol with appropriate monitoring is essential for success. The general management of the patient during the procedure is similar to that of patients receiving high-dose chemotherapy (who will have prolonged neutropenic periods).

Complication of haemopoietic stem-cell transplantion

Respiratory failure[10]

Respiratory failure is the commonest cause of death in patients undergoing bone marrow transplantation. Both CMV-induced interstitial pneumonia and the idiopathic pneumonia syndrome rarely occur in the early cytopenic phase posttransplantation. Haematological reconstitution with donor-type cells seems to be a prerequisite to the development of these pulmonary complications, suggesting a key role of immunological reactions. While CMV pneumonia can be effectively treated or prevented by ganciclovir, the idiopathic syndrome is usually fatal. Due to improved prophylaxis and therapy, lethal interstitial pneumonia due to *Pneumocystis carinii*, herpes simplex, varicella-zoster or *Toxoplasma gondii*, as well as lethal pneumonia caused by bacteria or *Candida* spp., are generally rare events. However,

Aspergillus species have emerged as frequent causative pathogens in lethal pneumonitis. Prolonged granulocytopenia and medication with corticosteroids are major risk factors for pulmonary aspergillosis, which is usually fatal. Prophylaxis may be achieved by sterile air supply during the hospital stay, and by prophylactic inhalation of amphotericin B thereafter. Pulmonary haemorrhage, as diagnosed by bronchoalveolar lavage, may develop due to the toxicity of the conditioning regimen, or may be secondary to infectious pneumonia of various kinds. Congestive heart failure or the application of cytokines may give rise to pulmonary oedema. Patients with hepatic veno-occlusive disease have a high risk of subsequent pulmonary complications.

Graft-versus-host disease[3,11]

GvHD continues to be a major complication after allogeneic bone marrow transplantation, especially with increasing use of unrelated and mismatched donors. The target of the immune response in GvHD has long been regarded to be histocompatibility antigens possessed by the host, but not the donor. However self antigens have been documented in GvHD, confirming that GvHD is more complex than simple alloreactivity. The effector mechanisms in GvHD have traditionally been regarded to be direct cytotoxicity by alloreactive T cells, but it now seems that cytokines play a central role in mediating many of the clinical and experimental manifestations of GvHD.

Nearly all patients with GvHD have a rash. Other classical features may include liver abnormalities and gut dysfunction. Inital therapy for low-grade disease is systemic corticosteroids. Therapy for more severe disease may include cyclosporin, antithymocyte globulin, methotrexate, psoralen with ultraviolet light or thalidomide.

Veno-occlusive disease of the liver[12]

Veno-occlusive disease is another major complication, predominantly seen in allogeneic transplants. The disorder is due to thrombotic occlusion in the small hepatic vessels, probably as a result of endothelial damage associated with high-dose chemotherapy. The problem manifests as weight gain, oedema, ascites, tender hepatomegaly and jaundice, and may proceed to liver failure. There is a high mortality in the more advanced forms. Prophylaxis with low-dose heparin or prostaglandins is useful. Treatment is predominantly supportive, with fluid management a critical aspect. Recent treatment with tissue plasminogen activator has been successful.

References

1. Williams JW, Beutler E, Erslev AJ and Lichtman MA (1994) *Hematology*, 5th edn. New York: McGraw-Hill.
2. Hoffman R, Benz EJ, Shattil SJ, Furie B and Cohen H (1995) *Hematology: Basic Principles and Practice*. New York: Churchill Livingstone.
3. Handin RI, Lux SE and Stossel TP (1995) *Blood: Principles and Practice of Hematology*. Philidelphia: JB Lippincott.
4. Frankel SR, Eardley A, Lauwers G, Weiss M and Warrell RP Jr (1992) The 'retinoic acid syndrome' in acute promyelocytic leukemia. *Ann Intern Med* **117**:292–296.
5. Anderson FC and Ness PM (1994) *Scientific Basis of Transfusion Medicine: Implications for Clinical Practice*. Philadelphia: WB Saunders.
6. Vose JM and Armitage JO (1995) Clinical applications of hematopoietic growth factors. *J Clin Oncol* **13**: 1023–1035.
7. Maschmeyer G, Link H and Hiddemann W (1994) Pulmonary infiltrations in febrile patients with neutropenia: risk factors and outcome under empirical antimicrobial therapy in a randomized multicenter study. *Cancer* **73**:2296–2304.
8. Armitage JO (1994) Bone marrow transplantation. *N Engl J Med* **330**:827–838.
9. McCarthy LJ, Danielson CFM, Cornetta K, Srour EF and Broun ER (1995) Autologous bone marrow transplantation. *Crit Rev Clin Lab Sci* **32**:67–119.
10. Quabeck K (1994) The lung as a critical organ in marrow transplantation. *Bone Marrow Transplant* **14**(suppl. 4):S19–S28.
11. Vogelsang GB and Hess AD (1994) Graft-versus-host disease: new directions for a persistent problem. *Blood* **84**:2061–2067.
12. McDonald GB, Hinds MS, Fisher LD *et al.* (1993) Veno-occlusive disease of the liver and multiorgan failure after bone marrow transplantation: a cohort study of 355 patients. *Ann Intern Med* **118**: 255–267.

Part XV

Transplantation

TA Buckley

Advances in transplant techniques and ICU management have improved 1-year survival to over 80% in heart transplants, 75% in liver transplants and 70–80% in kidney transplants.[1,2] The major obstacle to organ transplantation is the lack of suitable donors. Of patients awaiting a heart, lung or liver transplant, 15–20% die before a donor organ becomes available.[3] Also, only 15–20% of potential organ donors actually end up having their organs transplanted. Adoption of 'opting in' and presumed consent legislations, public awareness campaigns, better coordination of transplant organizations and retrieval of multiple organs from each donor will increase the availability of donor organs.[4–7] Thus ICUs today have to care for potential organ donors, and increasingly, impending brain-death patients are admitted to the ICU for optimal preservation of pre-harvest organs.[8]

Identification and assessment of potential donors

All patients with severely impaired and deteriorating neurological function should be considered as potential donors (e.g. patients with severe head injuries, intracerebral haemorrhage and primary brain tumours, and victims of cardiac arrests, drownings and poisoning). Identifying a patient as a potential

organ donor must not influence medical management before brain death is established. Contraindications to organ donation (Table 92.1) and criteria for specific organs (Table 92.2) should be identified early. Exclusion by age depends on the urgency of the need for the donor organs. Successful transplantations of

Table 92.2 Organ-specific donor criteria

Organ	Donor criteria for suitability of organs
Kidney	Age 2–70 years; absent renal disease and hypertension Avoid use of diuretics
Pancreas	Age 10–45 years; absent diabetes, pancreatitis or alcohol abuse
Liver	Age 1 month to 65 years; absent liver disease, gallstones or alcohol abuse Appropriate size-matching Prevent prolonged resuscitation and hypotension ($<70\,mmHg$) for more than 30 min
Heart	Age 1 month to 60 years Size matching $\neq 20\%$ MAP > 60 mmHg, CVP or PCWP < 12 mmHg, LVSWI > 15 g/m Inotrope dosage < 5 µg/kg per h.
Lungs	Age 1 month to 55 years; non-smokers; absent lung disease, barotrauma, lung contusions, fractured ribs, lung infiltrates, purulent secretions or pulmonary oedema; on mechanical ventilation for under 4 days Normal blood gases at low F_{IO_2}; good lung compliance Size-matching critical
Eyes	Absent ocular disease and trauma

MAP = Mean arterial pressure; CVP = central venous pressure; PCWP = pulmonary capillary wedge pressure; LVSWI = left ventricular stroke work index.

Table 92.1 General contraindications to organ donation

Age > 70 years
Malignancy (except primary cerebral tumours)
Juvenile-onset diabetes
Intravenous drug abuse
Severe multiple-organ dysfunction
Active tuberculosis
Systemic infection

Table 92.3 Information required by transplant teams

Age, sex, weight and approximate height

History of acute illness, including other injuries resulting in brain death

Clinical condition: periods of hypotension and resuscitation requirements

Previous medical history, including surgery, alcohol and smoking habits, medications, and allergies

Current condition: vital signs, urine output and peripheral perfusion

Current medications, particularly inotrope requirements

Current investigations: haemoglobin, white cell count, platelets, prothrombin time, activated partial thromboplastin time, serum electrolytes, glucose, urea and creatinine, liver function tests, arterial blood gases, chest X-ray, ECG and microbiology results

ECG = Electrocardiogram.

Table 92.4 Sequelae of brain death

Absence of brain reflexes
Impaired cardiovascular regulation
Impaired thermal regulation
Deranged hormone metabolism
Presence of spinal reflexes

kidneys from the extremes of age and livers from elderly donors have been reported.[9–11] Extracerebral malignancies and systemic infections[12] are absolute contraindications. Cardiac arrest is not a contraindication to heart donation if the resuscitation is not prolonged and an effective cardiac output is re-established.[13] The transplant team requires certain information about the donor to assess the suitability of organs, and to select appropriate recipients (Table 92.3). Activation of organ retrieval procedures occurs only after three conditions have been met:

1 Brain death must be established.
2 Relatives must have given formal consent for organ donation.
3 Notification must be made to, and agreement for organ donation obtained from, the coroner (medical examiner) if the case is pertinent to the coroner's office.

Investigations

Specific investigations are required to aid recipient selection and identify donor-transmissible infections. These include ABO blood group, human leukocyte antigen (HLA) tissue typing and serological tests for cytomegalovirus (CMV), *Toxoplasma*, Epstein–Barr virus, hepatitis virus and human immunodeficiency virus (HIV).

Management of the multiorgan donor

Following brain death certification, management emphasis changes from minimizing the neurological insult to preserving organ function. The pathophysiological sequelae of brain death (Table 92.4) manifest in dysfunction of various organs. During brain coning, there is an agonal period of intense autonomic activity associated with hypertension. This phase is short-lived and is followed by hypotension, the most common problem in organ donors. Hyperpyrexia may occur during the initial phase of brain injury, but hypothermia follows, due to metabolic depression. Hormone abnormalities include diabetes insipidus and depressed adrenocortical function. Spinal reflexes may be absent, or hyperactive with diaphoresis and muscle spasms. Management of the organ donor aims to achieve haemodynamic stability, maintain systemic perfusion pressure and treat physiological derangements, as discussed below.

Monitoring

Minimal monitoring requirements include hourly measures of core temperature, pulse and urine output. Continuous electrocardiogram (ECG) monitoring and pulse oximetry are mandatory. Intra-arterial pressure monitoring also enables frequent blood-gas analysis. Central venous pressure monitoring is necessary in haemodynamically unstable patients. A pulmonary artery catheter may be required, particularly if blood pressure and urine output fail to respond to fluid challenges at a central venous pressure of above 15 mmHg (2.0 kPa).

Cardiovascular abnormalities

Hypertension

Prior to brain death, there is intense adrenergic activity with intracranial hypertension and systemic arterial hypertension. Myocardial function may be impaired, resulting in left ventricular failure and pulmonary oedema.[14,15] Cardiac microinfarcts have been demonstrated,[16] which may be responsible for transplantation heart failure.[17] Esmolol hydrochloride, a short-acting β-blocker, can be used to ablate this hypertensive response.

Hypotension

Multiple factors cause hypotension in organ donors, the commonest being hypovolaemia (Table 92.5).

Table 92.5 Causes of hypotension in brain-dead patients

Volume depletion

Fluid restriction and inadequate replacement of essential and third-space fluid losses

Osmotic diuretics (i.e. mannitol)

Diabetes insipidus (low levels of antidiuretic hormone)

Hyperglycaemia (low levels of insulin)

Brainstem death

Loss of vasomotor control; decreased systemic vascular resistance and increased venous capacitance

Impaired left ventricular function

Catecholamine-induced

Hypoxia

Endocrine abnormalities (low triiodothyronine levels)

Hypothermia

Regardless of the cause, blood pressure should be raised to allow adequate tissue perfusion. A fluid challenge may indicate a hypovolaemic cause. Optimal fluid replacement regimens are controversial,[18] but should be determined by the type of fluid lost, and haemoglobin and serum electrolyte concentrations. Suitable regimens include crystalloids such as 4.3% dextrose/0.25% saline or 1/5 isotonic saline in 4% dextrose, colloids and packed red cells to maintain a haematocrit of 0.3. Rapid infusions of glucose-containing fluids should be avoided, because of potential hyperglycaemic osmotic diuresis. Goals for haemodynamic stabilization include a systolic blood pressure over 100 mmHg (13.3 kPa), mean arterial pressure over 70 mmHg (9.3 kPa) or a central venous pressure of 8 mmHg (1.1 kPa), with a sinus rhythm of under 100 beats/min. Overhydration may precipitate pulmonary oedema, liver congestion and cellular injury, and must be avoided.

Inotropic drugs may be used if hypotension persists after adequate fluid replacement. They should ideally be discontinued before organ retrieval, to avoid peripheral vasoconstriction and possible ischaemic end-organ injury. However, studies on the use of vasoactive drugs in organ donors are lacking. Choices of inotropes are infusions of dopamine (up to 10 µg/kg per min), dobutamine (up to 15 µg/kg per min), or adrenaline (up to 0.1 µg/kg per min). Isoprenaline may be useful in paediatric donors, because of their fixed stroke volume and rate-dependent cardiac output. α-Adrenergic vasopressors (e.g. metaraminol, phenylephrine or noradrenaline)

should be avoided, as they may cause severe peripheral vasoconstriction.[19] However, in patients with a low systemic vascular resistance, noradrenaline may be required to improve cardiac output. Good haemodynamic stability with normal liver and renal laboratory variables has been reported with combined administration of a pressor dose of vasopressin ($<1–2$ units/h) and low-dose adrenaline (<500 µg/h).[20,21]

Arrhythmias and ECG abnormalities

Abnormal ECG changes are frequent and may be of no pathological significance. They should not be confused with changes suggestive of myocardial ischaemia. Atrial or ventricular arrhythmias and various degrees of conduction block occur with varying frequency.[22] These may result from electrolyte and arterial blood-gas disorders, loss of the vagal motor nucleus, increased intracranial pressure, drug therapy, myocardial ischaemia, hypothermia or ventricular irritability from cardiac contusion. Appropriate treatment should be given. Bradycardia is not a problem unless it contributes to hypotension, and may be treated with adrenergic agents or temporary venous pacing. Conversely, arrhythmias may be exacerbated by inotropes. All brain-dead patients will eventually undergo terminal arrhythmias that are resistant to therapy. Paradoxical septal wall motion is common but is not a negative prognostic factor.

Respiratory dysfunction

Management aims for optimal oxygen delivery to vital organs with minimal cardiovascular depression. Measures include careful posturing of the patient, maintaining normocarbia and using adequate tidal volumes, low levels of positive end-expiratory pressure (PEEP), fractional inspired oxygen (Fio_2) of less than 0.60, and peak inspiratory pressures less than 30 cmH$_2$O (3.0 kPa). A higher Fio_2 may be used to avoid high levels of PEEP, peak airway pressure or mean intrathoracic pressure, all of which may reduce cardiac output and oxygen delivery. Alkalaemia from therapeutic hyperventilation may be present, with resultant fluxes of potassium and phosphorus and a leftward shift in the oxygen dissociation curve. The cause of a metabolic acidosis must be identified and corrected. Frequent arterial blood-gas analyses will allow assessment of oxygenation, ventilation and acid–base status. Hypoxaemia may result from pneumonia, pulmonary oedema, aspiration, atelectasis or barotrauma. Head-injured patients positioned with their heads elevated may develop orthostatic lung changes. In lung donors, the endotracheal tube must be sited at an appropriate level, so as to avoid injury to the tracheal anastomosis site. Aseptic respiratory toilet care must be observed.

Endocrine dysfunction

Impaired hormone release may result from hypothalamic–pituitary axis malfunction. Posterior pituitary dysfunction is common (77% incidence) but panhypothyroidism is less so.

Thyroid hormones

Serum thyroxine (T_4) and triiodothyronine (T_3) concentrations are decreased in experimental brain-dead animals.[16,23] Depletion of thyroid hormones has been reported in human organ donors.[17,24–26] However, concentrations of other hormones, except antidiuretic hormone arginine vasopressin (see below), are not decreased following brain death. This suggests that thyroid hormone depletion is due to a sick euthyroid syndrome rather than true hypothyroidism.[25–28] Thus, T_3 administration theoretically would be of no benefit. None the less, some studies have reported significant haemodynamic improvement with restoring T_3 concentrations to normal,[29–31] but other studies are contradictory.[24,32] In general, routine thyroid hormone replacement is not recommended.[17,23,25,27,28,32]

Cortisol

Serum cortisol concentrations decrease after brain death in experimental animals[16] and human donors.[28] However, routine donor replacement therapy prior to organ retrieval is not supported,[28] unless antemortem dexamethasone therapy has suppressed adrenal function. In these cases, cortisol administration may be indicated.

Insulin and hyperglycaemia

Pancreatic endocrine function is thought to be effective following brain death,[33] but mild to severe hyperglycaemia is a frequent complication. This is due to a combination of infusing glucose-containing fluids, reduced insulin secretion and increased circulating catecholamines. The subsequent increased extracellular osmolality, metabolic acidosis and ketosis result in intracellular dehydration, osmotic diuresis and electrolyte disturbances. Osmotic diuresis, if untreated, contributes to hypovolaemia, oliguria and cardiac instability. Control of hyperglycaemia is achieved with an insulin infusion at rates determined by serial blood glucose and ketone measurements. Blood glucose concentration should be maintained between 8 and 13 mmol/l. Unless the donor is an insulin-dependent diabetic, or requires continuous high-dose infusions of inotropes, small amounts of insulin (0.5–2.0 units/h) are usually sufficient.

Diabetes insipidus

Deficiency of antidiuretic arginine vasopressin is the most frequent hormone abnormality, occurring in 70–80% of brain-dead patients.[25,28,34] It results in an inappropriate, frequently massive urine output, independent of circulating blood volume, and presents as hypotonic polyuria (urine osmolality < 300 mmol/kg), hypernatraemia and hyperosmolality. Inadequately treated diabetes insipidus may also result in hypomagnesaemia, hypokalaemia, hypophosphataemia and hypocalcaemia. Hypovolaemia and electrolyte imbalances will result in haemodynamic instability. Treatment involves appropriate IV fluid and electrolyte replacement. Serum electrolytes and osmolality measurements should be monitored frequently.

In severe cases of diabetes insipidus (e.g. urine output exceeding 5–7 ml/kg per h), vasopressin may be required. The use of vasopressin is controversial, because of dose-dependent vasoconstriction,[35] a higher incidence of acute tubular necrosis and a lower rate of graft survival.[86] Aqueous vasopressin given subcutaneously, IM or IV has a short duration of action. Other forms of vasopressin include IM vasopressin tannate in oil 2.5–5.0 μg/day and synthetic desmopressin (1-D-amino-8-D-arginine vasopressin, DDAVP) as a nasal spray 10–20 μg/12 h. Their effects are cumulative, and determining the appropriate dose can often take several days; they are thus unsuitable in the brain-dead patient. Continuous low-dose infusions of vasopressin (0.5–6.0 units/h) have been used to reduce urine output to 1.5–3.0 ml/kg per h, with minimal vasoconstrictive effects in coronary, pulmonary and hepatic circulatory beds.[37,38] Alternatively, donors can be managed with IM or subcutaneous aqueous vasopressin 2–5 units, repeated every few hours to maintain urine output at 2–3 ml/kg. DDAVP IV 0.5–2.0 μg every 8–12 h appears to be as effective in brain-dead patients.[39] It has greater potency, less pressor activity and a longer duration of action than the natural hormone.

Electrolyte imbalance

Electrolyte abnormalities have been mostly discussed above. The cause of hyponatraemia is often difficult to ascertain and is frequently multifactorial, including alcohol intoxication, hyperglycaemia, renal dysfunction, cirrhosis, cardiac failure, adrenal insufficiency or hypothyroidism. Treatment is specific to the electrolyte derangement. Serum sodium should be maintained below 155 mmol/l and serum potassium above 3.5 mmol/l.

Hypothermia

A mild degree of hypothermia may benefit organ protection, but a core temperature under 32°C results in dysrhythmias, decreased cardiac contractility, vasoconstriction, decreased glomerular filtration, cold diuresis, thrombocytopenia and coagulopathy, and a left shift in the oxyhaemoglobin dissociation curve. Hypothermia should be anticipated and heat loss prevented. A core temperature above 35.5°C is a prerequisite to diagnose brain death. Use of warm ambient room temperatures (23–24°C), infusion fluid warmers, heated humidifiers and active warming systems (e.g. heat blankets) should be implemented.

Renal dysfunction

Hypotension results in acute tubular necrosis and reduced allograft survival. A donor urine output less than 100 ml in the hour preceding nephrectomy is associated with increased acute tubular necrosis in the recipient.[40] Optimal blood volume must be maintained. Oliguria in a well-hydrated patient is managed with low-dose dopamine infusion, intermittent IV frusemide and an infusion of mannitol 0.5 g/kg.

Haematological dysfunction

A bleeding diathesis may be consequent to release of tissue fibrinolytic and plasminogen activators from areas of ischaemic and necrotic brain.[41] Disseminated intravascular coagulation occurs in 28% of brain-dead donors.[34,42] Aetiological factors include shock and/or sepsis. It has been considered a contraindication to organ donation, but this view is challenged by recent successful liver and kidney donations.[43] Management includes infusion of platelets to maintain a platelet count above 30×10^9/l, provision of clotting factors until clinically evident bleeding ceases, and early procurement of organs.

Infection

Febrile donors must have full blood and sepsis investigations, including daily chest X-rays and sputum, urine, and blood cultures and sensitivities. Invasive lines, catheters and tubes must be inserted aseptically, and any unnecessary invasive device removed. Organ donation is still possible, provided systemic bacterial infections are eradicated with non-nephrotoxic antibiotics. There are no data to suggest that prophylactic antibiotics given to the donor will reduce infectious complications in the recipient.

Heart–lung and lung transplantations are less successful if tracheal aspirates of donors show fungi, significant bacteria and large numbers of polymorphonuclear cells.[44,45] Techniques to minimize airway colonization, such as aseptic suctioning, chest physiotherapy and use of systemic or aerosol antibiotics have not been evaluated.[46]

Serological screening for hepatitis B, HIV and CMV must be performed. CMV infection occurs more frequently (39–70%) after renal transplantation if CMV-positive donors are used for CMV-negative recipients.[47,48] However, its influence on posttransplantation mortality and morbidity is controversial.[49–51] In general, the CMV status of the donor and the recipient is not a detrimental prognostic factor for graft and patient survival in cadaveric kidney and heart transplantation.[52] Kidney transplantation with hepatitis B surface antigen (HBsAg)-positive donors has shown no HBsAg transmission in the short term,[53] and no major deleterious effects.[54] However, long-term survival is less with recipients who are HBsAg-positive, compared with recipients who are HBsAg-negative.[55] Use of hepatitis C virus-positive donors is, similarly, controversial. There is a variable rate of hepatitis C virus transmission to the recipient,[56,57] but appreciable serious infection may not occur.[58,59] Further studies and newer serological tests will clarify the situation in the future.

References

1. Alexander JW (1990) The cutting edge – a look at the future in transplantation. *Transplantation* **49**:237–240.
2. Editoral (1990) Organ donors in the UK – getting the numbers right. *Lancet* **335**:80–82.
3. Sheil AGR, McCauhgan GW, Thompson JF, Dorney SFA, Stephen MS and Bookallil MJ (1992) The first five years' clinical experience of the Australian National Liver Transplantation Unit. *Med J Aust* **156**:9–16.
4. Gore SM, Hinds CJ and Rutherford AJ (1989) Organ donation from intensive care units in England. *Br Med J* **299**:1193–1197.
5. Gentleman D, Easton J and Jennett B (1990) Brain death and organ donation in a neurosurgical unit: audit of recent practice. *Br Med J* **301**:1203–1206.
6. Gore SM, Ross Taylor RM and Wallwork J (1991) Availability of transplantable organs from brain stem dead donors in intensive care units. *Br Med J* **302**:149–153.
7. Gore SM, Armitage WJ, Briggs JD *et al.* (1992) Consensus on general medical contraindications to organ donation? *Br Med J* **305**:406–409.
8. Feest TG, Riad HN, Collins CH, Golby MGS, Nicholls AJ and Hamad SN (1990) Protocol for increasing organ donation after cerebrovascular deaths in a district general hospital. *Lancet* **335**:1133–1135.
9. Lloveras J (1991) The elderly donor. *Transplant Proc* **23**:2592–2595.
10. Sautner T, Gotzinger P, Wamser P, Gnant M, Steininger R and Muhlbacher F (1991) Impact of donor age on graft function in 1180 consecutive kidney recipients. *Transplant Proc* **23**:2598–2601.
11. Adams R, Astarcioglu I, Azoulay D *et al.* (1989) Age greater than 50 years is not a contraindication for liver donation. *Transplant Proc* **23**:2602–2603.
12. Slapak M (1986) The immediate care of potential donors for cadaveric organ transplantation. *Anaesthesia* **33**: 700–709.
13. De-Begona JA, Gundry SR, Razzouk AJ, Boucek MM, Kawauchi M and Bailey LL (1993) Transplantation of hearts after arrest and resuscitation: early and long-term results. *J Thorac Cardiovasc Surg* **106**:1196–1201.
14. Novitsky D, Wicomb WN, Rose AG, Cooper DKC and Reichart B (1987) Pathophysiology of pulmonary edema following experimental brain death in the Chacma baboon. *Ann Thorac Surg* **43**:288–294.

15. Malik AB (1985) Mechanisms of neurogenic pulmonary edema. *Circ Res* **57**:1–18.

16. Novitsky D, Wicomb WN, Cooper DKC, Rose AG, Fraser RC and Barnard CN (1984) Electrocardiographic, hemodynamic and endocrine changes occurring during experimental brain death in the Chacma baboon. *J Heart Transplant* **4**:63–69.

17. Macoviak JA, McDougall IR, Bayer MF, Brown M, Tazelaar H and Stinson EB (1987) Significance of thyroid dysfunction in human cardiac allograft procurement. *Transplantation* **43**:824–826.

18. Randell T, Orko R and Hockerstedt K (1990) Peroperative fluid management of the brain dead multiorgan donor. *Acta Anaesthesiol Scand* **34**:592–595.

19. Nishimura N and Sugi R (1984) Circulatory support with sympathetic amines in brain death. *Resuscitation* **12**:25–30.

20. Iwai A, Sakano T, Uenishi M, Sugimoto H, Yoshioka T and Sugimoto T (1989) Effects of vasopressin and catecholamines on the maintenance of circulatory stability in brain dead patients. *Transplantation* **48**:613–617.

21. Yoshioka T, Sugimoto H, Uenishi M *et al.* (1986) Prolonged hemodynamic maintenance by the combined administration of vasopressin and epinephrine in brain death: a clinical study. *Neurosurgery* **18**:565–567.

22. Logigram EL and Ropper AH (1985) Terminal electrocardiographic changes in brain dead patients. *Neurology* **35**:915–918.

23. Schwartz I, Bird S, Lotz Z, Innes CR and Hickman R (1993) The influence of thyroid hormone replacement in a porcine brain death model. *Transplantation* **55**:474–476.

24. Garcia-Fages LC, Cabrer C, Valero R and Manyalich M (1993) Hemodynamic and metabolic effects of substitutive triiodothyronine therapy in organ donors. *Transplant Proc* **25**:3038–3039.

25. Howlett TA, Keogh AM, Perry L and Touzel-Rees LH (1989) Anterior and posterior pituitary function in brainstem dead donors: a possible role for hormonal replacement therapy. *Transplantation* **47**:822–834.

26. Robertson KM, Hramiak IM and Gelb AW (1992) Endocrine changes and haemodynamic stability after brain death. *Transplant Proc* **21**:1197–1198.

27. Powner DJ, Hendrich A, Lagler RG, Ng RH and Madden RL (1990) Hormonal changes in brain dead patients. *Crit Care Med* **18**:702–708.

28. Gramm HJ, Meinhold H, Bickel U *et al.* (1992) Acute endocrine failure after brain death? *Transplantation* **54**:851–857.

29. Washida M, Okamoto R, Manaka D *et al.* (1992) Beneficial effect of combined 3,5,3′ triiodothyronine and vasopressin administration on hepatic energy status and systemic hemodynamics after brain death. *Transplantation* **54**:44–49.

30. Jeevanandam V, Todd B, Hellman S, Eldridge C, McClurken J and Addonizio VP (1993) Use of triiodothyronine replacement therapy to reverse donor myocardial dysfunction: creating a larger donor pool. *Transplant Proc* **25**:3305–3306.

31. Novitzky D, Cooper DKC, Chaffin JS, Greer AE, DeBault LE and Zuhdi N (1990) Improved cardiac allograft function following triiodothyronine therapy to both donor and recipient. *Transplantation* **49**:311–316.

32. Randell TT and Hockerstedt KAV (1993) Triiodothyronine treatment is not indicated in brain dead multiorgan donors: a controlled study. *Transplant Proc* **25**:1552–1553.

33. Masson F, Thicoipe M, Gin H *et al.* (1993) The endocrine pancreas in brain dead donors: a prospective study in 25 patients. *Transplantation* **56**:363–367.

34. Nygaard CE, Townsend RN and Diamond DL (1990) Organ donor management and organ outcome: a 6 year review from a level 1 trauma center. *J Trauma* **30**:728–732.

35. Hofbauer KG, Studer W, Wah SC, Michel JB, Wood JM and Stadler R (1984) The significance of vasopressin as a pressor agent. *J Cardiovasc Pharmacol* **6** (suppl): S429–S438.

36. Schneider A, Toledo-Pereyra LH, Zeichner W, Allaben R and Whitten J (1983) Effect of dopamine and pitressin on kidneys procured and harvested for transplantation. *Transplantation* **36**:110–111.

37. Levitt MA, Fleischer AS and Meislin HW (1984) Acute post traumatic diabetes insipidus: treatment with continuous intravenous vasopressin. *J Trauma* **24**:532–535.

38. Blaine EM, Tallman RD, Frolicher D, Jordan MA, Bluth LL and Howie MB (1984) Vasopressin supplementation in a porcine model of brain dead potential organ donors. *Transplantation* **38**:459–464.

39. Debelak L, Pollak R and Reckard C (1990) Arginine vasopressin versus desmopressin for the treatment of diabetes insipidus in the brain dead organ donor. *Transplant Proc* **22**:351–352.

40. Lucas BA, Vaughn WK, Spees EK and Sanfilippo F (1987) Identification of donor factors predisposing to high discard rates of cadaver kidneys and increased graft loss within one year post transplantation – SEOFF 1977–1982. *Transplantation* **43**:253–257.

41. Soifer BE and Gelb AW (1989) The multiple organ donor: identification and management. *Ann Intern Med* **110**:814–823.

42. Miner ME, Kaufman HH, Graham SH, Haar FH and Gildenberg PL (1982) Disseminated intravascular coagulation fibrinolytic syndrome following head injury in children: frequency and prognostic implications. *J Pediatr* **100**:687–691.

43. Gil-Vernet S, Martinez-Brotons F, Gonzalez C, Domenech P and Carreras M (1992) Disseminated intravascular coagulation in multiorgan donors. *Transplant Proc* **24**:33.

44. Zenati M, Dowling RD, Armitage JM *et al.* (1989) Organ procurement for pulmonary transplantation. *Ann Thorac Surg* **48**:882–886.

45. Harjula A, Starnes VA, Oyer PE, Jamieson SW and Shumway NE (1987) Proper donor selection for heart lung transplantation. *J Thorac Cardiovasc Surg* **94**:874–880.

46. Darby JM, Stein K, Grenvik A and Stuart SA (1989) Approach to management of the heartbeating 'brain dead' organ donor. *J Am Med Assoc* **261**:2222–2227.

47. Ludwin D, White N, Tsai S, Chernesky M, Achong M and Smith EKM (1987) Results of prospective matching for cytomegalovirus status in renal transplant recipients. *Transplant Proc* **19**:3433–3434.

48. Waltzer WC, Arnold AN, Anaise D *et al.* (1987) Impact of cytomegalovirus infection and HLA-matching on outcome of renal transplantation. *Transplant Proc* **19**:4077–4080.

49. Tenschert W, Dittmer R, Harfmann P *et al.* (1991) Vascular rejection of renal allografts is linked to CMV IgG, positive organ donor. *Transplant Proc* **23**:2641–2642.

50. Dunn DL, Mayoral JL, Gillingham KJ *et al.* (1991) Treatment of invasive cytomegalovirus disease in solid organ transplant patients with ganciclovir. *Transplantation* **51**:98–106.

51. von Willebrand E, Petterson E, Ahonen J and Hayry P (1986) CMV infection, class II antigen expression, and human kidney allograft rejection. *Transplantation* **42**:364–367.

52. Krishnan G, Vaughn WK, Capelli JP and Glass NR (1993) Positive donor/recipient CMV status is not a detrimental factor for renal allograft/patient survival. *Transplant Proc* **25**:1485–1486.

53. Bedrossian J, Akposso K, Metivier F, Moal MC, Pruna A and Idatte JM (1993) Kidney transplantations with HBsAg+ donors. *Transplant Proc* **25**:1481–1482.

54. Chan PCK, Lok ASF, Cheng IKP and Chan MK (1992) The impact of donor and recipient hepatitis B surface antigen status on liver disease and survival in renal transplant recipients. *Transplantation* **53**:128–131.

55. Gagnadoux MF, Guest G, Ronsse-Nussenzveig P, Mitsioni A and Broyer M (1993) Long term outcome of hepatitis B after renal transplantation during childhood. *Transplant Proc* **25**:1454–1455.

56. Pereira BJG, Milford EL, Kirkman RL *et al.* (1992) Prevalence of hepatitis C virus RNA in organ donors positive for hepatitis C antibody and in the recipients of their organs. *N Engl J Med* **327**:910–915.

57. Morales JM, Munoz MA, Castellano G *et al.* (1993) Impact of hepatitis C in long functioning renal transplants: a clinicopathological follow up. *Transplant Proc* **25**:1450–1453.

58. Aswad S, Obispo E, Mendez RG and Mendez R (1993) HCV+ donors: should they be used for organ transplantation? *Transplant Proc* **25**:3072–3074.

59. Roth D, Fernandez JA, Babischkin S *et al.* (1992) Detection of hepatitis C virus infection among cadaver organ donors: evidence for low transmission of disease. *Ann Intern Med* **117**: 470–475.

FH Hawker

Liver transplantation is now part of the therapy of irreversible end-stage liver disease. Introduced more as an experimental treatment in the 1960s, results have progressively improved, because of better patient selection, surgical techniques, immunosuppressive therapy and postoperative intensive care. Liver transplantation can now expect 80% 1 year and 70–80% long-term survival,[1,2] but this is achieved only by a highly motivated and efficient team.

Indications and selection for liver transplantation

Common indications for adults are shown in Table 93.1. Autoimmune diseases (e.g. chronic active hepatitis, primary sclerosing cholangitis and primary biliary cirrhosis) account for about 50% of candidates. Cirrhosis secondary to chronic infection with hepatitis B (HBV) or hepatitis C (HCV) may be an indication. However, transplantation in patients with HBV is controversial, as recurrent infection may cause loss of the allograft,[3] despite treatment with hepatitis B immune globulin postoperatively. HCV infection may also recur but reinfection is usually mild.[4] Results of transplantation for hepatic malignancy are generally poor,[5] because of recurrence of the primary tumour. Patients with alcoholic liver disease with a record of abstinence and good social support may be candidates. Liver transplantation for acute liver failure (ALF) and children is discussed below.

Patients are only considered for transplantation when the acute or chronic disease is advanced, and conventional therapies have failed. Those with a high risk of complications or a poor chance of success are excluded (Table 93.2). End-stage liver disease is commonly associated with cardiorespiratory, neurological and renal complications. Advanced multiorgan complications are usually contraindications to transplantation (although hepatic encephalopathy,[6] the hepatopulmonary syndrome[7] and the hepatorenal

Table 93.1 Possible indications for liver transplantation in adults

Autoimmune liver diseases
  Primary biliary cirrhosis
  Primary sclerosing cholangitis
  Chronic active hepatitis
Chronic viral infection
  Hepatitis B
  Hepatitis C
Fulminant hepatic failure
  Viral
  Drug-induced
  Other
Cryptogenic cirrhosis
Alcoholic cirrhosis
Unresectable hepatic malignancies
Budd–Chiari syndrome
Metabolic disorders
  Wilson's disease
  α_1-Antitrypsin deficiency
  Haemochromatosis
  Cystic fibrosis
  Haemophilia
  Hyperlipoproteinaemia
  Primary oxalosis

syndrome[8] may improve with transplantation), unless combined organ transplantation can be undertaken.[9,10] Patients at the extremes of age, i.e. who are very small (under 1 year old or less than 7–8 kg weight) or older than 60 years, generally have a poorer outcome. However, with careful selection, excellent results have been reported in both groups.[11,12]

The preoperative evaluation consists of tests to define structural abnormalities of the liver and biliary system (e.g. computed tomography (CT) scan, angiography and biliary radiology) and tests to assess

Table 93.2 Contraindications to liver transplantation

Disseminated infection*
Human immunodeficiency virus infection
Disseminated malignancy*
$Pa_{O_2} < 55$ mmHg (7.3 kPa)†
Active alcoholism
Extrahepatic manifestations of alcoholism
Severe psychiatric illness refractory to therapy
Irreversible cerebral injury from cerebral oedema‡

* Transplantation may be indicated if confined to the liver.
† Combined heart–lung–liver transplantation may be possible.
‡ Only relevant in patients with fulminant hepatic failure. Confirm with cerebral angiography or nuclear medicine scan.

cardiorespiratory, liver, renal and neurological function (e.g. electrocardiogram (ECG), chest X-ray, spirometry, echocardiography, haematological tests and plasma and urine biochemistry). Patients with chronic encephalopathy or a history of alcoholism have psychometric testing and brain CT scan.

Operative aspects

Donor liver

The usual procedure is orthotopic liver transplantation – the recipient's liver is removed and replaced by one from a brain-dead donor. Donors are unsuitable if there is human immunodeficiency virus (HIV), HBV or HCV infection, a history of intravenous drug or alcohol abuse, malignancy (except primary central nervous system tumours) and bacterial sepsis. Relative contraindications include age over 55 years, diabetes mellitus and other concurrent diseases, an incompatible ABO blood group, abnormal liver function tests and a history of haemodynamic instability. Acceptance of donors with relative contraindications depends on the urgency of the transplantation. Good early graft function in the recipient depends on the function of the donor liver, and quantitative tests (e.g. monoethylglycinexylidide, MEGX test) are used to select donors in some centres.[13]

Donor hepatectomy is usually performed at the donor hospital as part of multiple organ procurement. The liver graft is preserved by instillation of special solutions – the University of Wisconsin solution is most widely used.[14]

Operation

The recipient operation involves hepatectomy, revascularization of the donor liver, biliary tract reconstruction and securing of haemostasis. Venovenous bypass from the portal and femoral veins is often used in adults, because the inferior vena cava and portal vein are cross-clamped. Biliary reconstruction is usually end-to-end anastomosis of the donor and recipient bile ducts over a T-tube, but a side-to-side anastomosis or a choledochojejunostomy may also be performed. Heterotopic liver transplantation involves implanting the donor liver beneath the recipient's liver, which remains in place. This procedure has not been fully evaluated.

Major problems in anaesthetic management are the large volumes of blood and fluid replacement needed, coagulopathy, metabolic abnormalities, hypothermia and cardiovascular instability that frequently occur at revascularization. Skilled anaesthetic management greatly reduces the problems encountered in the ICU in the early postoperative period.

Postoperative management

The recipient almost always requires mechanical ventilation when admitted to ICU postoperatively. Close monitoring of cardiovascular, respiratory, renal, metabolic and haematological parameters is necessary. Any blood loss is measured from the intra-abdominal drains. If there is a biliary drain (T-tube), the colour, volume and consistency of bile are observed. Assessment of hepatic function at this stage also involves plasma concentrations of aspartate aminotransferase (AST), alanine aminotransferase (ALT), glucose, potassium and other electrolytes, and the international normalized ratio (INR) for prothrombin time. The hepatobiliary iminodiacetic acid (HIDA) scan is used routinely in some centres to screen for graft dysfunction.[15] It can assess hepatic perfusion, hepatocyte function (uptake of the tracer by hepatocytes) and biliary complications, such as leaks or strictures. Doppler ultrasound can be used to screen for hepatic arterial flow or rejection. The MEGX test has also been used to assess posttransplant liver function.[16]

Immunosuppressive therapy is started in the immediate postoperative period (Table 93.3). Cyclosporin is given IV. Doses depend on measured drug concentrations, and are influenced by renal and liver function. Cyclosporin can cause marked and immediate renal impairment; smaller doses may be necessary if renal function is poor. Excretion is exclusively dependent on bile flow, and may be impaired by significant cholestasis. Cyclosporin is given orally when gastrointestinal activity is established. If severe renal dysfunction precludes use of cyclosporin, OKT3 can be used. FK506 is a newer immunosuppressive drug with similar actions to cyclosporin, and is used instead in many centres. It has better oral bioavailability in the immediate postoperative period, and in the long term may lead to a slight decrease in chronic rejection.[17]

Table 93.3 Typical early immunosuppressive protocol

Immediately	Cyclosporin	10 mg/kg orally
postoperative	Methylprednisolone	500 mg IV
(optional)	Azathioprine	1 mg/kg IV
Postoperatively		
Day 1	Methylprednisolone	500 mg IV
	Azathioprine	1 mg/kg IV
	Cyclosporin	2 mg/kg IV
Day 2	Methylprednisolone	250 mg IV
	Azathioprine	1 mg/kg IV
	Cyclosporin	4 mg/kg IV
After day 2	Methylprednisolone reduced slowly to 20 mg by day 10	
	Azathioprine: maintain at 1 mg/kg orally	
	Cyclosporin: change to oral 12 mg/kg	

Table 93.4 Causes of allograft dysfunction

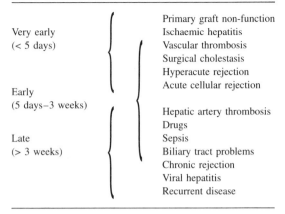

Very early (< 5 days)	Primary graft non-function
	Ischaemic hepatitis
	Vascular thrombosis
	Surgical cholestasis
	Hyperacute rejection
Early (5 days–3 weeks)	Acute cellular rejection
	Hepatic artery thrombosis
	Drugs
Late (> 3 weeks)	Sepsis
	Biliary tract problems
	Chronic rejection
	Viral hepatitis
	Recurrent disease

From McCaughan *et al.*,[59] with permission.

Postoperative complications

Intra-abdominal haemorrhage

This is uncommon. Intraperitoneal bleeding may occur from many sources, including mesenteric tears and vascular anastomoses. Reoperation is necessary if there is overt haemorrhage, but a slow ooze often resolves as allograft function improves over the first 24–48 h.

Ascites

This occurs commonly in patients with preoperative ascites, but may appear for the first time post-operatively. Causes include slow return of graft function (with delayed resolution of hypoalbuminaemia), interruption to the lymphatic drainage of the peritoneal cavity, and slowly resolving portal hypertension. Portal or hepatic venous thrombosis may be an occasional cause. Ascites itself is not a good indicator of graft function, and usually resolves over 4–6 weeks. However, its presence may predispose to intra-abdominal infection.

Allograft dysfunction

Allograft dysfunction may result from a number of causes (Table 93.4). Time of onset is important in the differential diagnosis. Primary graft dysfunction is characterized by absent or poor function of the allograft from the time of operation. In the extreme situation, there is progressive hypoglycaemia, coagulopathy, hyperkalaemia, acidosis and a rapid increase in plasma aminotransferase enzyme concentrations. There is usually poor bile output. Shock, renal failure and the acute respiratory distress syndrome (ARDS) are common accompaniments. Allograft dysfunction

is probably caused by preservation injury and/or prolonged cold ischaemia. When severe, treatment is urgent retransplantation. If intermediate in nature, then prostaglandin E_1 is given by infusion (up to 0.1 μg/kg per min). However, emergency retransplantation may be needed if there is no significant improvement within 24 h.

Hepatic artery thrombosis can result in a very similar clinical picture. If the diagnosis is established quickly by either Doppler studies or angiography, emergency reoperation should be undertaken to reestablish arterial patency. However, if the hepatic injury is progressive, urgent retransplantation is required. Hepatic artery thrombosis may also occur later after transplantation, when it can present as recurrent bacteraemia (secondary to hepatic abscess formation) or as a delayed biliary leak. Hepatic vein or portal vein thrombosis may present in the early postoperative period. Both can be associated with significant graft dysfunction and the onset of marked ascites.

Hyperacute rejection is uncommon.[18] It is heralded by a similar syndrome to primary graft non-function or hepatic artery thrombosis, and may occur after the patient has left the ICU.

Graft dysfunction occurring between 1 and 4 postoperative weeks is usually caused by acute cellular rejection. Biochemical markers are non-specific, and it can only be diagnosed reliably by liver biopsy. The triad of portal tract inflammation, endothelialitis and bile duct damage are sufficient to make the diagnosis. Usual therapy is a pulse of corticosteroids (1 g methylprednisolone on 3 successive days). If this is unsuccessful, or if there is early relapse, therapy using monoclonal antibody OKT3 is undertaken.[19] Between 60 and 80% of liver transplant recipients develop acute cellular rejection, and up to 30% may require OKT3 rescue therapy.

Biliary tract abnormalities occur in approximately 10% of recipients,[20] and may be technical complications, or result from preservation injury or hepatic artery thrombosis. Biliary strictures are more common than leaks. They are diagnosed by T-tube cholangiography, or, if the T-tube has been removed, by endoscopic or percutaneous cholangiography. Biliary tract strictures are usually managed by placement of an internal stent, and rarely require surgical reconstruction.

Cytomegalovirus (CMV) infection tends to occur approximately 4–6 weeks after transplantation, and can develop despite prophylaxis with high doses of acyclovir or ganciclovir. It is characterized by high fevers, generalized aches and pains, and often mild hepatitis. The diagnosis is best made by the detection of CMV early antigen in blood. Treatment is with ganciclovir (5 mg/kg twice daily).

Progressive cellular rejection results in interlobular bile duct damage to the graft, with severe cholestasis, but usually without significant hepatic necrosis. Affected patients develop progressive hyperbilirubinaemia, with high plasma concentrations of alkaline phosphatase and γ-glutamyltransferase. Retransplantation may be necessary. Recurrent hepatitis may also cause significant graft abnormalities at this stage in HBV-positive patients.

Cardiovascular complications

End-stage chronic liver disease is accompanied by a characteristic haemodynamic state, in which there is increased cardiac output and decreased systemic vascular resistance. This persists in the immediate postoperative period, although some normalization occurs in the first 3 days.[21] Most patients have normal myocardial function and life-threatening cardiovascular complications are uncommon.

Early after liver transplantation, hypotension is usually the result of inadequate volume replacement or bleeding. Hypertension develops in the majority of patients, and is a side-effect of cyclosporin therapy. As transplant recipients are frequently coagulopathic or thrombocytopenic, hypertension carries a high risk of intracranial bleeding, and must therefore be controlled aggressively.

Pulmonary complications

Most liver transplant recipients can be weaned from mechanical ventilation and extubated within the first postoperative day.

Pleural effusions

Pleural effusions occur commonly in the first postoperative week and are most often right-sided.[22] They usually resolve spontaneously. Drainage should only be considered if there is significant respiratory impairment. If effusions increase later than 3 days after transplantation, associated subdiaphragmatic pathology may be likely,[23] and an abdominal CT scan is needed.

Atelectasis

Atelectasis is common and usually involves the right basal areas. Treatment involves aggressive physiotherapy and occasionally bronchoscopy.

Pre-existing pulmonary pathology

Chronic liver disease may be associated with the hepatopulmonary syndrome (see Chapter 37). Mild to moderate hypoxaemia associated with intrapulmonary shunting of 20–30% does not usually result in important postoperative problems. However, in some patients, there is a transient deterioration in intrapulmonary shunting after transplantation that can be life-threatening.

Pulmonary hypertension is a less common but well-recognized accompaniment of chronic liver disease. Its reversibility after liver transplantation remains questionable. It is often regarded as a contraindication for liver transplantation, unless heart–lung transplantation can also be performed. Therapy to decrease pulmonary artery pressure with vasodilator drugs is logical, but of unproven value.

Acute respiratory distress syndrome

ARDS occurs in liver transplant recipients,[24] but the incidence appears to have decreased. Major precipitating factors are severe graft dysfunction and sepsis. When associated with acute rejection, ARDS has been reported to resolve after retransplantation.[25] It is treated conventionally.

Pulmonary infection

After the immediate postoperative period, the most common pulmonary complication is bacterial pneumonia, usually involving Gram-negative pathogens. The majority of infections occur in patients requiring long-term mechanical ventilation. Treatment is appropriate respiratory support, antibiotics and physiotherapy. Other potential causes of pneumonia include fungi (usually *Candida albicans*, but occasionally *Aspergillus*),[26] CMV and *Pneumocystis carinii*.

Renal impairment

Renal impairment may occur in as many as 90% of recipients, depending upon the definition used.[27] Overt renal failure requiring renal replacement therapy is very much less common. Causes include preoperative renal dysfunction, massive blood loss, poor early graft function, sepsis and, importantly, cyclosporin therapy. The severity of cyclosporin nephrotoxicity does not necessarily correlate with trough cyclosporin levels.[28] The mechanism appears to be renal vasoconstriction,[29] and the decreased renal perfusion is reflected by a low urinary sodium concentration. When renal dysfunction is present, cyclosporin doses should be reduced to the minimum necessary to prevent rejection (although, in reality, this minimum dose or blood concentration is unknown). In some centres, alternative immunosuppressive drugs are substituted until a diuresis is established. Other nephrotoxic drugs should be avoided.

If renal failure is unresponsive to preventive measures, renal replacement therapy may be necessary. Continuous dialysis methods are preferred. When the indication for dialysis is acute tubular necrosis from graft failure and/or sepsis, and multiorgan dysfunction is present, the mortality rate is high.

Infection

Infection will develop at some time in most liver transplant recipients.[30] Sepsis and multiorgan failure are together responsible for over half of deaths.[31] The high incidence is the result of preoperative deficient immunocompetence, complicated surgery, invasive procedures and monitoring, and postoperative immunosuppressive therapy. Specific risk factors include prolonged operation time, prolonged antibiotic therapy and gastrointestinal or vascular complications.

Most infections develop in the first 2 months. Early infections primarily involve the lungs, intra-abdominal structures, wounds, intravascular lines and urinary tract. Usual microorganisms are Gram-positive and Gram-negative aerobes. Later infections may be caused by fungi. Invasive candidiasis carries a high mortality, and appears to be particularly common in patients transplanted for ALF.

The most prevalent viral infection is CMV, usually presenting 1–4 months after transplantation, and is associated with fever, neutropenia and atypical lymphocytosis. Other signs reflect the organs affected. It is best diagnosed using culture techniques, such as detection of immediate-early antigen.[32] Symptomatic CMV infection is treated with ganciclovir. The most common adverse effect is neutropenia. Strategies for preventing CMV infection include giving only CMV-negative blood products in the perioperative period,[33] and CMV-specific immunoglobulin and ganciclovir or high-dose acyclovir prophylaxis.

In general, strict infection control measures must be enforced, including an antibiotic policy. A broadspectrum antibiotic is given intraoperatively and for 2–4 days after surgery. Some ICUs use prophylactic nystatin (by oral and nasogastric tube) to reduce fungal colonization of the upper gastrointestinal tract, and sometimes fluconazole or low-dose amphotericin B IV is used for prophylaxis against invasive fungal infection. Selective decontamination of the digestive tract may reduce the incidence of early infection and perhaps infection-associated morbidity and mortality.[34]

The treatment of infections follows conventional guidelines. When infections are life-threatening, it may be possible to withdraw immunosuppressive therapy temporarily, without developing immediate rejection.[35]

Neurological complications

Neurological complications occur more often after retransplant operations and in children, and can result in significant morbidity and mortality.[36] Reversible neurological complications include seizures (often due to cyclosporin toxicity with associated hypomagnesaemia),[37] and a spectrum of clinical features associated with cyclosporin neurotoxicity.[38] The most extreme forms are encephalopathy and cerebral white matter changes, sometimes associated with cortical blindness. Symptoms and signs resolve after reducing cyclosporin dosage. FK506 appears to have similar or more severe neurotoxic effects.[39]

Preoperative hepatic encephalopathy usually improves significantly after liver transplantation. Most patients transplanted with hepatic encephalopathy have ALF, and recovery of consciousness can take up to a week, especially if sedatives were used to control intracranial pressure preoperatively. Less severely encephalopathic patients can awaken much earlier. When hepatic encephalopathy develops or worsens postoperatively, serious causes of graft dysfunction should be investigated.

Other factors, such as electrolyte imbalance (especially hypernatraemia and hyponatraemia), uraemia, sepsis and drugs (particularly sedatives, cyclosporin and OKT3) may contribute to impaired consciousness in the recipient. Intracerebral haemorrhage is a rare but lethal complication, usually attributed to severe thrombocytopenia and hypertension. Other rare causes of neurological dysfunction include hypoxic encephalopathy, central pontine myelinolysis[40] and opportunistic infection (e.g. with CMV, herpes simplex, toxoplasmosis and *Cryptococcus*). Confusion, depression and frank psychosis occur in some patients. Peroneal nerve and brachial plexus lesions have been reported as a result of patient positioning on the operating table.[41]

Haematological complications

Coagulopathy

The INR and activated partial thromboplastin time (APTT) normalize rapidly when early graft function is good. If there is ischaemic injury, vascular complications or rejection, impaired hepatic synthesis of coagulation factors results in prolongation of the INR. Coagulopathy (e.g. disseminated intravascular coagulation, DIC) may occur with severe sepsis.

Treatment of coagulopathy involves assessment, treatment of the underlying cause and replacement of coagulation factors. In some circumstances, treatment is withheld, so that INR can be used to assess graft function.

Thrombocytopenia

Thrombocytopenia is common[42,43] and the lowest platelet counts occur 3–5 days postoperatively. Pre-operative thrombocytopenia, haemodilution from massive blood transfusion, DIC, bone-marrow suppression from immunosuppressive agents and uptake of platelets into the graft are contributing factors. Failure of the platelet count to improve spontaneously by the sixth postoperative day is a poor prognostic sign, but deaths caused directly by thrombocytopenia are unusual. Pancytopenia is far less common and occurs later in the postoperative course. Causes include immunosuppressive therapy and CMV infection, or its treatment with ganciclovir.

Haemolysis

Haemolysis may occur in recipients of ABO-incompatible grafts, and also in a proportion of patients receiving non-identical ABO-compatible grafts. It is usually mild, but may cause fever, anaemia, increasing jaundice and renal dysfunction.

Metabolic complications

Early metabolic complications include hypokalaemia, hypomagnesaemia, hyperglycaemia and metabolic alkalosis. Hypoglycaemia may occur if there is severe graft dysfunction. Metabolic acidosis persisting after the first few hours of ICU admission suggests significant hypovolaemia or graft dysfunction.

Liver transplantation for acute liver failure

Most patients with ALF have fulminant hepatic failure (FHF), which is discussed in Chapter 37. Liver transplantation has changed the focus of treatment. The spontaneous recovery rate with aetiologies other than paracetamol is 20–25%, whereas survival with liver transplantation is 68%.[44] Despite the lack of controlled trials, liver transplantation appears to benefit selected individual patients. Contraindications and death before donor availability limit its feasibility.[45] Some innovative techniques such as temporary auxiliary transplantation,[46] temporizing hepatectomy[47] and baboon-to-human liver transplantation[48] require evaluation.

In general, transplantation is indicated when survival is unlikely with medical treatment alone. Major issues are patient selection and support until a donor organ is found. Precise indications vary from centre

Table 93.5 Criteria for liver transplantation in acute liver failure (non-paracetamol induced)[49]

Prothrombin time > 100 s (INR > 6.5)
or any three of:
Age < 10 or > 40 years
Non-A, non-B hepatitis, halothane hepatitis or idiosyncratic drug reaction
Duration of jaundice before onset of encephalopathy > 7 days
Prothrombin time > 50 s (INR > 3.5)
Serum bilirubin > 300 μmol/l

INR = International normalized ratio.

to centre. The King's College criteria (Table 93.5)[49] have good positive predictive value.[50] Other tests, such as serial recording of sensory evoked potentials, may be useful prognostic indicators.[51]

In most cases, orthotopic liver transplant operation is performed. Surgery is generally less complicated than in patients with chronic liver disease, because portosystemic vascular collaterals are absent. The danger of worsening cerebral oedema and brainstem coning persists throughout the procedure. Elevations in intracranial pressure may persist into the postoperative period, especially if the graft does not function immediately. Although most patients recover normal neurological function after transplantation, failure to regain consciousness is reported (reflecting perioperative structural brain damage).

Postoperative management is similar to that for elective liver transplantation. The incidence of postoperative sepsis is high. Some units include amphotericin B prophylactically, because of the increased risk of fungal infection. Fulminant hepatitis B infection is not associated with graft reinfection.

Liver transplantation in children

Between 30 and 50% of liver transplant recipients are children.[52] Overall, surgery, ICU management and immunosuppression are similar, but specific problems arise from shortage of paediatric donors, difficulties with small-sized blood vessels, absent extrahepatic bile ducts, previous surgery and the psychological needs of chronically ill children and their families.

The most common reason for transplantation in children is biliary atresia when the Kasai procedure has failed. Metabolic disorders such as α_1-antitrypsin deficiency, Wilson's disease and tyrosinaemia are the next most frequent indication. ALF is the reason for transplantation in approximately 10% of recipients.

Preoperatively, nutritional assessment and support are particularly important. The child and family should be familiarized with the procedures and staff. Due to the shortage of paediatric donors, techniques of reducing adult donor livers are used[53] (e.g. split grafting of one liver to treat two small recipients[54] and grafting from living donors[55].

Venovenous bypass is rarely used in small children. The small hepatic artery may require complicated vascular reconstructions. In older children, the preferred biliary anastomosis is duct-to-duct reconstruction, but for most small children and for all cases of biliary atresia, a Roux-en-Y choledochojejunostomy is used. In general, surgical complications are more common in children (up to 30% of cases), and usually involve vascular and biliary anastomoses. The retransplantation rate is higher, especially in children under 1 year.[56]

Medical complications are similar to those for adults. One-year survival is approximately 75%. Only 2–4% of children who survive the first year die within the next 5 years.[57] The majority of children are home by 2 months posttransplantation.

Outcome of liver transplantation

Survival from liver transplantation is approximately 10% higher than a decade ago, with 80% 1-year and 70–80% 5–10-year survival. However, patients transplanted for ALF and chronic HBV infection have a slightly worse outcome. Also, even carefully selected patients with primary hepatocellular malignancy have 20–30% 2-year survival after transplantation. The most important intraoperative predictor of survival is blood loss; patients receiving over 10 units of red cells have decreased hospital survival.[58] Postoperative factors that predict short- or long-term survival are the severity and number of episodes of allograft rejection.

References

1. Gordon RD, Fung J, Tzakis AG *et al.* (1991) Liver transplantation at the University of Pittsburgh, 1984 to 1990. *Clin Transplant* 105–117.
2. Belle SH, Beringer KC, Murphy JB *et al.* (1991) Liver transplantation in the United States: 1988 to 1990. *Clin Transplant* 13–29.
3. Lake JR and Wright TL (1991) Liver transplantation for patients with hepatitis B: what have we learned from our results? *Hepatology* **13**:796–799.
4. McCaughan GW, Pau A, Parsons C, McGuiness PH, Gallagher ND and Sheil AGR (1992) Hepatitis C infection in liver transplant patients. *Transplant Proc* **24**:2256.
5. Calne R, Yamanoi A, Oura S and Kawamura M (1993) Liver transplantation for hepatocarcinoma. *Surgery Today* **23**:1–3.
6. Tarter RE, Switala J, Plail J, Havrilla J and Van Thiel DH (1992) Severity of hepatic encephalopathy before liver transplantation is associated with quality of life after liver transplantation. *Arch Intern Med* **152**:2097–2101.
7. Krowka MJ and Cortese DA (1994) Hepatopulmonary syndrome: current concepts in diagnostic and therapeutic considerations. *Chest* **105**:1528–1537.
8. Gonwa TA, Poplawski S, Paulsen W *et al.* (1989) Pathogenesis and outcome of hepatorenal syndrome in patients undergoing orthotopic liver transplant. *Transplantation* **47**:395–397.
9. Fung JJ, Makowka L, Griffin M, Duquesnoy R, Tzakis A and Starzl TE (1987) Successful liver–kidney transplantation in patients with preformed lymphocytotoxic antibodies. *Clin Transpl* **1**:187–194.
10. Wallwork J, Williams R and Calne RY (1987) Transplantation of liver, heart and lungs for primary biliary cirrhosis and primary pulmonary hypertension. *Lancet* **ii**:182–185.
11. Beath SV, Brook GD, Kelly DA *et al.* (1993) Successful liver transplantation in babies under 1 year. *Br Med* **307**:825–828.
12. Stieber AC, Gordon RD, Todo S *et al.* (1991) Liver transplantation in patients over 60 years of age. *Transplantation* **51**:271–284.
13. Potter JM, Hickman PE, Balderson G, Lynch SV and Strong R (1992) Lignocaine metabolism and MEGX production in the liver transplant donor. *Transplant Proc* **24**:198–199.
14. Kalayoglu M, Sollinger WH, Stratta RJ *et al.* (1988) Extended preservation of the liver for clinical transplantation. *Lancet* **i**:617–619.
15. Rossleigh MA, McCaughan GW, Gallagher ND *et al.* (1988) The role of nuclear medicine in liver transplantation. *Med J Aust* **148**:561–563.
16. Schroeder TJ, Gremse DA, Mansour ME *et al.* (1989) Lidocaine metabolism as an index of liver function in hepatic transplant donors and recipients. *Transplant Proc* **21**:2299–2301.
17. Wallemacq PE and Reding R (1993) FK506 (Tacrolimus) a novel immunosuppressant in organ transplantation: clinical, medical and analytical aspects. *Clin Chem* **39**:2219–2228.
18. Imagawa DK, Noguchi K, Iwaki Y and Busuttil RW (1992) Hyperacute rejection following ABO-compatible orthotopic liver transplantation. *Transplantation* **54**:1114–1117.
19. Goldstein RM, Husberg BS and Klintmalm GB (1993) OKT3 rescue for steroid-resistant rejection in adult liver transplantation. *Transplantation* **55**:87–91.
20. Greif F, Bronsther OL, Van Thiel DH *et al.* (1994) The incidence, timing, and management of biliary tract complications after orthotopic liver transplantation. *Ann Surg* **219**:40–45.
21. Glauser FL (1990) Systemic hemodynamic and cardiac function changes in patients undergoing orthotopic liver transplantation. *Chest* **98**:1210–1215.
22. Olutula PS, Hutton L and Wall WJ (1985) Pleural effusion following liver transplantation. *Radiology* **157**:594.

23. Spizarny DL, Gross BH and McLoud T (1993) Enlarging pleural effusion after liver transplantation. *J Thorac Imaging* **8**:85–87.

24. Takaoka F, Brown MR, Paulsen W, Ramsay MAE and Klintmalm GB (1989) Adult respiratory distress syndrome following orthotopic liver transplantation. *Clin Transplant* **3**:294–299.

25. Matuschak GM and Shaw BW Jr (1987) Adult respiratory distress syndrome associated with acute liver allograft rejection: resolution following hepatic retransplantation. *Crit Care Med* **15**:878–881.

26. Kusne S, Dummer JS, Singh N *et al.* (1988) Fungal infections after liver transplantation. *Transplant Proc* **20**:650–651.

27. McCauley J, Van Thiel DH, Starzl TE and Puschett JB (1990) Acute and chronic renal failure in liver transplantation. *Nephron* **55**:121–128.

28. Poplawski SC, Gonwa TA, Goldstein R, Husberg BS and Klintmalm G (1989) Renal dysfunction following orthotopic liver transplantation. *Clin Transplant* **3**:94–100.

29. Kahan BD (1985) Cyclosporine: the agent and its actions. *Transplant Proc* **17**:5–18.

30. Colonna JO, Winston DJ, Brill JE *et al.* (1988) Infectious complications in liver transplantation. *Arch Surg* **123**:360–364.

31. Park GR, Gomez-Arnau J, Lindop MJ, Klinck JR, Williams R and Calne RY (1989) Mortality during intensive care after orthotopic liver transplantation. *Anaesthesia* **44**:959–963.

32. Chou S (1990) Newer methods for diagnosis of cytomegalovirus infection. *Rev Infect Dis* **12**:S727–S736.

33. Singh N, Dummer JS, Kusne S *et al.* (1988) Infections with cytomegalovirus and other herpes viruses in 121 liver transplant recipients: transmission by donated organ and the effect of OKT3 antibodies. *J Infect Dis* **158**:124–131.

34. Gorensek MJ, Carey WD, Washington JA, Vogt DP, Broughan TA and Westveer MK (1993) Selective bowel decontamination with quinolones and nystatin reduces Gram-negative and fungal infections in orthotopic liver transplant recipients. *Cleve Clin J Med* **60**:139–144.

35. Manez R, Kusne S, Linden P *et al.* (1994) Temporary withdrawal of immunosuppression for life-threatening infections after liver transplantation. *Transplantation* **57**:149–164.

36. Lopez OL, Estol C, Colina I, Quiroga J, Imvertarza OC and Van Thiel DH (1992) Neurological complications after liver transplantation. *Hepatology* **16**:162–166.

37. Thompson CB, June CH, Sullivan KM and Thomas ED (1984) Association between cyclosporin neurotoxicity and hypomagnesaemia. *Lancet* **ii**:1116–1120.

38. De Groen PC, Aksamit AJ, Rakela J, Forbes GS and Krom RA (1987) Central nervous toxicity after liver transplantation. *N Engl J Med* **317**:861–866.

39. Mueller AR, Platz K-P, Bechstein W-O *et al.* (1994) Neurotoxicity after orthotopic liver transplantation. A comparison between cyclosporine and FK506. *Transplantation* **58**:155–169.

40. Estol CJ, Faris AA, Martinez AJ and Ahdab-Barmada M (1989) Central pontine myelinolysis after liver transplantation. *Neurology* **39**:493–498.

41. Moreno E, Gomez SR, Gonzalez I *et al.* (1993) Neurological complications in liver transplantation. *Acta Neurol Scand* **87**:25–31.

42. O'Grady JG (1992) Blood cell disorders after liver transplantation. *J Hepatol* **16**:1–3.

43. McCaughan GW, Herkes R, Powers B *et al.* (1992) Thrombocytopenia post liver transplantation: correlations with pre-operative platelet count, blood transfusion requirements, allograft function and outcome. *J Hepatol* **16**:16–22.

44. Bernuau J and Benhamou J-P (1991) Fulminant and subfulminant liver failure. In: McIntyre N, Benhamou J-P, Bircher J, Rizzetto M and Rodes J (eds) *Oxford Textbook of Clinical Hepatology.* Oxford: Oxford Medical Publications, p. 942.

45. Castells A Salmeron JM, Navasa M *et al.* (1993) Liver transplantation for acute liver failure: analysis of applicability. *Gastroenterology* **105**:532–538.

46. Boudjema K, Jaeck D, Simeoni U, Chenard MP and Brunot P (1993) Temporary auxiliary liver transplantation for subacute liver failure in a child. *Lancet* **342**:778–779.

47. Henderson A, Webb I, Lynch S, Kerlin P and Strong R (1994) Total hepatectomy and liver transplantation as a two stage procedure in fulminant hepatic failure. *Med J Aust* **161**:318–319.

48. Starzl TE, Fung J, Tzakis A *et al.* (1993) Baboon-to-human-liver transplantation. *Lancet* **341**:65–71.

49. O'Grady JG, Alexander GJM, Haylar KM and Williams R (1989) Early indicators of prognosis in fulminant hepatic failure. *Gastroenterology* **97**:439–445.

50. Pauwels A, Mostefa-Kara N, Florent C and Levy VG (1993) Emergency liver transplantation for acute liver failure: Evaluation of London and Clichy criteria. *J Hepatol* **17**:124–127.

51. Madl C, Grimm G, Ferenci P *et al.* (1994) Serial recording of sensory evoked potentials: a noninvasive prognostic indicator in fulminant liver failure. *Hepatology* **20**:1487–1494.

52. Scharschmidt BF (1984) Human liver transplantation: analysis of data on 540 patients from four centers. *Hepatology* **4**:955–1015.

53. Otte JB, de Ville de Goyet J, Sokal F *et al.* (1990) Size reduction of the donor liver is a safe way to alleviate the shortage of size-matched organs in pediatric liver transplantation. *Ann Surg* **211**:146–157.

54. Emond JC, Whitington PF, Thistlethwaite JR, Zucker AR and Broelsch CF (1990) Transplantation of two patients with one liver. Analysis of a preliminary experience with split liver grafting. *Ann Surg* **212**:14–22.

55. Strong RW, Lynch SV, Ong TH, Matsunami H, Koido Y and Balderson GA (1990) Successful liver transplantation from a living donor to her son. *N Engl J Med* **322**:1505–1507.

56. Salt A, Noble-Jamieson G, Barnes ND *et al.* (1992) Liver transplantation in 100 children: Cambridge and King's College Hospital series. *Br Med J* **304**:416–421.

57. Otte JB, de Ville de Goyet J, Alberti D *et al.* (1989) Liver transplantation in children: University of Louvain Medical School (Brussels) experience with the first 139 patients. *Clin Transplant* **4**:143–152.

58. Mor E, Jennings L, Gonwa TA *et al.* (1993) The incidence of operative bleeding on outcome in transplantation of the liver. *Surg Gynecol Obstet* **176**:219–227.

59. McCaughan GW, McDonald JA, Davies S and Painter DM (1989) Clinicopathological approach to human liver allograft dysfunction. *J Gastroenterol Hepatol* **4**: 467–477.

94 Heart and lung transplantation

JM Branch and GA Harrison

The first successful human heart transplant in the world was performed by Dr Christiaan Barnard in South Africa in 1967,[1] and in Australia by Dr Harry Windsor in 1968. Since then, successful cardiac transplantation programmes have been established worldwide, due to better immunosuppression, improved surgical techniques and ICU management, and earlier detection of rejection with endomyocardial biopsies.[2] Following the success of cardiac transplantation, lung and heart–lung transplantations have also been undertaken successfully in selected patients. Improved survival of these transplant recipients increases the likelihood that some will present to ICUs due to procedures or disorders which may be unrelated to the transplant. This chapter presents the principles of these transplants and management of these patients in ICU.

Cardiac transplantation

Despite the success of cardiac transplantation, donor availability remains a problem. Hence cardiac support measures are being investigated, such as pharmacological long-term management of heart failure, ventricular assist devices and cardiomyoplasty. Cardiomyoplasty involves wrapping a latissimus dorsi flap around the left ventricle. Muscular contraction of this flap is augmented by an implantable electronic pacemaker to enhance left ventricular contractility and performance.[3]

Paediatric cardiac transplantation has become more frequent for congenital heart disease and cardiomyopathy, even in infants under 2 months. However, the limited donor supply makes surgical correction the first option for most congenital lesions. The long-term outcome of paediatric cardiac transplantation is still being defined.[4]

Donors and recipients

As donor supply falls short of the number of patients requiring transplants, many potential donors are assessed for multiorgan retrieval. Criteria to select a cardiac donor are listed in Table 94.1. After brain death is confirmed, ICU management changes from that of 'minimizing neurological damage to maximizing total organ preservation'.[5] Care of potential donors is discussed in Chapter 92. Matching of a cardiac donor with a cardiac recipient is determined by weight within 80–120%, ABO blood group compatibility and negative lymphocyte cross-match. Support of the failing heart is discussed in Chapters 13 and 15. Criteria to select recipients are shown in Table 94.2.[6]

Table 94.1 Criteria to select cardiac transplant donors

General criteria
Age under 60 years
Brain death criteria fulfilled
Family consent obtained
Absence of infection
Absence of chest trauma
Absence of prolonged cardiac arrest
Minimal inotropic support
Hepatitis B-, C-negative and HIV-negative
No malignancy except primary cerebral tumour

Criteria for heart–lung donors in addition to the above
Absence of coronary artery disease
Normal cardiac function
No previous thoracic surgery
No pulmonary infection or trauma

HIV = Human immunodeficiency virus.

Table 94.2 Criteria to select cardiac transplant recipients

Clinical criteria

NYHA class III–IV patients with cardiomyopathy of viral, ischaemic, idiopathic or alcoholic aetiology or secondary to chemotherapeutic agents

Patients with intractable angina due to inoperable coronary artery disease

Exclusion criteria

Age greater than 65 years

Transpulmonary gradient (mean PAP – mean PCWP) > 15 mmHg (2.0 kPa) or PVR > 5.0 Wood units, not reducible with glyceryl trinitrate or sodium nitroprusside (these patients may need heart–lung transplant because of the high incidence of postoperative right ventricular failure)

Insulin-dependent diabetes mellitus with end-stage organ dysfunction.

Severe psychiatric disturbance or intellectual retardation

Current alcohol or drug abuse

Morbid obesity

Concurrent malignancy

Severe hepatic or renal disease, unrelated to cardiac disease (unless for combined organ transplant)

Immunodeficiency illness

Active systemic infection

NYHA = New York Heart Association; PAP = pulmonary arterial pressure; PCWP = pulmonary capillary wedge pressure; PVR = pulmonary vascular resistance.

The transplant procedure

Preoperative preparation of the recipient includes management of any psychosocial problems, physiotherapy, exercise and nutritional manipulation. Any associated medical problems are investigated and treated as necessary. Antibiotics, immunosuppressives and ganciclovir (if the donor is positive and the recipient negative for cytomegalovirus) are started according to local protocols.

The heart and other organs are usually obtained by distant procurement, preferably with a total ischaemic time of less than 6 h. Myocardium is preserved by infusion of hypothermic cardioplegia during procurement, and packaging in cold normal saline surrounded by ice after excision. The donor heart is excised at the atrial level, leaving the posterior atrial walls *in situ*, with the great vessels being excised 2–3 cm above the semilunar valves. The donor heart is sutured into the recipient with atrial anastomoses in sequence, a procedure which takes approximately 3–5 h.

Before induction of anaesthesia, the patient is given methylprednisolone 500 mg, azathioprine 3 mg/kg and an antibiotic (e.g. cephazolin 500 mg). After cardiopulmonary bypass, repeat doses of methylprednisolone and antibiotic are given, and isoprenaline is infused to maintain heart rate over 110 beats/min. An infusion of glyceryl trinitrate and/or sodium nitroprusside is started to lower systemic pressure and maintain central venous pressure (CVP) at 10 mmHg (1.33 kPa) and left atrial pressure (LAP) at 12 mmHg (1.60 kPa) or higher. Inotropes are continued for haemodynamic stability. Fresh frozen plasma (FFP) is given as required to help reverse the coagulation defect of pre-admission warfarin therapy.

Physiology and pharmacology of the denervated heart

At surgery, the sinoatrial (SA) node of the recipient is retained but does not activate the transplant heart across the suture line. The donor heart has its own SA node which is not innervated. It is often possible to discern 2 P waves on the electrocardiogram (ECG). The donor SA node controls the graft's rate. Hence, because of the absence of autonomic innervation, only drugs or manoeuvres that act directly on the heart will affect myocardial function. For example, the Valsalva manoeuvre or carotid sinus massage will not affect heart rate, but drugs such as adrenaline, noradrenaline and isoprenaline will exert a positive inotropic and chronotropic effect, and β-adrenergic blockers will depress myocardial function.[7] Quinidine and digitalis will influence conductivity through their direct effect only. The denervated heart retains its intrinsic control mechanisms, e.g. a normal Frank–Starling response to volume loading, normal conductivity and intact α- and β-adrenergic receptors (perhaps with enhanced responsiveness).

The coronary arteries retain their vasodilatory responsiveness to nitrates and metabolic demands. They can develop atherosclerosis in the long term, but the patient experiences no anginal pain with ischaemia or infarction because of the denervation.

Denervation results most importantly in an atypical response to exercise, hypovolaemia and hypotension. Any increase in cardiac output from increased heart rate or contractility depends on an increasing venous return and circulating catecholamines, and the response may be delayed. During exercise, muscle contraction increases venous return and the increased circulating catecholamines increase the heart rate. This is a gradual response and, as exercise ceases, the heart rate and cardiac output slowly fall as the catecholamine and the response levels decrease.[8,9] In pathological states, the transplanted heart is especially dependent on adequate filling volumes, and attention to preload is a critical initial management step.

The denervated heart is also sensitive to extremes of heart rate; arrhythmias are unusual but may cause serious haemodynamic problems. Cardiac arrhythmias can be atrial, junctional or ventricular, and may be a sign of rejection. These may resolve if the rejection is adequately treated. Occasionally, antiarrhythmic drugs that act directly on the conduction system (e.g. quinidine, disopyramide and procainamide) or electrical cardioversion are required.[10]

Verapamil and nifedipine have enhanced effects in the transplanted heart. Hypotension and bradycardia may be profound because of the absence of the normal cardiac sympathetic-mediated response to vasodilatation. Adenosine used for supraventricular tachycardias may induce asystole and cause profound hypotension in the transplanted heart.[11] Amiodarone has been used successfully for ventricular and atrial arrhythmias, but its mild negative inotropy and vasodilatation can cause hypotension. Lignocaine and phenytoin are effective in the treatment of ventricular arrhythmias.

Postoperative care

Uncomplicated patients are managed in the ICU for 3–5 days, and discharged from the next-stage ward in 10–14 days. An example of routine postoperative medications is given in Table 94.3. Important principles of early postoperative management are described below.

Maintaining optimal denervated heart function

Adequate heart rate (90–120 beats/min) and contractility are managed by an isoprenaline infusion

Table 94.3 Routine postoperative medications for the heart transplant recipient

Cephazolin 0.5 g/IV × 3 doses

Methylprednisolone 125 mg 8-hourly × 3 doses then 1 mg/kg per day and then a tapering dose

Ketoconazole 200 mg/day

Ranitidine 150 mg b.d. PO or IV 50 mg t.d.s.

Diltiazem 60 mg t.d.s. (control of blood pressure)

Bactrim DS – tab 2 × per week (*Pneumocystis* prophylaxis)

Cyclosporin b.d. or mane – dose depending on renal and hepatic function and serum concentrations (diltiazem and ketoconazole will augment serum cyclosporin concentrations)

Azathioprine 2 mg/kg IV or orally

Nystatin oral liquid 1 ml/q.i.d.

(5–15 µg/kg per min) and atrial or atrioventricular pacing, depending on the heart's underlying rhythm. Isoprenaline is weaned after 2–3 days, and heart rate is maintained by pacing if it falls below 90 beats/min. The donor heart rate will eventually develop a spontaneous rate of 70–90 beats/min.

An adequate preload is maintained by appropriate volume replacement based on LAP and CVP measurements. Vasodilators (glyceryl trinitrate, sodium nitroprusside, and isoprenaline) help to control filling pressures in the first 2–3 days whilst myocardial compliance is still reduced. These are weaned slowly to avoid sudden atrial and ventricular distension. Higher filling pressures may be required initially because of the postischaemic reduction in ventricular compliance. Therefore, CVP should be maintained at 4–10 mmHg (0.5–1.3 kPa) and LAP at 6–12 mmHg (0.8–1.6 kPa).

An appropriate afterload is achieved with vasodilators. Blood pressure should be controlled vigorously posttransplantation, to avoid headaches, visual disturbances and convulsions. Early control is undertaken with sodium nitroprusside to maintain a systolic arterial pressure of 120 mmHg (15.9 kPa) and mean arterial pressure of 70–85 mmHg (9.3–11.3 kPa) and reduce tension on suture lines. Later, sublingual nifedipine, diltiazem or angiotensin-converting enzyme inhibitors may be helpful.

Right ventricular afterload may also require attention. Sodium nitroprusside can be used to lower pulmonary vascular resistance if high, or if ischaemic injury causes moderate impairment of right ventricular function. Glyceryl trinitrate is also effective. Nitric oxide has been used successfully after cardiac transplantation to lower pulmonary vascular resistance. Prostacyclin is another possibility but often produces profound systemic vasodilatation and hypotension.

Removal of invasive lines and early mobility

Intravascular lines, drains, endotracheal tubes and catheters are removed as soon as possible, to reduce infection risk and encourage mobility. Patients sit in a chair on the first or second postoperative day and commence ambulation on the second or third day.

Insulin

An insulin infusion is routinely started for hyperglycaemia secondary to the stress response of surgery, methylprednisolone and insulin resistance from hypothermia. The infusion is weaned within 24–48 h.

Correction of coagulapathy

Further FFP is given if the prothrombin time is still prolonged. Platelets are required occasionally.

Management of renal function

Renal impairment may follow transplantation due to the effects of cardiopulmonary bypass, cyclosporin and any reduction in cardiac output. Strict fluid balance is mandatory. Diuretics (frusemide or ethacrynic acid) and dopamine (2.0–2.5 µg/kg per min) may be required.

Complications

Early postoperative complications

Postoperative hypotension may result from an inadequate heart rate (<100 beats/min), hypovolaemia (usually due to haemorrhage), tamponade, left and/or right ventricular failure, sepsis, and hyperacute or acute rejection (see below). Symptoms and signs of rejection can include fever, hypotension, lassitude, decreasing physical ability, shortness of breath, anorexia, nausea or vomiting, tachycardia, bradycardia, atrial arrhythmias, fluid retention, rapid weight gain >2 kg in 24 h, abdominal discomfort or pain and any other signs of cardiac failure. Other early postoperative complications include bleeding, atelectasis, pericardial and pleural effusions, and pulmonary oedema (from renal failure, sepsis, left ventricular failure or acute respiratory distress syndrome). Transplant patients can deteriorate rapidly; thus any of these symptoms and signs must be related to the transplant team.

Rejection

Rejection is graded histopathologically according to the type and degree of cellular infiltrate, presence of myocyte necrosis and presence of haemorrhage. Hyperacute rejection occurs rarely in the postoperative period due to ABO mismatch. It presents as acute ventricular failure secondary to diffuse myocardial intravascular thrombosis. Treatment of hyperacute rejection is retransplantation. Other rejection episodes are treated with equine antithymocyte globulin (ATG; if within 10 days of transplantation) or methylprednisolone IV (if after 10 days). OKT3 monoclonal antibody is also used in some centres. Long-term immunosuppression is with double therapy – azathioprine and cyclosporin – or triple therapy, with the addition of prednisolone.

One or more episodes of rejection is experienced by the majority of recipients within the first 3 months, and may occur as early as a few days postoperatively. The frequency of rejection episodes then decreases to negligible at 12–18 months. Immunosuppression is started preoperatively with cyclosporin A, azathioprine, methylprednisolone and sometimes ATG.

Early detection of rejection by endomyocardial biopsy is imperative. The first biopsy is generally performed 7–10 days posttransplant, then weekly for about 1 month, then fortnightly for another month

and, if there are no problems, monthly until 6 months postoperatively. Frequency is then decreased to a biopsy at 6 months, 9 months and at 1 year, and then only when indicated.

Late complications

These include:

1 *Infection*: The most common bacterial organisms are pneumococcus, *Staphylococcus*, *Escherichia coli* and *Pseudomonas*. Other common aetiological organisms are viral (i.e. herpes simplex, herpes zoster and cytomegalovirus (CMV), protozoan (*Pneumocystis carinii* and *Toxoplasma*), and fungal (*Aspergillus* and *Candida*).
2 *Malignancies*: Lymphoproliferative and skin cancers may occur from as early as 3 months after transplantation.
3 *Graft atherosclerosis* is a diffuse process related to donor age and high blood lipid concentrations unrelated to rejection.

Management of the cardiac transplant patient for non-cardiac surgery

The longer survival of cardiac transplant patients means that many will subsequently present for non-cardiac surgical procedures, which may or may not be related to the transplant. Most procedures are uneventful, provided care is taken regarding the physiological, pathological and pharmacological differences between the transplanted and non-transplanted individual.[11]

Both general and regional anaesthetic techniques have been safely used, and as long as there is no acute rejection, functional impairment of the heart is not a problem other than that imposed by denervation. It is important that adequate preload manipulation occurs, especially when drugs which suppress the sympathoadrenal system are used.[12] It is recommended that adequate volume replacement and vasopressors be used during spinal anaesthetic. Drugs which act directly on the heart (e.g. adrenaline and isoprenaline), in addition to vasoconstrictors (e.g. phenylephrine or metaraminol) should be readily available. Any drugs which depress the myocardium or cause ganglion blockade should be avoided. Those drugs which depend on an intact autonomic nervous system for their chronotropic effects will not affect the denervated heart (e.g. pancuronium, anticholinesterases or anticholinergics). If an arrhythmia develops and there is evidence of rejection, then quinidine, procainamide or cardioversion may be used. Cardioversion may result in asystole, so isoprenaline and pacing facilities should be available.

Strict attention to asepsis is mandatory because of the immune suppression. Prophylactic antibiotics should be employed. As soon as possible, all IV lines, urinary and nasogastric catheters and endotracheal tubes should be removed.

Knowledge of the side-effects of the immunosuppressive drugs is essential as they must be continued in the perioperative period. Cyclosporin A can result in hepatic and renal toxicity, hypertension and, rarely, gastrointestinal upsets, anaemia, leukopenia and thrombocytopenia. It must be given with milk or juice on the morning of the surgery. Azathioprine may produce hepatic dysfunction and bone-marrow suppression. Prednisolone may produce adrenal suppression, peptic ulceration, osteoporosis, cataracts, glaucoma and hyperglycaemia.

It is imperative to contact the hospital managing the transplant patient, requesting full details of myocardial function (e.g. last endomyocardial biopsy, echocardiography or gated heart pool scan). If there is any doubt regarding the rejection status, the patient should be referred back to that hospital for reassessment.

Heart–lung transplantation

The first heart–lung transplant (HLT) was performed in Stanford in 1981. HLT was then performed for both parenchymal lung disease and pulmonary hypertension. With the advent of single- or double-lung transplantations, there is overlap between indications for these procedures. The present indications for HLT are primary pulmonary hypertension, Eisenmenger's syndrome, end-stage suppurative pulmonary disease or end-stage bilateral lung disease associated with significant cardiac failure – generally right ventricular failure.[13]

Selection criteria

These are similar to those for heart transplantation, except that an elevated pulmonary vascular resistance tips clinical judgement towards HLT. Exclusion criteria for recipients are age over 45 years, high-dose corticosteroid therapy (relative contraindication), active bronchopulmonary fungal disease, and prior sternotomy, thoracotomy or mediastinal irradiation.[6] The criteria to select donors are listed in Table 94.4.

Table 94.4 Heart–lung transplantation – donor selection criteria

Age and ABO blood group compatibility as per heart donors

'Close size' lung match to restrictive problems or persistent residual space between lung and chest wall

Donor Pao_2 > 100 mmHg (13.3 kPa) on Fio_2 0.3 or > 300 mmHg (39.9 kPa) on Fio_2 1.0

Clear chest X-ray

The transplant procedure

In the donor operation, the heart–lung bloc is removed with the aorta divided as high as possible. The trachea is stapled and cut at a minimum of five rings above the carina, with the lungs half-inflated. The posterior pulmonary ligaments are then dissected. In the recipient operation, preservation of the vagus may be difficult, but preservation of phrenic and recurrent laryngeal nerves, with particular attention to haemostasis in the posterior mediastinum, is essential for the success of the operation. Many centres are now using aprotinin, a serine protease inhibitor, with good results to minimize blood loss in the HLT recipient.[13]

Postoperative care (see also lung transplantation, below)

This is similar to that for cardiac transplant patients, with some differences. The patient is without a bronchial arterial supply or pulmonary innervation. Lymphatic drainage of the lungs is lost. Thus patients are kept in a negative fluid balance in the early postoperative period. Aggressive physiotherapy is required, sometimes with bronchoscopic toilet to clear secretions, as denervation prevents reflex coughing of secretions below the anastomosis. Once secretions reach the native trachea, coughing will result. Daily peak flow estimations are performed. Immunosuppression is given as for cardiac transplantation. Cefotaxime is used instead of cephazolin, and other antibiotics may be required depending on the donor sputum culture. Lung function assessment, transbronchial lung biopsy and endomyocardial biopsies are used to assess rejection.

Complications

Bleeding may occur due to extensive dissection and systemic pulmonary collaterals in congenital heart disease. Other early complications include tracheal anastomotic dehiscence, acute reperfusion lung injury (i.e. pulmonary oedema) due to long ischaemic times or inadequate protection with the pulmonary 'plegia' solution (see below), and infection. Heart–lung recipients have three times as many infections as heart recipients, and this contributes significantly to their higher mortality rate. Infection is the major cause of mortality in the first 6 months, and rejection thereafter.

Single- or double-lung transplantation

Early work on single-lung transplantation (SLT) yielded only short-term survival.[14] However, subsequent successes by the Toronto group[15,16] encouraged the development of double-lung transplantation[17–19], initially by the *en bloc* method with tracheal anastomosis. The extensive dissection required in the recipient and the high incidence of anastomotic problems encouraged development of bilateral sequential lung transplantation (BSLT), which is the favoured method today. SLT is indicated for non-suppurative lung disease in a patient who does not have cardiac disease (e.g. emphysema from smoking or α_1-antitrypsin deficiency, or fibrosing alveolitis – either cryptogenic or secondary). Whilst these conditions can also be managed by BLST, SLT provides satisfactory results and makes more efficient use of a limited donor pool. BSLT is indicated for suppurative and/or bilateral lung disease (e.g. cystic fibrosis and bilateral bronchiectasis). The merits of BSLT or HLT for these conditions are controversial. With HLT, the recipient's heart may be used in a 'domino' procedure[20] – as a donor heart for a second recipient. Either BLST or a domino HLT allows the most efficient use of donor organs. Lung transplantation can be combined with kidney or liver transplantation.

Recipients are accepted for lung transplantation up to age 55 years. It is usually possible to perform SLT without cardiopulmonary bypass (CPB). The requirement for CPB is higher in BSLT (approximately 5–10%) because the first lung transplanted (usually the right) must immediately provide ventilation and gas exchange whilst the other side is transplanted. CPB increases the amount of operative blood loss and the volume of colloid required in the postoperative period. The incidence of 'wet' lungs, with X-ray appearances of capillary leak into the interstitial space of the lungs, is also increased.

Physiology of the denervated lungs

The lungs appear to remain permanently denervated. There is evidence that the bronchial artery circulation and lymphatic system regenerate after several weeks. Control of respiration is not affected by the loss of pulmonary afferent nerves. Regulation of breathing is through chest wall afferents. Patients regain spontaneous breathing early, and are usually able to be weaned off ventilation and extubated within 4–8 h.

Patients who were dependent on their hypoxic drive may take time to achieve normocarbia. Arterial blood gases otherwise tend to remain normal. On exercise, minute volume, tidal volume and respiratory rate are able to increase appropriately. Bronchomotor tone is retained.[21] Asthmatic subjects who are transplanted with non-asthmatic lungs do not experience asthma.[22] The ventilatory response to CO_2 eventually becomes normal,[23] and the pulmonary vascular response to hypoxia is retained.[24] Coronary–bronchial collaterals can open to restore vascularity to vessels previously supplied by the bronchial arteries. The cough response is lost below the anastomosis.

Postoperative care

Ventilation

Patients can regain spontaneous ventilation with an acceptable Pa_{CO_2}. This Pa_{CO_2} depends on the patient's preoperative level. With ventilation to limited peak inspiratory pressures between 35 and 40 cm H_2O (3.5–4.0 kPa), Pa_{CO_2} of most patients lies between 35 and 40 mmHg (4.6–5.3 kPa), but values between 60 and 70 mmHg (7.9–9.2 kPa) are common. Many patients who were chronically hypercarbic preoperatively show a remarkable tolerance to the cerebral effects of CO_2. Pa_{CO_2} values 80–100 mmHg (10.5–13.3 kPa) may be seen in such patients postoperatively without drowsiness, particularly when epidural analgesia is provided. These patients may take several weeks for their Pa_{CO_2} to fall below 40 mmHg (5.3 kPa).

Earlier fears that patients receiving SLT for emphysema would not be able to ventilate the transplanted lung due to mediastinal shift[25] have proved to be unfounded, unless an overwhelming implantation response or massive sputum retention occurs in the transplanted lung.

Gas transfer

All patients have an increased alveolar–arterial oxygen gradient ($A–a_{DO_2}$) following lung transplant, but it is usually possible to achieve a Pa_{O_2} of 100 mmHg (13.3 kPa) or greater on Fi_{O_2} 0.3–0.4 within a few postoperative hours. A low-level (5 cm H_2O – 0.5 kPa) positive end-expiratory pressure (PEEP) is not contraindicated, but must be used cautiously. There is uncertainty as to the impact of PEEP on the mediastinal position in SLT.

After extubation, standard techniques of oxygen therapy are used. In the first 48 h, gas transfer is monitored by frequent arterial blood gases, and thereafter by pulse oximetry. Continuous positive airway pressure (CPAP) at low levels (5.0–7.5 mmHg, 0.5–0.75 kPa) is not contraindicated, but is not usually required. It is generally avoided to avoid unnecessary pressure on the anastomosis.

The $A–a_{DO_2}$ in the immediate postoperative period may increase further due to the following complications, which may be difficult to distinguish from one another.

Implantation response

This manifests within a few hours. Infiltrates in the transplanted lung or lungs appear on chest X-ray, and the lungs may appear to be wet with increased peribronchial cuffing. In severe cases, a picture suggestive of severe acute respiratory distress syndrome is seen with widespread loss of translucency. There is an association between ischaemic time and the severity of the response, but clinically significant implantation response is difficult to predict in a given patient. Management comprises:

1 continued pressure-limited ventilation;
2 judicious use of low PEEP;
3 fluid restriction and diuretics as indicated by filling pressures, tissue perfusion and urinary output;
4 fibreoptic bronchoscopy to exclude retention of secretions;
5 limitation of vasodilators, e.g. glyceryl trinitrate, sodium nitroprusside or isoprenaline;
6 nitric oxide to redistribute blood to the best-ventilated alveoli.

Hyperacute rejection

This is fortunately rare. It usually results in acute graft failure with a very poor prognosis for recovery of function. Management requires continued massive respiratory support, including extracorporeal membrane oxygenation if necessary, but survival is unlikely.

Early rejection

Acute rejection of the transplanted lung occurs in almost all recipients in the first 3 months, but may occur very early in some recipients. Deterioration in Pao_2 and pulmonary infiltrates after 48–72 h should favour a suspicion of rejection rather than implantation response. It may be difficult to distinguish between early rejection and bacterial infection. Flexible bronchoscopic washings may be helpful and transbronchial biopsy is essential in doubtful cases. In many cases, a course of pulsed steroids is appropriate on suspicion whilst antibiotics are also given.

Sputum retention

Effective analgesia, aggressive physiotherapy and early mobilization are essential to minimize this problem. Secretions below the anastomoses do not elicit a cough reflex and voluntary coughing is important. The patient sits out of bed on the first or second postoperative day and becomes ambulant on the second or third day. Flexible bronchoscopy under topical anaesthesia is used to clear secretions in patients with ineffective cough due to various causes.

Pulmonary infection

Early pulmonary bacterial infection is common, and infection with other microorganisms can occur later. Fortunately, bronchitis is a more usual initial bacterial infective manifestation than pneumonia. Patients with resident microorganisms are given prophylactic antibiotics. Samples of the donor's pulmonary secretions are taken at the time of lung harvesting.[26] The recipient is given appropriate antibiotics when results of these cultures are known. Meanwhile, the recipient is given a broad-spectrum antibiotic with good penetrance into pulmonary tissues, e.g. cefotaxime. Prophylactic Bactrim is given to all patients (see

section on cardiac transplantation, above) and prophylactic ganciclovir is given to patients who have a CMV mismatch (i.e. positive donor and a negative recipient).

Circulation

Patients undergoing SLT or BSLT retain their own fully innervated heart. Primary haemodynamic problems are uncommon. Decisions on filling pressures are based on pulmonary artery pressure and CVP. Measurement of pulmonary artery occlusion pressure is avoided, due to concerns about the inflation of the balloon in a pulmonary artery anastomosis. Fluid replacement is usually restricted to replacement of drainage loss and maintenance fluids at 1 ml/kg per h. Patients who return from the operating room with marked vasodilatation (e.g. mean arterial pressure < 70 mmHg – 9.3 kPa and very warm hands and feet) are given metaraminol or noradrenaline by infusion. Secondary right ventricular failure may occur in hypoxia and pulmonary hypertension associated with severe implantation response or early rejection. Glyceryl trinitrate and sodium nitroprusside are traditional pulmonary vasodilators, but inhaled nitric oxide offers the advantage of reduced pulmonary vascular resistance and redistribution of blood to the best-ventilated alveoli without systemic vasodilatation.

Anastomoses

Ischaemic anastomotic ulceration is usually superficial, but occasionally deeper tissue loss eventually produces bronchial or tracheal stenosis requiring dilatation and/or stent insertion in the early months. Anastomotic dehiscence is rare but fatal. It may be preceded by fungal invasion of the anastomosis. Some centres wrap the anastomosis with an omental or intercostal muscle pedicle to improve anastomotic blood supply. Invaginating one airway into the other (telescope technique)[27] is now a more popular technique.

Fibreoptic bronchoscopy to inspect the anastomoses and remove residual secretions is performed at the conclusion of surgery or after return to the ICU. This is repeated on the third postoperative day and thereafter as indicated.

Analgesia

HLT is performed through a sternotomy incision. Pain is rarely severe and is easily managed with standard IV opioids. SLT is performed through a thoracotomy and BSLT through a bilateral thoracotomy or extended anterior butterfly incision. Pain after SLT or BSLT is best managed with a thoracic epidural analgesia. The catheter is inserted at the end of surgery, or when coagulation has returned to normal if CPB was used. A mixture of bupivacaine and fentanyl is infused at 2–10 ml/h.

Immunosuppression

Immunosuppression is the same as for HLT.

Nutrition

Many patients in chronic respiratory failure are in a poor nutritional state when assessed for lung transplantation. This is corrected by an exercise programme and optimal diet in the months before transplantation. Most patients undergoing SLT can begin oral fluids a few hours after extubation, and begin feeding on the second postoperative day. Patients undergoing BSLT present with more difficult problems. Those suffering from cystic fibrosis are prone to chronic nutritional deficiencies, and the operation may injure the vagus nerve so that gastric emptying is delayed. Therefore, early nutritional support by enteral feeding or total parenteral nutrition may be required.

Long-term complications

Obliterative bronchiolitis[28,29] which may be a manifestation of chronic rejection, may eventually lead to graft failure. Recurrent infections with *Pseudomonas* or methicillin-resistant *Staphylococcus* can be serious. After the first 6 weeks, infection with CMV or any fungus, yeast, protozoan or virus presents potential hazards. Chronic renal failure due to cyclosporin therapy may persist, but is not usually a major problem unless other complications occur. Most patients have a good quality of life with few complications.

Results of cardiopulmonary transplantation

Cardiac and lung transplantation generally produce good 1-year actuarial survival 85–90% for hearts and 75–85% for heart–lung. Different centres report 60–90% 1-year survival for lung transplantation. Two-year actuarial survival for cardiac transplantation is 80% and for heart–lung and lung transplantation is between 60 and 75%. Mortality is generally secondary to infection (sometimes during treatment for acute rejection), malignancy or the complications of possible chronic rejection, e.g. coronary artery disease in heart transplant recipients or obliterative bronchiolitis in lung transplant recipients.[6,30]

References

1. Barnard CN (1967) The operation. A human cardiac transplant: an interim report of a successful operation performed at Groote Schur Hospital, Capetown. *S Afr Med J* **41**:1271–1274.
2. Billingham ME (1981) Diagnosis of cardiac rejection by endomyocardial biopsy. *Heart Transplant* **1**:25.
3. Aggarnal A and Warltier D (1994) Adenosine: present uses future indications. *Curr Opin Anesthesiol* **7**:109–122.
4. Baum D, Bernstein D, Starres VA *et al.* (1991) Paediatric heart transplantation at Stanford: results of a 15 year experience. *Pediatrics* **88**:203–214.
5. Pickett JA, Wheeldon D and Oturo A (1994) Multiorgan transplantation: donor management. *Curr Opin Anesthesiol* **17**:80–83.
6. St Vincent's Cardiopulmonary Transplant Unit (1995) *Protocol Manual.* Sydney: St Vincent's Hospital.
7. Cannon DS and Graham AF (1973) Electrophysiological studies in the denervated transplanted human heart. *Circ Res* **32**:268–278.
8. Pope SE, Stinson EB, Daughters GT *et al.* (1980) Exercise response of the denervated heart in long term cardiac transplant recipients. *Am J Cardiol* **46**:213–218.
9. Banner NR and Yacoub MH (1990) Physiology of the orthotopic cardiac transplant recipient. *Semin Thorac Cardiovasc Surg* **2**:259–270.
10. Schroeder JS, Berke DK, Graham AF *et al.* Arrhythmias after cardiac transplantation. *Am J Cardiol* **33**:604–607.
11. Bexton RS, Nathan AW, Cory-Pearce R *et al.* (1984) Electrophysiological effects of nifedipine and verapamil in the transplanted human heart. *Heart Transplant* **3**:97–104.
12. Cooper DKC, Becerra EA, Novitsky D *et al.* (1986) Surgery in patients with transplanted hearts. Anaesthetic and operative considerations. *S Afr Med J* **70**:137–142.
13. Bricker SR and Sugden JC (1985) Anaesthesia for surgery in a patient with a transplanted heart. *Br J Anaesth* **57**:634–637.
14. Derom F, Barbier F, Ringoir S *et al.* (1971) Ten-month survival after lung homotransplantion in man. *J Thorac Cardiovasc Surg* **61**:835–846.
15. Toronto Lung Transplant Group (1986) Unilateral lung transplantation for pulmonary fibrosis. *N Engl J Med* **314**:1140–1145.
16. Grossman RF, Frost A, Zamal N *et al.* (1990) Results of single-lung transplantation for bilateral pulmonary fibrosis. *N Engl J Med* **322**:727–733.
17. Noirclerc MJ, Metras D, Vaillant A *et al.* (1990) Bilateral bronchial anastomosis in double lung and heart lung transplantations. *Eur J Cardiothorac Surg* **4**:314–317.
18. Bisson A and Bonette P (1992) A new technique for double lung transplantation: 'bilateral single lung' transplantation. *J Thorac Cardiovasc Surg* **103**:40–46.
19. Kaiser LR, Pasque MK, Trulock EP *et al.* (1991) Bilateral sequential lung transplantion: the procedure of choice for double lung replacement. *Ann Thorac Surg* **52**:438–446.
20. Yacoub MH, Banner NR, Khaghani A *et al.* (1990) Heart–lung transplantation for cystic fibrosis and subsequent domino heart transplantation. *J Heart Transplant* **9**:459–466.
21. Glanville AR, Theodore J, Baldwin JC *et al.* (1990) Bronchial responsiveness after human heart–lung transplantation. *Chest* **97**:1360–1366.
22. Corris PA and Dark JH (1993) Aetiology of asthma: lessons from lung transplantation. *Lancet* **341**:1369–1371.
23. Duncan SR, Kagawa FT, Chaplan SR *et al.* (1989) Respiratory control of heart–lung transplant recipients during CO_2 rebreathing. *Am Rev Respir Dis* **139**:A240.

24. Glanville AR, Baldwin JC, Hunt SA *et al.* (1990) Long-term cardiopulmonary function after human heart lung transplantation. *Aust NZ J Med* **20**:208–214.

25. Stevens PM, Johnson PC, Bell RL *et al.* (1970) Regional ventilation and perfusion after lung transplantation in patients with emphysema. *N Engl J Med* **282**:245–249.

26. Zenati M, Dowling RD, Drummer JS *et al.* (1990) Influence of the donor lung on development of early infections in lung transplant recipients. *J Heart Transplant* **9**:502–509.

27. Calhoon JH, Grover FL, Gibbons WJ *et al.* (1991) Single lung transplantation: alternative indication and technique. *J Thorac Cardiovasc Surg* **101**:816–824.

28. McGregor CG, Dark JH, Hilton CJ *et al.* (1989) Early results of single lung transplantation in patients with end-stage pulmonary fibrosis. *J Thorac Cardiovasc Surg* **98**:350–354.

29. de Hoyos AL, Patterson GA, Maurer JR *et al.* (1992) Pulmonary transplantation. Early and late results. *J Thorac Cardiovasc Surg* **103**:295–306.

30. Kriett JM and Kaye MP (1991) The registry of the international society for heart transplantation: 8th official report. *J Heart Lung Transplant* **10**: 491–491.

Part XVI

Monitoring and diagnostic procedures

JL Derrick and TE Oh

The ultimate aim of computerizing the ICU is to improve patient care. In this chapter we will look at technology which is currently being developed, as well as potential areas in which computers could assist staff in the modern ICU. In many cases, to achieve maximal benefit it will be necessary to change the way in which clinicians practise.

It is important to recognize the relative strengths of computers and their human users. Computers are particularly good at performing calculations on numeric data, whereas people are much better at pattern recognition. Computers are good at conducting organized searches of structured data, whereas people have the capacity for lateral thinking. Computers are consistent, and do not tire during long shifts, but are only as good as their underlying program. The optimal ICU should recognize and use the strengths of each, to maximize efficiency and improve patient outcome.

Types of computers

Mainframe computers

Mainframe computers are powerful and fast. They can be used to handle multiple tasks, linked to a number of peripheral stations (e.g. bed areas, reception and doctors' desks). They are, however, expensive, and any malfunction will jeopardize all computer-based operations.

Personal computers

Stand-alone personal computers offer advantages of low cost, portability and the isolation of a failure to a single replaceable unit. Personal computers do not need to run as fast as mainframe computers as the individual load is smaller, although modern personal computers are as fast as mainframe computers of a few years ago. Multiple personal computers can be connected together in a local area network (LAN) to enable sharing of information.

Task-dedicated microprocessors

Most modern electronic equipment uses microprocessors, e.g. infusion pumps, pulse oximeters, cardiac output and other monitors and ventilators. These devices can often be upgraded by changing their software.

System design

A common finding is that computerizing an ICU leads to an increased proportion of time spent in clerical duties.[1] Systems must be designed carefully to improve patient care. Important features are described below.

Human interface

Staff using intensive care computers come from a variety of backgrounds, and many visit the ICU infrequently, or work there for short periods of time. A computer system for the ICU needs to be designed to meet the needs of all of these individuals, and must be capable of being used by people with no prior computer experience. This requires a system which is flexible, intuitive and easy to use. In general, programs with a graphical user interface (GUI) are easier to use than ones with a text command line interface. Context-sensitive online help is essential. Data displays need to be designed to display data differently to meet the needs of different users. Colour displays are preferable to monochrome.

Capacity

The system must be designed with enough capacity to cope with peaks of usage, especially around the times of handover, and before and during rounds. It is also vital that admission and discharge of patients into and from the system should be made simple and fast, so as to interfere minimally with periods of peak staff activity. In particular, haemo-dynamic and respiratory data should be logged from the patient, even if staff have not yet had a chance to admit the patient formally. Data from remote systems should be downloaded and stored locally to improve speed of access, and to ensure availability in the event of hospital information system breakdown. If enough terminals are avail-able, multiple personal computers are less affected by peaks of activity than mainframe systems.

Data storage

Collected information needs to be stored on a regular basis to avoid data loss in the event of system malfunction. Storage devices include hard disk, magneto-optical drives, writable compact discs (CDs) and write-once-read many (WORM) drives. Modern data storage devices have large capacities which are necessary to store the large amount of information generated in the ICU. File size will vary according to rate of sampling. If values alone are stored, files would be expected to be about 50 kilobytes per hour at a 5 s sample rate. If waveforms are recorded, file size will expand to as much as several megabytes per hour. Digitized images such as computed tomography (CT) scans may require up to several megabytes to store. Data can be compressed to reduce storage requirements.

Breakdowns

All devices are subject to breakdown. Allowances need to be made both for failure of individual components, and also failure of external power supplies and hospital computer systems, when set-ting up a computerized ICU. If a device should fail, recorded data from that particular station must not be lost. This requires multiple simultaneous back-ups of data to be made on a regular basis. It is preferable if such workstations are modular and portable to allow for rapid replacement in event of failure. Power supplied to the computer system should be 'clean', and there should be a back-up supply in the event of hospital-wide power failure. If the entire system crashes it should automatically restart if possible.

Other factors

Electrical safety needs to be considered when using a computer system in the clinical environment.[2] If a mainframe computer is installed, other factors such as air conditioning and fire regulations will need to be addressed.[3] It will also be necessary to allocate space for storage and repair of computer equipment and work space for the systems engineer.

Data collection

The computer system must integrate data from multiple sources, including clinical observation, med-ical devices, laboratories and medical imaging.

Local devices

Currently, data from most medical devices such as monitors, ventilators and infusion pumps are usually transposed by hand to a flowsheet. Automated data collection should decrease transcription errors, and time spent in clerical activities. Data can be trans-mitted in analog or digital format.

Analog transmission

The voltage in the data wire is proportional to the value of the variable. This requires a data wire and a ground wire. Any analog-to-digital (A to D) converter is capable of downloading any analog signal. Each signal requires calibration, however, and there needs to be at least one channel allocated per variable. Pressure transducers are an example of a modern device using analog signals.

Digital transmission

Data are sent as a series of binary numbers, encoded by a fluctuating voltage. Commonly used serial transmission protocols include RS232C, RS232D and RS422. Digital transmission requires a ground wire and a transmission wire. A receiving wire is usually included to allow two-way communications between devices. Often other wires are used to signal things such as device status. Different manufacturers have interpreted the RS232 standard differently, so usually custom cables must be made for each device. Digital communication can transmit multiple variables over a single line, but format has not been standardized, so a separate interpreter must be written for each device. A new communications standard,[4,5] the medical infor-mation bus (MIB), is expected to improve this situation.

Patients in the ICU may not remain in their beds throughout their stay, so allowances need to be made for data collection during transport, and whilst they are in remote locations such as the CT scanner or the operating room. Possible solutions to this problem include a combination of transport monitors and laptop computers, or transport monitors with memory modules, which can be downloaded on return to the ICU.

Manual data entry

Manual data entry is more cumbersome than auto-mated data entry, and the system needs to be designed carefully to encourage use. Data entry devices include:

1 keyboards with or without a pointing device, such as a trackpad, a trackball or a mouse;
2 touch screens, often in combination with a keyboard or keywheel;
3 bar code readers;
4 voice recognition – considered to be the optimal entry method, but currently unreliable in noisy environments;
5 other devices such as light pens and graphics tablets.

Remote devices

Data from other hospital computers also need to be collected and integrated into the database. These include laboratory results, digitized images such as CT scans and X-rays, results of other investigations such as echocardiography or nuclear medicine, and surgical and anaesthetic data.

Future possibilities

Technology is currently available to put video and audio clips of the physical examination of the patient into the patient record.

Data processing

Raw data contain artefacts from automated collection and mistakes from manual entry. Artefacts can be removed or decreased by digital filtering. Mistakes can be decreased by good design of data entry software, and by alerting the user to unusual values as the data is being entered. Data can be enhanced by extraction of variables from complex signals, such as spectral edge from the electroencephalogram (EEG).

Display

Data collected need to be displayed in such a way as to be helpful to the clinician. It should be possible to display data as a trend, metaphor graphics,[6–8] or in tabular form to suit the task at hand. This approach can be used for laboratory as well as physiological data.

Variables which are not easily shown on a temporal display can also be displayed graphically by a bedside computer. Examples of this include flow–volume loops, and a patient's left ventricular function plotted on a Starling curve.[9]

Results such as chest X-rays, CT and magnetic resonance imaging (MRI) scans should be available at the bedside, as well as at the central desk. This allows for easier review of all results on routine rounds. It may also encourage the review of older films which are not usually kept on a traditional viewing box.[10]

Security

Provisions must be made to protect patient privacy, especially if information is to be made available to the hospital-wide computer system, or via 'dial-up' lines. Security measures include user identification and authentication, limitation of access according to need, audit trails of data access, timeouts on unused terminals, data encryption, protection of executable code, appointment of a security officer and procedures being put into place to handle security breaches and independent system audits.[11,12] Log-on codes should be changed on a regular basis. The computer system should ensure that obvious passwords are not chosen, e.g. date of birth or spouse's name. The use of caller ID to limit dial-up access to selected staff members is also possible, where available. Medical records created can be signed using public key cryptography digital signatures, to enhance medicolegal acceptability.[13,14]

Uses of computers

The many applications of computers in the ICU are discussed below. These uses and the interactions of ICU computers with other hospital and outside computer systems are shown diagrammatically in Figure 95.1

Record keeping

Records need to be kept for use in the ICU, after discharge to the ward and on subsequent admission. Current records are often designed for use in ICU, but ward staff find them difficult to interpret. One of the uses for the ICU computer is to print or display the same data in the optimal format for the task at hand. All data should be kept even after discharge, within the guidelines for electronic information storage laid down by local regulatory bodies.

Calculations

Some of the earliest uses for computers in intensive care have been to perform complex or time-consuming calculations.[15] These range from relatively simple calculations such as haemodynamic variables, including the cardiac output computer, respiratory[16,17] and laboratory values,[17,18] to more complicated calculations such as median frequency and spectral edge from the EEG. Many systems automatically calculate simple illness severity scores such as APACHE II[14] (see Chapter 2).

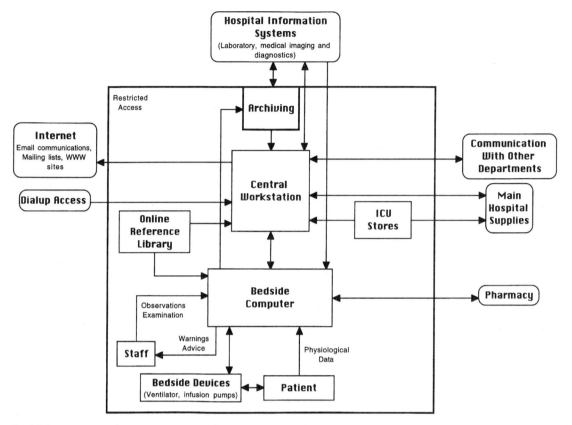

Fig. 95.1 An integrated ICU computer system. Computers at the bedside and central station are linked to hospital and outside systems. WWW = World Wide Web.

Early warning systems

With the large amount of data collected from critically ill patients, it is not surprising that important pieces of information are missed. Computers can be used to warn staff of impending problems. Currently the most common examples of such devices are alarms on monitors, which are triggered by a value transgressing a set limit. These are important in that they alert the staff to a potentially life-threatening situation, but suffer from the problem that they are only reacting once the problem has occurred. Setting the limits more closely increases the number of false alarms, and alarms which are frequently activated may then be ignored.[19,20]

A number of other early-warning systems have been tried or are in use. Computers have also been used to examine the morphology of recorded waveforms. An example of this is automatic arrhythmia detection,[21,22] although other waveforms such as arterial line tracings or respiratory waveforms are also amenable to analysis.[16,23] Trend analysis systems may detect significant changes in a patient's condition before the condition becomes criti-cal.[18,24,25] Intelligent alarm systems may integrate a number of variables, to give specific diagnoses and decrease false alarms.[23,26-28] In the future, the computer may be used to provide continuous real-time multivariate analysis to predict which patients are likely to deteriorate. At a more mundane level, they can also be used to flag patients who will require line changes or laboratory testing, who might have drug interactions, or whose antibiotic therapy is inappropriate.

Online help systems

These may range from simple references to artificial intelligence systems. Reference libraries and standar-dized treatment protocols can be made available at the bedside.[29,30] These libraries range from local resources, such as a CD-ROM, to references on World Wide Web sites. Computerized searches of journal articles via Medline can be helpful in searching for data on obscure diseases.

Intensive care mailing lists exist on the Internet, allowing for discussion of complex problems amongst a worldwide group of intensivists.

Expert systems encode the knowledge of experts into the computer. These can then be used to suggest diagnosis or treatment of various patients on the basis of haemodynamic, respiratory or laboratory data.[31-34] Such systems have the advantage of being available after hours, when less experienced clinicians may be in charge of the unit, and also help to keep management consistent. They do not, however, take autonomy away from staff, who are not constrained to take the advice given. Such systems require careful design, to ensure that data underlying the decision are valid rather than artefactual. Setting up these systems can be difficult, because of problems in defining even simple disease states, and because of differences in opinion between experts as to the best appropriate management.[35]

Control systems

Pharmacokinetics and pharmacodynamics may be altered radically and unpredictably in critically ill patients, making conventional dosage regimens inappropriate in the ICU. Concurrently administered drugs may make the net effect even more variable. Computers can be used to assist the clinician in administering drugs with potentially toxic effects.

A closed loop is where the effect of an intervention is used to adjust the level of intervention to achieve a constant effect. Computers have been used to control ventilation,[36-38] and also to administer hypotensive agents, blood, fluids, inotropes, anaesthetic agents, mannitol and muscle relaxants.[39-45] The aim of the controller is to minimize oscillations due to the lag time between measurement and intervention, and those introduced by outside disturbances. Algorithms used include servo (on/off), proportional integral derivative (PID), fuzzy logic and expert systems. Technical difficulties prevent some of these, such as muscle relaxant infusions, from being used routinely.[46,47]

Open loop refers to the use of known pharmacokinetic models to predict the required dosage of a drug to achieve a certain effect site or plasma concentration. Such techniques have been tried with antibiotics, anticonvulsants, antiarrhythmics, aminophylline and anticoagulants.[48-52]

Outcome prediction

Prolonged treatment in patients whose prognosis is hopeless is costly and may be distressing to both patient and relatives. It is desirable to be able to identify patients whose prognosis is hopeless early after admission, or even before admission. It may be necessary to decide which one of two or more deserving patients to admit to the ICU if bed space is limited. Doctors' and nurses' predictions are frequently incorrect.[53] Scores such as the APACHE II are poor predictors of individual outcome,[54] probably because of their relative simplicity. Computers can be

used to perform complex calculations on large amounts of data, and presumably should be able to predict outcome more accurately.[55-57] Even relatively simple computer models have been shown to be better predictors of outcome than by doctors and nurses.[53]

Quality assurance

Quality assurance and improvement are an integral part of modern medical practice. Instituting such a program using a paper-based record system is time-consuming and costly. If all data are kept in electronic format, this process can be simplified. The database can be used to generate general statistics, look for specific indicators, prospectively monitor for specific events, and also to review patient records retrospectively.[58] To implement such a system successfully, allowance needs to be made during the design and implementation of the data collection programs. If this is not done, the electronic record becomes no different from the paper record in ease of review.[59]

Communications

Currently most communication occurs using voice, either over the telephone or in person. Both disrupt activities of potentially higher priority in which staff may be engaged at the time. In addition, time is often wasted trying to contact members of other departments. Computer systems could be designed to decrease lost time by improving communications. These could include e-mail, automated message paging and communications scheduling by arranging a mutually acceptable time for communication between the two members of staff.

One application of e-mail could be for drug ordering. Digitally signed drug orders can be sent to pharmacy, as well as to the nursing staff caring for the patient. E-mail communications are not limited by distance. Using the Internet, it is possible to obtain opinions from other intensive care specialists on a given problem within a period of hours.

Current computer systems allow not only voice but also video communication, and can transmit other information (e.g. digitized CT and MRI scans) over telephone lines. This could allow earlier assessment and management of patients, as consulted specialists would not necessarily have to come to ICU in person before instituting a course of treatment.

Administration

Computers have been used to simulate staff requirements in the ICU.[60] Real-time assessment of patient numbers and requirements could be built into a computer system to give earlier warning of probable shortage of nursing staff for coming shifts.

Many commercial enterprises such as supermarkets currently use a computerized inventory to aid in ordering of stock. Such a system could be used to increase efficiency in the ICU by identifying items which will require replenishing, and also by identifying usage patterns, thus allowing for more efficient stocking of rarely used items. Currently, bar coding is not universal on items of medical equipment, which makes such a system more difficult to implement.

A complete computer database could be used for costing of individual patient care, and improved billing of these patients.

Education

Programs aimed at self-education are available in cardiovascular and respiratory physiology and pathology, applied pharmacology, mechanical ventilation and anatomy. These programs have the advantage of pacing themselves to the student, and are available at all hours. They can demonstrate problems or techniques which are difficult to show in a lecture, and allow the user to simulate conditions which would be dangerous in live patients. Using colour projectors, these programs and other multimedia-style presentations can be made to audiences at formal lectures.

Summary

Maintaining a large computer system requires knowledgable professionals on site to solve the myriad of day-to-day problems.[3,61] In the past, computer systems have been written by members of an institution to meet their own specific needs.[2,3,17,62–67] It is likely that more complex systems, such as the one outlined in this chapter, will require teams of computer programmers and biomedical engineers to develop and maintain, and will become the domain of private enterprise companies. The ultimate success of their systems, however, will depend upon the ease with which staff in intensive care can use the programs, and on the ability of the systems both to decrease staff workload and to improve patient care.

References

1. Bradshaw KE, Sittig DF, Gardner RM, Pryor TA and Budd M (1989) Computer-based data entry for nurses in the ICU. *MD Computing* **6**:274–280.
2. Friesdorf W, Gross-Alltag F, Konichezky S, Schwilk B, Fatroth A and Fett P (1994) Lessons learned while building an integrated ICU workstation. *Int J Clin Monit Comput* **11**:89–97.
3. Avila LS and Shabot MM (1988) Keys to the successful implementation of an ICU patient data management system. *Int J Clin Monit Comput* **5**:15–25.
4. Kennelly RJ and Wittenber J (1994) New IEEE standard enables data collection for medical applications. *Proc Annu Symp Comput Appl Med Care*, 531–535.
5. Shabot MM (1989) Standardised acquisition of bedside data: the IEEE p1073 medical information bus. *Int J Monit Comput* **6**:197–204.
6. Cole WG and Stewart JG (1993) Metaphor graphics to support integrated decision making with respiratory data. *Int J Clin Monit Comput* **10**:91–100.
7. Mrochen H, Hieronymi U and Meyer M (1991) Physiological profiles and therapeutic goals – graphical aids support quick orientation in intensive care. *Int J Clin Monit Comput* **8**:207–212.
8. Hekking M, Gelsema ES and Lindemans J (1994) A new representation of acid–base disturbances. *Int J Biomed Comput* **36**:209–221.
9. Dasta JF (1990) Computers in critical care: opportunities and challenges. *DICP* **24**:1084–1092.
10. Bellon E, Feron M, Marchal G *et al.* (1994) Design for user efficiency in a dedicated ICU viewing station. *Med Informatics* **19**:161–170.
11. Gostin LO, Turek-Brezina J, Powers M, Kozloff R, Faden R and Steinauer DD (1993) Privacy and security of personal information in a new health care system. *J Am Med Assoc* **270**:2487–2493.
12. Clemmer TP and Gardner RM (1992) Medical informatics in the intensive care unit: state of the art 1991. *Int J Clin Monit Comput* **8**:237–250.
13. Smith JP (1995) Authentication of digital medical images with digital signature technology. *Radiology* **194**:771–774.
14. Bleumer G (1994) Security for decentralized health information systems. *Int J Biomed Comput* **35** (suppl): 139–145.
15. Oh TE and Cameron P (1982) Bedside computer programs in the intensive care unit. *Anaesth Intens Care* **10**:217–222.
16. Klingstedt C, Ludwigs U, Baehrendtz S, Bokliden A and Matell G (1989) A microcomputer system for on-line monitoring of pulmonary function during artificial ventilation. *Int J Clin Monit Comput* **6**:99–107.
17. Salasidis R, Padjen AL and Fleiszer D (1991) Patient management in the ICU: the PDB system. *Proc Annu Symp Comput Appl Med Care*, 990–992.
18. Shabot MM, LoBue M, Leyerle BJ and Dubin SB (1990) Decision support alerts for clinical laboratory and blood gas data. *Int J Clin Monit Comput* **7**:27–31.
19. Lawless ST (1994) Crying wolf: false alarms in a pediatric intensive care unit. *Crit Care Med* **22**:981–985.
20. O'Carroll TM (1986) Survey of alarms in an intensive therapy unit. *Anaesthesia* **41**:742–744.
21. Alcover IA, Henning RJ and Jackson DL (1984) A computer-assisted monitoring system for arrhythmia detection in a medical intensive care unit. *Crit Care Med* **12**:888–891.
22. Oyama T, Ishihara H, Tanioka F, Matsuki A, Aida N and Ishii H (1987) Clinical application of arrhythmia analyzer in ICU. *Int J Clin Monit Comput* **4**:99–104.
23. Farrell RM, Orr JA, Kück K and Westenskow DR (1992) Differential features for a neural network bases anesthesia alarm system. *Biomed Sci Instrument* **28**:99–104.
24. Endresen J and Hill DW (1977) The present state of trend detection and prediction in patient monitoring. *Intensive Care Med* **3**:15–26.

25. Koski EM, Makivirta A, Sukuvaara T and Aarno K (1992) Development of an expert system for haemodynamic monitoring: computerized symbolization of on-line monitoring data. *Int J Clin Monit Comput* **8**:289–293.

26. Sukuvaara T, Koski EMJ, Makivirta A and Kari A (1993) A knowledge-based alarm system for monitoring cardiac operated patients – technical construction and evaluation. *Int J Clin Monit Comput* **10**:117–126.

27. Benis AM, Fitzkee HL, Jurado RA and Litwak RS (1980) Improved detection of adverse cardiovascular trends with the use of a two-variable computer alarm. *Crit Care Med* **8**:341–344.

28. Brunner JX, Westenskow DR and Zelenkov P. (1989) Prototype ventilator and alarm algorithm for the NASA space station. *J Clin Monit* **5**:90–99.

29. Henderson S, Crapo RO, Wallace CJ, East TD, Morris AH and Gardner RM (1992) Performance of computerized protocols for the management of arterial oxygenation in an intensive care unit. *Int J Clin Monit Comput* **8**:271–280.

30. Burridge PW, Skakun EN and King EG (1985) Evaluation of a computer-based clinical reference library in an ICU. *Crit Care Med* **13**:763–766.

31. Schwaiger J, Haller M and Finsterer U (1992) A framework for the knowledge-based interpretation of laboratory data in intensive care units using deductive database technology. *Proc Annu Symp Comput Appl Med Care*, 13–17.

32. Tong DA (1991) Weaning patients from mechanical ventilation. A knowledge-based system approach. *Comput Methods Programs Biomed* **35**:267–278.

33. Gill H, Ludwigs U, Matell G *et al.* (1990) Integrating knowledge-based technology into computer aided ventilation systems. *Int J Clin Monit Comput* **7**:1–6.

34. Groth T and Collinson PO (1993) Strategies for decision support for fluid and electrolyte therapy in the intensive care unit – approaches and problems. *Int J Clin Monit Comput* **10**:3–15.

35. Buchman TG (1995) Computers in the intensive care unit: promises yet to be fulfilled. *J Intensive Care Med* **10**:234–240.

36. Lampard DG, Coles JR and Brown WA (1973) Electronic digital computer control of ventilation and anaesthesia. *Anaesth Intensive Care* **1**:382–392.

37. Laubscher TP, Frutiger A, Fanconi S, Jutzi H and Bruner JX (1994) Automatic selection of tidal volume, respiratory frequency and minute ventilation in intubated ICU patients as start up procedure for closed loop controlled ventilation. *Int J Clin Monit Comput* **11**:19–30.

38. Dojat M, Brochard L, Lemaire F and Harf A (1992) A knowledge-based system for assisted ventilation of patients in intensive care units. *Int J Clin Monit Comput* **9**:239–250.

39. Blankenship HB, Wallace FD and Pacifico AD (1990) Clinical application of closed-loop postoperative autotransfusion. *Med Prog Technol* **16**:89–93.

40. Isaka S and Sebald AV (1993) Control strategies for arterial blood pressure regulation. *IEEE Trans Biomed Eng* **40**:353–363.

41. Meline LJ, Westenskow DR, Somerville A, Wernick RT, Jacobs J and Pace NL (1986) Evaluation of two adaptive sodium nitroprusside control algorithms. *J Clin Monit* **2**:79–86.

42. Schwilden H and Stoeckel H (1990) Effective therapeutic infusions produced by closed-loop feedback control of methohexital administration during total intravenous anesthesia with fentanyl. *Anesthesiology* **73**:225–229.

43. Schwilden H, Stoeckel H and Schuttler J (1989) Closed-loop feedback control of propofol anaesthesia by quantitative EEG analysis in humans. *Br J Anaesth* **62**:290–296.

44. O'Hara DA, Bogen DK and Noordergraaf A (1992) The use of computers for controlling the delivery of anesthesia. *Anesthesiology* **77**:563–581.

45. Price DJ, Dugdale RE and Mason J (1980) The control of ICP using three asynchronous closed loops. In: Shulman K (ed.) *Intracranial Pressure IV.* Heidelberg: Springer-Verlag, pp. 395–399.

46. Freebairn RC, Derrick JL, Gomersall CD, Young RJ and Joynt GM (1996) Oxygen delivery, oxygen consumption and pHi following vecuronium closed loop infusion in severe sepsis and septic shock. *Crit Care Med* (in press).

47. Sladen R (1995) Neuromuscular blocking agents in the intensive care unit. A two edged sword. *Crit Care Med* **23**:423–428.

48. Svec JM, Coleman RW, Mungall DR and Ludden TM (1985) Bayesian pharmacokinetic/pharmacodynamic forecasting or prothrombin response to warfarin therapy: preliminary evaluation. *Ther Drug Monit* **7**:174–180.

49. Burton ME, Brater DC, Chen PS, Day RB, Huber PJ and Vasko MR (1985) A bayesian feedback method of aminoglycoside dosing. *Clin Pharmacol Ther* **37**:349–357.

50. Rodman JH, Jelliffe RW, Kolb E *et al.* (1984) Clinical studies with computer-assisted initial lidocaine therapy. *Arch Intern Med* **144**:703–709.

51. Garcia MJ, Gavira R, Santos Buelga D and Bomingue-Gil A (1994) Predictive performance of two phenytoin pharmacokinetic dosing programs from nonsteady state data. *Ther Drug Monit* **16**:380–387.

52. Ilett KF, Nation RL, Oh TE and Silbert B (1983) Pharmacokinetic optimisation of aminophylline infusion requirements in critically ill asthmatic patients. *Clin Exp Pharmacol Physiol* **10**:713–717.

53. Chang RWS, Lee B, Jacobs S and Lee B (1989) Accuracy of decisions to withdraw therapy in critically ill patients: clinical judgment versus a computer model. *Crit Care Med* **17**:1091–1097.

54. Oh TE, Hutchinson RC, Short S, Buckley TA, Lin ES and Leung D (1993) Verification and use of the acute physiology and chronic health evaluation scoring system in a Hong Kong intensive care unit. *Crit Care Med* **21**:698–705.

55. Buchman TG, Kubos KL, Seidler AJ and Siegforth MJ (1994) A comparison of statistical and connectionist models for the prediction of chronicity in a surgical intensive care unit. *Crit Care Med* **22**:750–762.

56. Doig GS, Inman KJ, Sibbald WJ, Martin CM and Robertson JM (1993) Modelling mortality in the intensive care unit: comparing the performance of a back-propagation, associative-learning neural network with multivariate logistic regression. *Proc Annu Symp Comput Appl Med Care*, 361–365.

57. Tu JV and Guerriere MRS (1993) Use of a neural network as a predictive instrument for length of stay in the intensive care unit following cardiac surgery. *Comp Biomed Res* **26**:220–229.

58. Weissman C, Mossel P, Haimert S and King TC (1990) Integration of quality assurance activities into a computerized patient data management system in an intensive care unit. *Quality Rev Bull* **16**:398–403.

59. Abenstein JP, DeVos CB, Tarhan A and Tarhan S (1992) Eight years' experience with automated anesthesia record keeping: lessons learned – new directions taken. *Int J Clin Monit Comput* **9**:117–129.

60. Hashimoto F, Bell S and Marshment S (1987) A computer simulation program to facilitate budgeting and staffing decisions in an intensive care unit. *Crit Care Med* **15**:256–259.

61. Sainsbury DA (1993) An object-orientated approach to data display and storage: 3 years' experience, 25 000 cases. *Int J Clin Monit Comput* **10**:225–233.

62. Pryor TA, Gardner RM, Clayton PD and Warner HR (1983) The HELP system. *J Med Syst* **7**:87–102.

63. Ross DG, Ramayya P and Kulkarni V (1990) ABICUS: Aberdeen intensive care unit system. *Int J Clin Monit Comput* **7**:69–81.

64. Siegel JH and Coleman B (1986) Computers in the care of the critically ill patient. *Urol Clin North Am* **13**:101–117.

65. Hohnloser JH and Purner F (1992) PADS (patient archiving and documentation system): a computerized patient record with educational aspects. *Int J Clin Monit Comput* **9**:71–84.

66. Clevert HD, Schober HJ and Weiss H (1991) INTENSIV – Construction and structure of the knowledge-based PC system for the intensive care unit. *Klin Wochenschr* **69**(suppl 26):234–240.

67. van der Lei J and Derksen-Samson JF (1987) Neontal ICU system: experiences with AIDA. *Computer Methods Programs Biomed* **25**:315–320.

Haemodynamic monitoring

CD Gomersall and TE Oh

The intensivist can only manipulate the cardiovascular system in the critically ill patient with fluids and drugs, if the performance of the system in adequately monitored. Haemodynamic measurements are important to establish a precise diagnosis, determine appropriate therapy and monitor the response to that therapy. The extent of monitoring depends on how much data is required to optimize the patient's condition, and how precisely the data is to be recorded. Monitoring may be categorized into non-invasive, invasive and derived (i.e. indices are calculated from primary measurements). Nevertheless, monitors are not a substitute for careful clinical examination, and the most important monitor are the nurse and clinician.

Non-invasive cardiovascular monitoring

Electrocardiogram (ECG)

A specific lead can be used to view a known ischaemic area on the 12-lead ECG. For routine use, the CM5 lead monitors the anterolateral aspects of the left ventricle (LV), and gives over 80% detection of LV ischaemia with few problems in diagnosing arrhythmias. The right arm (RA) lead is attached to the manubrium, left arm (LA) lead to V5 position, and left leg (LL) lead to its usual position, and monitoring is set to lead I. The MCL1 (modified chest lead) is useful in patient with rhythm disturbances, as atrial activity and conduction defects are easily seen. LA lead is sited at the left subclavian position, LL at V1 position and RA as ground; the monitor is set to lead III.

Blood pressure

Most automated non-invasive blood pressure (NIBP) devices use an oscillotonometric technique.

Consequently, the most accurate pressure determined is mean arterial pressure (MAP). These devices tend to overestimate at low pressure and underestimate at high pressure, but 95% confidence limits are ± 15 mmHg (2 kPa) over the normotensive range. They can also give erroneous results in patients with arrhythmias (e.g. atrial fibrillation). Cuff width is the most important determinant of measurement accuracy. Too narrow cuffs tend to overestimate pressure, and those which are too wide tend to underestimate. Cuff width should be 40% of the mid-circumference of the limb. Complications associated with NIBP devices include ulnar nerve injury (usually with the cuff placed too low on the upper arm), limb oedema, petechiae and bruising, friction blisters and problems with fluid infusions.

Urine output

Although an index of renal perfusion only, urine output is often used as a guide to adequacy of cardiac output, as the kidney receives 25% of cardiac output. When renal perfusion is adequate, urine output will exceed 0.5 ml/kg per h. The use of diuretics (e.g. frusemide or dopamine)[1] abolishes its usefulness as a haemodynamic monitor.

Thoracic electrical bioimpedence

This is a non-invasive method of estimating cardiac output. Unfortunately, there is considerable doubt as to its accuracy.[2,3] One recent study reported a mean relative error compared to thermodilution measurement of only 16.6%, but this was associated with a large standard deviation (12.9%), indicating gross inaccuracy in some patients.[4]

Echocardiography and Doppler

These techniques are discussed in Chapter 21.

Table 96.1 Assessment of the resonant frequency and damping coefficient of arterial pressure monitoring systems

Start paper trace to make a paper record of the output of the transducer

Snap or flick the valve of the continuous flush system or flick the tubing connecting the cannula to the transducer. This will produce an interference square wave on the output trace

Repeat the process at least twice

Resonant frequency is the distance between successive peaks divided by the paper speed in millimetres per second

Damping is satisfactory if each snap test has at least two oscillation waves and if the ratio of successive amplitudes is three or greater

Table 96.2 Complications of invasive arterial pressure monitoring

Ischaemia distal to cannula
    Major sequelae associated with low cardiac output, shock, sepsis, prolonged cannulation, vasculitis and hyperlipidaemia

Exsanguination
    Flows through 18 FG cannula can cause blood loss of 500 ml/min

Spurious result

Infection

Intra-arterial injection of drugs

Invasive cardiovascular monitoring

Arterial pressure

Direct intra-arterial measurement may overestimate systolic pressure due to systolic overshoot. This is a result of the physical properties of the fluid–pressure transducer monitoring system, and can be overcome by increasing the damping of the system (e.g. by using a smaller gauge cannula-transducer tubing). However, increasing damping reduces the resonant frequency, and thus the sensitivity of the system. The system should have a resonant frequency of >30 Hz for heart rates up to 180 beats/min, and >20 Hz for rates up to 120 beats/min, while retaining sufficient sensitivity. The tubing should be non-compliant and < 1 m in length. Table 96.1 outlines a method to assess resonant frequency and damping. MAP is accurately monitored even if the system does not meet the above criteria.

Derived variables

A number of variables can be derived from analysis of the arterial pressure waveform. A rough approximation of stroke volume, and therefore cardiac output, can be obtained from the area under the systolic arterial pressure curve. However, correlation with cardiac output assessed by thermodilution is poor, and the method is not sufficiently reliable for clinical decision-making.[5]

Systolic time intervals are an indirect index of ventricular contractility. The pre-ejection period (PEP) is the interval from the onset of ventricular electrical activity (Q wave) to the ejection of blood from the ventricle. It consists of the electromechanical delay between the action potential and initiation of ventricular contraction, and the isovolumic contraction time. PEP is inversely proportional to ventricular contractility.

The arterial pressure trace can also be used to indicate adequacy of preload. In mechanically ventilated patients, positive intrathoracic pressure increases LV output (and systolic pressure) early in inspiration, which is followed a few heart beats later by a decrease. This variation in arterial pressure is exaggerated in the presence of reduced preload, and a significant correlation has been demonstrated between the systolic arterial pressure variations and end-diastolic area estimated with transoesophageal echocardiography[6]

Complications associated with invasive arterial pressure monitoring are listed in Table 96.2. The morbidity associated with arterial cannulation is less than that associated with five or more arterial punctures.

Central venous pressure (CVP)

CVP can be monitored using catheters inserted via the internal jugular, subclavian and femoral veins. Correct placement should be confirmed by observing pressure change with respiration, aspirating blood freely through the catheter, and a chest X-ray. Inferior vena cava pressure can be used as a guide to CVP in mechanically ventilated patients, provided that the tip of the catheter is close to the diaphragm.[7]

CVP is used as a guide to right ventricular filling. However, right ventricular preload is determined by end-diastolic volume (not pressure) and hence, an isolated CVP reading is of limited value without knowledge of ventricular compliance. Compliance varies from patient to patient, and with time in the same patient. Thus, dynamic changes in CVP are more useful than absolute values. If the CVP rises <3 mmHg (0.4 kPa) in response to a fluid challenge (e.g. 50–200 ml of colloid over 10 min), more volume loading may be required. If the CVP rises >7 mmHg (0.9 kPa), fluid loading is then probably maximal. However, should the CVP return to within 3 mmHg (0.4 kPa) of its original

Table 96.3 Analysis of central venous pressure waveform

Condition	Pressure changes	Waveform changes
Tricuspid regurgitation	Increased RA pressure	Prominent v wave, x descent obliterated, y descent steep
Right ventricular infarction	RA and RV pressures elevated. RAP does not fall and may rise in inspiration	Prominent x and y descents
Constrictive pericarditis	RA, RV diastolic, PA diastolic and occlusion pressures elevated and equalized. RAP may rise in inspiration	Prominent x and y descents
Pericardial tamponade	RA, RV diastolic, PA diastolic and occlusion pressures elevated and equalized. RAP usually falls in inspiration	y descent damped or absent

RA = Right atrial: RV = right ventricular: RAP = right atrial pressure: PA = pulmonary artery.

value within 10 min, the risk of pulmonary oedema is only moderate; nevertheless no further filling is required. In most patients, adequate right ventricular (RV) filling equates with adequate LV filling. This may not be so in lung disease with pulmonary hypertension, or in impaired RV func-

Table 96.4 Complications associated with central venous pressure monitoring

Associated with insertion
Pneumothorax/haemothorax
Arterial puncture
Air embolism
Arrhythmias (especially with Seldinger method)
Nerve injury (e.g. Horner's syndrome)
Mediastinal/pleural effusion
Chylothorax (left internal jugular/subclavian puncture)

Associated with use
Sepsis
Disconnection, leading to bleeding or air embolus
Pleural or pericardial effusion due to use of misplaced catheter

tion (e.g. severe sepsis and some patients with inferior myocardial infarction). Analysis of the CVP waveform may yield further information (Table 96.3). Complications associated with CVP monitoring are listed in Table 96.4.

Pulmonary artery catheter[8,9]

Although use of the pulmonary artery (PA) catheter has become common in the ICU, there is no conclusive evidence that it leads to decreased mortality.[10] However, in a substantial proportion of patients, it provides unexpected haemodynamic information, leading to a change in therapy.[11] The waveforms seen as the catheter passes through the heart and PA to the wedged position are shown in Figure 96.1. Normal pressures are given in Table 96.5.

Indications for a PA catheter are:

1 volume assessment and fluid management in impaired RV or LV function, or pulmonary hypertension;

Table 96.5 Pressures measured by a pulmonary artery catheter

Site	Pressure	
	mmHg	(kPa)
Right atrium: mean	–1–7	(0.13–0.93)
Right ventricle: systolic	15–25	(2.0–3.3)
Right ventricle: diastolic	0–8	(0–1.1)
Pulmonary artery: systolic	15–25	(2.0–3.3)
Pulmonary artery: diastolic	8–15	(1.1–2.0)
Pulmonary artery: mean	10–20	(1.3–2.6)
Pulmonary artery capillary wedge	6–15	(0.8–2.0)

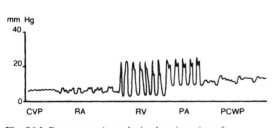

Fig. 96.1 Pressure tracings obtained on insertion of a pulmonary artery catheter. CVP = Central venous pressure; RA = right atrium; RV = right ventricle; PA = pulmonary artery; PCWP = pulmonary capillary wedge pressure.

Table 96.6 Pulmonary artery capillary wedge pressure as a poor reflection of left ventricular end-diastolic pressure – possible causes

Position of catheter tip outside West's zone III
Pulmonary venous obstruction
   Atrial myxoma
   Pulmonary fibrosis
   Vasculitis

Valvular heart disease
   Mitral stenosis (LAP > LVEDP)
   Mitral regurgitation (LAP > LVEDP)
   Aortic regurgitation and premature closure of aortic valve
   (LAP < LVEDP)

Markedly reduced pulmonary vascular bed
   Pneumonectomy
   Large pulmonary embolus

LAP = Left atrial pressure; LVEDP = left ventricular end-diastolic pressure.

2 cardiac output measurement;
3 mixed venous saturation measurement;
4 diagnosis of ventricular septal defect.

The PA catheter allows measurement of a number of pressures, including pulmonary artery capillary wedge pressure (PCWP), pulmonary artery pressure (PAP) and right atrial pressure (RAP).

Pulmonary artery occlusion pressure

PCWP approximates to LA pressure (LAP), which approximates to left ventricular end-diastolic pressure (LVEDP). It is thus related to left ventricular end-diastolic *volume* (LVEDV) in the same way CVP is related to right ventricular end-diastolic volume. Hence, PCWP may not reflect LVEDP in a number of conditions (Table 96.6). Pulmonary artery diastolic pressure (PADP) is closely related to PCWP except when the patient has pulmonary hypertension or is tachycardic. When heart rate exceeds 120 beats/min, there is insufficient time during diastole for venous run-off, so PADP may be spuriously high.

To obtain valid readings, the catheter tip must be in West's zone III portion of the lung (i.e. PAP > LAP > alveolar pressure; flow is independent of alveolar pressure). In mechanically ventilated patients, alveolar pressure is raised, and the boundary between zone III and zone II (i.e. PAP > alveolar pressure > LAP) will shift. This, similarly, occurs with lung disease. Hence, catheter-tip position on chest X-ray (i.e. anatomical position) may not reliably confirm siting within zone III. However, the following characteristics suggest that the tip is outside zone III:

1 PCWP tracing is smooth-looking.
2 PA diastolic pressure < PCWP.
3 PCWP increases >50% of change in alveolar pressure.
4 PCWP decreases >50% of a reduction in positive end-expiratory pressure (PEEP).

Blood should be easily aspirated from the tip with the catheter wedged, and should be arterialized. In patients with a markedly reduced vascular bed, wedging the balloon may reduce venous return sufficiently to underestimate both LAP and LVEDP.

LVEDV is determined by LV compliance and the transmural pressure. The latter can be obtained by LVEDP minus the pressure surrounding the heart (which approximates to intrapleural pressure). Intrapleural pressure is closest to zero at end-expiration; thus LVEDP is closest to transmural pressure at end-expiration.

As with CVP, analysis of the PCWP waveform may give some indication of cardiac pathology. Constrictive pericarditis and pericardial tamponade show the same abnormalities (but less clearly) as in the CVP trace. Mitral regurgitation may cause a large v wave, which may be confused with the PA waveform. The two can be distinguished by examining the timing of the waves relative to the T wave of the ECG. The peak of the PA systolic wave occurs within and the v wave occurs after the T wave. Large v waves may also be associated with mitral stenosis, congestive heart failure or ventricular septal defect.

Thermodilution cardiac output measurement

Injection of cold injectate into the right atrium causes a decrease in blood temperature monitored in the pulmonary artery. This decrease in temperature is inversely proportional to the extent of dilution of the injectate; the latter is directly related to cardiac output at time of injection. Cardiac output can thus be derived using the principle of indicator dilution. The decrease in blood temperature also depends on the injectate temperature and volume. The relationship of these factors to cardiac output is given by the Stewart–Hamilton equation:

$$Q = \frac{V(T_B - T_I) \, K_1 K_2}{T_B(t)dt}$$

where Q = cardiac output, V = volume injected, T_B = blood temperature, T_I = injectate temperature, K_1 and K_2 = computational constants and $T_B(t)dt$ = change in blood temperature as a function of time.

A colder injectate has a greater signal-to-noise ratio and better accuracy and precision. However, in most clinical situations 10 ml of injectate at room temperature provides an acceptable measurement. Smaller

Table 96.7 Causes of inaccuracy in thermodilution cardiac output measurements

Thermistor impinged on vessel wall, insulating it from cool injectate – suggested by unacceptable cardiac output curves or inadequate PA pressure tracings

Abnormal respiratory pattern

Intracardiac shunts

Tricuspid regurgitation

Cardiac arrhythmias which cause beat-to-beat variation in stroke volume

Injectate warmer than temperature recorded by computer (e.g. temperature recorded is that of ice bath, but injectate fluid has not cooled to that temperature; injectate is warmed by higher temperature of syringe or operator's hand)

Fluid being infused through side-arm of percutaneous sheath

Proximal injectate port lies within sheath

PA = Pulmonary artery.

injectate volumes can be used with acceptable results when volume overload is a concern. Careful filling of syringes is necessary to avoid errors from varying injectate volumes. Respiration affects cardiac output and PA temperature; measurements should ideally be made in the same phase of respiration. This is difficult, and in practice, an average of three evenly spaced measurements gives an accurate estimation of cardiac output. Causes of inaccuracy in measurements are listed in Table 96.7.[12] Cardiac index is derived using body surface area obtained from nomograms of height and weight.

Derived variables

A number of haemodynamic variables can be calculated from the measurements obtained with a PA

catheter (Table 96.8). Systemic vascular resistance index (SVRI) is used as a measure of LV afterload. Left ventricular stroke work index (LVSWI) can be used as a direct estimate of contractility, if preload remains constant (since a change in preload can increase LV stroke work without increasing contractility).

Mixed venous oxygen saturation (Svo_2)

This has been used as a measure of adequacy of tissue perfusion. Svo_2 varies directly with cardiac output, haemoglobin and Sao_2, and inversely with metabolic rate. Normal Svo_2 is 75% but decreases when oxygen delivery falls or tissue oxygen demand increases. When it decreases as low as 30%, oxygen delivery is insufficient to meet tissue oxygen demand, with potential anaerobic metabolism and lactic acidosis. Situations with increased Svo_2 are more difficult to interpret; sepsis, arteriovenous fistulae, cirrhosis, left-to-right cardiac shunts, cyanide poisoning, hypothermia and unintentional PA catheter wedging have all been reported as being associated with increased values. Increased Svo_2 reflects a failure of cells to take up and utilize oxygen. None the less, Svo_2 cannot be used in isolation to monitor tissue perfusion in sepsis due to varied factors. For example, a normal value may actually reflect a combination of low cardiac output and arteriovenous shunting. Svo_2 can be measured either continuously using a fibreoptic PA catheter, or from intermittent blood sampling from the distal lumen of the PA catheter. A co-oximeter is necessary, as calculated saturations produced by blood-gas machines are not accurate in the lower Svo_2 range.

Right ventricular ejection fraction pulmonary artery catheter

This utilizes a PA catheter with a rapid-response thermistor and an injection port that is designed to ensure uniform mixing of the iced injectate in the right atrium. The mean residual fraction (MRF) is

Table 96.8 Derived haemodynamic variables

Parameter	Formula	Normal range	Units
Stroke volume index (SVI)	CI/HR	35–70	ml/beat per m^2
Systemic vascular resistance index	(MAP–CVP)/CI × 79.92	1760–2600	dyn s/cm^5 per m^2
Pulmonary vascular resistance index	(PAP–PAOP)/CI × 79.92	44–225	dyn s/cm^5 per m^2
Left ventricular stroke work index	SVI × MAP × 0.0144	44–68	g m/m^2 per beat
Right ventricular stroke work index	SVI × PAP × 0.0144	4–8	g m/m^2 per beat
Oxygen delivery	CI × Cao_2 × 10	520–720	ml/min per m^2
Oxygen consumption	CI × (Cao_2 – Cvo_2) × 10	100–180	ml/min per m^2

CI = Cardiac index; HR = heart rate; MAP = mean arterial pressure; CVP = central venous pressure; PAP = pulmonary artery pressure; PAOP = pulmonary artery occlusion pressure; Cao_2 = arterial oxygen content; Cvo_2 = mixed venous oxygen content.

calculated over time by dividing the temperature change by the ECG R–R interval. The ejection fraction (RVEF) = 1 – MRF. End-diastolic volume can then be calculated from the stroke volume (cardiac output/heart rate) divided by RVEF. Reasonable estimates of RVEF can be obtained provided that there is no valve regurgitation or arrhythmias.[7]

Continuous thermodilution cardiac output

This uses infusion of heat from a filament in the right atrium rather than an injection of cold saline, and stochastic system identification to enhance the signal-to-noise ratio. The monitor gives the average cardiac output over the previous 3–6 min, updated every 30 s. Results appear to agree well with those obtained by bolus thermodilution.[13,14]

Pulmonary capillary pressure (PCP)

PCP is the major determinant in the formation of pulmonary oedema. It can be calculated in patients with normal lungs from the sum of PCWP and 40% of the difference between mean PAP and PCWP. This assumes that the ratio of pulmonary venous resistance to total pulmonary vascular resistance is 0.4, but may not be the case in patients with lung disease or injury.[15] When the PA catheter is occluded, the pressure distal to the balloon decreases from PAP to PCWP. The decrease is characterized by a fast, followed by a slow phase. The fast phase results from the cessation of PA blood flow distal to the occlusion, while the second phase results from the release of blood stored in the pulmonary capacitance vessels. The level to which the pressure decreases purely from cessation of PAP flow is PCP. Thus PCP can be calculated by extrapolating the slow phase back to the time of occlusion. This, however, requires knowledge of the precise time of occlusion. By using a double-port PA catheter (with a port at the tip and another 1 cm behind), the precise time of occlusion can be determined, i.e. the time when the two PAP curves abruptly diverge.[16]

Complications of PA catheters

Complications associated with PA catheters are listed in Table 96.9.[17] A catheter may not actually be knotted, despite a chest X-ray appearance to suggest this. Other catheters should be removed in reverse order in which they were inserted, and the chest X-ray repeated. If a true knot exists, an attempt is made to pull the knot into the introducer sheath, whereupon the sheath and catheter are removed. If a sheath is not present, the catheter is pulled as far back as possible, and a cut-down to vein under local anaesthesia is undertaken. When these attempts are unsuccessful (only 0.5%), exploration by a vascular surgeon is indicated.

Table 96.9 Complications associated with pulmonary artery (PA) catheters

Complications of central venous catheterization (see Table 96.4)
Complications of catheter insertion
Arrhythmias
Knotting/kinking
Valve damage
Perforation of pulmonary artery
Right bundle branch block
Complete heart block

Complications of catheter in PA
Thrombosis
PA rupture (may be difficult to diagnose)
Sepsis
Endocarditis
Pulmonary infarction
Arrhythmias
Air embolus (due to repeated attempts to fill ruptured balloon)

Risk factors for major morbidity (with PA rupture being the most important)
Pulmonary hypertension
Anticoagulation
In situ duration > 3 days

Fick principle

Application of the Fick principle to oxygen uptake in the lungs can be used to measure cardiac output. This method has traditionally been considered to be the 'gold standard' of cardiac output measurement. However, the preconditions for accurate measurement using the oxygen Fick method are not met in most ICU patients.[18] Use of modified CO_2 Fick methods results in greater agreement with thermodilution measurements.[19] A non-invasive CO_2 method is reported to be reliable in certain groups of patients.[20]

Transpulmonary indicator dilution

The principle of injecting an indicator into the right atrium, with measurement of its subsequently diluted concentration at the radial or femoral artery, was previously used to estimate cardiac output. A new system using this method is currently being studied to measure cardiac output, intrathoracic and total blood volume, and extravascular lung water.[21,22] The sensor can be combined with an intra-arterial catheter for blood pressure monitoring. Although it has a number of potential advantages, especially in children, the system had not been validated.

Regional blood flow

Gastric tonometry

Splanchnic perfusion is particularly sensitive to decreases in global oxygen delivery,[23,24] and the mucosal layer of the gut is particularly susceptible to ischaemia because of a countercurrent mechanism in the villi.[25] Therefore, monitoring gastric intramucosal pH may detect covert ischaemia. A semipermeable balloon filled with saline is passed into the stomach. CO_2 but not H^+ passes across the balloon membrane into saline. After an equilibration period, the saline is aspirated and the Pco_2 measured. An arterial blood sample is simultaneously taken to obtain calculated arterial bicarbonate. The values obtained are substituted into a modified Henderson–Hasselbalch equation, and a value for intramucosal pH is derived. There are, however, some theoretical shortcomings with gastric tonometry. The arterial bicarbonate may not be the same as intramucosal bicarbonate, particularly in the hypoperfused patient. Gastric intraluminal Pco_2 may not reflect intramucosal Pco_2, particularly with reflux of bicarbonate from the duodenum. The gut may not be hypoperfused in certain shock states (e.g. septic shock), and there are no villi in the stomach. Although low intramucosal pH values have been associated with a worse prognosis,[26] and therapy based on intramucosal pH has been shown to improve prognosis in certain patients,[27] more convincing studies on the benefits of gastric tonometry monitoring are required.

Jugular bulb oxygen saturation (Sjo₂)

Sjo_2 monitoring has been proposed as a method of identifying patients with mismatched cerebral oxygen metabolic rate ($CMRO_2$) and cerebral blood flow (CBF),[28] and has become widely used in neurosurgical intensive care.[29,30] Its use is based on the Fick principle, according to which the cerebral arterial–mixed venous oxygen difference ($AVDO_2$) is related to $CMRO_2$ and CBF in the following way:

$$AVDO_2 = CMRO_2/CBF$$

Assuming that arterial saturation, haemoglobin concentration and the affinity of haemoglobin for oxygen remain constant, the ratio of $CMRO_2/CBF$ is proportional to the cerebral mixed venous oxygen saturation. Sjo_2 is assumed to be equivalent to cerebral mixed venous oxygen saturation.

Sjo_2 monitoring has two major limitations. First, it reflects the adequacy of global cerebral oxygen delivery, and gives no indication of adequacy of regional cerebral oxygen delivery. Thus, a normal Sjo_2 is compatible with critical ischaemia in some parts of the brain and simultaneous luxury perfusion in others. Second, the results become difficult to interpret when increased oxy-

gen extraction can no longer compensate for reductions in oxygen delivery. In this situation, $CMRO_2$ falls and thus the Sjo_2 remains unchanged despite a fall in cerebral oxygen delivery.[31] Hence the role of Sjo_2 monitoring requires further evaluation.

References

1. Duke GJ, Briedis JH and Weaver RA (1994) Renal support in critically ill patients: low-dose dopamine or low-dose dobutamine? *Crit Care Med* **22**:1919–1925.
2. Clarke DE and Raffin TA (1993) Thoracic electrical bioimpedance measurement of cardiac output – not ready for prime time. *Crit Care Med* **21**:1111–1112.
3. Sageman WS and Amundsen DE (1993) Thoracic electrical bioimpedance measurement of cardiac output in post-aortocoronary bypass patients. *Crit Care Med* **21**:1139–1142.
4. Shoemaker WC, Wo CCJ, Bishop MH *et al.* (1994) Multicenter trial of a new thoracic electrical bioimpedance device for cardiac output estimation. *Crit Care Med* **22**:1907–1912.
5. Gratz I, Kraidin J and Afshar M (1993) Continuous cardiac output by pulse waveform. *Int Anesthesiol Clin* **31**:87–98.
6. Coriat P, Vrillon M, Perel A *et al.* (1994) A comparison of systolic blood pressure variations and echocardiographic estimates of end-diastolic left ventricular size in patients after aortic surgery. *Anesth Analg* **78**:46–53.
7. Joynt GM, Gomersall CD, Buckley TA *et al.* (1996) Comparison of intrathoracic and intra-abdominal measurements of central venous pressure. *Lancet* **347**:1155–1157.
8. Vender JS (1993) Clinical utilization of pulmonary artery catheter monitoring. *Int Anesthesiol Clin* **31**:57–85.
9. European Society of Intensive Care Medicine expert panel (1991) The use of the pulmonary artery catheter. *Intensive Care Med* **17**:I–VIII.
10. Eidelman LA, Pizov R and Sprung CL (1994) Pulmonary artery catheterization – at the crossroads? *Crit Care Med* **22**:543–545.
11. Mimoz O, Rauss A, Rekik N, Brun-Buisson C, Lemaire F and Brochard L (1994) Pulmonary artery catherization in critically ill patients: a prospective analysis of outcome changes associated with catheter-prompted changes in therapy. *Crit Care Med* **22**:573–579.
12. Boyd O, Mackay J, Newman P, Bennett ED and Grounds RM (1994) Effects of insertion depth and use of the sidearm of the introducer sheath of pulmonary artery catheters in cardiac output measurement. *Crit Care Med* **22**:1132–1135.
13. Boldt J, Menges T, Wollbrück M, Hammermann H and Hempelmann G (1994) Is continuous cardiac output measurement using thermodilution reliable in the critically ill patient? *Crit Care Med* **22**:1913–1918.
14. Yelderman ML, Ramsay MA, Quinn MD *et al.* (1992) Continuous thermodilution cardiac output measurement in ICU patients. *J Cardiothorac Vasc Anesth* **6**:270–274.

15. Collee CG, Lynch KE, Hill RD and Zapol WM (1987) Bedside measurement of pulmonary capillary pressure in patients with acute respiratory failure. *Anesthesiology* **66**:614–620.

16. Yamada Y, Komatsu K, Suzukawa M *et al.* (1993) Pulmonary capillary pressure measured with a pulmonary artery double-port catheter in surgical patients. *Anesth Analg* **77**:1130–1134.

17. Shah KB, Rao TK, Laughlin S *et al.* (1984) A review of pulmonary artery catheterization in 6245 patients. *Anesthesiology* **61**:271–275.

18. Taylor SH (1966) Measurement of the cardiac output in man. *Proc R Soc* **59**(suppl):35–53.

19. Mahutte CK, Jaffe MB, Chen PA, Sasse SA, Wong DH and Sassoon CSH (1994) Oxygen Fick and modified carbon dioxide Fick cardiac outputs. *Crit Care Med* **22**:86–95.

20. Neviere R, Mathieu D, Riou Y *et al.* (1994) Carbon dioxide rebreathing method of cardiac output measurement during acute respiratory failure in patients with chronic obstructive pulmonary disease. *Crit Care Med* **22**:81–85.

21. Hoeft A (1995) Transpulmonary indicator dilution: an alternative approach for hemodynamic monitoring. In: Vincent J-L (ed.) *Yearbook of Intensive Care and Emergency Medicine 1995*. Berlin: Springer Verlag, pp. 593–605.

22. Murdoch IA, Marsh MJ and Morrison G (1995) Measurement of cardiac output in children. In: Vincent J-L (ed.) *Yearbook of Intensive Care and Emergency Medicine 1995*. Berlin: Springer Verlag, pp. 606–614.

23. Lundgren O (1989) Physiology of the intestinal circulation. In: Marston A, Bulkley GB, Fiddian-Green RG and Haglund UH (eds) *Splanchnic Ischaemia and Multiple Organ Failure*. London: Edward Arnold, pp. 29–40.

24. Lundgren O and Haglund U (1978) The pathophysiology of the intestinal countercurrent exchanger. *Life Sci* **23**:1411–1422.

25. Fink MP, Fiallo V, Stein KL *et al.* (1987) Systemic and regional haemodynamic changes after intraperitoneal endotoxin in rabbits. Development of a new model of the clinical syndrome of hyperdynamic sepsis. *Circ Shock* **22**:73–81.

26. Doglio GR, Pusajo JF, Egurrola MA *et al.* (1991) Gastric intramucosal pH as a prognostic index of mortality in critically ill patients. *Cric Care Med* **19**:1037–1040.

27. Gutierrez G, Palizas F, Doglio G *et al.* (1992) Gastric intramucosal pH as a therapeutic index of tissue oxygenation in critically ill patients. *Lancet* **339**:195–199.

28. Dearden NM (1991) Jugular bulb venous oxygen saturation in the management of severe head injury. *Curr Opin Anaesth* **4**:279–286.

29. Sheinberg M, Kanter MJ, Robertson CS, Contant CF, Narayan RK and Grossman RG (1992) Continuous monitoring of jugular venous oxygen saturation in head-injured patients. *J Neurosurg* **76**:212–217.

30. Chan KH, Dearden NM, Miller JD, Andrews PJD and Midgley S (1993) Multimodality monitoring as a guide to treatment of intracranial hypertension after severe brain injury. *Neurosurgery* **32**:547–552.

31. Brown RW (1993) Continuous monitoring of cerebral haemoglobin oxygen saturation. *Int Anesthesiol Clin* **31**:141–158.

DR Hillman

The importance of respiratory function testing in the ICU is to identify and assess the severity of respiratory disease, and to monitor changes with time and treatment. Clinical history, examination, chest X-ray, arterial blood gases, and simple bedside tests, such as spirometry and measurement of maximum mouth pressures, usually provide sufficient data to manage the acute illness. However, more sophisticated tests allow very accurate definition of pulmonary functional impairment, thus providing a more complete assessment.

As many respiratory function tests require patient cooperation, assessment of critically ill patients is limited to those that can be adapted and/or are independent of patient cooperation (e.g. analysis of arterial blood or respired gas). This chapter presents commonly used tests, emphasizing their use in the critically ill where appropriate.

Lung volume and capacities (Fig. 97.1)

Tidal volume (V_T) is the volume of gas that moves into and out of the lungs with each breath. The volume of gas in the lungs at maximum inspiration is total lung capacity (TLC) and at maximum expiration is residual volume (RV). Vital capacity (VC) is the volume of gas between TLC and RV. Functional residual capacity (FRC) is the volume of gas in the lungs after a normal expiration. Inspiratory capacity (IC) is the volume of gas between TLC and FRC. Inspiratory reserve volume (IRV) is the volume of gas between TLC and normal end-inspiration. Expiratory reserve volume (ERV) is the volume of gas between FRC and RV.

Methods of measurement

Vital capacity and subdivisions

These volumes may be measured by spirometers, either wet or dry (e.g. wedge spirometer), elec-

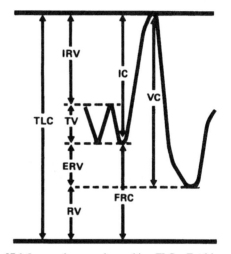

Fig. 97.1 Lung volumes and capacities. TLC = Total lung capacity; IRV = inspiratory reserve volume; TV = tidal volume; ERV = expiratory reserve volume; RV = residual volume; IC = inspiratory capacity; FRC = functional residual capacity; VC = vital capacity.

tronic flowmeters, where volume is derived by integration of the flow signal (see the section on ventilatory capacity, below) or the Wright respirometer[1] – a convenient but less accurate instrument which incorporates a flow-directed turbine, the revolutions of which are recorded on a dial via a series of gears (volume being inferred from flow).

Residual volume

RV is not part of respired volume, and cannot be measured by the above methods. It may be measured by gas dilution techniques[2,3] or body plethysmography.[4,5]

Table 97.1 Diseases which decrease vital capacity

Diseases of:
    Chest wall
    Respiratory muscles
    Nerve supply to above
    Pleura
    Lung parenchyma

Effusions
    Pleural
    Haemothorax
    Pneumothorax

Pulmonary congestion, fibrosis

Loss of lung tissue (e.g. lung resection)

Replacement of lung tissue (e.g. space-occupying lesions)

Premature airways closure (e.g. chronic obstructive airways disease)

Abdominal distension

Interpretation

At TLC, the expanding force exerted by the inspiratory muscles is exactly balanced by the elastic forces of the lung and chest wall, acting to recoil the respiratory system to a smaller volume. At RV, the force exerted by the expiratory muscles is exactly balanced by the opposing outward recoil of the chest wall and high flow resistance of the narrowed airways. Hence VC is determined by the power of the respiratory muscles, elastic properties of the chest wall and lung parenchyma, size and patency of the airways at low lung volumes, and size of the lung which varies with sex and body size. It is decreased in many diseases of the lung, chest wall and airways (Table 97.1).

Conditions diminishing VC may also diminish V_T if sufficiently severe. In the presence of adequate ventilatory drive, a decrease in V_T may be compensated for by an increase in respiratory rate. However if V_T is sufficiently small relative to dead space, pulmonary gas exchange will be adversely affected.

Serial measurements of VC and V_T are helpful in assessing the progress of patients with borderline respiratory function. In general, a V_T less than 5 ml/kg body weight and VC less than 15 ml/kg indicates a probable need for mechanical ventilatory support.

Lung elastic recoil is the major determinant of TLC, if gross respiratory muscle weakness is absent. Where decreased (e.g. in emphysema), TLC is increased; where increased (e.g. in pulmonary fibrosis), TLC is decreased. Similarly, decreased lung elastic recoil is associated with increased RV, and vice versa. Airways narrowing, whether due to loss of elastic support (e.g. emphysema) or to intrinsic disease of airways (e.g. asthma), is associated with an increased RV.

FRC is decreased in obesity, abdominal distension and in the presence of painful thoracic or abdominal wounds. If FRC is decreased to below closing volume (see below), significant intrapulmonary shunting will occur during quiet breathing.[6]

Ventilatory capacity

Ventilatory capacity is the maximal ability to move gas into and out of the lungs, and is usually quantified by measuring maximum expiratory flow rates. Maximum expiratory flow is determined by the elastic recoil of the lung and resistance of intrathoracic airways. It is greatest at high lung volumes, where elastic recoil is greatest and airways resistance is least, and progressively decreases throughout expiration. Except at the onset of expiration, maximal expiratory flow is largely independent of muscular effort. Beyond modest effort, a further increase in driving pressure is not accompanied by increased flow, because it is matched by a proportional increase in resistance due to compression of intrathoracic airways. Gross respiratory muscle weakness will, however, decrease maximum expiratory flow rates.

Methods of measurement

Maximum expiratory flow rates may be examined over the whole range of VC as the maximum expiratory flow volume (MEFV) curve[7] (Fig. 97.2).

At the bedside, maximum expiratory flow rates are commonly estimated by the forced expiratory volume in the first second of exhalation from TLC (i.e. FEV_1) or the peak expiratory flow rate (PEFR). The latter is relatively effort-dependent, and is less specific and reproducible than FEV_1. Other less commonly used measurements of ventilatory capacity include maximum mid expiratory flow rate and maximum breathing capacity.

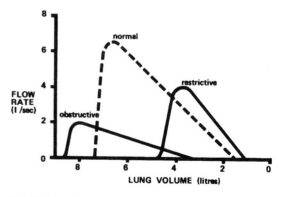

Fig. 97.2 Maximum expiratory flow volume curves, showing normal, obstructive and restrictive patterns.

The FEV_1 and the forced vital capacity (FVC, i.e. VC measured during forced expiration) may be measured with a wet or dry spirometer, or with an electronic flowmeter. The pneumotachograph is a very accurate, rapidly responsive flowmeter. It incorporates a resistance across which a pressure gradient develops with airflow through it. The magnitude of the gradient is proportional to flow rate, as long as flow is laminar. The gradient is measured with a differential pressure transducer, which is calibrated to produce a reading of flow. Other flowmeters include instruments that measure the change of temperature of a heated wire or thermistor by respired air.

PEFR may also be measured with such flowmeters. The Wright peak flow meter is another instrument used to measure PEFR. It measures the volume expired in the first 0.1 s of forced expiration, and gives a reading in litres per minute. While it is cheap, convenient and portable, the limitations of PEFR as a measure of ventilatory capacity (referred to earlier) must be recognized.

Interpretation

When FEV_1 is examined with FVC, two general disease patterns are seen – restrictive or obstructive. In restrictive diseases (e.g. chest-wall disease or pulmonary fibrosis), both FEV_1 and FVC are reduced, but the ratio of FEV_1 to FVC is normal or increased. In obstructive diseases (e.g. asthma or chronic obstructive airways disease) FEV_1 is reduced out of proportion to any reduction in FVC, so the ratio of FEV_1 to FVC is low. FEV_1 is normally 50–60 ml/ kg body weight, and is normally 70–83% of FVC. PEFR is also reduced in obstructive diseases, and in gross respiratory muscle weakness. PEFR is normally approximately 450–700 l/min in adult males and 300–500 l/min in females.

Examination of the complete MEFV curve reveals typical patterns for obstructive and restrictive disorders when compared with the normal for the patient's age, sex and size (Fig. 97.2). There may be mixed patterns. Improvement in maximal expiratory flow rates following bronchodilator administration helps distinguish asthma from irreversible air flow obstruction. The progress of diseases in which ventilatory capacity is impaired and their response to treatment can be conveniently and accurately followed by these measures. They also indicate the patient's ventilatory reserves, and are hence important in preoperative assessment.[8] In addition, upper airway obstruction produces abnormal patterns in maximum expiratory and inspiratory flow which help diagnosis and definition.[9]

Maximum mouth pressures

Maximum inspiratory (MIP) and expiratory (MEP) mouth pressures are useful measurements of the power, respectively, of inspiratory and expiratory muscles. MIP is usually measured during maximum inspiratory effort against an occluded airway at RV or FRC. Its normal value varies with age and sex,[10] exceeding –90 cm H_2O (–12 kPa) in young females and –130 cm H_2O (–17.3 kPa) in young males. A value less than –25 cm H_2O (–2.5 kPa) suggests that spontaneous ventilation will probably be inadequate.

Diaphragmatic function can be assessed by measuring the pressure developed across the diaphragm (transdiaphragmatic pressure, P_{di}) during spontaneous ventilation,[11] maximum inspiratory effort and phrenic nerve stimulation.[12] P_{di} is estimated from the difference between pleural and abdominal pressures, measured using balloon catheters placed in the mid-oesophagus and stomach respectively.

Distribution of ventilation

Normally, cessation of air flow at the end of expiration occurs almost simultaneously throughout the lung. In diffuse airways disease, the airways close irregularly and progressively as expiration proceeds. The evenness, or otherwise, of ventilation distribution may be assessed by two tests – single-breath nitrogen test and pulmonary nitrogen washout.

Single-breath nitrogen test[13] (Fig. 97.3)

The slope of the alveolar plateau (i.e. phase III) on slow exhalation after a single breath of 100% oxygen defines the evenness of ventilation distribution. Normally, the change in nitrogen concentration per 500 ml of expired air is less than 1.5% during phase III. Departure from this plateau (commencement of phase IV) defines the lung volume at which significant airways closure commences (i.e. closing volume). In the young, closing volume is equal to

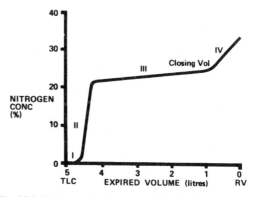

Fig. 97.3 Single-breath nitrogen test. Idealized tracing of expired nitrogen concentration during a slow exhalation from total lung capacity (TLC) to residual volume (RV) after a previous breath of 100% oxygen.

10% of VC. In the elderly, where the airways are less well-supported by surrounding elastic tissue, it may be up to 40% VC. Closing volume is increased in airways disease where the airways are narrowed (e.g. asthma or chronic bronchitis) or have decreased elastic support (e.g. emphysema). It is considered a sensitive measure of small airways disease. When closing volume exceeds FRC, significant shunting will occur during quiet breathing. An increase in closing volume following surgery is important in the genesis of postoperative hypoxaemia.[6]

Pulmonary nitrogen washout

In this test the subject is given 100% oxygen to breathe, having breathed room air. Maldistribution is indicated by a nitrogen concentration in the expired gas exceeding 2.5% after having breathed 100% oxygen for 7 min.

Gas transfer (diffusing capacity)[14]

The concept of gas transfer (TL) allows the ability of the lungs to transfer oxygen (from inspired air to the blood) to be quantified. In terms of oxygen transfer defects, reduced diffusing capacity of the alveolar–capillary membrane is much less important clinically than ventilation–perfusion mismatch. Hence the term transfer factor is preferred to the older term diffusing capacity because the test is of the lung's overall capacity to transfer gas.

The gas transfer factor for a gas x equals:

$$\frac{\text{Volume of gas } x \text{ taken up}}{\begin{array}{cc} \text{Alveolar pressure} & - \text{ Mean capillary pressure} \\ \text{of gas } x & \text{of gas } x \end{array}}$$

It is usually estimated for carbon monoxide (CO) because its rate of diffusion resembles that of oxygen, and it is so completely taken up by haemoglobin that the mean capillary pressure is effectively zero. The value is given in millilitres (of CO taken up) per minute per mmHg alveolar pressure CO. It is most commonly measured by the single-breath method[15] in ambulant patients. Although not commonly measured in the critically ill, the rebreathing method has been used to measure TL_{co} in ventilated patients.[16]

Interpretation

A number of factors affect the transfer of CO (Table 97.2).

The influence of reduced lung volume or unevenly distributed ventilation on TL may be corrected by dividing TL by the effective alveolar volume (VA), to yield TL/VA. VA is the the lung volume into which CO distributes during the measurement of TL. It is determined by gas dilution of helium, which is

Table 97.2 Factors influencing gas transfer for carbon monoxide

The epithelial–endothelial surface area (increasing with increasing size of subject)

The pulmonary capillary blood volume and haemoglobin concentration (increasing in polycythaemia and pulmonary capillary distension; decreasing with pulmonary embolism)

Rate of reaction of carbon monoxide with haemoglobin

Thickness of the alveolar–capillary membrane

Distribution of ventilation and ventilation–perfusion relationships

administered during the test, in a concentration of 10%, along with the 0.3% CO and air. In parenchymal lung disease characterized by destruction (e.g. emphysema) or by diffuse infiltration, both TL and TL/VA are decreased. In disease characterized by loss of long of lung tissue (e.g. fibrotic replacement) TL is decreased but TL/VA may be normal.

Lung mechanics

Mechanics is the science of the action of forces in producing motion or equilibrium. The major forces encountered by the respiratory muscles in performing their work of breathing are elastic recoil of the lung and chest wall, and the frictional resistance to flow, both tissue flow and air flow.

Elastic properties of lung and chest wall[17] (Fig. 97.4)

Measurement

The elastic properties of the lung are defined by the relationship of changes in lung volume (ΔVL) to the associated changes in transpulmonary pressure (ΔPL), measured during cessation of air flow. Similarly, the elastic properties of the chest wall are defined by the relationship of ΔVL to the associated changes in transthoracic pressure measured during cessation of air flow. These measurements are usually performed under static conditions, produced by momentary occlusion of the airway by a shutter during expiration. Interruption of air flow ensures that the measured pressure gradients only reflect elastic recoil forces, and not those associated with air flow (i.e. resistance). In measuring chest-wall elasticity, interruptions also allow the chest-wall musculature to be relaxed, as the measurement is otherwise meaningless.

The volume–pressure (VP) relationship of the lung is curvilinear. The VP curve may be examined between

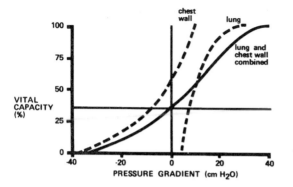

Fig. 97.4 Volume–pressure relationships of the lung and chest wall.

Interpretation

Lung compliance is decreased (i.e. the VP curve is displaced down and to the right) by pulmonary congestion, increased pulmonary smooth-muscle tone (e.g. after histamine administration), increased surface tension (e.g. decreased surfactant levels in neonatal respiratory distress syndrome), pulmonary fibrosis, infiltration or atelectasis and pleural fibrosis. Lung compliance is increased (i.e. VP curve displaced up and to the left) by pulmonary oligaemia, decreased pulmonary smooth-muscle tone (e.g. after β_2 agonists or prostaglandin F_2), augmented surfactant release (as may occur with lung distension provided by positive end-expiratory pressure) and destruction of lung tissue (e.g. emphysema).

TLC and FRC; both its shape and position are important in evaluating the elastic properties of the lung. A simple estimate of lung elasticity, lung compliance, is obtained by measuring the the slope of the linear portion of the curve – the litre above FRC.

Lung compliance (l/cm H_2O)

$$= \frac{\Delta VL \ (l)}{\Delta PL \ (cm \ H_2O)}$$

A measure of lung compliance (dynamic compliance) may also be obtained during uninterrupted respiration, by relating ΔVL to the ΔPL from end-expiration to end-inspiration, at which points air flow has momentarily ceased, and pressure gradient is representative of elastic recoil forces only. The measure of compliance may be standardized for variations in lung size, by dividing compliance by FRC. This is known as specific compliance (normal value = 0.04–0.07 l/cm H_2O/l).

Total respiratory system compliance is derived from lung and chest-wall compliance as follows:

$$\frac{1}{C_T} = \frac{1}{C_L} + \frac{1}{C_C}$$

where C_T = total compliance, C_L = lung compliance, and C_C = chest compliance.

A crude estimation of total compliance in ventilated patients is gained by dividing V_T by inspiratory pressure at cessation of inspiratory flow. This plateau can be obtained by using the ventilator's inspiratory hold facility if available, or momentarily occluding flow manually. The measurement is only reasonable if the patient is relaxed (i.e. heavily sedated and/or paralysed) so that chest-wall muscle tone is minimized.

Lung resistance

The total resistance of the lung is the sum of the airway resistance (>90%) and the tissue resistance (<10%). The respiratory resistance are usually measured at low flow rates. Assuming laminar flow,

Resistance (cm H_2O/l per s)

$$= \frac{Pressure \ gradient \ (cm \ H_2O)}{Flow \ (l/s)}$$

In the measurement of airway resistance, the relevant pressure gradient is that between the mouth and the alveoli. In the measurement of total lung resistance, it is that between the mouth and the pleural space. Flow is measured at the mouth with a pneumotachograph.

Several techniques have been developed to measure these pressure gradients.[18] In measuring airways resistance, alveolar pressure, which cannot be measured directly, has been derived using either the body plethysmograph or the interrupter method. Measurement of total lung resistance may be made by simultaneous recording of flow, mouth-to-intrapleural pressure gradient, and lung volume. The proportion of change in pressure attributable to lung volume change (i.e. compliance) is then subtracted. This subtraction method may be applied to estimate resistance in ventilated patients by dividing the difference between peak inspiratory pressure and plateau pressure at cessation of inspiratory flow, by the air flow at peak pressure.

These measurements of resistance are useful when precise assessment is required. However, for routine clinical purposes, measurements of maximum expiratory flow rates (in patients able to perform them), are an adequate guide to the degree of air flow obstruction.

Work of breathing

The work performed in overcoming the elastic, resistive and inertial forces generated by the lungs, chest wall and respiratory apparatus can be estimated by integrating inspiratory pressure change with respect to V_T. The product of pressure and volume has the same units as that of force and distance. Such measurements are useful in assessing the afterload on respiratory muscles, diagnosing specific abnormalities and monitoring the effects of treatment.[19] They also allow the breathing work imposed by various types of respiratory apparatus such as intermittent mandatory ventilation and continuous positive airways pressure system to be compared.[20]

Arterial blood gases and gas exchange

Measurement of arterial blood gases yields information on the patient's metabolic and respiratory state.

Hypoxaemia

With normal inspired oxygen tension and a normal cardiac output, hypoxaemia may be caused by hypoventilation ($Pa\text{CO}_2$ is increased) and by diffusion impairment, shunt and ventilation–perfusion inequality ($Pa\text{CO}_2$ is usually normal).

Hypoventilation

The many causes of hypoventilation include airways obstruction, increased stiffness or loss of structural integrity of the chest wall or pleural space, respiratory muscle disease, neuromuscular junction dysfunction due to drugs or disease, disease of the neural pathways and respiratory centre dysfunction due to drugs or disease.

Diffusion impairment

Diffusion impairment of the alveolar–capillary membrane is much less important than ventilation–perfusion inequality as a cause for arterial hypoxaemia, because of the reserves available.

Shunt

True shunts allow blood to reach the arterial system from the venous system without passing through the alveolar capillary bed. Examples are right-to-left intracardiac shunts, patent ductus arteriosus and intrapulmonary arteriovenous fistulae. Shunts through perfused but unventilated alveoli, are considered part of the spectrum of ventilation–perfusion inequality.

Ventilation–perfusion (V/Q) inequality

Normally, ventilation and perfusion of alveoli are reasonably well-matched throughout the lung. Mismatching of ventilation and perfusion results in inefficient gas exchange. The lung may be considered as a three-compartment model with;

1 ideal matching of ventilation and perfusion;
2 dead space, where the alveolus is well-ventilated but poorly perfused;
3 venous admixture (shunt) where the alveolus is poorly ventilated but well-perfused.

Three equations allow the *V/Q* inequality to be recognized and defined.

Alveolar gas equation

Alveolar $P\text{O}_2$ ($PA\text{O}_2$) is derived from the alveolar gas equation:

$$PA\text{O}_2 = \text{inspired } P\text{O}_2 - \frac{Pa\text{CO}_2}{\text{Respiratory quotient}}$$

where respiratory quotient normally approximates 0.8.

Normally, the difference between ideal $PA\text{O}_2$ and the arterial $P\text{O}_2$ ($Pa\text{O}_2$), i.e. the alveolar–arterial (or *A-a*) oxygen gradient, is less than 15 mmHg (2.0 kPa) in youth and 25 mmHg (3.3 kPa) in old age. This small difference is due to some venous admixture through the lungs, plus a small right-to-left shunt through bronchial veins and the thebesian veins of the coronary circulation. A larger *A-a* gradient in the absence of major right-to-left shunts is evidence that *V/Q* abnormality exists (see Appendix 4). The Bohr equation and the shunt equation allow that *V/Q* abnormality to be characterized.

Bohr equation

The Bohr equation calculates the proportion of the V_T which is unavailable for gas exchange (i.e. the physiological dead space, V_D).

$$\frac{V_D}{V_T} = \frac{Pa\text{CO}_2 - \text{mixed expired } P\text{CO}_2}{Pa\text{CO}_2}$$

Normally, V_D is approximately 30% V_T at rest. It consists predominantly of anatomical dead space, which is the volume of the conducting airways and does not participate in gas exchange. The balance of V_D is made up by alveoli that are ventilated but not perfused. In chronic lung disease, V_D may be greater than 50% V_T. It is also increased in old age, anaesthesia and controlled ventilation, especially with the use of large tidal volumes, high respiratory rates and short inspiratory times.

Shunt equation

This estimates the proportion of blood being shunted past poorly ventilated alveoli (Q_s) relative to total blood flow (Q_t).

$$\frac{Q_s}{Q_t} = \frac{C\acute{c}o_2 - Cao_2}{C\acute{c}o_2 - Cvo_2}$$

where $C\acute{c}o_2$ = end capillary O_2 content (calculated from PAo_2), Cao_2 = arterial O_2 content (calculated from Pao_2), Cvo_2 = mixed venue O_2 content (either calculated from mixed venous Po_2 measured from a pulmonary artery catheter or assumed to be 50 ml/l less than arterial O_2 content).

Oxygen delivery

The quantity of oxygen delivered to the tissues per minute is given by the product of cardiac output and arterial oxygen content:

$$= \text{Cardiac output (l/min)} \times [Sao_2 (\%) \\ \times \text{Hb (g/l)} \times 1.39 + Pao_2 \times 0.03]$$

where Sao_2 = arterial O_2 saturation and Hb = haemoglobin.

Note that normally each litre of blood contains approximately 200 ml O_2 combined with Hb and 3 ml dissolved O_2. Hence Sao_2 is a more important measure of O_2 carriage than Pao_2, and measurement of the concentration of *functional* Hb is necessary. While most arterial blood-gas analysers estimate Sao_2 from Pao_2, some directly measure it, along with measurement of Hb and abnormal Hb forms.

Fick equation

The Fick equation relates cardiac output, O_2 uptake and arteriovenous O_2 content difference ($Cao_2 - Cvo_2$) as follows:

$$\text{Cardiac output} = \frac{O_2 \text{ uptake}}{Cao_2 - Cvo_2}$$

It is most commonly applied in the ICU to calculate O_2 uptake from measurement of the other variables.

Hypercarbia and hypocarbia

The important interrelationships between $Paco_2$ and metabolic rate, alveolar ventilation, Pao_2 and arterial pH may be defined by three equations:

Alveolar ventilation equation

$$Paco_2 = \frac{\text{Metabolic rate}}{\text{Effective volume of breathing}}$$

This equation defines the relationship between the $Paco_2$ and its rates of production (i.e. metabolic rate) and elimination (i.e. effective breathing). An increase in the metabolic rate (e.g. fever, shivering or convulsions) increases CO_2 production. Decreased metabolic rate (e.g. hypothermia) decreases the arterial CO_2 production. Hypoventilation increases, and hyperventilation decreases $Paco_2$.

Alveolar gas equation:

$$Pao_2 = \text{inspired } Po_2 - \frac{Paco_2}{\text{Respiratory quotient}}$$

This equation defines the relationships between $Paco_2$ and PAo_2 and allows the *A-a* gradient to be estimated, as discussed earlier. The relationship between alveolar ventilation and Pao_2 is hyperbolic: hyperventilation, by eliminating CO_2, produces a small increase in PAo_2; hypoventilation allows $PAco_2$ to rise and may produce a dramatic decrease in PAo_2. Increasing the inspired Po_2 helps compensate for the hypoxia of hypoventilation, but in the patient dependent on hypoxic drive may produce further respiratory depression.

Henderson–Hasselbalch equation

$$pH = pK + \frac{\log \text{ arterial } [\, HCO_3^- \,]}{0.03 \times Paco_2}$$

This equation defines the relationship between arterial pH, $[HCO_3^-]$ and $Paco_2$. In acute CO_2 retention, as $Paco_2$ rises, pH falls. Conversely, with acute hyperventilation, $Paco_2$ falls and pH rises. Renal compensation occurs over several days, by the adjustment of $[HCO_3^-]$ so as to restore the ratio of arterial $[HCO_3^-]$ to arterial Pco_2 towards normal.

Non-invasive monitoring of blood gases (see Chapter 98)

Cutaneous oximetry

Pulse oximeters allow continuous non-invasive assessment of Sao_2 with sufficient accuracy for many clinical applications. Above an Sao_2 of 50% the method appears accurate to within 2%. It is unaffected by skin pigmentation. However, poor peripheral perfusion or abnormal forms of Hb introduce inaccuracies into the estimates.[21]

Cutaneous electrodes

Pao_2 and $Paco_2$ may be estimated using cutaneous electrodes. The skin is heated under an enclosed surface and the partial pressures of O_2 and CO_2 diffusing through the skin are measured using standard polarographic electrodes. The method is best suited to neonates where the correlation between transcutaneous and arterial partial pressures is good, except where peripheral circulation is compromised. The system responds slowly to Pa_{O_2} and Pa_{CO_2} changes, and hence is best suited to following trends.

Respired gas analysis

Analysis of expired gases can indirectly monitor Pa_{CO_2} concentration. A mass spectrometer or rapidly responsive capnometer is required. In lungs where ventilation is uniformly distributed and evenly matched to perfusion, end-tidal CO_2 ($P_{ET}CO_2$) reasonably reflects Pa_{CO_2}. $P_{ET}CO_2$ underestimates Pa_{CO_2} in the presence of significant shunt or dead space. Pulmonary emboli or decreased cardiac output are associated with a decrease in $P_{ET}CO_2$, because of decreased alveolar blood flow.[22] The slope of the alveolar plateau on the capnogram increases with increasing non-uniformity of distribution of ventilation; hence it reflects the presence of airway narrowing or other lung disease associated with inhomogeneous changes in the mechanical properties of the lungs.

Control of breathing

The control of respiration is assessed by measuring the ventilatory responses to hypercarbia[23] and hypoxia.[24] They do not distinguish disorders of central respiratory control (e.g. brainstem lesions, central nervous system-depressant drugs, and obtunded drive secondary to chronic hypoxaemia and/or hypercarbia) from disorders which severely impair ventilatory capacity (such that ventilatory response is inadequate despite increased respiratory centre activity).

Exercise testing[25]

Patients with mild lung dysfunction may have normal pulmonary function tests at rest, but reveal abnormalities when stressed by exercise. The presenting complaint may be low exercise tolerance, and exercise testing objectively measures the degree of abnormality, by measuring maximum acheived workload or oxygen uptake. Relating ventilatory responses, Sa_{O_2} and CO_2 output to workload and oxygen uptake, with electrocardiogram monitoring, pulmonary causes of exertional dyspnoea may be distinguished from other causes (e.g. cardiac disease or lack of general fitness). The degree of arterial O_2 desaturation with exercise is a sensitive indicator of parenchymal or pulmonary vascular disease. Comparing FEV_1 pre- and post-exercise allows exercise-induced asthma to be detected. These tests are only applicable to ambulant patients, but are useful in assessing recovery from acute lung injury.

Regional lung function

The tests referred to so far look at the respiratory system as a whole. Occasionally, it is useful to examine regional lung function. Physical signs and X-ray appearances, including bronchography and tomography, yield valuable information about regional lung function. Abnormalities of chest-wall movement may be measured using magnetometers, and diaphragmatic movements monitored by fluoroscopy. Quantitative lung scanning, using radioactive isotopes, allows the relative ventilation and perfusion of different lung regions to be determined. Inhalation of gas labelled with xenon 133 produces regional radioactivity proportional to regional ventilation. Injection of technetium 99-labelled albumen produces regional radioactivity proportional to local blood flow, and is used to detect pulmonary emboli. The multiple inert gas elimination technique is a method that allows ventilation–perfusion matching to be accurately assessed and has been used in the ICU.[26] However, its complexity has prevented its widespread application.

References

1. Wright BM (1955) A respiratory anemometer. *J Physiol* **127**:25.
2. Gilson JC and Hugh-Jones P (1948) The measurement of total lung volume and breathing capacity. *Clin Sci* **7**:185–216.
3. Hathirat S, Renzetti AD and Mitchell M (1970) Total lung capacity measured by helium dilution. *Am Rev Respir Dis* **102**:760–770.
4. Dubois AB, Botelho SY, Bedell GN, Marshall R and Comroe JH (1956) A rapid plethysmographic method for measuring thoracic gas volume. *J Clin Invest* **35**:322–326.
5. Mead J (1960) Volume displacement plethysmograph for respiratory measurements in human subjects. *J Appl Physiol* **15**:736–740.
6. Alexander JI, Spence AA, Parikh RK and Stuart B (1973) The role of airway closure in postoperative hypoxemia. *Br J Anaesth* **45**:34–40.
7. Hyatt RE and Black LF (1973) The flow–volume curve. *Am Rev Respir Dis* **107**:191–199.
8. Gass GD and Olsen GN (1986) Preoperative pulmonary function testing to predict postoperative morbidity and mortality. *Chest* **89**:127–134.
9. Acres JC and Kryger MH (1981) Upper airways obstruction. *Chest* **80**:207–211.
10. Black LF and Hyatt RE (1969) Maximal respiratory pressures: normal values and relationship to age and sex. *Am Rev Respir Dis* **99**:696–702.

11. Hillman DR and Finucane KE (1988) Respiratory pressure partitioning during quiet inspiration in unilateral and bilateral diaphragmatic weakness. *Am Rev Respir Dis* **137**:1401–1405.

12. Aubier M, Murciano D, Lecocguic Y *et al.* (1985) Bilateral phrenic nerve stimulation: a simple technique to assess diaphragmatic fatigue in humans. *J Appl Physiol* **58**:58–64.

13. Buist AS (1975) The single breath nitrogen test. *N Engl J Med* **293**:438–440.

14. Davies NJH (1982) What does the transfer of carbon monoxide mean? *Br J Dis Chest* **76**:105–241.

15. Ogilvie CM, Forster RE, Blakemore WS and Morton JW (1957) Measurement of diffusing capacity of the lung. *J Clin Invest* **36**:1–17.

16. Clark EH, Jones HA and Hughes JMB (1978) Bedside rebreathing technique for measuring carbon monoxide uptake by the lung. *Lancet* **1**:791–793.

17. Gibson GJ and Pride NB (1976) Lung distensibility. *Br J Dis Chest* **70**:143–184.

18. Cotes JE (1993) *Lung Function*, 5th edn. Oxford: Blackwell Scientific, pp. 166–174.

19. Banner MJ, Jaeger MJ and Kirby RR (1994) Components of the work of breathing and implications for monitoring ventilator-dependent patients. *Crit Care Med* **22**:515–523.

20. Hillman DR, Breakey JN, Lam M *et al.* (1987) Minimizing work of breathing with continuous positive airway pressure and intermittent mandatory ventilation. *Crit Care Med* **15**:665–670.

21. Taylor MB and Whitwam JG (1986) The current status of pulse oximetry. *Anaesthesia* **41**:943–949.

22. Weil MH, Bisera J, Trevino RP and Rackow EC (1985) Cardiac output and end-tidal CO_2. *Crit Care Med* **13**:907–909.

23. Read DJC (1969) A clinical method for assessing the ventilatory response to carbon dioxide. *Aust Ann Med* **16**:20–32.

24. Rebuck AS and Campbell EJM (1974) A clinical method for assessing the ventilatory response to hypoxia. *Am Rev Respir Dis* **109**:345–350.

25. Spiro SG (1977) Exercise testing in clinical medicine. *Br J Dis Chest* **71**:145–172.

26. Gillespie DJ, Didier EP and Rehder K (1990) Ventilation perfusion distribution after aortic valve replacement. *Crit Care Med* **18**:136–140.

Monitoring oxygenation

J Takala

Monitoring oxygenation is one of the most important aspects of monitoring the critically ill patient. To understand the pathophysiology of oxygenation disorders, it is convenient to divide the chain of oxygen transport into components. The different monitoring techniques may provide information on one or several components of oxygen transport and tissue oxygenation (Table 98.1). Ideally, monitoring should provide comprehensive information on each component, so that derangement at any point of the chain could be detected early, and treatment given before tissue hypoxia occurs.

The adequacy of oxygenation can be monitored by simple means (e.g. in uncomplicated postoperative patients). In contrast, all components of the oxygen transport system and their interactions have to be considered in patients with severe cardiovascular or respiratory failure.

Table 98.1 Components of oxygen transport and tissue oxygenation

Oxygen delivery from the inspiratory gases to the alveoli
Oxygenation of arterial blood
Delivery of oxygen to the tissues
Oxygen uptake
Oxygen in the mixed venous blood
Interaction of arterial oxygenation and mixed venous oxygenation
Lactate and intramucosal pH
Adequacy of tissue oxygenation and detection of hypoxia

Monitoring delivery of oxygen to alveoli

This is the most straightforward step in monitoring oxygenation. Alveolar partial pressure of oxygen

(PA_{O_2}) is a function of the barometric pressure (P_B), the inspired fraction of oxygen (Fi_{O_2}), the alveolar partial pressure of carbon dioxide (PA_{CO_2}, estimated as the arterial P_{CO_2}, Pa_{CO_2}) and, to a small extent, the respiratory quotient (RQ):[1]

$$PA_{O_2} = Fi_{O_2} \times (P_B - P_{WATER}) - Pa_{CO_2}$$
$$\times [1 - Fi_{O_2} \times (1 - RQ)]/RQ$$

where P_{WATER} is the partial pressure of fully saturated water vapour at body temperature (e.g. 47 mmHg or 6.3 kPa at 37°C).

Accordingly, excluding high altitudes, monitoring the delivery of oxygen to the alveoli can be performed by monitoring the Fi_{O_2}, once adequate ventilation has been verified either clinically, by end-tidal CO_2 monitoring (which gives an index of the PA_{CO_2}), or by blood-gas analysis.[2-4] An increased Fi_{O_2} will reduce the effect of Pa_{CO_2} on the PA_{O_2}. In practice, even severe hypercarbia rarely limits oxygenation, when Fi_{O_2} exceeds 0.30.

A more direct way to monitor PA_{O_2} is to monitor end-tidal P_{O_2} as an estimate of PA_{O_2}. Clinical experience on end-tidal P_{O_2} monitoring in intensive care is so far limited. It should be noted that the difference between the true alveolar and the end-tidal gas tensions will increase in the presence of marked ventilation–perfusion inequalities.[5,6] End-tidal P_{O_2} will then overestimate PA_{O_2} and end-tidal P_{CO_2} will underestimate PA_{CO_2}.

Monitoring oxygenation of arterial blood

The main proportion of oxygen in arterial blood is bound in haemoglobin. Blood oxygen content (Ca_{O_2}) is a function of haemoglobin concentration (Hb), the proportion of oxyhaemoglobin (haemoglobin oxygen saturation, Sa_{O_2}), and oxygen dissolved in plasma (a function of arterial oxygen partial pressure, Pa_{O_2}):

$$Ca_{O_2} \text{ (ml/l)} = 1.39 \times \text{Hb (g/l)} \times Sa_{O_2} + 0.03$$
$$\times Pa_{O_2} \text{ mmHg (or } + 0.2325$$
$$\times Pa_{O_2} \text{ kPa)}$$

At atmospheric pressure (excluding severe hypothermia and severe anaemia), usually less than 5% of the arterial oxygen content is dissolved in plasma. In severe hypothermia (e.g. during hypothermic cardiopulmonary bypass), the solubility of oxygen will markedly increase, and significant amounts of oxygen can be transported dissolved in plasma. It is evident from the above equation that haemoglobin concentration has a major impact on Ca_{O_2}.

Oxygenated and reduced haemoglobin are different in colour, i.e. they absorb and reflect light at different wavelengths. This is the physical basis for clinical cyanosis and the measurement of Sa_{O_2}. The bluish colour of reduced haemoglobin is the cause of clinical cyanosis. The presence of cyanosis indicates that 50 g/l or more of desaturated haemoglobin is present. The absence of cyanosis does not exclude severe hypoxaemia, as cyanosis will not be evident if haemoglobin concentration is low or capillary perfusion is poor.

Available methods for clinical monitoring of arterial blood oxygenation are blood-gas analysis (measurement of oxygen partial pressure and saturation) and pulse oximetry.[7,8] Continuous measurement of arterial blood gases using intravascular probes is rapidly developing, though clinical use is still very limited. Problems associated with continuous measurement of arterial blood gases have been shifts in calibration, clot formation and, importantly, costs.[9,10]

Pulse oximetry measures the saturation of blood in the arterial capillaries. Sensors can be placed on the fingertip, ear and forehead. Detection of capillary pulse is a prerequisite, and hence monitoring cannot be performed if severe vasoconstriction is present. The pulse oximeter measures the *effective* saturation, i.e. the percentage of normal haemoglobin that is oxygenated. It does not take into account the amount of methaemoglobin or carboxyhaemoglobin in the blood, and will overestimate the percentage of oxyhaemoglobin in total haemoglobin.[11] Pulse oximetry should be regarded rather as a trend monitor than a substitute for blood co-oximetry. As such, it is very useful in following changes in arterial oxygenation. The calibration curves for pulse oximeters are empirical, and tend to overestimate saturation in severe hypoxaemia. Differences between patients may exist. It is therefore important to establish the relationship between the saturation values measured by pulse oximetry and by co-oximetry, especially in the treatment of patients with severe hypoxaemia.

Since Sa_{O_2} is usually on the flat part of the oxyhaemoglobin dissociation curve, the position of the curve has little effect on the relationship between haemoglobin oxygen saturation and partial pressure. In severe hypoxaemia, the effect of the position of the dissociation curve will be magnified, and should be considered in evaluating saturation values.

Delivery of oxygen to tissues

Oxygen delivery to any tissue bed is the product of blood flow and Ca_{O_2}. For the whole body, oxygen delivery (Do_2) is equal to the product of cardiac output (CO) or cardiac index (CI) and Ca_{O_2}:

$$Do_2 \text{ (ml/min per m}^2)$$

$$= \text{CI (l/min per m}^2) \times Ca_{O_2} \text{ (ml/l)}$$

$$= \text{CI (l/min per m}^2) \times [1.39 \times \text{Hb (g/l)}$$
$$\times Sa_{O_2} + 0.03 \times Pa_{O_2}; \text{mmHg]}$$
$$(\text{or } + 0.2325 \times Pa_{O_2}; \text{kPa)}$$

Oxygen delivery to the tissues can be only very roughly evaluated clinically, since neither Ca_{O_2} nor CI can be reliably estimated without actual measurements.[12] Accordingly, a pulmonary artery catheter is necessary for the assessment and monitoring of oxygen delivery.

Measurement of cardiac output by the thermodilution method is fundamentally important in the monitoring of oxygen delivery.[12-15] The measurement is based on injection of fluid with a temperature lower than body temperature into the right atrium. The change in pulmonary artery blood temperature is measured at the catheter tip, and the area of the curve of temperature reduction is integrated. The area of the curve is proportional to the cardiac output. Cardiac output varies during the respiratory cycle.[14] Hence, the mean of several measurements spread randomly over the respiratory cycle should be obtained. The number of measurements depends on the observed variability: the higher the variability, the larger number of injections should be averaged. In practice, three to five injections are usually sufficient, if the variation between measurements is 10–15%. Recently, a technique for continuous monitoring of cardiac output by thermodilution has been introduced.[16] This is based on electronically generated small heat pulses delivered by a coil near the distal end of the catheter. Clinical experience is still limited.

Cardiac output can be monitored also with less invasive means, e.g. by ultrasound.[17] However, the great advantage of the pulmonary artery catheter is the simultaneous access to intravascular pressures and mixed venous blood, which will give important additional information (see below).

Monitoring oxygen uptake

Uptake of oxygen from arterial blood reflects the oxygen consumed by cellular metabolism. The fraction of oxygen uptake (Vo_2) of the amount of oxygen delivered (Do_2) is the oxygen extraction:

$$O_2 \text{ extraction} = Vo_2/Do_2$$

Oxygen extraction is never 100% in any tissue, and the extraction capability differs between various tissue beds. When Do_2 decreases and oxygen extraction reaches its maximum, Vo_2 becomes dependent on Do_2, an oxygen debt will develop in the tissue, and anaerobic metabolism with increased production of lactate will ensue.

Measurement of Vo_2 and its changes in response to therapy can be used to evaluate the adequacy of Do_2: a major increase (>15–20%) in Vo_2 in response to increased Do_2 suggests that Do_2 was insufficient. Measurement of Vo_2 is also valuable to evaluate arterial hypoxaemia. In the presence of increased venous admixture (physiological shunt), Vo_2 may have a substantial impact on arterial oxygenation (see the section on interaction of arterial oxygenation and mixed venous oxygenation, below).

Oxygen consumption can be either measured from expired gases or calculated from data obtained by the pulmonary artery catheter and arterial and mixed venous blood samples.[18] Modern gas exchange monitors have made continuous bedside measurement of Vo_2 possible in ICU. When proper calibration and control of the measurement conditions are assured, Vo_2 can be measured with high accuracy and reproducibility.[19–21] At Fio_2 exceeding 0.60–0.70, the gas exchange monitors progressively lose their accuracy.

Alternatively, Vo_2 can be measured using the Fick principle, as the product of cardiac output and the arterial–mixed venous oxygen content difference:

$$Vo_2 = CO \times (Cao_2 - Cvo_2)$$

This calculated Vo_2 is less accurate and has a larger variability than Vo_2 measured by the gas exchange monitors.[18] Nevertheless, it can be easily derived in any patient with a pulmonary artery catheter.

Monitoring mixed venous oxygenation

Mixed venous oxygenation is probably the best single indicator of the adequacy of whole-body oxygen transport. The mixed venous oxygen content represents the amount of oxygen that is left after perfusion of the capillary beds in the systemic circulation.[22] As such, it can be regarded as the oxygen reserve, or an indicator of the balance between oxygen delivery and consumption. It is the flow-weighted average oxygen content of the venous effluents from various tissues. This characteristic is also the main limiting factor in interpreting mixed venous oxygenation: severe tissue hypoxia in a tissue bed receiving only a small proportion of cardiac output will have little effect on mixed venous oxygen content, if the rest of the tissues are well-perfused. In the most common conditions associated with tissue hypoxia, mixed venous oxygen content, and especially its changes, will reflect the adequacy of oxygen delivery.[23,24]

A close look at the Fick equation for Vo_2 helps to interpret the mixed venous oxygen saturation (Svo_2) and partial pressure (Pvo_2):

$$Vo_2 = CO \times (Cao_2 - Cvo_2)$$
$$Cvo_2 = Cao_2 - Vo_2/CO$$
$$Cvo_2/Cao_2 = 1 - Vo_2/(Cao_2 \times CO) =$$
$$1 - Vo_2/Do_2$$

For most clinical conditions, the effect of dissolved oxygen on both arterial and venous oxygen content is small:

$$Cao_2 \text{ (ml/l)} = 1.39 \times Hb \text{ (g/l)} \times Sao_2 + 0.03$$
$$\times Pao_2 \text{ mmHg}$$
$$(\text{or} + 0.2325 \times Pao_2 \text{ kPa})$$

$$Cvo_2 \text{ (ml/l)} = 1.39 \times Hb \text{ (g/l)} \times Svo_2 + 0.03$$
$$\times Pao_2 \text{ mmHg}$$
$$(\text{or} + 0.2325 \times Pvo_2 \text{ kPa})$$

If the contribution of the dissolved oxygen is ignored, the equations for mixed venous oxygenation can be simplified further:

$$Svo_2/Sao_2 = 1 - Vo_2/Do_2$$
$$Svo_2 = Sao_2 - Vo_2/1.39 \times Hb \times CO$$

Accordingly, an increase in Vo_2 and a decrease in haemoglobin, cardiac output and arterial oxygenation will all reduce Svo_2.

There is no clear-cut safe level of Svo_2. In patients with chronic heart failure, levels below 50% are often tolerated well. In contrast, in acutely ill intensive care patients, tissue hypoxia may ensue at Svo_2 levels over 60%.[23,24] As a practical guide, an increased risk for tissue hypoxia should be considered in the acutely ill patient at Svo_2 <65%. A low Svo_2 should always prompt a suspicion of tissue hypoxia, whereas a normal Svo_2 does not guarantee adequate oxygenation in all organs, if vasoregulation is abnormal.

Changes in Svo_2 in response to therapy are more important than single values.[23,24] A rapidly decreasing Svo_2 should alert for an impending catastrophe. The changes can be monitored on-line using fibreoptic pulmonary artery catheters. These catheters use reflection spectrophotometry to measure saturation of mixed venous blood, and the measurement is calibrated against blood samples analysed by laboratory co-oximetry.[25,26]

Interaction of arterial oxygenation and mixed venous oxygenation

Venous oxygen content has very little effect on arterial oxygen content in normal lungs, since venous admixture (physiological shunt, Q_s/Q_t) is very small. When Q_s/Q_t increases, the impact of any Cvo_2 change on Cao_2 will be magnified. In the presence of large Q_s/Q_t, an increase in Vo_2, or a reduction of cardiac output or haemoglobin, can cause substantial arterial hypoxaemia. This is evident from the equation of Q_s/Q_t:

$$Q_s/Q_t = (Cco_2 - Cao_2)/$$
$$(Cco_2 - Cvo_2) \qquad \text{(equation 1)}$$

where Cco_2 is the pulmonary venous capillary oxygen content in normally ventilated and perfused alveoli. This can be rearranged and written as

$$Cao_2 = Cco_2 \times (1 - Q_s/Q_t)$$
$$+ Cvo_2 \times Q_s/Q_t \qquad \text{(equation (2)}$$

According to the Fick equation, Vo_2 is the product of cardiac output and arterial–mixed venous oxygen content difference, which can be rewritten as

$$Cvo_2 = Cao_2 - Vo_2/CO \qquad \text{(equation 3)}$$

By combining equations 2 and 3:

$$Cao_2 = Cco_2 - (Vo_2/CO)$$
$$\times (Q_s/Q_t)/(1 - Q_s/Q_t) \qquad \text{(equation 4)}$$

If the dissolved oxygen is ignored, equation 4 can be written as

$$Sao_2 = 1 - (Vo_2/CO \times Hb \times 1.39)$$
$$\times (Q_s/Q_t)/(1 - Q_s/Q_t) \qquad \text{(equation 5)}$$

Equation 4 demonstrates that arterial oxygenation (Sao_2) is directly related to cardiac output and haemoglobin, and inversely related to oxygen consumption. The effect of these variables on arterial oxygenation will be markedly magnified in the presence of large Q_s/Q_t.[6]

Lactate and intramucosal pH

Increased production of lactate is one of the early biochemical changes in tissue hypoxia. Indeed, increased blood concentrations of lactate are associated with increased morbidity and mortality in various clinical conditions. The production of lactate from pyruvate is necessary to maintain glycolysis under anaerobic conditions. In aerobic glycolysis, NADH is oxidized to NAD^+ via the respiratory chain. In order to maintain glycolysis when oxygen availability is reduced, NAD^+ must be regenerated via the lactate dehydrogenase (LDH) reaction, in which pyruvate accepts hydrogen from NADH to form NAD^+:

$$\text{Pyruvate} + \text{NADH} \xrightleftharpoons{\text{LDH}} \text{lactate} + NAD^+$$

Accordingly, the ratio of lactate to pyruvate is a better indicator of the redox state of the tissue than lactate alone.[27] Pyruvate measurements are currently not routinely available, while blood lactate can be promptly measured with modern lactate analysers. Tissue hypoxia should be suspected when blood lactate is increased, although moderately increased lactate concentrations may also result from increased aerobic glycolysis, inhibition of the pyruvate dehydrogenase enzyme and reduced metabolic clearance of lactate due to liver dysfunction. Despite the limitations, increased blood lactate concentrations should prompt an evaluation of adequate oxygenation.

Assessment of visceral tissue oxygenation by estimation of gastric intramucosal pH (pH_i) using gastric tonometry has recently been introduced to clinical practice.[28–30] The basic principle is that when intramucosal perfusion and oxygen demand are in imbalance, pH_i will decrease, as mucosal acidosis will reflect inadequate perfusion.[31] A special nasogastric tube with a CO_2-permeable silicone balloon in its tip is placed in the stomach. Saline injected into the balloon will approach within 90 min the same Pco_2 as that within the gastric mucosa. Saline Pco_2 is measured using a standard blood-gas analyser and, simultaneously, an arterial blood-gas sample is taken for the measurement of the actual arterial bicarbonate concentration. The gastric pH_i can then be calculated by applying a modified Henderson–Hasselbalch equation:

$$pH_i = 6.1 + \log \frac{\text{arterial } [HCO_3^-]}{Pco_2 \text{ (tonometer)} \times 0.03 \times K}$$

where K is a time-dependent equilibration constant provided by the manufacturer.

Clinical assessment of regional tissue oxygenation in critically ill patients with a tonometer is an attractive idea. Prolonged gastric mucosal acidosis measured with tonometry predicts poor prognosis in critically ill patients,[28-30] but its validity in assessing transient changes in response to therapy has not been established. The method is non-invasive, and theoretically easy to perform. Nevertheless, clinical use has revealed technical and physiological problems. Analysis of gastric P_{CO_2} with different blood-gas analysers contributes to errors in calculated gastric pH_i.[32,33] Back-diffusion of CO_2, generated by the reaction between secreted H^+ and HCO_3^-, can result in erroneously low values of pH_i.[34,35] Based on studies performed in healthy volunteers, H_2-blockers have been recommended to reduce the generation of intraluminal CO_2, and to improve the reproducibility of measurements of pH_i. This recommendation is controversial, since studies in critically ill patients suggest that the use of H_2-blockers has no effect on calculated gastric pH_i.[36] This is probably related to reduced gastric acid secretion, especially in patients with compromised visceral perfusion.

When variability of the method is minimized by meticulous handling of the sample and use of only one blood-gas analyser with verified capability to measure saline P_{CO_2}, a change in pH_i of 0.05 pH units can usually be regarded as significant. When normality of a pH_i value is considered, the type of blood-gas analyser and the use of H_2-blockade should be taken into account. In patients with an abnormal arterial pH, the pH gap (arterial $pH-pH_i$) is a more relevant variable.

Monitoring adequacy of tissue oxygenation

Monitoring adequacy of tissue oxygenation in intensive care is based on a comprehensive evaluation of the patient to exclude direct and indirect signs of tissue hypoxia. Sufficient arterial oxygen content, perfusion pressure and blood flow are necessary prerequisites for adequate oxygen delivery. The clinical evaluation should ensure that no signs of overt hypovolaemia or circulatory failure or untreated respiratory failure are present. The cardiac output should be able to maintain the peripheral tissues free from vasoconstriction.

The following criteria suggest that tissue hypoxia may be present in the acutely ill intensive care patient:

1 increased blood lactate concentrations with or without metabolic acidosis;
2 low Svo_2 (<60-65%), high oxygen extraction (>35-40%).
3 low Do_2: tissue hypoxia is likely if $Do_2 < 8-10$ ml/ kg per min, possible if $Do_2 = 10-15$ ml/kg per min, and unlikely if >15 ml/kg per min.
4 very low Vo_2 (<2.5-3.0 ml/kg per min).
5 gastric mucosal acidosis (normal values depend on the specific blood-gas analyser).

These guidelines are crude indicators only, and should always be put into perspective with the overall clinical status of the patient.

References

1. Nunn JF (1987) Principles of assessment of distribution of ventilation and pulmonary blood flow. In: Nunn JF (ed.) *Applied Respiratory Physiology*. London: Butterworths, pp. 177-183.
2. Nunn JF (1987) The minute volume of pulmonary ventilation. In: Nunn JF (ed.) *Applied Respiratory Physiology*. London: Butterworths, pp. 110-112.
3. Severinghaus JW (1989) Water vapor calibration errors in some capnometers: respiratory conventions misunderstood by manufacturers? *Anesthesiology* **70**:996-998.
4. Hoffman RA, Krieger BP, Kramer MR *et al.* (1989) End-tidal carbon dioxide in critically ill patients during changes in mechanical ventilation. *Am Rev Respir Dis* **140**:1265-1268.
5. Marshall BE, Marshall C, Frasch F and Hanson CW (1994) Role of hypoxic pulmonary vasoconstriction in pulmonary gas exchange and blood flow distribution. Basic science series: 1. Physiologic concepts. *Intensive Care Med* **20**:291-297.
6. Marshall BE, Hanson CW, Frasch F and Marshall C (1994) Role of hypoxic pulmonary vasoconstriction in pulmonary gas exchange and blood flow distribution. Basic science series: 2. Pathophysiology. *Intensive Care Med* **20**:379-389.
7. Scuderi PE, Macgregor DA, Bowton DL, Harris LC, Anderson R and James RL (1993) Performance characteristics and interanalyzer variability of Po_2 measurements using tonometered human blood. *Am Rev Respir Dis* **147**:1354-1359.
8. Yelderman M and New W (1983) Evaluation of pulse oximetry. *Anesthesiology* **59**:349-352.
9. Shapiro BA, Mahutte CK, Cane RD and Gilmour IJ (1993) Clinical performance of a blood gas monitor: a prospective, multicenter trial. *Crit Care Med* **21**:487-494.
10. Zimmerman JL and Dellinger RP (1993) Initial evaluation of a new intra-arterial blood gas system in humans. *Crit Care Med* **21**:495-500.
11. Severinghaus JW and Kelleher JF (1992) Recent developments in pulse oximetry. *Anesthesiology* **76**:1018-1038.
12. Nightingale P (1990) Practical points in the application of oxygen transport principles. *Intensive Care Med* **16**:173-177.
13. Pinsky MR (1990) The meaning of cardiac output. *Intensive Care Med* **16**:415-417.
14. Jansen JRC, Schreuder JJ, Settels JJ, Kloek JJ and Versprille A (1990) An adequate strategy for the thermomodulation technique in patients during mechanical ventilation. *Intensive Care Med* **16**:422-425.
15. Cunnion RE and Natanson CH (1994) Echocardiography, pulmonary artery catheterization, and radionuclide cineangiography in septic shock. *Intensive Care Med* **20**:535-537.

16. Boldt J, Menges T, Wollbrück M, Hammermann H and Hempelmann G (1994) Is continuous cardiac output measurement using thermodilution reliable in the critically ill patient? *Crit Care Med* **22**:1913–1918.

17. Wong DH, Tremper KK, Stemmer EA *et al.* (1990) Noninvasive cardiac output: simultaneous comparison of two different methods with thermodilution. *Anesthesiology* **72**:784–792.

18. Brandi LS, Grana M, Mazzanti T, Giunta F, Natali A and Ferrannini E (1992) Energy expenditure and gas exchange measurements in postoperative patients: thermodilution versus indirect calorimetry. *Crit Care Med* **20**:1273–1283.

19. Takala J, Keinänen O, Väisänen P and Kari A (1989) Measurement of gas exchange in intensive care: laboratory and clinical validation of a new device. *Crit Care Med* **17**:1041–1047.

20. Makita K, Nunn JF and Royston B (1990) Evaluation of metabolic measuring instruments for use in critically ill patients. *Crit Care Med* **18**:638–644.

21. Damask MC, Weissman C, Askanazi J, Hyman AI, Rosenbaum SH and Kinney JM (1982) A systematic method for validation of gas exchange measurements. *Anesthesiology* **57**:213–218.

22. Nelson LD (1987) Mixed venous oximetry. In: Snyder JV and Pinsky MR (eds) *Oxygen Transport in the Critically III*. Chicago: Year Book, pp. 235–248.

23. Weissman C and Kemper M (1991) The oxygen uptake–oxygen delivery relationship during ICU interventions. *Chest* **99**:430–435.

24. Ruokonen E, Takala J and Uusaro A (1991) Effect of vasoactive treatment on the relationship between mixed venous and regional oxygen saturation. *Crit Care Med* **19**:1365–1369.

25. Armaganidis A, Dhainaut JF, Billard JL *et al.* Accuracy assessment for three fiberoptic pulmonary artery catheters for Svo₂ monitoring. *Intensive Care Med* **20**:484–488.

26. Keinänen O, Takala J and Kari A (1992) Continuous measurement of cardiac output by the Fick principle: clinical validation in intensive care. *Crit Care Med* **20**:360–365.

27. Cone JB (1987) Monitoring of tissue oxygenation. In: Snyder JV and Pinsky MR (eds) *Oxygen Transport in the Critically III*. Chicago: Year Book, pp. 164–175.

28. Fiddian-Green RG and Baker S (1987) Predictive value of stomach wall pH for complications after cardiac operations: comparison with other monitoring. *Crit Care Med* **15**:153–156.

29. Maynard N, Bihari D, Beale R *et al.* (1993) Assessment of splanchnic oxygenation by gastric tonometry in patients with acute circulatory failure. *J Am Med Assoc* **270**:1203–1210.

30. Doglio GR, Pusajo JF, Egurrola MA *et al.* (1991) Gastric mucosal pH as a prognostic index of mortality in critically ill patients. *Crit Care Med* **19**:1037–1040.

31. Grum C, Fiddian-Green R and Pittenger G (1984) Adequacy of tissue oxygenation in the intact dog intestine. *J Appl Physiol* **56**:1065–1069.

32. Riddington D, Balasubramanian Venkatesh K, Clutton-Brock T and Bion J (1994) Measuring carbon dioxide tension in saline and alternative solutions: quantification of bias and precision in two blood gas analyzers. *Crit Care Med* **22**:96–100.

33. Takala J, Parviainen I, Siloaho M, Ruokonen E and Hämäläinen E. (1994) Saline Pco_2 is an important source of error in the assessment of gastric intramucosal pH. *Crit Care Med* **22**:1877–1879.

34. Heard SO, Helsmoortel CM, Kent JC, Shahnarian A and Fink MP (1991) Gastric tonometry in healthy volunteers: effect of ranitidine on calculated intramural pH. *Crit Care Med* **19**:271–274.

35. Kolkman J, Groeneveld A and Meuwissen S (1994) Effect of ranitidine on basal and bicarbonate enhanced intragastric Pco_2: a tonometric study. *Gut* **35**:737–741.

36. Maynard N, Atkinson S, Mason R, Smithies M and Bihari D (1994) Influence of intravenous ranitidine on gastric intramucosal pH in critically ill patients. *Crit Care Med* **22**:A79.

99	# Imaging techniques in intensive care

AB Kumar

Modern imaging techniques have developed at a very rapid rate in the last decade. An understanding of the applications and limitations of imaging examinations on critically ill patients is essential for their correct management. Like any investigation, the clinician should ask whether the right imaging technique is being performed for the problem at hand. Consultation with a radiologist will help in choosing the appropriate investigation. This chapter summarizes the most important techniques and their applications.

General considerations[1–5]

Most X-rays performed on the critically ill are done in the ICU using mobile equipment with the patient in a standard ward bed. As such, these films are suboptimal, which should be borne in mind when making comparisons with those taken in the radiology department or previous ICU films. Over-interpretation of subtle changes on chest X-rays due to a change in exposure or technique may lead to erroneous assumptions, e.g. a diagnosis of pulmonary oedema in particular.

When considering what imaging technique should be performed, the following questions should be asked:

1 What anatomical region needs imaging?
2 What type of imaging technique will give the most information?
3 What information do you expect to obtain from the investigation?
4 Where should the investigation be performed? Can the patient be safely moved to the radiology department for specialized films?

Adequate preliminary resuscitation of the critically ill, traumatized or hypoxic patient will reduce the morbidity and mortality related to the investigations. In addition, facilities for resuscitation in the radiology department should be freely available. No patient should leave the accident and emergency department or ICU for diagnostic investigations without attention to these issues (see Chapter 3). The development of specialized trauma radiology suites may facilitate the rapid investigation and management of acutely ill patients.

The chest X-ray (CXR) examination[5]

The CXR is the most commonly performed radiological investigation in the ICU. Patients, if possible, should be in the sitting or semi-erect position at full inspiration for the film. Common abnormalities are shown in Table 99.1.

Lobar collapse (Plates 3–6)

Collapse may involve entire lobes, segments or only subsegments; this is commonly termed atelectasis. When an entire lobe is collapsed, the following abnormalities often occur:

1 loss of lung volume;
2 displacement of fissures and vascular markings;
3 mediastinal and tracheal shift to the involved side;

Table 99.1 Common abnormalities seen in chest X-rays

Lobar collapse
Lobar consolidation
Barotrauma, especially pneumothorax
Pleural effusions
Pulmonary oedema
Pulmonary embolism or infarction
Abnormal positioning of invasive devices
Mediastinal abnormalities

4 diaphragmatic elevation or obscurity;
5 confluent density within lung substance;
6 rapid improvement following re-expansion.

Lower lobes are most commonly involved, due the pooling of secretions in dependent zones. Distinction between collapse, pleural effusion and consolidation may be difficult. The common causes of lobar collapse are sputum retention and malpositioning of the endotracheal tube (Plate 6). Less extensive areas of collapse may be recognized by plate-like bands of increased density within the lung parenchyma – so-called plate atelectasis. This lesion may also be produced by pulmonary embolism.

Lobar consolidation

Classic lobar consolidation is rarely seen in the critically ill patient. Lung infiltrates are often patchy and may be particularly hard to distinguish aetiologically. Coexistent collapse is common (Plate 3). In general, consolidation has the following features:

1 homogeneous shadowing, confined to segments and bounded by fissures, diaphragm, pleura and chest;
2 no loss of lung volume;
3 air bronchograms;
4 relative constancy from day to day.

The pattern of infiltration often bears little relationship to the likely pathogen, and may be unhelpful in defining the likely pathogen. Secretions or biopsy specimens should be examined for the presence of bacteria or other organisms.

Barotrauma[6] (Plates 7 and 8)

The commonest form of barotrauma is pneumothorax. Important diagnostic features include:

1 a white, visible air–lung interface;
2 mediastinal shift to the opposite side (in tension pneumothoraces);
3 hypertransradiancy of affected hemithorax (looks darker) and lack of lung markings crossing the air–lung interface.

Due to the preponderance of supine X-rays, an anterior or loculated pneumothorax may be missed if unsuspected. Loculated pneumothoraces are common where there has been previous pleural disease. Features of this lesion include:

1 diaphragmatic depression or inversion;
2 deep diaphragmatic sulcus medially or laterally;
3 clear organ borders, indicating an air–organ interface.

One should be careful about diagnosing pseudopneumothoraces (Plate 9). Since most ICU films are performed supine, the skin–film cassette interface may produce what looks like a pneumothorax. This is easily differentiated from a true pneumothorax by the presence of lung markings traversing the area, its bilaterality and the ill-defined nature of the lesion (i.e. not a clear air–lung interface). If a pneumothorax is suspected but not proven on a standard X-ray, a lateral decubitus film or thoracic computed tomographic (CT) scan may identify the lesion. In an emergency, a large-bore IV cannula or intercostal catheter should be inserted into the chest cavity without confirmatory X-ray.

Other less important forms of barotrauma are due to air leaking from major airways into the mediastinum or subcutaneous tissues. The characteristic feel of subcutaneous air (surgical emphysema) is noted (Plate 10) and is usually of no consequence. Its presence should prompt the exclusion of true pneumothorax. Occasionally, the degree of pharyngeal swelling produced by extravasated gas may make intubation difficult.

Pleural effusion (Plate 11)

The hallmarks of a pleural effusion include:

1 fluid meniscus;
2 homogeneous white density;
3 diaphragmatic and cardiac obscurity;
4 no loss of hemithoracic volume;
5 possible shift of the mediastinum away from a large effusion.

These criteria are best seen with the patient in the erect position. In the supine position, if mobile, the fluid tracks posteriorly, and a meniscus may not be seen. In this case, a ground-glass appearance to the hemithorax may give a clue. A lateral decubitus film should show a fluid level. Whilst ultrasound may help identify fluid, CT scanning is the preferred examination, as it will also demonstrate underlying lung pathology and possible sites for diagnostic aspiration.

Pulmonary oedema

One of the commonest pulmonary abnormalities is pulmonary oedema (Plate 12). This may be cardiac in origin, or non-cardiac (e.g. acute respiratory distress syndrome, ARDS; Plate 13). The distinction clinically is often difficult, even with the aid of the pulmonary artery catheter. Several radiological features in the erect CXR may help to differentiate these entities with a modest degree of certainty (Table 99.2).[7]

Table 99.2 Radiological features of cardiac and non-cardiac pulmonary oedema

Radiological feature	Cardiac	Non-cardiac
Distribution of blood flow	Upper zone increased	Normal
Distribution of infiltrates	Basal, hilar	Patchy
Width of vascular pedicle	Normal–wide	Normal
Pulmonary blood volume	Normal–increased	Normal
Peribronchial cuffing	Common	Rare
Septal lines	Common	Rare
Pleural effusions	Common	Rare
Air bronchograms	Rare	Common
Cardiac size	Enlarged	Normal

All criteria taken into account are highly predictive in discriminating the type of oedema present, although each in isolation has less value.

Pulmonary embolism (PE)

In the diagnosis of PE, the plain CXR serves primarily to exclude other pathology. Patchy areas of atelectasis are often seen in submassive PE, but are non-specific. Areas of infarction usually occur peripherally, but are uncommon, and may be confused with consolidation or collapse. Pulmonary oligaemia may be identified in massive PE as a segmental or lobar reduction in blood flow and relative lack of vascular shadowing in the affected areas. Distinction between this and other common pulmonary diseases (e.g. emphysema) make these signs non-specific. Other diagnostic procedures are more reliable (e.g. nuclear imaging). The definitive diagnosis is by a pulmonary angiogram. This is best performed within 48 h, and requires the patient be moved to the radiology department (see Chapter 30).

Positioning of invasive devices (Plates 4, 6 and 10)

Common invasive devices include endotracheal and nasogastric tubes, as well as central venous, pulmonary artery and aortic balloon pump lines. Malpositioning of these devices can lead to vascular erosion and inadvertent instillation of enteral feeds and other solutions into the bronchial tree.

The tip of the endotracheal tube (ETT) changes in position during neck movements. With the neck in extension the tip should be 7 ± 2 cm above the carina. In flexion, the tip should lie 3 ± 2 cm above this point. If the ETT is in too far, obstruction of the left main and/or right upper lobe bronchi may occur.[5]

The nasogastric tube ideally should be radiopaque and traced into the stomach. Occasionally, the tube can follow the ETT into the bronchi without any obvious clinical manifestation (Plate 4). Any difficulties with nasogastric tube placement should alert one to the possibility of malposition and a confirmatory CXR should be performed.

Complications of central venous catheters (CVC) include pneumothorax, cardiac arrhythmias, venous erosion into the mediastinum and erosion into the pericardium with acute tamponade. To avoid these, the tip of the CVC should be identified by CXR to be in the superior vena cava above the pericardial reflection, clearly separated from the vessel wall. Most cases of vascular erosion are associated with placement via the left subclavian, left jugular or antecubital approach (Plate 8). These should be avoided where possible.

Pulmonary artery catheters should be placed with the tip identified in a main pulmonary artery or large branch to avoid inadvertent pulmonary infarction. Clues to such malpositions include intermittent wedge pressure tracing and minimal air needed to wedge the catheter. Under these conditions, excessive balloon inflation may lead to rupture of the pulmonary artery.

Aortic counterpulsation balloon catheters should be placed with the tip just distal to the origin of the left subclavian artery. Like ETTs, catheter position can change with variation in posture.

Cardiac assessment

Cardiac size is difficult to assess on a mobile CXR. The technique used tends to exaggerate the cardiac size, and this can change from film to film quite dramatically. Occasional valvular calcification may be seen on the anteroposterior film, but is better detected with departmental studies and lateral projection. Pulmonary oedema may help identify heart disease. Cardiac structure and function are better assessed with ultrasound or radionuclide studies.

Mediastinal abnormalities

The mediastinum may be damaged in thoracic trauma, with consequent venous and aortic injury (Plate 14). Radiological signs raising the possibility of traumatic aortic dissection include:[8]

1 haemothorax;
2 fracture of the first three ribs;
3 pleural capping in apices (due to blood in pleural cavity in the supine position);
4 mediastinal widening;
5 loss of aortic knuckle;
6 depression of the left main bronchus;
7 deviation of the nasogastric tube to the right.

As a rule of thumb, if both first ribs are fractured, contrast aortography or CT scanning of the aorta is indicated. The absence of mediastinal haematoma on CT excludes major vascular injury (see Chapter 68).

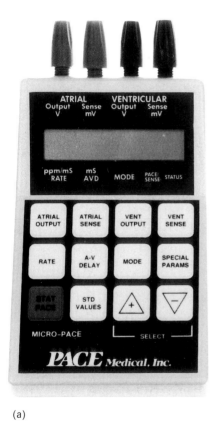

(a)

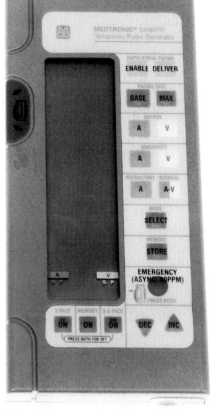

(b)

Plate 1 External DDD pacemakers. (a) Pace Medical (model 4553); (b) Medtronic (model 5346^DDD).

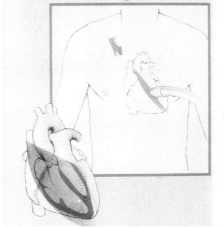

Parasternal Long Axis View

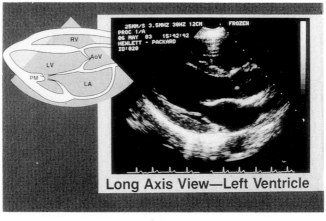

Long Axis View—Left Ventricle

(a)

Parasternal Short Axis Views

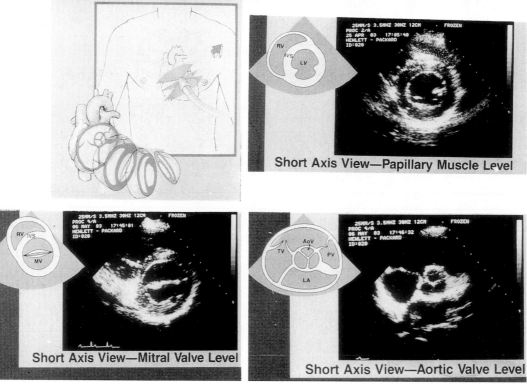

Short Axis View—Papillary Muscle Level

Short Axis View—Mitral Valve Level

Short Axis View—Aortic Valve Level

(b)

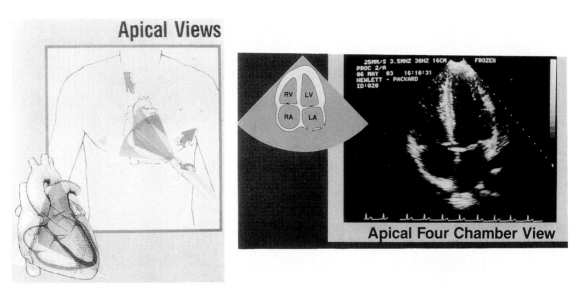

(c)

Plate 2 Two-dimensional transthoracic echocardiogram views. (a) Parasternal long-axis view; (b) parasternal short-axis view; (c) apical view. RV = Right ventricle; LV = left ventricle; AoV = aortic valve; PM = papillary muscle; LA = left atrium; IVS = interventricular septum; MV = mitral valve; TV = tricuspid valve; PV = pulmonary valve; LV = left ventricle. Ultrasound images courtesy of Hewlett-Packard.

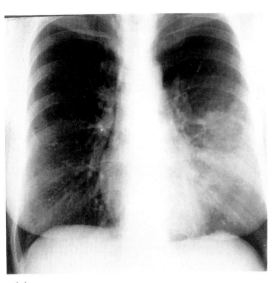

(a)

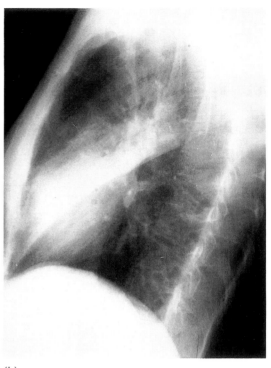

(b)

Plate 3 (a,b) Lingular lobe collapse/consolidation. The left heart border is obscured.

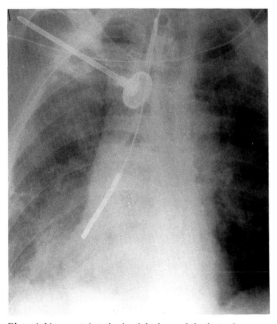

Plate 4 Nasogastric tube in right lower lobe bronchus.
There is an associated left lower lobe patchy consolidation
due to feeding through the tube.

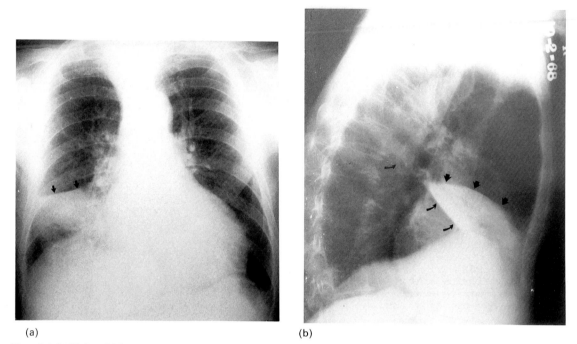

(a)   (b)

Plate 5 (a,b) Right middle lobe collapse and consolidation. Curved arrows indicate elevation of oblique fissure. Short straight arrows show depressed longitudinal fissure.

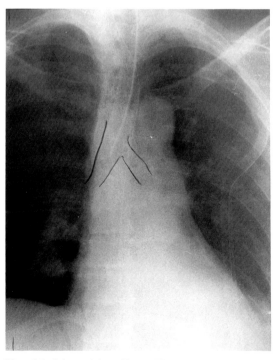

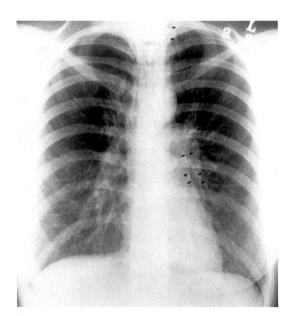

Plate 6 Left lower lobe collapse. The endotracheal tube is in the right main bronchus.

Plate 7 Mediastinal emphysema. Arrows show air tracking along the left pleuropericardial outline, crossing the aortic knuckle and into the neck.

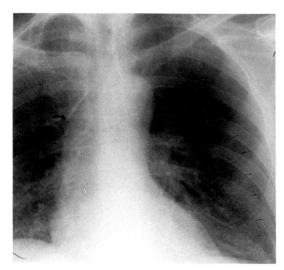

Plate 8 Left pneumothorax and malposition of the central venous catheter. Note the white line (short straight arrows) outlining the left side of the pneumothorax. The tip of the central line abuts the lateral wall of the superior vena cava (curved arrow). This is common when inserted from the left subclavian approach, and can cause vascular perforation.

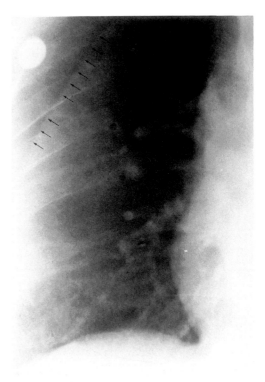

Plate 9 Pseudopneumothorax. Arrows outline the skin–film cassette interface. Vessels can be seen crossing this area.

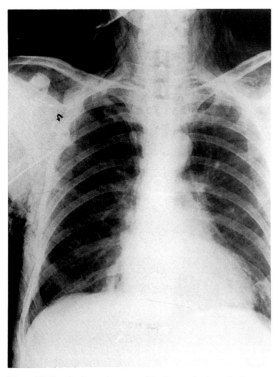

Plate 10 Surgical emphysema. Black streaks in soft tissues indicate air leak. Note that the intercostal catheter (curved arrow) lies subcutaneously outside the pleural cavity.

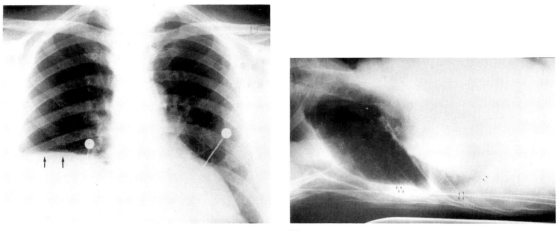

(a)   (b)

Plate 11 Right subpulmonary effusion. (a) Is it a raised diaphragm (vertical arrows)? (b) Free fluids is confirmed in the right decubitus position (short arrows).

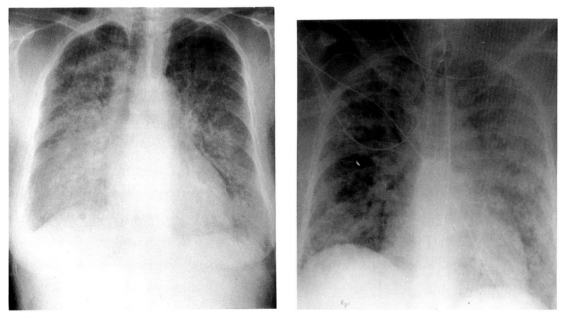

Plate 12 Cardiogenic pulmonary oedema. Note the small bilateral pleural effusion.

Plate 13 Non-cardiogenic pulmonary oedema. It is difficult to differentiate from cardiac oedema, but note the absence of radiologically detectable pleural fluid.

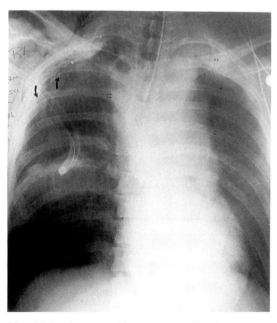

Plate 14 Aortic rupture. Short arrows outline the widened mediastinum. Curved arrows show right rib fracture associated with pneumothorax and surgical emphysema. Note the haemothorax at left apex (BB).

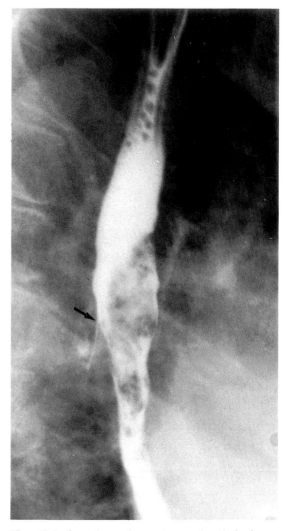

Plate 15 Perforated oesophagus. Arrows show leak of Gastrografin from a perforation secondary to nasogastric tube placement in an obstructed oesophagus (due to food bolus).

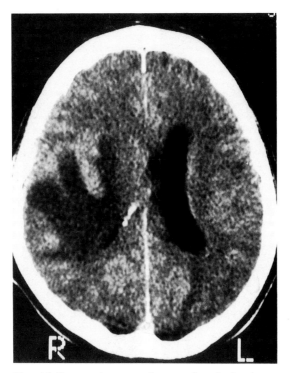

Plate 16 Computed tomography scan of cerebral oedema. Note the frond-like low-density areas in the right parietal lobe causing compression of the ipsilateral lateral ventricle and hydrocephalus of the opposite lateral ventricle.

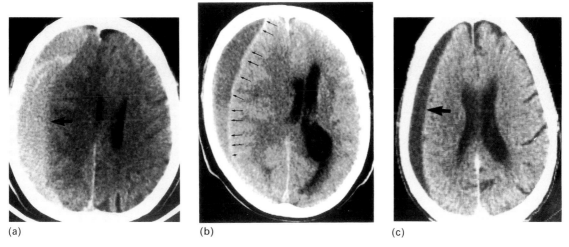

(a)　　　　　　　　　(b)　　　　　　　　　(c)

Plate 17 Subdural haematoma. (a) Dense collection of acute subdural haematoma. (b) Less dense collection of subacute haematoma and membrane enhancement. Note the space effect with shift across the midline of the lateral ventricles. (c) Low-density collection of chronic subdural haematoma.

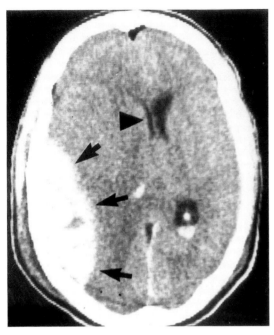

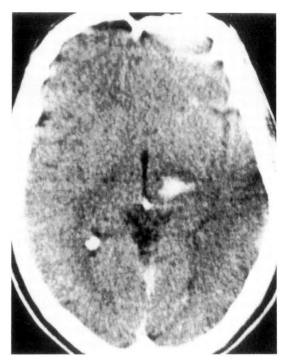

Plate 18 Extradural haematoma. Lentiform shape of an acute extradural collection (arrows). Note space effect (arrow head).

Plate 19 Intracerebral haemorrhage. Acute haemorrhage of left thalamus, commonly seen in hypertensives.

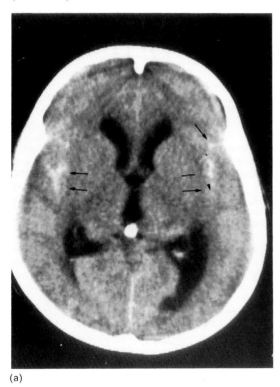

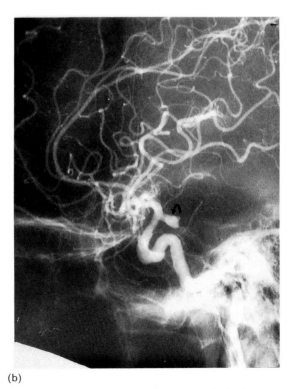

(a)

(b)

Plate 20 Subarachnoid haemorrhage. (a) Computed tomography scan shows fresh blood in sylvian cisterns. (b) Angiogram shows posterior communicating artery aneurysm as the cause of the event.

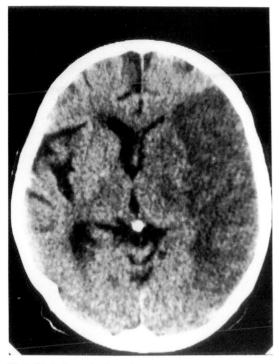

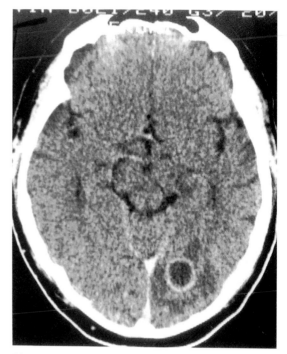

Plate 21 Left cerebral non-haemorrhagic infarct. Note the low-density area involving territory of the left middle cerebral artery with compression of the ipsilateral ventricle due to oedema.

Plate 22 Cerebral abscess; enhanced ring lesion in the left occipital lobe. This appearance cannot be differentiated from tumour.

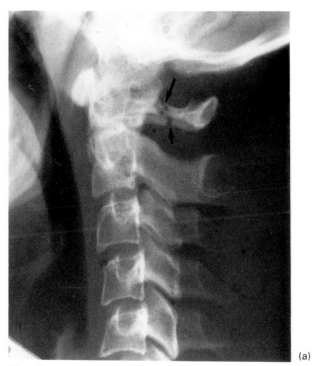

(a)

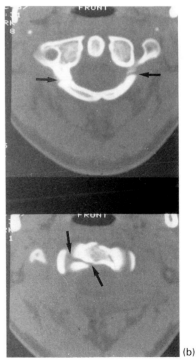

(b)

Plate 23 Cervical fracture. (a) Fracture of C2 lamina on the plain lateral film. (b) Computed tomography shows, in addition to this fracture, another one involving the vertebral body, making the fracture unstable.

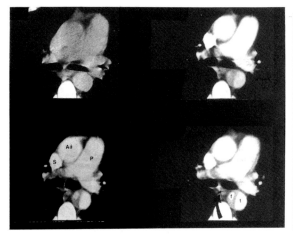

Plate 24 Thoracic aortic dissection. A dynamic scan through the aorta at the level of the pulmonary arteries, taken 5 s apart following intravenous contrast. s = Superior vena cava; Aa = ascending aorta; p = pulmonary conus; f = false lumen; t = true lumen in descending aorta.

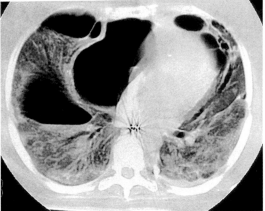

Plate 25 Computed tomography scan of patient with acute respiratory distress syndrome showing multiple loculated pneumothoraces not apparent on the chest X-ray shown in Plate 13.

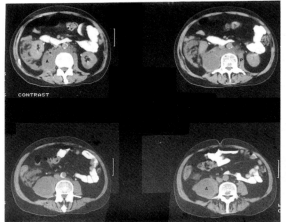

Plate 26 Computed tomography scan of psoas abscess. Note the larger right psoas muscle compared to the normal psoas (P). A = Abscess.

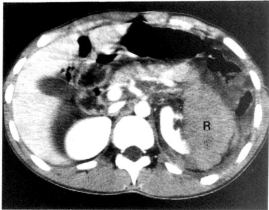

Plate 27 Computed tomography scan of left renal rupture. Note the contrast enhancing kidneys. There is a perinephric haematoma surrounding rupture (R).

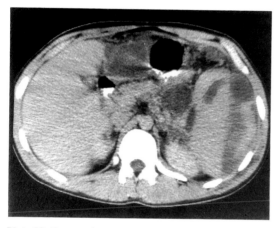

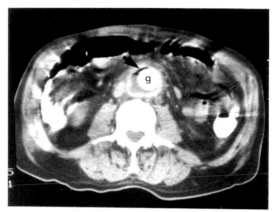

Plate 28 Computed tomography scan of splenic rupture. Note the low mixed density along the lateral aspect of a swollen spleen. This represents the vertical rupture line and associated haemorrhage.

Plate 29 Computed tomography scan of periaortic graft abscess. g = Blood in the lumen of graft. Arrow indicates gas in perigraft (native aorta).

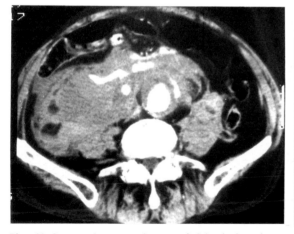

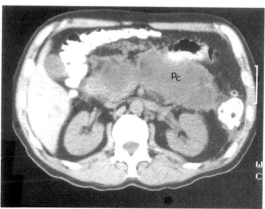

Plate 30 Computed tomography scan of abdominal aortic aneurysm rupture. Contrast (white areas) is seen leaking into the retroperitoneum.

Plate 31 Computed tomography scan of pancreatic pseudocyst (pc).

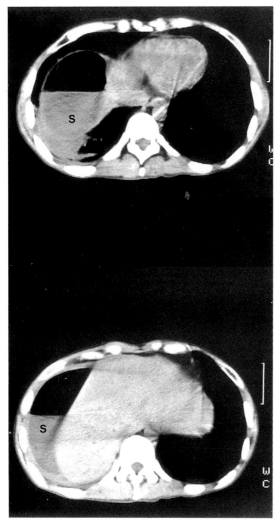

Plate 32 Computed tomography scan of subphrenic collection. Note the air–fluid level. s = Subphrenic abscess.

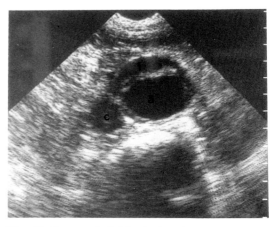

Plate 33 Ultrasound of abdominal aortic aneurysm. f = False lumen; a = true lumen; c = inferior vena cava.

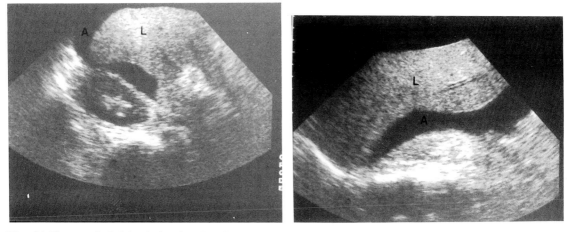

Plate 34 Ultrasound of abdominal ascites. L = Liver; A = ascites.

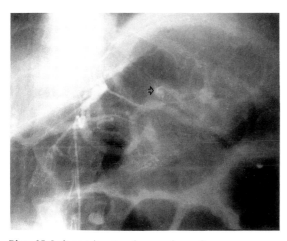

Plate 35 Left gastric artery haemorrhage. Open arrow shows pool of contrast extravasation from left gastric arterial branch (successfully embolized with gelfoam).

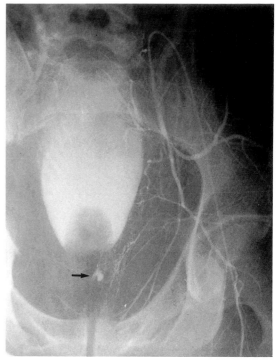

Plate 36 Pelvic haemorrhage. Note the multiple fractures of pubic rami and right acetabulum. Selective angiography shows pool of contrast arising from vesical artery laceration. The bladder is 'squeezed' by pelvic haematoma. Bleeding has been successfully embolized and controlled.

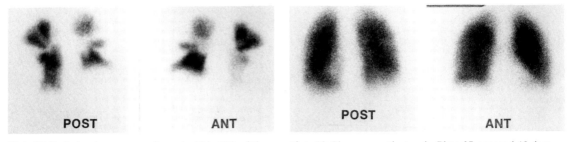

Plate 37 Perfusion lung scan performed within 12 h of the development of bilateral pleuritic chest pain. Multiple segmental perfusion defects, indicative of pulmonary emboli, are evident. POST = Posterior; ANT = anterior.

Plate 38 The same patient as in Plate 37, scanned 10 days later. Note the almost complete resolution of perfusion. POST = Posterior; ANT = anterior.

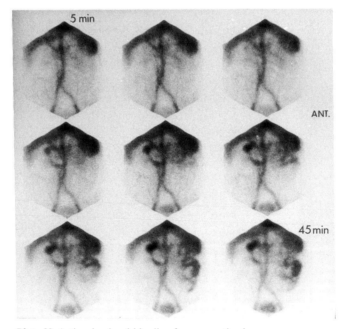

Plate 39 Active duodenal bleeding from a peptic ulcer, showing extravasation of technetium 99m-labelled red blood cells within the small intestine.

Contrast-enhanced radiography

Radiopaque contrast (intravenous or other) may enhance the sensitivity and specificity of conventional radiographs but, like any drug, may produce significant side-effects. These include:

1 anaphylaxis (with an approximate death rate 1:40 000);
2 renal failure, particularly in patients with volume depletion, with multiple myeloma, and diabetics with diabetic nephropathy;
3 extravasation into body cavities – related to type of contrast.

Attention to these possibilities, particularly the nephrotoxicity of some agents, will reduce morbidity related to their use. Newer, more expensive contrast agents may be less nephrotoxic, and worth discussing with a radiologist beforehand. Before these agents are given IV, one should ensure that the patient is adequately hydrated, as this will reduce the incidence of renal failure and possible post-procedural dehydration caused by the osmotic diuresis from the agents. Hydration should be maintained following the procedure.

Common IV contrast procedures include IV pyelography, angiography, venography and CT.

Other procedures involving (non-IV) contrast include Gastrografin swallow (Plate 15), which is useful to exclude an oesophageal or gastic perforation quickly, and cystography to exclude a ruptured bladder.

Computed tomography

CT scanning has revolutionized the investigation of head-injured patients. In addition, it may offer significant advantages in the identification of chest and abdominal pathology in the critically ill. The presence of metallic foreign bodies or movement interferes with image generation, and predictable degradation of picture quality can be anticipated. CT scanning, like any other imaging procedure, requires the patient to be haemodynamically stable, as he or she may be out of the ICU for a considerable period of time.

Cranial CT

CT of the head gives information about the brain substance and skull. Lesions well-delineated include:

1 cerebral oedema (Plate 16);
2 hemispheric shift and space effect (Plate 17);
3 hydrocephalus (Plate 16);
4 subdural haematomata (Plate 17);
5 extradural haematomata (Plate 18);

6 intracerebral haematomata (Plate 19);
7 subarachnoid haemorrhage (Plate 20);
8 non-haemorrhagic and haemorrhagic infarction (Plate 21);
9 skull fracture and foreign bodies (e.g. bullet wounds).

Detection of non-basal simple skull fractures can be extremely difficult and time consuming. Plain skull X-rays are more useful in this regard. CT, however, is very sensitive in detecting intracranial pathology, in contrast to plain skull X-rays, and will show the complications of skull fractures, which are more relevant in neurosurgical assessment.[9]

In general, most studies can be performed without IV contrast. If a cerebral tumour or abscess is suspected, contrast should be given, as small lesions may be missed (Plate 22). As a rule of thumb, intracranial fresh blood looks white, cerebrospinal fluid looks black, and oedema is darker than brain substance.

CT of cervical spine (Plate 23)

Specific regions of the cervical spine can be imaged whilst undergoing cranial CT, and should be considered when inadequate plain X-rays are obtained. This may reduce the time wasted identifying unstable cervical spine fractures. When the status of the cervical spine is unknown, full precautions should be undertaken to prevent spinal cord injury during patient transfer.

CT of thorax

Thoracic CT gives detailed anatomical information about most forms of thoracic pathology. In addition, it will discriminate between fluid and lung tissue accurately, and aid in the placement of pleural catheters. Contrast-enhanced CT aortography may identify dissection without the need for further investigation (Plate 24). In patients with poor pulmonary compliance and deteriorating lung function, a CT scan of the lungs can reveal significant information such as loculated pneumothoraces which can be easily missed on conventional supine chest X-ray (Plate 25). Chest CT scans have also been used to derive lung densities, lung tissue mass and percentage of aerated to non-aerated tissue,[10] to quantify lung bullae,[11] and to study lung structure in ARDS.[11] Used in this way, atelectasis in acute respiratory failure[10] and ARDS[12] has been demonstrated to be gravity-dependent.

CT of abdomen (Plates 26–32)

The sensitivity and specificity of CT in this region are dependent on the type of pathology suspected. CT will identify lesions in the liver, biliary tree and pancreas with a high degree of accuracy. The presence of a large, swollen pancreas on CT may help to prevent unnecessary laparotomy in an unstable patient with an acute abdomen. The retroperitoneal structures are also accurately assessed with CT. Intravenous contrast helps identify vascular structures and the renal parenchyma.

Pathology (e.g. abscess) within loops of bowel is notoriously difficult to identify with CT, and usually laparotomy is the investigation of choice. Reasons for the reduced sensitivity include the inability to introduce contrast within the lumen of the small and large bowel due to ileus or local pathology. It should be remembered that instillation of large volumes of contrast into the stomach may induce vomiting, resulting in pulmonary aspiration. In addition, contrast agents are hyperosmolar, causing transudation of fluid into the gut lumen in ileus.

CT of other sites

As an adjunct to conventional radiology, CT may aid in the identification of fractures and soft-tissue injuries. Major fractures of the face, spine and pelvis are well-delineated with CT. Metal fixtures and pins sometime preclude CT scanning of the affected region.

Ultrasound examinations (Plates 33 and 34)

Ultrasound examination is a non-invasive form of organ imaging, with considerable appeal. Its advantages include minimal risk to patients, no radiation exposure and good diagnostic specificity in selected types of pathology. The advent of portable ultrasound equipment has meant that these examinations may be carried out at the bedside, without the need to move the critically ill patient out of the ICU. An ultrasound examination is critically operator-dependent.

Ultrasound may help identify pathology in the following organs with a high degree of accuracy:

1 liver and biliary tree;
2 pancreas;
3 renal tract;
4 pelvic structures;
5 pleural, abdominal and pelvic fluid collections.

In general, ultrasound and CT are complementary investigations, and have increased diagnostic accuracy together in comparison to when used alone. Cardiac ultrasound is discussed in Chapter 21.

Therapeutic radiology (Plates 35 and 36)

An advantage of radiology includes the ability not only to identify pathology, but also to treat it. Specific instances include:

1 drainage of abscesses or other body fluids;
2 insertion of drains (e.g. percutaneous nephrostomy);
3 embolization of arteries to control haemorrhage.

Specifically, the percutaneous drainage of abscesses by insertion of catheters may be performed with the aid of CT or ultrasound. The major application of this technique is in the management of abdominal sepsis. If an abscess is loculated, the likelihood of complete percutaneous drainage is significantly reduced and may delay definitive surgical drainage. Drainage of subphrenic and intrahepatic abscesses, as well as insertion of percutaneous nephrostomies, is commonly performed.

Embolization of major arteries with gelfoam or other agents for the control of massive gastrointestinal or traumatic retroperitoneal or pelvic haemorrhage may be life-saving.[1,2] The role of barium studies is limited, and is not recommended if angiography is envisaged. With modern superselective angiography, bleeding as little as 0.5 ml/min may be detected. Infusion of vasopressors may control bleeding in 90% of cases. Embolization is only safe if there is good collateral supply (e.g. left gastric and gastroduodenal arteries). For lower gastrointestinal tract haemorrhage,[13] a double-contrast barium study should be performed at some stage when the patient is stable, to exclude specific lesions, such as diverticular disease, carcinoma or polyps (see Chapters 35 and 56).

The cervical spine

Correct management of trauma includes the identification of significant injury to the cervical spine (see Chapter 69). The unconscious or head-injured patient may not have any clinical evidence of this likelihood, and thus correct and complete radiological examination of the cervical spine is mandatory, to prevent spinal cord damage. A complete cervical spine X-ray series should, at a bare minimum, include views including T1 in both the anteroposterior and lateral projection. If possible, oblique views should be taken as well. The absence of an unstable fracture/dislocation can only be confidently excluded when the above films are taken. T1 may be particularly difficult to image in the bull-necked or muscular patient. Caudal traction applied to the arms during exposure may help, as may a 'swimmer's' view, with one arm raised above the head. The procedure should be discussed with the radiographer or radiologist.

Conventional tomography for ICU patients is now almost never used. If a fracture needs further evaluation, CT scanning is more appropriate and more cost-effective.

Magnetic resonance imaging

Magnetic resonance imaging has surpassed conventional CT scanning in the neurological patient. However, its place in the acute investigation of head injury is limited.[14] Further refinements in patient monitoring equipment will need to occur before this modality can be considered a routine investigation in the critically ill. CT scanning will remain the prime investigation in head injury for the immediate future.

References

1. Oddson TA, Johnrude IS, Jackson DC and Rice RP (1978) Acute gastrointestinal hemorrhage. *Radiol Clin North Am* **16**:123–133.

2. Keller FS and Rosch J (1988) Embolization of acute gastric and duodenal hemmorrhage. *Semin Interventional Radiol* **5**:25–38.

3. Sutton D (ed.) (1980) *Textbook of Radiology and Imaging*, 3rd edn. London: Churchill Livingstone.

4. Kreel L (ed.) (1971) *Outline of Radiology*. London: William Heinemann.

5. Umali CB and Smith EH (1985) The chest radiologic examination. In: Rippe JM, Alpert JS and Dalen JE (eds) *Intensive Care Medicine*, 1st edn. Boston: Little, Brown, pp. 483–510.

6. Buckner CB, Harman BH and Pallin JS (1988) The radiology of abnormal intrathoracic air. *Curr Probl Diagnostic Radiol* **27**:49–68.

7. Milne ENC, Pistolesi M, Miniati M and Giuntini C (1985) The radiological distinction of cardiogenic and non-cardiogenic edema. *Am J Radiol* **144**:879–894.

8. American College of Surgeons, Committee on Trauma (1984) *Advanced Trauma Life Support Course (Student Manual)*. Chicago: American College of Surgeons, pp. 78–79.

9. Thornbury JR, Masters SJ and Campbell JA (1987) Imaging recommendations for head trauma. *Am J Radiol* **149**:781–783.

10. Gattinoni L, Pelosi P, Vitale G, Pesenti A, D'Andrea L and Mascheroni D (1991) Body position changes redistribute lung computed density in patients with acute respiratory failure. *Anesthesiology* **74**:15–25.

11. Gattinoni L, Bombino M, Pelosi P *et al.* (1994) Lung structure and function in different stages of severe adult respiratory distress syndrome. *J Am Med Assoc* **271**:1772–1779.

12. Pelosi P, D'Andrea L, Vitale G, Pesenti A and Gattinoni L (1994) Vertical gradient of regional lung inflation in adult respiratory distress syndrome. *Am J Respir Crit Care* **149**:8–13.

13. Sebrechts C and Bookstein JJ (1988) Embolisation in the management of lower GI hemorrhage. *Semin Interventional Radiol* **5**:39–47.

14. National Health and Technology Advisory Panel (Australia) (1988) *Consensus Statement on Clinical Efficacy of Nuclear Magnetic Resonance Imaging*. Canberra: AIH.

FTA Lovegrove

Nuclear medicine investigations involve the use of short-lived radioactive isotopes to evaluate the function of particular organ systems.[1,2] The radioactive tracer may be introduced in specific chemical form (radiopharmaceutical) or tagged to a particular body component, such as the leukocyte or erythrocyte.[3] Imaging is performed with a γ-camera, and tomographs can be constructed with computer assistance. Non-imaging tests are performed on fluid samples (e.g. blood), or by using scintillation probes. Technetium 99m (^{99m}Tc) is the commonest isotope used because of its short half-life ($T_{\frac{1}{2}} = 6$ h) and the easily detected γ-ray energy (140 keV). The dose of radiation administered to patients is low, and the radiation-absorbed dose for most procedures is less than that of a conventional computed tomographic (CT) head scan. Repeated examinations incur an insignificant radiation burden. Likewise, the radiation dose to staff in the ICU is minimal. Potentially radioactive waste should be handled in gloves, to decrease radiation exposure further.

Where radioactive gases are used (e.g. ventilation lung scanning), special exhaust facilities are necessary. For most studies, no specific preparation is required. Patient studies are generally performed in multiple projections, for which transfer to a special imaging couch is recommended.

Modern nuclear medicine has a defined place in the investigation and management of the critically ill. The choice of which imaging test to perform (Table 100.1) will involve close liaison between clinician, radiologist and nuclear medicine physician. Often, a group of investigations will have to be performed. Consultation with individual specialists will ensure that the correct examination is carried out with a minimum of delay and hazard to the patient.

Neurological nuclear medicine studies

Cerebral blood flow

To assess cerebral blood flow in subarachnoid haemorrhage, an inhaled diffusible tracer such as xenon 133 allows flow to be assessed (in ml/min per 100 g brain tissue), using appropriate scintillation probes and computer analysis.[4] Hemispheric reduction in cerebral blood flow may be detected by this technique. However, localized flow reductions may be missed. Absence of cerebral blood flow is easily assessed using IV ^{99m}Tc exametazime (HMPAO) or diethylene tetraamine penta-acetic acid (DTPA) and a γ-camera. This technique can be used to corroborate a clinical diagnosis of brainstem death.[5–7] However, its use should be restricted to specific clinical situations where complicating factors exist (e.g. extreme hypothermia or head injury with detectable sedative drugs in serum). These situations are uncommon, as the diagnosis of brainstem death should be based primarily on clinical criteria (see Chapter 45).

Regional blood flow assessment, where the relative flow of one area is compared with another (e.g. in stroke[8] or epilepsy[9]) can be assessed using new brain-imaging agents, iodine 123 amphetamine, ^{99m}Tc HMPAO or ^{99m}Tc ethyl cysteinate dimer (ECD).[10–12] These techniques require computer reconstruction using a γ-camera capable of single-photon emission computed tomographic (SPECT) scanning.[13]

Space-occupying lesions

CT and magnetic resonance scans are the preferred imaging techniques in the assessment of cerebral tumour, abscess and fluid collections.

Table 100.1 Indications for nuclear medicine investigations in intensive care

Neurological

Cerebral blood flow	Spasm in subarachnoid haemorrhage
Regional blood flow	Stroke
	Epilepsy
Space-occupying lesions	Abscess
	Subdural haematoma
	Neoplasia

Respiratory

Perfusion/ventilation	Pulmonary embolus
Alveolar permeability	Acute respiratory distress syndrome

Cardiovascular

Ventricular function	Left and right heart failure
Left ventricular motion	Left ventricular dyskinesis, akinesis
Q_p/Q_s ratio	Left-to-right shunt
Systemic shunt	Right-to-left shunt
Thallium	Ischaemia
± Dipyridamole, adenosine or dobutamine	
± Exercise	
^{99m}Tc pyrophosphate	Myocardial damage

Skeletal

Three-phase bone scan	Infection
	Injury
	Infarction
	Muscle necrosis
Bone scan	Metastases

Renal

Perfusion	Acute tubular necrosis
	Acute cortical necrosis
	Vascular injury
Cortical function	Renal infarction
	Renal trauma

Infection

Gallium	Low-grade infection
	Chronic infection
	Associated prostheses
Labelled leukocytes	Acute soft-tissue infection
	Pelvis infection
	Inflammatory bowel disease

Liver, biliary

^{99m}Tc sulphur colloid	Space-occupying lesions
^{99m}Tc-IDA	Biliary anatomy, function, bile leaks
	Cholecystitis (acute or chronic)

Spleen

Labelled red cells	Trauma

Gastrointestinal

Labelled red cells	Bleeding

Respiratory nuclear medicine studies

Ventilation/perfusion abnormalities

Perfusion of the lungs is simply assessed by IV injection of ^{99m}Tc-labelled microspheres (or macro-aggregates of albumin; MAA). These are distributed to the lungs in proportion to blood flow. Preferential perfusion to the upper zones occurs in pulmonary venous hypertension (as in cardiac failure) and reduced perfusion occurs wherever ventilation is impaired, or where consolidation, collapse, fibrosis or congestion causes localized hypoxia (due to reflex hypoxic pulmonary vasoconstriction).

Pulmonary embolism[14–17] is diagnosed by the presence of segmental perfusion defects (Plates 37 and 38) in the appropriate clinical and radiological setting. The diagnosis is further substantiated by those areas of reduced perfusion having a normal ventilation pattern, assessed with aerosolized tracers or xenon 133.

Ventilation scanning in the critically ill can be difficult, if not impossible, especially when the patient is intubated. The ability for the patient to hold the breath is not required for the performance or interpretation of lung scans.

The diagnostic specificity of ventilation/perfusion ($\dot{V}/\dot{Q}$) lung scanning depends on patient factors, time between onset of illness and examination, and the pattern of abnormality seen on scan. The presence of pre-existing lung disease can make interpretation of $\dot{V}/\dot{Q}$ abnormalities difficult; the commonest problems are the presence of acute or chronic air flow obstruction and/or segmental atelectasis. A probability weighting (for pulmonary embolus) can be assigned to the patient after consideration of these issues.[18,19] Scans may be classified as low, intermediate or high probability for pulmonary embolism. Depending on this result the physician may proceed to impedence plethysmography, Doppler studies, lower limb venography or pulmonary angiography to define pathology. Iodine 131-labelled fibrinogen leg scanning detects thrombus distal to the popliteal fossa, but the significance of this entity is disputed, and probably of less importance than proximal thrombi (see Chapter 30).

Alveolar–capillary permeability

Alveolar permeability can be assessed by recording the clearance rate of ^{99m}Tc DTPA following aerosol inhalation. Permeability is increased in smokers and in diffuse alveolar damage associated with the acute respiratory distress syndrome (ARDS).[20,21]

Infection

Pulmonary inflammation and infection are best assessed by X-ray, but gallium 67 scanning may be used to localize the infective site.[22] In immunocompromised patients with *Pneumocystis carinii* pneumonitis, gallium scans are abnormal when standard chest X-rays are not.[23–26] The place of nuclear medicine techniques in pulmonary infection is, however, limited.

Cardiovascular nuclear medicine studies

Ventricular function

Left (LV) and right (RV) ventricular function may be assessed with nuclear medicine techniques.[27] Measurement of cardiac function depends on the tracer remaining in the blood for a sufficient time for measurement to be complete. If measurements are to be made only during initial transit through the heart, an agent which is subsequently cleared is adequate.[27] However, for most cardiac assessments, a blood pool label is preferred, and the most stable is ^{99m}Tc-labelled red cells.[27] Labelling of red cells is quick and efficient, performed in the laboratory (*in vitro*), patient (*in vivo*) or a combination ('*in vivtro*').

The *in vitro* label is most specific, but labelling efficiencies *in vivo* approach 90%. Accurate estimations of RV and LV ejection fractions are easily performed using portable γ-cameras in the ICU. Ventricular ejection fractions can be calculated by computing the total count rate at end-systole and diastole, having made the appropriate correction for the non-cardiac background.

Calculation of LV volumes and knowing the pulse rate allows derivation of stroke volume indices and cardiac output. Regular assessment of cardiac function by this method has been suggested by some to be invaluable in the management of the critically ill. Changes in ventricular function in these conditions may guide the appropriate fluid and inotrope combinations needed. Prognostic information may be obtained in the setting of acute myocardial ischaemia/ infarction, as well as acute and chronic heart failure.

Wall motion abnormalities

Whilst first-pass dynamics allow calculation of cardiac function, most cardiovascular nuclear medicine uses electrocardiographically gated studies and multiple projections with a γ-camera.[28] By collecting in multiple projections, regional wall motion abnormalities may define focal areas of hypo- or dyskinesis. Stress-induced wall motion abnormalities are an indicator of reversible myocardial ischaemia.

Cardiac perfusion

Perfusion imaging of the heart, utilizing thallium 201[29] or ^{99m}Tc methloxyisobutile isonitrile (MIBI)[30,31] will demonstrate perfusion defects indicative of myocardial ischaemia or infarction. Thallium concentrates in viable myocardium as a result of

active transport via the Na^+/K^+-ATPase system located in the cell membrane. Myocardial infarction appears as an area of low uptake at rest, which is unchanged following exercise. Reversible perfusion defects are seen in areas of ischaemic myocardium, induced by controlled exercise. Exercise thallium scanning increases the sensitivity and specificity of a standard 12-lead exercise electrocardiogram (ECG) in the detection and extent of coronary artery disease, especially where there is a pre-existing ECG abnormality (e.g. left bundle branch block) or where false-positive exercise ECGs are common (e.g. young women with mitral valve prolapse).

A thallium scan following IV administration of the coronary vasodilator dipyridamole has been shown to have similar specificity and sensitivity as exercise thallium scan.[32] This procedure has been used with success in the preoperative screening of patients undergoing major vascular surgery, and in the early phase following myocardial infarction, to determine the additional myocardium at risk, where the incidence of coexistent coronary artery disease is high and where limb claudication prevents a standard treadmill exercise ECG from being performed. Coronary vasodilatation can also be induced using adenosine,[33] and dobutamine[34] has been used to provide pharmacological stress when asthma prevents the safe use of dipyridamole or adenosine.

^{99m}Tc pyrophosphate is taken up preferentially in recently damaged myocardium, and may be seen as an area of increased uptake ('hot-spot' scanning).[35] The test should be performed within 2–6 days following infarction as it reverts to normal after 10 days. The resolution of the images generated is improved with SPECT. Hot-spot scanning is limited to cases where the diagnosis of myocardial infarction is delayed and difficult to make with standard criteria. Positive scans may also be seen following cardiac trauma and high-energy cardioversion, and in some left ventricular aneurysms.

Cardiac shunts

For the assessment of intracardiac shunt, first-pass studies can qualitatively evaluate left-to-right shunt from early recirculation of tracer through the lungs, or right-to-left shunt from tracer bypassing the lungs with increased uptake in the kidneys. Also, particularly with a left-to-right shunt, the shunt can be accurately quantitated in the range:

$$Q_p:Q_s = 1.3{-}3.0$$

where Q_p = pulmonary blood flow and Q_s = systemic blood flow.[36]

Blood volume

Blood volume is assessed by the use of chromium 51-labelled erythrocytes. The patient's red cells are labelled with chromium 51, reinjected and allowed adequate time to mix (at least 15 min, or longer if there is giant splenomegaly).[37] The number of counts in a known volume of sampled red cells is compared to the total counts injected, and the circulating red-cell volume is thus calculated.

Liver, spleen and gastrointestinal studies

Liver anatomy and function

Either reticuloendothelial (Kupffer cell) or parenchymal tracers may be used to assess liver function.[38] Liver anatomy is usually defined with CT or ultrasound scans, but liver abscess, cysts, benign or malignant tumours cause focal defects on technetium sulphur colloid scans; trauma can also be assessed. Hepatobiliary agents (Tc IDA agents) demonstrate parenchymal function and biliary excretion, and are valuable in the delineation of biliary leaks, partial biliary obstruction or cystic duct obstruction associated with acute cholecystitis.[39-41] These investigations may complement endoscopy, ultrasound, CT and laparotomy in the management of the acute abdomen. With the appropriate clinical picture of acute cholecystitis, the sensitivity of cholescintigraphy in confirming the diagnosis approaches 100%. False-positive cholescintigrams may be seen in alcoholic liver disease, chronic cholecystitis, cholelithiasis and in patients receiving parenteral nutrition, because of prolonged fasting.[42-44]

Spleen imaging

The spleen may be imaged separately using ^{99m}Tc sulphur colloid or, preferably, heat-damaged ^{99m}Tc-labelled red cells, which sequester in the spleen rapidly after injection, corresponding to local blood supply. The high spleen-to-background ratio makes this test ideal for identifying small areas of splenic trauma, and the technique is especially suited in the absence of active spleen bleeding, when the patient is haemodynamically stable.[45]

Gastrointestinal bleed

Where active gastointestinal haemorrhage cannot be localized by endoscopy, the extravasation of labelled red blood cells (^{99m}Tc-RBC) will be discernible, when bleeding rates are in excess of 0.1 ml/min (Plate 39; see Chapter 35). Because bleeding may be intermittent, the test may need to be prolonged over at least 1 h. Broad localization of the bleeding site is of value, even when radiographic contrast angiography is being considered. Contrast angiography is less sensitive, even when selective angiography can be undertaken.[46,47]

Infection

Focal infection, not demonstrable by conventional imaging techniques, may be identified with the aid of either gallium 67 citrate (a non-specific but sensitive indicator of inflammation)[48] or indium 111 or ^{99m}Tc-labelled leukocytes.[49] With gallium scanning, the tracer physiologically accumulates in the liver, spleen and colon, making assessment of these areas difficult. The taking of multiple images up to 48 h after injection of the tracer may be required. For chronic low-grade infection, gallium 67 is likely to yield abnormal images. Bone and joint infections require comparison with standard ^{99m}Tc methylene diphosphonate bone scans.[50] Similarly, intrahepatic abscesses should be compared with a standard ^{99m}Tc liver scan.

More acute soft-tissue infections, inflammatory bowel disease and pelvic inflammation are better assessed using radiolabelled leukocytes.[51] Leukocyte studies have the advantage of being completed on the same day as requested, but the technique is less sensitive for chronic infection and requires a laboratory which is skilled and equipped for the preparation of labelled cells.

Renal nuclear medicine studies

Renal perfusion

The radiopharmaceuticals used for most renal studies are ^{99m}Tc DTPA, a chelate preferentially excreted by glomerular filtration, and ^{99m}Tc MAG3, which also has tubular excretion and gives better contrast in impaired renal function.

Demonstration of preserved renal blood flow in the setting of oliguria and rising serum creatinine is strongly suggestive – although not absolutely diagnostic – of acute tubular necrosis.[52] Absence of renal perfusion in the anuric patient signifies irreversible cortical necrosis, which may aid prognostication and future management.[53]

The sequelae of renal vascular damage secondary to trauma can be assessed, but its place in acute investigation/management is limited. Abdominal CT, angiography and laparotomy are currently the favoured investigations. More specific renal cortical pharmaceuticals such as ^{99m}Tc dimercaptosuccinic acid (DMSA) or ^{99m}Tc gluconate allow assessment of focal cortical abnormalities.[54]

Musculoskeletal nuclear medicine studies

Bone scans

The use of bone scanning to detect alterations in musculoskeletal blood flow, soft tissue and bone metabolism, dominates most nuclear medicine departments.[55,56] The bone scan is performed to evaluate focal alteration in metabolism, and complements standard X-ray definition of anatomy. The initial pattern of blood flow and tissue phase is assessed at the time of injection of ^{99m}Tc methylene diphosphonate (MDP). Reduced uptake is seen in infarction, the early phase of avascular necrosis (the late phase may show increased uptake due to a healing reaction) and a minority of tumours, multiple myeloma being the commonest. Most tumours are associated with increased uptake, due to a remodelling reaction.

In osteomyelitis, there is an early increase in blood flow, with focal increased uptake of tracer within 1–2 days of onset. Rarely, an initial scan may be negative. A repeat scan in 4–5 days may show the lesions. Unfortunately, standard ^{99m}Tc MDP bone scanning fails to differentiate between osteomyelitis and bone healing. The addition of gallium 67 scanning helps solve this clinical problem.[57] The pattern in septic arthritis is less specific, with diffuse periarticular uptake being enhanced in most cases, and reduced regional uptake occurring when the joint has increased intraarticular pressure.

Undisplaced fracture, such as femoral neck or trochanter fracture, and insufficiency fractures of the pelvis show increased blood flow and uptake within 2–5 days. In flat bones (skull), uptake is much less because of the lack of a healing reaction in the absence of stress.

Muscle necrosis

Necrosis of skeletal muscle is associated with increased soft-tissue uptake of all bone-scanning agents. However, ^{99m}Tc imidodiphosphonate or pyrophosphate may be more appropriate soft-tissue phase radiopharmaceuticals.[58]

References

1. Murray IPC and Ell PJ (eds) (1995) *Nuclear Medicine in Clinical Diagnosis and Treatment*, vols 1 and 2. Edinburgh: Churchill Livingstone.
2. Maisey MN, Britton KE and Gilday DL (eds) *Clinical Nuclear Medicine*, 2nd edn. London: Chapman and Hall.
3. Sampson CB (ed.) (1994) *Textbook of Radiopharmacy*, 2nd edn. Amsterdam: Gordon and Breach Science.
4. Mountz JM, McGillicuddy JT, Wilson MW, Bartold SP and Siegel EM (1991) Pre and post operative cerebral blood flow changes in subarachnoid haemorrhage. *Acta Neurochirurg* **109**:30–33.
5. Wilson K, Gordon L and Selby JB (1993) The diagnosis of brain death with technetium 99m HMPAO. *Clin Nucl Med* **18**:428–434.
6. Goodman JM, Heck LL and Moore BD (1985) Confirmation of brain death with portable isotope angiography: a review of 204 consecutive cases. *Neurosurgery* **16**:492–497.
7. Adelstein W (1994) Confirmation of brain death using 99m technetium HMPAO. *J Neurosci Nursing* **26**:118–120.
8. Shimosegawa T, Hatazawa J, Inugami A *et al.* (1994) Cerebral infarction within 6 hours of onset: prediction of completed infarction with technetium-99m-HMPAO SPECT. *J Nucl Med* **35**:1097–1103.
9. Kuikka JT and Berkovic SF (1994) Localisation of epileptic foci by single photon emission tomography with new radiotracers. *Eur J Nucl Med* **21**:1173–1174.
10. Kuhl DE, Barrio JR, Hung SC *et al.* (1982) Quantifying local cerebral blood flow by N isoprofile P [I 123] iodoamphetamine (IMP) tomography. *J Nucl Med* **23**:196–203.
11. Morreti JM, Tamgac F, Weinmann P *et al.* (1994) Early and delayed brain SPECT with technetium 99m ECD and iodine 123 IMP in subacute strokes. *J Nucl Med* **35**:1444–1449.
12. Leveille J, Demonceau G and Walovich RC (1992) Intrasubject comparison between technetium 99m ECD and technetium 99m HMPAO in healthy human subjects. *J Nucl Med* **33**:480–484.
13. Holman BL and Devous MD Snr (1992) Functional brain SPECT: the emergence of a powerful clinical method. *J Nucl Med* **33**:1888–1904.
14. Wellman HN (1986) Pulmonary thromboembolism: current status report on the role of nuclear medicine. *Semin Nucl Med* **16**:236–274.
15. PIOPED investigators (1990) Value of the ventilation/perfusion scan in acute pulmonary embolism: results of the prospective investigation of pulmonary embolism diagnosis (PIOPED). *J Am Med Assoc* **263**:2753–2759.
16. Broaddus C and Matthay MA (1986) Pulmonary embolism. Guide to diagnosis treatment and prevention. *Postgrad Med* **79**:340–343.
17. Biello DR, Mattar AG, McKnight RC and Segal BA (1979) Ventilation-perfusion studies in suspected pulmonary embolism. *Am J Venography* **133**:1033–1037.
18. Hull RD, Hirsch J, Carter CJ *et al.* (1983) Pulmonary angiography, ventilation lung scanning, and venography for clinically suspected pulmonary embolism with abnormal perfusion lung scan. *Ann Intern Med* **98**:891.
19. Murray IPC (1991) Clinical experience with technegas. *Clin Nucl Med* **16**:247–250.
20. Coates G and O'Brodovich H (1986) Measurement of pulmonary permeability with technetium-99m DTPA aerosol. *Semin Nucl Med* **16**:275–284.
21. Coates G, O'Brodovich H and Dolobich M (1988) Lung clearance of technetium 99mTc DTPA in patients with acute lung injury and pulmonary oedema. *J Thorac Imaging* **3**:21–27.
22. Picard C, Meignan M, Ross J *et al.* (1987) Technetium-99m DTPA aerosol and gallium scanning in acquired immune deficiency syndrome. *Clin Nucl Med* **12**:501–506.
23. Kramer EL, Sanger JJ, Garay SM *et al.* (1987) Gallium-67 scans of the chest in patients with acquired immune deficiency syndrome. *J Nucl Med* **28**:1107–1114.
24. Bitran J, Bekerman C, Weinstein R *et al.* (1987) Patterns of gallium 67 scintigraphy in patients with acquired immunodeficiency syndrome and the AIDS related complex. *J Nucl Med* **28**:1103–1106.

25. Woolfenden JM, Carrasquillo JA, Larson SM *et al.* (1987) Acquired immunodeficieincy syndrome: Ga-67 citrate imaging. *Radiology* **162**:383–387.

26. Stevens DA and Allegra JC (1986) Gallium accumulation in early *Pneumocystis carinii* infection. *South Med J* **79**:1148–1151.

27. Strauss HW and Pitt B (eds) (1979) *Cardiovascular Nuclear Medicine*, 2nd edn. St Louis: Mosby, pp. 109–20, 121–124, 136–139.

28. Purvall DG, Byrom E, Lamb W *et al.* (1983) Detection and quantification of regional wall motion abnormalities using phase analysis of equilibrium gated cardiac studies. *Clin Nucl Med* **8**:315–321.

29. Beller GA (1994) Myocardial perfusion imaging with thallium 201. *J Nucl Med* **35**:674–680.

30. Kiat H, Maddahi J, Troy LT *et al.* (1989) Comparison of technetium 99m methoxyisobutyl isonitryle and thallium 201 for evaluation of coronary artery disease by planar and tomographic methods. *Am Heart J* **1017**:1–11.

31. Heo J, Wolmer I, Kegel and Iskandrian AS (1994) Sequential dual isotope SPECT imaging with thallium 201 and technetium 99m sestamibi. *J Nucl Med* **35**:549–553.

32. Iskandrian AS (1991) Single photon emission computer tomographic thallium imaging with adenosine, dipyridamole and exercise. *Am Heart J* **122**:279–284.

33. Iskandrian AS (1994) Adenosine myocardical perfusion imaging. *J Nucl Med* **35**:737–739.

34. Verani MS (1994) Dobutamine myocardial perfusion imaging. *J Nucl Med* **35**:737–739.

35. Taki J, Taki S, Ichiyanagi K *et al.* (1992) Acute subendocardial infarction with diffuse intense Tc^{99m} PYP uptake and minimal Tl^{201} abnormality. *Clin Nucl Med* **17**:643–645.

36. Askenazi J, Ahnberg DS, Korngold E *et al.* (1976) Quantitative radionuclide angiocardiography. Detection and quantitation of left to right shunts. *Am J Cardiol* **37**:382.

37. Polycove M and Tono M (1988) Blood volume. In: Gottschalk A, Hoffer PB and Potchen EJ (eds) *Diagnostic Nuclear Medicine*, vol. II. Baltimore, MD: Williams & Wilkins, pp. 690–698.

38. Oppenhelm BE, Wellman HN and Hoffer PB (1988) Liver imaging. In: Gottschalk A, Hoffer PB and Potchen EJ (eds). *Diagnostic Nuclear Medicine*, vol. II. Baltimore MD: Williams & Wilkins, pp. 538–565.

39. Shapiro MJ, Luchtefeld WB, Kurzweil S, Kaminski DL, Durham RM and Mazuski JE (1994) Acute acalculous cholecystitis in the critically ill. *Am Surgeon* **60**:335–339.

40. Watson A, Better N, Kalff V, Nottle P, Scelwyn M and Kelly MJ (1994) Cholecystokinin (CCK)-HIDA scintigraphy in patients with suspected gall bladder dysfunction. *Australasian Radiol* **38**:30–33.

41. Bouchier IAD (1984) Imaging procedures to diagnose gallbladder disease. *Br Med J* **288**:1632–1633.

42. Shuman WP, Gibbs P, Rudd TG and Malk LA (1982) PIPIDA scintigraphy for cholecystitis: false positives in alcoholism and total parenteral nutrition. *Aust J Radiol* **138**:1–5.

43. Poter T, McClain CJ and Shafter RB (1983) Effect of fasting and parenteral alimentation on PIPIDA scintigraphy. *Dig Dis Sci* **28**:667–691.

44. Welssmann HS, Gltedman ML, Wilk PJ *et al.* (1982) Evaluation of the post-operative patient with 99mTc IDA cholescintigraphy. *Semin Nucl Med* **12**:27–57.

45. Fischer KC, Eraklis AP, Rosselio P and Treves S (1978) Scintigraphy in the follow up of paediatric splenic trauma treated without surgery. *J Nucl Med* **19**:3–9.

46. McKusick KA, Froelich J, Callaghan RJ *et al.* (1981) Tc^{99m} red blood cells for detection of gastrointestinal bleeding: experience with 80 patients. *Am J Roentgenol*, **137**:1113–1118.

47. Maurer AH, Rodman MS, Vitti RA *et al.* (1992) Gastrointestinal bleeding: improved localisation with cine scintigraphy. *Radiology* **185**:187–192.

48. Goshen E, Zwas T, Sadan M and Kronenberg J (1994) The combined use of classified bone and gallium scans in the management of frontal sinusitis. *Nucl Med Commun* **15**:361–366.

49. Kim EE, Haynie TP, Podoloff DA *et al.* (1989) Radionuclide imaging in the evaluation of osteomyelitis and septic arthritis. *Crit Rev Diag Imaging* **29**:257–305.

50. Laughlin RT, Sinha A, Calhoun JH and Mader JT (1994) Osteomyelitis. *Curr Opin Rheumatol* **6**:401–407.

51. Gagliardi PD, Hoffer PV and Rosenfield AT (1988) Correlated imaging in abdominal infection: an algorhythmic approach using nuclear medicine, ultrasound and computer tomography. *Sem Nucl Med* **18**:320–334.

52. Maisey MN, Britton KE and Gilday DL (eds) *Clinical Nuclear Medicine*, 2nd edn. London: Chapman & Hall.

53. Britton KE, Maisey MN and Hilson AJ (1990) Renal radionuclide studies. In: Maisey MN, Britton KE and Gilday DL (eds) *Clinical Nuclear Medicine*, 2nd edn. London: Chapman & Hall, pp. 91–100.

54. Mountford PJ and Cokely AJ (1995) Radiolabelled agents for the localisation of infection. In: Murray IPC and EII PJ (eds) *Nuclear Medicine in Clinical Diagnosis and Treatment*. Edinburgh: Churchill Livingstone, pp. 129–140.

55. Parekh JS and Teates CD (1992) Emergency nuclear medicine. *Radiol Clin North Am* **30**:455–474.

56. Matin P (1988) Basic principles of nuclear medicine techniques for detection and evaluation of trauma and sports medicine injuries. *Semin Nucl Med* **18**:90–112.

57. Gupta NC and Prezio JA (1988) Radionuclide imaging in osteomyelitis. *Sem in Nucl Med* **18**:287–299.

58. Matin P, Lang G, Carretta RF and Simon T (1983) Scintigraphic evaluation of muscle damage following extreme exercise. *J Nucl Med* **24**:308–311.

Part XVII

Paediatric intensive care

101 | The critically ill child

AW Duncan

The chapters on paediatric intensive care are intended to help intensivists outside specialized paediatric centres manage common paediatric emergencies. They should be read with relevant adult chapters, as there are areas of common interest. Some common neonatal emergencies are also presented.

Differences of neonates and infants from adults render them susceptible to critical illness and alter their response to disease processes. Most aspects of organ monitoring and support in adult ICUs have been modified for use in children, and are applicable to even the smallest infants.

The major differences between paediatric and adult patients are described below.

Adaptation

Dramatic physiological adaptation takes place as the fetus adjusts to extrauterine life. Many changes are incomplete until some time after birth; until then, reversion to fetal physiology may occur. This particularly applies to the cardiorespiratory events at birth and the subsequent development of a transitional pattern of circulation (persistent fetal circulation: see below).

Growth and development

There is progressive growth and development of all organ systems throughout childhood. 'Small-body technology' has evolved to cope with the technical aspects of paediatric critical care. Some aspects of growth are non-linear, and contribute to the reduced cardiorespiratory reserve of the infant. Physiological differences that influence disease processes and their management are discussed in respective chapters in this section.

Maturation

At birth, the immaturity of many systems and biochemical processes alters the response to patho-physiological stress and drugs. Thermoregulation, immune function and renal function are immature at birth, even in the full-term infant. Such immaturity is magnified in the premature infant (e.g. surfactant deficiency in the lung causing hyaline membrane disease, and liver glucuronyl transferase deficiency causing jaundice).

Diverse pathophysiological states

Developmental anomalies, inborn errors of metabolism, susceptibility to infection and various accidents and trauma provide a wide spectrum of paediatric critical illnesses. The response to these illnesses is modified by various aspects of adaptation, growth and development and maturation.

Paediatric intensive care

The development of separate paediatric ICUs recognized the unique problems and requirements of critically ill children. The paediatric ICU (PICU) should not be seen in isolation, but as part of a tertiary paediatric centre, with well-defined pre-hospital care, emergency medical services and retrieval teams. Minimum standards should be adopted. In general, a PICU should provide:

1 a specialist trained in paediatric intensive care available at short notice;
2 a range of paediatric subspecialty support;
3 immediately available junior medical staff with advanced life support skills;
4 nursing staff with experience in paediatric intensive care;
5 allied health professionals and ancillary support staff;
6 specialized advanced life support equipment for children ranging in age from neonates to adolescents;

7 24-h laboratory, radiological and pharmacy services;

8 a purpose-built PICU, recognizing the special physical and emotional needs of critically ill children and their families;

9 programme for teaching, continuing education, research and quality assurance.

Neonatal ICUs have their own particular requirements.

Cardiorespiratory events at birth

During intrauterine life, 60% of blood returning to the right atrium passes directly through the foramen ovale into the left ventricle and ascending aorta. As most of this blood is from the umbilical arteries, the heart and brain are perfused with better-oxygenated blood. Pulmonary vascular resistance (PVR) is high, and most of the blood reaching the right ventricle passes through the ductus arteriosus to the descending aorta. Only 10% of right ventricular output passes to the lungs which, although non-functional, require a blood supply for nutrition, growth and development of the lung vasculature.

At birth, closure of the umbilical vessels increases systemic vascular resistance (SVR) and lung expansion leads to the dramatic fall in PVR. Pulmonary blood flow increases, leading to a rise in left atrial pressure and functional closure of the foramen ovale. The ductus arteriosus subsequently constricts and eventually thromboses.

Following the dramatic fall in PVR at birth, there is a gradual regression in muscularization of the pulmonary arterioles over the following weeks to months. This regression is prevented if high pulmonary blood flow occurs, due to congenital heart lesions (e.g. ventricular septal defect, large patent ductus arteriosus and truncus arteriosus) or lesions associated with persistent hypoxaemia (e.g. transposition of great vessels). With these lesions, progression to irreversible pulmonary vascular disease may occur at an early age.

Persistent fetal circulation

Haemodynamic adaptation at birth may be delayed or reversed by a number of factors. Persistent pulmonary hypertension and patency of the fetal channels result in right-to-left shunting through the foramen ovale and ductus arteriosus. A vicious cycle may develop, with increasing hypoxaemia and acidosis, increased PVR and further shunting. Unless the underlying disturbance is treated and the pulmonary hypertension corrected, progression to death is likely. Pulmonary circulation pathophysiology is probably related to abnormalities of endogenous nitric oxide production, and manipulation of this agent is proving useful in therapy.

Causes of persistent fetal circulation

A fetal pattern circulation may persist due to:

1 low lung volume states (e.g. hyaline membrane disease and perinatal asphyxia);
2 pulmonary hypoplasia (e.g. diaphragmatic hernia and Potter's syndrome);
3 meconium aspiration syndrome;
4 chronic placental insufficiency;
5 perinatal hypoxia and acidosis from any cause;
6 sepsis (e.g. group B streptococcal infection);
7 hyperviscosity syndrome.

Clinical features

Hypoxaemia disproportional to the degree of respiratory distress is typical of persistent fetal circulation and suggests the possibility of congenital cyanotic heart disease. In cases without significant lung disease, echocardiography may be necessary to exclude a structural cardiac lesion. Severe respiratory distress is present in cases secondary to pulmonary disease. Differential cyanosis (i.e. increased cyanosis affecting the lower limbs when compared with the head, neck and right arm) may be seen with right-to-left shunting at ductal level. This may be confirmed by simultaneous pre- and postductal arterial blood sampling or transcutaneous Po_2 monitoring.

Treatment

It is important to treat the underlying cause (e.g. surfactant therapy for hyaline membrane disease) in addition to therapy to reduce PVR. The main steps employed are:

1 maintenance of high inspired oxygen. Alveolar oxygen tension is an important determinant of pulmonary arteriolar resistance. Sudden reductions in inspired oxygen may increase shunting through fetal channels (so-called flip-flop phenomenon);
2 correction of low lung volume states with continuous positive airway pressure (CPAP) or positive-pressure ventilation with positive end-expiratory pressure (PEEP);
3 correction of both metabolic and respiratory acidosis;
4 deliberate hyperventilation using muscle relaxants to lower $Paco_2$ and generate a respiratory alkalosis. This manoeuvre is limited by lung immaturity and risk of barotrauma. Rapid rates of ventilation (> 60 breaths/min) may prove beneficial;
5 maintenance of systemic arterial pressure with volume expanders and inotropic agents, to reduce the pressure gradient favouring ductal shunting;

6 isovolaemic haemodilution with colloid, if indicated, to reduce hyperviscosity;
7 administration of pulmonary vasodilators, e.g. inhaled nitric oxide,[1] and IV tolazoline, nitroglycerin and prostaglandin E;
8 some centres have successfully employed extracorporeal membrane oxygenation (ECMO) in this situation.

Thermoregulation in the newborn

Human body temperature is maintained within narrow limits. This is achieved most easily in the thermoneutral zone – the range of ambient temperature within which the metabolic rate is at a minimum. Once ambient temperature is outside the thermoneutral zone, heat production (shivering or non-shivering thermogenesis) or evaporative heat loss processes are required to maintain body temperature within normal limits. Regulatory mechanisms are less effective in the neonate (there is no shivering or sweating), who is otherwise disadvantaged by a high surface area to body weight ratio and lack of subcutaneous tissue.

The thermoneutral zone is higher in premature infants, and falls with increasing postnatal age. Oxygen consumption is minimal with an environmental or abdominal skin temperature of 36.5°C. Oxidation of brown fat found in the interscapular and perirenal areas (non-shivering thermogenesis) is the major source of heat production when 'cold-stressed'. This process is mediated by noradrenaline.

Alteration of body temperature above or below normal leads to increased or decreased metabolism respectively. Attempts by the body to maintain body temperature within normal limits are associated with increased metabolism and cardiorespiratory demands. Radiation is a major source of heat loss in the neonate, and is effectively minimized by double-walled incubators or by servo-controlled radiant heaters. The latter allows better access to critically ill babies for monitoring and procedures. Cold stress *per se* increases neonatal mortality. In the presence of respiratory or cardiac disease, it may lead to decompensation.

Immunology of the infant

The immunological system consists of:

1 non-specific mechanisms, including phagocytosis and the inflammatory response;
2 specific immune responses, consisting of cell-mediated (T-cell) and humoral (B-cell) systems (see Chapter 59). These two components are intimately related and both may be abnormal in the newborn infant.

The inflammatory response of the newborn is attenuated. Febrile response to infection may be lacking, and both cellular (chemotaxis and phagocytosis) and humoral (complement activity and opsonization) responses may be impaired. Cell-mediated immunity is completely absent in infants born without thymic function (DiGeorge syndrome). In the normal newborn, however, T-cell function appears to be quite well-developed. Rejection of skin allografts is slower in the newborn, but this seems to be related mainly to the attenuated inflammatory response.

The B-cell system, responsible for antibody production, is immature at birth. The neonate has passive immunity against some infections, because of transplacental transfer of maternal antibodies. Natural immunity is acquired as a result of immunoglobulin A (IgA) in breast milk, and protects against some acquired gastrointestinal infections. Overall, the immaturity and inexperience of the immune system result in a markedly increased susceptibility to infection in the first 6 months of life.

Resuscitation of the newborn

Some newborn infants fail to adapt from fetal to extrauterine life, and require immediate cardiopulmonary and cerebral resuscitation. The Apgar scoring system (Table 101.1) scored after 1 min, remains the most widely accepted method of assessment. The best Apgar score is 10 and the worst is zero. There is an inverse relationship between the Apgar score and the degree of hypoxia and acidosis. It has been suggested that the 5-min score is a guide to ultimate prognosis,

Table 101.1 Apgar scoring system

Score	0	1	2
Heart rate	Absent	<100 beats/min	>100 beats/min
Respiratory effort	Absent	Weak cry	Strong cry
Muscle tone	Limp	Some flexion	Active motion
Reflex irritability (in response to catheter in nose)	No response	Grimace	Grimace and cough or sneeze
Colour	Blue, pale	Body pink, extremities blue	Pink

but this is questioned. Collection of sequential scores must not delay the institution of resuscitation.

Birth asphyxia

The causes of birth asphyxia may be:

1 placental failure – acute or chronic (e.g. toxaemia, diabetes and antepartum haemorrhage);
2 drug depression due to maternal analgesics or sedatives administered immediately prior to delivery;
3 obstetrical complications (e.g. difficult forceps, breech, caesarean section, and prolapsed cord);
4 fetal conditions (e.g. multiple births and prematurity);
5 postnatal problems (e.g. respiratory distress immediately after birth from any cause).

Management

The principles of resuscitation are identical to those employed in other situations. Resuscitation must be started immediately after delivery. Although some cerebral insult may have occurred *in utero* or intrapartum, secondary insults from postpartum asphyxia must be avoided.

Babies suffering mild asphyxia immediately before birth with Apgar scores between 5 and 7 usually respond to stimulation and gentle suction to the nose, mouth and pharynx, although oxygen therapy is occasionally required. Babies with moderate asphyxia (Apgar 3–4) usually respond to bag-and-mask ventilation with oxygen. Acid–base status should be determined, and sodium bicarbonate administered to restore pH > 7.25. Severely asphyxiated infants (Apgar 0–2) need urgent cardiopulmonary resuscitation (CPR). After airway suction, bag-and-mask ventilation should be followed by rapid orotracheal intubation and positive-pressure ventilation with oxygen. Fear of complications of oxygen therapy must not mitigate against the administration of 100% oxygen at this stage. If the liquor contains thick meconium, it is vital that the pharynx and trachea be suctioned prior to the onset of respiration or application of positive pressure. Meconium aspiration syndrome is a preventable condition that is often difficult to manage.

Venous access via umbilical or peripheral veins must be established immediately, and followed by the administration of 1–2 mmol/kg of sodium bicarbonate. Subsequent buffer therapy should be based on arterial acid–base status if available. Rapid or excessive infusions of hypertonic solutions (e.g. sodium bicarbonate or hypertonic dextrose) or volume expanders may precipitate intracranial haemorrhage, particularly in premature infants.

Asphyxiated infants are usually volume-depleted at birth, and blood pressure should be restored with colloids immediately (10 ml/kg in the first instance). External cardiac massage and additional drug therapy (see below) should be employed, if necessary, to restore cardiac rhythm. Post resuscitative care to maintain cerebral perfusion pressure, correct abnormal serum biochemistry and control seizures is required to prevent secondary cerebral insults.[2] Myocardial dysfunction may occur secondary to asphyxia. Dopamine or dobutamine (5–10 μg/kg per min) may prove useful.

The orotracheal tube should be changed to nasotracheal to enable secure fixation, once some physiological stability is attained. Radiological confirmation of tube position should be made as soon as possible. Endobronchial intubation is a particular risk in the premature infant with a short trachea.

Approximate nose to mid-trachea (T2) distances are:

1 28 weeks' gestation – 7 cm;
2 33 weeks' gestation – 9 cm;
3 term infant – 10.5 cm.

Cardiorespiratory arrest in children

The vast majority of children lack intrinsic myocardial disease, and cardiac arrest is the end-result of hypoxaemia and acidosis. The most common predisposing causes are rapidly progressive upper airway obstruction (e.g. epiglottitis), near drowning, sudden infant death syndrome, pneumonia, sepsis, gastroenteritis and major trauma. Such children invariably arrest in asystole, and this should be assumed if an electrocardiogram (ECG) is not immediately available.

Ventricular fibrillation (VF) may be anticipated in the following situations:

1 congenital heart disease;
2 cardiomyopathies;
3 myocarditis;
4 poisoning (e.g. tricyclic antidepressant ingestion);
5 hereditary prolongation of QT interval (Romano–Ward syndrome).

Assessment

Cardiac arrest is diagnosed in a child who is unconscious, apnoeic and has no palpable pulse. The carotid pulse is the best pulse to assess in children. Assessment of heart sounds with a precordial stethoscope or palpation of the apex beat is useful in neonates and small infants.

Management

The ABCs of resuscitation (see Chapter 7) must be modified according to the patient's size.

Airway

Anatomical differences between the infant and adult make airway obstruction more likely and maintenance more difficult. The infant has a large head, a short neck and a relatively large tongue. Excessive neck flexion or extension may compromise the airway. Pressure exerted on the soft tissues of the neck, and hence on the tongue, may obstruct the airway. The airway is best made patent by opening the mouth and using jaw thrust. Mouth-to-mouth or mouth-to-nose and mouth-expired air resuscitation may be used depending on the size of the child. Children are prone to gastric distension, particularly if the airway is partially obstructed. Rapid tracheal intubation should be performed by an experienced person without delay. Tracheal tube size and length are deduced from age or weight (Table 101.2). Care is taken to avoid accidental extubation or endobronchial intubation.

Cardiac massage

The technique of cardiac massage is outlined in Table 101.3. The heart lies behind the mid-sternum, at which point massage should be concentrated. Due to the relative organomegaly of the infant and the compressible nature of the chest wall, cardiac massage applied to the lower sternum risks rupturing the liver or spleen. Massage and ventilation rates recommended for both one- and two-person resuscitations are given in Table 101.4 External cardiac compression is likely to be less effective in complex congenital heart disease and valvular incompetence. When cardiac arrest occurs following open heart surgery, open cardiac massage should be attempted if there is no rapid response to closed chest massage.

Treatment of asystole

The child with asystole can often be restored to sinus rhythm with effective resuscitation, even after 45–60

Table 101.2 Paediatric resuscitation table

Age (years)	Birth	1	2	3	4	5	6	7	8	9	10	11	12	13
Weight (kg)	3	5	10		15		20		25		30	35		40
Adrenaline IV/1 in 10 000 0.1 ml/kg (up to 1 ml/kg per dose if no response) via ETT 1:1000 0.1 ml/kg (ml)	1	1			1.5		2		2.5		3	3.5		4
Sodium bicarbonate 8.4% 2 ml/kg stat (ml)	6	10	20	25	30		40		50		60	70		80
Sodium bicarbonate 8.4% 1 ml/kg per 10-min arrest time (ml)	3	5	10		15		20		25		30	35		40
Lignocaine 1% 0.1 ml/kg (1 mg/kg, then 20–40 µg/kg per min) (ml)	0.5	1			1.5		20		2.5		3	3.5		4
Calcium chloride 10% 0.2 ml/kg (maximum 10 ml) (ml)	1	1	2		3		4		5		6	7		8
Calcium gluconate 10% 0.5 ml/kg (maximum 20 ml) (ml)	2	3	5	7			10				15			20
Volume expansion. Initially 10 ml/kg, repeat × 2–3 if required (ml)	30	50	100	125	150		200		250		300	350		400
ETT internal diameter (mm)	3.0	3.5	4.0	4.5	5.0		5.5		6.0		6.5		7.0	
ETT (oral) length at lip (cm)	8.5	11	12	13	14		15		16		17		18	
ETT (nasal) length at nose (cm)	10.5	14	15	16	17		19		20		21		22	
Cardioversion: atrial arrhythmia 1 J/kg (J)	3	5	10		15		20		25		30	35		40
Cardioversion: ventricular arrhythmia 5 J/kg (J)	15	20			75		100		125		150	175		200

ETT = Endotracheal tube.

873

Table 101.3 Technique of cardiac massage

Victim	Site	How	Rate/min	Depth
Adult	Lower half of sternum	Two hands	60	5 cm
Child to 8 years	Middle of sternum	One hand	75	2.5 cm
Infant to 1 year	Middle of sternum	Two fingers or thumbs	100	1–2.5 cm

min of cardiac arrest. Poor outcome is highly likely, however, due to hypoxic brain damage. With brief arrests, cardiac massage and oxygenation alone are often adequate to restart the heart. Sodium bicarbonate to correct acidosis and adrenaline are additional therapy. These are given according to estimated body weight (Table 101.2). The usual initial dose of adrenaline is 0.01 mg/kg and should be increased to 0.1 mg/kg if there is inadequate response. If blood gases are unavailable, sodium bicarbonate is given empirically, according to the estimated duration of arrest. Failure to restart the asystolic heart reflects either residual acidosis or a prolonged period of anoxia. Bicarbonate and adrenaline should be repeated as long as resuscitation attempts are continued. It is uncommon for adrenaline to precipitate VF in children; the transient tachycardia produced is rarely a problem.

The use of calcium chloride or gluconate in resuscitation is contentious.[3,4] Calcium increases blood pressure by increasing contractility and/or peripheral resistance, and may be useful after restoration of a normal rhythm.[5] Concern exists that it may cause or exacerbate myocardial (and cerebral) reperfusion injury, and may cause heart block. The recommendation for its use in asystole and electromechanical dissociation was withdrawn by the American Heart Association in 1986.[6] The use of calcium in resuscitation is still recommended in hyperkalaemia, hypocalcaemia (including citrate toxicity) and calcium-channel blocker intoxication.

Treatment of ventricular fibrillation

Spontaneous reversion of VF sometimes occurs in children with effective CPR. DC countershock must be administered urgently in those who do not revert immediately. The recommended output is 5 J/kg. If reversion does not occur with two DC shocks, adrenaline should be administered to increase SVR, improve coronary perfusion and the response to DC shock. Lignocaine 1 mg/kg may improve the response to defibrillation. It may be repeated in a dose of 0.5 mg/kg. VF secondary to poisoning with tricyclic antidepressants may prove refractory to this therapy. This relates to the quinidine-like effect of these drugs and, for this reason, phenytoin 15 mg/kg prior to DC shock has proved beneficial.[7]

Vascular access

Venous access may be difficult, particularly in the collapsed, hypovolaemic or hypothermic child. The external jugular vein may be prominent when usual sites are inaccessible. Cannulation of central veins, apart from the femoral route, is hazardous even in ideal situations, and should not be attempted during cardiac arrest in small children and babies. Three alternatives may be considered: intraosseous infusion, intracardiac injection or endotracheal instillation.

Table 101.4 Cardiopulmonary resuscitation ratios and rates

Operators	*1* *15 Compressions* *2 Ventilations*		*2* *5 Compressions* *1 Ventilation*	
	Child	Infant	Child	Infant
Seconds/cycle	12	10	4	3
Cycles/min	5	6	15	20
Compression/min	75	90	75	100
Ventilations/min	10	12	15	20

Intraosseous infusion[8]

This involves infusion into bone marrow – a non-collapsible venous system in direct communication with the circulation. The technique is simple and quick to learn. A metal needle with a trocar (e.g. disposable intraosseous needle, Cook, Illinois, USA) is used to penetrate the thin cortex of the upper tibia in the first year of life, and the iliac crest in older children. In dogs, drugs infused this way reach the central circulation as rapidly as those injected into a central vein. The effect of equal doses of adrenaline given by the intraosseous and IV routes is identical in shocked dogs. Volume expanders need to be given by syringe to gain rapid access to the central circulation. This is best achieved using a 10-ml syringe with a three-way tap in the IV tubing.

Intraosseous infusion has been successfully used in CPR.[9] Osteomyelitis is a potential complication, and conventional venous access should be established after resuscitation. Compartment syndromes requiring limb amputation have also been described recently,[10] resulting from needle misplacement in muscle or influx of fluids into muscle through another bone perforation. Careful placement, close observation of the limb and early removal of needle are necessary.

Intracardiac injection

Intracardiac injection reliably delivers drugs to the central circulation, but is unsuitable to correct hypovolaemia. The injection can be made using a subxiphoid approach aiming towards the left shoulder, or through the left fourth intercostal space, aiming directly posteriorly. This latter technique is easy to perform and easier to teach, but has a risk of lacerating the left anterior descending coronary artery. Stopping massage and ventilation during needle insertion and aspirating blood before injection should lessen the risk of intramyocardial injection. Other complications include pneumothorax and cardiac tamponade.

Endotracheal instillation

Endotracheal instillation is at best a poor substitute for the above methods. Blood concentrations of drugs are lower, and certain drugs (e.g. bicarbonate and calcium) will cause direct lung damage if given by this route. Adrenaline, lignocaine and atropine may be diluted in saline (newborn 1 ml, infants and preschool children 3 ml and older children 5 ml). The dose of adrenaline should be twice the calculated IV dose. The drugs should be delivered in diluted form into the bronchi through a catheter passed down the endotracheal tube.

Outcome of paediatric cardiac arrest

The prognosis of paediatric cardiorespiratory arrest is poor. Unless hypothermic, the vast majority of children who present to an emergency department without vital signs either die or, if resuscitated, survive with severe neurological impairment.[11–13] The outcome of children resuscitated before admission is somewhat better, and may justify advanced life support in the pre-hospital setting.[14,15] In previously normal children, cardiac arrest occurs either as a result of lethal traumatic injury or as a consequence of prolonged hypoxia and acidosis. In children with structurally abnormal hearts, CPR is inefficient and usually ineffective. The outcome of cardiorespiratory arrest within hospital is better.[16] Respiratory arrest alone followed by rapid resuscitation also has a more favourable outcome, particularly when it occurs within the hospital setting.[17,18] Poor prognostic features include location of arrest (in-hospital compared with out of hospital, operating theatre compared with general ward), absent vital signs on admission, need for more than one dose of adrenaline[12] and severe acidosis (pH < 7.0).[19] A more favourable outcome is associated with in-hospital arrest, extreme bradycardia as the presenting arrhythmia, successful resuscitation with only ventilation, oxygen and closed chest massage, and a duration of CPR less than 15 min.[16] Provided that the child is normothermic, consideration should be given to ceasing active resuscitation if it is not successful within 25 min.

Paediatric monitoring

Technology has allowed most aspects of adult monitoring to be applied to neonatal and paediatric practice. The ideal paediatric haemodynamic and respiratory monitoring system should:

1 be non-invasive, painless and readily interfaced with the child;
2 constitute minimal risk to the child;
3 provide specific data relevant to the child's status that are reproducible and readily understood;
4 respond rapidly to changes in cardiorespiratory status;
5 provide continuous visual and/or auditory display of data;
6 have appropriate alarms;
7 have facilities for recording data;
8 be inexpensive and require low maintenance.

Arterial cannulation

Arterial cannulation is routine practice in paediatric intensive care, even in infants weighing < 1 kg. It is indicated in all critically ill infants for continuous blood pressure monitoring and accurate blood-gas sampling. In the neonate, difficult 'stabs' may lead to significant errors in Pao_2 and $Paco_2$. The use of umbilical arterial catheters is avoided whenever possible, because of vaso-occlusive complications (e.g. lower limb ischaemia, renal thrombosis, necrotizing enterocolitis and paraplegia).

Peripheral arteries used include radial, ulnar, brachial, femoral, posterior tibial and dorsalis pedis. Radial and ulnar or posterior tibial and dorsalis pedis vessels must never be cannulated sequentially in the same limb. The safety of brachial and femoral cannulation lies in the presence of rich collateral vessels around the elbow and hip joints. Arterial lines are kept patent by continuous flushing with 1–2 ml/h of heparinized normal saline (5 units heparin/ml flushing solution) or 5% dextrose. Complications include distal ischaemia, infection, retrograde embolization and haemorrhage. Retrograde embolization occurring with flushing is a particular risk in the small infant, depending on the length and volume of vessel, and volume and speed of injection. In a 1.5-kg infant, as little as 0.5 ml of fluid injected rapidly into the right radial artery will reach the cerebral circulation. Haemorrhage from accidental disconnection can be significant because of the relatively small blood volume. Meticulous fixation is therefore required.

Central venous, pulmonary artery and left atrial pressure monitoring

Central venous pressure

All routes of central venous cannulation are applicable to infants and children, and must be within the skills of paediatric intensivists.[11] Catheters utilizing the Seldinger technique have greatly increased successful placement. Multilumen catheters are useful when infusing multiple drugs and for parenteral nutrition. Catheter sepsis is a risk, and relates to duration of catheterization, age and use of inotropic agents. The need for prolonged venous access warrants frequent catheter changes, or surgical implantation of a central venous device (e.g. Infusaport, Broviac or Hickman catheter). Umbilical venous cannulation and passage of the catheter through the sinus venosus to the right atrium are useful in neonatal emergencies.

Pulmonary artery (PA) pressure

PA pressure monitoring using flow-directed 4 and 5 FG catheters is feasible even in neonates. It is, however, invasive, technically more difficult, and has greater risks than in the adult. It is rarely required in the neonate, as the pulmonary circulation and response to therapy can usually be gauged indirectly from the magnitude of right-to-left shunting. Systemic levels of PA pressure are usually found in neonates with severe lung disease.

The major indication for PA pressure monitoring is following surgery for congenital heart disease

(e.g. repair of ventricular septal defect with pulmonary hypertension, truncus arteriosus and obstructed total anomalous pulmonary venous drainage). A catheter is inserted directly into the PA at the time of surgery. It is most useful in guiding weaning from mechanical ventilation.

Left atrial pressure

Left atrial pressure monitoring is also required after open heart surgery for congenital heart disease, by means of a catheter placed in the left atrium during surgery.

Cardiac output measurement

Cardiac output determination can be performed in small children by dye dilution, thermodilution or Doppler techniques. Unfortunately, errors are substantial, and the first two techniques are invasive, intermittent and only repeatable within finite limits. Interpretation of results is made difficult or impossible in the presence of intracardiac shunts or valvular incompetence. The dye curve may, in fact, be useful in demonstrating residual intracardiac shunts. Calculation of derived variables is only as accurate as the flow measurement.

Temperature monitoring

Temperature monitoring is important in neonatal and paediatric intensive care. Prevention of cold stress requires accurate measurement of core and skin temperature. Core–toe–ambient temperature gradients provide a sensitive index of cardiac output and peripheral perfusion, and are useful in managing fever. Toe temperature normally lies between core temperature (tympanic or oesophageal) and ambient temperature. The toe–core temperature gradient increases with low cardiac output or vasoconstriction from any cause. Toe temperature is a useful guide to the efficacy of vasodilator therapy.

Pulse oximetry

Pulse oximetry provides continuous non-invasive measurement of arteriolar saturation (Sao_2) and rapidly indicates hypoxaemia. Accurate information is given:

1 when the oxyhaemoglobin dissociation curve is shifted to the left (e.g. fetal haemoglobin and alkalosis) or to the right (e.g. sickle-cell disease and acidosis);

2 in the presence of carboxyhaemoglobin (functional saturation is accurate);

3 with severe desaturation (e.g. cyanotic heart disease);

4 with anaemia (haemoglobin concentrations above 5 g/dl);

5 when skin is pigmented.

Errors occur with extreme hypoperfusion, excessive movement and rapidly changing ambient light. A range of sensors are now available to monitor children of all ages.

Transcutaneous Po_2 and Pco_2 monitoring

Oxygen and carbon dioxide diffuse through well-perfused skin from the superficial capillary network, and can be measured using modified polarographic and glass electrodes respectively. The electrodes are heated to 43–45°C to arterialize the capillary blood and maximize capillary blood flow. Under optimal conditions, there is good correlation between arterial (Pao_2) and transcutaneous gas tensions ($Ptco_2$). Hence continuous monitoring of blood-gas tensions is possible in a non-invasive way. The $Ptco_2$–Pao_2 gradient and the output of the heating element have been used as indices of microcirculation. The accuracy of these devices is mainly confined to the neonatal period.

Drug infusions

All drugs used in cardiovascular and respiratory support are administered according to body weight; accurate delivery is crucial. Accurate drug infusions require accurate devices, of which syringe pumps are the most useful. Potentially lethal errors in calculating drug dilutions are minimized by the use of dose/dilution/infusion rate guidelines (Table 101.5).[20]

Pain relief in children

Management of pain in children has received inadequate attention and has tended to be underestimated and undertreated. Infants and children are often unable or unwilling to complain of pain. In the past, some believed that the neonate could not perceive pain. It is now clear that even neonates possess all the anatomical and neurochemical systems necessary for pain perception, and exhibit physiological and behaviour responses to pain.[21] Stress responses associated with pain may increase morbidity and mortality in critically ill patients. Analgesia can be provided by opioid infusions, local blocks and regional techniques in children of all ages. Painful procedures in the ICU must always be accompanied by appropriate analgesia (see Chapter 79).

Neonatal and paediatric emergency transport

Care of critically ill neonates and children necessitates the use of specialized retrieval services linked to neonatal and paediatric ICUs. Retrieval services should offer facilities for specialist consultation in addition to secondary transport. Careful audit of such services is necessary to improve patient outcome.[22] The aim of retrieval services is to extend the intensive care facility to peripheral hospitals, allowing stabilization by experienced personnel prior to rapid transport to a regional centre in the most appropriate vehicle (see Chapter 3). Special considerations such as thermoregulation and oxygen monitoring must be provided for in neonatal transport. Well-designed neonatal emergency transport services have resulted in significant reductions in morbidity and mortality.

Outcome of paediatric intensive care

Depending on admission criteria, mortality in paediatric ICUs ranges from 5 to 15%. If patients with pre-existing severe disabilities are excluded, the majority of survivors have a normal or near-normal life expectancy. A number of scoring systems have been developed or modified for paediatric application to predict ICU mortality. These scoring systems allow comparison between different ICUs, internal audits over time, evaluation of therapeutic interventions and analysis of cost benefit. Such scoring systems include the paediatric risk of mortality score (PRISM), the modified injury severity scale (MISS), paediatric trauma score (PTS) and the modified Glasgow coma scale.

Compared with adult intensive care, children with equivalent therapeutic intervention scores (TISS) have a lower in-hospital and 1-month mortality.[23] In addition, non-survivors do not consume a disproportionate amount of resources. Whilst multiple organ failure increases mortality, the prognosis is considerably better than for adults.[24] There is evidence that mortality is lower in specialist paediatric ICUs,[25] and that paediatric ICUs with a larger workload are likely to perform better than those looking after fewer children. General hospitals should therefore have facilities for urgent resuscitation of children prior to early transport to a specialized paediatric ICU. Unless unavoidable, critically ill children, particularly those requiring mechanical ventilation, should not be cared for in an adult ICU for longer than 24 h. The American Academy of Pediatrics, the Society of Critical Care Medicine, the British Paediatric Association and the Australian National Health and Medical Research Council have all stated that children should receive intensive care in specialist paediatric units.

Table 101.5 Calculation of drug infusion dilutions:

1 Select desired drug dosage to be delivered in μg/kg per min.
2 Select infusion rate of syringe pump in ml/h (from centre of table)
3 Calculate number of milligrams of drug to be mixed in 50-ml syringe
  e.g.: 10-kg child, 0.1–2 μg/kg per min, infusion 1–20 ml/h: put 0.3 ml/kg (= 3 mg) in 50 ml

μg/kg per min	0.15 mg/kg in 50 ml	0.3 mg/kg in 50 ml	0.6 mg/kg in 50 ml	1.5 mg/kg in 50 ml	3 mg/kg in 50 ml	6 mg/kg in 50 ml	15 mg/kg in 50 ml	30 mg/kg in 50 ml	60 mg/kg in 50 ml
0.05	1	ml/h							
0.1	2	1	ml/h						
0.2	4	2	1						
0.3	6	3	1.5						
0.4	8	4	2	ml/h					
0.5	10	5		1					
0.6	12	6	3						
0.7	14	7							
0.8	16	8	4						
0.9	18	9			ml/h				
1	20	10	5	2	1				
1.5		15		3	1.5	ml/h			
2		20	10	4	2	1			
3				6	3	1.5			
4			20	8	4	2	ml/h		
5				10	5		1		
6				12	6	3			
7				14	7				
8				16	8	4			
9				18	9		ml/h		
10				20	10	5	2	1	
12					14	7			
14					14	7			
15					15		3	1.5	ml/h:
20					20	10	4	2	1
25							5		
30						15	6	3	1.5
40						20	8	4	2
50							10	5	
100							20	10	5
150								15	
200								20	10

Drug labels (right-hand side brackets):
Noradrenaline; Morphine; Adrenaline isoprenaline; Salbutamol; Tolazoline; Nitroglycerin-Tridilset; Dopamine; Dobutamine; Ketamine; Nitroprusside Max. hours of infusion (10, 8, 7, 7, 6); Lignocaine; Thiopentone.

References

1. Kinsella JP, Neish SR, Dunbar ID *et al.* (1993) Clinical responses to prolonged treatment of persistent pulmonary hypertension of the newborn with low doses of inhaled nitric oxide. *J Pediatr* **123**:103–108.

2. Fletcher J, Shann F and Duncan AW (1987) The dangers of premature extubation after severe birth asphyxia. *Aust Paediatr J* **23**:27–29.

3. Steuven HA, Thompson BM, Aprahamian C, Tonsfeldt DJ and Kastenson EH (1985) Lack of effectiveness of calcium chloride in refractory asystole. *Ann Emerg Med* **14**:630–632.

4. Steuven HA, Thompson BM, Aprahamian C, Tonsfeldt DJ and Kastenson EH (1985) The effectiveness of calcium chloride in refractory electromechanical dissociation. *Ann Emerg Med* **14**:626–629.

5. Drop LJ (1985) Ionized calcium, the heart and hemodynamic function. *Anesth Analg* **64**:432–451.

6. Standards and guidelines for cardiopulmonary resuscitation and emergency care. *J Am Med Assoc* 1986; **255**:2841–3044.

7. Uhl JA (1981) Phenytoin: the drug of choice in tricyclic antidepressant overdose? *Ann Emerg Med* **10**:270–274.

8. Rosetti VA, Thompson BM, Miller J *et al.* (1985) Intraosseous infusion: an alternative route of pediatric intravascular access. *Ann Emerg Med* **14**:885–888.

9. Saccheti AD, Linkenheimer R, Liberman M *et al.* (1989) Intraosseous drug administration: successful resuscitation from asystole. *Pediatr Emerg Care* **5**:97–98.

10. Moscati R and Moore GP (1990) Compartment syndrome with resultant amputation following intraosseous infusion. *Am J Emerg Med* **8**:470–471.

11. Biggart MJ and Bohn DJ. (1990) Effect of hypothermia and cardiac arrest on outcome of near-drowning accidents in children. *J Pediatr* **117**:179–183.

12. Barzilay Z, Someleh E, Sagy M and Boichis H (1988) Pediatric cardiopulmonary resuscitation outcome. *J Med* **19**:229–241.

13. O'Rourke PP (1986) Outcome of children who are apneic and pulseless in the emergency room. *Crit Care Med* **14**:466–468.

14. Hickey RW, Cohen DM, Strausbaugh S and Dietrich AM (1995) Pediatric patients requiring CPR in the prehospital setting. *Ann Emerg Med* **25**:495–501.

15. Quan L, Wentz KR, Gore EJ and Copass MK (1990) Outcome and predictors of outcome in pediatric submersion victims receiving prehopsital care in King County, Washington. *Pediatrics* **86**:586–593.

16. Nichols DG, Kettrick RG, Swedlow DB *et al.* (1986) Factors influencing outcome of cardiopulmonary resuscitation in children. *Pediatr Emerg Care* **2**:1–5.

17. Gillis J, Dickson D, Rieder M, Steward D and Edmonds J (1986) Results of inpatient pediatric resuscitation. *Crit Care Med* **14**:469–471.

18. Zaritsky A, Nadkarni V, Getson P and Kuehl K (1987) CPR in children. *Ann Emerg Med* **16**:1107–1111.

19. Fiser DH and Wrape V (1987) Outcome of cardiopulmonary resuscitation in children. *Pediatr Emerg Care* **3**:235–238.

20. Shann F (1983) Continuous drug infusions in children: a table for simplifying calculations. *Crit Care Med* **11**:462–463.

21. Anand KJS and Hickey PR (1987) Pain and its effects in the human neonate and fetus. *N Engl J Med* **317**:1321–1329.

22. Henning R and McNamara V (1991) Difficulties encountered in transport of the critically ill child. *Pediatr Emerg Care* **7**:133–137.

23. Yeh TS, Pollack MM, Holbrook PR, Fields AI and Ruttiman UE (1982) Assessment of pediatric intensive care – application of the Therapeutic Intervention Scoring System. *Crit Care Med* **10**:497–500.

24. Wilkinson JD, Pollack MM, Ruttiman UE, Glass NL and Yeh TS (1986) Outcome of pediatric patients with multiple organ system failure. *Crit Care Med* **14**:271–274.

25. Pollack MM, Alexander SR, Clarke N *et al.* (1991) Improved outcomes from tertiary center pediatric intensive care: a statewide comparison of tertiary and nontertiary care facilities. *Crit Care Med* **19**:150–159.

AW Duncan

Upper respiratory tract obstruction (URTO) is a common cause of respiratory failure in infants and children. This reflects the frequency of upper respiratory tract disorders, presence of narrow airways and the compliant nature of the chest wall. The majority of children with critical airway obstruction are otherwise healthy, and expert management results in a normal life expectancy. Improper management has dire consequences.

Anatomical differences and clinical relevance

Differences in the anatomy and function of the airway are important considerations in airway maintenance, laryngoscopy and intubation. In the newborn, the nose contributes approximately 42% of total airways resistance – considerably less than the adult's 63%. Thus infants are obligatory nose-breathers. The epiglottis is longer, U-shaped and floppy, and may need to be lifted with a straight-bladed laryngoscope for visualization of the larynx and intubation. The larynx is higher in the neck (C3–4) in the neonate, and has an anterior inclination.[1] It descends over the first 3 years of life, and again at puberty, to lie opposite C6. The length of the trachea varies from 3.2 to 7.0 cm in babies weighing less than 6 kg. Accurate positioning of tracheal tubes is required to prevent accidental extubation and endobronchial intubation. The narrowest part of the airway until puberty is the cricoid ring. This part of the airway is most vulnerable to trauma and swelling. The narrow cricoid ring also dictates tube size, and allows use of uncuffed tubes in infants and children.

Pathophysiology

Although the ratio of airway diameter to body weight is relatively large in the infant, in absolute terms airway diameter is small, and a minimal reduction causes a devastating increase in airway resistance. For example, the diameter of the newborn's cricoid ring is 5 mm. A 50% reduction in radius will result in turbulent flow, and increases the pressure (and work) required to maintain breathing 32-fold.[2]

Symptoms and signs vary with the level of obstruction, the aetiology and the age of the child. Airway obstruction may be either extrathoracic or intrathoracic. Extrathoracic obstruction increases during inspiration and is characterized by inspiratory stridor and prolongation of inspiration. Intrathoracic obstruction of both large and small airways increases during expiration, and is characterized by expiratory stridor, prolonged expiration, wheeze and air trapping. Biphasic stridor is characteristic of mid tracheal lesions. These features mirror the intrapleural and airway pressure changes of the respiratory cycle (Fig. 102.1). Retraction of the chest wall reflects the negative intrapleural pressures generated and the compliant chest wall. Large negative intrapleural pressures are also transmitted to the interstitium of the lung, and may result in pulmonary oedema.[3,4] Cor pulmonale may develop secondary to chronic obstruction, hypoxia and pulmonary hypertension.[5,6]

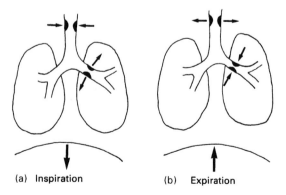

(a) Inspiration   (b) Expiration

Fig. 102.1 Dynamics of (a) extrathoracic and (b) intrathoracic airways obstruction.

Clinical presentation

Stridor is noisy breathing due to turbulent air flow. It is the cardinal feature of URTO. Parents complain that their child has noisy breathing and is 'sucking its chest in'. The pitch and timing of stridor provide information about the degree and level of obstruction.

Voice sounds may also be informative. Nasal obstruction results in hyponasality. Oropharyngeal obstruction may cause 'hot potato' voice. Supra-glottic obstruction is characterized by a muffled voice. Children with glottic lesions may be hoarse or aphonic.

Retraction of chest wall develops as obstruction progresses. Retraction is less prominent in older children, as chest-wall structure stabilizes. As obstruction worsens, the work of breathing increases and the accessory muscles become active. The alae nasi (vestigial muscles of ventilation) begin to flare. Fever increases minute volume and magnifies any degree of obstruction. Whereas infants and older children can maintain an increased work of breathing, premature infants and neonates rapidly fatigue, and many develop apnoeic episodes.[7,8]

Auscultation over the neck and larynx may identify the site obstruction. A foreign body in the airway may produce a mechanical or slapping sound. Decreased or absent breath sounds may occur with greater degrees of obstruction. Chronic URTO is a cause of failure to thrive, chest deformity (pectus excavatum) and cor pulmonale.[5,6] Some infants present with recurrent chest infections, and abnormal posturing (head retraction) may be a feature.

Initially, the child with airway obstruction exhibits tachypnoea and tachycardia. If obstruction is severe and persistent, exhaustion eventually occurs, and the child exhibits decreased respiratory effort, decreased stridor and breath sounds, restlessness, cyanosis, pallor and eventually bradycardia.

Aetiology

A classification of the causes of URTO is presented in Table 102.1. The neonatal causes are predominantly due to congenital structural lesions. Acute inflammatory lesions, foreign bodies and trauma predominate in older infants and children (see below).

Diagnosis

The cause of URTO can often be determined from the history and clinical features. Radiographic examination of the upper and lower airways with antero-posterior and lateral views may show soft-tissue swelling or the presence of foreign bodies.[9] Air shadows may indicate fixed stenotic or compressive lesions. In significant respiratory distress, these should be undertaken in the ICU rather than the radiology department.

Table 102.1 Causes of upper airway obstruction in children

Level	Newborn	Older infant and child
Nasal	Choanal atresia	
Oropharyngeal	Facial malformations, e.g. Pierre Robin syndrome, Treacher Collins syndrome Macroglossia Cystic hygroma Vallecular cyst	Macroglossia/post-glossectomy Angioedema Retropharyngeal abscess Tonsillar and adenoidal hypertrophy Obstructive sleep apnoea
Laryngeal	Infantile larynx Bilateral vocal cord palsy Congenital subglottic stenosis Subglottic haemangioma Laryngeal web Laryngeal cysts	Acute laryngotracheobronchitis Croup Bacterial tracheitis Acute epiglottitis Post-intubation oedema and stenosis Laryngeal papillomata Laryngeal foreign body Inhalation burns Caustic ingestion External trauma
Tracheal	Tracheomalacia Vascular ring	Foreign body Anterior mediastinal tumours (lymphoma)

Previously, barium swallow and aortography have been used to confirm the diagnosis of vascular compression of the trachea. Computed tomography (CT) has assumed importance in the assessment of fixed lesions such as intrinsic stenosis and extrinsic compression. Magnetic resonance imaging (MRI) and CT with contrast are useful to assess vascular anomalies.[10] Tracheobronchography may provide excellent anatomical delineation of the proximal tracheobronchial tree.

Direct visualization of the airway may be necessary, and may also prove therapeutic (e.g. removal of a foreign body). Nasoscopy, flexible fibreoptic and rigid laryngoscopy and bronchoscopy all have a place in assessing the paediatric airway. Investigation of the child's airway should only be undertaken in specialized centres by experienced endoscopists, radiologists and anaesthetists.

Blood-gas determination is rarely used. It is dangerous practice to await respiratory failure before intervention. Mild hypoxaemia only may be present until fatigue, hypoventilation, cyanosis and hypercapnoea occur. Pulse oximetry may provide useful warning information.

Specific airway obstructions

Epiglottitis

Epiglottitis is a life-threatening supraglottic lesion caused almost exclusively by *Haemophilus influenzae* type B. The prevalence of epiglottitis will fall as *H. influenzae* vaccination increases. Occasional cases are caused by streptococci, staphylococci or pneumococci. The diagnosis is usually obvious from history and clinical features. There is an acute onset of high fever, toxaemia and noisy breathing. The child adopts a characteristic posture, preferring to sit with the mouth open, drooling saliva. The tongue is often proptosed and immobile. Cough is usually absent. These features are the legacy of an intensely painful pharynx. Due to the accompanying septicaemia, the severity of illness often appears out of proportion to the degree of airway obstruction. Typically, a low-pitched inspiratory stridor is present, accompanied by a characteristic expiratory snore. Atypical cases with cough and without fever may obscure the diagnosis.

Sudden total obstruction is not infrequent, and may be precipitated by examination of the pharynx, the supine position or stressful procedures (e.g. cannula insertion). When the diagnosis is in doubt, a lateral X-ray of the neck in the sitting position should be taken in the ICU. Examination of the pharynx must not be undertaken unless personnel and facilities are available for immediate intubation.

Management

Parenteral antibiotics

Third-generation cephalosporins are the preferred antibiotics because of emerging resistances to ampicillin and, to a lesser extent, chloramphenicol. Appropriate regimens include cefotaxime 200 mg/kg per day IV for 5 days, or ceftriaxone 100 mg/kg IV statim followed by 50 mg/kg IV after 24 h. Children receiving cefotaxime may be changed to oral chloramphenicol once sensitivities are available and oral intake is tolerated.

Relief of airway obstruction

All but the mildest cases require an artificial airway. Nasotracheal intubation is the optimal treatment,[11] although tracheostomy is a satisfactory alternative, depending on the available personnel. Anaesthesia for relief of airway obstruction is described below. A tube of size appropriate to age is chosen (see Chapter 109). Extubation can be undertaken when fever subsides and the child no longer appears toxic. Most cases can be extubated in less than 18 h. Only those complicated by pulmonary oedema, pneumonia or cerebral hypoxia (from delayed therapy) will require intubation for longer than 24 h. It is not necessary to re-examine the larynx prior to extubation. Nebulized adrenaline is of no benefit in this condition and may aggravate the situation.[12] Pulmonary oedema, when it occurs, is due to airway obstruction, septicaemia and increased lung capillary permeability.[3,13,14] It is managed conventionally.

Prophylaxis

Most invasive infections due to *H. influenzae* occur in children under 5 years of age. The risk of infection in close contacts is about 500 times higher than in the general population. It is thus recommended that members (including adults) of any household with *H. influenzae* type B infection and with another child under 4 years should be given prophylactic antibiotics. The accepted regimen is rifampicin 20 mg/kg daily (maximum 600 mg) for 4 days (see Chapter 64). An alternative is a single dose of ceftriaxone 100 mg/kg IM.

Croup

Croup or acute laryngotracheobronchitis is due to inflammation and oedema of the glottic and sub-lottic regions. The narrowest part of the child's upper airway is the subglottic region, the point at which critical narrowing occurs. Retained secretions due to the bronchitic component may compound the obstruction. Three subgroups are recognized: viral croup, spasmodic croup and bacterial tracheitis.

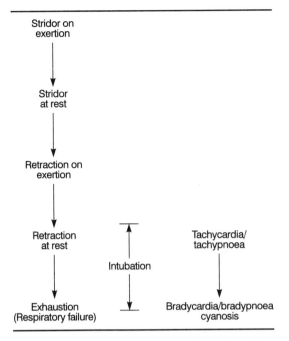

Fig. 102.2 Features of progressive upper airway obstruction.

Viral croup

Viral croup, most commonly due to parainfluenza virus, respiratory syncytial virus and rhinovirus, is characterized by a coryzal prodrome, low-grade fever, harsh barking (croupy) cough and hoarse voice. Progression of airway obstruction in severe cases is presented in Figure 102.2.

Spasmodic croup

Spasmodic or recurrent croup occurs in children with an allergic predisposition.[15,16] It usually develops suddenly, often at night, and without prodromal symptoms. Endoscopy reveals pale, watery oedema of the subglottic mucosa. Such children probably represent part of the asthma spectrum and wheeze may be a feature.

Bacterial tracheitis

Bacterial tracheitis is uncommon but should be suspected in children with croup accompanied by high fever, leukocytosis and copious purulent secretions.[17] There is a significant risk of sudden complete obstruction. *Staphylococcus aureus* is usually the cause, although *H. influenzae* and group A *Streptococcus* have also been isolated.

Croup is uncommon under 6 months of age, and an underlying structural lesion such as subglottic sten-

osis or haemangioma with superimposed infection should be suspected. Endoscopy is warranted with a prior history of stridor or if symptoms persist.

Management

1 *Minimal disturbance* is important, as handling will increase minute ventilation, oxygen consumption and signs of obstruction.
2 *Adequate hydration*: Oral fluid intake must be encouraged to avoid dehydration. Gavage feeding is contraindicated, and IV fluids may occasionally be necessary. Overhydration must also be avoided. Hyponatraemia and convulsions due to inappropriate antidiuretic hormone secretion have been observed with prolonged, severe airway obstruction.
3 *Oxygen therapy* may mask signs of respiratory failure, but should be given to treat hypoxaemia. Its use can be guided by pulse oximetry (i.e. keep Sao_2 >90%). Oxygen administration may further stress the young child. The need for oxygen therapy is often an indication for intubation.
4 *Corticosteroids* have dramatically reduced the requirement for intubation in children with croup. They are effective in both viral and spasmodic croup.[18,19] Steroids will also shorten the duration of intubation and increase the success rate of extubation.[20,21] The dose of dexamethasone is 0.6 mg/kg statim (maximum 10 mg) followed, if necessary, by 0.15 mg/kg 6-hourly. In very distressed children it is best administered IM to ensure absorption. Inhaled steroids are also effective in milder cases.[22]
5 *Humidification* of inspired gases was the mainstay of supportive care for decades. Controlled studies showing efficacy are lacking. A study by Bourchier *et al.* failed to demonstrate benefit and its use has been abandoned in many centres.[23]
6 *Nebulized adrenaline* will usually provide temporary relief of acute obstruction.[24] Historically, racemic adrenaline (a 2.25% solution, i.e. 1:88 L-adrenaline) for use in asthma was employed. Indications for adrenaline nebulization are:

(a) acute laryngotracheobronchitis, where relief usually lasts 1–2 h, but may be longer if secretions are expelled. It is debatable whether the natural history of the disease is altered. If given prior to induction, it will facilitate inhalational anaesthesia for intubation;
(b) spasmodic croup, where one or two inhalations may obviate the need for intubation;
(c) postendoscopy or intubation oedema, where the benefit is often dramatic;
(d) transport, where administration will render the child safe for interhospital transfer.

The empirical dose is 0.05 ml/kg diluted to 2 ml with saline, and nebulized with oxygen. A strong

Table 102.2 Nasotracheal tube size in croup

Age	Size
Less than 6 months	3.0 mm
6 months to 2 years	3.5 mm
2–5 years	4.0 mm
Over 5 years	4.5 mm

preparation (1%) of the L-isomer can also be used. The same mass of L-adrenaline is provided by 0.5 ml/kg of the standard 1:1000 solution of adrenaline, and this is equally effective.

7 *Antibiotics* are indicated only for bacterial tracheitis where anti-staphylococcal cover is recommended.

8 *Mechanical relief of airway obstruction*: This requirement has been greatly reduced by early use of steroids. The need for tracheal intubation is indicated by increasing tachycardia, tachypnoea and restlessness. A Sa_{O_2} persistently less than 90% is another reason for concern. One should not wait for the development of bradycardia, bradypnoea, cyanosis, exhaustion and respiratory failure. Blood gases are not a useful guide for intubation. Nasotracheal intubation is preferred. An orotracheal tube, size ID 1 mm less than that predicted by age (Table 102.2), is first inserted under anaesthesia (see below). A stylet is used to overcome the resistance of the subglottic region. The tube is changed to a nasotracheal tube immediately after aspiration of secretions.

Extubation is performed when the child is afebrile, secretions have diminished and a leak is audible around the tube with coughing or positive pressure (25 cm H_2O or less). The duration of intubation averages 5 days. Children under 1 year old have a higher incidence of intubation and a longer duration of intubation. Reintubation may be required in some cases. Tracheostomy is a suitable alternative for some situations, although complications are more significant.

Other supraglottic lesions

Retropharyngeal abscess, tonsillitis, peritonsillar abscess, infectious mononucleosis and Ludwig's angina may all mimic epiglottis. Local features will usually indicate the diagnosis. A retropharyngeal abscess can be detected by palpation and is obvious on a lateral X-ray of the neck. Airway relief, antibiotics, drainage and, rarely, neck incision form the basis of treatment for these disorders. A nasopharyngeal tube is often useful in supraglottic lesions. Tonsillectomy, although best performed electively, is occasionally indicated in the acute phase. Steroids

appear to be effective in infectious mononucleosis and the response is rapid.

Tonsillar and adenoidal airway obstruction

The conservative approach to tonsillectomy and adenoidectomy has led to an increased incidence of hypertrophy and chronic upper airway obstruction in some children.[25] Such children may present with severe, acute exacerbations due to intercurrent infection (e.g. tonsillitis). They may present in a toxic state with drooling, thereby mimicking acute epiglottitis. Obstruction is most marked during sleep. In the most severe cases, it may be necessary to relieve the obstruction with a nasotracheal tube or a nasopharyngeal tube positioned beyond the tonsillar bed. Tonsillectomy and adenoidectomy are generally contraindicated in the acute phase, because of increased risk of bleeding, but are performed when infection has settled.

Obstructive sleep apnoea syndrome

Obstructive sleep apnoea (OSA) syndrome is characterized by intermittent upper airway obstruction during sleep, with heavy snoring, stertorous breathing and an abnormal, irregular respiratory pattern.[26] Frequent episodes of chest-wall motion with inadequate air flow (hypopnoea) or absent air flow (obstructive apnoea) are a feature. These episodes are most frequent during rapid eye movement sleep. They are accompanied by variable degrees of oxygen desaturation. OSA may be associated with enlarged tonsils and adenoids, a large uvula or long soft palate, macroglossia, retrognathia or various neurological disorders. Obesity is a common finding.

If OSA is severe and protracted, cardiac and pulmonary decompensation may occur. Chronic hypoxia and hypercarbia lead to pulmonary hypertension and cor pulmonale.[5,6] There may also be evidence of left ventricular failure and pulmonary oedema. Urgency of treatment is dictated by the mode of presentation. Critically ill children may require immediate relief of airway obstruction (nasopharyngeal or nasotracheal tube), oxygen therapy, diuretics and digitalization. Antibiotics are indicated if there is bacterial superinfection. Surgical intervention is required after stabilization. Tonsillectomy and adenoidectomy are often dramatically beneficial. They are best removed even when not grossly enlarged. Other surgical procedures such as uvulopalatopharyngoplasty or tracheostomy may be required when this fails. The use of nocturnal continuous positive airway pressure (CPAP) or nasopharyngeal intubation is rarely feasible in young children.

Pierre Robin syndrome

This consists of a posterior cleft palate, retrognathia and relative macroglossia. It is a cause of airway obstruction, feeding difficulties and failure to thrive in the newborn. Differential growth eventually reduces the significance of the deformity. Acute airway obstruction may be relieved by nursing the infant in the prone position or by passage of a nasopharyngeal tube.[27] Occasionally, nasotracheal intubation or tracheostomy is required. Tongue–lip anastomosis is sometimes beneficial.

Cystic hygroma

Although often conspicuous at birth, cystic hygroma is a relatively rare cause of upper airway obstruction in infancy. The tumours consist of masses of dilated lymphatic channels. They usually occur in the neck and may involve tissues of the tongue and larynx. Occasionally, extension into the mediastinum occurs. Airway obstruction may be due to infection or haemorrhage into the lesion. Surgical excision has been the mainstay of treatment, although complete removal is difficult and recurrence is common. Treatment using sclerosing therapy with bleomycin emulsion is now used.[28] In severe cases, long-term tracheostomy is required.

Inhalation burns

Respiratory complications are the major cause of mortality in children who are burnt. Direct airway burns or inhalation of products of combustion may lead to rapidly progressive oedema. The situation may be compounded by small airway and lung injury. Early intubation is strongly recommended prior to an emergency situation developing. Tracheal tube fixation may be problematic with extensive facial burns.

Subglottic stenosis

Neonates with congenital subglottic stenosis may present with severe obstruction requiring intubation at birth. Other infants present with persistent stridor or recurrent croup due to superimposed infection. Subglottic stenosis may also occur as a complication of intubation, or as the result of pressure, mucosal ischaemia and healing by fibrosis. Prolonged intubation or tracheostomy may be required. Surgical techniques such as the cricoid split procedure or laryngotracheoplasty may be required to enlarge the airway.

Subglottic haemangioma

Haemangiomata are common in infancy and occur in many parts of the body. Subglottic lesions often present in the second or third month of life and owe their importance to the anatomical location. Stridor is usually both inspiratory and expiratory. A hoarse cry is indicative of vocal cord involvement. Obstruction may be severe and is aggravated by crying, struggling or superimposed infection. Cutaneous haemangiomata are present in 50%, and provide a clue to diagnosis. Definitive diagnosis rests on endoscopy. The natural history is of spontaneous resolution between the first and second years of life. Meanwhile, tracheostomy or repeated intubation may be indicated to cover periods of obstruction. Encouraging results are being obtained with laser surgery. Steroids are of dubious benefit.

Foreign body or choking

A foreign body must be suspected in any acute obstruction occurring in an infant or child between 6 months and 2 years of age. A foreign body lodged in the pharynx results in gagging, respiratory distress and facial congestion. Laryngeal impaction usually produces stridor, a distressing cough and aphonia. Sudden total obstruction may occur. Symptoms usually develop while the child is playing or eating.

The technique for removal of a pharyngolaryngeal foreign body without equipment in infants and children is controversial and difficult. The American Academy of Pediatrics has made recommendations to cover various ages.[29] Gravity should be utilized by placing the child prone, straddled over your arm with the head down and a hand supporting the jaw. Four back blows between the shoulder blades should be administered. If this fails, chest thrusts or finger sweep across the pharynx should be attempted. There is some risk that the latter manoeuvre may impact the foreign body in the larynx. Abdominal thrusts (the Heimlich manoeuvre) are not recommended in infants but may be useful in children older than 1 year. Expired air resuscitation should be attempted in an emergency, although the risk of gastric distension is great. The best method of removal is extraction under direct vision using a laryngoscope, forceps, suction or finger.

Tracheal or bronchial foreign bodies produce persistent cough and wheeze, and recurrent pneumonia. A foreign body lodged in the upper oesophagus may compress the trachea and present with either acute or, more commonly, persistent stridor. Radiopaque materials are easily shown radiologically, but both anteroposterior and lateral views may be necessary. Barium studies may prove useful for nonradiopaque material in the oesophagus. Treatment is removal at bronchoscopy or oesophagoscopy.

Anterior mediastinal tumours

Anterior mediastinal tumours, such as lymphoma, may compress the trachea or bronchi, causing symptoms such as dry cough, stridor or wheeze. Airway compression may become severe enough to cause hyperinflation or atelectasis. Pleural effusion is common and may add to the respiratory distress. Symptoms may be aggravated by the supine position, especially during anaesthesia for a biopsy procedure.

This is particularly likely in patients with superior vena caval syndrome. Postural symptoms or findings on flow–volume loops may allude to this risk. Sudden complete obstruction that cannot be bypassed by a standard tracheal tube has been described. The use of armoured tubes or a rigid bronchoscope may be required. Consideration should be given to leaving the tracheal tube *in situ* postoperatively until corticosteroids and chemotherapy reduce the tumour mass.

Anaesthesia for relief of airway obstruction

Inhalational induction and anaesthesia with oxygen and halothane is the preferred technique for intubation. The use of muscle relaxants is hazardous if the ability to maintain a patent airway is doubtful. Important points are:

1 A prepared induction should be undertaken with efficient suction apparatus, a range of tracheal tubes and suitable stylets. One must be prepared to intubate without deep anaesthesia if sudden obstruction occurs.
2 Inhalational anaesthesia is slow in upper airway obstruction and lower airways disease.
3 Induction in the sitting position is advocated with epiglottitis. The child is laid flat after induction and prior to intubation.
4 CPAP or assisted ventilation will reduce obstruction and hasten induction. Care must be taken not to distend the stomach.
5 Laryngoscopy is performed, and the child intubated only when adequate depth of anaesthesia is achieved (approximately 8–10 min of 4% halothane in oxygen).
6 Orotracheal intubation is quickest and safest, and should be performed initially. After good tracheal toilet, the tube is changed to a nasotracheal one.

Care of nasotracheal tube

Successful management of URTO in children requires optimal care of nasotracheal intubation. Such children must always be nursed in an ICU. The nasotracheal tube must be positioned at the level of the clavicular heads (T2) on an anteroposterior chest X-ray. Length of tube from 1 to 6 years of age (in centimetres measured at the nose) is given by age in years + 13 cm. A meticulous technique of fixation must be employed to prevent accidental extubation.

Adequate humidification is difficult in the active child. It is, nevertheless, important to prevent obstruction of narrow tubes by inspissated secretions. Lightweight heat and moisture exchangers (HME), e.g. Thermovent (Gibeck) and Humidvent (Portex), are very useful.[30] The HME should be changed every 24 h to reduce contamination and increased resistance. Oxygen supplementation can be provided, if necessary. Some children will tolerate connection of a humidified T-piece.

Effective bagging and tracheal toilet is vital, and should be repeated until the airway is clear. Instillation of saline (0.5–1.0 ml) prior to suction may be necessary to remove secretions. Light sedation is used to improve tolerance of the tracheal tube and to reduce the risk of self-extubation. Midazolam 0.1–0.2 mg/kg statim followed by continuous infusion (0.05–0.2 mg/kg per h) is effective. Arm restraints may also be advisable, particularly in very young children. Signs of obstruction are usually relieved by intubation. Mild retraction may persist due to high fever and increased minute ventilation in the presence of a smaller than predicted tube. Fibreoptic bronchoscopy can be performed to confirm patency. The tracheal tube must be changed or removed if there is doubt about its patency.

Nasogastric tube feeding should be commenced in children who require intubation longer than 24 h.

Tracheostomy

Tracheostomy remains a life-saving procedure and must be undertaken if tracheal intubation is impossible or if appropriate equipment or personnel to facilitate intubation is unavailable. For chronic airway problems, it is more comfortable, allows better nasopharyngeal toilet, and permits the child to leave the ICU and eventually return home. It is best performed under tracheal anaesthesia with the neck extended. A longitudinal slit is made through the second and third tracheal rings without removal of cartilage. Stay sutures in the tracheal wall lateral to the incision aid recannulation if accidental dislodgment occurs prior to formation of a well-defined tract (after 4 days). A postoperative chest X-ray should be obtained to check the position of the tip of the tracheostomy tube and to exclude pneumothorax.

Care of a newly created tracheostomy is similar to that of an endotracheal tube, with the additional problem of some discomfort and blood in the airway. The first tracheostomy tube change is usually performed between 5 and 7 days.

Cricothyrotomy

A wide-bore plastic IV cannula (14- or 16-gauge) passed into the trachea via the cricothyroid membrane may be life-saving, if alternative procedures are unavailable. This should be performed with the neck extended as for tracheostomy. A system of connection to a low-pressure oxygen supply must be planned in advance. One method is to attach the hub of the cannula to the sleeve of a plastic 2–3 ml syringe (without plunger), to an adaptor from a 7.5 mm OD tracheal tube, and then to a breathing circuit (e.g. Jackson Rees modification of Ayres T-piece).

References

1. Westhorpe RN (1987) The position of the larynx in children and its relationship to the ease of intubation. *Anaesth Intens Care* **15**:384–388.
2. Badgwell JM, McLeod ME and Friedberg J (1987) Airway obstruction in infants and children. *Can J Anaesth* **34**:90–98.
3. Sofer S, Bar-Ziv J and Scharf SM (1984) Pulmonary edema following relief of upper airway obstruction. *Chest* **86**:401–403.
4. Stalcup SA and Mellins RB (1977) Mechanical forces producing pulmonary edema in acute asthma. *N Engl J Med* **297**:592–596.
5. Cox MA, Schiebler GL, Taylor WJ, Wheat MW and Krovetz LJ (1965) Reversible pulmonary hypertension in a child with respiratory obstruction and cor pulmonale. *J Pediatr* **67**:192–197.
6. Luke MJ, Mehrizi A, Folger GM and Rowe RD (1966) Chronic nasopharyngeal obstruction as a cause of cardiomegaly, cor pulmonale, and pulmonary oedema. *Pediatrics* **37**:762–768.
7. Keens TG, Bryan AC, Levinson H and Ianuzzo CD (1978) Development pattern of muscle fibre types in human ventilatory muscles. *J Appl Physiol: Respir Environ Exercise Physiol* **44**:909–913.
8. Muller NL and Bryan AC (1979) Chest wall mechanics and respiratory muscles in infants. *Pediatr Clin North Am* **26**:503–516.
9. Kushner DC and Harris GBC (1978) Obstructing lesions of the larynx and trachea in infants and children. *Radiol Clin North Am* **16**:181–194.
10. Siegel MJ, Nadel SN, Glazer HS and Sagel SS (1986) Mediastinal lesions in children. Comparison of CT and MR. *Radiology* **160**:241–244.
11. Butt W, Shann F, Walker C, Williams J, Duncan A and Phelan P (1988) Acute epiglottitis: a different approach to management. *Crit Care Med* **16**:43–47.
12. Kissoon N and Mitchell I (1985) Adverse effects of racemic epinephrine in epiglottitis. *Pediatr Emerg Care* **1**:143–144.
13. Soliman MG and Richer P (1978) Epiglottitis and pulmonary oedema in children. *Can Anaesth Soc* **25**:270–275.
14. Travis KW, Todres DI and Shannon DC (1977) Pulmonary edema associated with croup and epiglottitis. *Pediatrics* **59**:695–698.
15. Zach M, Erben E and Olinsky A (1981) Croup, recurrent croup, allergy and airways hyper-reactivity. *Arch Dis Child* **56**:336–341.
16. Zach MS, Schnall RP and Landau LI (1980) Upper and lower airway hyper-reactivity in recurrent croup. *Am Rev Respir Dis* **121**:979–983.
17. Jones R, Santos JI and Overall JC (1979) Bacterial tracheitis. *J Am Med Assoc* **242**:721–726.
18. Super DM, Cartelli NA, Brooks LJ, Lembo RM and Kumar ML (1989) A prospective randomized double-blind study to evaluate the effect of dexamethasone in acute laryngotracheitis. *J Pediatr* **115**:323–329.
19. Koren G, Frand M, Barzilay Z and MacLeod SM (1983) Corticosteriod treatment of laryngotracheitis in spasmodic croup in children. *Am J Dis Child* **137**:941–944.
20. Tibballs J, Shann FA and Landau FI (1992) Placebo controlled trial of prednisolone in children intubated for croup. *Lancet* **340**:745–748.
21. Freezer N, Butt W and Phelan P (1990) Steroids in croup: do they increase the incidence of successful extubation? *Anaesth Intens Care* **18**:224–228.
22. Klassen TP, Feldman ME, Watters LK, Sutcliffe T and Rowe PC (1994) Nebulized budesonide for children with mild to moderate croup. *N Engl J Med* **331**:285–289.
23. Bourchier D, Dawson KP and Fergusson DM (1984) Humidification in viral croup: a controlled trial. *Aust Paediatr J* **20**:289–291.
24. Jordan WS, Graves CL and Elwyn RA (1970) New therapy for postintubation laryngeal edema and tracheitis in children. *J Am Med Assoc* **212**:585–588.
25. Check WA (1982) Does drop in tonsillectomies and adenoidectomies pose new issue of adeno-tonsillar hypertophy? *J Am Med Assoc* **247**:1229–1230.
26. Guilleminault C, Tilkian A and Dement WC (1976) The sleep apnea syndromes. *Ann Rev Med* **27**:465–484.
27. Heaf DP, Helms PJ, Dinwiddie MB and Mathew DJ (1982) Nasopharyngeal airways in Pierre Robin syndrome. *J Pediatr* **100**:698–703.
28. Tanaka K, Inomata Y, Utsunomiya H *et al.* (1990) Sclerosing therapy with bleomycin emulsion for lymphangioma in children. *Pediatr Surg Int* **5**:270–273.
29. American Academy of Pediatrics committee on accident and poison prevention (1988) First aid for the choking child, 1988. *Pediatrics* **81**:740–742.
30. Duncan A (1985) Use of disposable condenser humidifiers in children. *Anaesth Intens Care* **13**:330.

Acute respiratory failure in children

AW Duncan

Established or imminent respiratory failure is the commonest reason for admission to neonatal and paediatric ICUs. Respiratory failure is frequently a consequence of pathology primarily affecting other organ systems, e.g. congenital heart disease or central nervous system (CNS) disturbances. The high incidence of respiratory failure, particularly in the first year of life, is due to a lower respiratory reserve.

Predisposing factors

Respiratory function must equate with metabolic demands. Oxygen consumption in the neonate is approximately 7 ml/kg per min (3–4 ml/kg per min in the older child and adult). Fever, illness, and restlessness dramatically increase demands; in apnoea, Pa_{CO_2} rises at twice the rate of normal. The lower respiratory reserve in infants and neonates is due to the following.

Structural immaturity of the thoracic cage[1]

The ribs are short and horizontal, and the bucket motion that increases the anteroposterior and lateral dimensions of the thorax is minimal. Thus, the infant is dependent on diaphragmatic displacement of abdominal contents to increase the length and volume of the thorax. Ribcage structure and function alter between 12 and 18 months, possibly related to assumption of an upright posture. Any impairment of diaphragmatic function (e.g. abdominal distension) may precipitate respiratory failure.

The chest wall is soft and provides a poor fulcrum for respiratory effort. Retraction of bony structures and soft tissues occurs with reduced lung compliance and increased airway resistance. Infant intrapleural pressure is −1 to −2 cm H_2O (−0.1 to −0.2 kPa) compared with −5 to −10 cm H_2O (−0.5 to −1.0 kPa) in the adult. This is due to the higher compliance of the chest wall (which tends to collapse in) and a lower elastic recoil of the lung. The result is an increased

tendency to airway closure, atelectasis and intra-pulmonary shunting.

In the neonate, the diaphragm and intercostal muscles have a lower percentage of type 1 (slow twitch and high oxidative) muscle fibres, and therefore fatigue more readily. Increased respiratory work is poorly sustained and may culminate in apnoea.[2]

Infant airways

Although relatively large compared with the adult, airways of infants in absolute terms are small and more prone to obstruction. Trachea and bronchiole diameters of a 3-kg neonate are one-third and one-half, respectively, those of a 60-kg adult. However, any oedema will have a more profound effect on airway resistance in the infant.

Increased susceptibility to infection

The immaturity and inexperience of the immune system result in a markedly increased susceptibility to infection in the first 6 months of life. Both cell-mediated (T-cell) and humoral (B-cell) systems may be impaired.

Immature development of the respiratory system

Premature infants in particular may have surfactant deficiency, with alveolar instability, atelectasis, intrapulmonary shunting and reduced lung compliance.

Immaturity of respiratory control

Inadequate respiratory drive from immaturity of the respiratory centre is a factor leading to apnoeic spells, particularly in premature infants. Opioid analgesics are associated with greater respiratory depression.

Congenital abnormalities

Defects of the respiratory system or associated organs (e.g. heart) often present with respiratory failure shortly after birth.

Perinatal asphyxia or injuries

Asphyxia or intracranial haemorrhage associated with birth may result in seizures and respiratory depression.

Clinical presentation

Respiratory distress is manifested by tachypnoea, distortion of the chest wall (i.e. sternal and rib retraction, recession of intercostal, subcostal and suprasternal spaces) and use of accessory muscles (e.g. flaring of alae nasi and use of neck muscles).

In *young infants*, lethargy, pallor, apnoea, bradycardia and hypotension may be the first signs of hypoxia. The physiological anaemia of infancy may delay recognition of cyanosis, and major signs are those of CNS and cardiovascular depression. Increased work of breathing, marked by tachypnoea and chest-wall retraction, is poorly sustained; bradypnoea and apnoea are evidence of respiratory fatigue. Expiratory grunting represents an attempt to maintain a positive expiratory airway pressure to prevent airway closure and alveolar collapse, the equivalent of pursed-lip breathing in the adult.

The *older child* with acute hypoxia, like the adult, demonstrates tachypnoea, tachycardia, hypertension, mental confusion and restlessness prior to CNS and cardiovascular depression. Sweating occurs with CO_2 retention – a feature lacking in the newborn.

In the *newborn*, the effects of hypoxia may be compounded by the development of pulmonary hypertension and reversion to a transitional circulation, with right-to-left shunting through a patent ductus arteriosus and foramen ovale. If untreated, increasing hypoxaemia, progressive acidosis and death may occur.

Clinical examination of the chest should be performed routinely. It is, however, of limited value in the neonate, as breath sounds may be transmitted uniformly throughout the chest, even in the presence of tension pneumothorax, lobar collapse or endobronchial intubation. Chest X-ray is an essential part of assessment.

Aetiology

Acute respiratory failure may result from upper or lower airway obstruction, alveolar disease, pulmonary compression, neuromuscular disease or injury (Table 103.1). Upper respiratory tract obstruction is discussed in Chapter 102.

Tracheomalacia, tracheal stenosis and vascular compression

Instability of the tracheal wall is most commonly associated with oesophageal atresia, tracheo-oesophageal fistula and various vascular anomalies. The most common causes of vascular compression are a double aortic arch and the complex of a right-sided aortic arch, left ductus arteriosus and an aberrant left subclavian artery. These produce a true vascular ring, with encirclement of the trachea and oesophagus. Anterior tracheal compression may also be due to an anomalous innominate artery. Lower tracheomalacia or tracheal stenosis may occur in association with an anomalous left pulmonary artery. The problem may extend to the major bronchi (bronchomalacia).

Division of the vascular ring and ligation or repositioning of the aberrant vessel, while removing the cause of obstruction, do not immediately re-establish normal airway dimensions or stability. Although severity of symptoms may be alleviated by surgery, problems may persist for some years. Tracheomalacia may sometimes be stabilized by a prolonged period of nasotracheal intubation or tracheostomy with continuous positive airway pressure (CPAP). Tracheopexy, which suspends the anterior tracheal wall from the posterior sternal surface and great vessels, is occasionally useful.

Meconium aspiration syndrome

Meconium aspiration is seen in 0.3% of live births, and is most common in term or post-term infants. There is usually a history of fetal distress in labour, or prolonged and complicated delivery. Asphyxia during labour results in the expulsion of meconium into the liquor. With the first few breaths, material in the upper airway (i.e. amniotic fluid, meconium, vernix and squames) is inhaled, obstructing small airways and producing atelectasis and obstructive emphysema. Meconium also causes a chemical pneumonitis. With recovery, the aspirated material is absorbed and phagocytosed.

Clinical signs include tachypnoea, retraction and cyanosis. The chest may become hyperexpanded and pneumomediastinum or pneumothorax are frequent complications. Pulmonary hypertension and persistent fetal circulation are common.

The chest X-ray confirms the diagnosis, with coarse mottling and streakiness radiating from the hila. Lungs are over-expanded, with flattened diaphragms and an increase in the chest anteroposterior diameter. The condition is largely preventable if the airway can be aspirated rapidly and completely following delivery of the head, before the first breath.

Most of these infants require oxygen therapy. Severely affected ones require conventional

Table 103.1 Causes of respiratory insufficiency in infancy and childhood

Site	Neonate	Older infant and child
Upper airway obstruction	See Chapter 102	
Lower airway obstruction		
Tracheal	Tracheomalacia	Foreign body
	Vascular anomalies	
	Tracheal stenosis	Mediastinal tumour
Bronchial	Bronchomalacia	Foreign body
Bronchiolar	Meconium aspiration	
	Lobar emphysema	Acute viral bronchiolitis
Disorders of lung function		
	Aspiration syndromes	Pneumonia
		Cystic fibrosis
	Hyaline membrane disease	
	Bronchopulmonary dysplasia	Aspiration syndromes
	Perinatal pneumonia	
	Massive pulmonary haemorrhage	Congenital heart disease
	Pulmonary oedema	Near-drowning
	Pulmonary hypoplasia	Trauma
	Diaphragmatic hernia	Burns
		Acute respiratory distress syndrome
Pulmonary compression		
	Diaphragmatic hernia	Pneumothorax
	Pneumothorax	Pleural effusion
	Repaired exomphalos or gastroschisis	Empyema
Neurological and muscular disorders	Diaphragmatic palsy	Poisoning
	Birth asphyxia	Meningitis
	Convulsions	Encephalitis
	Apnoea of prematurity	Status epilepticus
		Trauma
		Guillain–Barré syndrome
		Envenomation

mechanical ventilation (CMV), which may be difficult because of the high pressures required, unevenness of ventilation, and danger of pneumothorax. Extracorporeal membrane oxygenation (ECMO) has been shown to be effective in some infants.[3,4] Promising results are being achieved with inhaled nitric oxide, sometimes in association with high-frequency ventilation.[5] Cerebral effects of severe intrapartum asphyxia contribute to some deaths.

Lobar emphysema

Most cases (70%) present in the first month of life, with tachypnoea, wheezing, grunting and cough. Signs include hyperresonance, decreased air entry and deviation of the trachea and heart away from the affected lobe. There may be asymmetry of the chest due to bulging of the affected hemithorax. Cyanosis may be associated with periods of increased respiratory distress.

Radiologically, the affected lobe is over-distended with compression and deviation of the surrounding structures. The pathogenesis is unknown in over 50%; 25% have localized bronchial cartilaginous dysplasia; the remainder have obstruction of a lobar bronchus from a mucous plug, redundant mucosa, aberrant vessels or localized stenosis. Lobectomy is often required. Care must be taken with positive airway pressure, because of the risk of further overdistension.

Aspiration pneumonia

In the newborn, aspiration may result from pharyngeal incoordination or lack of protective reflexes, due to prematurity, birth asphyxia or intracranial haemorrhage. It is particularly likely to occur with abnormalities of the alimentary tract, such as oesophageal atresia, tracheo-oesophageal fistula and oesophageal reflux. Large and small airways obstruction and pneumonia may occur.

Hyaline membrane disease

This is due to deficiency of lung surfactant. Predisposing factors are prematurity, maternal diabetes, intranatal asphyxia and elective caesarean section. Surfactant production is also inhibited by postnatal hypoxia and acidosis. Lack of surfactant results in alveolar instability, atelectasis, intrapulmonary shunting and increased work of breathing.

Clinical signs appear shortly after birth and consist of tachypnoea, chest-wall retraction, expiratory grunting and a progressive increase in oxygen requirements. The chest X-ray reveals a reticulogranular pattern (ground-glass appearance) with air bronchograms. In uncomplicated cases, the disease is self-limiting and resolves in 4–5 days. Respiratory failure may require increasing inspired oxygen concentrations (Fio_2), CPAP, intermittent mandatory ventilation (IMV) or CMV. CPAP is known to improve oxygenation, the pattern and regularity of respiration, retard the progression of the disease and reduce morbidity.

Instillation of surfactant into the trachea has been shown to improve oxygenation and compliance (despite some initial deterioration) and reduce the risk of pneumothorax, early mortality and morbidity.[6-8] Surfactant therapy may increase the risk of lesser degrees of intracranial haemorrhage, particularly in very-low-birthweight infants. Two types of surfactant are used, synthetic (Exosurf) and bovine (Survanta) or porcine (Curosurf).

Bronchopulmonary dysplasia

Bronchopulmonary dysplasia may occur in survivors of neonatal lung disease. Its occurrence correlates with lung immaturity, high airway pressures and barotrauma. It is a cause of chronic respiratory failure in infancy, and occasionally progresses to cor pulmonale and death in the first 2 years of life. Prolonged low-flow home oxygen therapy may be necessary to reduce this risk.

Pneumonia

Perinatal pneumonia may occur as a result of transplacental spread of a maternal infection, prolonged rupture of membranes, passage through an infected birth canal or cross-infection in the nursery. The immunoparetic state of the newborn and the need for invasive procedures increase the risk.

Clinical and radiological features may be indistinguishable from hyaline membrane disease. Antibiotics (e.g. penicillin and gentamicin) should be given until negative cultures exclude the diagnosis. The most common organisms include group B haemolytic streptococcus, *Escherichia coli*, *Pseudomonas aeruginosa*, *Klebsiella pneumoniae* and *Staphylococcus aureus*. Group B haemolytic streptococcus infection is frequently associated with septic shock and persistent fetal circulation. Failure to suspect group B haemolytic streptococcus infections (and hence treat promptly with penicillin) will result in poor outcome. Multiresistant staphylococcal and Gram-negative bacillary infections must be suspected in longer-stay patients in neonatal ICUs.

Most pneumonia in infants and young children is of viral origin. Viruses commonly implicated are respiratory syncytial virus (RSV), influenza A1, A2 and B, and parainfluenza types 1 and 3. Adenovirus and rhinovirus are less common causes. The spectrum of illness is wide. Many infants and children have cough, fever and tachypnoea, with X-ray evidence of patchy consolidation, all of which resolve rapidly. Occasionally, infants develop life-threatening respiratory illness with extensive pneumonic changes and marked tissue necrosis. Permanent lung damage with bronchiolitis obliterans and pulmonary fibrosis may occasionally complicate severe adenoviral pneumonia.

Bacterial pneumonia also occurs. Pneumococcal pneumonia is common and usually responds dramatically to appropriate antibiotic therapy. Staphylococcal pneumonia is relatively uncommon, but may result in life-threatening respiratory failure, and is often associated with complications (e.g. empyema, pneumatocele, tension pneumothorax and suppuration in other organs). Aspiration of an effusion may be useful for diagnostic purposes. Tube thoracostomy or rib resection may be necessary to treat empyema. In severe cases with bronchopleural fistula, surgical resection of the necrotic area offers the best chance of survival.

Pneumonia due to *Haemophilus influenzae* may also occur and be associated with epiglottitis, meningitis, pericarditis or middle-ear disease.

Gram-negative pneumonia is seen mostly in infants with debilitating conditions who are hospitalized for prolonged periods. It is a particular risk for patients in ICUs with endotracheal or tracheostomy tubes. Other opportunistic infections, such as *Pneumocystis carinii*, *Candida albicans*, *Aspergillus* and cytomegalovirus, may occur in immune deficiency states.

Massive pulmonary haemorrhage

This usually presents as acute cardiorespiratory collapse, accompanied by outpouring of blood-stained fluid from the trachea, mouth and nose. It is seen in association with severe birth asphyxia, hyaline membrane disease, congenital heart disease, erythroblastosis fetalis, coagulopathy and sepsis. Hypoxia is often a precipitating factor. The condition is believed to represent haemorrhagic pulmonary oedema due to acute left ventricular failure. Treatment is that of the underlying condition with oxygenation, CMV and correction of any coagulation disturbance.

Pulmonary oedema

Pulmonary oedema in the newborn period is due mostly to congenital heart disease, especially coarctation of the aorta, patent ductus arteriosus, critical aortic stenosis and, rarely, obstructed total anomalous pulmonary venous drainage. Pulmonary oedema due to circulatory overload may also occur in erythroblastosis foetalis, the placental transfusion syndrome, or as a result of inappropriate fluid therapy.

Clinical features are those of respiratory distress in the newborn period, but specific features of congenital heart lesions may be evident. There is a spectrum of severity, from tachypnoea with a widened alveolar–arterial oxygen gradient to life-threatening respiratory failure requiring urgent support. Chest X-ray usually shows an enlarged heart (except in total anomalous pulmonary venous drainage) and a ground-glass appearance fanning out from the hilar regions.

Pulmonary hypoplasia

This is seen most often with congenital diaphragmatic hernia, but bilateral pulmonary hypoplasia may also occur in association with renal agenesis or dysgenesis (Potter's syndrome), in babies with severe rhesus isoimmunization, and in the presence of chronic amniotic fluid leak. It may also present as an isolated malformation. Unilateral hypoplasia can occur as an isolated anomaly or in association with cardiovascular defects.

Diaphragmatic hernia

Congenital diaphragmatic hernia (usually left-sided) results in respiratory failure, partly due to lung compression but mainly related to the associated lung hypoplasia (both ipsilateral and contralateral). The disturbance of pulmonary function ranges from mild to severe. In severe cases, life-threatening respiratory distress is present from birth, with cyanosis, intercostal retraction, mediastinal displacement, and poor or absent breath sounds on the affected side. The abdomen is usually scaphoid, due to much of its usual contents being in the chest. Chest X-ray shows loops of bowel in the affected hemithorax, with pulmonary compression and mediastinal displacement to the contralateral side.

Neonates presenting in the first 4 h of life have major degrees of lung hypoplasia and have a mortality of 50% despite maximal supportive therapy. Those presenting after 4 h of age should all survive. CMV may be complicated by tension pneumothorax and bronchopleural fistula on either side. Pulmonary hypertension with persistent fetal circulation and difficulties of CMV present major challenges. Some centres use ECMO[3,4] or high-frequency ventilation in these infants. Nitric oxide may be a useful pulmonary vasodilator in this condition.[5] Prolonged ventilatory support is often required but the outlook of survivors is excellent.

Pneumothorax

Spontaneous pneumothorax may occur in normal newborns associated with the birth process, or secondary to hyaline membrane disease or meconium aspiration. Tension pneumothorax is particularly likely to occur when CMV is required with immature lungs, lung hypoplasia, non-uniform lung disease (e.g. staphylococcal pneumonia) and diseases characterized by air trapping (e.g. meconium aspiration, bronchiolitis and asthma).

Tension pneumothorax should be suspected with any sudden deterioration of an infant on a ventilator. Classical signs are evident in older children, but are of limited value in neonates. Abdominal distension due to depression of the diaphragm or unilateral chest hyperexpansion are useful signs. Transillumination of the thorax is a sensitive guide in infants weighing less than 2.5 kg. A chest X-ray is mandatory, but should be preceded by needle aspiration or drainage if the infant's condition is critical. Pre-existing pulmonary interstitial emphysema in one lung may also point to the side of the pneumothorax.

Repaired exomphalos or gastroschisis

Complete repair of abdominal wall defects may cause marked elevation of intra-abdominal pressure when the intestines are enclosed in a poorly developed peritoneal cavity. The diaphragm is elevated, compressing the lungs. In addition, compression of the inferior vena cava may lead to peripheral oedema, reduced cardiac output and oliguria. The associated paralytic ileus may further increase intra-abdominal pressure.

Disturbed lung function with inadequate gas exchange may require postoperative ventilation for several days. With large defects, it may be necessary to house the abdominal contents in a prosthesis, to allow gradual reduction into the abdominal cavity.

Diaphragmatic palsy

Phrenic nerve palsy is a relatively common complication of cardiothoracic surgery. It occasionally occurs as a congenital abnormality or may result from birth trauma. Paralysis and paradoxical movement of the affected diaphragm lead to reduced lung and tidal volumes, hypoxaemia and increased work of breathing. A chest X-ray taken without positive airway pressure reveals the elevated hemidiaphragm. Screening with ultrasound or fluoroscopy confirms the paradoxical movement.

Paralysis of the hemidiaphragm may cause respiratory failure in infants, particularly if associated with another disorder affecting lung function. Problems are greatest in children under 3 years, due to the poor stability of the chest wall. CPAP may be an effective method of increasing lung volume, stabilizing the ribcage and reducing paradoxical movement. Surgical plication of the diaphragm is usually effective in cases that fail to resolve with conservative management.

Birth asphyxia

Birth asphyxia may result from placental failure, obstetric difficulties or maternal sedation. The resulting central respiratory depression, convulsions, intracerebral haemorrhage, meconium aspiration and persistence of fetal circulation contribute to respiratory failure. The Apgar score at 1 min is an objective means of evaluating the degree of asphyxia; the score at 5 min is a guide to prognosis. Delayed spontaneous respiration (> 5 min) is also a poor prognostic sign. Further postnatal hypoxaemia, hypercapnia and brain ischaemia must be avoided. Severely asphyxiated infants need CMV after delivery, with correction of acidosis and hypovolaemia; inotropic drugs may be needed to maintain cerebral blood flow. It is important to prevent hypoglycaemia and control convulsions.

Convulsions

Convulsions in the newborn are most frequent in the first 3 days of life. They are commonly due to birth asphyxia, trauma, intracranial haemorrhage and metabolic abnormalities such as hypoglycaemia or hypocalcaemia and meningitis. Seizures in older children commonly occur with fever, idiopathic epilepsy, CNS infection, poisoning, trauma and metabolic disturbances (e.g. hypoglycaemia and hypocalcaemia).

Generalized seizures may cause respiratory failure from airway obstruction, aspiration, apnoea or central respiratory depression. During grand mal seizures, ventilation may be inadequate, and oxygen consumption and CO_2 production may be increased by associated muscle activity. Anticonvulsant drugs may further depress respiration.

Initial management consists of ensuring a clear airway, adequate oxygenation and ventilation, and administering anticonvulsants. Oxygen should be given, because cerebral and total body oxygen consumption are increased, and it is difficult to assess adequacy of ventilation. Urgent control of seizures is important, as protracted seizures longer than 1 h may result in permanent neurological sequelae, even if hypoxaemia is avoided. Chapter 107 discusses pharmacological control of seizures. The underlying cause must then be determined and treated.

Apnoea of prematurity

Recurrent apnoeic episodes (> 20 s) are common in premature infants, and relate to immaturity of the brainstem, hypoxia, altered chemoreceptor respon-

siveness, diaphragmatic fatigue and the active (rapid eye movement) sleep state. Underlying causes such as hyaline membrane disease, hypoglycaemia, aspiration, sepsis, anaemia and intracranial haemorrhage should be sought. Mild episodes revert spontaneously or with tactile stimulation. Severe episodes may require bag-and-mask ventilation. Apnoeic episodes may be reduced or prevented by theophylline or caffeine (central respiratory stimulants) or CPAP. IMV is necessary in some cases.

Many premature infants also suffer obstructive or mixed (central and obstructive) apnoea, both disorders of respiratory and airway musculature control. The infant airway is easy to collapse, and this is aggravated by neck flexion. Ex-premature infants may develop recurrent apnoea with intercurrent infection or following general anaesthesia and surgical procedures. This risk may persist until a post-conceptual age of 46 weeks, and demands close monitoring.[9] The risk may be greater in infants with a history of apnoeic episodes, bronchopulmonary dysplasia, anaemia or neurological disease. This is remarkably responsive to theophylline or caffeine loading. Maintenance therapy is often unnecessary.

Status asthmaticus

Asthma is the commonest reason for admission to most paediatric hospitals. Asthma is an inflammatory disease affecting the airways. Airway obstruction is due to mucosal oedema, mucus plugging and bronchiolar muscle spasm. Under 2 years of age, bronchiolar muscle is poorly developed, and muscle spasm is probably of less importance, with less response to bronchodilator therapy.

Clinical and radiological features and management of asthma in small children are similar to that in adults (see Chapter 32). Blood-gas estimation is indicated for any child with acute severe asthma, if pulsus paradoxus greater than 20 mmHg (2.6 kPa) is present, or if the child fails to respond to optimal drug therapy. Hypoxaemia is the usual finding, and is the main cause of morbidity and mortality. High inspired oxygen therapy is therefore important. Hypocapnia in response to hypoxic drive is the rule; normocapnia or a rising $Pa\text{co}_2$ are signs of worsening asthma or fatigue, and require increased medical therapy or CMV.

Nebulized β_2-sympathomimetic amines, IV aminophylline and corticosteroids form the mainstay of drug therapy; maximal therapy should be introduced early. Salbutamol is nebulized with oxygen as 0.05 mg/kg of 0.5% solution diluted to 4 ml with sterile water, given 2–4-hourly initially, or more frequently in severe cases. A greater and more sustained response may be achieved by more frequent or continuous salbutamol nebulization.[10] Children under 9 years have increased metabolism, and require higher doses of theophylline (0.85 mg/kg per h, equivalent to an aminophylline infusion of 1.1 mg/kg per h). Serum concentrations should be measured (therapeutic range is 60–110 μmol/l). Continuous infusion of salbutamol has been shown to reduce the need for CMV. It should be added when Pa_{CO_2} is rising or is greater than 60 mmHg (8 kPa), as an infusion of 1 μg/kg per min and increased every 20 min until Pa_{CO_2} decreases by about 10%, or a maximum dose of 14 μg/kg per min is reached.

Metabolic acidosis may occur as a result of hypoxaemia and increased work of breathing. Cautious bicarbonate therapy is recommended to improve cardiovascular function and bronchomotor responsiveness to theophylline and sympathomimetic agents. Isoprenaline and theophylline may both override pulmonary hypoxic vasoconstrictor responses and worsen hypoxaemia. Salbutamol is believed to be preferable in this respect.

Particular attention should be paid to fluid balance. Dehydration may lead to inspissation of secretions, but the risks of inappropriate antidiuretic hormone (ADH) secretion and pulmonary oedema must be noted.[11,12]

With aggressive medical therapy, the need for CMV should be rare. Its use should be based predominantly on clinical features rather than solely on blood-gas analysis. It should not, however, be withheld out of fear of difficulties. CMV may worsen air trapping and lead to hypotension or pneumothorax. Controlled hypoventilation (permissive hypercapnia) with a long expiratory time is advocated to minimize airway pressures and air trapping. A trial of PEEP may be justified to reduce intrinsic (auto) PEEP and air trapping.

Acute viral bronchiolitis

Most cases of bronchiolitis occur in the first 6 months of life and are caused by RSV. Cough, low-grade fever, tachypnoea and wheeze are the cardinal signs. Some infants, particularly ex-premature, develop apnoeic episodes. The chest is hyperinflated with rib retraction and widespread crepitations. Clinical features are due to small airways obstruction from oedema and exudate.

Management consists of minimal handling and oxygen therapy. If respiratory distress is marked, feeds should be withheld and fluids administered IV. Progression of the disease leads to exhaustion and respiratory failure in 1–2% of cases. CPAP[13] and/or aminophylline therapy[14] are reported to reduce the work of breathing, lower Pa_{CO_2} and eliminate recurrent apnoea. CMV is required in some cases, particularly when other problems (e.g. congenital heart disease) are present. High airway pressures may be required, increasing the risk of pneumothorax. The antiviral agent Ribaviran is difficult to administer and has not been shown to improve outcome.[15] Bacterial coinfection is common, and justifies the use of broad-spectrum antibiotics in severe cases.[16]

Respiratory failure secondary to congenital heart disease[17]

Infants with congenital heart disease may develop respiratory failure for a number of reasons.

Type of cardiac lesion

Congenital heart lesions producing acute respiratory failure fall into four main groups.

1 *Left heart obstruction* (e.g. critical aortic stenosis, interrupted aortic arch and coarctation of aorta). In this group, left ventricular failure leads to pulmonary oedema and respiratory failure.
2 *Large left-to-right shunts* (e.g. ventricular septal defect and patent ductus arteriosus). Respiratory failure in this group with excessive pulmonary blood flow results from volume overloading of the left ventricle, with pulmonary oedema, small airways obstruction, bronchial compression or intercurrent infection. Correction of the defect is associated with improved lung mechanics.[18]
3 *Hypoxaemic lesions,* where:
   (a) there is obstruction to pulmonary blood flow (e.g. tetralogy of Fallot and critical pulmonary stenosis);
   (b) the pulmonary and systemic circuits are in parallel (e.g. transposition of the great vessels);
   (c) there is complete mixing of systemic and pulmonary venous blood (e.g. single ventricle and truncus arteriosus).
   In lesions associated with reduced pulmonary blood flow, lung compliance is high. High-pressure ventilation may further impede pulmonary blood flow, leading to increased hypoxaemia and, occasionally, CO_2 retention. Those with increased pulmonary blood flow have problems of reduced lung compliance and air trapping (due to small airways disease and bronchial compression) in addition to hypoxaemia (due to mixing).
4 *Vascular lesions* associated with compression or stenosis of large airways (e.g. vascular rings and anomalous left pulmonary artery).

Intercurrent infection

Recurrent pneumonia and bronchiolitis are common in infants with congenital heart disease, particularly those associated with high pulmonary blood flow.

Postoperative

Respiratory failure may occur following repair of cardiac lesions due to low cardiac output state and pulmonary oedema, acute respiratory distress syndrome (ARDS), lobar collapse, pneumonia, phrenic nerve palsy, respiratory depressant drugs, abdominal distension and ascites.

Near-drowning

Respiratory failure after near-drowning may result from aspiration pneumonitis or CNS depression from hypoxic–ischaemic encephalopathy. Acute gastric dilatation (associated with the immersion or resuscitation) is common and may be a contributing factor. Pulmonary oedema may be secondary to water and particulate matter inhaled, or to chemical pneumonitis from aspiration of gastric contents. Secondary infection occasionally leads to necrotizing pneumonia. Prophylactic antibiotics are not of proven benefit, but there are reports of fulminant ARDS associated with pneumococcal infection after immersion.[19] Broad-spectrum antibiotic therapy should be administered early if there is significant pulmonary disease. Ongoing therapy should be guided by culture of tracheal aspirate.

Patients with both fresh- and salt-water drowning are usually hypovolaemic, hypoxic and acidotic at the time of admission. Oxygen therapy is mandatory, even in so-called dry drowning. Resuscitation usually requires volume expansion, correction of acidosis and inotropic support (see Chapter 71). Immersion hypothermia may afford some protection to the brain. Complete rewarming should not be undertaken until circulatory resuscitation is achieved. Resuscitation attempts should be sustained in the presence of severe hypothermia. CMV produces a dramatic improvement in gas exchange.

Trauma

Respiratory failure may follow trauma to the brain, spinal cord, chest or abdomen (see Chapter 108). High spinal cord injuries may be difficult to detect in the presence of severe brain injury. Presence of rhythmic flaring of the alae nasi without accompanying respiratory excursion is a useful sign (Duncan's sign). As the chest wall is compliant, severe pulmonary contusion can occur from blunt trauma with minimal chest-wall injury. Fractured ribs, haemothorax and pneumothorax may all precipitate respiratory failure. Clinical signs of a ruptured diaphragm are easily confused with a tension pneumothorax, making chest X-ray mandatory in resuscitation. CMV will effectively displace abdominal contents from the thorax and improve gas exchange prior to surgery.

Acute gastric dilatation is almost invariable in the traumatized child, and may itself exacerbate respiratory failure. Emergency decompression with a wide-bore gastric tube improves cardiorespiratory function and reduces the risk of aspiration.

Acute respiratory distress syndrome

ARDS may occur in children of all ages from a variety of lung insults. ARDS is characterized by respiratory distress or failure, diffuse pulmonary infiltrates, reduced pulmonary compliance and

hypoxaemia, in the presence of a known precipitating cause. In children, common causes include shock from any cause, pneumonia with septicaemia, near-drowning, aspiration and pulmonary contusion (see Chapter 29).

Poisoning

Accidental poisoning is a common but preventable cause of respiratory failure in the first 4 years of life. Deliberate overdose is seen in children beyond 8 years. Tricyclic antidepressants, antihistamines, anticonvulsants and benzodiazepines form the commonest CNS-depressant drugs ingested. Convulsions may aggravate the situation (see Chapter 77).

Meningitis and encephalitis

Meningitis is common in the early years of life. After the neonatal period, the usual causative organisms are *Haemophilus influenzae*, *Neisseria meningitidis* and *Streptococcus pneumoniae*. Rapid diagnosis and appropriate antibiotic therapy form the cornerstone of treatment. Respiratory failure is mainly associated with uncontrolled convulsions, altered conscious state or raised intracranial pressure (ICP). Encephalitis may also cause unconsciousness and raised ICP. Associated problems are upper airway obstruction, pulmonary aspiration and central respiratory depression. Encephalitis is usually viral in origin and may be complicated by hyperpyrexia, convulsions and cerebral oedema.

Guillain–Barré syndrome

This is the most common polyneuritis in childhood. The onset may be rapid, with respiratory failure occurring within 48 h. Intervention is based on clinical assessment of cough reflex and bulbar function, a measured vital capacity < 15 ml/kg, and evidence of hypoxaemia (Sao_2 < 90%). An elevated $Paco_2$ is a late feature, suggesting a vital capacity in the tidal range, i.e. < 5–7 ml/kg. CMV is usually necessary if intubation is required. Unless rapid recovery is anticipated, early tracheostomy is advocated for patient comfort and communication. The condition is often improved by the early use of plasmapheresis or IV immunoglobulin therapy. Muscle pain may require analgesic relief (see Chapters 48 and 107).

Envenomation

Some animal venoms, such as those of some snakes, ticks and the blue-ringed octopus, are neurotoxic and may cause muscle weakness and respiratory insufficiency. The Sydney funnel web spider causes widespread acetylcholine release and symptoms similar to anticholinesterase poisoning. These symptoms include intense salivation, lacrimation, sweating, laryngeal and muscle spasm and pulmonary oedema. Paralysis due to tetrodotoxin may rapidly follow puffer-fish ingestion. In Australia and many other countries, specific antivenom therapy is available for most potentially lethal envenomations. Supportive therapy is required until antivenom is administered and recovery occurs.

Management of acute respiratory failure

In some cases, definitive treatment of the underlying cause will lead to resolution of respiratory failure (e.g. relief of upper airway obstruction or reversal of drug depression). Where this is not possible, mechanical ventilatory support is required until the underlying process has resolved.

General measures

General nursing care

Skilled one-to-one nursing is vital. It is a major difference between general and paediatric ICUs.

Thermal environment

Maintenance of body temperature is of major importance. The immature newborn is particularly vulnerable to cold stress, which increases metabolism, rapidly depletes carbohydrate stores and causes cardiorespiratory deterioration. In a normal newborn, oxygen consumption may rise threefold on exposure to environmental temperatures of 20–25°C. Conditions are optimal when the abdominal skin temperature is 36–36.5°C.

The most satisfactory devices to maintain temperature homeostasis are servo-controlled infrared-heated open cots. These allow for observation of and access to the exposed infant. In an incubator, the environmental temperature is less stable and access is difficult. Double-glazed incubators reduce radiant heat loss. Older infants and children can be nursed in standard cots and beds.

Posture

Neonates are best nursed prone with the hips and knees flexed and the head turned regularly. This posture may abolish apnoeic episodes in premature infants. It also decreases gastric emptying time, making aspiration of vomitus less likely. However, if the neonate is unstable and interventions are likely, the supine position is preferred. Older infants and young children are usually nursed in the position they find most comfortable. Provided cardiovascular function is stable, the semi-upright posture is encouraged, because of improved respiratory function.

Physiotherapy

The role of conventional chest physiotherapy with posturing, percussion and vibration in the paediatric ICU setting is unproven. Physiotherapy must be applied cautiously in children with cardiovascular instability or raised ICP. Chest compression and vibration in the newborn may result in rib fractures and possibly intracranial damage. Physiotherapy may cause a significant fall in Pao_2; Fio_2 should be increased beforehand. In infants, periodic gentle pharyngeal suction removes pharyngeal secretions and may stimulate coughing. Effective bagging, tracheal suction and positioning are the most useful techniques in the intubated patient.

Fluid therapy

Oral feeding should be suspended with severe respiratory distress, because of the difficulty in oxygen administration and the risk of abdominal distension, vomiting and aspiration. Nasogastric feeding may be cautiously employed in infants with mild to moderate respiratory distress.

Lung and airway disease is often associated with increased secretion of ADH, leading to fluid retention. Increased airway pressure (e.g. CMV and CPAP) may also increase ADH secretion. Efficient humidification via a tracheal or tracheostomy tube prevents insensible loss from the airway, and diminishes fluid requirements. Most patients with acute lung disease benefit from some degree of fluid restriction. Fluid balance and biochemical status must be monitored carefully. In prolonged respiratory failure, it is essential to minimize wasting of the respiratory muscles and to provide energy for increased work of breathing. High-calorie oral or nasogastric feeding may be tolerated. Parenteral nutrition is particularly useful when fluid restriction is necessary, and should be commenced early if prolonged interruption to enteral feeding is likely.

Monitoring and assessment

Repeated clinical observation by skilled staff is necessary to detect early signs of hypoxia, increasing respiratory distress, or onset of fatigue. Deterioration may represent a progression of disease state, development of fatigue or the presence of complications. Monitoring of cardiorespiratory parameters and respiratory therapy is imperative for optimal respiratory care.

Blood gases
Measurement of blood gases and acid–base status is essential in cardiorespiratory assessment. Arterial blood is obtained from an indwelling cannula or by direct puncture of peripheral arteries. The latter may be distressing to the child. Results from difficult collections may not accurately reflect the true blood-

gas status. Topical anaesthesia using Emla cream should be considered for non-urgent percutaneous sampling.

Peripheral arterial cannulation is routine practice in paediatric intensive care, even in infants weighing less than 1 kg. It allows continuous blood pressure monitoring and reduces sampling errors. The radial, ulnar, brachial, femoral, posterior tibial and dorsalis pedis arteries are suitable. Cannulation by cut-down should be considered when the percutaneous method fails. Radial and ulnar or posterior tibial and dorsalis pedis vessels must not be cannulated in the same limb, even at different times, because of the danger of distal limb ischaemia. The safety of brachial and femoral cannulation lies in the collateral vessels around the elbow and hip joints. Complications of arterial cannulation include distal ischaemia, infection, haemorrhage and retrograde embolization when the cannula is flushed.

In the neonate with acute respiratory failure, a preductal vessel, such as the right radial artery, should be used. Preductal sampling is important, because it indicates the Pao_2 of blood perfusing the retina. Knowledge of the Fio_2 is essential to interpret information from all forms of oxygen monitoring.

Pulse oximetry

Pulse oximetry provides valuable information about the state of oxygenation (i.e. Sao_2) on a continuous basis (see Chapter 98). It is applicable to children of all sizes and can obviate the need for arterial cannulation in some cases. Surprising degrees of desaturation, undetectable clinically, may be identified and treated. Ideally, pulse oximetry should be available and utilized with every critically ill child.

Capnography

Measurement of end-tidal CO_2 in the intubated patient provides a continuous guide to the adequacy of alveolar ventilation. In severe lung disease, the value does not reflect arterial Pco_2 (due to a wide alveolar–arterial gradient). It may still provide valuable trend information, and is useful to detect sudden reductions in cardiac output.

Chest X-ray

Clinical examination of the thorax may be misleading in the small infant and serial chest X-rays form a vital part of assessment. Anteroposterior supine films usually provide the necessary information. Lateral or decubitus views may be useful to localize lung pathology, or to confirm air or fluid collections. Examination should look for focal or generalized lung disease, pleural effusions, air leak phenomena, the size and shape of the cardiac contour and the position of invasive devices. The tracheal tube should be level with the second thoracic vertebra or the ends of the clavicles, and take account of the neck posture. A change from extension to flexion may advance the endotracheal tube by 1 cm in the term neonate. As the trachea in the neonate is only 4 cm long, accurate placement is critical. Multiple chest X-rays may be required with rapidly changing clinical situations.

Transillumination

Transillumination of the thorax with a fibreoptic light source is a useful technique to detect pneumothorax in infants under 2.5 kg. Transillumination occurs on the side of the pneumothorax, but does not quantify the amount of air present. Bilateral pneumothoraces may cause confusion. In severe pulmonary interstitial emphysema, increased transillumination may be seen. A chest X-ray should be performed to confirm the pneumothorax if time permits.

Vital capacity and maximum inspiratory force

In diseases such as Guillain–Barré syndrome, measurements of vital capacity and maximum inspiratory force are useful in cooperative children. A vital capacity < 15 ml/kg or a maximum inspiratory force of less than –25 cm H_2O (–2.5 kPa) are indications for intubation and assisted ventilation. These parameters are also useful to guide weaning.

Specific measures

Oxygen therapy[20]

Mode of administration is guided by patient size and required Fio_2. Neonates requiring less than 40% oxygen can be nursed in an incubator. Plastic headboxes are used to deliver higher concentrations to neonates and infants. Older infants and children can be nursed in oxygen cots, provided Fio_2 under 0.4 is adequate. Cot opening results in an immediate fall in oxygen concentration, which takes a considerable time to return to its prescribed setting.

Older children tolerate appropriately sized facemasks, but Fio_2 is rarely known. Masks incorporating a reservoir bag will deliver high concentrations in small children. Restless children do not tolerate facemasks and oxygen delivery becomes intermittent. A single catheter in the post nasal space (1–2 l/min) is then an effective method of delivery. Fio_2 then depends on flow rate, size of the nasopharynx, mouth-breathing and peak inspiratory flow rate. A flow rate of 150 ml/kg per min provides Fio_2 about 0.5 in children under 2 years.[21] Effective humidification is difficult, and drying of mucosa and secretions may be a problem.

Therapeutic procedures, physiotherapy and handling may all increase oxygen consumption and lead to hypoxaemia and deterioration. Timing of these manoeuvres is important and a prior increase in Fio_2 may be justified.

Complications of oxygen therapy in neonates

Retrolental fibroplasia

Retinal vessels of premature infants are susceptible to vasoconstrictive effects of high arterial oxygen tension. Visual impairment is due to retinal fibroproliferative changes or to subsequent retinal detachment. While the absolute safe maximal level and duration of hyperoxia are unknown, Pao_2 between 50 and 80 mmHg (6.6 and 10.6 kPa) is recommended.

Bronchopulmonary dysplasia

The development of chronic pulmonary insufficiency in mechanically ventilated neonates correlates best with peak inspiratory pressures and other evidence of barotrauma. Pulmonary oxygen toxicity is probably a factor. Chronic hypoxaemia is a factor in the development of cor pulmonale.

Intubation

Tracheal intubation relieves airway obstruction, and allows accurate control of inspired oxygen, application of positive airway pressure and tracheal toilet. Nasotracheal intubation is preferred, as it allows better fixation. Implant-tested polyvinyl chloride tubes may be left in place indefinitely. For long-term use, however, tracheostomy is indicated. Disadvantages of nasotracheal intubation include bypassing nasal humidifying mechanisms, increased airway resistance, risk of subglottic stenosis, impaired cough reflex, loss of physiological positive end-expiratory pressure (PEEP) and impaired pulmonary defence mechanisms. In neonates, risk of laryngeal injury correlates with duration of intubation and number of attempts. The correct tracheal tube size permits a small leak when a positive pressure of less than 25 cm H_2O (2.5 kPa) is applied (see Chapter 109). Exceptions to this rule are in:

1 neonates: for unknown reasons, absence of leak rarely results in complications;
2 croup, where a smaller tube than predicted for age is passed, and a subsequent leak indicates resolution of subglottic oedema;
3 mechanical ventilation with low-compliance lungs, where an airtight seal may be required for effective ventilation – a risk of subglottic stenosis occurs;
4 infants with Down's syndrome, who frequently have subglottic narrowing.

Mechanical ventilatory support

Mechanical ventilation[22]

Paediatric ventilators are discussed in Chapter 109. The risks of barotrauma and oxygen toxicity demand that specific ventilator settings be prescribed for rate, peak inspiratory pressure, PEEP, CPAP, flow rate, inspiratory time, minute volume and inspired oxygen.

If pulmonary function progressively deteriorates, a stepwise increase of each setting should be considered. The least toxic alternative should be undertaken first (e.g. increasing Fio_2 is probably a safer alternative than increasing PEEP). Unless contra-indicated, a PEEP of 3–5 cmH$_2$O (0.3–0.5 kPa) is recommended in all ventilated infants to prevent airway closure. PEEP in brain injuries should be titrated against ICP. Removing or reducing PEEP must be considered if there is evidence of barotrauma. Increased PEEP demands a similar increase in peak inspiratory pressure if the same tidal volume is to be maintained. Mean airway pressure is the main determinant of oxygenation. It is dependent on rate, peak inspiratory pressure, flow rate, inspiratory time and PEEP.

In general, slow ventilatory rates (e.g. neonates 30 breaths/min, infants under 12 months 25 breaths/min, children 16–20 breaths/min) and an inspiratory time of about 1.0 s provide optimal gas exchange. Infants under 1 kg may benefit from faster ventilatory rates with an inspiratory time of about 0.8 s. Short inspiratory times may, however, be associated with loss of lung volume and increased intrapulmonary shunting. Recruitment of alveoli is important after suction and disconnection of bagging.

Continuous positive airway pressure[23]

CPAP applies a constant pressure gradient to the spontaneously breathing patient via a special circuit. The T-piece system requires a fresh gas flow of two to three times the predicted minute ventilation to prevent rebreathing. For CPAP to be well-sustained, either flow rate must exceed peak inspiratory flow or a reservoir bag must be incorporated into the system.

Nasotracheal intubation is the safest and most efficient method of applying CPAP, although nasal cannulae or a single nasopharyngeal tube may be used. These latter techniques rely on neonates being obligatory nose-breathers; positive pressure is lost during crying or mouth-breathing, and abdominal distension may occur. Blood-gas sampling during mouth-breathing may lead to errors in oxygen therapy. The stomach should be decompressed continuously with a nasogastric tube.

Benefits of CPAP are the following:

1 CPAP increases functional residual capacity (FRC), recruits alveoli, promotes alveolar stability and reduces intrapulmonary shunt. An increased Pao_2 results and allows a reduction in Fio_2.
2 CPAP promotes the stability of large and small airways. This splinting effect is useful in airway obstruction, bronchomalacia and tracheomalacia. CPAP has also been recommended in croup, bronchiolitis and even asthma.
3 In neonates, CPAP may abolish or reduce apnoeic episodes and improve the rhythmicity of spontaneous breathing. Physiological amounts of CPAP

(2–5 cm H_2O, 0.2–0.5 kPa) should be applied to intubated children whenever practical to prevent airway closure.

CPAP may reduce cardiac output or cause baro-trauma. Increased ADH secretion and fluid retention are also seen, although the exact mechanism is disputed. If CPAP results in hyperinflation it may also increase pulmonary vascular resistance and right ventricular afterload. This effect is often balanced by the beneficial effect of CPAP in preventing atelectasis, optimizing lung volume and thereby reducing pulmonary vascular resistance.

Sedation

Sedation should be used to reduce restlessness and discomfort, and to minimize the work of breathing. In the brain-injured, sedation prevents coughing, straining and unwanted autonomic responses. Heavy sedation (± relaxants) is recommended, provided supervision and monitoring facilities are adequate (see Chapter 105).

Complications

Complications of mechanical ventilatory support include:

1 *Reduced cardiac output.* Circulatory effects of increased airway pressure seem to be less marked in young children.[24] Nevertheless, volume expansion (e.g. with 10–20 ml/kg of colloid) may be required at the start of CMV, particularly if muscle relaxants are employed;

2 *Barotrauma* may present as:
(a) *pulmonary interstitial emphysema* with gas in the lung interstitium, outside the alveoli. This is deleterious to gas exchange and is not amenable to drainage. It may produce intrapulmonary tension and mediastinal shift. Unfortunately, the initiating factor, positive pressure, may need to be increased further to restore gas exchange. It is a forerunner of pneumothorax. Management is to limit or remove positive pressure as early as possible. Occasionally, needle or thoracotomy decompression may be required;
(b) *pneumothorax*;
(c) *pneumomediastinum*;
(d) *tension pneumopericardium* occasionally occurs in neonates on ventilation and may require decompression by needle aspiration or limited sternotomy and drainage;
(e) *pneumoperitoneum*, where a differential diagnosis from ruptured viscus may be difficult. Occasionally, drainage is required to reduce intra-abdominal tension and respiratory embarrassment.

Mechanical ventilation must be approached cautiously if air leak is a particular risk (e.g. in immature lungs and diseases characterized by air trapping). Often, permissive hypercapnia can be tolerated, provided that oxygenation, perfusion and acid–base balance are acceptable.

Weaning

Weaning commences when the underlying process has resolved sufficiently, the cardiovascular system is stable and the child is awake or active. It is unlikely to be successful if an Fio_2 over 0.5 or peak airway pressures greater than 25 cm H_2O (2.5 kPa) are required. PEEP or CPAP should be reduced to 5 cm H_2O (0.5 kPa) or less prior to extubation. The rate of weaning is determined by the underlying pathology and the expected response. Progression through IMV and CPAP is usually advised. Attention to the status of all organ systems must be meticulous, and some degree of fluid restriction is usually indicated. Other forms of circulatory support such as inotropic agents and vasodilators should be maintained during the weaning period. Increased work of breathing places additional demands on the cardiovascular system and may divert blood flow from other vital organs. The patient should be fasted and the abdomen decompressed prior to extubation. A period of fasting before and after long-term intubation is recommended (e.g. 24 h), to allow for return of laryngeal competence.

High-frequency ventilation (HFV)

HFV now generally refers to ventilation at respiratory rates greater than 4 Hz, with tidal volumes close to or less than anatomical dead space. Methods of HFV most commonly used are high-frequency jet ventilation, high-frequency flow interruption and high-frequency oscillation. When combined with PEEP, all three can produce adequate oxygenation and CO_2 removal in infants, children and adults with restrictive lung disease, often using lower peak and mean airway pressures than in CMV.

Studies in preterm infants have not demonstrated improvement in mortality, morbidity or long-term lung function with HFV, compared with conventional ventilation. There is, however, renewed interest in the use of HFV combined with nitric oxide therapy as an alternative to ECMO in the newborn period. The role of HFV is not yet settled, but there have been many favourable case reports of its use, especially in severe pulmonary air leak.

References

1. Muller NL and Bryan AC (1979) Chest wall mechanics and respiratory muscles in infants. *Pediatr Clin North Am* **26**:503–526.
2. Keens TG, Bryan AC, Levison H and Ianuzzo CD (1978) Developmental pattern of muscle fibre types in human ventilatory muscles. *J Appl Physiol Respir Environ Exercise Physiol* **44**:909–913.

3. O'Rourke PP, Crone RK, Vacanti JP *et al.* (1989) A prospective randomised study of extracorporeal membrane oxygenation (ECMO) and conventional medical therapy in neonates with persistent pulmonary hypertension of the newborn. *Pediatrics* **84**:957–963.

4. Extracorporeal Life Support Organization (ELSO) (1994) *National Registry*. Ann Arbor, MI: ELSO.

5. Kinsella JP, Neish SR, Dunbar ID *et al.* (1993) Clinical responses to prolonged treatment of persistent pulmonary hypertension of the newborn with low doses of inhaled nitric oxide. *J Pediatr* **123**:103–108.

6. Stevenson D, Walther F, Long W *et al.* (1992) Controlled trial of a single dose of synthetic surfactant at birth in premature infants weighing 500–699 grams. *J Pediatr* **120**:S3–S12.

7. Long W, Corbet A, Cotton R *et al.* (1991) A controlled trial of synthetic surfactant in infants weighing 1250 g or more with respiratory distress syndrome. *N Engl J Med* **325**:1696–1703.

8. Bose C, Corbet A, Bose G *et al.* (1990) Improved outcome at 28 days of age for very low birth weight infants treated with a single dose of a synthetic surfactant. *J Pediatr* **117**:947–953.

9. Sims C and Johnson CM (1994) Postoperative apnoea in infants. *Anaesth Intens Care* **22**:40–45.

10. Robertson CF, Smith F, Beck R and Levison H (1985) Response to frequent low doses of nebulized salbutamol in acute asthma. *J Pediatr* **106**:672–674.

11. Baker JW, Yerger SY and Segar WE (1976). Elevated plasma antidiuretic hormone levels in status asthmaticus. *Mayo Clin Proc* **51**:31–34.

12. Stalcup SA and Mellins RB (1977) Mechanical forces producing pulmonary edema in acute asthma. *N Engl J Med* **297**:592–596.

13. Beasley JM and Jones SEF (1981) Continuous positive airway pressure in bronchiolitis. *Br Med J* **283**:1506–1508.

14. Mezey AP (1985) Treatment of respiratory failure associated with acute bronchiolitis. *Am J Dis Child* **139**:650–651.

15. Smith DW, Frankel LR, Mathers LH *et al.* (1991) A controlled trial of aerosolized ribavirin in infants receiving mechanical ventilation for severe respiratory syncytial virus infection. *N Engl J Med* **325**:24–29.

16. Korppi M, Leinonen M, Koskela M *et al.* (1989) Bacterial coinfection in children hospitalized with respiratory syncytial virus infections. *Pediatr Infect Dis J* **8**:687–692.

17. Lister G and Talner NS (1981) Management of respiratory failure of cardiac origin. In: Gregory GA (ed.) *Respiratory Failure in the Child. Clinics in Critical Care Medicine*. New York: Churchill Livingstone, pp. 67–87.

18. Lanteri CJ, Kano S, Duncan AW and Sly PD (1996) Changes in respiratory mechanics in children undergoing cardiopulmonary bypass. *Am J Respir Crit Care Med* **152**: 1893–1900.

19. Vernon DD, Banner W, Cantwell P *et al.* (1990) *Streptococcus pneumoniae* bacteremia associated with near drowning. *Crit Care Med* **18**:1175–1176.

20. Oh TE and Duncan AW (1988) Oxygen therapy. *Med J Aust* **149**:141–146.

21. Shann F, Gatchalian S and Hutchinson R (1988) Nasopharyngeal oxygen in children. *Lancet* **1**:1238–1240.

22. Henning R (1986) Clinical applications of mechanical ventilation. *Anaesth Intens Care* **14**:267–280.

23. Duncan AW, Oh TE and Hillman DR (1986) PEEP and CPAP. *Anaesth Intens Care* **14**:236–250.

24. Clough JB, Duncan AW and Sly PD (1994) The effect of sustained positive airway pressure on derived cardiac output in children. *Anaesth Intens Care* **22**:30–34.

104 | Paediatric fluid and electrolyte therapy

FA Shann

Children need a much higher intake of water and electrolytes per kilogram of body weight than adults. This makes children more susceptible to dehydration if they have abnormal losses of water or a reduced intake. On the other hand, an inability to excrete a water load, due to immature kidneys (in neonates) or high levels of antidiuretic hormone (ADH), means that many children in ICUs can easily become overhydrated. Fluid and electrolyte problems in paediatric intensive care and neonates have been well-reviewed.[1–5]

Water

The full-term neonate is 80% water. This figure falls to about 60% by 12 months of age, and then remains almost constant throughout childhood. The average IV fluid requirements for children in bed are shown in Tables 104.1 and 104.2. Substantial modification to these intakes will often be necessary (Table 104.3). For example, if a 14-kg child (maintenance fluid of 50 ml/h; Table 104.2) sustains a head injury and has evidence of high levels of ADH (maintenance fluid × 0.7),[6] is ventilated with humidified gas (maintenance × 0.75),[7] is paralysed (basal state, maintenance × 0.7), and is maintained at a rectal temperature of 36°C (maintenance −12%), then the actual maintenance fluid requirement is (50 × 0.7 × 0.75 × 0.7) − 12% = 16 ml/h. Even less water should be given initially if

Table 104.1 Intravenous fluid requirements in infants

Age	Fluid requirements
Day 1 of life	2 ml/kg per h
Day 2 of life	3 ml/kg per h
Day 3 of life	4 ml/kg per h

Table 104.2 Intravenous fluid requirements in children

<10 kg	100 ml/kg per day
10–20 kg	1000 ml + (50 ml/kg per day for each kg over 10 kg)
>20 kg	1500 ml + (20 ml/kg per day for each kg over 20 kg)

Weight (kg)	ml/h	Weight (kg)	ml/h
10	40	30	70
12	45	35	75
14	50	40	80
16	55	50	90
18	60	60	95
20	65	70	100

the child is overhydrated, or if mild dehydration is considered desirable. In very small children, all fluid administered has to be taken into account, including the volume of drugs (bicarbonate, dextrose and antibiotics) and flushes used to clear IV lines (after blood sampling or administration of drugs).

Estimates of water requirements in Tables 104.1–104.3 are only approximate, and water balance must be monitored closely in any child in intensive care. Unfortunately, regular accurate weighing of very sick children is often impractical, and hydration has to be assessed by skin turgor, urine output (minimum 0.5–1.0 ml/kg per h), urine osmolality (maximum 600 mosmol/kg), serum sodium, central venous pressure and arterial blood pressure.

Very frequent monitoring is required in very-low-birthweight babies. There is controversy about the degree of dehydration that is acceptable in these infants[4,8–10] Higher fluid intakes allow a higher calorie intake, but may increase the incidence of patent ductus arteriosus (PDA), heart failure and

Table 104.3 Modifications to fluid intake

	Adjustment
Decrease	
Humidified inspired air	× 0.75
Basal state (e.g. paralysed)	× 0.7
High ADH (IPPV, brain injury)	× 0.7
Hypothermia	−12% per °C
High room humidity	× 0.7
Renal failure	× 0.3 (+ urine output)
Increase	
Full activity + oral feeds	× 1.5
Fever	+12% per °C
Room temperature >31°C	+ 30% per °C
Hyperventilation	× 1.2
Neonate	
Preterm (1–1.5 kg)	× 1.2
Radiant heater	× 1.5
Phototherapy	× 1.5
Burns	
First day	+ 4% per 1% area burnt
Subsequently	+ 2% per 1% area burnt

ADH = Antidiuretic hormone; IPPV = intermittent positive-pressure ventilation.

bronchopulmonary dysplasia.[4] In hyaline membrane disease (HMD), improvement in lung function is preceded by diuresis.[11] Frusemide therapy may increase survival in HMD by initiating diuresis[4,12] or by some other mechanism.[13] One study suggests that frusemide may increase the incidence of PDA,[14] but a meta-analysis suggests that this is not the case.[4]

In a child with oliguria following a severe ischaemic or hypoxic insult (e.g. birth asphyxia, drowning or cardiac arrest), it may be helpful to measure urinary sodium.[15] In oliguria due to acute tubular necrosis, where restriction of fluid intake may be necessary, the urine sodium is usually more than 40 mmol/l. In oliguria due to hypovolaemia, the urine sodium is usually less than 20 mmol/l.

Sodium and potassium

In the first 1 or 2 days of life, small preterm babies often have poor urine output and high transcutaneous fluid losses. They are therefore prone to hypernatraemia and hyperkalaemia, and such infants should usually be given 5% or 10% dextrose without sodium or potassium. From 2 days of age, 2–4 mmol/kg per day of sodium and potassium will usually be sufficient, but much higher intakes of sodium may be required in some preterm neonates due to their impaired renal conservation of sodium.

Table 104.4 Doses and formulae in paediatric fluid and electrolyte therapy

Albumin 25%	Undiluted: 2–4 ml/kg 5% in 5% dextrose or saline: 10–20 ml/kg
Bicarbonate	Under 5 kg: base excess × weight (kg) × ½ (give ½ of this) Over 5 kg: base excess × weight (kg) × ⅓ (give ½ of this)
Blood volume	85 ml/kg in neonate 70 ml/kg in older children
Calcium	Chloride 10% (0.7 mmol/ml Ca^{2+}): maximum 0.2 ml/kg IV stat, requirement 1.5 ml/kg per day Gluconate 10% (0.22 mmol/ml Ca^{2+}): maximum 0.5 ml/kg IV stat, requirement 5 ml/kg per day
Dextrose	For hypoglycaemia: 1 ml/kg 50% dextrose IV In neonate: 4 mg/kg per min (2.4 ml/kg per h 10% dextrose) day 1, increasing to 8 mg/kg per min (up to 12 mg/kg per min with hypoglycaemia) For hyperkalaemia: 0.1 u/kg insulin and 2 ml/kg 50% dextrose IV stat
Magnesium	Chloride 0.48 g/5 ml (1 mmol/ml Mg^{2+}: 0.4 mmol (0.4 ml)/kg per dose slow IV 12-hourly Sulphate 50% (2 mmol/ml Mg^{2+}): 0.4 mmol (0.2 ml)/kg per dose slow IV 12-hourly
Mannitol	0.25–0.5 g/kg per dose IV (1–2 ml/kg of 25%) 2-hourly, provided serum osmolality <330 mosmol/kg
Packed cells	10 ml/kg raises Hb 3 g%, 1 ml/kg raises PCV 1%
Potassium	Maximum 0.5 mmol/kg per h Requirement 2–4 mmol/kg per day. 1 g KCl = 13.3 mmol K^+. Hyperkalaemia: see dextrose
Sodium	Depletion: ml 20% NaCl = weight × 0.2 (140-serum Na^+). Requirement 2–6 mmol/kg per day, 1 g NaCl = 17.1 mmol/Na^+
Urine	Minimum acceptable is 0.5–1.0 ml/kg per h

Hb = Haemoglobin; PCV = packed cell volume

Hyponatraemia may be due to poor renal conservation of sodium, a low sodium intake (e.g. breast milk), diuretic therapy, high levels of ADH (e.g. with central nervous system (CNS) disease, intermittent positive pressure ventilation (IPPV) or lung disease) or excessive water intake. Hyponatraemia causes ileus, hypotension, listlessness and convulsions. Hyponatraemia due to sodium deficit should be corrected by administration of sodium (Table 104.4). Hyponatraemia due to water excess should be treated with restriction of water intake and, if symptomatic, can be corrected by administration of sodium (Table 104.4) and frusemide 0.5 mg/kg IV; the serum sodium should be increased by no more than 2 mmol/l per h to 125 mmol/l, then restored to normal very slowly over 48–72 h.[16]

Hypernatraemia may be due to administration of large amounts of sodium (e.g. sodium bicarbonate) or to dehydration from a large insensible fluid loss (e.g. caused by radiant heaters or phototherapy), diarrhoea, osmotic diuresis (e.g. caused by glycosuria) or inadequate fluid intake. With hypernatraemic dehydration, shock should be treated with rapid IV infusion of 10–20 ml/kg of 5% albumin or isotonic (0.9%) saline. The water deficit should then be corrected very slowly (over 48 h or longer) to prevent cerebral oedema. Peritoneal dialysis or plasma filtration may be indicated for severe hypernatraemia without dehydration.

The concentration of potassium in the serum depends on pH as well as the total body potassium (which is usually about 50 mmol/kg). A child may have hypokalaemia without a deficit of total body potassium in the presence of alkalosis and, conversely, there may be a large deficit of potassium without hypokalaemia in the presence of acidosis. Potassium should never be infused at more than 0.5 mmol/kg per h, and it should not normally be given to a patient with severe oliguria or anuria.

Calcium, magnesium and phosphate

Hypocalcaemia in children usually occurs in sick neonates in the first 2 days of life, in infants of diabetic mothers, exchange transfusion with citrated blood (temporary effect only), magnesium deficiency and infants of about a week of age fed cows' milk (which is of high phosphate content). Hypocalcaemia and hypomagnesaemia cause jitters, tetany, cardiac arrhythmias, and convulsions – doses of calcium and magnesium are given in Table 104.4. Normal IV maintenance requirements in infants are 1 mmol/kg per day of calcium and 0.3 mmol/kg per day of magnesium.

Rickets is very common in small preterm babies, particularly those fed solely on breast milk. There is increasing evidence that this can be prevented by giving extra phosphorus (in particular) and calcium,[17] as well as the usual supplement of vitamin D.

Standard paediatric maintenance solution[1]

In the first 1 or 2 days of life, it is usual to give plain 5% or 10% dextrose if IV fluid therapy is required. Thereafter, a solution that is usually satisfactory is 5% or 10% dextrose with 40 mmol/l of sodium chloride (quarter normal saline) and 20 mmol/L of potassium chloride. Maintenance solution is an unfortunate term, since these solutions do not provide maintenance calorie or protein requirements (see the section on parenteral nutrition, below).

Dehydration and shock

Weight loss is the best guide to the degree of dehydration, if a recent weight is known. Many of the commonly used clinical signs of dehydration in children are inaccurate, and this leads to dehydration being diagnosed when it is not present, and to overestimation of its degree.[18] Clinical signs of mild to moderate dehydration in children are decreased peripheral perfusion (as shown by pallor or reduced capillary return), deep breathing and decreased skin turgor. These signs become apparent with only 3–4% dehydration.[18]

In children with shock, IV access may be difficult. In these circumstances, parenteral fluid can be given rapidly into the bone marrow, which is an intravascular compartment.[19] The usual sites chosen are the junction of the upper and middle third of the tibia (0–12 months of age), the medial malleolus (1–5 years) and the iliac crest (over 5 years). A 0.9-mm (20-gauge) lumbar puncture needle or an intraosseous needle can be used; the needle is held perpendicular to the bone and pushed in *gently* with a rotary motion about its long axis – a slight decrease in resistance will be felt as the needle enters the medulla.

Shock should be treated with an initial bolus of 20 ml/kg of 5% albumin, followed by further boluses of 10–20 ml/kg of fluid until the intravascular volume has been restored.[20] There are benefits in using 5% albumin (a colloid) rather than a crystalloid to restore intravascular volume in shock.[20]

After shock has been corrected with a rapid infusion of fluid, the remainder of the deficit is replaced over the next 24–48 h (while giving maintenance requirements at the same time). Standard maintenance solution (see above) is usually appropriate. Thus a 5-kg child with 10% dehydration from diarrhoea (i.e. 500 ml deficit) might receive 100 ml of isotonic saline rapidly to restore the circulation, leaving a 400 ml deficit to be replaced over 24 h. If the maintenance requirement is 500 ml/day, then the child should be given a further 900 ml of fluid in the next 24 h (i.e. 40 ml/h) in addition to the initial 100 ml. Further fluid losses should be replaced with an appropriate fluid (Table 104.5).

Table 104.5 Composition of some body fluids in children

Fluid	Na^{2+} mmol/l	K^+ mmol/l	Cl^- mmol/l	HCO_3^- mmol/l	Other
Gastric fluid	20–80	10–20	100–150	0	H^+ 30–120
Bile	140–160	3–15	80–120	15–30	
Pancreatic fluid	120–160	5–15	75–135	10–45	Basal state
Jejunal fluid	130–150	5–10	100–130	10–20	
Ileal fluid	50–150	3–15	20–120	30–50	
Diarrhoeal fluid	10–90	10–80	10–110	20–70	
Sweat					
Normal	10–30	3–10	10–35	0	
Cystic fibrosis	50–130	5–25	50–110	0	
Burn exudate	140	5	110	20	Protein 30–50 g/l
Saliva	10–25	20–35	10–30	2–10	Unstimulated

With hypernatraemic dehydration, shock should be treated as above, with rapid infusion of 10–20 ml/kg of 5% albumin in isotonic saline. The remaining deficit should then be replaced *slowly* (over at least 48 h), to prevent cerebral oedema.[2,3] It has been traditional to use 0.45% saline (with dextrose and potassium) for this slow replacement phase, but the rate of replacement is probably much more important than the type of fluid used; standard maintenance solution is satisfactory, provided it is given slowly.

In dehydration due to pyloric stenosis, there is a deficit of water, hydrogen ion, chloride and potassium. Initial resuscitation should be with rapid infusion of 10–20 ml/kg of isotonic saline, then 0.45% saline in 5% dextrose with 20–40 mmol/l of potassium chloride should be given.

Oedema

Oedema is common in children in ICU. It may be due to prematurity,[21] excess water intake, high levels of ADH (from CNS disease, IPPV or lung disease), capillary leak (due to the effects of hypoxia, ischaemia, acidosis or sepsis), heart failure, renal failure or hypoalbuminaemia. Several possible causes are often present in a child, and it can be difficult to decide which is the most important.

Children with oedema and high levels of ADH will have a serum osmolality less than 270 mosmol/kg (with hyponatraemia) and a urine osmolality greater than 270 mosmol/kg. The appropriate treatment is fluid restriction. However, in children with oedema due to capillary leak, fluid restriction and attempts to remove water (with diuretics or dialysis) are unlikely to cure the oedema, and often cause hypovolaemia. Indeed, large amounts of fluid (e.g. blood and concentrated albumin) may be needed to preserve the intravascular volume in these children; the oedema will only disappear when the capillary damage resolves.

Parenteral nutrition[22,23]

Maintenance solution is an unfortunate medical term, particularly when small children are concerned. A solution of 5% dextrose with sodium and potassium chloride provides maintenance amounts of water, sodium, potassium and chloride, but little or no calories, protein, trace elements or vitamins. For example, 100 ml/kg per day of 5% dextrose provides 20 kcal/kg per day (84 kJ/kg per day), which is only 20% of the requirement of a normal infant (let alone a child with increased calorie requirements). It has been estimated that although an adult has the energy reserve to survive for about a year on 3 l of 10% dextrose a day, a small preterm infant will survive only 11 days on 75 ml/kg per day of 10% dextrose.[24]

Many children in ICUs are unable to absorb adequate amounts of food from the gut, and their nutritional reserves are small, so they often need parenteral nutrition. However, parenteral nutrition is difficult to administer and dangerous in small children. Such patients should be referred to a specialist paediatric unit as soon as possible.

The usual requirements for amino acids, dextrose and fat in parenteral nutrition in children are shown in Table 104.6. The amino acids (Vamin in neonates, Synthamin in older children) can be mixed with dextrose in the pharmacy department to make a nutrient solution. A standard nutrient solution might provide 4 mmol/kg per day of sodium, 3 mmol/kg per day of potassium, and 7.5 mmol/day of calcium and phosphate (with up to 12 mmol/l for neonates). The standard solution should also contain 4 mmol/l of magnesium, 0.2 μmol/kg per day of manganese, 3 μmol/kg per day of zinc, 0.5

Table 104.6 Approximate requirements in paediatric parenteral nutrition

	Total fluid ml/kg per day*	Amino acids (g/kg per day) Day			Dextrose (g/kg per day) Day			Fat (Nutralipid) (g/kg per day) Day				Total calories (kcal) needed (1 kcal = 4.2 kJ)
		1	2	3+	1	2	3+	1	2	3	4+	
Neonates	100	1.5	2	2	10	10–15	15–20	1	2	3	3	100/kg
Under 10 kg	100	1.5	2	2	10	10	15–20	1	2	3	3	100/kg
10–15 kg	90	1	1.5	2	5	10	15	1	2	3	3	1000 + (50/kg over 10 kg)
15–20 kg	80	1	1.5	1.5–2	5	10	10–15	1	2	2	3	1000 + (50/kg over 10 kg)
20–30 kg	65	1	1	1–2	5	10	10–15	1	1.5	2	2.5	1500 + (20/kg over 20 kg)
30–50 kg	50	1	1	1–2	5	5–10	10	1	1.5	1.5	2	1500 + (20/kg over 20 kg)

*One ml/kg per day of fluid is needed for each kcal/kg per day; for adjustments to requirements, see Table 104.3. [Total kcal/kg per day equals g/kg per day of (amino acids × 4) + (dextrose × 4) + (fat × 10).]

μmol/kg per day of copper, 0.04 μmol/kg per day of iodide, 0.005 μmol/kg per day of chromium, 20 μg/l of hydroxycobalamin, 2 mg/l of phytomenadione, 1 mg/l of folic acid and a multivitamin preparation. For short-term nutrition, the solution need not provide fluoride, iron or vitamins A, D and E, but multivitamins (e.g. MVI paediatric) paediatric should be given to children on long-term parenteral nutrition. Fat can be given as a 20% emulsion (Nutralipid or Intralipid), either through a separate IV line or alternating with the nutrient solution. Nutrient solutions for paediatric use contain high concentrations of calcium, magnesium and phosphorus, and they should not be mixed with the fat emulsion, even in a Y-connection placed just before the cannula.

In a child on parenteral nutrition, it is important that abnormal fluid losses (Table 104.5) should be replaced with an appropriate solution (in addition to the nutrient solution), and that parenteral nutrition should always be introduced and withdrawn slowly. A dislodged IV cannula should be replaced immediately in a child on parenteral nutrition, to prevent rebound hypoglycaemia. If nutrient solution is not available at any time, it should be replaced with an infusion of a similar amount of dextrose (e.g. 20% dextrose with 40 mmol/l of sodium chloride and 20 mmol/l of potassium chloride).

Children on parenteral nutrition are liable to develop hyperglycaemia (with glycosuria and dehydration), hypoglycaemia, sepsis, extravasation of solutions with necrosis of tissue, thrombocytopenia, hypoproteinaemia, electrolyte imbalance, acidosis, anaemia, hyperlipaemia, uraemia and cholestatic jaundice. Frequent, careful monitoring is essential (Table 104.7). Initially, monitoring may need to be more frequent than suggested in Table 104.7, partic-

Table 104.7 Monitoring in paediatric parenteral nutrition

Daily: inspect IV site, electrolytes, acid/base, serum lipaemia (reduce Intralipid rate if lipaemia is significant).

Twice weekly: haemoglobin (transfuse if anaemia develops), platelets, proteins.

Weekly: creatinine, MG^{2+}, Ca^{2+}, phosphate, bilirubin, aspartate aminotransferase.

Dextrostix (or BM test) of blood 8 hourly until the dextrose intake is stable.

Clinitest (or BM test) of urine 8 hourly (reduce dextrose intake if more than trace).

Weigh frequently (daily if possible).

ularly in preterm babies. Monitoring can be less frequent once a child is stabilized on parenteral nutrition.

References

1. Winters RW (ed.) (1973) *The Body Fluids in Pediatrics*. Boston: Little Brown.
2. Finberg L, Kravath RE and Hellerstein S (1993) *Water and Electrolytes in Pediatrics: Physiology, Pathophysiology and Treatment*, 2nd edn. Philadelphia: Saunders.
3. Paschall JA and Melvin T (1993) Fluid and electrolyte therapy. In: Holbrook PR (ed.) *Textbook of Pediatric Critical Care*. Philadelphia: Saunders, pp. 653–702.
4. Bell EF (1992) Fluid therapy. In: Sinclair JC and Bracken MB (eds) *Effective Care of the Newborn Infant*. Oxford: OUP, pp. 59–71.

5. El-Dahr SS and Chevalier RL (1990) Special needs of the newborn infant in fluid therapy. *Pediatr Clin North Am* **37**:323–336.

6. Bouzarth WF and Shenkin HA (1982) Is "cerebral hyponatraemia" iatrogenic? *Lancet* **1**:1061–1062.

7. Sousulski R, Polin RA and Baumgart S (1983) Respiratory water loss and heat balance in intubated infants receiving humidified air. *J Pediatr* **103**:307–310.

8. Lorenz JM, Kleinman LI, Kotagal UR and Reller MD (1982) Water balance in very low-birth-weight infants: relationship to water and sodium intake and effect on outcome. *J Pediatr* **101**:423–432.

9. Baumgart S, Langman CB, Sosulski R, Fox WW and Polin RA (1982) Fluid, electrolyte, and glucose maintenance in the very low birth weight infant. *Clin Pediatr* **21**:199–206.

10. Oh W (1982) Fluid and electrolyte therapy and parenteral nutrition in low birth weight infants. *Clin Perinatol* **9**:637–643.

11. Engle WD, Arant BS, Wiriyathian S and Rosenfeld CR (1983) Diuresis and respiratory distress syndrome: physiologic mechanisms and therapeutic implications. *J Pediatr* **102**:912–917.

12. Green TP, Thompson TR, Johnson DE and Lock JE (1983) Diuresis and pulmonary function in premature infants with respiratory distress syndrome. *J Pediatr* **103**:618–623.

13. Najak ZD, Harris EM, Lazzara A and Pruitt AW (1983) Pulmonary effects of furosemide in preterm infants with lung disease. *J Pediatr* **102**:758–763.

14. Green TP, Thompson TR, Johnson DE and Lock JE (1983) Furosemide promotes patent ductus arteriosus in premature infants with the respiratory distress syndrome. *N Engl J Med* **308**:743–748.

15. Harrington JT and Cohen JJ (1975) Measurement of urinary electrolytes – indications and limitations. *N Engl J Med* **293**:1241–1243.

16. Ayus JC, Krothapalli RK and Arieff AL (1987) Treatment of symptomatic hyponatraemia and its relation to brain damage. *N Engl J Med* **317**:1190–1195.

17. Specker BL, DeMarini S and Tsang R (1992) Vitamin and mineral supplementation. In: Sinclair JC and Bracken MB (eds) *Effective Care of the Newborn Infant.* Oxford: OUP, pp. 161–177.

18. Mackenzie A, Barnes G and Shann F (1989) Clinical signs of dehydration in children. *Lancet* **1**:605–607.

19. Spivey WH (1987) Intraosseous infusion. *J Pediatr* **111**:639–643.

20. Scheinkestel CD, Tuxen DV, Cade JF and Shann F (1989) Fluid management of shock in critically ill patients. *Med J Aust* **150**:508–517.

21. Wu PYK, Rockwell G, Chan L, Wang S and Udani V (1981) Colloid osmotic pressure in newborn infants: variations with birth weight, gestational age, total serum solids, and mean arterial pressure. *Pediatrics* **68**:814–819.

22. Kerner JA (ed.) *Manual of Pediatric Parenteral Nutrition.* New York: Wiley.

23. Heird WC (1993) Parenteral support of the hospitalised child. In: Suskind RM and Lewinter-Suskind L (eds) *Textbook of Pediatric Nutrition,* 2nd edn. New York: Raven Press, pp. 225–238.

24. Heird WC, Driscoll JM, Schullinger JN, Grebin B and Winters RW (1972) Intravenous alimentation in pediatric patients. *J Pediatr* **80**:351–372.

105 | Sedation and analgesia in children

GJ Knight

It is generally acknowledged that all children, including preterm infants, feel and remember pain and discomfort.[1,2] Provision of adequate sedation and analgesia should, therefore, be a priority in the management of all critically ill children.

Indications and benefits

Pain in the paediatric ICU may be surgical in origin, or due to the underlying illness or to procedures (e.g. central venous catheterization, lumbar puncture and removal of drains). Sedation is frequently necessary to allow a child to tolerate an endotracheal tube and mechanical ventilation. It may also be needed to allow sleep in a brightly lit, noisy environment. As young children are unlikely to cooperate during investigations such as an echocardiograph or computed tomographic (CT) scan, sedation is often necessary to prevent excessive movement.

Apart from humane benefits, sedation and analgesia can suppress non-advantageous physiological responses to noxious stimuli. Analgesic suppression of the marked post-surgery stress response has been associated with significant improvements in post-operative morbidity and mortality.[3-5] Sedation and analgesia have also been shown to blunt pulmonary hypertensive responses to stimulation in children with labile pulmonary vasculature.[6]

Assessment

Adequacy of pain relief and sedation is dependent on an accurate assessment of the degree of discomfort. This may be particularly difficult in the critically ill child for many reasons. The patient may be preverbal, developmentally delayed, intubated and/or paralysed, or simply uncooperative. Thorough assessment requires careful and frequent consideration of a number of factors. These include the nature of the noxious stimulus, variations in physiological parameters such as heart rate and blood pressure, and interpretation of subjective clues, such as facial expressions and posture. Parental interpretations of a child's expressions should also be considered. In older children self-reporting measurement scales may be useful and a number of methods have been developed to measure pain[7,8] (see Chapter 78). Although these tools are useful, they are only part of the overall assessment of discomfort.

Management

Supportive measures

The management of discomfort, anxiety and pain may take many forms. It can begin prior to the child's admission to intensive care, through orientation to the unit and explanation of a procedure and its expected course. Parental presence is important to allay anxiety and fear. Close attention should also be paid throughout a child's admission to physiological factors that may cause distress (e.g. hunger). Despite these supportive measures, many paediatric patients require a pharmacological form of analgesia or sedation.

Paediatric pharmacological considerations

Differences in drug handling between children and adults should be considered. Drug distribution, rates of drug metabolism and relative organ blood flows differ in children, particularly infants. These differences may result in greater concentrations of free drug and differing volumes of distribution. Neonates have relatively larger total body water, extracellular fluid volume, blood volume and cardiac output, and significantly less body fat than adults.[9-11] Their blood–brain barrier is less efficient and allows more ready entry of some drugs to the brain. Mixed-function oxidases mature quickly to adult levels by 6 months of age, and acetylation and glucuronidation mechanisms mature by about 3 months.[12,13] Renal blood flow and glomerular filtration rate are low in the immediate neonatal period. However, both increase significantly in the first 2–3 days, and reach adult values by 5 months.[14,15] Tubular secretory capacity reaches adult levels by 6 months of age.[13] In general, drug metabolism and clearance are relatively mature by 6 months of age.

Specific sedative agents (Table 105.1)

Midazolam

Midazolam is water-soluble, has rapid onset and generally does not produce haemodynamic instability in children. Dose-related respiratory depression has, however, been documented.[16] Metabolism is mature by 6 months of age.[17] A continuous infusion is usually effective, particularly in combination with an opioid, to facilitate mechanical ventilation. Midazolam is also useful, in bolus doses, to sedate patients for uncomfortable procedures, such as echocardiography and cardioversion. Accumulation can occur during an infusion and lead to delayed wakening. This is more likely in patients with liver dysfunction.

The standard IV sedative dose is 0.1–0.2 mg/kg. A continuous infusion (50–200 µg/kg per h) administered in combination with morphine (10–40 µg/kg per h) provides satisfactory sedation for the patient on mechanical ventilation. Midazolam has been reported as the sole sedative agent for ventilated patients, although the initial dose of 24 µg/kg per h is unlikely to be adequate.[18,19] Nasal administration of midazolam (0.2 mg/kg) can be useful in children who do not have established IV access and in whom oral agents are not appropriate.[20] The oral route (0.5 mg/kg) may also be useful.

Ketamine

Ketamine is a dissociative anaesthetic agent with analgesic and amnesic properties. Cardiovascular disturbance is minimal. Biotransformation occurs by the microsomal enzyme system. Thus there is little

metabolism in the newborn.[21] Clearance is less and elimination half-life is greater in infants than in older children and adults.[22] Preterm infants, to a postconceptual age of 51 weeks, are at increased risk of postanaesthetic apnoea.[23] Concomitant use of an antisialogogue, such as glycopyrrolate, helps control the increase in respiratory tract secretions often seen with ketamine. The unpleasant emergent phenomena, seen frequently in adults, are reported less often in children. Studies indicate that they can be controlled by the concurrent administration of benzodiazepines.[24,25]

An initial IV dose of 1–2 mg/kg is usually adequate to induce deep sedation. Prolonged sedation for ventilated children has been achieved with a continuous infusion of 10–15 µg/kg per min.[26] Ketamine (1–2 mg/kg) supplemented by midazolam (0.1 mg/kg) is an effective sedative regimen for painful procedures.

Propofol

Propofol is a rapidly acting anaesthetic agent that has been used for short and longer-term sedation in paediatric intensive care.[27] The half-life decreases with age, probably due to development of metabolizing capacity and increasing hepatic blood flow.[28] Rapid emergence from sedation is propofol's most attractive property. It has been safely used for short-term sedation in the spontaneously breathing patient, by using small induction doses of 1 mg/kg, followed by intermittent smaller doses.[29] Its role has been extended to that of sole sedating agent for ventilated children. However, a number of problems have been reported with such infusions, including neurological disorders and death from myocardial failure and metabolic acidosis.[30,31] All the children who died had respiratory disease and were given relatively high doses. Although lipaemia was noted, the lipid load was not excessive by normal standards for parenteral nutrition, and the pathogenesis of these complications remains unclear. Seizures have been reported in the withdrawal phase following the use of propofol as a sedative in adult intensive care.[32] Thus, as a result of these problems, propofol should be limited to short-term sedation of the ventilated child. It can be useful to provide sedation, whilst the effects of a longer-acting opioid/benzodiazepine infusion wear off. Long-term sedation with propofol cannot be recommended until further studies of safety are available.

Thiopentone

Thiopentone is useful as an anaesthetic induction agent, although its hypotensive effects limit its use in shocked patients. The standard dose is 5 mg/kg, reduced to 2–3 mg/kg when hypotension is a risk. Thiopentone is rarely used to manage acute brain injury, but is occasionally useful, as an infusion, to

Table 105.1 Doses of commonly used sedative and analgesic drugs

Drug	Bolus dose	Infusion rate
Morphine	0.1–0.2 mg/kg	10–40 µg/kg per h
Pethidine	1.0–1.5 mg/kg	100–300 µg/kg per h
Fentanyl	1–2 µg/kg	1–10 µg/kg per h
Midazolam	0.1–0.2 mg/kg	50–200 µg/kg per h
Ketamine	1–2 mg/kg	10–15 µg/kg per min[26]

manage refractory status epilepticus and difficult cases of raised intracranial pressure.

Chloral hydrate

Chloral is an effective oral hypnotic and sedative agent with no analgesic effect. The hypnotic dose is 50 mg/kg, and appropriate sedation can be achieved with lower doses. Gastric irritation can be a problem in some children. Toxic doses can produce depression of respiration and cardiac contractility. There is some evidence that it may not be suitable in acutely wheezing infants.[33] Despite a major disadvantage of delayed onset, chloral can be usefully given before procedures, and it can be used effectively to induce nocturnal sleep.

Opioids

Morphine

Morphine is the most frequently used analgesic agent in paediatric intensive care, and is commonly used with a benzodiazepine in children on mechanical ventilation. By 6 months of age, clearance and half-life (2 h) are at adult values.[34] Morphine's active metabolite is renally excreted, and can accumulate in renal failure. Marked variation in pharmacokinetics in the neonatal period has been demonstrated, but infants over 1 month of age eliminate morphine efficiently, and should not be more sensitive to respiratory depression than adults.[34,35]

The standard IV dose is 0.1–0.2 mg/kg, and an infusion rate of 10–30 μg/kg per h has been shown to be safe for postoperative pain relief in spontaneously breathing patients.[36] With careful titration of dose to effect, higher rates can safely be administered, particularly to the child on mechanical ventilation. Patient-controlled analgesia devices delivering fixed doses of opioid with or without a background infusion can be used successfully by the majority of school-aged children, and may occasionally be appropriate in intensive care[37] (see Chapter 79).

Histamine-related side-effects, in particular nasal itch, may warrant a change of opioid. Pethidine is generally suitable, and the equipotent dose is 10-fold that of morphine.

Fentanyl and alfentanil

Fentanyl has theoretical advantages over morphine in certain situations, because of its rapid onset and its systemic and pulmonary haemodynamic stability. Termination of the effects of a single dose is by redistribution, and the elimination half-life does not change significantly through childhood.[38] After prolonged infusion, unchanged fentanyl is returned to the circulation from peripheral compartments, resulting in a prolonged terminal elimination half-life of approximately 21 h.[39] Clearance of fentanyl is more rapid in neonates and infants compared to adults, and does not change with time during continuous infusion.[38,39] Fentanyl is useful as an anaesthetic agent in patients with labile pulmonary vasculature, as it can blunt changes in pulmonary vascular resistance seen with stimulation.[6] However, it does not prevent the increase in pulmonary vascular pressure caused by hypoxia.[6,40]

The effective dose for painful procedures is 1–2 μg/kg. Even large anaesthetic doses of 30–50 μg/kg produce minimal haemodynamic changes.[6] Infusions of 1–5 μg/kg per h produce effective sedation in neonates on mechanical ventilation;[41] 1–10 μg/kg/per h is required to provide analgesia in older children. Tolerance, noted in both neonates an older children, can develop rapidly, and adjustment of the infusion rate may be necessary.[42] Fentanyl's short duration of action makes it suitable for use in epidural regimens.

Alfentanil, because of its shorter duration of action, may have advantages for analgesia or sedation for very short procedures.

Drug withdrawal syndromes

Opioid withdrawal is now a more frequently recognized problem, and occurs particularly following prolonged high-dose infusions.[43] Katz *et al.*[44] reported that a fentanyl infusion for longer than 5 days had greater than 50% incidence of withdrawal symptoms; the risk was strongly linked to the total drug dose. Symptoms include poor feeding, agitation, diarrhoea and sweating. When an opioid is combined with a benzodiazepine, withdrawal symptoms involving dystonic posturing may be attributed to the benzodiazepine component.[45] Careful attention to weaning an infusion can minimize symptoms and signs. Pharmacological management is occasionally required, and drugs used include methadone, benzodiazepines and clonidine.[44,46] Concerns about withdrawal problems should not preclude the provision of adequate sedation or analgesia.

Inhaled agents

Nitrous oxide

Nitrous oxide is a potent analgesic agent. It is useful in intensive care during short painful procedures such as removal of surgical drains. It is unsuitable for repeated or continuous use because of toxicity.

Isoflurane

Isoflurane has been used for long-term sedation in intensive care in adults.[47] As elimination is independent of hepatic and renal mechanisms, there are theoretical advantages in many critically ill patients. However, an association between isoflurane sedation in children and neurological abnormalities has been reported.[48] These abnormalities, although reversible, were a considerable clinical problem.

Local anaesthesia

Local anaesthesia can produce effective analgesia without systemic effects. In the intensive care setting it can be used as the sole method of analgesia or to supplement IV agents. Metabolism of local anaesthetic agents is reduced in infants less than 6 months of age.[49] Toxicity, rarely seen in children, is related to the dose and rapidity of absorption (which is dependent on local blood flow).[50]

Emla

Emla, an emulsion of lignocaine and prilocaine, is effective in reducing the pain associated with percutaneous procedures.[51] It needs to be applied to the skin 60 min beforehand, and is thus not suitable for urgent procedures. Systemic absorption of the prilocaine component and subsequent methaemoglobinaemia can occur.[52] Neonates, because of their relative deficiency of methaemoglobin reductase, are particularly at risk, and Emla should not be used in this group.

Nerve blocks

Femoral nerve blockade is a simple technique that produces effective analgesia in cases of femoral shaft fracture. A single injection is effective for approximately 3 h, and a technique has been developed to provide long-term analgesia.[53] Bupivacaine (0.125%) is infused continuously at 0.2–0.3 ml/kg per h through a fine catheter placed adjacent to the femoral nerve. This technique is useful in trauma patients with a coexistent head injury, as it can decrease opioid requirements.

Intercostal blocks have been described after thoracotomies and liver transplants in children.[54] Continuous infusions via an intercostal catheter can be effective. The dose must be carefully limited, because the relatively high blood flow to the area increases the risk of toxicity.

Epidurals

Caudal, lumbar and thoracic epidural anaesthesia provide effective control of postoperative pain in children, and epidural analgesia has been applied in the management of paediatric trauma.[49,55–57] Epidural administration of morphine has been shown to be effective in children following abdominal and cardiac surgery. Epidural opioids are associated with a decrease in the slope of the CO_2 response curve, and close observation in the ICU for the first 24 h is advisable.

References

1. Anand KJS and Hickey PR (1987) Pain in the foetus and neonate. *N Engl J Med* **317**:1321–1329.
2. McGrath PJ and Craig KD (1989) Developmental and psychological factors in children's pain. *Paediatr Clin North Am* **36**:823–836.
3. Anand KJS and Ward-Platt MP (1988) Neonatal and pediatric responses to anaesthesia and operation. *Int Anaesthesiol Clin* **26**:218–225.
4. Anand KJS and Hickey PR (1992) Halothane–morphine compared with high dose sufentanil for anaesthesia and postoperative analgesia in neonatal cardiac surgery. *N Engl J Med* **326**:1–9.
5. Anand KJS, Sippell WG and Aynsley-Green A (1987) Randomised trial of fentanyl anaesthesia in preterm neonates undergoing surgery: effects on the stress response. *Lancet* **1**:243–248.
6. Hickey P, Hansen DD, Wessell DL, Lang P, Jonas RA and Elixson EM (1985) Blunting of stress response in the pulmonary vasculature of infants by fentanil. *Anesth Analg* **64**:1137–1142.
7. McGrath PA, deVeber L and Haarn M (1985) Multidimensional pain assessment in children. In: Fields H, Dubner R and Cervero F (eds) *Advances in Pain Research and Therapy*, vol. 9. New York: Raven Press, pp. 387–393.
8. Wong D and Baker C (1988) Pain in children: comparison of assessment scales. *Paediatric Nursing* **14**:9–17.
9. Friis-Hansen B (1971) Body composition during growth. In vivo measurements and biochemical data correlated to differential anatomical growth. *Pediatrics* **47**:264–274.
10. Widdowson EM (1981) Changes in body composition during growth. In: Davis JA and Dobbing J (eds) *Scientific Foundations of Paediatrics*. London: Heinemann, pp. 330–342.
11. Friis-Hansen B (1983) Water distribution in the foetus and newborn infants. *Acta Paediatr Scand* **305**(suppl):7–11.
12. Nitowsky HM, Matz L and Berzofsky JA (1966) Studies on oxidative drug metabolism in the full term newborn infant. *J Pediatr* **69**:1139–1149.
13. Gladtke E (1979) The importance of pharmacokinetics for paediatrics. *Eur J Paediatr* **131**:85–91.
14. Arant BS Jr (1978) Developmental patterns of renal functional maturation compared in the human neonate. *J Pediatr* **92**:705–712.
15. Leake RD and Trystad CW (1977) Glomerular filtration rate during the period of adaptation to extrauterine life. *Pediatr Res* **11**:959–962.
16. Forster A, Morel D, Bachmann M and Gemperle M (1982) Ventilatory effects of various doses of IV midazolam assessed by a noninvasive method in healthy volunteers. *Anesthesiology* **57**:A480.
17. Lloyd-Thomas AR and Booker PD (1986) Infusion of midazolam in paediatric patients after cardiac surgery. *Br J Anaesth* **58**:1109–1115.
18. Silvani DL, Rosen DA and Rosen KR (1988) Continuous midazolam infusion for sedation in the paediatric intensive care unit. *Anesth Analg* **67**:286–288.

19. Durbin CG (1994) Sedation in the critically ill patient. *New Horizons* 2:64–74.

20. Wilton N, Leigh J, Rosen D and Pandit U (1988) Preanaesthetic sedation of preschool children using intranasal midazolam. *Anesthesiology* 69:927–975.

21. Chang T and Glazko T (1974) Biotransformation and metabolism of ketamine. *Int Anesthesiol Clin* 12:157–177.

22. Cook DR and Davis PJ (1993) Paediatric anaesthesia pharmacology. In: Lake CH (ed.) *Paediatric Cardiac Anaesthesia*. Norwalk, CT: Appleton & Lange, pp. 119–150.

23. Welborn LG, Rice LJ, Hannallah RS, Broadman LM, Ruttiman UE and Fink R (1990) Postoperative apnoea in former preterm infants: prospective comparison of spinal and general anaesthesia. *Anesthesiology* 72:838–842.

24. Rita L and Seleny FL (1974) Ketamine hydrochloride for paediatric premedication II. Prevention of post anaesthetic excitement. *Anesth Analg* 53:380–382.

25. Green SM, Nakamura R and Johnson NE (1990) Ketamine sedation for paediatric procedures. Part 1. A prospective series. *Ann Emerg Med* 9:1024–1032.

26. Tobias JD, Martin LD and Wetzel RC (1990) Ketamine by continuous infusion for sedation in the paediatric intensive care unit. *Crit Care Med* 18:819–821.

27. Norreslet J and Wahlgren C (1990) Propofol infusion for sedation in children. *Crit Care Med* 18:890–892.

28. Jones RDM, Chan K and Andrew LJ (1990) Pharmacokinetics of propofol in children. *Br J Anaesth* 65:661–667.

29. Paschall A, Braner DAV and Portland OR (1993) Sedation with propofol in the PICU. *Crit Care Med* 21:S150.

30. Trotter C and Serpell MG (1992) Neurological sequelae in children after prolonged propofol infusion. *Anaesthesia* 47:340–342.

31. Parker TJ, Stevens JE, Rice ASC *et al.* (1992) Metabolic acidosis and fatal myocardial failure after propofol infusion in children: five case reports. *Br Med J* 305:613–616.

32. Valente JF, Anderson GL, Branson RD *et al.* (1994) Disadvantages of prolonged propofol sedation in the critical care unit. *Crit Care Med* 22:710–712.

33. Mallol J and Sly PD (1988) Effect of chloral hydrate on arterial oxygen saturation in wheezy infants. *Paediatr Pulmonol* 5:96–99.

34. McRori TI, Lynn AM, Nespecca MK, Opheim KE and Slattery JT (1992) The maturation of morphine clearance and metabolism. *Am J Dis Child* 146:972–976.

35. Bhat R, Chari, Gulati A, Aldana O, Velamati R and Bhargava H (1990) Pharmacokinetics of a single dose of morphine during the first week of life. *J Pediatr* 117:477–481.

36. Lynn A, Opheim K and Tyler D (1984) Morphine infusion after paediatric surgery. *Crit Care Med* 12:863–866.

37. Gaukroger PP (1993) Patient controlled analgesia in children. In: Schechter NL, Berde CB and Yaster M (eds) *Pain in Infants, Children and Adolescents*. Baltimore, MD: Williams & Wilkins, pp. 203–211.

38. Johnson KL, Erickson JP, Holley FO and Scott JC (1984) Fentanyl pharmacokinetics in the paediatric population. *Anesthesiology* 61:A441.

39. Katz R and Kelly WH (1993) Pharmacokinetics of continuous infusions of fentanyl in critically ill children. *Crit Care Med* 21:995–1000.

40. Vacanti JP, Crone PK, Murphy JP *et al.* (1984) The pulmonary haemodynamic response to perioperative anaesthesia in the treatment of high risk infants with congenital diaphragmatic hernia. *J Pediatr Surg* 19:672–679.

41. Truog RD and Anand KJS (1989) Management of pain in the perioperative neonate. *Clin Perinatol* 16:61–78.

42. Arnold JH, Truog RD, Scavone JM and Fenton T (1991) Changes in the pharmacodynamic response to fentanyl in neonates during continuous infusion. *J Pediatr* 119:639–643.

43. Anand KJS and Arnold J (1994) Opioid tolerance and dependence in infants and children. *Crit Care Med* 22:334–342.

44. Katz R, Kelly WH and Hsi A (1994) Prospective study on the occurrence of withdrawal in critically ill children who receive fentanyl by continuous infusion. *Crit Care Med* 22:763–767.

45. Bergman I, Steeves MG and Thompson A (1991) Reversible neurological abnormalities associated with prolonged midazolam and fentanyl infusion. *J Pediatr* 119:644–648.

46. Tobias JD, Deshpande JK and Gregory DF (1994) Outpatient therapy of iatrogenic drug dependency following prolonged sedation in the paediatric intensive care unit. *Intensive Care Med* 20:504–507.

47. Breheny FX and Kendall PA (1992) Use of isoflurane for sedation in intensive care. *Crit Care Med* 20:1062–1064.

48. Kelsall AWR, Ross-Russell R and Herrick MJ (1994) Reversible neurological dysfunction following isoflurane sedation in paediatric intensive care. *Crit Care Med* 22:1032–1034.

49. Yaster M and Maxwell LG (1989) Paediatric regional anaesthesia. *Anesthesiology* 70:324–338.

50. Covino BG (1986) Pharmacology of local anaesthetic agents. *Br J Anaesth* 58:701–716.

51. Sims C (1991) Thickly and thinly applied lignocaine–prilocaine cream prior to venepuncture in children. *Anaesth Intensive Care* 19:343–345.

52. Frayling IM, Addison GM, Chattergee K and Meakin G (1990) Methaemoglobinaemia in children treated with lignocaine–prilocaine cream. *Br Med J* 301:153–154.

53. Johnson CM (1994) Continuous femoral nerve blockade for analgesia in children with femoral nerve fractures. *Anaesth Intensive Care* 22:281–283.

54. Shelly MP and Park GR (1987) Intercostal nerve blockade for children. *Anaesthesia* 42:541–545.

55. Dalens B, Tanguy A and Haberer J-P (1986) Lumbar epidural anaesthesia for operative and postoperative pain relief in infants and children. *Anesth Analg* 65:1069–1073.

56. Attia J, Ecoffey C, Sandouk P, Gross JB and Samii K (1986) Epidural morphine in children: pharmacokinetics and CO_2 sensitivity. *Anesthesiology* 65:590–594.

57. Shapiro L, Jedeiken RJ, Shalev D and Hoffman S (1984) Epidural morphine analgesia in children. *Anesthesiology* 61:210–212.

106 Shock and cardiac disease in children

RD Henning

Most cases of shock in childhood are due to hypovolaemia or sepsis (Table 106.1). The causes and complications of shock differ from those of adults, because the spectrum of childhood disease is different: abdominal sepsis, pancreatitis and obstructive vascular disease are uncommon in childhood. Most cases of septic shock in children with cancer are due to neutropenia and immune suppression after chemotherapy or bone marrow transplantation. Other considerations in children are given below.

Table 106.1 Causes of shock in childhood, with specific examples on the right

Hypovolaemia	
Bleeding	External, GI tract, body cavity, haematoma
Water and electrolyte loss	
Bowel	Vomiting, diarrhoea, ileus
Renal	Diuretic, diabetes mellitus, diabetes insipidus
Skin	Burns, heat stroke
Plasma loss (capillary leak)	Sepsis, burns, anaphylaxis, post cardiac arrest
Distributive	
Sepsis	
Anaphylaxis	
Drugs	e.g. barbiturates, phenothiazines
Neurogenic	Injury to brainstem or high cervical spine
Cardiogenic	
Structural congenital heart disease	
Arrhythmia	Heart block, supraventricular tachycardia
Myocardial hypoxia/ischaemia	
Global hypoxia	e.g. SIDS, near-drowning
Myocardial ischaemia	Kawasaki, anomalous left coronary artery
Cardiomyopathy	
Metabolic	Storage diseases, muscular dystrophies, maternal diabetes
Endocardial fibroelastosis	
Infective	Bacteria, enteroviruses
Valvular heart disease	Congenital, infective endocarditis, rheumatic, traumatic
Sepsis	
Drug intoxication	e.g. tricyclic antidepressants, calcium antagonists, narcotics
Tamponade	Bleeding, uraemia, right heart failure
Combined	Sepsis, drugs, pancreatitis, post cardiac arrest

GI = Gastrointestinal; SIDS = sudden infant death syndrome.

Smaller body fluid compartments

A small volume of blood or diarrhoeal fluid may represent a large percentage loss of blood or extracellular fluid volume in an infant.

Immature immune system under 5 years

In the first 6 months of life, immature and permeable gut, lung and skin barriers, low complement, immunoglobulin M (IgM) and IgA concentrations, and poor neutrophil migration and phagocyte function increase susceptibility to severe bacteraemias.[1] Antibody response to bacterial capsular polysaccharide antigens (e.g. *Pneumococcus* and *Haemophilus*) remains poor until 5 years of age. Low IgG concentrations and immunological naivety predispose to frequent viral infection in the first 5 years.[2] Reduced production of some cytokines (e.g. tumour necrosis factor (TNF) and interleukin-4 (IL-4)[3,4] in infants may alter the features and duration of the shock syndrome.

Microbiology

In the newborn, septic shock is most often caused by Gram-negative bacilli, *Staphylococcus aureus*, group B β-haemolytic streptococci, *Listeria monocytogenes* or enteroviruses. In childhood, pneumococcus and meningococcus, Gram-negative bacilli and *S. aureus* are usually responsible. *Haemophilus influenzae* still causes septicaemia in non-immunized children under 5 years.

Severe congenital abnormalities

Children with congenital heart disease, multiple congenital abnormalities, inborn errors of metabolism and the inherited immunodeficiencies are prone to develop cardiogenic, hypovolaemic or septic shock.

Pathophysiology

The pathophysiology of shock is described in Chapter 14. Features peculiar to childhood include the following.

Immature cardiovascular system[5]

The maximum force and velocity of myocardial contraction are less in infancy, because the immature heart has fewer myofilaments and less myofibrillar adenosine triphosphate (ATP) per unit cross-sectional area, and the myofibrils and cytoskeleton are less efficiently aligned for force development. Heart rate is therefore the main influence on cardiac output in infancy. The diastolic compliance of the infant heart is poor, and ventricular interdependence is greater than that of adults. Consequently, the response to volume loading is less, and the depression of left ventricular output by pulmonary hypertension is greater.

Beat-to-beat control of calcium release from sarcoplasmic reticulum is less than in adults, because calcium uptake, storage and release are less, and extracellular fluid calcium concentration has a greater effect on contractile force and velocity.

Autonomic innervation

The development of cardiac sympathetic innervation in infants is incomplete; myocardial noradrenaline stores are smaller than in adults. Thus, response to severe stress is bradycardia rather than tachycardia as in the adult, and the infant heart is relatively refractory to dopamine.

The numbers and sensitivity of myocardial adrenergic receptors are greater than in the adult. Hence the contractile response of the infant heart to α-agonist drugs is much greater.[6] Phosphodiesterase inhibitors such as amrinone depress contractility in the immature heart.[7]

Response to hypoxia and ischaemia

Myocardial cell survival and rate of recovery of performance after periods of hypoxia or ischaemia are greater in infants, because of lower rates of energy demand and ATP consumption or efflux, as well as higher cell glycogen reserves.[8]

The infant with sphanchnic ischaemia is more likely to develop bowel mucosal damage and leakage of endotoxin and bacteria, because its plasma concentration of platelet-activating factor (PAF), acetylhydrolase and levels of catalase and reduced glutathione in the colonic mucosa are low.[9]

Clinical presentation of shock in childhood

Hypovolaemic shock

A history of blood or fluid loss and signs of haematoma, external bleeding or dehydration may be present. Signs of homeostatic compensation usually precede hypotension, which tends to occur late (after loss of 15–20% of blood volume) and precipitously in young children. Compensatory signs include increasing tachycardia, tachypnoea and narrow pulse pressure. In severe shock of any cause, signs of multiple organ hypoperfusion (e.g. cool, mottled extremities, slow capillary refill, oliguria of under 0.5 ml/kg per h urine, lethargy or coma and an increasing metabolic acidosis) are found. Plasma lactate is high, and bleeding due to disseminated intravascular coagulation and liver dysfunction may occur in the first 6 h. In early shock, these changes are reversible by plasma volume expansion with boluses of 10 ml/kg blood, colloid or normal saline, repeated as necessary.

Failure to respond to such treatment indicates refractory shock requiring more aggressive treatment (see below).

Cardiogenic shock

Tachycardia, hypotension, poor pulses and signs of poor organ perfusion are usually present. Cardiomegaly and a gallop rhythm may be found. Chest rales and tachypnoea indicate left heart failure, while hepatomegaly develops rapidly, and is a more reliable sign of right heart failure than a raised jugular venous pressure (JVP) (which may be hard to detect in infants). Signs of specific heart lesions (e.g. murmurs or cyanosis, absent femoral pulses in aortic coarctation, skull, liver or renal bruits of arteriovenous fistulae, and arrhythmias) may indicate the cause of the shock. Investigation should include urgent chest X-ray, electrocardiogram (ECG), echocardiography and in some cases cardiac catheterization.

Septic shock

Septic infants younger than 6 months present with a hypodynamic circulation, low cardiac output and cool extremities. However, early septic shock in older children is similar to that in adults: tachycardia, tachypnoea and hypotension are accompanied by warm extremities, wide pulse pressure and increased cardiac output. Lethargy, oliguria and metabolic acidosis deteriorate. As shock progresses, myocardial depression by bacterial toxins and cytokines[10] decreases cardiac output, resulting in worsening hypotension, decreased pulse pressure and cool mottled extremities. Capillary leakage caused by PAF, TNF, IL-1 and IL-2[11] causes hypovolaemia and reduced oxygen delivery to tissues. Peripheral oedema exacerbates cellular hypoxia by increasing the diffusion distances for oxygen between capillaries and cells.

Distributive shock

The main features are vasodilatation and hypovolaemia due to plasma leakage from capillaries. The extremities are warm and pink; blood pressure is low and pulse pressure is wide. There is tachycardia, oliguria and stupor.

Management

The child's airway, breathing and circulation should be secured during the initial assessment. The priorities in management are given below.

Adequate perfusion of brain and heart

This requires systolic and diastolic blood pressures 80% of normal for age (Table 106.2), ach-

Table 106.2 Normal blood pressure and heart rate in childhood

Age	Blood pressure (mmHg (kPa))	Heart rate (beats/min)
Birth	75/40 (10.0/5.3)	125
1 year	95/60 (12.6/8.0)	120
2 years	96/60 (12.8/8.0)	110
6 years	98/60 (13.0/8.0)	100
10 years	110/70 (14.6/9.3)	90
14 years	118/75 (15.7/10.0)	80

ieved by aggressive early blood volume expansion and by inotropic drugs. In distributive shock, IV infusion of vasoconstrictors such as noradrenaline (0.05–0.50 μg/kg per min into a central vein) may be needed to maintain adequate coronary and cerebral perfusion pressure. The conscious state is the best index of adequate cerebral perfusion, while improved coronary perfusion is shown by rising blood pressure with falling atrial pressures.

Gas exchange

Early mechanical ventilation secures adequate oxygenation and pH of arterial blood. Mechanical ventilation reduces work of breathing and muscle oxygen demand, diverting the limited cardiac output away from muscles to vital organs. Airway pressures and tidal volumes should be limited to the minimum needed, as impaired venous return from positive-pressure ventilation may exacerbate hypotension.

Adequate perfusion of kidneys, liver and gut

Bowel and liver ischaemia in a shocked child greatly increases the risk of bacteraemia and endotoxaemia of bowel origin,[12] and reduces detoxification of drugs and toxic metabolites. Hypovolaemia and low cardiac output must be corrected. Vasoconstrictor drugs should be reduced or stopped as early as possible. Urine output greater than 0.5 ml/kg per h with a normal plasma creatinine concentration are the best indices of adequate renal perfusion. Adequacy of splanchic perfusion is shown by gastric pH 7.32 (calculated by Henderson–Hasselbalch equation from arterial HCO_3^- and gastric P_{CO_2} sampled from an intragastric balloon)[13] or by a gastric–arterial P_{CO_2} difference of 12 or less. Blood volume expansion and inotropic drugs such as dobutamine and low-dose dopamine (2 μg/kg per min) are used to improve renal and splanchnic perfusion.

Adequate perfusion of muscle and other tissues

Improvement of circulation to these tissues may require further volume expansion and infusion of vasodilators (e.g. sodium nitroprusside or milrinone) in shock states where myocardial depression is prominent, provided an adequate blood pressure can be sustained. The usefulness of supranormal levels of oxygen delivery in adults[14] is debated (see Chapter 22). No such prospective studies have been performed in children.

Methods of treatment

Optimal preload

IV fluid is given in aliquots of 10 ml/kg blood or colloid, or 20 ml/kg crystalloid. Administration of further aliquots is titrated against changes in blood pressure, homeostatic responses such as heart rate and skin vasoconstriction (i.e. skin warmth and colour, and nailbed capillary return), and indices of organ perfusion (i.e. urine output, conscious state, serum pH and lactate). Heart and liver size are used to assess hypervolaemia. If more than 20 ml/kg colloid is given, central venous pressure and sometimes cardiac output and pulmonary capillary wedge pressure (PCWP) should be monitored. Their therapeutic gains must be weighed against the risks of catheterization, especially in infants. The presence of hypovolaemic shock implies a blood volume deficit greater than 30 ml/kg.

Increased contractility

Inotropic drugs are infused, initially at high doses (e.g. dopamine or dobutamine 10–20 μg/kg per min), reducing the dose when possible. Aggressive early measures to improve cardiac output may reduce the duration and complications of shock. Children often need higher doses than adults because of increased myocardial oxygen demand, although catecholamines increase body oxygen consumption by increasing futile fat cycling.[15] Dopamine also suppresses prolactin, thyroid-stimulating hormone and growth hormone secretion in infants and children.[16]

If reduced cardiac output is due to systemic or pulmonary vasoconstriction, dobutamine or a phosphodiesterase inhibitor (e.g. milrinone or enoximone) may be used instead of dopamine. Dobutamine and dopamine down-regulate β-adrenergic receptors, and dopamine depletes myocardial noradrenaline stores. If the cardiac index is poor, especially after 24–48 h of infusion of either drug, the combination of myocardial α-receptor stimulation by low-dose noradrenaline (0.05–0.20 μg/kg per min) and vasodilatation with sodium nitroprusside may improve myocardial performance, while infusion of 10% calcium gluconate (0.2–0.5 ml/h) can increase blood pressure and cardiac output in infants with heart failure. Serum ionized calcium should be monitored.[17]

Afterload reduction in cardiogenic shock

Vasoconstrictors and blood transfusion (to achieve a haemoglobin concentration of 120 g/l) may be required to ensure adequate coronary and cerebral perfusion pressure. If blood pressure is adequate, cardiac output may be improved by afterload reduction. Short-acting drugs such as sodium nitroprusside are preferred. Inhaled nitric oxide (NO) via the ventilator circuit may improve cardiogenic shock due to pulmonary hypertension after cardiac surgery, and in persistent pulmonary hypertension of the newborn.[18] Infusion of vasodilators such as nitroglycerin, prostaglanclin E (PGE), prostacyclin (PGI_2) and sodium nitroprusside reduces systemic as well as pulmonary vascular resistance. These drugs are easier to administer than NO, but are less effective pulmonary vasodilators, and often cause systemic hypotension.

Investigations

After appropriate samples are taken for investigations (Table 106.3), possible sepsis is treated aggressively with appropriate antibiotics, replacement of invasive lines and drainage of collections.

Table 106.3 Investigation of shock in children

All shocked children
Arterial blood gases
Plasma electrolytes, creatinine, glucose
Haemoglobin, platelet count, total and differential white cell count
Blood group (hold serum)

If the cause of shock is unknown
Exclude sepsis:
   Several sets of blood cultures, percutaneous and via vascular catheters
   Culture and Gram stain pus
   Urine cultures, MSU or suprapubic aspirate
   Urine, stool, nasopharyngeal aspirate for virology
   CSF bacterial and viral culture plus PCR for specific organisms
   Urine bacterial antigens
To exclude cardiogenic shock: echocardiography, ECG, cardiac catheter
Drug screen: urine; gastric aspirate; blood
Metabolic screen: urinary amino acids and organic acids, plasma ammonia and glucose

---

MSU = midstream urine; CSF = cerebrospinal fluid; PCR = polymerase chain reaction; ECG = electrocardiogram.

Supportive measures

These include administration of platelets and fresh frozen plasma in consumptive coagulopathy, use of corticosteroids in the Waterhouse–Friderichsen syndrome, and early commencement of renal support with haemofiltration or peritoneal dialysis in established acute renal failure.

Controversial measures

1 *Correction of metabolic acidosis*: Administration of $NaHCO_3$ reduces myocardial intracellular pH, myocardial performance and cardiac output in adult humans and animals, but not in newborn animals.[19] $NaHCO_3/Na_2CO_3$ mixtures raise both intracellular and extracellular pH,[20] increase cardiac output and reduce pulmonary vascular resistance in some patients with systemic acidosis.[21]

2 *High-dose steroids after antibiotics started*: No benefits were found in two large multicentre trials.[22] Steroids before the first antibiotic dose in children with septic shock are being studied.[23]

3 *Naloxone*: No useful effect on haemodynamics or survival has been reported.[24]

4 *Antiendotoxin antibodies* have not been found to be useful in clinical trials.[25]

5 *PAF antagonist Ginkgolide B* reduced mortality in a large controlled trial of adults with Gram-negative sepsis.[26]

6 *Anti-TNF and anti IL-1* treatment has not yet been shown conclusively to be useful in human trials, despite promising animal studies.[25]

7 *Circulatory support with extracorporeal membrane oxygenation (ECMO)* was associated with 50% survival in 9 children who were moribund with septic shock.[27]

8 *Granulocyte transfusion, exchange transfusion, plasma exchange*: There are no convincing human trials, but favourable case reports of use in neonates and children[28,29] and animal models[30] have appeared.

Heart failure in children

In cardiac failure, cardiac output is insufficient to meet the metabolic needs of the tissues without developing abnormally high atrial pressures.[31] The main causes are:

1 *Preload*:
   (a) *excessive* (i.e. volume loading, e.g. systemic arteriovenous malformation and large ventricular septal defect (VSD) or
   (b) *inadequate* (e.g. mitral stenosis and pericardial tamponade);
2 *excessive afterload* (pressure loading, e.g. pulmonary hypertension and aortic stenosis);

Table 106.4 Common causes of heart failure from infancy to adolescence

Heart failure presenting at birth
Birth asphyxia
Sepsis
Severe anaemia (hydrops fetalis)
Obstructive left-sided lesions presenting after closure of the ductus arteriosus (e.g. coarctation, aortic stenosis, interrupted aortic arch)
Arrhythmias, congenital SVT or heart block
Aortopulmonary window, truncus arteriosus
Systemic AV fistula (e.g. liver, brain or kidney)
Congenital cardiomyopathy

Heart failure presenting in the first 8 weeks of life
Large left-to-right shunts (e.g. VSD, PDA, total anomalous pulmonary venous drainage) cause heart failure as pulmonary vascular resistance decreases
Bronchopulmonary dysplasia (causing pulmonary hypertension)
Infiltrative cardiomyopathy
Anomalous origin of left coronary artery
Hypothyroidism

Heart failure presenting later in childhood[46]
Congenital heart disease
   Eisenmenger syndrome, Ebstein's anomaly
   VSD with or without aortic regurgitation
   Systemic AV valve regurgitation
Congenital heart disease: postoperation
   Fontan procedure
   Obstructed prosthetic valve
   Post-ventriculotomy (e.g. Fallot's tetralogy)
   Coronary artery injury
   Imperfect myocardial preservation during bypass
   Valve regurgitation after aortic or pulmonary valvotomy
   Large Blalock–Taussig shunt or aortopulmonary collaterals
Cardiomyopathy
   Infective, infiltrative, neuromuscular disease
   Asphyxia (e.g. near-drowning)
   Ischaemia (e.g. Kawasaki disease)
   Acute hypertension (e.g. glomerulonephritis, haemolytic–uraemic syndrome)
   Severe polycythaemia (haematocrit $\geq$ 70%)
   Toxic: acute (e.g. tricyclic antidepressant, verapamil, flecainide)
   Toxic: chronic (e.g. anthracycline)
   Cor pulmonale (e.g. sickle cell, thalassaemia)
   Valvular (e.g. postrheumatic, infective endocarditis, trauma)
   Metabolic
   Arrhythmia (e.g. SVT, complete heart block)
   Heart transplant rejection

SVT = Supraventricular tachycardia; AV = arteriovenous; VSD = ventricular septal defect; PDA = patent ductus arteriosus.

3 *inadequate contractility* (e.g. myocarditis and asphyxia);
4 *heart rate*:
   (a) *too fast* (e.g. supraventricular tachycardia and atrial flutter);
   (b) *too slow* (e.g. heart block).

Many conditions which impair ventricular contractility also reduce ventricular diastolic compliance, resulting in reduced ventricular filling and high atrial pressures (Table 106.4). Pure diastolic dysfunction is uncommon in childhood.

Presenting signs

In childhood, heart failure may present with growth failure. Feeding is slow and may cause sweating and dyspnoea. Useful signs are tachypnoea, cardiomegaly, hepatomegaly, gallop rhythm, tachycardia and cool mottled extremities. There may be clinical and X-ray signs of lung congestion, oedema and air trapping (probably due to bronchial mucosal oedema and seen in large left-to-right shunts such as VSDs). In infants, the JVP is an unreliable sign; the liver enlarges rapidly as heart failure deteriorates, and oedema is non-pitting and located in the eyelids and the dorsum of the hands and feet.[32]

Investigations

After a detailed history and examination, investigations include:

1 *chest X-ray*;
2 *electrocardiogram (ECG) and echocardiography examination* (for structural abnormality, valve stenosis or regurgitation, chamber size, wall thickness and fractional shortening, and pericardial fluid);
4 *cardiac catheterization* when indicated to quantify shunts, measure pressures and demonstrate anatomy;
5 *others* as indicated (e.g. blood gases, serum digoxin, viral culture of stool, urine and throat swabs, urine screen for amino acids and ketoacids, and myocardial biopsy).

Management

The development of heart failure in infancy is an emergency requiring urgent hospitalization.[33] Management includes the following:

1 *Correct precipitating factors* (e.g. fever, infection, anaemia or hypertension).

2 *Correct the underlying cause* (e.g. repair aortic coarctation, replace a regurgitant valve, treat an arrhythmia or infection).
3 *Support systemic circulation* and reduce systemic and pulmonary venous congestion:
   (a) Give oxygen therapy by mask.
   (b) Reduce preload with diuretics, fluid and salt restriction, head elevation and administration of venodilatator drugs (e.g. nitroglycerin (GTN) infusion). Preload reduction may depress cardiac output in acute correctable lesions which obstruct ventricular inflow (e.g. cardiac tamponade).
   (c) Reduce afterload with infusion of GTN or sodium nitroprusside or with oral phenoxybenzamine, angiotensin-converting enzyme (ACE) inhibitors or prazosin. ACE inhibitors reduce mortality in early and late heart failure by improving ventricular performance and inhibiting myocardial remodelling.[33] Vasodilators must be used cautiously in obstructive left-sided lesions to avoid myocardial ischaemia (due to reduced aortic diastolic pressure with high ventricular end-diastolic pressure and ventricular wall hypertrophy). Vasodilators may exacerbate volume loading in VSD or aortopulmonary shunts.
   (d) Increase contractility[34] with digoxin orally or dopamine or dobutamine (2.5–20 µg/kg per min) IV. Milrinone infusion (250–750 ng/kg per min) improves cardiac output in the short term by reducing afterload and increasing contractility.
4 *Mechanical ventilation* improves myocardial performance by improving gas exchange and reducing acidaemia, work of breathing and left ventricular afterload.[35] Sedation and muscle relaxants reduce metabolic rate and the cardiac output needed to meet metabolic demands.
5 *Ventricular assist devices* (VAD) in very severe but reversible cardiac failure can maintain life for days to weeks pending ventricular recovery.[17] When severe respiratory failure complicates severe heart failure, ECMO may be needed.[36] Aortic balloon counterpulsation is less feasible in small children than in adults.

Congenital heart disease (CHD)

Management of a critically ill child with congenital heart disease (CHD) before a definitive structural diagnosis is made depends on the mode of presentation. All such children should be referred immediately to a paediatric cardiac centre. Management of acute postoperative deterioration depends on the underlying condition, nature of surgery and cause of deterioration.

CHD in children may present in the following ways.

Shock in the first few days of life

The commonest CHD causes are obstructive lesions of the left heart, including coarctation of the aorta with or without VSD, aortic stenosis, and hypoplastic left heart (HLH). Differential diagnosis includes cardiomyopathy, systemic arteriovenous malformation (AVM), septicaemia, anaemia and supraventricular tachycardia.

In left-sided obstructive lesions, shock develops as the ductus arteriosus closes. All pulses (or femoral pulses only, in the case of coarctation) are decreased or absent. Tachycardia, tachypnoea, oliguria, cool mottled extremities, metabolic acidosis, hepatomegaly, cardiomegaly and pulmonary oedema are often present. Murmurs are often absent.

Emergency management consists of PGE_1 infusion (5–25 ng/kg per min, to provide aortic blood flow from the pulmonary artery by opening the ductus arteriosus), dopamine infusion, $NaHCO_3$ given slowly to correct metabolic acidosis and mechanical ventilation (to reduce work of breathing, maintain normocarbia and prevent apnoea due to the PGE_1). Hypocarbia and a high Fio_2 should be avoided. They reduce pulmonary vascular resistance and divert blood to the lungs, thereby reducing systemic blood flow. Normoglycaemia and normocalcaemia should be maintained.

Acyanotic heart failure

In the first week of life

Coarctation, aortic stenosis, cardiomyopathy (including obstructive cardiomyopathy in the infant of a diabetic mother) and endocardial fibroelastosis, anaemia, septicaemia, overtransfusion and systemic AVM can present as heart failure. Signs include poor feeding, tachycardia, tachypnoea, sweating, hepatomegaly, cardiomegaly, alar flaring, wheezing and expiratory grunt. Femoral pulses may be absent in coarctation, and bruits are audible in skull, liver or kidneys in AVM.

Emergency management includes oxygen, diuretics, fluid restriction (to 50% of maintenance) and digoxin. In severe failure, mechanical ventilation and inotropic drug infusion are started, and the child is transferred to a paediatric cardiac unit.

After 2–8 weeks of age

Systolic murmurs and signs of heart failure appear in infants with lesions such as VSD, patent ductus arteriosus, aortopulmonary window and common atrioventricular canal due to the physiological decreases of haemoglobin concentration and pulmonary vascular resistance at this time. Emergency management includes diuretics, digoxin and oxygen given via a headbox. Transfusion (to haemoglobin 130–140 g/l) may reduce left-to-right shunt. If these measures fail

to control heart failure, surgery is often needed, preceded if necessary by mechanical ventilation and inotropic drug infusion.

Cyanosis

Pao_2 greater than 150 mmHg (20 kPa) breathing 100% oxygen almost completely rules out cyanotic CHD.[37] Most cyanotic CHD have a Pao_2 less than 60 mmHg (7.98 kPa). An urgent chest X-ray is mandatory. Cyanosis occurs when:

(a) pulmonary blood flow is reduced (e.g. pulmonary atresia);
(b) pulmonary and systemic circulations are separate (e.g. transposition of the great arteries);
(c) in lesions causing mixing of saturated and unsaturated blood in the heart.

Cyanosis with pulmonary oligaemia on chest X-ray

This is usually pulmonary or tricuspid valve atresia or stenosis, or tetralogy of Fallot. Deep cyanosis is present, often without murmurs or with a pulmonary ejection murmur. Tachypnoea may be present. Chest X-ray shows concavity in the pulmonary artery segment of the left heart border.

Emergency management

1 *In the newborn*: PGE_1 infusion (5–25 ng/kg per min) is used to open the ductus arteriosus and increase pulmonary blood flow. Fio_2 of 0.5 gives a small increase in oxygen delivery, and $NaHCO_2$ is used to correct a metabolic acidosis. Gentle assisted ventilation is needed if PGE_1 causes apnoea. The lungs are very compliant and high airway pressures further reduce lung blood flow. The haemoglobin concentration should be kept at 120–150 g/l by transfusion if necessary. The child needs urgent echocardiographic diagnosis and most need a Blalock–Taussig shunt.
2 *Beyond 1 month*: If the Pao_2 is less than 30 mmHg (4.0 kPa), or if cyanotic spells occur in a child with tetralogy of Fallot despite oral propranolol, an urgent Blalock–Taussig shunt is needed. Urgent treatment in such a patient consists of a high Fio_2, knee–chest position, IV morphine and infusion of colloid 10–20 ml/kg. If these measures fail, then propranolol 0.05 mg/kg IV may be needed to reduce right-to-left shunting across the VSD (by reducing contractility and increasing systemic vascular resistance). Inotropic drugs and vasodilators should be avoided.

Cyanosis with pulmonary plethora or oedema in the newborn

The commonest cardiac lesions are transposition of the great arteries (TGA), single ventricle, HLH, truncus arteriosus and total anomalous pulmonary venous drainage (TAPVD). Signs include tachypnoea, tachycardia, cardiomegaly and hepatomegaly. A murmur may be present. Differential diagnosis includes lung disease, group B streptococcal sepsis and persistent pulmonary hypertension of the newborn.

Emergency management

Acidaemia should be corrected and Fio_2 should be high. If heart failure is present, mechanical ventilation and dopamine or dobutamine infusion are used. PGE_1 infusion (5–25 ng/kg per min) is used in all cases except when a small heart accompanies cyanosis and pulmonary oedema. These signs suggest TAPVD with obstruction of the pulmonary veins, in which PGE_1 will exacerbate the pulmonary oedema. Assessment at a paediatric cardiac centre is needed urgently. A child with TGA needs balloon atrial septostomy and the other lesions need urgent surgery.[38]

Arrhythmias in children

Sinus bradycardia (Table 106.2)

Predisposing conditions include hypoxaemia, acidosis, hypotension, high intracranial pressure and cardiac surgery (especially the Fontan and Senning operations).

Management

Correct any reversible cause. Atropine (20 μg/kg) or isoprenaline infusion (0.1–0.5 μg/kg per min) may be used if the sinoatrial node is damaged.

Bradycardia–tachycardia (sick sinus) syndrome[17]

Predisposing conditions are:

1 congenital atrial anomalies (e.g. Ebstein's anomaly and atrioventricular canal defects);
2 extensive atrial surgery (e.g. Fontan and Senning operations).

Management

Atrial pacing followed by propranolol, digoxin, amiodarone, sotalol or quinidine.

Atrioventricular block[39]

Predisposing conditions include congenital cardiomyopathy, myocarditis, post cardiac surgery, vasculitic conditions (e.g. rheumatic fever or maternal systemic lupus erythematosus), and carbamazepine or tricyclic overdose.

Management

Management involves temporary pacing via a transoesophageal or transvenous lead followed by implantation of a permanent pacemaker. Sodium bicarbonate 1–3 mmol/kg is given for tricyclic overdose. Drug removal in overdoses is enhanced with activated charcoal or plasmapheresis if necessary.

Supraventricular tachycardia

Re-entrant supraventricular tachycardia

Predisposing conditions are accessory pathways in Wolff–Parkinson–White and Lown–Ganong–Levine (no short PR interval or δ wave) syndrome, sometimes associated with congenital defects (e.g. Ebstein's anomaly, tricuspid atresia and atrioventricular canal defects), post cardiac surgery, myocarditis, drugs, sepsis, acidosis and adrenaline infusion.[40]

Management

1 Infants
  (a) vagal stimulation (e.g. gag and ice water on face);
  (b) neostigmine 10 μg/kg per min to a maximum of 50 μg/kg (atropine must be readily available);
  (c) adenosine by rapid IV bolus 0.05 mg/kg (maximum 3 mg) increasing by 0.05 mg/kg (maximum 3 mg) every 2 min to a maximum of 0.25 mg/kg (maximum 12 mg);[41]
  (d) overdrive atrial pacing via transoesophageal, transvenous or epicardial leads;[42]
  (e) DC cardioversion 1 J/kg;
  (f) amiodarone, procainamide or propafenone;[17,43]
  (g) digoxin is useful provided Wolff–Parkinson–White syndrome is absent;
  (h) verapamil causes profound myocardial depression and should be avoided.[17]
2 Child – as above: verapamil 0.1 mg/kg IV over 30 min may be used.

Junctional ectopic tachycardia (JET)

Atrioventricular dissociation and ventricular rate 160–290 beats/min is seen on an ECG from oesophageal and epicardial pacing leads.[17] Predisposing conditions include post cardiac surgery, especially when myocardial function is poor, and after Fontan operation or surgery near the atrioventricular node (e.g. repair of VSD or common atrioventricular canal).

Management

1 Propafenone 1–2 mg/kg IV is given over 3 min or infused at 4–8 μg/kg per min if JET recurs.[43]
2 Induce hypothermia to 34–35°C for 2–3 days with 12-hourly normothermia to allow assessment.[17]

3 Amiodarone infusion 25 μg/kg per min is given for 4 h, then 5–15 μg/kg per min (maximum 1.2 g/24 h).

Ventricular ectopic beats (VEBs) and tachycardia (VT)[44]

VT is uncommon in childhood but may present as syncope, poor feeding (in infants) or heart failure. The QRS axis on ECG is different from that of the underlying sinus rhythm. QRS duration is usually (but not always) prolonged (>0.08 s). Supraventricular tachycardia with aberrant conduction is very rare in childhood: more than 90% of wide-complex tachycardia in children are VT. Fusion or captive beats, atrioventricular dissociation and new bundle branch block also favour the diagnosis of VT.

Predisposing conditions are congenital heart lesions and their surgery (e.g. aortic and subaortic stenosis), myocardial ischaemia, mitral valve prolapse, myocarditis, cardiomyopathy, long QT syndrome, blunt chest trauma, hypokalaemia or hypomagnesaemia and drug toxicity.

Emergency management

1 Correct any electrolyte abnormalities.
2 Give oxygen by mask.
3 A vasoconstrictor may abolish VT or ventricular fibrillation (VF) in aortic stenosis by increasing the coronary perfusion pressure.
4 Enhance drug removal if there is drug toxicity (e.g. by digitalis Fab antibodies).
5 Magnesium chloride 0.4 mmol/kg is given 12-hourly slowly IV.
6 Lignocaine is given IV (1 mg/kg bolus then 20–50 μg/kg per min).
7 Bretylium IV is administered (5–10 mg/kg over 1 h, then 5–20 μg/kg per min).
8 Maintenance dose is quinidine 12 mg/kg stat, then 6 mg/kg 6-hourly orally, or phenytoin 4 mg/kg 8-hourly orally.

Arrhythmias in tricyclic overdoses

Most arrhythmias are sinus tachycardia, multifocal VEBs, VT (torsade de pointes), VF, supraventricular tachycardia or heart block.

Management[45]

Drug removal is accelerated with gastric lavage and charcoal. Blood is alkalinized to maintain pH at 7.45–7.50 with $NaHCO_2$ 1–3 mmol/kg. Additional sodium loading to increase the serum sodium by 2–3 mmol/kg may suppress arrhythmias. Class 1A and 1C antiarrhythmic drugs exacerbate the arrhythmias by their membrane-stabilizing effects and are contraindicated. Magnesium chloride 0.4 mmol/kg 12-hourly IV, isoprenaline infusion or pacing are used

to control torsade de pointes. Verapamil, β-blockers and amiodarone may be tried for supraventricular tachycardia and bretylium for VEBs. Pacing is used for heart block.

References

1. Roberton DM (1994) The immunodeficient child. In: Robinson MJ and Roberton DM (eds) *Practical Paediatrics*, 3rd edn. Melbourne: Churchill Livingstone, pp. 316–325.
2. Sorensen RU and Moore C (1994) Immunology in the pediatrician's office. *Pediatr Clin North Am* **41**:691–714.
3. Parkman R (1991) Cytokines and T-lymphocytes in pediatrics. *J Pediatr* **118**:S21–S23.
4. Harris MC, Costarino AT, Sullivan JS *et al.* (1994) Cytokine elevations in critically ill infants with sepsis and necrotizing enterocolitis. *J Pediatr* **124**:105–111.
5. Anderson PAW (1992) Physiology of the fetal, neonatal and adult heart. In: Polin RA and Fox WW (eds) *Fetal and Neonatal Physiology*. Philadelphia: WB Saunders, pp. 722–758.
6. Heitmiller ES, Zahka KG and Rogers MC (1992) Developmental physiology of the cardiovascular system. In: Rogers MC (ed.) *Textbook of Pediatric Intensive Care*, 2nd edn. Baltimore, MD: Williams & Wilkins, pp. 383–422.
7. Ross-Ascuitto N, Ascuitto R, Chen V and Downing SE (1987) Negative inotropic effects of amrinone in the neonatal piglet heart. *Cric Res* **61**:847–852.
8. Williams CE, Mallard C, Tan W and Gluckman PD (1993) Pathophysiology of perinatal asphyxia. *Clin Perinatol* **20**:305–325.
9. Crissinger KD, Grisham MB and Granger DN (1989) Developmental biology of oxidant-producing enzymes and antioxidants in the piglet intestine. *Pediatr Res* **25**:612–616.
10. Moldawer LL (1994) Biology of proinflammatory cytokines and their antagonists. *Crit Care Med* **22**: S3–S7.
11. Bone RC (1994) Sepsis and its complications: the clinical problem. *Crit Care Med* **22**:S8–S11.
12. Van Camp JM, Tomaselli V and Coran AG (1994) Bacterial translocation in the neonate. *Curr Opin Pediatr* **6**:327–333.
13. Mythen MG and Webb AR (1994) Intra-operative gut mucosal hypoperfusion is associated with increased postoperative complications and cost. *Intensive Care Med* **20**:99–104.
14. Yu M, Levy MM, Smith P, Takiguchi SA, Miyasaki A and Myers SA (1993) Effect of maximizing oxygen delivery on morbidity and mortality rates in critically ill patients: a prospective, randomized, controlled study. *Crit Care Med* **21**:830–838.
15. Chioléro R, Flatt J-P, Revelly J-P and Jéquier E (1991) Effects of catecholamines on oxygen consumption and oxygen delivery in critically ill patients. *Chest* **100**:1676–1684.
16. Van den Berghe G, de Zegher F and Lauwers P (1994) Dopamine suppresses pituitary function in infants and children. *Crit Care Med* **22**:1747–1753.

17. Castañeda AR, Jonas RA, Mayer JE and Hanley FL (1994) *Cardiac Surgery of the Neonate and Infant.* Philadelphia: WB Saunders, pp. 65–107.

18. Tibballs J (1993) Clinical applications of gaseous nitric oxide. *Anaesth Intens Care* 21:866–871.

19. Sessler D, Mills P, Gregory G, Litt L and James T (1987) Effects of bicarbonate on arterial and brain intracellular pH in neonatal rabbits recovering from hypoxic lactic acidosis. *J Pediatr* 111:817–823.

20. Shapiro JI, Whalen M, Kucera R, Kindig N, Filley G and Chan L (1989) Brain pH responses to sodium bicarbonate and Carbicarb during systemic acidosis. *Am J Physiol* 256:H1316–H1321.

21. Leung JM, Landow L, Franks M *et al.* for the SPI Research Group (1994) Safety and efficacy of intravenous Carbicarb in patients undergoing surgery: comparison with sodium bicarbonate in the treatment of mild metabolic acidosis. *Crit Care Med* 22:1540–1549.

22. Bone RC, Fisher CJ, Clemmer TP, Slotman GJ, Metz CA and Balk RA (1987) A controlled clinical trial of high-dose methylprednisolone in the treatment of severe sepsis and septic shock. *N Engl J Med* 317:653–658.

23. Saez-Llorens X and McCracken GH (1993) Sepsis syndrome and septic shock in pediatrics: current concepts of terminology, pathophysiology and management. *J Pediatr* 123:497–508.

24. De Maria A, Craven DE, Heffernan JJ, McIntosh TK, Grindlinger GA and McCabe WR (1985) Naloxone versus placebo in treatment of septic shock. *Lancet* i:1363–1365.

25. Suffredini AF (1994) Current prospects for the treatment of clinical sepsis. *Crit Care Med* 22: S12–S18.

26. Dhainaut J-FA, Tenaillon A, Le Tulzo Y *et al.* (1994) Platelet-activating factor receptor antagonist BN 52021 in the treatment of severe sepsis: a randomized double-blind placebo-controlled, multicenter clinical trial. *Crit Care Med* 22:1720–1728.

27. Beca J and Butt W (1994) Extracorporeal membrane oxygenation for refractory septic shock in children. *Pediatrics* 93:726–729.

28. Barzilay E, Kessler D, Berlot G, Gullo A, Geber D and Ben Zeev I (1989) Use of extracorporeal supportive techniques as additional treatment for septic-induced multiple organ failure patients. *Crit Care Med* 17:634–637.

29. Cairo MS, Worcester C, Rucker R *et al.* (1987) Role of circulating complement and polymorphonuclear leukocyte transfusion in treatment and outcome in critically ill neonates with sepsis. *J Pediatr* 110:935–941.

30. Stein B, Pfenninger E, Grunert A, Schmitz JE and Hudde M (1990) Influence of continuous haemofiltration on haemodynamics and central blood volume in experimental endotoxic shock. *Intensive Care Med* 16:494–499.

31. Braunwald E (1994) Heart failure. In: Isselbacher KJ, Braunwald E, Wilson JD, Martin JB, Fauci AS and Kasper DL (eds) *Harrison's Principles of Internal Medicine*, 13th edn. New York: McGraw-Hill, pp. 998–1009.

32. Wilkinson JL (1994) Heart disease in infancy and childhood. In: Robinson MJ and Roberton DM (eds) *Practical Paediatrics*, 3rd edn. Melbourne: Churchill Livingstone, pp. 382–390.

33. Cohn JN (1994) Has the problem of heart failure been solved? *Am J Cardiol* 73:40C–43C.

34. Armstrong PW and Moe GW (1994) Medical advances in the treatment of congestive heart failure. *Circulation* 88:2941–2952.

35. Miro AM and Pinksy MR (1991) Hemodynamic effects of mechanical ventilation. In: Grenvik A, Downs JB, Räsänen J and Smith R (eds) *Mechanical Ventilation and Assisted Respiration: Past, Present and Future.* New York: Churchill Livingstone, pp. 73–89.

36. Klein MD and Whittlesey GC (1993) Extracorporeal membrane oxygenation therapy for cardiac disease. In: Arensman RM and Cornish JD (eds) *Extracorporeal Life Support.* Boston: Blackwell Scientific Publications, pp. 302–319.

37. Victorica BE (1993) Cyanotic newborns. In: Gessner IH and Victorica BE (eds) *Pediatric Cardiology: A Problem Oriented Approach.* Philadelphia: WB Saunders, pp. 97–109.

38. Freedom RM, Smallhorn JF and Trusler GA (1992) Transposition of the great arteries. In: Freedom RM, Benson LN and Smallhorn JF (eds) *Neonatal Heart Disease.* London: Springer-Verlag, pp. 179–212.

39. Epstein ML (1993) Disturbances of cardiac rhythmn. In: Gessner IH and Victorica BE (eds) *Pediatric Cardiology: A Problem Oriented Approach.* Philadelphia: WB Saunders, pp. 167–181.

40. Ludomirsky A and Garson A (1990) Supraventricular tachycardia. In: Gillette PC and Garson A (eds) *Pediatric Arrhythmias: Electrophysiology and Pacing.* Philadelphia: WB Saunders, pp. 380–426.

41. Ralston MA, Knilans TK, Hannon DW and Daniels SR (1994) Use of adenosine for diagnosis and treatment of tachyarrhythmias in pediatric patients. *J Pediatr* 124:139–143.

42. Dick M, Scott WA, Serwer GS *et al.* (1988) Acute termination of supraventricular tachyarrhythmias in children by transesophageal atrial pacing. *Am J Cardiol* 61:925–927.

43. Paul T and Janousek J (1994) New antiarrhythmic drugs in pediatric use: propafenone. *Pediatr Cardiol* 15:190–197.

44. Meldon SW, Brady WJ, Berger S and Mannenbach M (1994) Pediatric ventricular tachycardia: a review with three illustrative cases. *Pediatr Emerg Care* 10:294–300.

45. Pimentel L and Trommer L (1994) Cyclic antidepressant overdoses: a review. *Emerg Med Clin North Am* 12:533–547.

46. Artman M, Parrish MD and Graham TP (1983) Congestive heart failure in childhood and adolescence: recognition and management. *Am Heart J* 105:471–480.

GJ Knight and P Swan

Neurological emergencies (including traumatic head injury) are the most common life-threatening emergencies in children (Fig. 107.1). The incidence of sudden infant death syndrome (SIDS) has decreased in Australia recently.[1] However, in infancy SIDS remains the most common cause of death, other than congenital and perinatal causes. In childhood, trauma, particularly neurotrauma, accounts for 50% of deaths. The pathophysiology, clinical features, treatment and outcome of these acute neurological illnesses are influenced by several important differences between adults and children. These differences include response to injury, developmental maturity and capacity for growth.

Pathophysiology of brain injuries in children

Brain injuries are usually caused by a primary event (e.g. trauma, ischaemia, infection or metabolic disturbance) and are frequently accompanied by secondary injurious changes (e.g. oedema, alteration of cerebrovascular autoregulation, tissue hypoxia or other cytotoxic events). It is believed that neuronal damage or death at the time of the primary injury, particularly in cases of trauma and ischaemia, is unlikely to be influenced by therapy after the event. However, secondary neuronal disturbances may be prevented by appropriate treatment and avoidance of iatrogenic complications.

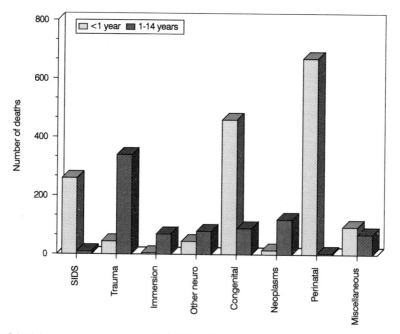

Fig. 107.1 Causes of death in Australian children in 1993.[1] SIDS = Sudden infant death syndrome.

Features of brain injury particular to the paediatric patient are described below.

Diffuse cerebral swelling

Diffuse brain swelling in the absence of oedema is a frequent early finding in severe paediatric head trauma due apparently to generalized cerebral vaso-dilatation.[2] It often resolves in 1–2 days if there is no other significant brain injury. However, in more severe primary neuronal impact damage accompanied by multifocal petechial haemorrhage, diffuse cerebral swelling, with the development of vasogenic oedema, may relentlessly progress over a period of several days.

Cerebral blood flow

The difference between arterial blood pressure and intracranial pressure (ICP) is the cerebral perfusion pressure (CPP). Following injury in which auto-regulation is disturbed, CPP becomes the major determinant of cerebral blood flow, particularly in the more severely damaged parts. Arterial hypotension or intracranial hypertension is likely to cause further cerebral damage by reducing CPP. In addition, venous distension will lower CPP, and may contribute to further cerebral insults in low cardiac output states. The ideal CPP in infancy is unknown, because normal blood pressure is lower than in adults and varies with age. In general, treatment is directed at maintaining CPP above 50 mmHg (6.7 kPa).

In conditions where vasogenic oedema occurs (e.g. trauma, severe hypoxic–ischaemic states and menin-gitis), arterial hypertension may increase extrava-scular shift of fluid and worsen brain swelling. None the less, treatment to lower arterial pressure (e.g. with vasodilators) may interfere with homeostatic mecha-nisms and should be used cautiously.

Hypovolaemia

Children have small blood volumes and commonly develop hypovolaemia from scalp bleeding or intra-cranial haemorrhage. For example, hypovolaemia will develop in a 5-kg infant (blood volume of 400 ml) following a blood loss of only 100 ml.

Relative growth

The child's short stature and relatively large head confer a number of risks. The toddler's head is at the level of a motor vehicle front, and isolated severe head injury is subsequently common following pedestrian injury in this age group. The neck muscles are relatively weak in infancy and they support a large head. This renders the brain prone to decelera-tion injury in motor vehicle accidents and cases of domestic violence. Shaking an infant by the shoulders snaps the head to and fro, leading to compression of brain tissue and rupture of delicate bridging sub-arachnoid veins.

Bone development[3]

The skull bones in the first year of life are thin, with open sutures and open fontanelles. Beyond 2 years, skull sutures close and the cranial vault thickens. Thus, in young children, there is less bony protection from high-impact trauma, but the non-rigid skull may expand somewhat to decompress expanding lesions partially.

Undiagnosed coma

An ordered approach to diagnosis and treatment is required for a child with depressed consciousness of unknown cause. This approach must consider com-mon life-threatening and rare treatable diseases (Table 107.1).

Initial management

Management should always begin with a rapid assessment and prompt treatment of inadequacies of airway, ventilation and circulation. Venous access is obtained and blood drawn for routine tests, including immediate measurement of blood sugar. If hypogly-

Table 107.1 Causes of coma in children

Structural	*Metabolic*
Trauma	*Post-ictal*
Accidental	*Infection*
Non-accidental	*Meningitis*
	Encephalitis
Hydrocephalus	*Drugs and toxins*
Blocked CSF shunts	*Hypoxia–ischaemia*
Haemorrhage	*Circulatory shock*
AVM	*Biochemical*
Aneurysms	Electrolyte disorders
Tumour	*Sodium/water*
Tumour	Calcium
Infection	Magnesium
Abscess	Acid–base disturbance
	Hypoglycaemia
	Hyperthermia
	Hepatic failure
	Haemolytic–uraemic syndrome
	Inborn errors of metabolism
	Reye's syndrome

Common causes are those in italics.
CSF = Cerebrospinal fluid; AVM = arteriovenous malformations.

caemia is demonstrated or cannot be excluded, 1 ml/kg of 50% (or 2 ml/kg of 25%) glucose should be given IV. During this initial phase, the level of coma is assessed and examination undertaken to detect localizing signs, including meningism. Concurrently, relevant details of the present and past history are obtained.

Following this initial phase (10–15 min) the likely diagnosis is often apparent, and the appropriate investigations and treatment will be clear. A detailed neurological and general physical examination should subsequently be performed to detect any deterioration. If the diagnosis is unclear, examination is directed at eliciting further diagnostic clues. Multiple factors may compound to produce coma (e.g. a child with severe gastroenteritis may have hyperthermia, hyponatraemic dehydration, metabolic acidosis and hypovolaemic shock).

Controlled ventilation

The indications for ventilation are:

1 apnoea, respiratory failure or poor airway control;
2 rapidly worsening coma;
3 progressively raised ICP (i.e. bradycardia, hypertension, fluctuating pupillary light reflexes and emerging localized signs such as oculovestibular or corticospinal tract dysfunction).

Once ventilation is instituted, the stomach is emptied via a gastric tube. Pulse rate and blood pressure should be checked every 5 min. Raised ICP should be considered in any case of rapidly progressive coma. Once diagnosed, this problem is managed with moderate hyperventilation and possibly head elevation to 30°. Mannitol (0.25 g/kg IV) is given. Long-acting muscle relaxants are used if necessary, to facilitate ventilation and prevent straining. Further neurological assessment is, however, then precluded and monitoring by way of computed tomographic (CT) scan and ICP measurement should be considered.

Cranial CT

A CT scan is required in comatose children with localizing signs, and in those without an apparent diagnosis. Even if the general condition does not warrant controlled ventilation, CT in childhood is often best performed under general anaesthesia. Unwanted movement will cause poor-quality images, and sedation alone may place the patient at risk of hypoventilation and/or aspiration. If a mass lesion is present, neurosurgical advice should be obtained immediately. CT defines intracranial haemorrhage as well as lumbar puncture (LP) in most cases and has less associated risk.

Lumbar puncture

LP should be performed when there is reasonable suspicion of meningitis or encephalitis. When there is evidence of raised ICP, LP should be deferred until a CT scan is reviewed and the pressure controlled. In children with a bulging patent fontanelle, reduction in tension of the fontanelle following ventilation provides a means of safely timing LP. As well as standard analyses and culture of cerebrospinal fluid (CSF), polymerase chain reaction (PCR) can be performed to provide evidence of herpes simplex virus infection rapidly.[4,5]

Additional useful investigations

These include arterial blood-gas estimations, electrolytes, urea and creatinine, liver function tests, serum ammonia, serum and CSF lactate and urinalysis. Screening of blood and urine will exclude common poisons and drug intoxications.

Specific treatment

Treatment is generally guided by the clinical signs and results of investigations. Herpes simplex encephalitis can present in many ways, and is not excluded by an absence of pleocytosis. Acyclovir should therefore be considered in any patient in whom herpes simplex encephalitis cannot be confidently excluded.

Prolonged seizures

The most common cause of prolonged seizures in children are:

1 epilepsy associated with first presentation, anticonvulsant withdrawal or intercurrent illness, often with fever;
2 prolonged febrile convulsion;
3 central nervous system infection (i.e. meningitis and encephalitis);
4 metabolic disturbance (e.g. hypoglycaemia, hyponatraemia and hypocalcaemia);
5 trauma.

Management

The initial management is as described; seizures must be stopped to avoid metabolic and ischaemic neuronal damage. Specific drug treatment includes the following:

Benzodiazepines

Diazepam and lorazepam are the most useful agents. Diazepam is given initially as 0.2 mg/kg IV, and repeated up to a total dose of 0.5 mg/kg. It is given per rectum if venous access cannot be secured. Excessive sedation and respiratory depression occur with larger doses and must be dealt with effectively. Lorazepam (0.05–0.10 mg/kg IV) has been shown to be effective in children and neonates.[6,7] It has advantages over diazepam as it has a longer half-life and causes less respiratory depression.[8] Clonazepam is also effective.

Phenytoin

Phenytoin is given as 20 mg/kg IV over 30 min, followed by a maintenance dose (4 mg/kg 8-hourly past the neonatal period). Phenytoin causes minimal sedation or respiratory depression.

Thiopentone

Thiopentone 2–5 mg/kg slowly IV, then 1–5 mg/kg per h by continuous infusion into a central vein, is given if the above measures are ineffective. Thiopentone administration necessitates endotracheal intubation and mechanical ventilation, and possibly inotropic drugs to counter its myocardial depressant effects. Blood concentrations need to be monitored during prolonged use. Seizures are only controlled by anaesthetic doses, and other agents need to be introduced as interval therapy. These drugs include phenobarbitone, carbamazepine, valproic acid and vigabatrin.

The patient must be protected from injury during seizures. Severe respiratory and metabolic acidosis are common, and are best managed by rapid control of the seizure and adequate ventilation and oxygenation. Topical cooling may be useful, as normothermia raises the seizure threshold. Once seizures are controlled, the cause should be sought. LP and CT scan should reveal evidence of most bacterial and viral infections as well as structural lesions. When the diagnosis remains unclear, viral encephalitis or metabolic encephalopathy should be considered. Herpes simplex is notorious for atypical presentations in children. Early use of acyclovir in this disease confers markedly reduced morbidity and mortality.[9] Its use is therefore justified in febrile patients with persistent seizures of unknown cause.

Bacterial meningitis

Pathology

The major route of infection is haematogenous spread from the nasopharynx. Meningitis may also be a local complication of a neural tube defect, dermoid sinus, middle ear infection or head trauma involving a paranasal sinus. Causative organisms are usually *Haemophilus influenzae* type b, *Neisseria meningitidis* or *Streptococcus pneumoniae*. The incidence of childhood bacterial meningitis has fallen markedly since the introduction of vaccination programmes against *H. influenzae*.[10–12] Unusual organisms may be seen in immunocompromised patients, and neonates are affected by Gram-negative organisms and group B streptococci.

Pathological changes include a purulent meningeal exudate, infective vasculitis in superficial layers and localized infarction in severe cases. Delayed changes include subdural effusions and communicating hydrocephalus.

Clinical features

The classical findings of fever, headache, altered conscious state, photophobia and neck stiffness occur, but may be absent in infants and following seizures. Younger children often present with only generalized signs of illness. Focal or protracted seizures, and seizures developing beyond the fourth day, are all associated with increased risks of permanent neurological sequelae.[13] There may be features of septic shock, particularly in meningococcal infection. A slowly evolving history in association with focal signs points to the possibility of tuberculous meningitis.[14]

Management

Resuscitation is vital and must include adequate restoration of intravascular volume. Once achieved, fluid intake is restricted to one-third maintenance water requirements, as inappropriate secretion of antidiuretic hormone nearly always occurs. If excessive hypotonic fluids are given, hyponatraemia may develop rapidly, which may lead to seizures, cerebral oedema and death. The timing of LP should be carefully considered when there is any suspicion of raised ICP. Antigen testing using latex particle agglutination has proven useful in rapidly diagnosing the three common pathogens.

Broad-spectrum antibiotic therapy should begin with penicillin (60 mg/kg 4-hourly) and a third-generation cephalosporin (cefotaxime 50 mg/kg 6-hourly or ceftriaxone 100 mg/kg daily). When sensitivities are known, therapy is rationalized. Treatment duration depends on the clinical state and the causative organism. Uncomplicated cases of meningococcal infection require 7 days of therapy. Cases of *Haemophilus* and pneumococcal meningitis require at least 10 days.[13] Dexamethasone has been shown to reduce the neurological sequelae following *Haemophilus* meningitis, and is now widely used in bacterial meningitis,[15] as 0.4 mg/kg 12-hourly for 2 days.[16] If possible, it should be administered prior to the first dose of antibiotics.

Prophylactic therapy is required for every household member in cases of meningococcal infection and *Haemophilus* infection when there is another child under 5 years in the household who is unimmunized. Rifampicin 10 mg/kg b.d. for 2 days (meningococcal) or for 4 days (*Haemophilus*) with a maximum daily dose of 600 mg is appropriate. Neonates require 10 mg/kg per day. Pregnant women can be effectively managed with a single IM dose of ceftriaxone (250 mg). Ciprafloxacillin has also been used.[17]

Profound coma, prolonged seizures and persistent focal neurological signs may indicate infarction, oedema, subdural effusion or venous sinus thrombosis. A CT examination will help define patients requiring surgical intervention and also those who might benefit from ICP monitoring.

Encephalitis

Common causes of encephalitis include *Mycoplasma*, enteroviruses, cytomegalovirus and herpes, Epstein–Barr and respiratory viruses (adenovirus and parainfluenza). The most significant causes worldwide are the insect-transmitted arbovirus encephalitides, including Australian, Japanese B and St Louis. These can cause profound coma and are associated with a significant incidence of residual neurological deficit.

Presenting symptoms of encephalitis include seizures, focal neurological deficits in the setting of an acute febrile illness, confusion and coma. Meningeal irritation may not be obvious. CSF analysis may show a moderate pleocytosis; rarely, this may consist predominantly of neutrophils in the early phase. Herpes simplex is the most important diagnosis because it is treatable. Electroencephalogram (EEG), CT and magnetic resonance imaging (MRI) are helpful in making the diagnosis. PCR on CSF may also aid rapid diagnosis. Acyclovir used early improves outcome, and should be commenced when the diagnosis is suspected.[9] Outcome in viral encephalitis is worse in herpes simplex and adenovirus infections, and in infants under 12 months.[18]

Non-traumatic intracranial haemorrhage

Non-traumatic intracranial haemorrhage is uncommon in children. However, it must be considered in the differential diagnosis in children with sudden severe headache or unexplained coma. Arteriovenous malformations (AVM) are a commoner cause of haemorrhage in children than aneurysms (Table 107.2).

Presenting features are similar to those seen in adults, and include sudden severe headache, obtundation and occasionally seizures. Diagnosis can usually be made by CT scan and LP is only indicated if doubt remains following the CT. Raised ICP, if present, is managed in the usual manner. A mass lesion or acute obstructive hydrocephalus requires neurosurgical assessment. Following diagnosis of a haemorrhage, further investigations may be required to clarify the

Table 107.2 Aetiology of spontaneous intracranial haemorrhage in children

Vascular malformations	Most common
Arteriovenous malformations	
Capillary telangiectasia	
Cavernous malformation	
Venous malformation	
Aneurysm	Rare
Berry	
Mycotic	
Posttraumatic	
Coagulopathy	
Thrombocytopenia	Rare if platelets $> 20 \times 10^9/l$
Haemophilia	
Anticoagulant therapy	
Tumours	
Gliomas	
Hypertension	Rare

underlying cause. These include coagulation profile and platelet count. MRI and angiography may detect an underlying vascular malformation or tumour. Definitive surgery or endovascular treatment of an AVM can be planned once the underlying lesion has been defined. A period of close observation is required, even of a stable patient, as children may be at greater risk of rebleeding from an AVM than adults.[19] Therapies (e.g. calcium-channel blockers) to prevent vasospasm in adults following aneurysm rupture may be applicable to children in the rare instances of aneurysmal haemorrhage.

Hypoxaemic–ischaemic encephalopathy

Aetiology

The most common causes of hypoxaemic–ischaemic encephalopathy outside the neonatal period are:

1 near-miss SIDS;
2 immersion;
3 accidents, including drug ingestion, child abuse and strangulation.

Pathology

The brain depends on an uninterrupted supply of oxygen and glucose to produce, via aerobic glycolysis, sufficient high-energy adenosine triphosphate (ATP) to maintain neuronal membrane and synthetic function. Under anoxic conditions, anaerobic glycolysis occurs, producing lactic acid but less ATP (by 18 times). As ATP stores are virtually nil, rapid neuronal failure ensues. If ischaemia accompanies hypoxia, there is associated failure of both substrate delivery and metabolic waste removal, which amplifies the cellular insult. Ischaemia produces coma in less than 10 s and cerebral damage in as little as 2 min.

Following restoration of cerebral blood flow, there is a period of relative hyperaemia followed by relative hypoperfusion. Animal studies suggest that blood flow during this phase of post-ischaemic hypoperfusion is determined by the metabolic needs of the brain.[20] Cytotoxic cerebral oedema may develop, but significant elevation of ICP is unusual, unless ischaemia and damage are profound.

Management

The principles of therapy are similar to other brain injuries. It is mandatory to provide rapid cardiopulmonary resuscitation (CPR) and prevent secondary insults. In cases of out-of-hospital cardiac arrest, full resuscitation must be attempted while the history is sought. The stomach may contain large volumes of water and air following immersion and subsequent resuscitative efforts, and should be drained. Haemodynamic disturbance may develop because of primary cardiac dysfunction or hypovolaemia secondary to bowel fluid loss (ischaemic diarrhoea). Pulmonary aspiration of water or gastric contents is also common, although in 10–15% of children early laryngospasm causes 'dry drowning'. Comatose patients with hyper- or hypotonia and a Glasgow coma scale < 8 are probably best managed by mechanical ventilation, sedation and paralysis for 1–2 days, although benefits are unproven. The role of ICP monitoring is limited, as correlation between ICP and outcome is poor.[21] Barbiturate coma and induced hypothermia are also of no proven value, and increase the risk of sepsis.[22] Hyperglycaemia has been associated with a worse prognosis in experimental situations, and it should be actively treated (see Chapter 44).

Prognosis

The major determinants of recovery are:

1 ischaemic time;
2 cerebral metabolic rate;
3 quality of resuscitation.

In immersion injuries, full recovery may be possible despite prolonged ischaemia if sufficient cerebral cooling has occurred. The onset of ischaemia may be delayed by bradycardia with preferential cerebral flow (diving reflex) in young children. In general, survival from out-of-hospital cardiac arrest is unlikely, even with expert CPR, if asystole is present on arrival at hospital.[23,24] The exception is the hypothermic child following immersion, and prolonged CPR is justified in this situation. If cardiac output is present on arrival, recovery is likely in those presenting with flexion or extension to pain. Normo-

thermic patients who present apnoeic, flaccid and unresponsive to pain are likely to die or have serious neurological deficits. This group is prone to further deterioration several days after the insult, with progression of cerebral oedema.[21] Residual neurological deficits present at the end of the first week are less likely to improve following ischaemic injury than following head injury.

Guillain–Barré syndrome (GBS)

Clinical features

GBS is the most common cause of acute motor paralysis in children. Although most patients develop ascending, symmetrical arreflexic weakness, GBS may present insidiously with lethargy or loss of motor milestones in the young child. Sensory loss is usually minimal and transient. Pain in the back and legs, possibly neurogenic in origin, is common and may be the presenting feature.[25] The pain may be severe and is often difficult to control. Papilloedema and encephalopathy occasionally occur.[26] The complications of deep venous thrombosis and thromboembolism are not common problems in children.

Management

Adequate respiratory care is the basis of minimizing morbidity and mortality in GBS. Admission criteria to the ICU include respiratory failure, bulbar palsy, severe autonomic disturbance or rapidly progressive weakness. Up to one-third of patients require ventilatory support. Ideally, mechanical ventilation should be undertaken electively. Early indications are increased work of breathing, fatigue, poor cough and progressive bulbar palsy. Hypercarbia is a late sign and should be avoided. Poor cooperation limits the usefulness of forced vital capacity as a test in childhood. Once mechanically ventilated, many patients require some degree of hyperventilation to prevent 'air hunger'. Although nasotracheal intubation is satisfactory initially, a tracheostomy should be performed if recovery is delayed. This will improve comfort and allow speech via pressure-controlled ventilation and an air leak around the tube. During recovery, successful weaning is unlikely unless vital capacity exceeds 12 ml/kg and maximum negative inspiratory force is at least 20 cm H_2O (2 kPa). Intermittent mandatory ventilation may promote fatigue, and progressively lengthened periods of spontaneous ventilation interspersed with a 'rest on the ventilator' and full ventilation at night are often better tolerated. Pressure support ventilation is also useful during weaning.

Autonomic dysfunction is an important cause of morbidity and mortality in children with GBS.[26] Serious cardiac arrhythmias may be provoked by airway manipulation or induction of anaesthesia, particularly in the presence of hypoxia. Fluctuating blood pressure, urine retention and gut dysfunction also occur.

Plasmapharesis reduces the duration of ventilation required in adults[27,28] and small studies support its use in children.[29,30] Intravenous immunoglobulin (IVIG) is as effective as plasma exchange in adults[31] (see Chapter 48). In a study in children IVIG 1 g/kg for 2 days was apparently as effective as daily plasma exchanges of 200–250 ml/kg.[32] IVIG has significant potential advantages over plasmapharesis, particularly in small children in whom venous access and large fluid volume shifts may cause difficulties. Also, the need for skilled staff limits the use of plasmapharesis to major centres. Both therapies have been used concurrently, although the benefit of the combination has not been proven. The indications for either form of therapy are rapid progression, respiratory insufficiency or weakness to the point of being unable to walk unassisted.

The problems of long-term ventilation in a conscious patient compounded by emotional immaturity, speech failure, fear of procedures and family disruption make the management of patient and family extremely difficult. A sensitive team approach is essential.

Prognosis

The prognosis in acute GBS may be better for children than adults. Full recovery is likely if the time from maximal deficit to onset of recovery is less than 18 days. Complete recovery, despite a longer plateau phase, has, however, been reported.[33] Good recovery can occur in patients who have required ventilation and the need for ventilation may not be a poor prognostic factor in children.[26] Those presenting with a subacute course are at risk of relapses and permanent motor deficits.

Table 107.3 Biochemical markers, representative conditions and some further investigations of metabolic disorders that present as coma

Biochemical marker	Representative conditions	Differentiating features
Hypoglycaemia	Organic acidurias	Marked metabolic acidosis
		Specific urinary acids
	Reye syndrome	Elevated transaminases
		Normal bilirubin
	Fat oxidation defects	
	Medium-chain acyl coenzyme A	Non-ketotic hypoglycaemia
	dehydrogenase deficiency (MCAD)	Urine dicarboxylic acids
Ketoacidosis	Diabetes mellitus	Hyperglycaemia
	Organic aciduria	Marked metabolic acidosis
	Methylmalonic	Specific urinary acids
	Propionic acidaemia	
Lactic acidosis	Mitochondrial encephalomyopathies	Lactate/pyruvate ratio
Respiratory chain disorders	Enzyme analysis	
	Pyruvate carboxylase deficiency	
	MERRF/MELAS	Myopathy
Hyperammonaemia (2–3 times normal)	Reye syndrome	Muscle biopsy
		Elevated transaminases
		Normal bilirubin
	Urea cycle defects	
	Ornithine transcarbamylase	X-linked
		Urine orotic acid
	Carbamyl phosphate synthetase	
	Fat oxidation defects	
	MCAD	Non-ketotic hypoglycaemia
		Urine dicarboxylic acids
	Carnitine-palmitoyl transferase deficiency	Urine dicarboxylic acids
	Systemic carnitine deficiency	Muscle weakness
		Urine dicarboxylic acids
	Organic acidurias	Marked metabolic acidosis
		Specific urinary acids

MERRF = Mitochondrial encephalopathy with ragged red fibres; MELAS = mitochondrial encephalopathy, lactic acidosis, stroke-like episodes.

Metabolic encephalopathy (including Reye's syndrome)[34,35]

About 0.1% of babies have an inborn error of metabolism. Acute encephalopathy is one of the many ways neurometabolic diseases present in childhood. In general, acute presentations occur in the neonatal period and early infancy. Symptoms are often vague and include lethargy, poor feeding and vomiting. Older infants and children more commonly present with a chronic encephalopathy, with features that may include seizures, long-tract signs, visual impairment and loss of milestones.

Diagnosis

A careful history and examination may elicit clues. Family history and history of drug exposure are extremely important. Valproate, in particular, has been associated with a Reye-like illness. The following investigations allow a broad categorization and direct further detailed investigations: blood-gas analysis, blood sugar, serum ammonia, serum lactate, urine metabolic screen and urine ketones. Lactic acidosis and hypoglycaemia can occur in a number of disease states, including sepsis, hypoxaemia and poisoning. Table 107.3 indicates the biochemical features of some of the more common conditions, and how initial non-specific abnormalities may guide further investigations. One condition may have a number of associated biochemical abnormalities.

Assessment

Metabolic coma can be staged using Lovejoy's classification for Reye's syndrome[36] (Table 107.4).

Management

Initial management is largely supportive. Metabolic derangements such as acidosis and hypoglycaemia are corrected. Acute intracranial hypertension is managed with mechanical ventilation and ICP mon-

Table 107.4 Staging in metabolic encephalopathy

Stage	Coma	Pain response	Reflexes
1	Lethargy	Normal	Normal
2	Combative	Variable	Pupils sluggish
3	Coma	Decorticate	Pupils sluggish
4	Coma	Decerebrate	Pupils sluggish Abnormal oculocephalic
5	Coma	Flaccid	No pupil response Absent oculocephalic

Adapted from National Institutes of Health modification of Lovejoy.[36]

itored to maintain CPP above 50 mmHg (6.7 kPa). Mannitol may be useful in the acute setting. Hyperammonaemia should be managed with limited protein intake initially. In certain circumstances, increasing ammonia metabolism using agents such as biotin, hydroxycobalamin, arginine and sodium benzoate may be appropriate.[35]

Reye's syndrome and Reye-like illness

Reye's syndrome is a rare disorder occurring almost exclusively in children, and is characterized by an acute encephalopathy, with brain swelling and fatty degeneration of viscera, especially the liver. Typically, the patient presents with intractable vomiting followed by progressive encephalopathy. There is an association with aspirin use and a preceding varicella infection. Diagnosis can be made when a compatible history accompanies hyperammonaemia and elevation of serum hepatocellular enzymes to at least twice normal, but with a normal bilirubin concentration. Hypoglycaemia occurs in patients under 2 years. Management consists of correcting hypoglycaemia, neurological monitoring and management of ICP.

A wide range of conditions have been described that mimic typical Reye's syndrome closely – 10% of cases originally described as Reye's syndrome in the UK between 1981 and 1991 were subsequently found to be inherited metabolic disorders.[37] A careful approach is mandatory to ensure detection of inherited disorders.

Spinal trauma[38–40]

Incidence

Paediatric spinal trauma is relatively rare, comprising <5% of all spinal injuries. Approximately 5% of children with severe head trauma will have a cervical spine injury. Injuries will occur at more than one spinal level in at least 16% of all children.

Aetiology

The commonest causes of paediatric spinal trauma are motor vehicle accidents (either as a pedestrian or passenger) and falls (especially diving accidents). Sports-related injuries are uncommon.

Pathophysiology

The patterns of spinal injury in children differ from those in adults. Spinal cord injury without radiographic abnormality (SCIWORA) occurs almost exclusively in children (20–60% of spinal cord injuries). It is associated with a high incidence of complete neurological deficit. Spinal injury in the first decade occurs almost exclusively in the first two cervical segments, with either atlantoaxial rotatory subluxation, bony or ligamentous injuries, or

SCIWORA and severe cord injury. Atlantoaxial rotatory subluxation is rarely associated with deficit; the uncommon high cervical fractures are less likely to be associated with permanent neurological deficit than ligamentous injury.[40] As the bony spine matures, the pattern of injury becomes more adult-like, with lower cervical and thoracic injuries seen in the second decade. A high proportion of children who die following motor vehicle trauma, particularly those with immediate cardiorespiratory arrests or who die before arrival at hospital, have disruption of the spinal cord above C3. This is most often at the cervicomedullary junction.[41]

Clinical features

The immediate effects of spinal cord damage are similar at any age. Frequently associated head injury renders clinical assessment extremely difficult; confirmation of cord injury is sometimes delayed. Clues to diagnosis in the unconscious patient include:

1 flaccidity, immobility and arreflexia below the level of the lesion;
2 hypoventilaion with paradoxical chest movement, if intercostal muscles are paralysed and the phrenic nerves are intact (in the absence of airway obstruction);
3 apnoea, with rhythmic flaring of the alae nasi if the lesion is above C3;
4 hypotension, with inappropriate bradycardia and cutaneous vasodilatation below the level of injury, due to absent spinal sympathetic outflow. Significant hypotension becomes more likely the higher the lesion, the younger the patient, and if other major injuries are present;
5 priapism, which frequently occurs.

There may be visible or palpable evidence of trauma to the spine and surrounding soft tissues. including retropharyngeal or retrolaryngeal haematomas. Spinal shock is common, with temporary complete loss of function. As this resolves after 3–5 days, reflexes progressively return, usually starting with bulbocavernosus and anal reflexes. Incomplete lesions, including the Brown-Séquard cord hemisection, and anterior and central cord syndromes may become apparent at this stage.

Investigations

Resuscitation, including emergency intubation, should not be delayed to perform X-rays. The entire spinal column should, however, subsequently be X-rayed to demonstrate the presence of subluxation, fractures or dislocations. CT may produce better definition of injuries, showing cord involvement by haematomas, bone fragments and foreign bodies. In cases of SCIWORA, metrizamide myelography with CT examination may reveal cord injury with soft-tissue or disc involvement and dural tears. MRI is also useful in both the acute setting and in assessment at later stages.[42] Somatosensory evoked potentials may be useful to evaluate the integrity of the spinal cord, particularly in the comatose patient.

Management

Achieving control of airway, ventilation and circulation is always of first priority. If tracheal intubation is indicated and neck stability is unknown, skilled assistance is necessary to immobilize the head and neck, particularly to prevent neck extension. Because of the sympathectomized state in high cord injuries, hypovolaemia is very poorly tolerated, though a relatively low blood pressure can be expected even after hypovolaemia is corrected. As up to 20% of patients will have multiple trauma, many will require major surgical procedures, during which the spinal cord must remain protected. If muscle relaxants are required 2–3 days following injury, suxamethonium, which may cause fatal hyperkalaemia, should be avoided.

Use of steroids is controversial. Results of a controlled study in adults, which are applicable to children, demonstrated that high-dose methylprednisolone administered within 8 h of injury (30 mg/kg initially followed by 5.4 mg/kg per h for the following 23 h) improved outcome, in those with incomplete as well as apparently complete deficits.[43]

As with brain injuries, preventing secondary neuronal damage is extremely vital. Adequate perfusion of the cord should be ensured, as autoregulation of blood flow is lost after trauma. Immobilization is usually maintained by skull tongs with axial traction or external bracing. Operative intervention is controversial with little evidence of neurological improvement from decompressive surgery. Laminectomy and decompression in children with complete cord injuries carry a significant mortality. General supportive care requires meticulous attention to each body system. A specialized spinal injuries unit should be consulted early for optimal rehabilitation, which requires a team of orthopaedic and/or neurosurgeons, rehabilitation specialists, nurses, physiotherapists, psychiatrists, social workers and school teachers.

Prognosis

The prognosis of all spinal injuries in children may be better than in adults. In one series of 113 children with spinal injuries,[38] 55 had no neurological deficit. Of the 38 patients with incomplete deficits, 23 made a complete recovery and 11 improved.[38] Twenty children had complete cord injuries; of these, 4 improved and 3 died. In another smaller series, 44% had neurological deficits and 11% were immediate, complete and permanent. SCIWORA was seen in 21% and 4 of these 18 children had a permanent, complete deficit.[40]

References

1. Australian Bureau of Statistics (1993) *Deaths: Cause by Sex and Age Group, 1993*. Canberra: Australian Government Printers.

2. Bruce DA, Raphaely RC, Goldbert Al *et al.* (1979) Pathophysiology, treatment and outcome following severe head injuries in children. *Child's Brain* **5**:174–191.

3. Mann KS, Chan KH and Yue CP (1986) Skull fractures in children: their assessment in relation to developmental skull changes and acute intracranial hematomas. *Child's Nervous System*. **2**:258–261.

4. Aurelius E, Johansson B, Skoldenberg B, Staland A and Forsgren M (1991) Rapid diagnosis of herpes simplex virus encephalitis by nested polymerase chain reaction assay of cerebrospinal fluid. *Lancet* **337**:189–192.

5. Troendle-Atkins J, Demmler GJ and Buffone GJ (1993) Rapid diagnosis of herpes simplex encephalitis by using polymerase chain reaction. *J Pediatr* **123**:376–380.

6. Lacey DJ, Singer WD, Horwitz SJ and Gilmore H (1986) Lorazepam therapy of status epilepticus in children and adolescents. *J Pediatr* **108**:771–774.

7. Maytal J, Novak GP and King KC (1991) Lorazepam in the treatment of neonatal seizures. *J Child Neurol* **6**:319–323.

8. Chiulli DA, Terndrup TE and Kanter RK (1991) The influence of diazepam or lorazepam on the frequency of endotracheal intubation in childhood status epilepticus. *J Emerg Med* **9**:13–17.

9. Wasiewski WW and Fishman MA (1988) Herpes simplex encephalitis: the brain biopsy controversy. *J Pediatr* **11**:575–578.

10. Mclntyre PB, Chey T and Smith WT (1995) The impact of vaccination against invasive *Haemophilus influenzae* type b disease in the Sydney region. *Med J Aust* **162**:245–248.

11. Adams WG, Deaver KA, Cochi SL *et al.* (1993) Decline of childhood *Haemophilus influenzae* type b (Hib) disease in the Hib vaccine era. *J Am Med Assoc* **269**:221–226.

12. Peltola H, Kilpi T and Antitila M (1992) Rapid disappearance of *Haemophilus influenzae* type b meningitis after routine childhood immunisation with conjugate vaccines. *Lancet* **340**:592–594.

13. Feigin R (1992) Bacterial meningitis beyond the neonatal period. In: Feigin R and Cherry J (eds) *Textbook of Paediatric Infectious Diseases*. Philadelphia: WB Saunders, pp. 410–428.

14. Smith MHD, Starke JR and Marquis JR (1992) Tuberculosis and opportunistic mycobacterial infections. In: Feigin R and Cherry J (eds) *Textbook of Paediatric Infectious Diseases*. Philadelphia: WB Saunders, pp. 1321–1362.

15. McCracken GH and Label MH (1989) Dexamethasone treatment for bacterial meningitis in infants and children. *Am J Dis Child* **143**:287–289.

16. Schaad UB, Lips U, Gnehm HE, Blumberg A, Heinzer I and Wedgwood J (1993) Dexamethasone therapy for bacterial meningitis. *Lancet* **342**:457–461.

17. Gaunt PN and Lambert BE (1988) Single dose ciprofloxacin for the eradication of pharyngeal carriage of *Neisseria meningitidis*. *J Antimicrob Chemother* **21**:489–496.

18. Koskiniemi M and Vaheri A (1989) Effect of measles, mumps, rubella vaccination on pattern of encephalitis in children. *Lancet* **1**:31–34.

19. Stein BM and Wolpert SM (1980) Arteriovenous malformation of the brain II: current concepts and treatment. *Arch Neurol* **37**:69–75.

20. Michenfelder JD and Milde JH (1990) Post-ischaemic canine cerebral blood flow appears to be determined by cerebral metabolic needs. *J Cereb Blood Flow Metab* **10**:71–76.

21. Sarnaik AP, Preston G, Lieh-Lai M and Eisenbrey AB (1985) Intracranial perfusion pressure in near-drowning. *Crit Care Med* **13**:224–227.

22. Bohn DJ, Biggar WD, Smith CR, Conn AW and Barker GA (1986) Influence of hypothermia, barbiturate therapy and intracranial pressure monitoring on morbidity and mortality after near-drowning. *Crit Care Med* **14**:529–534.

23. O'Rourke PP (1986) Outcome of children who are apnoeic and pulseless in the emergency room. *Crit Care Med* **14**:466–468.

24. Schindler MB, Cox PN, Jarvis A and Bohn DJ (1995) Factors influencing outcome from out of hospital paediatric cardiopulmonary arrest. *Anaesth Intens Care* **23**:381–383.

25. Manners PJ and Murray KJ (1992) Guillain–Barré syndrome presenting with severe musculoskeletal pain. *Acta Paediatr* **81**:1049–1051.

26. Cole GF and Matthew DJ (1987) Prognosis in severe Guillain–Barré syndrome. *Arch Dis Child* **62**:288–291.

27. The Guillain–Barré study group (1985) Plasmapharesis and acute Guillain–Barré syndrome. *Neurology* **35**:1096–1104.

28. The French cooperative group on plasma exchange in Guillain–Barré syndrome (1987) Efficiency of plasma exchange in Guillain–Barré syndrome: role of replacement fluids. *Ann Neurol* **22**:753–761.

29. Jansen PW, Perkin RM and Ashwal S (1993) Guillain–Barré syndrome in childhood: natural course and efficacy of plasmapharesis. *Pediatr Neurol* **9**:16–20.

30. Lamont PJ, Johnston HM and Berdoukas VA (1991) Plasmapharesis in children with Guillain–Barré syndrome. *Neurology* **41**:1928–1931.

31. Van der Meche FGA, Schmitz PIM and Dutch Guillain–Barré study group (1992) A randomised trial comparing intravenous immune globulin and plasma exchange in Guillain–Barré syndrome. *N Engl J Med* **326**:1123–1129.

32. Vajsar J, Sloane A, Wood E and Murphy EG (1994) Plasmapharesis vs intravenous immunoglobulin treatment in childhood Guillain–Barré syndrome. *Arch Pediatr Adolesc Med* **148**:1210–1212.

33. Briscoe DM, McMeniman LB and O'Donohoe NV (1987) Prognosis in Guillain–Barré syndrome. *Arch Dis Child* **62**:733–735.

34. Neville BGR (1993) Paediatric neurology. In: Walton J (ed.) *Brain's Diseases of the Nervous System*. Oxford: Oxford Medical Publications, pp. 453–477.

35. Chaves-Carballo E (1992) Detection of inherited neurometabolic disorders. A practical clinical approach. *Pediatr Clin North Am* **39**:801–819.

36. National Institutes of Health conference on Reye's syndrome (1981) Diagnosis and treatment of Reye's syndrome. *J Am Med Assoc* **246**:2441.

37. Green A and Hall S (1992) Investigation of metabolic disorders resembling Reye's syndrome. *Arch Dis Child* **67**:1313–1317.

38. Hadley MN, Zabramski MD, Browner CM, Rekate H and Sonntag VKH (1988) Paediatric spinal trauma. Review of 122 cases of spinal cord and vertebral column injuries. *J Neurosurg* **68**:18–24.

39. Ruge JR, Sinson GP, McLone DG and Cerullo LJ (1988) Pediatric spinal injury: the very young. *J Neurosurg* **68**:25–30.

40. Birney TJ and Hanley EN (1989) Traumatic cervical spine injuries in childhood and adolescence. *Spine* **14**:1277–1282.

41. Swan PK, Bohn DJ, Sides CA and Armstrong P (1987) Cervical spine damage associated with severe head injury in the paediatric patient: implications for airway management. *Anaesth Intens Care* **15**:115–116.

42. Kerslake RW, Jaspan T and Worthington BS (1991) Magnetic resonance imaging of spinal trauma. *Br J Radiol* **64**:386–402.

43. Bracken MB, Shepard MJ, Collins WF *et al.* (1990) A randomised controlled trial of methylprednisone or naloxone in the treatment of acute spinal-cord injury. *N Engl J Med* **322**:1405–1411.

NT Matthews

Trauma is the leading cause of death in children over 1 year old, and the third leading cause under 1 year after sudden infant death syndrome and congenital abnormalities.[1] Causes of trauma and patterns of injury are determined by age-related behaviour: falls and assaults are most common in younger children, while motor vehicle accidents are more common in older children. In general with paediatric trauma, blunt trauma with multiorgan injury is more likely.

As with adults (see Chapter 65), there are three peak mortality periods after injury: *minutes* at the scene, from airway obstruction, bleeding and injuries received; *hours* during transport and resuscitation from airway obstruction, aspiration, bleeding and head injury; and *days to weeks* later from head injury or complications. None the less, there are differences from adults in injury patterns, pathophysiology and management (see below). Paediatric trauma requires resources and coordinated efforts[2] to reduce mortality and morbidity, and this has been successfully demonstrated in Sweden.[3]

Head injury

Significant head injury occurs in 50% of children admitted with blunt trauma. The cause of the injury is determined by behaviour patterns, which change with age (see above). Head injury is commonly due to falls and assaults in infants, and motor vehicle accidents (including bicycle-related injuries) in older children.

Assessment

The Glasgow coma scale (GCS) requires different interpretation in children, where scores tend to be more subjective and prone to misinterpretation. When using the original GCS described for adults, children under 5 years are unable to score normally for verbal and motor responses. Normal aggregate scores for age are 9 at 6 months, 11 at 12 months, and 13–14 at 5 years. This has led to attempts to modify the scale

by either changing the scoring assessment signs, or by reducing the total score (i.e. eliminating some response categories).[4] The latter does not allow for comparison of outcome data.

An example of a commonly used scale modified for infants is shown in Table 108.1. However, difficulties remain as regards the accuracy and reproducibility of GCS for infants. Clinical assessment must also look for signs and symptoms of brain swelling or raised intracranial pressure (ICP; Table 108.2).

Management

The aims of therapy are to maintain adequate cerebral blood flow, while preventing secondary ischaemic injury and herniation from raised ICP. Deterioration in level of consciousness and the appearance of signs of herniation must be rapidly recognized. Airway, oxygenation and respiration should be optimized and intubation performed when the airway is compromised. Hypotension is most likely from blood loss (especially from scalp lacerations) and not brain injury, and the systemic circulation must be maintained. Controlled ventilation with muscle relaxation and sedation should be instituted in the presence of hypoventilation, seizures and signs of raised ICP (see below). Hyperthermia should be avoided with a servo-controlled cooling blanket, while mild hypothermia (to 35°C) reduces cerebral oxygen consumption. Cerebral venous return should be optimized by neutral head positioning. Cerebral perfusion pressure may be best with the bed flat.[5]

Treatment of seizures with phenytoin (20 mg/kg IV) provides less central nervous system depression than barbiturates or benzodiazepines. Monitoring for seizures to guard against resulting increases in cerebral blood flow is difficult in the paralysed patient. Systems for continuous electroencephalogram monitoring are complex to interpret at the bedside and provide limited information. Posttraumatic seizures are more common under 2 years of age.[6]

Table 108.1 Glascow coma scale modified for infants

Glascow coma scale			*Glascow coma scale modified for infants*		
Activity	*Best response*	*Scale*	*Activity*	*Best response*	*Scale*
Eye opening	Spontaneous	4	*Eye opening*	Spontaneous	4
	To speech	3		To speech	3
	To pain	2		To pain	2
	None	1		None	1
Verbal	Oriented	5	*Verbal*	Coos, babbles	5
	Confused	4		Irritable cries	4
	Inappropriate words	3		Cries to pain	3
	Non-specific sounds	2		Moans to pain	2
	None	1		None	1
Motor	Obeys commands	6	*Motor*	Spontaneous activity	6
	Localizes pain	5		Withdraws to touch	5
	Withdraws to pain	4		Withdraws to pain	4
	Abnormal flexion	3		Flexion to pain	3
	Extensor response	2		Extension to pain	2
	None	1		None	1

Continuous measurement of jugular venous oxygen saturation (Sjo_2) via fibreoptic reflection oximetry can identify global cerebral hypoperfusion and ischaemia.[7] However, its use in children is subject to technical difficulties, mainly related to catheter position.

Diagnostic investigations

Supportive investigations can be performed while emergency assessment and therapy proceed. These include pH and acid–base, serum glucose, osmolality, electrolytes, calcium, magnesium and phosphate, complete blood profile and blood cross-match. X-rays of skull and cervical spine (both anteroposterior and lateral views), chest and pelvis are needed. Ultrasound of the skull, where the fontanelle is open, measures ventricular size, and can detect intracranial haemorrhage. It is useful for repeated assessment in the unstable patient. A cranial computed tomography (CT) scan in stable patients is useful to exclude surgically treatable lesions, to assess the size of cerebrospinal fluid (CSF) spaces, including the basal cisterns, to detect herniation and shift, and to show the presence of hyperaemia, oedema, intracerebral haematomas, contusion and fractures. A normal CT scan does not exclude raised ICP. The following are poor prognostic signs:

1 subdural haemorrhage (as an indication of severe trauma and damage to underlying brain tissue);
2 ablated basal cisterns and midline shift;
3 reversal of grey/white differentiation.

Cerebral perfusion pressure (CPP)

Maintenance of CPP in children is important and has significant implications. CPP depends on the difference between systemic blood pressure and ICP. These values vary with age. In particular, blood pressure assumes great importance in the younger age group, where physiological systolic pressures are lower, being 85 mmHg (11.3 kPa) at 6 months, 95 mmHg (12.6 kPa) at 2 years, and 100 mmHg (13.3 kPa) at 7 years.[8] In addition, normal ICP is lower,[9] being up to 5 mmHg (0.67 kPa) at 2 years and up to 10 mmHg (1.3 kPa) at 5 years. Thus, in younger age groups, relative hypotension has a more profound effect on

Table 108.2 Signs of raised intracranial pressure

Depressed level of consciousness
Changes in respiratory pattern, blood pressure and pulse rate
Increased head circumference (less than 18 months' age)
Full or bulging fontanelle
Motor weakness
Cranial nerve palsies
Decorticate or decerebrate posturing
Vomiting
Headache
Papilloedema (late)

Table 108.3 Mechanisms of raised intracranial pressure

Increased intracranial blood volume
    Intracranial bleeding (e.g. epidural, subdural, subarachnoid, intracerebral)
    Cerebral hyperaemia (in the first 1–2 days postinjury)[12]
    Increased cerebral blood flow (increased $Pa\text{CO}_2$, decreased $Pa\text{O}_2$, convulsions)

Cerebral oedema (after day 2)[13]

Hydrocephalus (late, from subarachnoid haemorrhage)

Table 108.4 Physiological compensatory mechanisms for raised intracranial pressure in children

Displacement of CSF to distensible spinal subarachnoid space

Compression of intracranial venous system

Increased CSF reabsorption

Reduced CSF production

Stretching of dura, unfused skull bones and skin (less than 18 months' age)

CSF = Cerebrospinal fluid.

CPP and outcome;[10] hypotension may be the main cause of cerebral ischaemia. Therapy should aim to sustain CPP over 70 mmHg (9.3 kPa),[11] with maintaining normal blood volume and adequate blood pressure (with pressor agents if required). A CPP less than 40 mmHg (5.3 kPa) reduces the likelihood of intact survival.

Intracranial pressure

Mechanisms of raised ICP in childhood trauma are listed in Table 108.3.[12,13] If ICP remains persistently raised and uncompensated, cerebral ischaemia and herniation result. This herniation can be cingulate, uncal (temporal lobe), cerebellar tonsillar, upward cerebellar (posterior fossa hypertension) or transcalvarian (through vault defects). Signs of herniation are as for raised intracranial pressure (Table 108.2).

Measurement of ICP

As with adults, measurement of ICP is indicated when intracranial hypertension has developed or is likely to develop (e.g. GCS 8 or less), or where signs are hidden by muscle relaxation. However, measurement in children can be more difficult. Subdural catheters and intracranial transducers are widely used, but require careful placement in children. Subarachnoid bolts, such as the Richmond screw, need special threads to maintain stability in thin cranial bone, are difficult to insert under 12 months of age, and fail at high pressures. Ventricular catheters allow removal of CSF to reduce ICP, but are difficult to insert when ventricles are small, and readings are difficult to interpret when ventricles collapse. Non-invasive applanation devices over the anterior fontanelle allow trend recording of pressure in neonates,[14] but have not been widely accepted. Development of new strain-gauge technology will allow easier and more meaningful measurement of ICP (including intracerebral pressure).

    Increased ICP above 40 mmHg (5.3 kPa) indicates poor outcome.[15] However, regional pressure and perfusion are not linked to total cerebral blood flow,

and focal oedema affects local cerebral blood flow despite normal limits of ICP and CPP.

Reduction of raised ICP

Several mechanisms allow physiological compensation for raised ICP in children (Table 108.4). In the child under 18 months of age, a gradual increase in intracranial volume is achieved by an increase in head circumference. Measurement of this circumference is important, because this compensation can delay recognition of clinical signs and diagnosis in emerging intracranial pathology. The important factor in the rate of change in compliance and ICP is the elasticity of the dura, which is dependent on the rate of change in intracranial volume.

    Hyperventilation is effective in lowering raised ICP. However, excessive hyperventilation may cause cerebral ischaemia, and $Pa\text{CO}_2$ should be maintained between 35 and 40 mmHg (4.7–5.3 kPa). Weaning from hyperventilation should be slow, to minimize rebound rises in ICP.[16] Fluid restriction is helpful, provided circulating blood volume is maintained. Mannitol (0.25–0.50 g/kg IV slowly) reduces raised ICP by increasing the osmotic gradient across the intact blood–brain barrier and reducing cerebral oedema.[17] Its effects may also be due to reduced blood viscosity and induced cerebral vasoconstriction. Serum osmolality should be monitored to avoid hyperosmolar states. Frusemide (1 mg/kg) reduces cerebral water and CSF production, but excessive diuresis from mannitol or frusemide may compromise the circulation. CSF drainage is possible if a ventricular drain is *in situ*. Initial studies of surgical decompression in head trauma were not encouraging, but recent studies have shown improved results in unremitting focal oedema.[18,19]

Outcome in head injury

When comparing outcome with adults, the data are inconsistent. Various series show better outcome than for adults,[20] poor outcome in those under 2 years,[21] and no difference between adults and children for blunt trauma.[22] Somatosensory evoked potentials are reliable predictors of outcome in children.[23]

Brain death

Criteria for brain death are the same as for adults, although the ANZICS report[24] recommends that children under 2 months require longer observation times (which are not stipulated). Time must be allowed for relatives to come to terms with the diagnosis, and organ donation should be discussed wherever possible. Having relatives watch the physical examination for brainstem testing is helpful.

Spinal cord injury

Anatomical differences in children under 8 years render their spines more mobile and subject to stress. The cervical spine in this age group has less muscular support. Its ligaments and joint capsules are more flexible, and facet joints more horizontal. In addition, the relatively large head mass increases momentum, with the fulcrum of mobility at C2–C3 as opposed to C4–C5 in the adult. Thus paediatric cervical spine injuries tend to be above C4. The use of car seat belts has led to an increase in lumbar spinal cord injury in children.[25]

Assessment

Assessment can be difficult in the clinical examination of neurological deficits in the young child, and in the interpretation of radiological investigations. Despite improved detection of abnormalities with combined X-ray and CT scan examinations,[26] spinal cord injury without obvious radiological abnormality (SCIWORA) may be present.[27] Sensory evoked potentials can be a valuable adjunct to diagnosis. Spinal cord injury can only be dismissed after imaging assessments (which may include magnetic resonance imaging in the non-acute setting) and careful and repeated examination of the lucid patient. Delayed onset of spinal neurological signs has been reported in children.[28]

Management

From the time of injury, the spine should be assumed to be unstable until proved otherwise. Immobilization is necessary from the time of injury in the presence of:

1 signs or symptoms suggesting neurological spinal deficit;
2 a history of loss of consciousness;
3 altered mental status;
4 history of a high-speed accident or significant fall (including diving);
5 significant head or chest trauma.

It is often difficult to decide whether the spinal-injured child is initially best cared for in a paediatric ICU or a specialized spinal unit. This decision will be ultimately determined on the age of the child and the stability of the spine. Certainly, infants should not be managed in adult spinal units, whereas for older children, expertise in spinal care may be more important. However, once spinal column stability and surgical fixation have been achieved, children are best managed in paediatric facilities. Ongoing care is complex, and requires a multidisciplinary approach. Attention to pressure areas, bladder and bowel care and training, nutrition and prevention of contractures is essential. Symptoms of hypercalcaemia (e.g. vomiting, anorexia, nausea and malaise) can be distressing and difficult to control. Depression is common is adolescents.

With high spinal cord injury, chin-operated battery-powered wheelchairs, portable ventilators and computer-activated environment control devices allow for relative independence and a functional lifestyle.

Thoracic trauma

Despite a low incidence in children, thoracic trauma is usually associated with multiorgan injury and high mortality.[29] The mechanism of injury is almost entirely related to motor vehicle accidents, with penetrating trauma being uncommon. The child's small size and more elastic chest wall allow transmission of more kinetic energy to intrathoracic structures, with a high incidence of pulmonary contusion without rib fractures or flail chest. Despite this, the incidence of pneumothorax with or without tension can be high.[30]

As for adults, life-threatening injuries which require immediate intervention are upper airway obstruction, tension pneumothorax, open pneumothorax, flail chest, pericardial tamponade and massive haemothorax (see Chapter 68). Potentially life-threatening injuries are airway rupture, pulmonary contusion, ruptured aorta, diaphragmatic rupture, oesophageal perforation and myocardial contusion. Angiography is the method of choice in diagnosing aortic rupture in children.[31]

Abdominal trauma

Abdominal trauma is usually associated with blunt trauma and multiple organ injury, predominantly with injury to liver and spleen. However, massive haemorrhage, hollow viscus perforation and renal tract injury also need to be recognized. The abdominal wall and thoracic cage of children provide less protection to

Table 108.5 Indications for laparotomy in abdominal trauma

Profound hypovolaemia
Persistent haemorrhage
Penetrating injury
Gastrointestinal perforation
Signs of peritonism
Pancreatic injury

---

intra-abdominal organs. Also, the liver and spleen are relatively large and more exposed below the rib cage. Forces need not be excessive to cause rupture of either organ.

Improvements in radiological imaging techniques have allowed blunt abdominal trauma to be managed conservatively in children.[32] This approach requires appropriate monitoring and supervision in a paediatric setting, with an awareness of the need for urgent intervention, e.g. laparotomy (Table 108.5). CT scan assessment with intraluminal and IV contrast aids this non-operative approach. It allows examination of solid organs and renal tract, and detection of intra-peritoneal blood and free air. Diagnostic peritoneal lavage is only indicated when the source of continued bleeding is undetermined, or where a prolonged procedure or observation period is anticipated, but CT scan is not available.

Non-accidental injury

Non-accidental injuries to children include physical assault, sexual and emotional abuse and neglect, (especially inadequate supervision and deprivation of nutrition and medical care). Injuries resulting from intentional assault can be difficult to diagnose, unless a high index of awareness is maintained.

With regard to the history, suspicion should be raised when:

1 the cause of the injury cannot be explained;
2 there is discrepancy between the volunteered history and the sustained injury, especially when the child's stage of development is taken into account;
3 there is a history of repeated injuries;
4 it is alleged that the injury is self-sustained;
5 there is a delay in seeking care.

Physical examination should be thorough, to establish a pattern of injury. Multiple bruises in differing stages of development can be separately estimated for age.[33] Patterns for burns are typical for forced immersion in hot water (with sparing of the groin area), and from cigarettes. Suspicion should be raised where cerebral trauma is associated with retinal haemorrhages, subdural haematomas or fractures. Retinal haemorrhages are typical of head-shaking, but are also caused by cardiopulmonary resuscitation.[34] A whole-body X-ray series and bone scan will detect fractures in differing stages of healing from multiple assaults.

Whenever non-accidental injury is suspected or diagnosed, a multidisciplinary approach is required by a specialized child protection unit to deal with medical and legal issues, and with counselling. Urgent intervention may be necessary where the safety of other siblings is threatened.

Transport

The outcome of trauma in remote locations is optimal, when advice, pre-hospital stabilization and transport are provided by teams based in tertiary paediatric ICUs.[35] Secondary insults occur more frequently when paediatric-trained personnel are not used for transport.[36] A referral and retrieval infra-structure which links a tertiary centre and outlying areas within the region is necessary. Local health care providers must have sufficient skills to stabilize any critically ill child adequately. The transport team must offer a level of care during the stabilization and transport phases that is equivalent to that of the receiving paediatric ICU.

References

1. Klauber MR, Barrett-Conner E, Marshall LF and Bowers SA (1981) The epidemiology of head injury: a prospective of an entire community – San Diego County, California, 1978. *Am J Epidemiol* **113**:500–509.
2. National Road Trauma Advisory Council (1993) *Report of the Working Party on Trauma Systems*. Canberra: Australian Government Publishing Service.
3. Bergman AB and Rivara FP (1991) Sweden's experience in reducing childhood injuries. *Pediatrics* **88**:69–74.
4. Simpson D and Reilly P (1982) Paediatric coma scale (letter). *Lancet* **2**:450.
5. Rosner MJ and Cotey IB (1986) Cerebral perfusion pressure, intracranial pressure and head elevation. *J Neurosurg* **65**:636–641.
6. Hahn YS, Chyung C, Barthel MJ, Bailes J, Flannery AM and McLone DG (1988) Head injuries in children under 36 months of age. Demography and outcome. *Childs Nerv Syst* **4**:34–40.
7. Dearden NM and Midgley S (1993) Technical considerations in continuous jugular venous oxygen saturation measurement. *Acta Neurochir Suppl Wien* **59**:91–97.
8. Horan MJ (1987) Report of the second task force on blood pressure in children. *Pediatrics* **79**:1–25.
9. Welch K (1980) The intracranial pressure in infants. *J Neurosurg* **52**:693–699.
10. Raju TN, Vidyasagar D and Papazafiratou C (1981) Cerebral perfusion pressure and abnormal intracranial

waveforms: their relation to outcome in birth asphyxia. *Crit Care Med* 9:449–453.

11. Chan KH. Dearden NM, Miller JD, Andrews PJ and Midgley S (1993) Multimodality monitoring as a guide to treatment of intracranial hypertension after severe brain injury. *Neurosurgery* 32:547–552.

12. Bruce DA, Alavi A, Bilaniuk L, Dolinskas C, Obrist W and Uzzell B (1981) Diffuse cerebral swelling following head injuries in children: the syndrome of 'malignant brain edema'. *J Neurosurg* 54:170–178.

13. Snoek JW, Minderhoud JM and Wilmink JT (1984) Delayed deterioration following mild head injury in children. *Brain* 107:15–36.

14. Colditz PB, Williams GL, Berry AB and Symonds PJ (1988) Fontanelle pressure and cerebral perfusion pressure: continuous measurement in neonates. *Crit Care Med* 16:876–879.

15. Longfitt TW and Gennarelli TA (1982) Can the outcome from head injury be improved? *J Neurosurg* 56:19–25.

16. Havill JH (1984) Prolonged hyperventilation and intra-cranial pressure. *Crit Care Med* 12:72–74.

17. Stephenson HE, Safar P, Arfors KE *et al.* (1988) Treatment potentials for reversing clinical death. *Crit Care Med* 16:1034–1042.

18. Gower DJ, Lee KS and McWorter JM (1988) Role of subtemporal decompression in severe closed head injury. *Neurosurgery* 23:417–422.

19. Katayama Y, Tsubokawa S, Miyazaki T, Kawamata T and Yoshino A (1990) Oedema fluid formation within contused brain tissue as a cause of medically uncontrollable elevation of intracranial pressure: the role of surgical therapy. *Acta Neurochir* 51(suppl):308–310.

20. Bruce DA, Raphaely RC, Goldberg Al *et al.* (1979) Pathophysiology, treatment and outcome following severe head injury in children. *Childs Brain* 5:174–191.

21. Mahoney WJ, D'Souza BJ, Haller JA, Rogers MC, Epstein MH and Freeman JM (1983) Long-term outcome of children with severe head trauma and prolonged coma. *Pediatrics* 71:756–762.

22. Eichelberger MR, Mangubat EA, Sacco WS, Bowman LM and Lowenstein AD (1993) Comparative outcomes of children and adults suffering blunt trauma. *J Trauma* 28:430–434.

23. Taylor MJ and Farell EJ (1989) Comparison of the prognostic utility of veps and seps in comatose children. *Pediatr Neurol* 5:145–150.

24. Australian and New Zealand Intensive Care Society (1993) *Statement and Guidelines on Brain Death and Organ Donation. A Report of the ANZICS Working Party on Brain Death and Organ Donation.* Melbourne: ANZICS.

25. Newman KD, Bowman LM and Eichelberger MR (1990) The lap belt complex: intestinal and lumbar spine injury in children. *J Trauma* 30:1133–1140.

26. Borock EC, Gabram SGA, Jacobs LM *et al.* (1991) A prospective analysis of a two-year experience using computed tomography as an adjunct for cervical spine clearance. *J Trauma* 31:1001–1006.

27. Dickman CA, Rekate HL, Sonntag VKH and Zabramski JM (1989) Pediatric spinal trauma: vertebral column and spinal cord injuries in children. *Pediatr Neurosci* 15:237–256.

28. Pang D and Wilberger JE (1982) Spinal cord injury without radiological abnormalities in children. *J Neurosurg* 57:114–129.

29. Peclet MH, Newman KD, Eichelberger MR *et al.* (1990) Thoracic trauma in children: an indicator of increased mortality. *J Pediatr Surg* 25:961–966.

30. Nakayama DK, Ramenofsky ML and Rowe MI (1989) Chest injuries in childhood. *Ann Surg* 210:770–775.

31. Spouge AR, Burrows PE, Armstrong D *et al.* (1991) Traumatic aortic rupture in the pediatric population: role of plain films, CT and angiography in the diagnosis. *Pediatr Radiol* 21:324–328.

32. Erin S, Shandling B, Simpson J and Stephens C (1978) Nonoperative management of traumatised spleen in children. *J Pediatr Surg* 13:117–119.

33. Wilson EF (1977) Estimation of the age of cutaneous contusions in child abuse. *Pediatrics* 60:750–752.

34. Goetting MG and Sowa B (1990) Retinal haemorrhage after cardiopulmonary resuscitation in children: an etiological re-evaluation. *Pediatrics* 89:585–588.

35. Johnson CM and Gonyea MT (1993) Transport of the critically ill child. *Mayo Clin Proc* 68:982–987.

36. McNab JM (1991) Optimal escort for interhospital transport of pediatric emergencies. *J Trauma* 31:205–209.

J Tibballs

This chapter discusses the use of equipment and the performance required in paediatric and neonatal intensive care. Examples of equipment are given but exhaustive lists are not intended.

Intubation and ventilation

Endotracheal tube

Tube types

Polyvinyl chloride or Silastic tubes are suitable for long-term intubation. They should be cuffless and be of the Magill type – curved but neither preformed nor of variable diameter. Preformed tubes (e.g. Rae and Childs) make suction difficult, and automatically stipulate length in relation to diameter and circumference. Tubes of non-uniform diameter (e.g. Cole and Oxford) may damage the vocal cords, and do not prevent endobronchial intubation. Radio-opacity is necessary for correct positioning. Cuffs on tubes may damage subglottic tracheal mucosa, and reduce the tube diameter which would otherwise be available for gas flow. All tubes should have length markings and a Murphy eye, i.e. a side aperture at the distal end, allowing gas to flow if the tip abuts against the tracheal wall.

Tube size

Correct selection of size is necessary to avoid pressure-induced ischaemia/ulceration of tracheal mucosa and to limit aspiration around the tube. The correct size should allow a small leak on application of moderate inflation pressure (25 cm H_2O, 2.5 kPa) but also enable adequate pulmonary inflation and expiration. When lung compliance is poor, it is permissible to use a cuffless tube without a leak to achieve lung inflation. A selection of sizes, one larger and one smaller than the anticipated size, should be available at intubation. Tube sizes according to body weight and age are given in Table 109.1, and a rough

Table 109.1 Endotracheal tube sizes (internal diameter) according to body weight or age

Body weight/age	Size (mm)
Newborn (< 1 kg)	2.5
Newborn (1.0–3.5 kg)	3.0
1–6 months	3.5
6–12 months	4.0
1–2 years	4.5
3–4 years	5.0
5–6 years	5.5
6–7 years	6.0
8–9 years	6.5
9–10 years	7.0
11–12 years	7.5
12–15 years	8.0

guide for internal diameter size in the child is age (in years/4) + 4 mm.

High-volume low-pressure cuffed tubes may be used after puberty when the cricoid region of the trachea has enlarged and is no longer a narrow region at special risk. The cuff should be inflated with the minimum volume of air necessary to maintain a seal and checked every 4–6 h.

Tube length

The endotracheal tube tip should be located in the mid-trachea so that the risks of accidental extubation and endobronchial intubation are minimized. Correct positioning of the tube should always be checked by auscultation in the axillae, by chest X-ray immediately after intubation and daily thereafter.[1] At intubation, visualization of the length of the tube passed through the cords should be a guide only, since the tube advances when the head

Table 109.2 Nasotracheal tube length for premature neonates

Birth weight (g)	Gestation (weeks)	Length (cm)
750	25	7.0
1000	27	7.5
1500	31	8.0
1700	32	8.5
2000	34	9.0
2200	35	9.5
2500	36	10.0
2800	37	10.5
3200	39	11.0
3500	40	11.0

is released from extension as the laryngoscope is removed.[2]

The length of nasotracheal tubes can be chosen initially on the basis of weight or gestation in premature neonates (Table 109.2) and on the basis of age for infants and small children (Table 109.3). A guide to length in the older child is given by the formula: (age in years/2 + 15 cm). Oral endotracheal tubes should be likewise located with care in the mid-trachea. A guide to correct length is given by the formula: (age in years/2 + 12 cm). The length of insertion of both nasal and oral endotracheal tubes should be documented or marked on the tube.

Laryngoscopes

The adult curved Macintosh blade is suitable for all paediatric patients except neonates and infants, in whom a straight blade is needed to displace the relatively large epiglottis anteriorly from the laryngeal inlet. A straight flat blade, e.g. Miller (size 0 or 1) or Seward blade or a straight blade with a medial flange (Magill, Robertshaw, Oxford or Wisconsin) is

Table 109.3 Nasotracheal tube length correlated with age for infants and small children

Age	Length (cm)
Newborn (term)	11.0
6 months	12.0
1 year	14.0
2 years	16.0

equally suitable for this purpose. The latter blades displace the tongue medially and give a better view of the larynx, but leave less room for instrumentation with a sucker, introducer or forceps.

Resuscitator 'bagging' circuits

Manual pulmonary inflation is often necessary via a mask or endotracheal/tracheostomy tube. Two types of devices are available: flow-inflated and self-inflated bags.

Flow-inflated bags

This is exemplified by Ayre's T-piece. Gas flow must exceed 220 ml/kg per min for children and 3 l/min for infants, to prevent rebreathing during manual ventilation. It is possible to control precisely the concentration of inspired oxygen, which is an advantage, especially for the premature neonate at risk of oxygen-induced retrolental fibroplasia. However, considerable experience is necessary to provide adequate ventilation without barotrauma in the intubated neonate. The circuit has neither a valve nor any pressure-relief device. A pressure gauge should be incorporated in the circuit.

Self-inflated bags

This is exemplified by the Laerdal infant, child and adult resuscitators. Rebreathing is prevented by a series of one-way valves. A pressure-relief valve (infant and child size) opens at 35 cm H_2O (3.5 kPa). A pressure monitor can be incorporated in the circuit.[3] Supplemental oxygen is added to the ventilation bag with or without attachment of a reservoir bag, whose movement also serves as a visual monitor of tidal volume during spontaneous ventilation. The delivered oxygen concentration is dependent on the flow rate of oxygen, use of the reservoir bag and the state of the pressure relief valve (whether open or closed). With use of the reservoir bag and oxygen flow greater than the minute ventilation, 100% oxygen is delivered. However, the delivered gas is only 50% oxygen when the reservoir bag is not used, despite oxygen flow rate at twice minute ventilation. At an oxygen flow rate of 10 l/min to the infant resuscitator bag, the delivered gas is 85–100% oxygen without the use of the reservoir bag. Other self-inflated bags include the Combibag, Ambu, AirViva and HanauLife (see Chapters 7 and 27).

Suction catheters

Sizes 5, 6, 8, 10 and 12 FG should be available. The suction catheter should be large enough to remove secretions (Table 109.4) but not too large to occlude the endotracheal/tracheostomy tube lumen. Satinfinish types are preferable.

Table 109.4 Recommended suction catheters

ID (mm) of ETT or tracheostomy	Recommended suction catheter (FG)
2.5	5
3.0	6
3.5–5.5	8
6.0–6.5	10
7.0 and larger	12

ID = Internal diameter; ETT = endotracheal tube.

Masks

Masks should facilitate an airtight seal on the face with additional minimal dead space. For neonates, Rendell-Baker Soucek masks (sizes 0 and 1) or Bennett masks (sizes 1 and 2) are suitable. For infants and small children, the larger Rendell-Baker Soucek masks (sizes 2 and 3) or small masks with inflatable rims, such as CIG (sizes 2 and 3) or MIE (sizes 0 and 1), are suitable. For older children, masks with inflatable rims are preferred.

Oropharyngeal airways

A range of Guedel airways (sizes 000, 00, 0, 1, 2 and 3) constructed of polyvinyl chloride with a metal insert should be available. An airway which is too small may be occluded by the surface of the tongue, while an airway which is too large may enter the oesophagus. The correct size, when placed alongside the cheek, extends from the centre of the lips to the angle of the mandible. Nasopharyngeal airways are available for the older child, but any size can be constructed from an endotracheal tube.

Ventilators

Some ventilators are designed specifically for neonates and infants. A few adult ventilators are also satisfactory. In addition to general requirements of ventilators (see Chapter 27), the paediatric ventilator should have:

1 rapid response time for gas flow during spontanous respiratory effort;
2 low circuit volume, compliance and resistance;
3 inspiratory time adjustment independent of the inspiratory: expiratory ratio;
4 electronic display of inspiratory pressure wave;
5 capability for a ventilation rate up to 60 breaths/min (excluding capability for high-frequency ventilation);
6 variable gas flow up to 2–3 l/kg per min;
7 a light-weight circuit;
8 minimal dead space within the ventilator and circuit;
9 accurate measurement of low tidal volume;

For paediatric patients, the most useful classification of ventilators (and guide to use) is one of either a volume-preset or a pressure-preset mode of inspiration. Volume-preset ventilators are suitable for conditions in which lung compliance and resistance are variable. In these circumstances, the generated peak inspiratory pressure is a valuable observation. However, volume-preset ventilators do not compensate for leaks from the ventilator–patient circuit. Neonates and infants have small tidal volumes (5–50 ml), and are therefore prone to alveolar hypoventilation with variable air leaks around the endotracheal tube and from the ventilator–humidifier circuit. Moreover, the internal compliance and compressible volume of the circuit may exceed the tidal volume. Small tidal volumes are difficult to set and maintain when the lung compliance and resistance are abnormal.[4] Examples of ventilators which can be operated in a volume-preset mode are the Baby Bird, Bear Cub BP2001, Bourns LS, Sechrist V-100B, Veriflow, Servovent, Siemens-Elema Servo 900C, Drager Evita 2 and Ohmeda Logic 03N2.

Most neonatal ICUs have ventilators which are used as pressure-preset or pressure-limited. Examples are Bourns BP200, Bear Cub BP2001, Sechrist V-100B, Healthdyne 105, 200, Campbell, Vickers Neovent, Bio-med MVP-100, Amsterdam MK3, Siemens-Elema Servo 900C, Newport E100i and Infrasonics Infant Star ventilator. Pressure-preset ventilation in newborn infants with hyaline membrane disease achieves adequate oxygenation with minimal barotrauma.[5] The pressure-preset mode is more appropriate than volume-preset inspiration for neonates and infants 0.5–5.0 kg body weight, because there is some compensation for leaks from the patient–ventilator circuit. This compensation is better with pressure generators than with flow generators. Pressure generators deliver a variable flow dependent on lung and airway characteristics.

Ventilators which are flow generators deliver a constant flow, and do not compensate for leaks in the ventilator–patient circuit. When such ventilators have imposed a pressure limitation, there is likewise no compensation for changes in compliance and resistance. Although theoretically undesirable, this type of ventilator with flow generation, pressure limitation and time cycling is commonly used because of the relative ease of operation. Relatively large leaks may severely compromise tidal volume, mean airway pressure and oxygenation. Large leaks may also delay attainment of preset pressure until late in the inspiratory cycle. Thus, it is helpful to display the inspiratory waveform electronically. Gas flow should be set above 2 l/kg per min to achieve the preset pressure early in the inspiratory period. This flow rate is also suitable for peak inspiratory flow rate during spontaneous respiratory effort with intermittent mandatory ventilation. With use of these ventilators, both the flow rate and the pressure limitation must be specified, since pressure limitation is achieved by controlling a leak from the circuit. Pressure in the circuit should be monitored in close proximity to the endotracheal tube. Changes in endotracheal tube resistance from encrustation or kinking have a major adverse effect on tidal volume.[6]

Improvements in conventional ventilatory management of newborns are observed with a new generation of ventilators which utilize changes in airway pressure, airway gas flow or abdominal movement to trigger inspiration, and which have ultrashort trigger delays.[7] Previously, ventilators were unable to cope with the very short inspiratory times (mean 0.31, SD 0.06 s[8]) of newborns with respiratory distress syndrome. Patient-triggered ventilation (PTV) permits synchronous ventilation with better gas exchange, prevents the patient fighting the ventilator and reduces the need for neuromuscular paralysis.[9,10] Examples are the Bear Cub II infant ventilator system (flow trigger), Draeger babylog 8000 (flow trigger), infrasonics Infant Star ventilator with Star Sync module (abdominal movement trigger), VIP Bird infant/paediatric ventilator (pressure and flow trigger) and the Siemens Servo 300 (pressure and flow trigger).

High-frequency oscillatory ventilation (HFOV) at 15 Hz has been shown to achieve better gas exchange with less barotrauma than conventional mechanical ventilation in infants with respiratory distress.[11,12] Examples of high-frequency oscillators are the Sensor Medics 3100 and 3100A and the Humming series models, of which the latest is Atom Humming V. The latter also offers a synchronized intermittent mandatory ventilation mode.

Oxygen therapy and monitoring

Oxygen catheters

Sizes 6, 8 and 10 FG should be available and placed in the same nostril as the nasogastric tube, to limit airway resistance. Size 6 FG is suitable for neonates, 8 FG for infants and small children and 10 FG for older children. Nasal cannulae (two-pronged) are not recommended. Excessive flow may cause gastric distension. Flow rate for infants should be regulated by a low-flow meter, graduated 0–2.5 l/min.

Oxygen masks

The performance of masks is discussed in Chapter 22. Masks are not well-tolerated by the infant or small child; oxygen catheters are preferable.

Head boxes and incubators

A clear Perspex head box is the best way of administering a high concentration of oxygen to the unintubated neonate and infant. Precise oxygen therapy is possible but rebreathing, heat loss and desiccation are potential problems. To avoid rebreathing, a large flow rate (10–12 l/min) of fresh gas with predetermined oxygen content should be introduced. The practice of introducing a low flow rate of 100% oxygen into a head box (to gain a lesser concentration) may cause hypercarbia. If 100% oxygen is the only compressed gas available, lesser concentrations of oxygen may be attained without rebreathing by using a flow of 100% oxygen and a Venturi device. The relatively large capacity of an incubator precludes the attainment of a high concentration of oxygen, but limited oxygen therapy (e.g. 40%) can be achieved.

Oxygen analysers

These are essential to regulate oxygen therapy via incubator or head box. The devices utilize either a polarographic electrode or a galvanic cell (microfuel cell) as oxygen sensor. The polarographic types require a source of power (battery or mains), are more expensive to buy (but cheaper to run), and have a faster response time.[13] An incorporated alarm is recommended. The sensing electrode should be placed close to the patient's head.

Transcutaneous gas analysers

The invention of a miniaturized heated Clark electrode and the Stower Severinghaus CO_2 electrode has enabled measurement of transcutaneous oxygen ($Ptco_2$) and carbon dioxide ($Ptcco_2$) tension. The technique enables continuous monitoring and has become firmly established in the critical care of infants, children[14] and neonates.[15,16] Transcutaneous gas tensions equate well with arterial gas tensions. However, Pao_2 is underestimated by $Ptco_2$ during mild hyperoxaemia in neonates.[17] Transcutaneous gas values are dependent on both arterial gas tensions and on blood flow. During normovolaemia with adequate flow, $Ptco_2$ reflects Pao_2 and $Ptcco_2$ reflects $Paco_2$. However, during circulatory failure, a reduction in $Ptco_2$ reflects a reduction in flow, provided Pao_2 is normal.[18] Likewise, during circulatory failure, $Ptco_2$ exceeds $Paco_2$ and is flow-dependent.[19] Transcutaneous monitors available are the Radio-meter TCM2 (O_2), TCM20 (CO_2), Critikon 8030 and 8010 (O_2), Dragerwerk oxycapnometer S (O_2) and (CO_2), Kontron 820, 830 and 632 (O_2), Novametric TCO2M818 (O_2) and (CO_2), Biochem Sensomat PO2 and Roche O_2. In these models, $Ptco_2$ and $Ptcco_2$ are estimated by different electrodes.

Continuous-pulse oximetry (see Chapter 98) has evolved to be an integral part of monitoring in neonatal and paediatric intensive care. Transcutaneous pulse oximetry is more convenient than transcutaneous partial pressure measurement. Each patient should have a pulse oximeter. The value of pulse oximetry is detection of hypoxaemia, not hyperoxaemia, which requires blood or transcutaneous partial pressure measurement. The accuracy of pulse oximetry at low partial pressure (<70 mmHg, 9.3 kPa) is doubtful. Numerous devices are available.

Blood-gas analysers

In many neonatal and paediatric conditions, frequent blood-gas analysis is essential for optimal management. A blood-gas analyser utilizing small volumes (< 0.2 ml) is essential. The instrument should be located within or near the ICU, so that tests can be performed and the results known without delay.

Apnoea monitors

Infant apnoea is often due to upper airway obstruction, seizures or gastro-oesophageal reflux,[20] although it may be idiopathic and is commonly associated with prematurity. Short apnoeic spells (<15 s) are normal during sleep and feeding. Significant apnoea is associated with bradycardia, cyanosis and hypotonia. The detection and treatment of apnoea in intensive care are dependent on cardiovascular monitoring and constant nursing observation. In the home or ward, where observation is less than that available in the ICU, apnoea may be detected by the use of a pressure sensor in a pad or mattress under the infant, or by impedance pneumography, in which diaphragmatic movement causes a change in resistance between two electrodes on the skin. Apnoea of central origin is detected early by these devices but obstructive apnoea, resulting in paradoxical respiratory effort, is detected late. Some devices incorporate electrocardiogram monitoring and rely upon bradycardia as evidence of hypoxaemia, which is a useful but late sign in obstructive apnoea, when both hypoxaemia and movement of the diaphragm are present. False-positive alarms are not uncommon.

Thermoregulation

Radiant heaters and incubators

Adequate temperature regulation is essential in neonates and infants to avoid cold stress, and to maintain a thermoneutral environment.[21] Numerous heaters and incubators are available with special features for transport, resuscitation, intensive care and regular ward nursing. Open-type radiant heaters (e.g. Ohio nc, Atom, Drager, Air Shields, Ameda, Medix, Mediprema and Medishields) are more suitable for use in intensive care. The ideal radiant heater should incorporate:

1 servo-controlled overhead heating device with alarm for overheating;
2 a facility for phototherapy;
3 an open tiltable bed of adequate area;
4 clear Perspex removable/hinged sides;
5 adequate illumination;
6 adjustable height;
7 facility for X-ray examinations.

Additional features may include facilities for bottled oxygen, positive pressure, resuscitation and suction equipment.

Incubators are less suitable for use in intensive care because of limited access, but are better for transportation. Heating is via a conductive mattress. Double-walled infant incubators (e.g. Air Shields C-100, Ohio IC) reduce heat loss, attain preset temperature rapidly, do not produce excessive air currents or sound levels, and do not permit carbon dioxide accumulation.[22] Oxygen therapy and mechanical ventilation are possible with both types of units, but are technically easier with an open-cot radiant heater.

Humidifiers

Adequate humidification of ventilator circuits is of utmost importance in the paediatric patient. The relatively narrow endotracheal and tracheostomy tubes are prone to encrustation and blockage. Insensible water and heat loss are prevented with adequate humidification. Hot water bath humidifiers incorporated in adult ventilator circuits (see Chapter 28) are suitable for paediatric patients. However, the circuits have an internal compliance and a compressible volume which produce errors in both volume-preset and pressure-preset ventilators. Ideally, the compliance should not exceed 1.0 ml/cm H_2O for patients less than 10 kg body weight.[23] A water trap must be incorporated to prevent 'rain-out' in the delivery tube being aspirated.

Condenser-type humidifiers should only be used for short periods (e.g. for transport) and only when the dead space of the device is not significant. Unheated bubble humidifiers have limited applicability. The heated aerosol generator types (e.g. Puritan) are preferable for the administration of oxygen via facemask, nasal catheter or T-piece.

Miscellaneous equipment

Infusion devices

Numerous electromechanical devices have been developed to overcome the deficiencies of gravity-fed IV infusion sets. They enable constant and accurate infusion of predetermined volumes. These devices have wide clinical application and are used to control the administration of potent drugs, hormones and parenteral nutrition. Performance and application are variable.[24,25]

Flow regulators

With these devices (e.g. Dial-A-Flow and Helix), flow is manually regulated. They are simple, cheap, easy to adjust and are more suited to infusion at high flow rates. However, they do not overcome the main deficiencies of gravity-fed IV giving sets, such as the effects of venous pressure and fluid viscosity. Their accuracy is poor at low flow rates, and they are not suitable for administration of concentrated potent drugs.

Drip controllers

These devices utilize standard giving sets and regulate the drip rate by a photoelectric cell sensor and servo-loop. They eliminate the effect of venous pressure, but the drip size (hence flow) may vary considerably. Examples are IVAC 230, IMED 350, Schoch Dignifuse, Arcomed Diginfusa 3000, Intercare Infutec 400, Vickers Treonic C30 and Medix 200–201 and peristaltic pumps IVAC 530, IMED 915 and Medishield IVO.

Volumetric pumps

These regulate flow rate by delivering a pre-measured bolus under pressure. In some the delivery is not smooth. They utilize disposable closed cassettes. The risk of air pumping is minimal and alarms indicate infusion failure. High (up to 999 ml/h) and low flow rates (1 ml/h) are possible. Examples are IVAC 630, 560, 1500, IMED 922, 960/965, Valleylab 6000B, Critikon 2100A, Arcomed Volumed 4000, AVI 270, TOP 3100, Intercare Infutec 500/1000, Exactavol, TAL 121 and Fresenius Inca PT/ST.

Syringe pumps and drivers

These are suitable for infusion of potent drugs in concentrated form at very low rates (< 0.5 ml/h). They are mains electricity- and/or battery-powered. The latter are suitable for use during transport and miniaturized models are suitable for ambulant use. These devices are suitable for IV, intra-arterial, intramuscular, subcutaneous infusion or enterogastric feeding, being particularly suitable for use in neonates and infants. They are not suited to infusion of large volumes and offer no safeguard against extravasation unless an overpressure alarm is incorporated. Generally, the pumps utilize specified syringes unless recalibrated. Some syringe brands do not run smoothly. Examples are Nipro SP-150, IVAC P1000, Vickers IP4, Fresenius 30, 50, Injectomat series, Harvard 2620, Atom Medcor 235, Pye M516, Sage

242A, TOP 5100, GF Phoenix, Graseby range and Auto-Syringe range.

Indirect measurement of blood pressure

Measurement of blood pressure in the critically ill neonate and infant is important in cardiovascular monitoring. Continuous direct intra-arterial measurement is preferred in cardiovascular instability, but adequate monitoring can be achieved with Doppler ultrasonography (e.g. Roche Arteriosonde) or with microprocessor analysis of oscillometric signals (e.g. Critikon Dinamap, Nippon-Colin, Ohio NIMP, Narco Scientific and Vita-Stat, Kenz BPM). The latter devices provide time-automated analysis of systolic, diastolic and mean blood pressure, as well as heart rate at specified intervals. Some portable monitoring devices provide additional data, such as invasive pressure measurement, electrocardiogram, heart rate, pulse oximetry, capnography, respiratory rate and temperature (e.g. Nellcor Propaq, Datascope Passport, Schiller Argus TM-7, S & W Diascope, BCI 6100). Continuous non-invasive measurement of blood pressure may be measured with the Ohmeda Finapres non-invasive blood pressure monitor. Blood pressure measured with these non-invasive devices correlates well with simultaneous measurement by direct intra-arterial measurement in neonates,[26] infants and children.[27] Generally, systolic pressure is underestimated by only 2–4 mmHg (0.3–0.5 kPa), while the diastolic pressure is overestimated by a similar amount. Venostasis[28] and radial nerve compression are occasional complications.

Nasogastric tubes

These are mandatory in all intubated and/or ventilated patients as aids to prevent aspiration, and are a useful means of providing nutrition and medication. A range of sizes should be available: 5–6 FG for neonates, 8 FG for infants, 10 FG for small children, and 12 FG for larger children.

References

1. Greenbaum DM and Marcshall KE (1982) The value of routine daily chest X-rays in intubated patients in the medical intensive care unit. *Crit Care Med* **10**:29–30.
2. Bosman YK and Foster PA (1977) Endotracheal intubation and head posture in infants. *South Afr Med J* **52**:71–78.
3. Kaufmann GW and Hess DR (1982) Modification of the infant Laerdal resuscitation bag to monitor airway pressure. *Crit Care Med* **10**:112–113.
4. Simbruner G and Gregory GA (1981) Performance of neonatal ventilators: the effects of changes in resistance and compliance. *Crit Care Med* **9**:509–514.
5. Reynolds EOR and Taghizadeh A (1974) Improved prognosis of infants mechanically ventilated for hyaline membrane disease. *Arch Dis Child* **49**:505.

6. Abrahams N, Fisk GC, Vonwiller JB and Grant GC (1975) Evaluation of infant ventilators. *Anaesth Intens Care* **3**:6–11.

7. Greenough A and Milner AD (1992) Respiratory support using patient triggered ventilation in the neonatal period. *Arch Dis Child* **67**:69–71.

8. South M and Morley CJ (1992) Respiratory timing in intubated neonates with respiratory distress syndrome. *Arch Dis Child* **67**:446–448.

9. Hird MF and Greenough A (1991) Patient triggered ventilation using a flow triggered system. *Arch Dis Child* **66**:1140–1142.

10. Cleary JP, Bernstein G, Mannino FL and Heldt GP (1995) Improved oxygenation during synchronized intermittent mandatory ventilation in neonates with respiratory distress syndrome: a randomized, crossover study. *J Pediatr* **126**:407–411.

11. Ogawa Y, Miyasaka K, Kawano T *et al.* (1993) A multicenter randomized trial of high frequency oscillatory ventilation as compared with conventional mechanical ventilation in preterm infants with respiratory failure. *Early Hum Dev* **32**:1–10.

12. HiFO study group (1993) Randomized study of high-frequency oscillatory ventilation in infants with severe respiratory distress syndrome. *J Pediatr* **122**:609–619.

13. Cole AGH (1983) Small oxygen analysers. *Br J Hosp Med* **29**:469–471.

14. Monaco F and McQuitty GC (1982) Continuous transcutaneous oxygen and carbon dioxide monitoring in the pediatric ICU. *Crit Care Med* **10**:765–766.

15. Peabody JL, Gregory G, Willis MM and Tooley WH (1978). Transcutaneous oxygen tension in sick infants. *Am Rev Respir* **118**:83–87.

16. Monaco F and McQuitty GC (1981) Transcutaneous measurement of carbon dioxide partial pressure in sick neonates. *Crit Care Med* **9**:756–768.

17. Martin RJ, Robertson SS and Hopple MM (1982). Relationship between transcutaneous and arterial oxygen tension in sick neonates during mild hyperoxaemia. *Crit Care Med* **10**:670–672.

18. Tremper KK, Shoemaker WC, Shippy CR and Nolan LS (1981) Transcutaneous oxygen monitoring of critically ill adults with and without low flow shock. *Crit Care Med* **9**:706–709.

19. Tremper KK, Shoemaker WC, Shippy CR and Nolan LS (1981). Transcutaneous P_{CO_2} monitoring on adult patients in the ICU and operating room. *Crit Care Med* **9**:752–755.

20. Brown LW (1984) Home monitoring of the high-risk infant. *Clin Pediatr* **11**:85–100.

21. Hull D and Chellappah G (1983) On keeping babies warm. In: Chiswick ML (ed.) *Recent Advances in Perinatal Medicine.* Edinburgh: Churchill Livingstone, pp. 153–168.

22. Bell EF and Rios GR (1983) Performance characteristics of two double-walled infant incubators. *Crit Care Med* **11**:663–667.

23. Holbrook PR, Taylor G, Pollak MM *et al.* (1980) Adult respiratory distress syndrome in children. *Pediatr Clin North Am* **27**:677–685.

24. Shyam VSR and Tinker J (1981). Recent developments in infusion devices. *Br J Hosp Med* **25**:69–75.

25. Dickenson JR (1983) Syringe pumps. *Br J Hosp Med* **29**:187–191.

26. Lui K, Doyle PE and Buchanan N (1982) Oscillometric and intra-arterial blood pressure measurements in the neonates: a comparison of methods. *Aust Pediatr J* **18**:32–34.

27. Savage JM, Dillon MJ and Taylor JFN (1979) Clinical evaluation and comparison of the infrasonde, arteriosonde and mercury sphygomomanometer in measurements of blood pressure in children. *Arch Dis Child* **54**:184–189.

28. Showman A and Betts EK (1981) Hazard of automatic noninvasive blood pressure monitoring. *Anesthesiology* **55**:717–718.

J Tibballs

POISONING

Epidemiology[1]

The peak incidence of poisoning in childhood is among 1–3-year-olds. It usually occurs in the home when the child ingests a prescribed or over-the-counter medication or a household product. This mode of poisoning is called accidental but is usually the result of inadequate supervision or improper storage of poisons. Mortality is very low, and any required hospitalization is usually brief (1–3 days). Occasionally, poisoning in childhood is truly accidental, part of child abuse or iatrogenic, as when a parent mistakes medications at home or when hospital staff commit errors in drug administration. Self-poisoning in older children is usually with an intention to manipulate their psychosocial environment or commit suicide, or is the result of substance abuse. All circumstances of poisoning require remedial action.

Options for treatment

The options for treatment after presentation at hospital are to discharge home, observe for a short duration in the emergency department, provide nursing care or to treat medically. The problem is to match the intensity of treatment to the severity of the poisoning, thereby avoiding inappropriate treatment. The intensity of treatment should be determined by the observed and expected effects of the poison, the amount ingested and the interval between ingestion and presentation.

Principles of management

The four basic principles of management of suspected poisoning are:

1 support vital functions;
2 confirm the diagnosis;

3 remove the poison from the body;
4 administer an antidote.

Individual poisons may require specific measures[2] (see Chapter 77). Few poisons have antidotes.

The vast majority of childhood poisoning is by ingestion. Choosing the correct gastrointestinal decontamination technique is crucial to uncomplicated recovery. The choices are induced emesis, gastric lavage, activated charcoal administration, whole-bowel irrigation or a combination of techniques. The efficacy, indications, contraindications and disadvantages and complications of these techniques are given in Table 110.1, and a management plan is presented in Figure 110.1.

A crucial point in the management plan is initial differentiation of patients into states of full consciousness or less than full consciousness. Traditionally, management has depended on judging whether the gag reflex is present, but this is rarely tested and is a crude test of laryngeal competence. Since aspiration pneumonitis is a common feature of poisoning, it is prudent to regard all obtunded patients as having incompetent reflexes. Such patients should not be induced to vomit, undergo gastric lavage or whole-bowel irrigation, or given activated charcoal without protecting the airway. The decision to attempt removal should always be made in reference to two facts: first, that the vast majority of childhood poisonings recover with no treatment, and second, that aspiration pneumonitis is more serious than most poisonings. Occasionally, removal from the circulation by charcoal haemoperfusion, plasma filtration or haemofiltration is indicated (see Chapter 77).

Induced emesis

Administration of syrup of ipecacuanha causes vomiting in a high percentage of children within 30 min. However, its efficacy in removing gastric

Table 110.1 Techniques of gastrointestinal decontamination in children

	Induced emesis	*Gastric lavage*	*Activated charcoal*	*Bowel irrigation*
Efficacy	Good within minutes. Poor after 1 h	Good within minutes. Poor after 1 h	Good within minutes. Moderate at 1 h	Good
Indications	Early presentation of minor poisoning. Domiciliary first aid	Serious or potentially serious effects. Gastric stasis	Universal antidote	Delayed presentation. Slow-release preparations. Irretrievable substance (e.g. disc battery). Poison not adsorbed by charcoal
Contraindications	Less than full consciousness. Corrosives, hydrocarbons, petrochemicals	Less than full consciousness. Corrosives, hydrocarbons, petrochemicals	Less than full consciousness. Ileus	Less than full consciousness. Ileus
Disadvantages, complications	Hyperemesis. Mimics poisoning. Delayed effect. Delays discharge. Creates work	Aspiration pneumonitis. Water intoxication. Invasive – trauma common	Constipation. Fluid and electrolyte imbalance. Charcoal pneumonitis (high fatality). Not adsorbed: metals, corrosives, pesticides, petrochemicals.	

contents is poor. Solids are retained in the stomach or propelled into the duodenum.[3] Approximately 50–65% of ingested experimental drug is removed if ipecac is given after 5 min[4] but only 2–38% if given at 30 or 60 min.[5-8] Ipecac has some problems:

1 The incidence of hyperemesis is 17%.
2 Aspiration pneumonitis may occur even in the fully conscious.[10]
3 Vomiting may mimic the effects of a poison.
4 The onset of vomiting may be delayed, which is hazardous if loss of consciousness occurs.

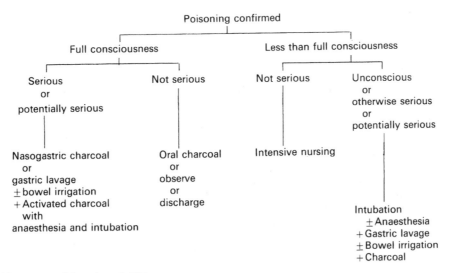

Fig. 110.1 Management of the poisoned child.

Critics of induced emesis claim that the technique merely creates work, delays discharge from the emergency department,[11] increases complications[12] and does not benefit the patient who presents more than 1 h after ingestion.[13] Emesis should not be induced if a corrosive, hydrocarbon or petrochemical has been ingested. Induced emesis has largely been abandoned by emergency departments, but may be indicated if a child presents early after a minor poisoning, in lieu of oral/nasogastric charcoal administration.

Gastric lavage

Experimental studies of the efficacy of gastric lavage reveal that the drug absorption is reduced by 90% at 5 min,[14] but only by 8–32% at 1 h after ingestion.[5,7] Efficacy is poor because even large-bore tubes cannot remove tablets, and lavage encourages propulsion into the duodenum.[3] In symptomatic patients, gastric lavage alone compared to gastric lavage plus administered activated charcoal increased aspiration and did not alter the duration of intubation or the stay in the emergency department or ICU.[15] Gastric lavage has been shown not to be beneficial unless performed within 1 h of ingestion.[13] It is contraindicated in less than full consciousness without airway protection, and after ingestion of corrosives, hydrocarbons or petrochemicals. Complications include aspiration pneumonitis, water intoxication, minor trauma to oropharynx (gastro-oesophageal perforation occurs rarely) and intrabronchial instillation of lavage fluid. Infants and children never cooperate for gastric lavage, thus increasing the risks of complications and psychological trauma.

If lavage is indicated, rapid-sequence induction of anaesthesia with intubation is advised. A lubricated tube of diameter similar to an appropriate-sized endotracheal tube should be used, and correct placement confirmed. Small volumes (1–2 ml/kg) of warm tap water may be used to lavage until clear returns are obtained. Most water should be retrieved.

Activated charcoal

Activated charcoal is rightly regarded as a universal antidote, and is superior to induced emesis and gastric lavage in treating symptomatic patients.[10,13,15] It reduces absorption of ingested experimental drugs by 85–98% when administered 5 min after ingestion,[4,16] by 40–75% at 30 min[4] and by 30–50% at 60 min.[8,16] Repeated doses enhance the elimination of many drugs and are particularly useful in slow-release preparations. A suitable single dose is 1–2 g/kg. A multiple-dose regimen for children is 1–2 g/kg stat, followed by 0.25–0.50 g/kg 4–6-hourly. An alternative regimen is 0.25–0.50 g/kg hourly for 12–24 h.[17] It is contraindicated if ileus is present and in a less than fully conscious patient, unless the airway is protected (i.e. tracheal intubation). Aspiration of

charcoal causes severe and often fatal pneumonitis and bronchiolitis obliterans. Constipation is common after charcoal, but bowel obstruction is rare. Addition of a laxative (e.g. sorbitol or magnesium sulphate) is not recommended. Although laxatives decrease transit time through the gut, efficacy of the charcoal is reduced, and life-threatening fluid and electrolyte imbalance may occur.[18] Activated charcoal does not adsorb metals, corrosives, hydrocarbons or petrochemicals.

Whole-bowel irrigation

Irrigation of the bowel with a solution of polyethylene glycol and electrolytes is effective in reducing absorption of experimental drug by 24–67% 1 h after ingestion,[19,20] and up to 73% 4 h after ingestion.[21] It is contraindicated in less than full consciousness or the presence of an ileus. The solution is adsorbed by activated charcoal, necessitating prior administration in a combined technique. Whole-bowel irrigation is most useful in delayed presentations, ingestion of slow-release preparations, irretrievable substances (e.g. disc batteries) and poisons not adsorbed by charcoal. A suitable regimen is 30 ml/kg per h for 4–8 h.

ENVENOMATION

Envenomation may occur from a wide variety of creatures in Australia and elsewhere.[22,23] Among children, the most frequent causes are bites by snakes and spiders. Particular difficulties are encountered in the management of snake envenomation in small children. These are an uncertain history, obscure signs and a large venom to body weight ratio.

Snake bite

The most dangerous species in Australia are from the genera of Brown, Tiger, Taipan, Death Adder, Black and Copperhead. Although antivenoms are widely available, deaths still occur.[24,25] Common principal toxins are neurotoxins and procoagulants, with the exception that Death Adders do not have a significant procoagulant effect. The predominant neurotoxic effects are neuromuscular paralysis with respiratory failure and bulbar palsy. The procoagulants (i.e. prothrombin activators) cause disseminated intravascular coagulation (DIC), with depletion of clotting factors and defibrination with subsequent haemorrhage. Other toxins are haemolysins, anticoagulants (weak) and rhabdomyolysins. Occasionally the effect of a single toxin may be the sole feature of envenomation (e.g. coagulopathy). Renal failure may occur secondary to hypotension, DIC, haemolysis and rhabdomyolysis.

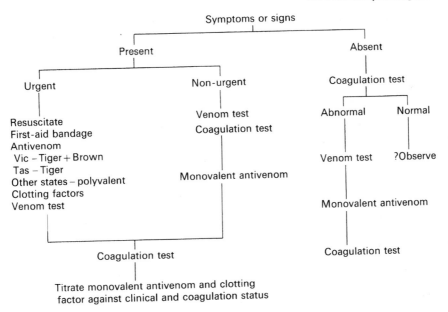

Fig. 110.2 Management of childhood 'snake bite'.

Symptoms and signs of envenomation

The bite site is typically identifiable by puncture marks, scratches or localized oedema, bruising or haematoma. Occasionally, the bite site may be inseparable from minor trauma commonly found on limbs of young children. Reliable symptoms within an hour of envenomation are headache, nausea or vomiting and abdominal pain.[26] Reliable early neurotoxic signs are ptosis, dysphonia, dysphagia, facial muscle weakness, diplopia and blurred vision. Advanced neurological effects are limb, trunk and respiratory muscle weakness. Spontaneous haemorrhage may occur from mucous membranes and needle puncture sites, or into solid organs. Cardiorespiratory failure occurs within several hours, but may be accelerated after massive envenomation from multiple bites.

Management

Although envenomation does not always accompany snake bite, every bite should be regarded as serious. Sometimes snake bite is suspected even though a snake was not observed. Diagnosis rests on clinical signs, a test of coagulation and an immunoassay of venom in biological fluid and from the bite site. A plan of management is given in Figure 110.2.

Suspected envenomation

Envenomation is confirmed in approximately 20% of children presenting to hospital with 'snake bite'. Although neither symptoms nor signs of envenoma-

tion may be present, a test of coagulation should be performed in all patients. Coagulopathy is a reliable test of envenomation,[26] except in a location where a bite from a Death Adder is a possibility. Routine coagulation tests such as prothrombin time, activated partial thromboplastin time, serum fibrinogen and fibrin degradation products can be used. If these cannot be done, a skin bleeding time or a whole-blood clotting time will suffice. If coagulopathy is present, a venom test or irrefutable herpetological evidence should be used to select the correct antivenom. A positive test of a washing from a bite site identifies the snake, but a positive test of urine (preferred) or blood also confirms envenomation. If a pressure-immobilization bandage is in place, it may be removed after ensuring that antivenom is available (see Chapter 75).

Definite envenomation

Envenomation is confirmed in approximately 50% of children after an observed snake bite. Clinically diagnosed envenomation or isolated coagulopathy requires treatment with IV antivenom. Supportive measures and tests include:

1 airway maintenance and mechanical ventilation;
2 infusion of blood, coagulation factors (fresh frozen plasma and cryoprecipitate) and platelets;
3 application of a pressure-immobilizing first-aid bandage to retard the absorption of venom into the blood stream.[27] The existing bandage must not be removed until antivenom has been administered;
4 venom test of urine, blood and bite site;

5 coagulation tests, full blood examination, serum electrolytes and creatinine, urine, haemoglobin and myoglobin.

Antivenom therapy

Antivenom is needed for clinically obvious envenomation and for otherwise symptomless coagulopathy which may cause serious haemorrhage. A knowledge of the distribution of snake species is helpful to aid in the interpretation of a coagulation test and the choice of antivenom. However, it is dangerous to guess the identification of a snake or to rely upon unverified identification, since antivenoms have limited cross-species efficacy. Occasionally, venom may be detected in the urine but neither clinical nor coagulopathic effects are apparent, in which case antivenom may be withheld.

Wherever possible, species-specific monovalent antivenom should be used to limit the risk of adverse reaction. Available antivenoms are Brown snake, Tiger snake, Taipan, Death Adder, Black snake and polyvalent antivenom – a mixture of the monovalent antivenoms – and a sea snake antivenom. If the species of snake cannot be determined or the need for antivenom is urgent, antivenom according to location is selected (e.g. Brown and Tiger snake in Victoria, Tiger snake in Tasmania, polyvalent elsewhere). Sea snake envenomation is treated with sea snake antivenom or Tiger snake antivenom. The antivenom is infused over 30 min, but faster in severe envenomation.

Premedication with adrenaline 0.005 mg/kg SC 5–10 min before the first dose of antivenom is advised, to prevent or ameliorate anaphylaxis. Because of the risk of cerebral haemorrhage in the presence of a coagulopathy, and hypertension induced by adrenaline, adrenaline should not be given IV or IM as a premedication.[28] Additional adrenaline should be at hand to treat anaphylaxis. An antihistamine and a steroid may also be given to a victim with known allergy to equine protein, although antihistamines may confound the signs of an adverse reaction. A course of steroids should be given after multiple doses of monovalent antivenom, or after polyvalent antivenom. The dose of antivenom cannot be reliably predicted because the amount of venom injected during snake bite varies considerably. The majority of paediatric envenomations resolve after several ampoules, but a few require many ampoules.

The antivenom is titrated against repeated clinical examinations and coagulation tests. Antivenom is not a clotting factor, but it permits restoration of endogenous clotting factors. Failing this, clotting factors should be administered. Thrombocytopenia may occur. Venoms do not have thrombolytic effects, and the presence of fibrin degradation products signifies endogenous thrombolysis. Additional antivenom should be administered before transfusion of blood and clotting factors, to prevent haemolysis and further consumptive coagulopathy.

Red back spider bite

Bites by the female of this species in children produces a similar syndrome to that observed in adults, with severe local pain, erythema, oedema and sweating about the bite site. The main systemic effects include regional lymph node pain, sweating, hypertension, abdominal pain and nausea and vomiting. Persistent or severe local pain and systemic effects are indications for IM antivenom in approximately 20% of envenomations.[29] The slow onset of respiratory failure is a possibility, but has not been observed since introduction of antivenom.

References

1. Tibballs J (1989) Epidemiology of acute poisoning. *Med Int* **61**:2496–2498.
2. Ellenhorn MJ and Barceloux DG (1988) *Medical Toxicogy.* Amsterdam: Elsevier.
3. Saetta JP, March S, Gaunt ME and Quinton DN (1991) Gastric emptying procedures in the self-poisoned patient: are we forcing gastric content beyond the pylorus? *J R Soc Med* **84**:274–276.
4. Neuvonen PJ, Vartiainen M and Tokola O (1983) Comparison of activated charcoal and ipecac syrup in prevention of drug absorption. *Eur J Clin Pharmacol* **24**:557–562.
5. Tenenbein M, Cohen S and Sitar DS (1987) Efficacy of ipecac-induced emesis, orogastric lavage, and activated charcoal for acute drug overdose. *Ann Emerg Med* **16**:838–841.
6. Curtis RA, Barone J and Giacona N (1984) Efficacy of ipecac and activated charcoal/cathartic. *Arch Intern Med* **144**:48–52.
7. Danel V, Henry JA and Glucksman E (1988) Activated charcoal, emesis, and gastric lavage in aspirin overdose. *Br Med J* **296**:1507.
8. McNamara RM, Aaron CK, Gemborys M and Davidheiseer S (1989) Efficacy of charcoal cathartic versus ipecac in reducing serum acetaminophen in a simulated overdose. *Ann Emerg Med* **18**:934–938.
9. Czajka PA and Russell SL (1985) Nonemetic effects of ipecac syrup. *Pediatics* **75**:1101–1104.
10. Albertson TE, Derlet RW, Foulke GE, Minguillon MC and Tharratt SR (1989) Superiority of activated charcoal alone with ipecac and activated charcoal in the treatment of acute toxic ingestions. *Ann Emerg Med* **18**:56–59.
11. Kornberg AE and Dolgin J (1991) Pediatric ingestions: charcoal alone versus ipecac and charcoal. *Ann Emerg Med* **20**:648–651.
12. Foulke GE, Albertson TE and Derlet RW (1988) Use of ipecac increases emergency department stays and patient complication rates. *Ann Emerg Med* **17**:402.

13. Kulig K, Bar-Or D, Cantrill SV, Rosen P and Rumack BH (1985) Management of acutely poisoned patients without gastric emptying. *Ann Emerg Med* **14**:562–567.

14. Auerbach PS, Osterich J, Braun O *et al.* (1986) Efficacy of gastric emptying: gastric lavage versus emesis induced with ipecac. *Ann Emerg Med* **15**:692–698.

15. Merigan KS, Woodard M, Hedges JR, Roberts JR, Stuebing R and Rashkin MC (1990) Prospective evaluation of gastric emptying in the self-poisoned patient. *Am J Emerg Med* **8**:479–483.

16. Neuvonen PJ and Elonen E (1980) Effect of activated charcoal on absorption and elimination of phenobarbitone, carbamazepine and phenylbutazone in man. *Eur J Clin Pharmacol* **17**:51–57.

17. Ohning BL, Reed MD and Blumer Jl (1986) Continuous nasogastric administration of activated charcoal for the treatment of theophylline intoxication. *Pediatr Pharmacol* **5**:241–245.

18. Palatnick W and Tenenbein M (1992) Activated charcoal in the treatment of drug overdose. *Drug Safety* **7**:3–7.

19. Smith SW, Ling LJ and Halstenson CE (1991) Whole bowel irrigation as a treatment for acute lithium overdose. *Ann Emerg Med* **29**:536–539.

20. Tenenbein M, Cohen S and Sitar DS (1987) Whole bowel irrigation as a decontamination procedure after acute drug overdose. *Arch Intern Med* **147**:905–907.

21. Kirshenbaum LA, Mathews SC, Sitar DS and Tenenbein M (1989) Whole-bowel irrigation versus activated charcoal in sorbitol for the ingestion of modified-release pharmaceuticals. *Clin Pharmacol Ther* **46**:264–271.

22. Sutherland SK (1983) *Australian Animal Toxins.* Oxford: Oxford University Press.

23. Covacevich J, Davie P and Pearn J (1987) *Toxic Plants and Animals.* Brisbane: Queensland Museum.

24. Sutherland SK (1992) Deaths from snake bite in Australia, 1981–1991. *Med J Aust* **157**:740–745.

25. Henderson A, Baldwin LN and May C (1993) Fatal brown snake (*Pseudonaja textilis*) envenomation despite the use of antivenom. *Med J Aust* **158**:709–710.

26. Tibballs J (1992) Diagnosis and treatment of confirmed and suspected snake bite. *Med J Aust* **156**:270–274.

27. Howarth DM, Southee AE and Whyte IM (1994) Lymphatic flow rates and first-aid in simulated peripheral snake or spider envenomation. *Med J Aust* **161**:695–700.

28. Tibballs J (1994) Premedication for snake antivenom. *Med J Aust* **160**:4–7.

29. Mead HJ and Jelinek GA (1993) Red-back spider bites to Perth children, 1979–1988. *J Paediatr Child Health* **29**:305–308.

Part XVIII

Appendices

I Blood chemistry

S = serum
P = plasma
HWB = heparin whole blood

α_1 Acid glycoprotein (S)		0.5–1.4 g/l
Aldosterone (S)		Supine – 140–530 pmol/l
		Erect – 220–970 pmol/l
Ammonia (P) to lab without delay		4–50 μmol/l
Amylase (S or P)		70–300 U/l
α_1 Antitrypsin (S or P)		2.1–4.0 g/l
Aspartate aminotransferase (AST) (P)		6–42 U/l
Bicarbonate (P)		22–32 mmol/l
Bilirubin (total) (S or P)		3–17 μmol/l
Bilirubin (direct) (S or P)		2–9 μmol/l
Caeruloplasmin (S or P)		0.20–0.60 g/l
Calcium (S or P)		2.25–2.65 mmol/l
Carotene (S or P)		1.0–4.8 μmol/l
Chloride (S or P)		98–108 mmol/l
Cholesterol (S or P)		3.1–6.5 mmol/l
Copper (S or P)		11–23 μmol/l
Cortisol (S or P)	8–9 am	300–800 nmol/l
	4–5 pm	100–600 nmol/l
Creatinine (P)		50–120 μmol/l
Creatinine clearance		> 1.3 ml/s
Creatinine kinase (P)		20–130 U/l
Creatinine kinase isoenzymes – qualitative		
Digoxin (S)	toxic	> 2 μg/l
Effective thyroxine ratio (ETR) (S)		0.90–1.09
FSH (S) Male		3–19 U/l
Female follicular		5–20 U/l
Mid-cycle		15–30 U/l
Luteal		5–15 U/l
Post-menopausal		50–100 U/l
Glucose (fasting) (fluoride) (P)		3.9–6.2 mmol/l
γ-Glutamyl-transferase (γ GT) (P)	F	7–30 U/l
	M	10–50 U/l
Growth hormone (fasting, resting) (S)	Male	< 6 mU/l
	Female	< 16 mU/l
	Child	< 10 mU/l

Insulin (fasting) (S)		3–28 mU/l
Iron (S or P) (1) Iron	M	14–31 μmol/l
8–10 am	F	11–29 μmol/l
(2) Iron binding capacity	M	41–70 μmol/l
	F	37–77 μmol/l
Lactate (special collection)		0.3–1.3 mmol/l
LDH (S or P)		< 80 U
Lead (HWB)		< 2 μmol/l
Lithium (S) not plasma		0.8–1.2 mmol/l
		(therapeutic range)
Magnesium (S or P)		0.7–1.1 mmol/l
Oestriol (pregnancy) (S)		Depends on gestation
Osmolality (S or P)		275–295 mosm/kg
Phosphatase		
A. Prostatic (S or P)		0–4 U/l
(stabilize plasma with 5 mg/ml of NaHSO₄ or freeze)		
B. Alkaline (S or P)		100–350 U/l
Phosphate (inorganic) (P)		0.8–1.4 mmol/l
Porphyrins (red cell) (HWB)		< 1.2 μmol/l
Potassium (P)		3.4–5.0 mmol/l
Prolactin (S) (resting)		25 μg/l
Proteins		
A. (1) Total (S)		63–78 g/l
(2) Albumin (S)		35–45 g/l
B. Electrophoresis (S) not plasma:		
Albumin		35–45 g/l
α₁ Globulin		2–4 g/l
α₂ Globulin		5–9 g/l
β Globulin		6–10 g/l
γ Globulin		8–16 g/l
Pyruvate (special collection)		30–80 μmol/l
Renin (special tubes – keep blood cold)		
100–180 mmol Na intake –		
Supine (6 h)		< 0.58 ng/s/l
Upright (4 h)		0.28–1.25 ng/s/l
Sodium (P)		134–146 mmol/l
Thyroxine (S)		60–150 nmol/l
Transferrin (S or P)		2.1–3.5 g/l
Triglyceride (fasting) (P)		1.80 mmol/l
Tri-iodothyronine (S)		1.3–2.9 nmol/l
TSH (S)		1–11 mU/l
Urea (P)		3.0–8.0 mmol/l
Uric acid (P)	M	0.18–0.48 mmol/l
	F	0.12–0.42 mmol/l
Zinc (P)		12–20 μmol/l

II URINE

AA = 20 ml 50% acetate
d   = 24 h collection
Sp = spot urine

Aldosterone (d, AA)		14–55 nmol/d
ALA (delta amino laevulinic acid) (Sp or d, AA)	Sp:	< 50 μmol/l
	d:	10–50 μmol/d
Amylase (Sp or d, NO ACID)	Sp:	< 900 U/l
	d:	100–1000 U/d
Calcium (d, AA)		< 7.5 mmol/d

Catecholamines and derivatives (d, 20 ml 50% HCL):

1. HMMA (VMA) Hydroxymethoxymandelic acid	< 35 μmol/d
2. Metadrenaline	< 5.6 μmol/d
3. Catecholamine	<1.6 μmol/d

Copper (d, AA)   < 1.6 μmol/d
Coproporphyrin (collect 24 hr urine into 8 g sodium carbonate)   < 245 nmol/d
Creatinine (d, AA)   10–20 mmol/d
5 Hydroxyindole-acetic acid (5-HIAA) (d, AA)   5–37 μmol/d
Hydroxyproline (d, AA)   < 0.35 mmol/d
                                                         (gelatin-free diet)
Indican (d, AA)   0.04–0.36 mmol/d
Lead (d, AA)   0.4 μmol/d
Magnesium (d, AA)   2.0–6.6 mmol/d
Melanin (fresh Sp)   Qualitative
Oestriol (in pregnancy) (d, AA)   50–160 μmol/d
                                                         at 36 weeks' gestation
Osmolality (Sp)   300–1300 mosm/kg
Oxalate (d, AA)   < 300 μmol/d
Phosphorus (d, AA)   10–42 mmol/d
Porphobilinogen (fresh Sp)   Qualitative
Potassium (d or Sp, AA)   25–100 mmol/d
Protein (d or Sp, AA)   0.02–0.06 g/d
Sodium (d or Sp, AA)   40–210 mmol/d

Steroids (d, AA):

1. 17-Oxosteroids	M	28–80 μmol/d
	F	14–60 μmol/d
2. 17-Hydroxy corticosteriods	M	14–70 μmol/d
	F	7–50 μmol/d

Urea (d or Sp, AA)   170–500 mmol/d
Uric acid (d, 8 g sodium carbonate)   < 3.6 mmol/d
                                                         (purine-free diet)
Urobilinogen (fresh Sp)   Qualitative
Uroporphyrin (collect as for Coproporphyrin)   < 50 nmol/d
Xylose absorption:
  Xylose excretion in 5 h   > 27 mmol
  Plasma value at 2 h   1.7–3.4 mmol/l

III FAECES

Fat (3 d collection)	< 5 g/l
Porphyrins (single stool)	
Coproporphyrins	< 30 nmol/g dry wt
Protoporphyrins	< 135 nmol/g dry wt

IV CSF

Protein	0.15–0.45 g/l
Glucose	2.7–4.2 mmol/l
IgG	< 0.05 g/l
IgG:Total protein ratio	5–14%

<table>
<tr><td>**Appendix 2**</td><td># Système International (SI) units</td></tr>
</table>

Appendix 2	# Système International (SI) units

BASIC SI UNITS

Physical quantity	Name	Symbol
Length	Metre	m
Mass	Kilogram	kg
Time	Second*	s
Electric current	Ampere	A
Thermodynamic temperature	Kelvin	K
Luminous intensity	Candela	cd
Amount of substance	Mole	mol

*Minute (min), hour (h) and day (d) will remain in use although they are not official SI units.

PREFIXES

Factor	Name	Symbol	Factor	Name	Symbol
10^{18}	Exa-	E	10^{-18}	Atto-	a
10^{15}	Peta-	P	10^{-15}	Femto-	f
10^{12}	Tera-	T	10^{-12}	Pico-	p
10^{9}	Giga-	G	10^{-9}	Nano-	n
10^{6}	Mega-	M	10^{-6}	Micro-	μ
10^{3}	Kilo-	k	10^{-3}	Milli-	m
10^{2}	Hecto-	h	10^{-2}	Centi-	c
10^{1}	Deca-	da	10^{-1}	Deci-	d

DERIVED SI UNITS

Quantity	SI units	Symbol	Expression in terms of SI base units or derived units
Frequency	Hertz	Hz	$1\,Hz = 1$ cycle/s $(1\ s^{-1})$
Force	Newton	N	$1\,N = 1\ kg.m/s^2$
Work, energy, quantity of heat	Joule	J	$1\,J = 1\ N.m\ (1\ kg.m^2.s^{-2})$
Power	Watt	W	$1\,W = 1$ J/s $(1\ J.s^{-1})$
Quantity of electricity	Coulomb	C	$1\,C = 1$ A.s
Electric potential, potential difference, tension, electromotive force	Volt	V	$1\,V = W/A\ (1\ W.A^{-1})$
Electric capacitance	Farad	F	$1\,F = 1$ A.s/V $(A.sV^{-1})$
Electric resistance	Ohm	Ω	$1\,\Omega = 1$ V/A $(1\ V.A^{-1})$
Flux of magnetic induction, magnetic flux	Weber	Wb	$1\,Wb = 1$ V.s
Magnetic flux density, magnetic induction	Tesla	T	$1\,T = 1\ Wb/m^2\ (1\ Wb.m^{-2})$
Inductance	Henry	H	$1\,H = 1$ V.s/A $(V.s.A^{-1})$
Pressure	Pascal	Pa	$1\,Pa = 1\ N/m^2\ (1\ N.m^{-2})$ $= 1\ kg/m^2.s^2\ (1\ kg.m^{-1}.s^{-2})$

The litre (1) ($10^{-3}\ m^3 = dm^3$), though not official, will remain in use as a unit of volume as also will the dyne (dyn) as a unit for force (1 dyn = 10^{-5} N).

PRESSURE MEASUREMENTS

		Conversion factors	
		Old to SI	*SI to old*
SI unit	*Old unit*	*(exact)*	*(approx.)*
kPa	mm Hg	0.133	7.5
kPa	1 standard atmosphere (approx 1 Bar)	101.3	0.01
kPa	cm H_2O	0.0981	10
kPa	lbs/sq in	6.894	0.145

HAEMATOLOGY

			Conversion factors	
Measurement	*SI unit*	*Old unit*	*Old to SI*	*SI to old*
Haemoglobin (Hb)	g/dl	g/100 ml	Numerically	equivalent
Packed cell volume	No unit*	Per cent	0.01	100
Mean cell Hb conc	g/dl	Per cent	Numerically	equivalent
Mean cell Hb	pg	uug	Numerically	equivalent
Red cell count	Cells/litre	Cells/mm^3	10^6	10^{-6}
White cell count	Cells/litre	Cells/mm^3	10^6	10^{-6}
Reticulocytes	Per cent	Per cent	Numerically	equivalent
Platelets	Cells/litre	Cells/mm^3	10^6	10^{-6}

* Expressed as decimal fraction.

pH   **H$^+$**

pH	*nmol/litre*
6.80	158
6.90	126
7.00	100
7.10	79
7.20	63
7.25	56
7.30	50
7.35	45
7.40	40
7.45	36
7.50	32
7.55	28
7.60	25
7.70	20

Respiratory physiology symbols and normal values

SYMBOLS

Primary

C Concentration of gas in blood
F Fractional concentration in dry gas
f Frequency of respiration (breaths/min)
P Pressure or partial pressure
Q Volume of blood
Q̇ Volume of blood per unit time
R Respiratory exchange ratio
S Saturation of haemoglobin with O_2
V̇ Volume of gas per unit time

Secondary symbols for gas phase

A Alveolar
B Barometric
D Dead space
E Expired
I Inspired
L Lung
T Tidal

Secondary symbols for blood phase

a arterial
c capillary
ć end-capillary
i ideal
v venous
v̄ mixed venous
⁻ above any symbol denotes a mean value
· above any symbol denotes a value per unit time

NORMAL VALUES

1. Blood

  (a) *Arterial*

pH	:	7.36–7.44	(H^+ = 44 – 36 nmol/l)
PaO_2	:	85–100 mm Hg	(11.3–13.3 kPa)
$PaCO_2$	:	36–44 mm Hg	(4.8–5.9 kPa)
O_2 content	:	20–21 vols%	(8.9–9.4 nmol/l)
CO_2 content	:	48–50 vols%	(21.6–22.5 nmol/l)

  (b) *Venous*

pH	:	7.34–7.42	(H^+ = 38–46 nmol/l)
PO_2	:	37–42 mm Hg	(5–5.6 kPa)
PCO_2	:	42–50 mm Hg	(5.6–6.7 kPa)
O_2 content	:	15–16 vols%	(6.7–7.2 mmol/l)
CO_2 content	:	52–54 vols%	(23.3–24.2 mmol/l)

2. Gases

(a) *Inspired air*

O_2	:	20.93%	
PIO_2	:	149 mm Hg	(19.9 kPa)
N	:	79.04%	
PIN_2	:	563 mm Hg	(75 kPa)
CO_2	:	0.03%	

(b) *Expired air*

O_2	:	16–17%	
PEO_2	:	113–121 mm Hg	(15–16 kPa)
N	:	80%	
PEN	:	579 mm Hg	(77 kPa)
CO_2	:	3–4%	
$PECO_2$	:	21–28 mm Hg	(2.8–3.7 kPa)

3. Ventilation:perfusion

(a) *Alveolar–arterial oxygen gradient*:
   5–20 mm Hg   (0.7–2.7 kPa) breathing air
   25–65 mm Hg   (3.3–8.6 kPa) breathing 100% oxygen

(b) *Venous admixture* ($\dot{Q}_S:\dot{Q}_T$): 5% of cardiac output

(c) *Right to left physiological shunt*: 3% of cardiac output

(d) *Anatomical dead space*: 2 ml/kg body weight

(e) *Dead space: tidal volume ratio* $V_D:V_T$): 0.25–0.4 or $33 + \dfrac{Age}{3}$ per cent

4. Lung volumes

Approximate values in adults are listed. Values are less in smaller subjects and in females.

Tidal volume	:	500 ml or 7 ml/kg
Inspiratory capacity	:	3.6 litres
Inspiratory reserve volume	:	3.1 litres
Expiratory reserve volume	:	1.2 litres
Functional residual capacity	:	2.4 litres
Residual volume	:	1.2 litres
Total lung capacity	:	6.0 litres
Vital capacity	:	4.8 litres

or 2.5 1/sq m body surface or 2.5 1/m height in males
   2.0 1/sq m body surface or 2.0 1/m height in females
or 65–75 ml/kg

5. Lung mechanics

(a) *Peak expiratory flow rate*   :   450–700 l/min (males)
                                              :   300–500 l/min (females)

(b) *Forced expiratory volume in 1 sec* (FEV$_1$)   :   70–83% of vital capacity

(c) *Compliance* (approximate values)   :

   (i) Lung compliance (C_L)   :

		Static	Dynamic
conscious (erect)	:	200 ml/cm H_2O	180 ml/cm H_2O
paralysed anaesthetized (supine)	:	160 ml/cm H_2O	80 ml/cm H_2O

   (ii) Chest wall compliance (C_{CW})   :   200 ml/cm H_2O

   (iii) Total compliance (C_T):

conscious (erect)	:	150 ml/cm H_2O	100 ml/cm H_2O
*paralysed anaesthetized (supine)	:	74 ml/cm H_2O	56 ml/cm H_2O

(d) *Airways resistance*   :
   conscious   :   0.6–3.2 cm H_2O/l/sec
   sedated, partially paralysed and ventilated (includes resistance of endotracheal tube and catheter mount): 10–15 cm H_2O/l/sec

(e) *Work of breathing*:   0.3–0.5 kg m/min
   or oxygen consumption of 0.5–1 ml/l ventilation

*Compliance values would be lower for the sedated, partially paralysed, ventilated patient in the Intensive Care Unit,
i.e. Effective dynamic compliance = 40–50 ml/cm H_2O

6. Cardiovascular – pressures in kPa are given within brackets

(a)	Cardiac index	: 2.5–3.6 l/min/m^2
(b)	Stroke volume	: 42–52 ml/m^2
(c)	Ejection fraction	: 0.55–0.75
(d)	End diastolic volume	: 75 ± 15 ml/m^2
(e)	End systolic volume	: 25 ± 8 ml/m^2
(f)	Left ventricular stroke work index	: 30–110 g-m/m^2
(g)	Left ventricular minute work index	: 1.8–6.6 kg-m/min/m^2
(h)	Oxygen consumption index	: 110–150 ml/l
(i)	Right atrial pressure	: 1–7 mm Hg (0.13–0.93)
(j)	Right ventricular systolic pressure	: 15–25 mm Hg (2.0–3.3)
(k)	Right ventricular diastolic pressure	: 0–8 (0–1)
(l)	Pulmonary artery systolic pressure	: 15–25 mm Hg (2.0–3.3)
(m)	Pulmonary artery diastolic pressure	: 8–15 mm Hg (1–2)
(n)	Pulmonary artery mean pressure	: 10–20 mm Hg (1.3–2.7)
(o)	Pulmonary capillary wedge pressure	: 6–15 mm Hg (0.8–2.0)
(p)	Systemic vascular resistance	: 770–1500 dyne-s/cm^5
		: 77–150 kPa-s/l
(q)	Pulmonary vascular resistance	: 20–120 dyne-s/cm^5
		: 2–12 kPa-s/l
(r)	Systolic time intervals – see Chapter 96, Haemodynamic Monitoring.	

RESPIRATORY EQUATIONS

(a) *Oxygen consumption* (250 ml/min)
Oxygen consumption = amount of oxygen in inspired gas minus amount in expired gas

i.e. $\qquad \dot{V}O_2 = (VI \times FIO_2) - (\dot{V}E \times F\bar{E}O_2)$

(b) *Carbon dioxide production* (200 ml/min)
Volume CO_2 eliminated in expired gas = expired gas volume times CO_2 concentration in mixed expired gas

i.e. $\qquad \dot{V}CO_2 = \dot{V} \times F\bar{E}CO_2$

As expired volume is made up of alveolar and dead space gas,

$$\dot{V}CO_2 = (\dot{V}A \times FACO_2) + (\dot{V}D \times FICO_2)$$

As $FICO_2$ is negligible, especially if there is no rebreathing,

$$\dot{V}CO_2 = \dot{V}A \times FACO_2$$

or $\qquad FACO_2 = \dfrac{\dot{V}CO_2}{\dot{V}A}$

or $\qquad PACO_2 \text{ (mmHg)} = \dfrac{\dot{V}CO_2 \text{ (ml/min STPD)}}{\dot{V}A \text{ (1/min BTPS)}} \times 0.863$

or $\qquad PACO_2 \text{ (kPa)} = \dfrac{\dot{V}CO_2 \text{ (mmol/min)}}{\dot{V}A \text{ (1/min BTPS)}} \times 2.561$

STPD: Standard temperature (0°C) and pressure (760 mm Hg or 101.35 kPa) dry gas
BTPS: Body temperature and ambient pressure, saturated with water vapour

(c) *Physiological dead space*

Bohr's equation, $\qquad \dfrac{V_D}{V_T} = \dfrac{PACO_2 - P\bar{E}CO_2}{PACO_2}$

or $\qquad \dfrac{V_D}{V_T} = \dfrac{PaCO_2 - P\bar{E}CO_2}{PaCO_2}$

(d) *Alveolar oxygenation*

$$PAO_2 = PIO_2 - \frac{PaCO_2}{R} \text{ where R is the Respiratory Quotient (normally 0.8)}$$

$$PAO_2 = PIO_2 - PACO_2 \frac{(PIO_2 - P\bar{E}O_2)}{(P\bar{E}CO_2)}$$

or

$$PAO_2 = PIO_2 - PACO_2 \left(FIO_2 + \frac{1 - FIO_2}{R} \right).$$

when $FIO_2 = 1.0$ (patient breathing 100% oxygen),
then PAO_2 = (PB – saturated water vapour pressure) – $PACO_2$
    = (PB – 47) – $PaCO_2$

(e) *Venous admixture*

$$\frac{\dot{Q}_S}{\dot{Q}_T} = \frac{C\acute{c}O_2 - CaO_2}{C\acute{c}O_2 - C\bar{v}O_2}$$

$$= \frac{(PAO_2 - PaO_2) \times 0.0031}{CaO_2 + (PAO_2 - PaO_2) \times 0.0031 - C\bar{v}O_2}$$

$$= \frac{(PAO_2 - PaO_2) \times 0.0031}{(PAO_2 - PaO_2) \times 0.0031 + 5} \text{ (simplified)}$$

(f) *Fractional inspired oxygen concentration*

$$FIO_2 = \frac{O_2 \text{ flow in l/min} + (\text{Air flow in l/min} \times 0.21)}{\text{Total } O_2 + \text{Air flows in l/min}}$$

(g) *Henderson–Hasselbalch equation*

$$pH = pK_A + \log \frac{(HCO_3^-)}{(CO_2)}$$

$$pH = 6.1 + \log \frac{(HCO_3^- \text{ in mmol/l})}{(PCO_2 \text{ in mm Hg}) \times 0.03}$$

$$[H^+] \text{ nmol/l} = 24 \times \frac{(PCO_2 \text{ in mm Hg})}{(HCO_3^- \text{ in mmol/l})}$$

$$[H^+] \text{ nmol/l} = 180 \times \frac{(PCO_2 \text{ in kPa})}{(HCO_3^- \text{ in mmol/l})}$$

CARDIOVASCULAR EQUATIONS

(a) *Mean blood pressure* (BP = DBP + 1.3 (SBP – DBP))
(b) *Rate pressure product* (RPP) = P × SBP
(c) *Body surface area* (BSA) in m² = $(Ht)^{0.725} \times (Wt)^{0.425} \times 71.84 \times 10^{-4}$

(d) **Cardiac Index* (CI) = $\dfrac{CO}{BSA}$ = ml/min/m²

(e) *Stroke volume* (SV) = $\dfrac{\text{CO}}{\text{P}}$ = ml/beat

(f) **Stroke volume index* (SVI) = $\dfrac{\text{SV}}{\text{BSA}}$ = ml/beat/m^2

(g) **Left ventricular stroke work index* (LVSWI) = (BP − PCWP) (SVI) (0.0136) = g-m/m^2/beat

(h) *Systemic vascular resistance* (SVR) = $\dfrac{\text{BP} - \text{RAP}}{\text{CO}}$ resistance units

    (Multiply × 79.9 to convert to absolute resistance units, dynes sec cm^{-5})

(i) *Pulmonary vascular resistance* (PVR) = $\dfrac{\text{PAP} - \text{PCWP}}{\text{CO}}$ resistance units

    (Multiply × 79.9 to convert to absolute resistance units, dynes sec cm^{-5})

(j) *Left ventricular pre-ejection period* (PEP) = QS$_2$ − LVET m sec

(k) *Other systolic time index ratios* may easily be calculated:

$$\frac{1}{\text{PEP}^2} \text{ and } \frac{\text{PEP}}{\text{LVET}}$$

*For interpatient comparisons and reference standards, the 'index' term, output normalized to body surface, may be used when

SBP	= systolic blood pressure in mm Hg
DBP	= diastolic blood pressure in mm Hg
P	= heart rate in beats/min
Ht	= height in cm
Wt	= weight in kg
CO	= cardiac output in ml/min
PCWP	= pulmonary capillary wedge pressure in mm Hg
RAP	= right atrial pressure in mm Hg
PAP	= mean pulmonary artery pressure in mm Hg
LVET	= left ventricular ejection time in m sec
QS$_2$	= total electromechanical systole in m sec

RENAL EQUATIONS

(a) *Standard creatinine clearance* (ml/min/1.73 m^2)

$$= \frac{\text{urine creatinine (mmol/l)}}{\text{serum creatinine (mmol/l)}} \times \text{urine volume (ml/min)} \times \frac{1.73}{\text{body surface area (m}^2)}$$

(b) *Per cent filtered Na$^+$ excreted*

$$= \frac{\text{urine Na}^+ \text{ (mmol/l)}}{\text{serum Na}^+ \text{ (mmol/l)}} \times \frac{\text{serum creatinine (mmol/l)}}{\text{urine creatinine (mmol/l)}} \times 100$$

(c) *Free water clearance* (ml/min)

$$= \text{urine vol (ml/min)} - \frac{\text{urine osmolality (mosm/kg)}}{\text{plasma osmolality (mosm/kg)}} \times \text{urine vol (ml/min)}$$

(d) *Additional calculated parameters*:

(i) $\dfrac{\text{urine}}{\text{plasma}}$ osmolality ratio

(ii) $\dfrac{\text{urine}}{\text{serum}}$ creatinine ratio

(iii) $\dfrac{\text{blood urea}}{\text{serum creatinine}}$ ratio

(iv) $\dfrac{\text{urine}}{\text{Plasma}}$ urea ratio

(v) urinary Na^+ and K^+ excretion (mmol)

(vi) $\dfrac{\text{urinary } Na^+}{\text{urinary } K^+}$ ratio

Plasma drug concentrations and American nomenclature

PLASMA DRUG LEVELS

Drug	Normal or therapeutic concentration mg/l	Toxic concentration mg/l	Lethal or potentially lethal concentration mg/l
Acetazolamide	10–15	–	–
Acetohexamide	21–56	–	–
Acetone	–	200–300	550
Aluminium	0.13	–	–
Aminophylline (Theophylline)	10–20	20	–
Amitriptyline	50–200 μg/l	400 μg/l	10–20
Ammonia	500–1700	–	–
Amphetamine	20–30 μg/l	–	2
Arsenic	0.0–20 μg/l	1.0	15
Barbiturates			
Short-acting	1	7	10
Intermediate-acting	1–5	10–30	30
Phenobarbitone	15	40–70	80–150
Benzene	–	any measurable	0.94
Beryllium	Tissue levels generally used (lung & lymph)	–	–
Boric acid	0.8	40	50
Bromide	50	0.5–1.5 g/l	2 g/l
Brompheniramine	8–15 μg/l	–	–
Cadmium	0.1–0.2 μg/l	50 μg/l	–
Caffeine	–	–	100
Carbamazepine	6–12	12	–
Carbon monoxide	1% saturation of Hb	15–35% saturation of Hb	50% saturation of Hb
Carbon tetrachloride	–	20–50	–
Chloral hydrate	10	100	250
Chlordiazepoxide	1.0–2.0	6	20
Chloroform	–	70–250	390
Chlorpromazine	0.3	1–2	3–12
Chlorpropamide	30–140	–	–
Codeine	25 μg/l	–	–
Copper	1–1.5	5.4	–
Cyanide	0.15	–	5
DDT	13 μg/l	–	–
Desipramine	0.59–1.4	–	10–20
Dextropropoxyphene	50–200 μg/l	5–10	57
Diazepam	0.5–2.5	5–20	50

Drug	Normal or therapeutic concentration mg/l	Toxic concentration mg/l	Lethal or potentially lethal concentration mg/l
Dieldrin	1.5 μg/l	–	–
Digitoxin	20–35 μg/l	–	320 μg/l
Digoxin	1–2 μg/l	2–9 μg/l	–
Dinitro-o-cresol	–	30–40 μg/l	75
Diphenhydramine	5	10	–
Disopyramide	3–7	–	–
Ethosuximide	40–80	–	–
Ethyl chloride	–	–	400
Ethylene glycol	–	1.5 g/l	2–4 g/l
Fluoride	0.5	–	2
Gentamicin	5–8	10–12	–
Glutethimide	1–5	10–30	30–100
Gold (sodium aurothiomalate)	3–6	–	–
Hydrogen sulphide	–	–	0.92
Hydromorphone (Dihydromorphinone)	–	–	0.1–0.3
Imipramine	0.1–0.3	0.7	2
Iron	500 (erythrocytes)	6 (serum)	–
Lead	0.05–1.3	1.3	–
Lignocaine	2–4	6	–
Lithium	0.8–1.2 mmol/l	1.5 mmol/l	4 mmol/l
LSD (lysergic acid diethylamide)	–	1–4 μg/l	–
Magnesium	0.7–1.1 mmol/l	–	–
Manganese	0.15	4.6	–
Meprobamate	10	100	200
Mercury	60–120 μg/l	–	–
Methadone	480–860 μg/l	2	4
Methanol	–	200	890
Methapyrilene	2 μg/l	30–50	50
Methaqualone	1–2	5–30	30
Methsuximide	2.5–7.5	–	–
Methylamphetamine	–	5	40
Methyprylone	10	30–60	100
Mexiletine	0.6–2.5	–	–
Morphine	0.1	–	0.5–4
Nickel	0.41	–	–
Nicotine	–	10	5–52
Nitrofurantoin	1.8	–	–
Nortriptyline	50–200 μg/l	400 μg/l	10–20
Orphenadrine	–	2	4–8
Oxalate	2	–	10
Papaverine	1	–	–
Paracetamol	5–25	30	250 at 4 h 50 at 12 h
Paraldehyde	50	200–400	500
Paramethoxy-amphetamine (PMA)	–	–	2–4
Pentazocine	0.1–1	2–5	10–20
Perphenazine	–	1	–
Pethidine	600–650 μg/l	5	30
Phenacetin	5–25	30	400
Phencyclidine	–	0.5	1
Phensuximide	10–19	–	–

Drug	Normal or therapeutic concentration mg/l	Toxic concentration mg/l	Lethal or potentially lethal concentration mg/l
Phenylbutazone	100	–	–
Phenytoin (Dilantin)	8–20	30	100
Phosphorus	Concentration in tissues usually used	–	–
Primidone	10	50–80	100
Probenecid	100–200	–	–
Procainamide	3–8	10	–
Prochlorperazine	–	1	–
Promazine	–	1	–
Propoxyphene	0.1–1	5–20	57
Propranolol	0.025–0.1	–	8–12
Propylhexedrine	–	–	2–3
Quinidine	3–6	10	30–50
Quinine	–	–	12
Salicylate (acetylsalicylic acid)	100–350	350–400	500
Strychnine	–	2	9–12
Sulphadiazine	80–150	–	–
Sulphafurazole	90–100	–	–
Sulphaguanidine	30–50	–	–
Sulthiame	4–10	–	–
Theophylline	10–20	20	–
Thioridazine	1–1.5	10	20–80
Tin	0.12	–	–
Tobramycin	5–8	10–12	–
Tolbutamide	53–96	–	–
Toluene	–	–	10
Tribromoethanol	–	–	90
Tricyclics	50–200 µg/l	400 µg/l	10–20
Trimethobenzamide	1.0–2.0	–	–
Valproate	50–100	–	–
Warfarin	1.0–10	–	–
Zinc	0.68–1.36	–	–
Zoxazolamine	3–13	–	–

AMERICAN NOMENCLATURE

Drug	American equivalent	Drug	American equivalent
Adrenaline	Epinephrine	Methohexitone	Methohexital
Amethocaine	Tetracaine	Methylamphetamine	Methamphetamine
Cinchocaine	Dibucaine	Methyprylone	Methyprylon
Corticotrophin	Corticotropin	Noradrenaline	Norepinephrine, Levarterenol
Desferrioxamine	Deferoxamine	Orciprenaline	Metaproterenol
Dextropropoxyphene	Propoxyphene	Oxybuprocaine	Benoxinate
Dihydromorphinone	Hydromorphone	Paracetamol	Acetaminophen
Ergometrine	Ergonovine	Pethidine	Meperidine
Frusemide	Furosemide	Phenobarbitone	Phenobarbital
Hydrallazine	Hydralazine	Salbutamol	Albuterol
Hyoscine	Scopolamine	Thiopentone	Thiopental
Isoprenaline	Isoproterenol	Thyroxine	Levothyroxine
Lignocaine	Lidocaine		
Meclozine	Meclizine		
Mepivacaine	Carbocaine		

REFERENCES

1. Koch-Weser J. Serum drug concentrations as therapeutic guides. N Engl J Med 1972, 287:227–31.
2. Winek CL. Tabulation of therapeutic, toxic and lethal concentrations of drugs and chemicals in blood. Clin Chem 1976, 22:832–6.
3. Richens A, Warrington S. When should plasma drug levels be monitored? Curr Therapeutics 1979, 20:167–85.
4. Koch-Weser J. The serum level approach to individualization of drug dosage. Eur J Clin Pharm 1975, 9:1–8.
5. Davies DS, Prichard BNC. Biological Effects of Drugs in Relation to their Plasma Concentrations. London, Macmillan, 1973.

Index